MYLES TEXTBOOK FOR MIDWIVES

V. Ruth Bennett BA RGN RM MTD is a Senior Lecturer at the Royal College of Midwives. She spent 10 years teaching midwives at the Nazareth Hospital, Israel and had held posts as Midwife Teacher and Senior Midwife Teacher before her present appointment. She has been instrumental in developing advanced courses for midwives and has an interest in continuing education for all practitioners.

Linda K. Brown BA RGN RSCN RM MTD is Course Director for the Diploma in Professional Studies in Midwifery at the Distance Learning Centre of the South Bank University, London. After experience as Midwife Teacher in Swindon she spent four years at the University of Surrey where she was involved with advanced midwifery courses, including the MSc in Advanced Midwifery Practice, and with Midwife Teacher education.

For Churchill Livingstone

Publisher Mary Law
Project Editor Dinah Thom
Indexer Liza Weinkove
Design Design Resources Unit
Production Controller Mark Sanderson, Neil Dickson
Sales Promotion Executive Hilary Brown

TWELFTH EDITION

MYLES TEXTBOOK FOR MIDWIVES

Edited by

V. RUTH BENNETT BA RGN RM MTD
LINDA K. BROWN BA RGN RSCN RM MTD

Foreword by

MARY E. UPRICHARD OBE RGN RSCN RM MTD
Director of Midwifery Education,
Northern Ireland College of Midwifery, Belfast

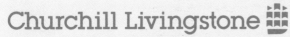

Churchill Livingstone

EDINBURGH LONDON MADRID MELBOURNE NEW YORK AND TOKYO 1993

CHURCHILL LIVINGSTONE
Medical Division of Longman Group UK Limited

Distributed in the United States of America by Churchill
Livingstone Inc., 650 Avenue of the Americas, New York,
N.Y. 10011, and by associated companies, branches and
representatives throughout the world.

First edition 1953   Seventh edition 1971
Second edition 1956   Eighth edition 1975
Third edition 1958   Ninth edition 1981
Fourth edition 1961   Tenth edition 1985
Fifth edition 1964   Eleventh edition 1989
Sixth edition 1968   Twelfth edition 1993

ISBN 0-443-04581-X

British Library of Cataloguing in Publication Data
A catalogue record for this book is available from the British
Library.

Library of Congress Cataloging in Publication Data
Myles textbook for midwives. — 12th ed./edited by V. Ruth
  Bennett, Linda K. Brown; foreword by Mary E. Uprichard.
      p.   cm.
    Includes index.
    ISBN 0-443-04581-X
    1. Obstetrics. 2. Midwives. I. Myles, Margaret F.
  II. Bennett, V. Ruth. III. Brown, Linda K. IV. Title:
  Textbook for midwives.
    [DNLM: 1. Midwifery. WQ 165 M9971 1993]
  RG524.M985 1993
  618.2—dc20
  DNLM/DLC
  for Library of Congress   93-3748

Printed in Great Britain by Bath Press Colourbooks, Glasgow

The
publisher's
policy is to use
**paper manufactured
from sustainable forests**

Foreword

The four years since the publication of the 11th edition of *Myles Textbook for Midwives* has been a period which has witnessed unprecedented and far reaching changes which have impinged in so many ways on the provision of maternity care and the work of the midwife.

In the UK the health service has been undergoing the most profound changes since the founding of the National Health Service. Central to the changes has been the introduction of the contracting process with the development of the Purchaser Provider Management Structures. Concurrent with this has been greater emphasis on cost and efficiency and effectiveness and total quality management.

In addition, major reform of midwifery education has resulted in programmes of midwifery education both pre and post registration at diploma and graduate level, with midwifery education linking, and in some instances, integrating with the higher education sector.

These changes with their emphasis on continuity, control and choice, with the mother being the centre of the maternity service, are being reflected in maternity care provision throughout the world. They provide great challenges for the midwife and will serve as a catalyst in the further development of innovative midwife led maternity care.

This 12th edition of *Myles Textbook for Midwives*, with several of the chapters written by new authors, has been extensively amended to take account of these changes. This edition uses even more research based findings than its predecessor. Chapters are well referenced and often useful addresses and further reading are given. Many of the chapters are perhaps better structured with clever use of headings throughout and helpful abstracts and introductions are often given. Reader activities have been included at the end of each chapter instead of at the end of the book as previously.

Two new chapters have been included: one on 'Ethics in Midwifery', a most welcome addition in view of major societal changes and ongoing technological advances; the other, 'Quality Assurance in Maternity Care', is also timely given the major emphasis on total quality management in health care. Both are by authors well qualified to comment and write on the subjects.

This up-to-date revised text, with the additional chapters, should ensure its enduring usefulness as a major text for students of midwifery at all levels.

Mary E. Uprichard OBE

Preface

This 12th edition follows the successful format of its immediate predecessor. The legacy left by its original author, Mrs Margaret Myles, has been valued and where the material still applies it has been incorporated into the present book. Although it has been extensively revised and re-written by 20 or so authors, it is still a challenge to meet the standard that she originally set.

Midwifery has continued to move forward in the years since the 11th edition was published. The use of references and further reading has proved a welcome innovation and this has been strengthened and extended in the new edition. This harmonises with the changes in the structure of midwifery courses and the fact that most midwifery schools have been absorbed into larger Colleges of Nursing and Midwifery linked to Universities. Student midwives are no longer asked to sit a national examination, so the chapter of specimen questions has become unnecessary; instead reader activities are suggested at the end of each chapter. It is hoped that these will be valued by qualified midwives as well as those who are undergoing a programme of education towards qualification.

Changes in the National Health Service have brought in new management ideas and the practice of audit and quality assurance has become an integral part of midwifery. A new chapter addresses this and should help the midwife to assess her own performance as well as to work with colleagues to achieve a high standard of care for her clients.

At the other end of the scale, practitioners are increasingly being challenged about the moral issues bound up with practice. Events frequently leave the midwife wondering what is the right way forward and how she should exercise her responsibility in her relationship with the woman in her care, and often the woman's family as well. A chapter on ethics for midwives explores the theories that abound in this field and tries to lead the midwife to a framework which will help decision-making while being true to the philosophy of midwifery in contrast to that of medicine.

The present edition continues to benefit from the writing of new authors and many chapters have undergone extensive revision and rewriting in order to make them as informative as possible for the reader.

In undertaking the revision of the textbook it has always been our prime concern to remember that the midwife is but the servant of the mothers whom she cares for and that she needs her knowledge and skill in order to achieve, in the measure that it is possible, a satisfying outcome for her clients. One of the greatest compliments that the 11th edition received was that the attitude that it conveyed towards the mother was noticeably softer, more respectful and desirous of giving her the choice and control that she wants. We have tried to retain that principle and to reinforce it in this 12th edition. It is our hope that this book will help midwives to practise their skill and art reflectively and responsibly.

Godalming 1993
V.R.B.
L.K.B.

General Acknowledge-ments

The volume editors wish to record their appreciation for the foundation work of chapter authors who contributed to the 11th edition of this book and whose material has been updated and adapted for the 12th edition. These include:

Joanne M. Alexander
Margaret Arnold
Ruth Bevis
Nina Firth
Elaine Healey
Ruth Preston.

They also wish to thank the various critics and correspondents who made constructive suggestions for alterations and improvements to the text and diagrams. They warmly acknowledge the support and encouragement of many colleagues, friends and well-wishers who have in countless ways enabled the present, as well as the previous, edition to be prepared and without whom the job would never have been accomplished.

Contributors

Jo M. Alexander PhD RGN RM MTD FPCert
Lecturer in Midwifery, University of
Southampton, UK

Janet Asherson BA RGN RM HV
Currently doing VSO, Nepal; Former Health
Visitor, Swindon, UK

Jean A. Ball MSc DipN RGN RM
Senior Teaching Fellow, Nuffield Institute for
Health Service Studies, University of Leeds, UK

Thelma Bamfield BA(Hons) SCM ADM MTD
Midwifery Tutor, Birmingham and Solihull
College of Midwifery, Birmingham, UK

V. Ruth Bennett BA RGN RM MTD
Senior Lecturer, Royal College of Midwives,
London, UK

E. Anne Bent MBE RGN RM MTD
Formerly UKCC Professional Officer
(Midwifery)

Ruth Bevis RGN RM HV ADM
Part-time Practice Nurse/Midwife, London, UK

Tricia Murphy-Black PhD MSc RGN RM RCNT
Midwife Member, National Board for Scotland;
Research Fellow, Nursing Research Unit,
University of Edinburgh, UK

Eileen M. Brayshaw DipPhys MCSP SRP FETC
Superintendent Physiotherapist, St James's
University Hospital, Leeds, UK

Linda K. Brown BA RGN RSCN RM MTD
Course Director for Diploma in Professional

Studies in Midwifery, South Bank University, London, UK

Patricia Cassidy RGN RM DipN(Lond) MTD
Midwifery Tutor, Glasgow College of Nursing and Midwifery, Glasgow, UK

Jean Davies RN RM MSc (Health and Social Research)
Community Midwife, Newcastle upon Tyne, UK

Chloe Fisher SRN SCM MTD
Clinical Specialist in Infant Feeding, John Radcliffe Hospital, Oxford, UK

Deborah Hughes BA(Hons) MA RGN RM ADM
Has recently completed Postgraduate Diploma in Education at Manchester University, UK

Lea E. Jamieson BEd(Hons) RGN RM MTD
Head of Midwifery and Women's Health Studies, Normanby College, King's College, London, UK

Rosemary Jenkins RGN RM MTD DMS MBIM
Director of Professional Affairs, Royal College of Midwives, London, UK

E. Sarah Kelly BEd(Hons) SRN SCM MTD
Senior Lecturer, Royal College of Midwives, London, UK

Margaret A. Lang RGN SCM RSCN
Senior Midwife Manager, Borders General Hospital, Melrose, UK

Victoria M. Lewis PGCEA ONC SRN RM ONC
Lecturer (Midwifery), Nightingale and Guy's College of Health, London, UK

Carmel A. Lloyd PGCEA SRN SCM ADM
Lecturer (Midwifery), Nightingale and Guy's College of Health, London, UK

Johnanna Matthew BA RGN RM MTD MN
Course Leader – Professional Development Midwifery, Glasgow College of Nursing and Midwifery, Glasgow, Member UKCC, UK

Maureen M. Michie RGN RM RSCN MTD
Midwifery Teacher, Glasgow College of Nursing and Midwifery, Glasgow, UK

Jean Proud SRN SCM MTD
Midwife Teacher, Mid Trent College of Nursing and Midwifery, Nottingham; Former Midwife in Charge of Obstetric Ultrasound, Peterborough District Hospital, Peterborough, UK

Sarah Rankin BEd(Hons) RN RM MTD
Professional and Academic Supervisor, Midwifery and Continuing Education Studies, Bethlehem University, Faculty of Nursing and Midwifery, West Bank, Israel; Former Education Officer, English National Board for Nursing, Midwifery and Health Visiting, UK

Sarah Roch RGN RM MTD FPACert
Head of Midwifery Education/Assistant Principal, Department of Midwifery Education, Southampton University College of Nursing and Midwifery; Member UKCC, UK

Carolyn Roth BA SRN SCM ADM MTD
Senior Lecturer, Midwifery Studies, South Bank University, London, UK

Jennifer Sleep BA SRN SCM MTD
Director of Nursing and Midwifery Research, Berkshire College of Nursing and Midwifery, Reading, UK

Anne Thompson BEd(Hons) RGN RM MTD
Senior Lecturer, Royal College of Midwives, London, UK

Elizabeth Thomson BA(Hons) RGN RSCN RM RCNT RNT
Nurse Teacher, Glasgow College of Nursing, Glasgow, UK

Valerie Thomson SRN SCM ADM PGCEA
Postgraduate Diploma in the Practice of Higher Education
Vice Principal, Continuing Nursing and Midwifery Studies, Princess Alexandra and Newham College of Nursing and Midwifery, London, UK

Valerie J. Tickner RGN RM MTD Diploma in Counselling Skills
Director of Education, Royal College of Midwives, London, UK

Elizabeth Torley BA RGN RSCN RCNT RNT
Nurse Teacher, Glasgow College of Nursing, Glasgow, UK

Josephine A. Williams SRN SCM DipN(Lond) ADM
Midwifery Manager, Royal Sussex County Hospital, Brighton, UK

Contents

1

Introduction

The midwife

V. RUTH BENNETT   LINDA K. BROWN

MIDWIVES AND WOMEN

Women throughout the ages have depended upon a skilled person, usually another woman, to be with them during childbirth. That person is the midwife, literally 'with woman'. Her skill is based on a mixture of art and science, art because it requires her to be able to understand the woman's needs, to encourage her and build her confidence, science because it demands a high degree of knowledge and decision-making ability. It is this thorough grounding in knowledge and experience that allows the midwife to refrain from taking control away from the mother while being at hand to step in where assistance is needed. Commitment to caring for the woman will lead the midwife to offer continuity wherever this is possible and to see through her responsibility to the individual mother.

Recent investigation into the maternity services in the United Kingdom (House of Commons 1992) established that women place a high premium on continuity, control and choice. Midwives see birth as a social event as opposed to a medical one and it is part of their remit to preserve this normal family context for women even when there are deviations from physiological expectations. Developments in patterns of the provision of care have led to schemes such as team midwifery and a renewal of interest in community-based practice (Hughes 1992, Melia et al 1991). A desire to see midwifery get back to its roots and detach itself from undue influence by nursing has resulted in an increase in pre-registration ('direct entry') midwifery education programmes (see Ch. 47).

Definition of the midwife

Over 20 years ago a definition of the midwife was jointly developed by the International Confederation of Midwives (ICM) and the International Federation of Gynaecology and Obstetrics (FIGO). In 1990, at the Kobe Council Meeting, ICM amended the definition which was later ratified by FIGO (in 1991) and the World Health Organization (in 1992).

DEFINITION OF THE MIDWIFE

A midwife is a person who, having been regularly admitted to a midwifery educational programme, duly recognized in the country in which it is located, has successfully completed the prescribed course of studies in midwifery and has acquired the requisite qualifications to be registered and/or legally licensed to practise midwifery.

She must be able to give the necessary supervision, care and advice to women during pregnancy, labour and the postpartum period, to conduct deliveries on her own responsibility and to care for the newborn and the infant. This care includes preventative measures, the detection of abnormal conditions in mother and child, the procurement of medical assistance and the execution of emergency measures in the absence of medical help. She has an important task in health counselling and education, not only for the women, but also within the family and the community. The work should involve antenatal education and preparation for parenthood and extends to certain areas of gynaecology, family planning and child care. She may practise in hospitals, clinics, health units, domiciliary conditions or in any other service.

(International Confederation of
Midwives 1992)

The concept of the midwife as an independent practitioner in her own right is one that is precious to those within the profession but not always fully understood. The midwife may diagnose pregnancy and various conditions related to it, give certain drugs without prescription (see Ch. 42) especially during labour and the postnatal period and retain responsibility for the total care of a childbearing woman as long as events remain within the range of normality. She is entitled to call upon medical assistance if it is required but is also empowered to undertake emergency measures pending the doctor's arrival.

AN INDEPENDENT PRACTITIONER

The competent midwife is able to carry out a wide range of skills. Some of her tasks overlap with those of the nurse, while others are similar to those of the obstetrician and paediatrician.

Skills of the midwife

The Midwives' Rules (UKCC 1991) detail the outcomes which programmes of midwifery education must achieve (Rule 33(3)). They encompass not only skills and duties but ability to appreciate the woman's background and the effect this may have on her well-being and that of her baby. The midwife takes responsibility for her own actions but also may initiate care by others and is able to function in a multi-professional team. Keeping up to date is an essential aspect of practice and she must work within legislation governing the profession. Her wise judgement is applied to decisions for care and also takes into account ethical principles (see Ch. 51).

Promotion of health. The midwife has an excellent opportunity to teach families about healthy living through parent education (see Ch. 9) both before and after the birth of the baby. Advice about health care needs to take into account the influence of social factors and to be given in the context of a political awareness and cultural understanding regarding her clients. Society is today composed of people from many religious and cultural backgrounds, some of whom may speak languages which are not the native tongue of the midwife. The use of link workers and interpreters may help to bridge the gap and to make health education accessible to all without offending sensibilities.

Assessment. Health is not simply an absence of disease and especially not a judgement about the 'normality' of a person. Health is not an impossible ideal nor even a potential that a person could reach if she followed a healthy lifestyle. It depends on context and on relationships and on the trust that a person can place in her body and herself (Benner & Wrubel 1989). The midwife needs a deep perception of the influence of emotions and of the meaning of events for an individual in the light of that person's understanding and the priorities which emanate from her experience. Physical factors are obviously important but other dimensions are equally essential to consider when assessing the well-being of a mother and her child.

Managing care. Midwifery is a balance between giving care and affirming the woman's ability to care for herself. The midwife must be competent to diagnose pregnancy and carry out examinations of the woman and her baby in order to assess their condition. She plans whatever care is necessary and sees that it is implemented. Very often, it will be the woman herself who will administer the care and the midwife treats her as an equal, if not the senior partner (Ashton 1992), in planning. The midwife's responsibility continues as she evaluates the effectiveness of the plan which has been carried out and changes it as necessary. The care has implications for the whole family and all aspects of their situation must be considered.

Independent action. The midwife is the expert in normal midwifery and has an obligation to care for mothers and babies. In emergency situations she is trained, while summoning medical aid, to take immediate steps to treat mother or baby and to continue to give care while help is on the way.

Initiating the action of others. The midwife is never in a position to relinquish care of a mother and baby (except to another midwife or in order to transfer care at the end of the postnatal period). She may, however, have need of the expertise and intervention of other disciplines. The obstet-

rician and general practitioner should be her closest allies and may be called upon to give aid when deviations from normal arise. Similarly, the paediatrician is available for the care of the baby. Dietitians, physiotherapists, social workers and health visitors are among other professionals to whom the midwife may refer in appropriate circumstances.

Undertaking care prescribed by a doctor. The duty to administer care and treatment prescribed by a registered medical practitioner goes beyond simply following instructions. The midwife is expected to interpret orders and, if necessary, question or challenge. There may be circumstances in which she has to urge the doctor to take action and others in which she may caution restraint. When a midwife has called in a doctor, the responsibility for the problem becomes that of the doctor, and she must follow medical orders, but there remains a duty to continue caring for the mother and baby even when the doctor has taken charge.

Communication. The skilful midwife develops effective communication with her clients, her colleagues and those in other disciplines. This will involve enabling them to express their wishes and views and exercising empathy towards them. Counselling skills are important tools which contribute to this and Chapter 49 discusses these more fully.

Research awareness. As midwifery research grows year by year, it becomes increasingly important for the competent midwife to be alert to new knowledge that has been established by research and to develop a questioning and reflective attitude towards her own practice. There is a wealth of literature and resources now available to help midwives to know what has been established by systematic enquiry. More and more midwives are ready to investigate questions by undertaking their own local studies and audit procedures. Chapter 50 will help midwives to understand the research process and to evaluate research reports while Chapter 52 gives a guide to quality control and audit.

A team member. Being an independent practitioner goes hand in hand with membership of the multi-professional team which exists to care for mothers and babies. The midwife must take the trouble to understand the roles of her colleagues and to develop harmonious relationships with them.

Keeping the law. The practice of a midwife is controlled by law. Midwives must have an understanding of the requirements of the legislation relevant to the practice of midwifery. In the United Kingdom the Nurses, Midwives and Health Visitors Acts 1979 and 1992 are the basis of this legislation (see Ch. 48); other Acts of Parliament that are relevant include the Congenital Disabilities (Civil Liabilities) Act 1976, the Data Protection Act 1984, the Births and Deaths Registration Acts and Public Health Acts (see Ch. 43) and the Acts regulating the prescription and use of drugs (see Ch. 42).

Ethical issues. Certain codes and standards are agreed by the profession, and midwives, like nurses and health visitors, are bound by the Code of Professional Conduct (UKCC 1992a). This includes matters such as maintaining confidentiality, maintaining and improving one's own professional competence while acknowledging any limitations, and working with clients in such a way as to foster their independence and respect them as unique individuals. The practitioner is enjoined to report circumstances which would jeopardise standards of practice or which would endanger the safe and appropriate care of clients or the health and safety of colleagues. The midwife may find herself in a situation where her own values are challenged and she has to assist parents in choices which involve moral judgements. Chapter 51 provides a framework in which she may consider such difficult decisions.

Assignment of duties to others. The midwife may not delegate any of her midwifery responsibilities to a non-midwife (although a registered medical practitioner may appropriately give midwifery care). She will often, however, have need of the assistance of other staff such as nurses, health care assistants and auxiliaries and perhaps of family members, especially the partner of her client. She may assign appropriate duties to such helpers, but retains the responsibility to supervise and monitor any tasks that she has asked them to undertake.

Responsibilities of the midwife

The unique status of the midwife brings tremendous satisfaction and reward: it also demands that she is accountable for her actions and it lays upon her great responsibility.

Competence. Each midwife has a responsibility to maintain professional competence. The sphere of her practice is clearly laid down in the Midwives' Rules (UKCC 1991) and A Midwife's Code of Practice (UKCC 1989) and is subject to the principles of the Code of Professional Conduct (UKCC 1992a). As midwifery practice develops, there may be occasion to integrate new skills into the range of those that midwives use in order to meet the needs of mothers and babies. Some of these will be required by all midwives and in due course will become part of the normal preparation of midwives during their basic training programmes in the way that perineal repair has done in recent years; others will be specific to midwives practising in certain settings, for example a midwife may (with appropriate study and experience) add ultrasonography to her skills in order to provide an additional service to women attending antenatal clinics. The UKCC (1992b) has published a booklet entitled *The Scope of Professional Practice* to guide practitioners in judging when this scope may appropriately be adjusted.

The supervisor of midwives has a special responsibility in regard to maintaining standards of midwifery practice (see Ch. 48). Part of her responsibility is to ensure that all midwives are fully competent and that they notify their intention to practise year by year. If any midwife lacks appropriate education the supervisor has a duty to ensure that this is arranged in order to maintain the midwife's skills and to protect the public.

Responsibility to keep records. Rule 42 (UKCC 1991) requires the midwife to keep detailed records which must be made 'as contemporaneously as is reasonable', in other words, as near the event as possible. Records must be in a form acceptable to the employer and approved by the Local Supervising Authority. A midwife in independent practice will discuss the format of her records with her supervisor of midwives.

The midwife's record is distinct from that of the doctor although she may contribute to the medical record, especially during pregnancy. She must keep records of the midwifery history (see Ch. 10) and of all antenatal examinations which she makes. During labour, records of observations, examinations and care are essential and it is here that it is particularly important to enter details promptly, because events move on so rapidly (see Chs 11 and 12). A register of controlled drugs is kept for the purpose of monitoring the issue and use of drugs of addiction. The midwife's register of births is usually kept communally by hospital midwives but individually by a community midwife. The fact that several midwives may make entries in a shared record does not absolve the individual midwife from entering all details of her own observations and care personally. Postnatal records are equally important and must be made at the time of each attendance (UKCC 1989 Section 7.1; see also Ch. 16).

Maternity units use a wide variety of records and notes, including those which are designed to be entered into a computer and others which are appropriate to the midwifery process or to varying styles of individualised care.

All records that are made by a midwife must be preserved for a period of not less than 25 years. The reason for this is that the record may be needed for the midwife's protection in cases of litigation or allegations of professional misconduct. Under the Congenital Disabilities (Civil Liabilities) Act 1976, a child may sue for damages where he has suffered as a result of negligence during his mother's pregnancy or labour and this litigation may be delayed as long as 21 years after the events involved. Scottish law makes similar provisions.

Responsibility to the family. As midwives are involved with very intimate aspects of the life of a family, they have a special duty to practise with absolute integrity. Confidentiality is of prime importance. Sensitive, private matters must be handled with delicacy and the midwife should value each individual without censure for beliefs or standards which may be at variance with her own. This does not mean that she does not use her judgement; she should constantly assess the needs of the mother and child within the family and may perceive a need for education or for warning of danger or for intervention on behalf of

an unprotected member such as a child at risk of abuse.

In order to offer the best care possible, the midwife needs to keep her knowledge and skills up to date. She may tap resources beyond her own if the family requires other support such as that of a social worker.

Society is subject to constant change and the midwife is challenged to be flexible in order to adapt to change as it occurs. Whatever the circumstances 'a woman will need to be physically safe, psychologically satisfied and morally unoffended during pregnancy and childbirth.' (Royal College of Midwives 1987).

Responsibility to the profession. Midwives have a responsibility for the image of their profession. For all to keep moving forward, each individual must be sufficiently committed to play an active role in order to preserve standards and improve care. For some this will mean initiating change or trying experiments, for others it will mean following in the footsteps of the innovators.

Professional involvement includes awareness of the activities of professional organisations and statutory bodies. Current journals should be read as a matter of course; discussion documents are often circulated for consultation and comment and it is vital that midwives respond to requests for their opinions. All should become members of professional organisations; some must be ready to accept office locally and nationally. Every midwife should use her vote in statutory body elections; a few are needed who have developed the knowledge and expertise to stand for election and become members of those bodies.

Drawing midwifery issues to the attention of the public may necessitate use of the media and midwives should be ready to write to the newspapers or to take part in broadcast features when appropriate. There are some occasions when the best course of action is to lobby Members of Parliament, and midwives made good use of the opportunity to do this during the hearings of the Select Committee on Health which culminated in the Winterton report (House of Commons 1992).

Midwives need not be afraid of making their voices heard. Responsible exercise of these means of activating those in power has in the past help-ed to achieve a better service for mothers and babies.

Responsibility to society. The midwife needs to act as a responsible citizen. She may be in a position to highlight areas of concern such as social deprivation, poor housing, racial prejudice, the effects of violence or the progress of epidemics or prevalent infections such as AIDS or tuberculosis. Her response in such circumstances may be to warn, to mobilise resources or to offer active care.

Midwives enjoy the trust of the public. Each midwife should value that trust and earn its continuation.

The rewards of being a midwife

The birth of an individual baby is unique and unrepeatable. The midwife is enormously privileged to share that event and contribute her skill to its accomplishment. If she has been fortunate enough to have known and worked with the family throughout pregnancy, or even before, she will derive great satisfaction from the continuity of care, especially if she can also assist with the integration of the baby into the family. Continuity is also much appreciated by the mother and adds to her feeling of security.

Sometimes things do not go so well and the baby dies before birth or soon after. At these times the midwife is treading on delicate ground as she shares the pain of the parents' loss, but she may earn their gratitude for her support if she has been able to use her skills to comfort them and accept their feelings of grief (see Ch. 49).

There is a delight for the midwife in developing and perfecting the skills of her art and in preparing her mind in the science of midwifery for possible contingencies. Many of her skills are gained through experience and adapted to individual mothers and babies through her judgement of circumstances. There are few instances where she is not working as a partner with the mother and helping her to achieve competence in her own abilities. On occasion, the midwife is in the position of acting to avert disaster and when life is saved the relief is overwhelming.

MIDWIFERY AROUND THE WORLD

The circumstances of midwifery care are as varied as the many different societies and geographical features in the world. Many developed countries offer sophisticated training for midwives and a comprehensive midwifery service to women and families, from before pregnancy to the end of the postnatal period. There is, however, a failure by governments in some countries, both in the developed and the developing world, to recognise midwifery as a profession. This situation leads either to midwives practising illegally or to women having the choice between care from an obstetrician, which could be an expensive option, and untrained help. The hazards of being attended by an untrained person or of birth being completely unattended are all too real.

The education of midwives may be a distinct training or be combined with nurse training or follow registration as a nurse: where there is no legal status for midwives it may be entirely informal. Standards of training are not only related to the length of the course but also to available resources. Rainy seasons, road conditions and the availability of transport, food and safe water all affect the working lives of midwives and students. Libraries may be a luxury item with essentials such as paper and pencils in sporadic supply. The inclusion of essential life-saving skills are not necessarily a feature of basic training.

Midwifery care in many countries begins before pregnancy, extends through antenatal, intrapartum and postnatal periods and continues on to immunisation programmes and the general care of the child until school age. The midwife's role includes family planning advice and care for the mother and also incorporates aspects which are assigned to dietitians and physiotherapists in developed countries.

Personnel with whom midwives work and liaise include not only obstetricians and paediatricians, with whom midwives in the developed world are familiar, but also faith healers, traditional medicine-men and the elders of villages. Without the sanction of these respected people in the villages it may not be permissible to seek the necessary care for the women. To be acceptable to the village communities the midwife will be expected to follow traditional methods of care. These may be healthy and beneficial but they may entail the use of harmful substances or practices. Technological advances may feature in care and prove advantageous; alternatively they may be improperly applied and therefore prove detrimental.

Friendship between midwives is demonstrated in many ways and crosses geographical limits and the barriers of sex and race. Midwives in developed countries are seeking to rediscover the simplicity of 'natural childbirth' whilst those in developing countries are seeking to improve the status and education of women alongside the provision of safe midwifery care and the adoption of some of the technological advances which may benefit mothers in their care. It is the responsibility of midwives to seek a balance between the extremes of care which are available, depending on local circumstances and resources.

European Community Midwives' Directive
In spite of variety within the EC, a common Directive (80/155/EEC Article 4) defines the activities of the midwife.

Safe motherhood
The Safe Motherhood Initiative began in Nairobi in 1987 and has as its target the halving of maternal mortality by the year 2000. While the developed world enjoys mortality rates that are almost negligible (see Ch. 43), this is not true for developing countries where an appallingly high toll of deaths is attributed to poverty, low status for women, female illiteracy, inadequate primary health care and poor communication networks (International News 1987). Midwives are actively playing a part in supporting the Initiative through the International Confederation of Midwives (ICM) network and the establishment of an International Day of the Midwife (IDN) each May to raise awareness throughout the world. At the celebration of the first IDN in 1991, ICM declared the intent of midwives to not only reduce mortality among mothers but to improve the quality of life for women whose health is damaged

Member States shall ensure that midwives are at least entitled to take up and pursue the following activities:
- to provide sound family planning information and advice;
- to diagnose pregnancies and monitor normal pregnancies; to carry out examinations necessary for the monitoring of normal pregnancies;
- to prescribe or advise on the examinations necessary for the earliest possible diagnosis of pregnancies at risk;
- to provide a programme of parenthood preparation and a complete preparation for childbirth including advice on hygiene and nutrition;
- to care for and assist the mother during labour and to monitor the condition of the fetus in utero by the appropriate clinical and technical means;
- to conduct spontaneous deliveries, including where required an episiotomy and in urgent cases a breech delivery;
- to recognise the warning signs of abnormality in the mother or infant which necessitate referral to a doctor and to assist the latter where appropriate; to take the necessary emergency measures in the doctor's absence,* in particular the manual removal of the placenta possibly followed by manual examination of the uterus;
- to examine and care for the new-born infant; to take all initiatives which are necessary in case of need and to carry out where necessary immediate resuscitation;
- to care for and monitor the progress of the mother in the postnatal period and to give all necessary advice to the mother on infant care to enable her to ensure the optimum progress of her new-born infant;
- to carry out the treatment prescribed by a doctor;
- to maintain all necessary records.

* In present day practice in the United Kingdom the midwife should not normally find herself in a position where medical aid is not available for such a grave emergency as manual removal of the placenta.

as a result of childbearing (ICM 1991). Among the measures that are needed to combat such ill-health are safe water and avoidance of heavy work in pregnancy as well as family spacing and the education of girls. Midwives have been identified as a group which has been overlooked as a resource with great potential for achieving appropriate care at the primary level, and initiatives have been taken for educating midwives for safe motherhood.

AN EDUCATED PRACTITIONER

Since the middle of this century midwives in the UK have enjoyed the privilege of statutory periodic refreshment and have attended approved courses every 5 years. In recent times the scope and range of refresher courses has widened and various alternatives are available such as 1-week residential courses, 2-week practical courses and single study days which can be accumulated. Equally important, however, is the need to read and reflect on a continuous basis, to use books and journals, discuss cases with peers, encourage colleagues (Hunt 1991) and implement changes that are tested by the use of research (Downe 1991). The range of advanced courses is growing each year, many midwives are acquiring diplomas and Bachelor's and Master's degrees and a few have earned doctorates through high quality research. The UKCC, in its PREP (post-registration education and practice) Project has indicated that all practitioners must in future demonstrate their continuing education by keeping a professional profile of learning throughout their careers; the renewal of their registration will depend on being able to demonstrate that they have been developing their knowledge during the previous 3 years.

The UKCC's Code of Professional Conduct states, 'As a registered ... midwife ... you are personally accountable for your practice and, in the exercise of your professional accountability,

must: maintain and improve your professional knowledge and competence;'. The midwife who takes this statement seriously will become the skilled person on whom a mother depends and she will take joy in providing a service which will satisfy her clients.

Acknowledgement

The chapter authors wish to express gratitude to Miss Joan Walker, Secretary-General of the International Confederation of Midwives, 10 Barley Mow Passage, Chiswick, London W4 4PH for advice and assistance with the preparation of this chapter and for drafting the section about international midwifery.

REFERENCES

Ashton R 1992 Who can speak for women? Nursing Times 88(29); 70

Benner P, Wrubel J 1989 The primacy of caring. Addison-Wesley, California

Downe S 1991 The midwife as practitioner: midwifery standards — uniformity or quality? Midwives Chronicle 104(1236): 2–3

House of Commons 1992 Health Committee: second report: maternity services. HMSO, London

Hughes D 1992 Midwifery care for the poor MIDIRS. Midwifery Digest 2: 1

Hunt S 1991 Continuing education for midwives — a woman's right. Midwives Chronicle 104(1236): 6–7

International Confederation of Midwives 1991 Statement of intent. Cited in: Midwives Chronicle 104(1242): 192

International Confederation of Midwives 1992 Definition of the midwife. Ref 90/1/PP, ICM, London

International News 1987 Safe motherhood. Midwifery 3(2): 97–98

Melia R J et al 1991 Consumers' views of the maternity services: implications for change and quality assurance. Journal of Public Health Medicine 13(2): 120–126

Royal College of Midwives 1987 Towards a healthy nation. RCM, London

United Kingdom Central Council for Nursing, Midwifery and Health Visiting 1989 A midwife's code of practice. UKCC, London, reprinted 1991

United Kingdom Central Council for Nursing, Midwifery and Health Visiting 1991 Midwives rules. UKCC, London

United Kingdom Central Council for Nursing, Midwifery and Health Visiting 1992a Code of professional conduct. UKCC, London

United Kingdom Central Council for Nursing, Midwifery and Health Visiting 1992b The scope of professional practice. UKCC, London

2

Anatomy and Physiology

2

The reproductive organs

V. RUTH BENNETT LINDA K. BROWN

Woman is first and foremost a person and, when she bears a child, a mother. Many societies define her through her fertility and her body is adapted for this by its shape and function. The midwife needs to be familiar with the anatomical features of the woman and to understand the processes of reproduction but must never forget the social significance of childbearing or that a woman's body is unique, personal and private. It should be approached only with permission and with respect.

FEMALE PELVIS

Functions

The primary function of the pelvic girdle is to allow movement of the body, especially walking and running.

It permits the person to sit and kneel. The woman's pelvis is adapted for childbearing, and because of its increased width and rounded brim women are less speedy.

The pelvis transmits the weight of the trunk to the legs, acting as a bridge between the femurs. This makes it necessary for the sacro-iliac joint to be immensely strong and virtually immobile. It also takes the weight of the sitting body onto the ischial tuberosities.

The pelvis affords protection to the pelvic organs and, to a lesser extent, to the abdominal contents. The sacrum transmits the cauda equina and

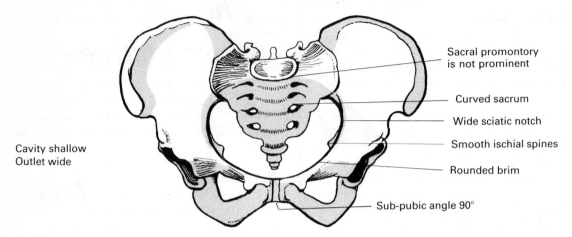

Sacral promontory
is not prominent

Curved sacrum

Wide sciatic notch

Smooth ischial spines

Rounded brim

Cavity shallow
Outlet wide

Sub-pubic angle 90°

Fig. 2.1
Normal female pelvis.

distributes the nerves to the various parts of the pelvis.

The gynaecoid pelvis

The gynaecoid is regarded as the true female pelvis because its characteristics give rise to no difficulties in childbirth, providing the fetus is of normal size. A knowledge of pelvic anatomy is needed for the conduct of labour as one of the ways to estimate the progress made is by assessing the relationship of the fetus to certain pelvic landmarks. A midwife must be competent to recognise a normal pelvis in order to be able to detect deviations from normal and refer them to the doctor.

Pelvic bones

There are four pelvic bones:

- two innominate ('nameless') or hip bones
- one sacrum
- one coccyx.

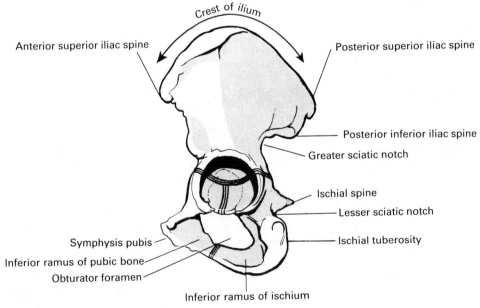

Crest of *ilium*

Anterior superior iliac spine

Posterior superior iliac spine

Posterior inferior iliac spine

Greater sciatic notch

Ischial spine

Lesser sciatic notch

Symphysis pubis

Ischial tuberosity

Inferior ramus of pubic bone

Obturator foramen

Inferior ramus of ischium

Fig. 2.2
Innominate bone showing important landmarks.

Innominate bones

Each innominate bone is composed of three parts:

The ilium is the large flared-out part. When the hand is placed on the hip it rests on the iliac crest which is the upper border. At the front of the iliac crest can be felt a bony prominence known as the anterior superior iliac spine.

A short distance below it is the anterior inferior iliac spine. There are two similar points at the other end of the iliac crest, namely the posterior superior and the posterior inferior iliac spines. The concave anterior surface of the ilium is the iliac fossa.

The ischium is the thick lower part. It has a large prominence known as the ischial tuberosity on which the body rests when sitting. Behind and a little above the tuberosity is an inward projection, the ischial spine. In labour the station of the fetal head is estimated in relation to the ischial spines.

The pubic bone forms the anterior part. It has a body and two oar-like projections, the superior ramus and the inferior ramus. The two pubic bones meet at the symphysis pubis and the two inferior rami form the pubic arch, merging into a similar ramus on the ischium. The space enclosed by the body of the pubic bone, the rami and the ischium is called the obturator foramen.

The innominate bone contains a deep cup to receive the head of the femur. This is termed the acetabulum. All three parts of the bone contribute to the acetabulum in the following proportions: two-fifths ilium, two-fifths ischium and one-fifth pubic bone.

On the lower border of the innominate bone are found two curves. One extends from the posterior inferior iliac spine up to the ischial spine and is called the *greater sciatic notch*. It is wide and rounded. The other lies between the ischial spine and the ischial tuberosity and is the *lesser sciatic notch*.

The sacrum

The sacrum is a wedge-shaped bone consisting of five fused vertebrae. The upper border of the first sacral vertebra juts forward and is known as the sacral promontory. The anterior surface of the sacrum is concave and is referred to as the *hollow of the sacrum*. Laterally the sacrum extends into a *wing* or *ala*. Four pairs of holes or foramina pierce the sacrum and, through these, nerves from the cauda equina emerge to supply the pelvic organs. The posterior surface is roughened to receive attachments of muscles.

The coccyx

The coccyx is a vestigial tail. It consists of four fused vertebrae, forming a small triangular bone.

Pelvic joints

There are four pelvic joints:

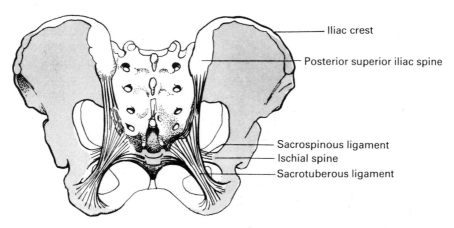

Fig. 2.3
Posterior view of the pelvis to show ligaments.

Iliac crest

Posterior superior iliac spine

Sacrospinous ligament
Ischial spine
Sacrotuberous ligament

- one symphysis pubis
- two sacro-iliac joints
- one sacrococcygeal joint.

The symphysis pubis is formed at the junction of the two pubic bones which are united by a pad of cartilage.

The sacro-iliac joints are the strongest joints in the body. They join the sacrum to the ilium and thus connect the spine to the pelvis.

The sacrococcygeal joint is formed where the base of the coccyx articulates with the tip of the sacrum.

In the non-pregnant state there is very little movement in these joints, but during pregnancy endocrine activity causes the ligaments to soften, which allows the joints to give. This may provide more room for the fetal head as it passes through the pelvis. The symphysis pubis may separate slightly in later pregnancy. If it widens appreciably, the degree of movement permitted may give rise to pain on walking. The sacro-iliac joints allow a limited backward and forward movement of the tip and promontory of the sacrum sometimes known as nodding of the sacrum. The sacrococcygeal joint permits the coccyx to be deflected backwards during the birth of the head.

Pelvic ligaments

Each of the pelvic joints is held together by ligaments:

- interpubic ligaments at the symphysis pubis

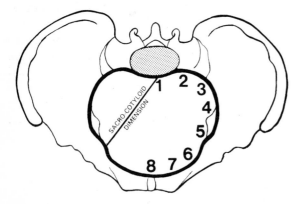

Fig. 2.4
Brim or inlet of female pelvis.

- sacro-iliac ligaments
- sacrococcygeal ligaments.

There are two other ligaments important in midwifery:

- sacrotuberous ligament
- sacrospinous ligament.

The sacrotuberous ligament runs from the sacrum to the ischial tuberosity and the sacrospinous ligament from the sacrum to the ischial spine. These two ligaments cross the sciatic notch and form the posterior wall of the pelvic outlet.

The true pelvis

The true pelvis is the bony canal through which the fetus must pass during birth. It has a brim, a cavity and an outlet.

The pelvic brim

The brim is round except where the sacral promontory projects into it. The promontory and wings of the sacrum form its posterior border, the iliac bones its lateral borders and the pubic bones its anterior border. The midwife needs to be familiar with the fixed points on the pelvic brim which are known as its landmarks. Commencing posteriorly these are (see Fig. 2.4):

- sacral promontory (1)
- sacral ala or wing (2)
- sacro-iliac joint (3)
- iliopectineal line which is the edge formed at the inward aspect of the ilium (4)
- iliopectineal eminence which is a roughened area formed where the superior ramus of the pubic bone meets the ilium (5)
- superior ramus of the pubic bone (6)
- upper inner border of the body of the pubic bone (7)
- upper inner border of the symphysis pubis (8).

Diameters of the brim
Three diameters are measured:

The anteroposterior diameter is a line from the sacral promontory to the upper border of the symphysis pubis. When the line is taken to the uppermost point of the symphysis pubis it is called the anatomical conjugate and measures 12 cm; when it is taken to the posterior border of the upper surface, which is about 1.25 cm lower, it is called the obstetrical conjugate and measures 11 cm. The reason for this is that the obstetrical conjugate represents the available space for passage of the fetus (see Fig. 2.5). The term *true conjugate* may be used to refer to either of these measurements and the midwife should take care to establish which is meant.

The diagonal conjugate is also measured anteroposteriorly from the lower border of the symphysis to the sacral promontory. It may be estimated per vaginam as part of a pelvic assessment and should measure 12–13 cm (Fig. 2.6).

The oblique diameter is a line from one sacro-iliac joint to the iliopectineal eminence on the opposite side of the pelvis and measures 12 cm. There are two oblique diameters. Each takes its name from the sacro-iliac joint from which it arises, that is, the left oblique diameter arises from the left sacro-iliac joint.

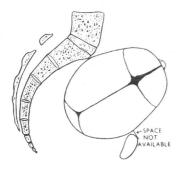

Fig. 2.5
Fetal head negotiating the narrow obstetrical conjugate.

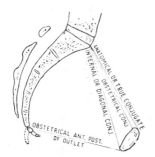

Fig. 2.6
Median section of the pelvis showing anteroposterior diameters.

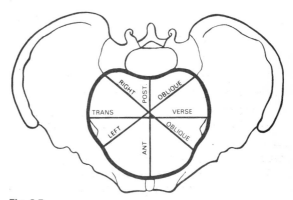

Fig. 2.7
View of pelvic inlet showing diameters.

The transverse diameter is a line between the points furthest apart on the iliopectineal lines and measures 13 cm.

Certain structures pass through the pelvic brim which may affect the space available for the fetus, for instance, the descending colon enters the pelvis near the left sacro-iliac joint.

Another dimension is described, the *sacrocotyloid*. It passes from the sacral promontory to the iliopectineal eminence on each side and measures 9–9.5 cm. Its importance is concerned with posterior positions of the occiput when the parietal eminences of the fetal head may become caught (see Ch. 26).

The pelvic cavity

The cavity extends from the brim above to the outlet below. The anterior wall is formed by the pubic bones and symphysis pubis and its depth is 4 cm. The posterior wall is formed by the curve of the sacrum which is 12 cm in length. Because there is such a difference in these measurements the cavity forms a curved canal. Its lateral walls are the sides of the pelvis which are mainly covered by the obturator internus muscle.

The cavity is circular in shape and although it is not possible to measure its diameters exactly, they are all considered to be 12 cm.

The pelvic outlet

Two outlets are described: the anatomical and the obstetrical. The anatomical outlet is formed by the lower borders of each of the bones together

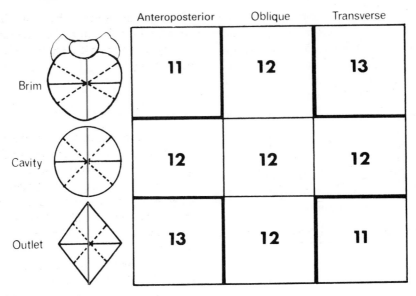

	Anteroposterior	Oblique	Transverse
Brim	11	12	13
Cavity	12	12	12
Outlet	13	12	11

Fig. 2.8
Measurements of the pelvic canal in centimetres.

with the sacrotuberous ligament. The obstetrical outlet is of greater practical significance because it includes the narrow pelvic strait through which the fetus must pass. The narrow pelvic strait lies between the sacrococcygeal joint, the two ischial spines and the lower border of the symphysis pubis. The obstetrical outlet is the space between the narrow pelvic strait and the anatomical outlet. This outlet is diamond-shaped. Its three diameters are as follows:

The anteroposterior diameter is a line from the lower border of the symphysis pubis to the sacrococcygeal joint. It measures 13 cm. As the coccyx may be deflected backwards during labour, this diameter indicates the space available during delivery.

The oblique diameter is said to be between the obturator foramen and the sacrospinous ligament, although there are no fixed points. The measurement is taken as being 12 cm.

The transverse diameter is a line between the two ischial spines and measures 10–11 cm. It is the narrowest diameter in the pelvis.

The false pelvis

This is the part of the pelvis situated above the pelvic brim. It is formed by the upper flared-out portions of the iliac bones and protects the abdominal organs, but is of no significance in obstetrics.

Pelvic inclination

When a woman is standing in the upright position, her pelvis is on an incline. The anterior superior iliac spines are immediately above the symphysis pubis in the same vertical plane. The brim is tilted and if the line joining the sacral promontory and the top of the symphysis pubis were to be extended, it would form an angle of 60° with the horizontal floor. Similarly if a line joining the centre of the sacrum and the centre of the symphysis pubis were to be extended, the resultant angle with the floor would be 30°. The angle of inclination of the outlet is 15° (see Fig. 2.9). When the woman is in the recumbent position the same angles are made with the vertical, which should be kept in mind when carrying out an abdominal examination.

Pelvic planes
These are imaginary flat surfaces at the brim, cavity and outlet of the pelvic canal at the levels of the lines described above.

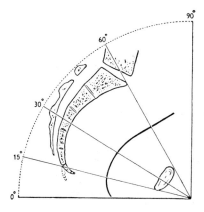

Fig. 2.9
Median section of the pelvis showing the inclination of the planes and the axis of the pelvic canal.

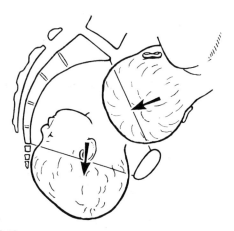

Fig. 2.10
Fetal head entering plane of pelvic brim and leaving plane of pelvic outlet. ·

Axis of the pelvic canal

A line drawn exactly half-way between the anterior wall and the posterior wall of the pelvic canal would trace a curve known as the curve of Carus.

The midwife needs to become familiar with this concept in order to make accurate observations on vaginal examination and to facilitate the birth of the baby.

The four types of pelvis

Classically pelves have been described as falling into four categories according to the shape of the brim. Of much more importance, however, is the individual woman's pelvic capacity and whether it is adequate for the passage of the child she is carrying (Williams et al 1989). It is a common saying that the fetal head is the best pelvimeter.

The gynaecoid pelvis, as described above, is the ideal pelvis for childbearing. Its main features are the rounded brim, the generous fore-pelvis (the part in front of the transverse diameter), straight side walls, a shallow cavity with a broad, well-curved sacrum, blunt ischial spines, a wide sciatic notch and a pubic arch of 90°. It is found in women of average build and height with a shoe size of 4 or larger.

The android pelvis is so called because it resembles the male pelvis. Its brim is heart-shaped with a narrow fore-pelvis, and has a transverse diameter which is towards the back. The side walls converge, making it a funnel shape with a deep cavity and a straight sacrum. The ischial spines are prominent and the sciatic notch is narrow. The angle of the pubic arch is less than 90°. It is found in short and heavily-built women who have a tendency to be hirsute. This type of pelvis predisposes to an occipitoposterior position of the fetal head and is the least suited to child bearing.

Table 2.1
Features of the four types of pelvis

Features	Gynaecoid	Android	Anthropoid	Platypelloid
Brim	rounded	heart-shaped	long oval	kidney-shaped
Fore-pelvis	generous	narrow	narrowed	wide
Side walls	straight	convergent	divergent	divergent
Ischial spines	blunt	prominent	blunt	blunt
Sciatic notch	rounded	narrow	wide	wide
Sub-pubic angle	90°	<90°	>90°	>90°
Incidence	50%	20%	25%	5%

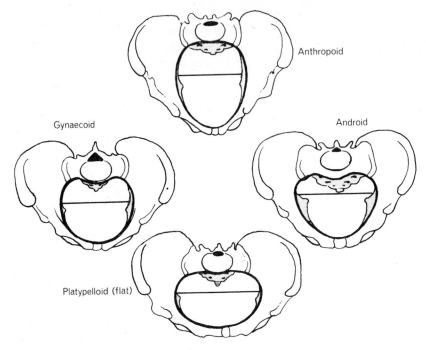

Fig. 2.11
Characteristic inlet of the four types of pelvis.

The anthropoid pelvis has a long, oval brim in which the anteroposterior diameter is longer than the transverse. The side walls diverge and the sacrum is long and deeply concave. The ischial spines are not prominent and the sciatic notch is very wide, as is the sub-pubic angle. Women with this type of pelvis tend to be tall, with narrow shoulders. Labour does not usually present any difficulties, but a direct occipito-anterior or occipitoposterior position is often a feature.

The platypelloid pelvis is flat, with a kidney-shaped brim in which the anteroposterior diameter is reduced and the transverse increased. The side walls diverge, the sacrum is flat and the cavity shallow. The ischial spines are blunt, and the sciatic notch and the sub-pubic angle are both wide. The head must engage with the sagittal suture in the transverse diameter, but usually descends through the cavity without difficulty.

PELVIC FLOOR

The pelvic floor is formed by the soft tissues which fill the outlet of the pelvis. The most important of these is the strong diaphragm of muscle slung like a hammock from the walls of the pelvis. Through it pass the urethra, the vagina and the anal canal.

Functions

The pelvic floor supports the weight of the abdominal and pelvic organs. Its muscles are responsible for the voluntary control of micturition and defaecation and play an important part in sexual intercourse. During childbirth it influences the passive movements of the fetus through the birth canal and relaxes to allow its exit from the pelvis.

Muscle layers

The superficial layer is composed of five muscles:

— *The external anal sphincter* surrounding the anus and attached behind by a few fibres to the coccyx.
— *The transverse perineal muscles* pass from the ischial tuberosities to the centre of the perineum.

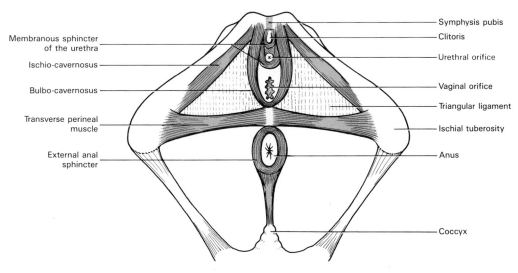

Membranous sphincter of the urethra

Ischio-cavernosus

Bulbo-cavernosus

Transverse perineal muscle

External anal sphincter

Symphysis pubis

Clitoris

Urethral orifice

Vaginal orifice

Triangular ligament

Ischial tuberosity

Anus

Coccyx

Fig. 2.12
Superficial layer of the pelvic floor.

— *The bulbocavernosus muscles* pass from the perineum forwards around the vagina to the corpora cavernosa of the clitoris just under the pubic arch.
— *The ischiocavernosus muscles* pass from the ischial tuberosities along the pubic arch to the corpora cavernosa.
— *The membranous sphincter of the urethra* is composed of muscle fibres passing above and below the urethra and attached to the pubic bones. It is not a true sphincter.

The deep layer is composed of three pairs of muscles which together are known as the levator ani muscles. They are so called because they lift or elevate the anus. Each levator ani muscle (left and right) consists of the following:

— *The pubococcygeus muscle* passes from the pubis to the coccyx, with a few fibres crossing over in the perineal body to form its deepest part.
— *The iliococcygeus muscle* passes from the

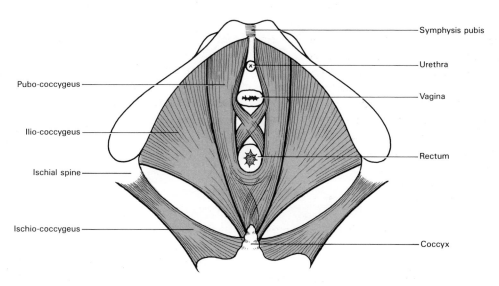

Pubo-coccygeus

Ilio-coccygeus

Ischial spine

Ischio-coccygeus

Symphysis pubis

Urethra

Vagina

Rectum

Coccyx

Fig. 2.13
Deep layer of the pelvic floor.

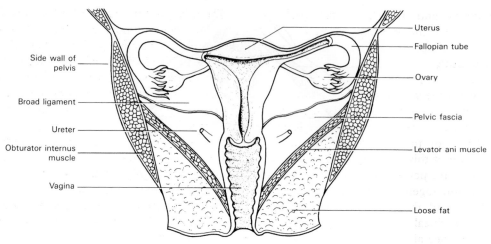

Fig. 2.14
Coronal section through the pelvis.

fascia covering the obturator internus muscle (the white line of pelvic fascia) to the coccyx.
— *The ischiococcygeus muscle* passes from the ischial spine to the coccyx, in front of the sacrospinous ligament.

Between the muscle layers, and also above and below them, there are layers of pelvic fascia. This is loose areolar tissue which is used like packing material in the spaces. The tissue that fills the triangular space between the bulbocavernosus, the

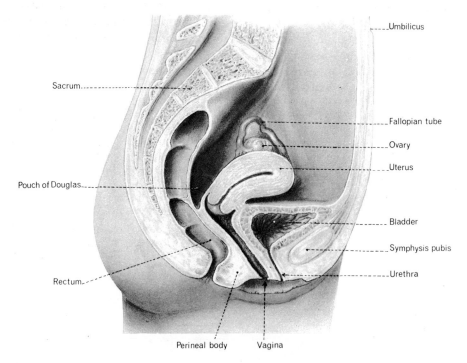

Fig. 2.15
Sagittal section of the pelvis.

ischiocavernosus and the transverse perineal muscles is known as the *triangular ligament*.

The perineal body

This is a pyramid of muscle and fibrous tissue situated between the vagina and the rectum. It is made up of fibres from muscles described above. The apex, which is the deepest part, is formed from the fibres of the pubococcygeus muscle which cross over at this point; the base is formed from the transverse perineal muscles which meet in the perineum, together with the bulbocavernosus in front and the external anal sphincter behind. The perineal body measures 4 cm in each direction. (See also Chapters 14 and 40 for the perineum in labour and for pelvic floor exercises.)

THE VULVA

This term applies to the external female genital organs. It consists of the following structures:

The mons pubis or **mons veneris** ('mount of Venus') is a pad of fat lying over the symphysis pubis. It is covered with pubic hair from the time of puberty.

The labia majora (greater lips) are two folds of fat and areolar tissue, covered with skin and pubic hair on the outer surface. They arise in the mons veneris and merge into the perineum behind.

The labia minora (lesser lips) are two thin folds of skin lying between the labia majora. Anteriorly they divide to enclose the clitoris; posteriorly they fuse, forming the fourchette.

The clitoris is a small rudimentary organ corresponding to the male penis. It is extremely sensitive and highly vascular and plays a part in the orgasm of sexual intercourse.

The vestibule is the area enclosed by the labia minora in which are situated the openings of the urethra and the vagina.

The urethral orifice lies 2.5 cm posterior to the clitoris. On either side lie the openings of Skene's ducts, two small blind-ended tubules 0.5 cm long running within the urethral wall.

The vaginal orifice is also known as the introitus of the vagina and occupies the posterior two-thirds of the vestibule. The orifice is partially closed by the hymen, a thin membrane which tears during sexual intercourse or during the birth of the first child. The remaining tags of hymen are known as the carunculae myrtiformes because they are thought to resemble myrtle berries.

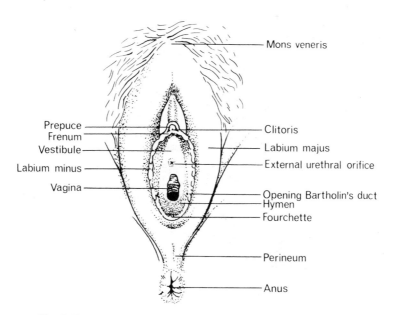

Fig. 2.16
Female external genital organs.

Bartholin's glands are two small glands which open on either side of the vaginal orifice and lie in the posterior part of the labia majora. They secrete mucus which lubricates the vaginal opening.

The vulval blood supply

This comes from the internal and the external pudendal arteries. The blood drains through corresponding veins.

Lymphatic drainage

This is mainly via the inguinal glands.

Nerve supply

This is derived from branches of the pudendal nerve.

THE VAGINA

Functions

The vagina is a passage which allows the escape of the menstrual flow, receives the penis and the ejected sperm during sexual intercourse and provides an exit for the fetus during delivery.

Position

It is a canal running from the vestibule to the cervix, passing upwards and backwards into the pelvis along a line approximately parallel to the plane of the pelvic brim.

Relations

A knowledge of the relations of the vagina is essential for the accurate examination of the pregnant woman and her safe delivery.

Anterior. In front lie the bladder and the urethra which are closely connected to the anterior vaginal wall.

Posterior. Behind, the pouch of Douglas, the rectum and the perineal body each occupy approximately one-third of the posterior vaginal wall.

Lateral. Beside the upper two-thirds are the pelvic fascia and the ureters which pass beside the cervix, while beside the lower third are the muscles of the pelvic floor.

Superior. Above the vagina lies the uterus.

Inferior. Below the vagina lie the external genitalia.

Structure

The posterior wall is 10 cm long while the anterior wall is only 7.5 cm in length because the cervix projects at a right angle into its upper part.

The upper end of the vagina is known as the vault. Where the cervix projects into it, the vault forms a circular recess which is described as four arches or fornices. The posterior fornix is the largest of these because the vagina is attached to the uterus at a higher level behind than in front. The anterior fornix lies in front of the cervix and the lateral fornices lie on either side. The vaginal walls are pink in appearance and thrown into small folds known as rugae. These allow the vaginal walls to stretch during intercourse and childbirth.

Layers

The lining is made of squamous epithelium.

Beneath the epithelium lies a layer of vascular connective tissue.

The muscle layer is divided into a weak inner coat of circular fibres and a stronger outer coat of longitudinal fibres.

Pelvic fascia surrounds the vagina, forming a layer of connective tissue.

Contents

There are no glands in the vagina. It is, however, moistened by mucus from the cervix and a transudate which seeps out from the blood vessels of the vaginal wall.

In spite of the alkaline mucus, the vaginal fluid is strongly acid (pH 4.5) due to the presence of lactic acid formed by the action of Döderlein's bacilli on glycogen found in the squamous epithelium of the lining. These lactobacilli are normal inhabitants of the vagina. The acid deters the growth of pathogenic bacteria.

Blood supply

This comes from branches of the internal iliac artery and includes the vaginal artery and a descending branch of the uterine artery. The blood drains through corresponding veins.

Lymphatic drainage
This is via the inguinal, the internal iliac and the sacral glands.

Nerve supply
This is derived from the Lee Frankenhäuser plexus.

THE UTERUS

Functions
The uterus exists to shelter the fetus during pregnancy. It prepares for this possibility each month and following pregnancy it expels the uterine contents.

Position
It is situated in the cavity of the true pelvis, behind the bladder and in front of the rectum. It leans forward, which is known as *anteversion*; it bends forwards on itself, which is known as *anteflexion*. When the woman is standing this results in an almost horizontal position with the fundus resting on the bladder.

Relations

Anterior. In front of the uterus lie the uterovesical pouch and the bladder.

Posterior. Behind the uterus are the recto-uterine pouch of Douglas and the rectum.

Lateral. On either side of the uterus are the broad ligaments, the fallopian tubes and the ovaries.

Superior. Above the uterus lie the intestines.

Inferior. Below the uterus is the vagina.

Supports
The uterus is supported by the pelvic floor and maintained in position by several ligaments of which those at the level of the cervix are the most important.

The transverse cervical ligaments fan out from the sides of the cervix to the side walls of the pelvis. They are sometimes known as the cardinal ligaments or Mackenrodt's ligaments.

The uterosacral ligaments pass backwards from the cervix to the sacrum.

The pubocervical ligaments pass forwards from the cervix, under the bladder, to the pubic bones.

The broad ligaments are formed from the folds of peritoneum which are draped over the fallopian tubes. They hang down like a curtain and spread from the sides of the uterus to the side walls of the pelvis.

The round ligaments have little value as a support but tend to maintain the anteverted position of the uterus. They arise from the cornua of the uterus in front of and below the insertion of each fallopian tube and pass between the folds of the broad ligament, through the inguinal canal to be inserted into each labium majus.

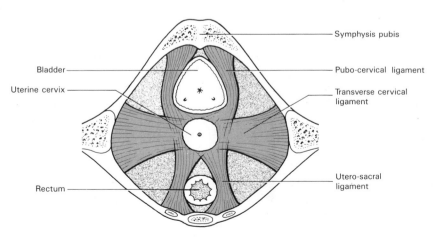

Fig. 2.17
Supports of the uterus.

The ovarian ligaments also begin at the cornua of the uterus but behind the fallopian tubes and pass down between the folds of the broad ligament to the ovaries.

It is helpful to note that the round ligament, fallopian tube and the ovarian ligament are very similar in appearance and arise from the same area of the uterus. This makes careful identification important when tubal surgery is undertaken.

Structures

The non-pregnant uterus is a hollow, muscular, pear-shaped organ situated in the true pelvis. It is 7.5 cm long, 5 cm wide and 2.5 cm in depth, each wall being 1.25 cm thick. The cervix forms the lower third of the uterus and measures 2.5 cm in each direction.

The uterus consists of the following parts:

The body or corpus makes up the upper two-thirds of the uterus and is the greater part.

The fundus is the domed upper wall between the insertions of the fallopian tubes.

The cornua are the upper outer angles of the uterus where the fallopian tubes join.

The cavity is a potential space between the anterior and posterior walls. It is triangular in shape, the base of the triangle being uppermost.

The isthmus is a narrow area between the cavity and the cervix, which is 7 mm long. It enlarges during pregnancy to form the lower uterine segment.

The cervix or neck protrudes into the vagina. The upper half, being above the vagina, is known as the supravaginal portion while the lower half is the infravaginal portion.

The internal os (mouth) is the narrow opening between the isthmus and the cervix.

The external os is a small round opening at the lower end of the cervix. After childbirth this becomes a transverse slit.

The cervical canal lies between these two ora and is a continuation of the uterine cavity. This canal is shaped like a spindle, narrow at each end and wider in the middle.

Layers

The uterus has three layers, of which the middle muscle layer is by far the thickest.

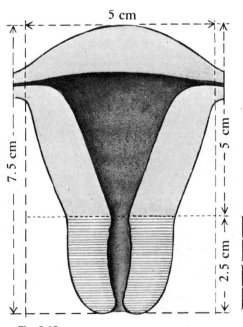

Fig. 2.18
Measurements of the uterus.

The endometrium forms a lining of ciliated epithelium (mucous membrane) on a base of connective tissue or stroma.

In the uterine cavity this endometrium is constantly changing in thickness throughout the menstrual cycle (see Ch. 3). The basal layer does not alter, but provides the foundation from which the upper layers regenerate. The epithelial cells are cubical in shape and dip down to form glands which secrete an alkaline mucus.

The cervical endometrium does not respond to the hormonal stimuli of the menstrual cycle to the same extent. Here the epithelial cells are tall and columnar in shape and the mucus-secreting glands are branching racemose glands. The cervical endometrium is thinner than that of the body and is folded into a pattern known as the arbor vitae (tree of life). This is thought to assist the passage of the sperm.

The myometrium, or muscle coat, is thick in the upper part of the uterus and is more sparse in the isthmus and cervix. Its fibres run in all directions and interlace to surround the blood vessels and lymphatics which pass to and from the endometrium. The outer layer is formed of longitudinal fibres which are continuous with those of the fallopian tube, the uterine ligaments and the vagina.

In the cervix the muscle fibres are embedded in collagen fibres which enable it to stretch in labour.

The perimetrium is a double serous membrane, an extension of the peritoneum, which is draped over the uterus, covering all but a narrow strip on either side and the anterior wall of the supravaginal cervix from where it is reflected up over the bladder.

Blood supply

The uterine artery arrives at the level of the cervix and is a branch of the internal iliac artery. It sends a small branch to the upper vagina, and then runs upwards in a twisted fashion to meet the ovarian artery and form an anastomosis with it near the cornua. The ovarian artery is a branch of the abdominal aorta, leaving near the renal artery. It supplies the ovary and fallopian tube before joining the uterine artery. The blood drains through corresponding veins.

Lymphatic drainage

Lymph is drained from the uterine body to the internal iliac glands and also from the cervical area to many other pelvic lymph glands. This provides an effective defence against uterine infection.

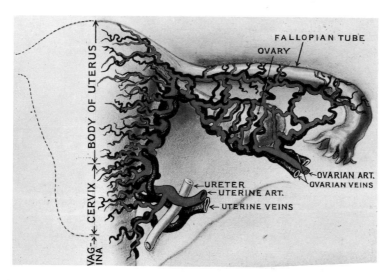

Fig. 2.19
Blood supply of uterus, fallopian tubes and ovaries.

Nerve supply

This is mainly from the autonomic nervous system, sympathetic and parasympathetic, via Lee Frankenhäuser's plexus or pelvic plexus.

THE FALLOPIAN TUBES OR UTERINE TUBES

Functions

The fallopian tube propels the ovum towards the uterus, receives the spermatozoa as they travel upwards and provides a site for fertilisation. It supplies the fertilised ovum with nutrition during its continued journey to the uterus.

Position

The fallopian tubes extend laterally from the cornua of the uterus towards the side walls of the pelvis. They arch over the ovaries, the fringed ends hovering near the ovaries in order to receive the ovum.

Relations

Anterior, posterior and superior. The peritoneal cavity and the intestines.

Lateral. The side walls of the pelvis.

Inferior. The broad ligaments and ovaries lie below the tubes.

Medial. The uterus lies between the two fallopian tubes.

Supports

The fallopian tubes are held in place by their attachment to the uterus. The peritoneum folds over them, draping down below as the broad ligaments and extending at the sides to form the infundibulopelvic ligaments.

Structure

Each tube is 10 cm long. The lumen of the tube provides an open pathway from the outside to the peritoneal cavity. The uterine tube has four portions:

The interstitial portion is 1.25 cm long and lies within the wall of the uterus. Its lumen is 1mm wide.

The isthmus is another narrow part which extends for 2.5 cm from the uterus.

The ampulla is the wider portion where fertilisation usually occurs. It is 5 cm long.

The infundibulum is the funnel-shaped fringed end which is composed of many processes known as fimbriae. One fimbria is elongated to form the ovarian fimbria which is attached to the ovary.

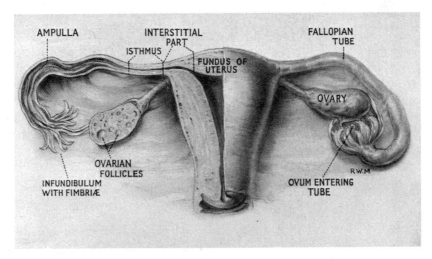

Fig. 2.20
Fallopian tube in section. Note the ovum entering the fimbriated end.

Layers

The lining is a mucous membrane of *ciliated cubical epithelium* which is thrown into complicated folds known as plicae. These folds slow the ovum down on its way to the uterus. In this lining are goblet cells which produce a secretion containing glycogen to nourish the ovum.

Beneath the lining is a layer of **vascular connective tissue**.

The muscle coat consists of two layers, an inner circular layer and an outer longitudinal layer, both of smooth muscle. The peristaltic movement of the fallopian tube is due to the action of these muscles.

The tube is covered with **peritoneum** but the infundibulum passes through it to open into the peritoneal cavity.

Blood supply

This is via the uterine and ovarian arteries, returning by the corresponding veins.

Lymphatic drainage is to the lumbar glands.

Nerve supply is from the ovarian plexus.

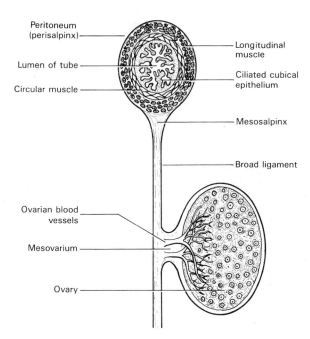

Fig. 2.21
Cross-section of fallopian tube.

Peritoneum (perisalpinx)
Lumen of tube
Circular muscle
Longitudinal muscle
Ciliated cubical epithelium
Mesosalpinx
Broad ligament
Ovarian blood vessels
Mesovarium
Ovary

THE OVARIES

Functions

The ovaries produce ova and the hormones oestrogen and progesterone.

Position

They are attached to the back of the broad ligament within the peritoneal cavity.

Relations

Anterior. The broad ligaments.
Posterior. The intestines.
Lateral. The infundibulopelvic ligaments and the side walls of the pelvis.
Superior. The fallopian tubes.
Medial. The uterus and the ovarian ligament.

Supports

The ovary is attached to the broad ligament but is supported from above by the ovarian ligament medially and the infundibulopelvic ligament laterally.

Structure

The ovary is composed of a medulla and cortex, covered with germinal epithelium.

The medulla. This is the supporting framework which is made of fibrous tissue and the ovarian blood vessels, lymphatics and nerves travel through it. The hilum where these vessels enter lies just where the ovary is attached to the broad ligament and this area is called the mesovarium.

The cortex. This is the functioning part of the ovary. It contains the ovarian follicles in different stages of development, surrounded by stroma. The outer layer is formed of fibrous tissue known as the tunica albuginea. Over this lies the germinal epithelium, which is a modification of the peritoneum.

The cycle of the ovary is described in Chapter 3.

Blood supply

The blood supply is from the ovarian arteries and drains by the ovarian veins. The right ovarian vein joins the inferior vena cava, but the left returns its blood to the left renal vein.

Lymphatic drainage is to the lumbar glands.
Nerve supply is from the ovarian plexus.

MALE REPRODUCTIVE SYSTEM

The scrotum

Function

The scrotum forms a pouch in which the testes are suspended outside the body. It lies below the symphysis pubis and between the upper parts of the thighs behind the penis.

Structure

It is formed of pigmented skin and has two compartments, one for each testis.

The testes

Function

They are the male gonads and produce spermatozoa and testosterone. Testosterone is responsible for the secondary sex characteristics. It also joins with follicle stimulating hormone (FSH) to promote production of sperm.

Position

The testes are situated in the scrotum. In order to achieve their proper function they must be kept below body temperature, and this is why they are situated outside the body.

Structure

Each testis is 4.5 cm long, 2.5 cm wide and 3 cm thick.

Layers

Tunica vasculosa. This is an inner layer of connective tissue containing a fine network of capillaries.

Tunica albuginea. This is a fibrous covering, ingrowths of which divide the testis into 200–300 lobules.

Tunica vaginalis. This is the outer layer which is made of peritoneum brought down with the descending testis when it migrated from the lumbar region in fetal life. The duct system is highly intricate:

The seminiferous ('seed-carrying') tubules are where spermatogenesis, or production of sperm, takes place. There are up to three of them in each lobule. Between the tubules there are

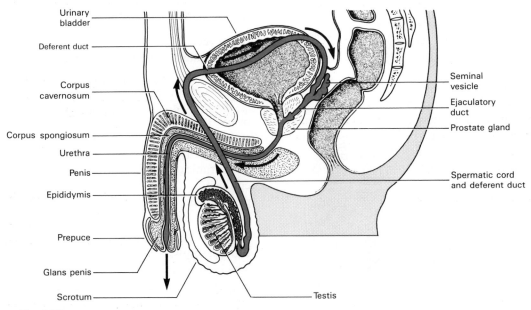

Fig. 2.22
Male reproductive system.

interstitial cells which secrete testosterone. The tubules join to form a system of channels which lead to the epididymis.

The epididymis is a comma-shaped, coiled tube which lies on the superior surface and travels down the posterior aspect to the lower pole of the testis, where it leads into the deferent duct or vas deferens.

The spermatic cord

Function
The spermatic cord transmits the deferent duct up into the body, along with other structures. The function of the deferent duct is to carry the sperm to the ejaculatory duct.

Position
The cord passes upwards through the inguinal canal, where the different structures diverge. The deferent duct then continues upwards over the symphysis pubis and arches backwards beside the bladder. Behind the bladder it merges with the duct from the seminal vesicle and passes through the prostate gland as the ejaculatory duct to join the urethra.

Structure
The spermatic cord consists of the deferent duct, the testicular blood vessels, lymph vessel and nerves.

Blood supply
The testicular artery, a branch of the abdominal aorta, supplies the testis, scrotum and attachments. The testicular veins drain in the same manner as the ovarian veins (see above).

Lymphatic drainage is to the lymph nodes round the aorta.

Nerve supply is from the 10th and 11th thoracic nerves.

The seminal vesicles

Function
The production of a viscous secretion to keep the sperm alive and motile.

Position
The seminal vesicles are two pouches situated posterior to the bladder.

Structure
They are 5 cm long and pyramid shaped. They are composed of columnar epithelium, muscle tissue and fibrous tissue.

The ejaculatory ducts
These small muscular ducts carry the spermatozoa and the seminal fluid to the urethra.

The prostate gland

Function
It produces a thin lubricating fluid which enters the urethra through ducts.

Position
It surrounds the urethra at the base of the bladder, lying between the rectum and the symphysis pubis.

Structure
It is 4 cm long, 3 cm wide and 2 cm deep. It is composed of columnar epithelium, a muscle layer and an outer fibrous layer.

The bulbo-urethral glands
These are two very small glands which produce yet another lubricating fluid which passes into the urethra just below the prostate gland.

The penis

Functions
It carries the urethra which is a passage for both urine and semen. During sexual excitement it stiffens (an erection) in order to be able to penetrate the vagina and deposit the semen near the woman's cervix.

Position
The root lies in the perineum, from where it passes forward below the symphysis pubis. The

lower two-thirds is outside the body in front of the scrotum.

Structure

There are three columns of erectile tissue:

The corpora cavernosa are two lateral columns, one on either side and in front of the urethra.

The corpus spongiosum is a posterior column which contains the urethra. The tip is expanded to form the glans penis.

The lower two-thirds of the penis is covered in skin. At the end, the skin is folded back on itself above the glans penis to form the prepuce which is a movable double fold. The penis is extremely vascular and during an erection the blood spaces fill and become distended.

The male hormones

The control of the male gonads is similar to the female, but it is not cyclical. The hypothalamus produces gonadotrophin-releasing factors. These stimulate the anterior pituitary gland to produce follicle-stimulating hormone (FSH) and luteinising hormone (LH). FSH acts on the seminiferous tubules to bring about the production of sperm, while LH acts on the interstitial cells which produce testosterone.

Testosterone is responsible for the secondary sex characteristics, namely deepening of the voice, growth of the genitalia and growth of hair on the chest, pubis, axilla and face.

Formation of the spermatozoa

Production of sperm begins at puberty and continues throughout adult life. Spermatogenesis takes place in the seminiferous tubules under the influence of FSH and testosterone. The process of maturation is a lengthy one and takes some weeks. The mature sperm are stored in the epididymis and the deferent duct until ejaculation. If this does not happen they degenerate and are reabsorbed. At each ejaculation, 2–4 ml of semen is deposited in the vagina. The seminal fluid contains about 100 million sperm per ml, of which 20–25% are likely to be abnormal. The remainder move at a speed of 2–3 mm per minute. The individual spermatozoon has a head, a body and a long, mobile tail which lashes to propel the sperm along. The tip of the head is covered by an acrosome which contains enzymes to dissolve the covering of the ovum in order to penetrate it.

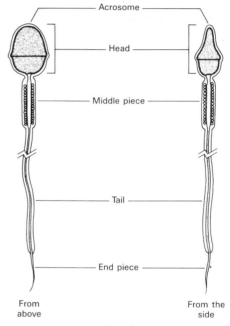

Fig. 2.23
Spermatozoon.

REFERENCE

Williams P L et al 1989 Gray's anatomy, 37th edn. Churchill Livingstone, Edinburgh

FURTHER READING

Hinchliff S, Montague S (eds) 1988 Physiology for nursing practice. Baillière Tindall, London

Johnson M, Everitt B 1988 Essential reproduction, 3rd edn. Blackwell Scientific Publications, Oxford

3

Hormonal cycles: fertilisation and early development

V. RUTH BENNETT   LINDA K. BROWN

The biological cycles of a woman follow a monthly pattern and have a profound influence on her life and behaviour. When a woman is sexually active and no fertility control is used, recurring pregnancies will intervene and may obliterate the pattern for most of her fertile life. These cycles are first described without this interruption.

The hypothalamus is the ultimate source of control and it governs the anterior pituitary gland by hormonal pathways. The anterior pituitary gland in turn governs the ovary by hormones. Finally the ovary produces hormones which control changes in the uterus. All the changes occur simultaneously and in harmony. A woman's moods may change along with the cycle and emotional influences can alter the cycle because of the close relationship between the hypothalamus and the cerebral cortex.

THE OVARIAN CYCLE

The ovarian cortex contains 200 000 primordial follicles at birth. Some of these become cystic and are then known as Graafian follicles. From puberty onwards, certain follicles enlarge and one matures each month to liberate an ovum.

Graafian follicle. The ovum is situated àt one end of the Graafian follicle and is encircled by the narrow *perivitelline space*. Surrounding this lies a clump of cells called the *discus proligerus*, the cells of which radiate outwards to form the *corona*

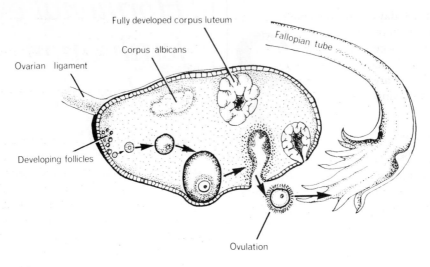

Fig. 3.1
The life cycle of a Graafian follicle.

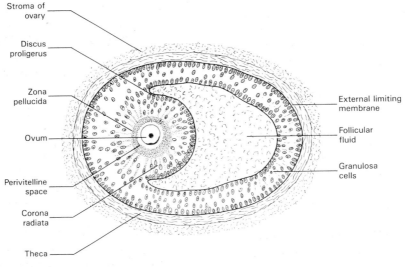

Fig. 3.2
A ripe Graafian follicle.

radiata. The innermost cells of the corona are very clear and are referred to as the *zona pellucida.* The whole follicle is lined with granulosa cells and contains follicular fluid. The outer coat of the follicle is the *external limiting membrane* and around this lies an area of compressed ovarian stroma known as the *theca.*

Under the influence of follicle-stimulating hormone (FSH) the Graafian follicle matures and moves to the surface of the ovary. At the same time it swells and becomes tense, finally rupturing to release the ovum into the fimbriated end of the fallopian tube which is cupped underneath the ovary in readiness. This is ovulation. Some women feel pain at this time; this may be related to a small loss of blood into the peritoneal cavity and is termed mittelschmerz. The empty follicle is known as the corpus luteum (yellow body).

Corpus luteum. After ovulation the follicle collapses, the granulosa cells enlarge and proliferate over the next 14 days and the whole structure becomes irregular in outline and yellow in colour. Unless pregnancy occurs, the corpus luteum will then atrophy and become the *corpus albicans* (white body). The ovary contains a number of these white bodies in varying stages of degeneration.

Ovarian hormones

Oestrogen. This comprises a number of compounds including oestriol, oestradiol and oestrone. They are produced under the influence of FSH by the granulosa cells and the theca in increasing amounts until the degeneration of the corpus luteum when the level falls.

The effects of oestrogen are widespread. It is responsible for the secondary sex characteristics such as the female shape, the growth of the breasts and the uterus and the female distribution of hair. It influences the production of cervical mucus and the structure of the vaginal epithelium. This in turn encourages the growth of Döderlein's bacilli which are responsible for the acidity of the vaginal fluid. During the cycle oestrogen causes the proliferation of the uterine endometrium. It inhibits FSH and encourages fluid retention.

Progesterone. This with related compounds is produced by the corpus luteum under the influence of LH. They only act on tissues which have previously been affected by oestrogen.

The effects of progesterone are mainly evident during the second half of the cycle. It causes secretory changes in the lining of the uterus, when the endometrium develops tortuous glands and an enriched blood supply in readiness for the possible arrival of a fertilised ovum. It causes the body temperature to rise by 0.5°C after ovulation and gives rise to tingling and a sense of fullness in the breasts prior to menstruation.

The changes caused by progesterone in pregnancy are listed in Chapter 8.

Relaxin is a hormone which has been measured in human blood and is at its maximum level between weeks 38 and 42 of pregnancy. It originates in the corpus luteum and is known to relax the pelvic girdle, to soften the cervix and to suppress uterine contractions. Although it reduces oxytocin release it does not affect the increasing number of oxytocin receptors in the myometrium. The presence of these receptors is a more important factor in labour than the actual level of oxytocin (Steer 1990).

PITUITARY CONTROL

Under the influence of the hypothalamus which produces gonadotrophin-releasing hormone (GnRH), the anterior pituitary gland (adenohypophysis) secretes two gonadotrophins, follicle-stimulating hormone (FSH) and luteinising hormone (LH). GnRH is released in a series of pulses about an hour apart and the gonadotrophins likewise are secreted in a pulsatile manner (Johnson & Everitt 1988). This appears to be crucial to the normal pattern of the menstrual cycle.

FSH causes several Graafian follicles to develop and enlarge, one of them more than all the others. FSH stimulates the granulosa cells and theca to secrete oestrogen. The level of FSH rises during the first half of the cycle and when the oestrogen level reaches a certain point its production is stopped.

LH is produced when the anterior pituitary stops producing FSH. As the LH rises and the FSH falls, the follicle ruptures and ovulation occurs. The corpus luteum develops under the influence of LH and it produces both oestrogen and progesterone. LH is produced for 14 days after which FSH reappears and the cycle begins again.

Prolactin is also produced in the anterior pituitary gland, but it does not play a part in the control of the ovary. If produced in excessive amounts, however, it will inhibit ovulation, a phenomenon which occurs naturally during breast feeding (see Ch. 33).

THE UTERINE CYCLE OR MENSTRUAL CYCLE

Although each woman has an individual cycle which varies in length, the average cycle is taken to be 28 days long and recurs regularly from puberty to the menopause except when pregnancy intervenes. The first day of the cycle is the day on which menstruation begins. There are three main phases and they affect the tissue structure of the endometrium, controlled by the ovarian hormones.

The menstrual phase, characterised by vaginal bleeding, lasts for 3–5 days. Physiologically this is the terminal phase of the menstrual cycle when the endometrium is shed down to the basal layer

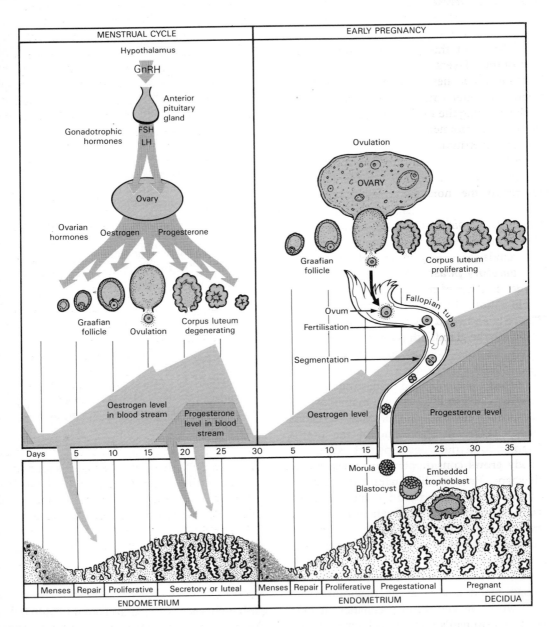

Fig. 3.3
MENSTRUAL CYCLE (*left half*). Diagrammatic representation of the action of the gonadotrophic hormones on the ovary and of the ovarian hormones on the endometrium.
EARLY PREGNANCY (*right half*). Diagrammatic representation showing ovulation, fertilisation, decidual reaction and embedding of the fertilised ovum.

along with blood from the capillaries and with the unfertilised ovum.

The proliferative phase follows menstruation and lasts until ovulation. Sometimes the first few days while the endometrium is reforming are described as the *regenerative phase*. This phase is under the control of oestrogen and consists of the regrowth and thickening of the endometrium. At the completion of this phase the endometrium consists of three layers:

A basal layer lies immediately above the myometrium, about 1 mm in thickness. This layer never alters during the menstrual cycle. It contains all the necessary rudimentary structures for building up new endometrium.

A functional layer which contains tubular glands and is 2.5 mm thick. This layer changes constantly according to the hormonal influences of the ovary.

A layer of cuboidal ciliated epithelium covers the functional layer. It dips down to line the tubular glands.

The secretory phase follows ovulation and is under the influence of progesterone and oestrogen from the corpus luteum. The functional layer thickens to 3.5 mm and becomes spongy in appearance because the glands are more tortuous.

Puberty

This is the period in life during which the reproductive organs undergo a surge in development and reach maturity. The first signs are breast development and the appearance of pubic hair. The body grows considerably and takes on the female shape. Puberty culminates in the onset of menstruation, the first period being called the *menarche*. The first few cycles are not usually accompanied by ovulation so that conception is unlikely before a girl has been menstruating for a year or two.

Menopause

The end of a woman's reproductive life is characterised by the gradual cessation of menstruation, the periods first becoming irregular and then ceasing altogether. This is often accompanied by physical symptoms like hot flushes and emotional changes such as mood swings. There is an increased tendency to obesity and in the following years signs of aging will appear. These changes are due to a fall in the production of oestrogen because the ovary is no longer able to respond to pituitary gonadotrophins. The sexual drive may not be diminished but some women find it difficult to accept that they are no longer fertile. The usual age for the menopause is between 45 and 50 years but it should not be assumed that it is complete until 2 years have elapsed since the last period. In the intervening months the woman should continue to use contraception if appropriate.

FERTILISATION

Following ovulation, the ovum, which is about 0.15 mm in diameter, passes into the fallopian tube and is moved along towards the uterus. The ovum, having no power of locomotion, is wafted along by the cilia and by the peristaltic muscular contraction of the tube. At this time the cervix, under the influence of oestrogen, secretes a flow of alkaline mucus that attracts the spermatozoa. At intercourse about 300 million sperm are deposited in the posterior fornix of the vagina. Those that reach the loose cervical mucus survive to propel themselves towards the fallopian tubes while the remainder are destroyed by the acid medium of the vagina. More will die on the journey through the uterus and only thousands reach the fallopian tube where they meet the ovum, usually in the ampulla. It is only during this journey that the sperm finally become mature and capable of releasing the enzyme, hyaluronidase, which allows penetration of the zona pellucida and the cell membrane surrounding the ovum. Many sperm are needed for this to take place but only one will enter the ovum. After this, the membrane is sealed to prevent entry of any further sperm and the nuclei of the two cells fuse. The sperm and the ovum each contribute half the complement of chromosomes to make a total of 46. The sperm and ovum are known as the male and female *gametes*, the fertilised ovum as the *zygote*.

Neither sperm nor ovum can survive for longer than 2 or 3 days and fertilisation is most likely to occur when intercourse takes place not more than 48 hours before or 24 hours after ovulation. It therefore follows that conception will take place about 14 days before the next period is due.

DEVELOPMENT OF THE FERTILISED OVUM

When the ovum has been fertilised, it continues its passage through the fallopian tube and reaches the uterus 3 or 4 days later. During this time segmentation or cell division takes place and the fertilised ovum divides into 2 cells, then into 4, then 8, 16 and so on until a cluster of cells is formed known as the *morula* (mulberry). These

divisions occur quite slowly, about once every 12 hours. Next, a fluid-filled cavity or *blastocele* appears in the morula which now becomes known as the *blastocyst*. Around the outside of the blastocyst there is a single layer of cells known as the *trophoblast* while the remaining cells are clumped together at one end forming the *inner cell mass*. The trophoblast will form the placenta and chorion, while the inner cell mass will become the fetus and the amnion. On its journey, the ovum is nourished by glycogen from the goblet cells of the fallopian tubes and later the secretory glands of the uterus.

When the blastocyst first tumbles into the uterus, it lies free for 2 or 3 more days. The trophoblast, especially the part which lies over the inner cell mass, then becomes quite sticky and adheres to the endometrium. It begins to secrete substances

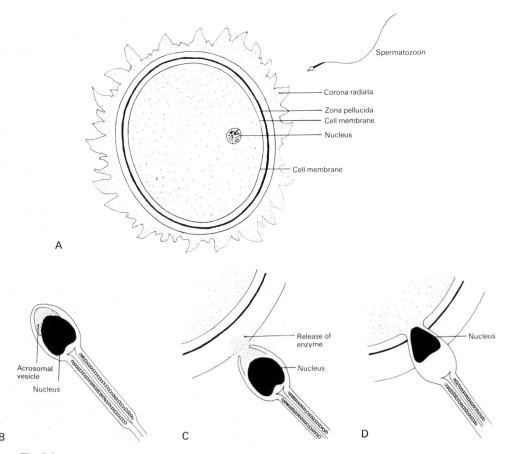

Fig. 3.4
Fertilisation. Diagrammatic representation of the fusion of the ovum and the spermatozoon.

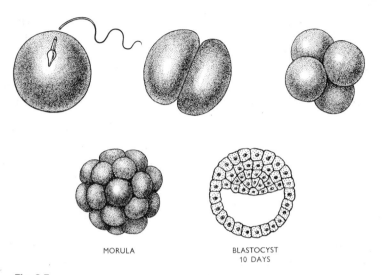

MORULA

BLASTOCYST
10 DAYS

Fig. 3.5
Diagrammatic representation of the development of the fertilised ovum.

which digest the endometrial cells, allowing the blastocyst to become enbedded in the endometrium. *Embedding*, sometimes known as *nidation* (nesting), is normally complete by the 11th day after ovulation and the endometrium closes over it completely, the only evidence of the presence of the blastocyst being a small bulge on the surface.

The decidua

This is the name given to the endometrium during pregnancy. From the time of conception the increased secretion of oestrogens causes the endometrium to grow to four times its non-pregnant thickness. The corpus luteum also produces large amounts of progesterone which stimulate the secretory activity of the endometrial glands and increase the size of the blood vessels. This accounts for the soft, vascular, spongy bed in which the fertilised ovum implants. Three layers are found:

The basal layer lies immediately above the myometrium. It remains unchanged in itself but regenerates the new endometrium during the puerperium.

The functional layer consists of tortuous glands which are rich in secretions. The stroma cells are enlarged in what is known as the decidual reaction. This affords a defence against

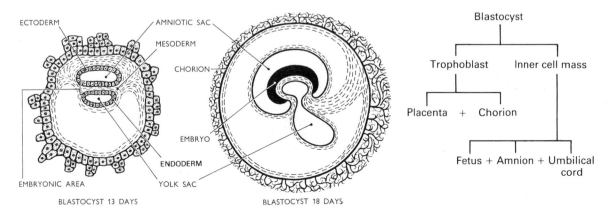

Fig. 3.6
The development of the blastocyst.

excessive invasion by the syncitiotrophoblast and limits its advance to the spongy layer. The advantage of this is that it provides a secure anchorage for the placenta and allows it access to nutrition and oxygen but as soon as the baby is born, separation can occur (see Ch. 15).

The compact layer forms the surface of the decidua and is composed of closely packed stroma cells and the necks of the glands.

The blastocyst embeds within the spongy layer and different areas of decidua are identified according to their relationship to it.

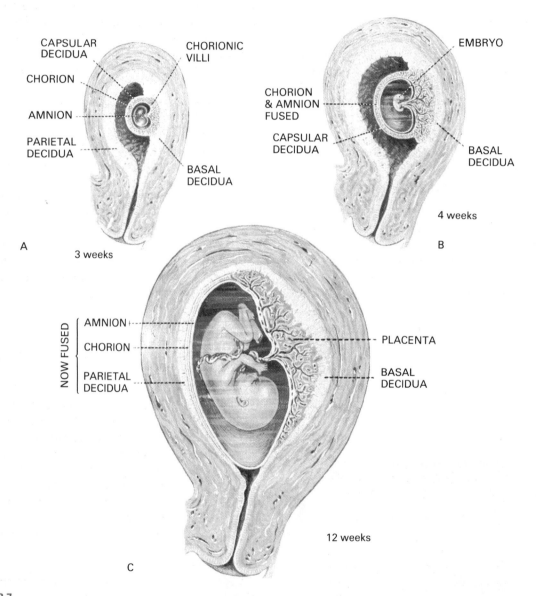

Fig. 3.7
The developing embryo.
(A) (3 weeks) Showing the amniotic sac, surrounded by chorion which is covered with capsular decidua.
(B) (4 weeks) The amnion is in contact with the chorion. The placenta is seen embedded in the basal decidua.
(C) (12 weeks) The capsular decidua has thinned out and atrophied. The chorion is attached to the parietal decidua.
(After Williams, *American Journal of Obstetrics and Gynecology*.)

The decidua underneath the blastocyst is termed the *basal decidua*, that which covers it is the *capsular decidua*, and the remainder is called the *parietal* (or the *true*) *decidua*. Eventually, as the embryo grows and fills the uterine cavity, the capsular decidua meets and fuses with the parietal decidua.

The trophoblast

Small projections begin to appear all over the surface of the blastocyst, becoming most prolific at the area of contact. These trophoblastic cells differentiate into layers, the outer syncitiotrophoblast (syncitium), the inner cytotrophoblast and below this a layer of mesoderm or primitive mesenchyme.

The syncitiotrophoblast is composed of nucleated protoplasm which is capable of breaking down tissue as in the process of embedding. It erodes the walls of the blood vessels of the decidua, making the nutrients in the maternal blood accessible to the developing organism.

The cytotrophoblast is a well-defined single layer of cells which produces a hormone known as human chorionic gonadotrophin (HCG). This is responsible for informing the corpus luteum that a pregnancy has begun. The corpus luteum continues to produce oestrogen and progesterone. Progesterone maintains the integrity of the decidua so that shedding does not take place. In other words, menstruation is suppressed. The high level of oestrogen suppresses the production of FSH.

The mesoderm consists of loose connective tissue. There is similar tissue in the inner cell

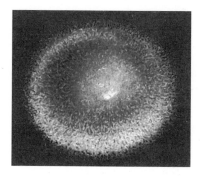

Fig. 3.8
Ovum in early pregnancy covered with chorionic villi.

mass and the two are continuous at the point where they join in the body stalk.

Further development of the trophoblast is discussed in Chapter 4.

The inner cell mass

While the trophoblast is developing into the placenta, which will nourish the fetus, the inner cell mass is forming the fetus itself. The cells differentiate into three layers, each of which will form particular parts of the fetus.

The ectoderm mainly forms the skin and nervous system.

The mesoderm forms bones and muscles and also the heart and blood vessels, including those which are in the placenta. Certain internal organs also originate in the mesoderm.

The endoderm forms mucous membranes and glands. The three layers together are known as the embryonic plate. Two cavities appear in the inner cell mass, one on either side of the embryonic plate.

The amniotic cavity lies on the side of the ectoderm. The cavity, which is filled with fluid, gradually enlarges and folds round the embryo to enclose it. The amnion forms from its lining. It swells out into the chorionic cavity (formerly the blastocele) and eventually obliterates it when the amniotic and chorionic membranes come into contact. Details of the amniotic fluid are found in Chapter 4.

The yolk sac lies on the side of the endoderm and provides nourishment for the embryo until the trophoblast is sufficiently developed to take over. Part of it contributes to the formation of the primitive gut; the remainder resembles a balloon floating in front of the embryo until it atrophies and becomes trapped under the amnion on the surface of the placenta. After birth, all that remains of the yolk sac is a vestigial structure in the base of the umbilical cord, known as the vitelline duct.

The embryo

This name is applied to the developing offspring after implantation and until 8 weeks after conception. During the embryonic period all the organs and systems of the body are laid down in rudimentary form so that at its completion they have simply to grow and mature for a further 7 months. The conceptus is known as a *fetus* during this time (see Ch. 5).

REFERENCES

Johnson M, Everitt B 1988 Essential reproduction, 3rd edn. Blackwell Scientific Publications, Oxford

Steer P J 1990 Endocrinology of parturition. In: Franks S (ed) Clinical endocrinology and metabolism. Vol 4 No 2 June. Baillière Tindall, London

FURTHER READING

Herbert R A 1988 Reproduction In: Hinchliff S, Montague S (eds) Physiology for nursing practice. Baillière Tindall, London

4

The placenta

V. RUTH BENNETT   LINDA K. BROWN

The placenta is a remarkable organ. Originating from the trophoblastic layer of the fertilised ovum itself, it links closely with the mother's circulation to carry out functions which the fetus is unable to perform for itself during intra-uterine life. The survival of the fetus depends upon its integrity and efficiency.

DEVELOPMENT

Initially the ovum appears to be covered with a fine, downy hair, which consists of the projections from the trophoblastic layer (see Ch. 3). These proliferate and branch from about 3 weeks after fertilisation, forming the chorionic villi. The villi become most profuse in the area where the blood supply is richest, that is, in the basal decidua. This part of the trophoblast is known as the chorion frondosum and it will eventually develop into the placenta. The villi under the capsular decidua, being less well nourished, gradually degenerate and form the chorion laeve (bald chorion) which is the origin of the chorionic membrane.

The villi erode the walls of maternal blood vessels as they penetrate the decidua, opening them up to form a lake of maternal blood in which they float. The opened blood vessels are known as sinuses, the areas surrounding the villi as blood spaces. The maternal blood circulates slowly, enabling the villi to absorb food and

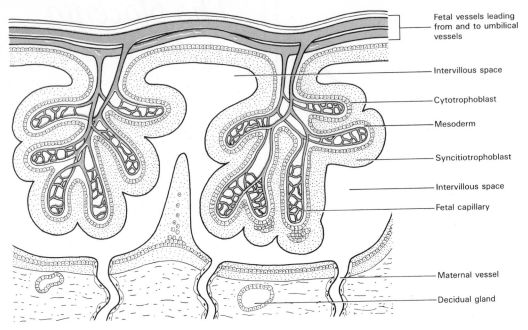

Fetal vessels leading from and to umbilical vessels

Intervillous space

Cytotrophoblast

Mesoderm

Syncitiotrophoblast

Intervillous space

Fetal capillary

Maternal vessel

Decidual gland

Fig. 4.1
Diagram to show chorionic villi.

oxygen and excrete waste. These are known as the nutritive villi. A few villi are more deeply attached to the decidua and are called anchoring villi.

Each chorionic villus is a branching structure arising from one stem. Its centre consists of mesoderm and fetal blood vessels, and branches of the umbilical artery and vein. These are covered by a single layer of cytotrophoblast cells and the external layer of the villus is the syncitiotrophoblast. This means that four layers of tissue separate the maternal blood from the fetal blood and make it impossible for the two circulations to mix unless any villi are damaged.

The placenta is completely formed and functioning from 10 weeks after fertilisation. In its early stages it is a relatively loose structure, but becomes more compact as it matures. Between 12 and 20 weeks' gestation the placenta weighs more than the fetus because the fetal organs are insufficiently developed to cope with the metabolic processes of nutrition. Later in pregnancy some of the fetal organs, such as the liver, begin to function, so the cytotrophoblast and the syncitiotrophoblast gradually degenerate.

Circulation through the placenta

Fetal blood, low in oxygen, is pumped by the fetal heart towards the placenta along the umbilical arteries and transported along their branches to the capillaries of the chorionic villi. Having absorbed oxygen the blood is returned to the fetus via the umbilical vein.

The maternal blood is delivered to the placental bed in the decidua by spiral arteries and flows into the blood spaces surrounding the villi. It is thought that the direction of flow is similar to a fountain; the blood passes upwards and bathes the villus as it circulates around it and drains back into a branch of the uterine vein. An alternative theory is that it flows in a similar manner to a whirlpool.

THE MATURE PLACENTA

Functions

Respiration. As pulmonary exchange of gases does not take place in the uterus the fetus must obtain oxygen and excrete carbon dioxide through the placenta. Oxygen from the mother's haemoglobin passes into the fetal blood by simple

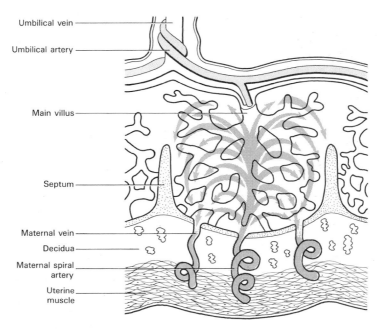

Umbilical vein

Umbilical artery

Main villus

Septum

Maternal vein

Decidua

Maternal spiral artery

Uterine muscle

Fig. 4.2
Blood flow around chorionic villi.

diffusion and similarly the fetus gives off carbon dioxide into the maternal blood.

Nutrition. The fetus needs the same nutrients as anyone else. Amino acids are required for body building, glucose for energy, calcium and phosphorus for bones and teeth, and iron and other minerals for blood formation. Food for the fetus derives from the mother's diet and has already been broken down into simpler forms by the time it reaches the placental site. The placenta is able to select those substances required by the fetus, even depleting the mother's own supply in some instances. It can also break down complex nutrients into compounds which can be used by the fetus. Protein is transferred across the placenta as amino acids, carbohydrate as glucose and fats as fatty acids. Water, vitamins and minerals also pass to the fetus. Fats and fat-soluble vitamins (A, D and E) only cross the placenta with difficulty and mainly in the later stages of pregnancy. The amino acids are actively transported across the placenta so that the level in the fetal blood is always higher than that in the maternal blood.

Storage. The placenta metabolises glucose, stores it in the form of glycogen and reconverts it to glucose as required. The placenta can also store iron and the fat-soluble vitamins.

Excretion. The main substance excreted from the fetus is carbon dioxide. Bilirubin will also be excreted as red blood cells are replaced relatively frequently. There is very little tissue breakdown apart from this and the amounts of urea and uric acid excreted are very small.

Protection. The placenta provides a limited barrier to infection. With the exception of the treponema of syphilis and the tubercle bacillus, few bacteria can penetrate. Viruses, however, can cross freely and may cause congenital abnormalities, as in the case of the rubella virus (see Ch. 22). It may be assumed that drugs will cross to the fetus although there are exceptions, for example heparin. Some drugs are known to cause damage, though many will be harmless and others are positively beneficial, such as antibiotics administered to a pregnant woman with syphilis.

Towards the end of pregnancy small antibodies, immunoglobulins G (IgG), will be transferred to the fetus, and these will confer immunity on the baby for the first 3 months after birth. It is important to realise that only those antibodies which the mother herself possesses can be passed on.

Endocrine. *Human chorionic gonadotrophin (HCG).* This is produced by the cytotrophoblastic layer of the chorionic villi. Initially it is present in very large quantities, peak levels being achieved between the 7th and 10th weeks, but it gradually reduces as the pregnancy advances. HCG forms the basis of the many pregnancy tests which are available, as it is excreted in the mother's urine. Its function is to stimulate the growth and activity of the corpus luteum.

Oestrogens. As the activity of the corpus luteum declines, the placenta takes over the production of oestrogens, which are secreted in large amounts throughout pregnancy. The fetus provides the placenta with the vital precursors for the production of oestrogens. The amount of oestrogen produced (measured as urinary or serum oestriol) is an index of fetoplacental well-being.

Progesterone. This is made in the syncitial layer of the placenta in increasing quantities until immediately before the onset of labour when its level falls. It may be measured in the urine as pregnanediol.

Human placental lactogen (HPL). HPL has a role in glucose metabolism in pregnancy. It appears to have a connection with the activity of human growth hormone, although it does not itself promote growth. As the level of HCG falls, so the level of HPL rises and continues to do so throughout pregnancy. Monitoring the level of HPL with the intention of assessing placental function has been disappointing in predicting fetal outcome.

Appearance of the placenta at term

The placenta is a round, flat mass about 20 cm in diameter and 2.5 cm thick at its centre. It weighs approximately one-sixth of the baby's weight at term, although this proportion may be affected by the time at which the cord is clamped due to the varying amounts of fetal blood retained in the vessels.

The maternal surface. Maternal blood gives this surface a dark red colour and part of the basal decidua will have been separated with it. The surface is arranged in about 20 lobes which are separated by sulci (furrows), into which the decidua dips down to form septa (walls). The lobes are made up of lobules, each of which contains a single villus with its branches. Sometimes deposits of lime salts may be present on the surface, making it slightly gritty. This has no clinical significance.

The fetal surface. The amnion covering the fetal surface of the placenta gives it a white, shiny appearance. Branches of the umbilical vein and arteries are visible, spreading out from the insertion of the umbilical cord which is normally in the centre. The amnion can be peeled off the surface, leaving the chorionic plate from which the placenta has developed and which is continuous with the chorion.

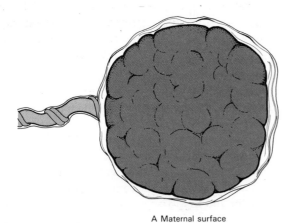
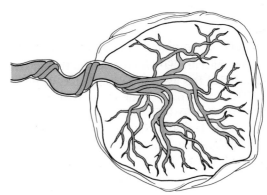

A Maternal surface   B Fetal surface

Fig. 4.3
The placenta at term.

The fetal sac

The fetal sac consists of a double membrane. The outer membrane is the chorion which lies under the capsular decidua and becomes closely adherent to the uterine wall. The inner membrane is the amnion which contains the amniotic fluid. As long as it remains intact, the fetal sac protects the fetus against ascending bacterial infection.

Chorion. This is a thick, opaque, friable membrane derived from the trophoblast. It is continuous with the chorionic plate which forms the base of the placenta.

Amnion. This is a smooth, tough, translucent membrane derived from the inner cell mass. It is thought to have a role in the formation of the amniotic fluid.

AMNIOTIC FLUID

Functions

The fluid distends the amniotic sac and allows for the growth and free movement of the fetus. It equalises pressure and protects the fetus from jarring and injury. The fluid maintains a constant temperature for the fetus and provides small amounts of nutrients. In labour, as long as the membranes remain intact, the amniotic fluid protects the placenta and umbilical cord from the pressure of uterine contractions. It also aids effacement of the cervix and dilatation of the uterine os, particularly where the presenting part is poorly applied.

Origin

The source of amniotic fluid is thought to be both fetal and maternal. It is secreted by the amnion, especially that which covers the placenta and umbilical cord. Some fluid is exuded from maternal vessels in the decidua and some from fetal vessels in the placenta. Fetal urine also contributes to the volume from the 10th week of gestation onwards.

Volume

The total amount of amniotic fluid increases throughout pregnancy until 38 weeks' gestation when there is about 1 litre. It then diminishes slightly until term when approximately 800 ml remains. However, there are very wide variations in the amount. If the total amount exceeds 1500 ml, the condition is known as polyhydramnios, and if less than 300 ml, the term oligohydramnios is applied. Such abnormalities are often associated with congenital malformations of the fetus. The normal fetus swallows amniotic fluid but if anything interferes with swallowing, an excessive amount of fluid will accumulate. Similarly, if the fetus is unable to pass urine, the amount of fluid will be reduced (see Ch. 38).

Constituents

Amniotic fluid (also termed liquor amnii) is a clear, pale straw-coloured fluid consisting of 99% water. The remaining 1% is dissolved solid matter including food substances and waste products. In addition the fetus sheds skin cells, vernix caseosa and lanugo into the fluid. Abnormal constituents of the liquor, such as meconium in the case of fetal distress, may give valuable diagnostic information about the condition of the fetus. Aspiration of amniotic fluid for examination is termed amniocentesis (see Ch. 41).

The umbilical cord

The umbilical cord or *funis* extends from the fetus to the placenta and transmits the umbilical blood vessels, two arteries and one vein. These are enclosed and protected by Wharton's jelly, a gelatinous substance formed from mesoderm. The whole cord is covered in a layer of amnion continuous with that covering the placenta.

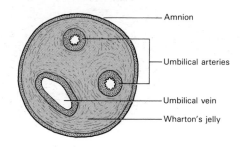

Fig. 4.4
Cross-section through the umbilical cord.

The length of the average cord is about 50 cm. This is sufficient to allow for delivery of the baby without applying any traction to the placenta. A cord is considered to be short when it measures less than 40 cm. There is no specific agreed length for describing a cord as too long, but the disadvantages of a very long cord are that it may become wrapped round the neck or body of the fetus or become knotted; either event could result in occlusion of the blood vessels, especially during labour. True knots should always be noted on examination of the cord, but they must be distinguished from false knots which are lumps of Wharton's jelly on the side of the cord and are not significant.

ANATOMICAL VARIATIONS OF THE PLACENTA AND THE CORD

Succenturiate lobe of placenta. This is the most significant of the variations in conformation of the placenta. A small extra lobe is present, separate from the main placenta, and joined to it by blood vessels which run through the membranes to reach it. The danger is that this small lobe may be retained in utero after delivery, and if it is not removed, it may lead to infection and haemorrhage. The midwife must examine every placenta for evidence of a retained succenturiate lobe — a hole in the membranes with vessels running to it.

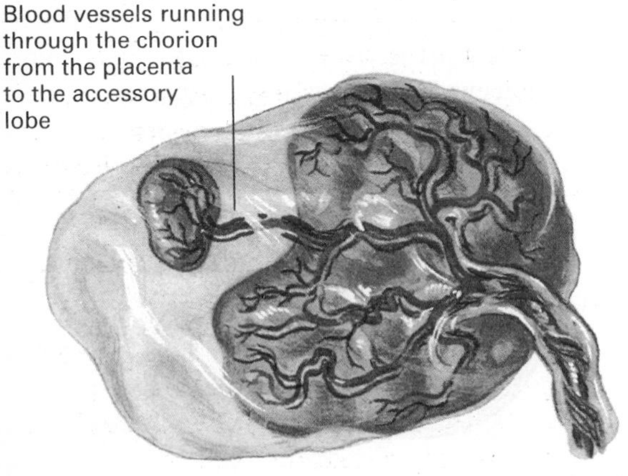

Circumvallate placenta. In this situation an opaque ring is seen on the fetal surface. It is formed by a doubling back of the chorion and amnion and may result in the membranes leaving the placenta nearer the centre instead of at the edge as usual.

Battledore insertion of the cord. The cord in this case is attached at the very edge of the placenta in the manner of a table tennis bat. It is unimportant unless the attachment is fragile.

Velamentous insertion of the cord. The cord is inserted into the membranes some distance from the edge of the placenta. The umbilical vessels run through the membranes from the

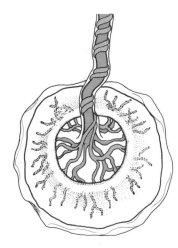

Fig. 4.6
Circumvallate placenta.

Blood vessels running through the chorion from the placenta to the accessory lobe

Fig. 4.5
Succenturiate lobe of placenta.

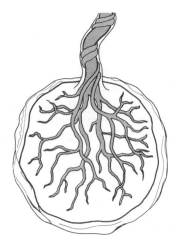

Fig. 4.7
Battledore insertion of the cord.

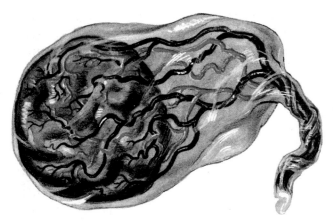

Fig. 4.8
Velamentous insertion of the cord.

cord to the placenta. If the placenta is normally situated, no harm will result to the fetus, but the cord is likely to become detached upon applying traction during active management of the third stage of labour.

If the placenta is low-lying, the vessels may pass across the uterine os. The term applied to the vessels lying in this position is vasa praevia. In this case there is great danger to the fetus when the membranes rupture and even more so during artificial rupture, as the vessels may be torn, leading to rapid exsanguination of the fetus. If the onset of haemorrhage coincides with rupture of the membranes, fetal haemorrhage should be assumed and delivery expedited. It is possible to distinguish fetal blood from maternal blood by Singer's alkali-denaturation test, although, in practice, time is so short that it may not be possible to save the life of the fetus. If the fetus survives, the baby's haemoglobin should be estimated after birth.

Bipartite placenta. Two complete and separate lobes are present, each with a cord leaving it. The bipartite cord joins a short distance from the two parts of the placenta. This is different from the two placentae in a twin pregnancy, where there are also two umbilical cords, but these do not join at any point. Where there is a succenturiate lobe, the vessels are attached to the placenta directly and never join the cord.

A tripartite placenta is similar but with three distinct lobes.

Except for the dangers noted above these varieties of conformation have no clinical significance.

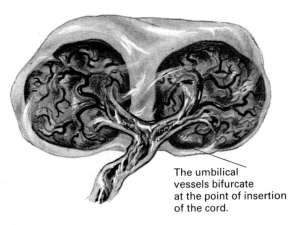

The umbilical vessels bifurcate at the point of insertion of the cord.

Fig. 4.9
Bipartite placenta.

Reader Activities

- Next time you examine a placenta, remove a piece of tissue, for example one lobe. Wash it thoroughly under running water to remove the maternal blood and decidua. Float it in clear water to observe the fronds and delicate structure of the villi.
- Compare a series of placental weights with the birthweights of the corresponding babies, working out the percentage or fraction in each case. Note whether the cord was clamped immediately or whether pulsation was allowed to cease first or if the placental blood was drained out before expulsion; observe any correlation. You might try weighing placentae before and after blood has been drained out via the cord.

FURTHER READING

Fox H 1978 Pathology of the placenta. Saunders, London

Fox H 1991 A contemporary view of the human placenta. Midwifery 7 (1 March): 31–39

Johnson M, Everitt B 1988 Essential reproduction, 3rd edn. Blackwell Scientific Publications, Oxford

Llewellyn-Jones D 1990 Fundamentals of obstetrics and gynaecology. Vol 1 Obstetrics, 5th edn. Faber, London

The fetus

V. RUTH BENNETT   LINDA K. BROWN

The midwife needs to have an understanding of fetal development in order to estimate the approximate age of a baby born before term. It is also helpful to know the outline of organogenesis in order to appreciate the ways in which developmental abnormalities arise. When making reference to the age at which various prenatal events happen, it is important to distinguish between menstrual age (the time since the first day of the last menstrual period) and the conceptional age (the interval since fertilisation). Embryologists use the latter while those involved with the pregnant woman tend to use the former.

The time-scale of the pregnancy is important. Figure 5.1 illustrates the comparative lengths of the different periods involved. The interval from the beginning of the last menstrual period (LMP) until conception is not strictly part of the pregnancy, although the as yet unfertilised ovum is already being prepared for release. For clinical purposes it is convenient to regard the pregnancy as beginning at the LMP because this is usually the only definitive date available. The midwife should be aware that an individual woman may know the exact date of conception and will rightly consider this as the beginning of her pregnancy.

For the first 3 weeks following conception the term fertilised ovum or zygote is used. From 3–8 weeks after conception it is known as the embryo and following this it is the fetus until birth when it becomes a baby. Although when speaking to mothers the fetus in utero may be referred to as a baby the midwife should use the correct terminology during professional discussions and in her records.

Summary of development

0–4 weeks after conception
Rapid growth
Formation of the embryonic plate (see Ch. 3)
Primitive central nervous system forms
Heart develops and begins to beat
Limb buds form.

4–8 weeks
Very rapid cell division
Head and facial features develop
All major organs laid down in primitive form
External genitalia present but sex not distinguishable
Early movements
Visible on ultrasound from 6 weeks.

8–12 weeks
Eyelids fuse
Kidneys begin to function and the fetus passes urine from 10 weeks
Fetal circulation functioning properly
Sucking and swallowing begin
Sex apparent
Moves freely (not felt by mother)
Some primitive reflexes present.

12–16 weeks
Rapid skeletal development — visible on X-ray
Meconium present in gut
Lanugo appears
Nasal septum and palate fuse.

16–20 weeks
'Quickening' — mother feels fetal movements
Fetal heart heard on auscultation
Vernix caseosa appears
Fingernails can be seen
Skin cells begin to be renewed.

20–24 weeks
Most organs become capable of functioning
Periods of sleep and activity
Responds to sound
Skin red and wrinkled.

24–28 weeks
Survival may be expected if born
Eyelids reopen
Respiratory movements.

28–32 weeks
Begins to store fat and iron
Testes descend into scrotum
Lanugo disappears from face
Skin becomes paler and less wrinkled.

32–36 weeks
Increased fat makes the body more rounded
Lanugo disappears from body
Head hair lengthens
Nails reach tips of fingers
Ear cartilage soft
Plantar creases visible.

36–40 weeks after conception (38–42 weeks after LMP)
Term is reached and birth is due
Contours rounded
Skull firm.

FETAL ORGANS

Some aspects of the development of fetal organs and their physiology are of special relevance to the midwife because of their effect on the newborn baby. A brief outline is given of the most important.

Blood
The origin of fetal blood is from the inner cell mass, along with all the other organs of its body. The fetus will inherit the genes which determine its blood group from both its parents and its ABO group and Rhesus factor may therefore be the same or different from those of its mother.

The fetal haemoglobin (Hb) is of a different type from adult haemoglobin and is termed HbF. It has a much greater affinity for oxygen and is found in greater concentration (18–20 g/dl at term). The reason for this is that oxygen must be obtained from the mother's blood in the placental site where the oxygen tension is lower than in the atmosphere. Towards the end of pregnancy the fetus begins to make adult-type haemoglobin (HbA).

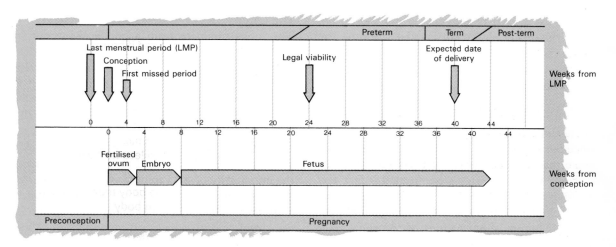

Fig. 5.1
Menstrual age, conceptional age and prenatal events.

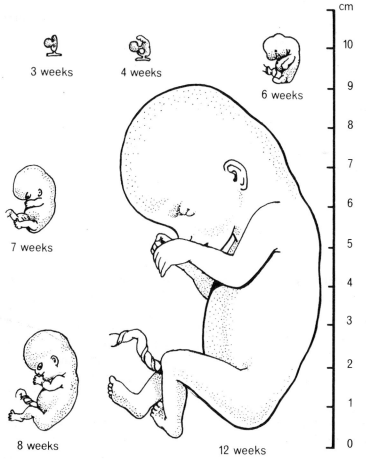

Fig. 5.2
Sizes of embryos and fetus between 3 and 12 weeks' gestation.

In utero the red blood cells have a shorter life span, this being about 90 days by the time the baby is born.

The renal tract

The kidneys begin to function and the fetus passes urine from 10 weeks' gestation. The urine is very dilute and does not constitute a route for excretion, since the mother eliminates waste products which cross the placenta. It is worth noting that the superior vesical arteries arise from the first few centimetres of the hypogastric arteries which lead to the umbilical arteries, so that if a single umbilical artery is found, abnormalities of the renal tract are suspected.

The adrenal glands

The fetal adrenal glands produce the precursors for placental formation of oestriols. They are also thought to play a part in the initiation of labour, although the exact mechanism is not fully understood (see Ch. 11; also Johnson & Everitt 1988).

The liver

The fetal liver is comparatively large in size, taking up much of the abdominal cavity, especially in the early months. From the 3rd to the 6th month of intra-uterine life, the liver is responsible for the formation of red blood cells, after which they are mainly produced in the red bone marrow and the spleen.

Towards the end of pregnancy iron stores are laid down in the liver.

The alimentary tract

The digestive tract is mainly non-functional before birth. It forms from the yolk sac as a straight tube, later growing out into the base of the umbilical cord and subsequently rotating back into the abdomen. Sucking and swallowing of amniotic fluid containing shed skin cells and other debris begins about 12 weeks after conception. Most digestive juices are present before birth and they act on the swallowed substances and discarded intestinal cells to form meconium. This is normally retained in the gut until after birth when it is passed as the first stool of the newborn.

The lungs

The lungs originate from a bud growing out of the pharynx which subdivides again and again to form the branching structure of the bronchial tree. The process continues after birth until about 8 years of age when the full number of bronchioles and alveoli will have developed. It is mainly the immaturity of the lungs which reduces the chance of survival of infants born before 24 weeks' gestation, due to the limited alveolar surface area, the immaturity of the capillary system in the lungs and the lack of adequate surfactant. Surfactant is a lipoprotein which reduces the surface tension in the alveoli and assists gaseous exchange. It is first produced from about 20 weeks' gestation and the amount increases until the lungs are mature at about 30–34 weeks. At term the lungs contain about 100 ml of lung fluid. About one-third of this is expelled during delivery and the rest is absorbed and carried away by the lymphatics and blood vessels as air takes its place.

There is some movement of the thorax from the 3rd month of fetal life and more definite respiratory movements from the 6th month.

The central nervous system

This is derived from the ectoderm. It folds inwards by a complicated process to form the neural tube which is then covered over by skin. This process is occasionally incomplete, leading to open neural tube defects.

The skin

From 18 weeks after conception the fetus is covered with a white, creamy substance called *vernix caseosa*. This protects the skin from the fluid and from any friction against itself. At 20 weeks the fetus will be covered with a fine downy hair called *lanugo* and at the same time the head hair and eyebrows begin to form. Lanugo is shed again from 36 weeks and a full-term infant has little left.

Fingernails develop from about 10 weeks but the toenails not until about 18 weeks. By term the nails usually extend beyond the fingertips but length of the nails is an unreliable guide to maturity.

THE FETAL CIRCULATION

The key to understanding the fetal circulation is the fact that oxygen is derived from the placenta. In addition the placenta is the source of nutrition and the site of elimination of waste. At birth there is a dramatic alteration in this situation and an almost instantaneous change must occur. Therefore all the postnatal structures must be in place and

ready to take over. There are several temporary structures in addition to the placenta itself and the umbilical cord and these enable the fetal circulation to take place while allowing for the changes at birth.

The umbilical vein leads from the umbilical cord to the underside of the liver and carries blood rich in oxygen and nutrients. It has a branch which joins the portal vein and supplies the liver.

The ductus venosus (from a vein to a vein) connects the umbilical vein to the inferior vena

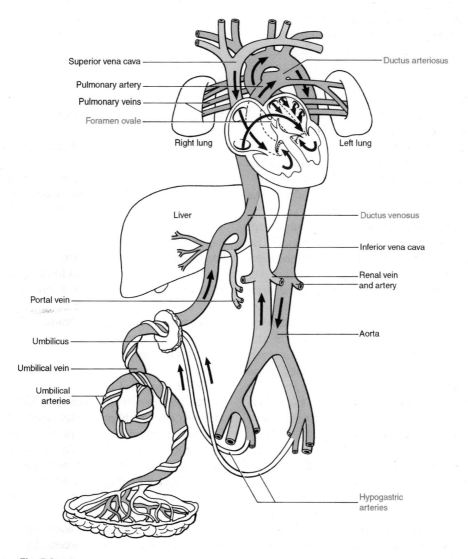

Fig. 5.3
A diagram of the fetal circulation. The arrows show the course taken by the blood. The temporary structures are labelled in colour.

cava. At this point the blood mixes with deoxygenated blood returning from the lower parts of the body. Thus the blood throughout the body is at best partially oxygenated.

The foramen ovale (oval opening) is a temporary opening between the atria which allows the majority of blood entering from the inferior vena cava to pass across into the left atrium. The reason for this diversion is that the blood does not need to pass through the lungs since it is already oxygenated.

The ductus arteriosus (from an artery to an artery) leads from the bifurcation of the pulmonary artery to the descending aorta, entering it just beyond the point where the subclavian and carotid arteries leave.

The hypogastric arteries branch off from the internal iliac arteries and become the umbilical arteries when they enter the umbilical cord. They return blood to the placenta.

The blood takes about half a minute to circulate and takes the following course.

From the placenta, blood passes along the umbilical vein through the abdominal wall to the under surface of the liver. This is the only vessel in the fetus which carries unmixed blood. The ductus venosus carries blood to the inferior vena cava where it mixes with blood from the lower body. From here the blood passes into the right atrium and most of it is directed across through the foramen ovale into the left atrium. Following its normal route it enters the left ventricle and passes into the aorta. The heart and brain each receive a supply of relatively well oxygenated blood since the coronary and carotid arteries are early branches from the aorta. The arms also benefit via the subclavian arteries which is why they are more developed than the legs at birth.

Blood collected from the upper parts of the body returns to the right atrium in the superior vena cava. This blood is depleted of oxygen and nutrients. This stream of blood crosses the stream entering from the inferior vena cava and passes into the right ventricle. The two streams remain separate due to the shape of the atrium but there is a mixing of 25% of the blood allowing a little oxygen and food to be taken to the lungs through the pulmonary artery. This is necessary for their development. However, only a small amount of the blood entering the pulmonary artery is required by the lungs. The remainder passes through the ductus arteriosus to the aorta. Blood continues along the aorta and, although low in oxygen, has sufficient to supply the remaining body organs and legs. The internal iliac arteries lead into the hypogastric arteries which return blood to the placenta via the umbilical arteries. The remaining blood supplies the lower limbs and returns to the inferior vena cava.

Adaptation to extra-uterine life

At birth the baby takes a breath and blood is drawn to the lungs through the pulmonary arteries. It is then collected and returned to the left atrium via the pulmonary veins resulting in a sudden inflow of blood. The placental circulation ceases soon after birth and so less blood returns to the right side of the heart. In this way the pressure in the left side of the heart is greater while that in the right side of the heart becomes less. This results in the closure of a flap over the foramen ovale which separates the two sides of the heart and stops the blood flowing from right to left.

With the establishment of pulmonary respiration the oxygen concentration in the blood stream rises. This causes the ductus arteriosus to constrict and close. For as long as the ductus remains open after birth, blood flows from the high-pressure aorta towards the lungs, in the reverse direction to that in fetal life.

The cessation of the placental circulation results in the collapse of the umbilical vein, the ductus venosus and the hypogastric arteries.

These immediate changes are functional and those related to the heart are reversible in certain circumstances. Later they become permanent and anatomical. The umbilical vein becomes the *ligamentum teres*, the ductus venosus the *ligamentum venosum* and the ductus arteriosus the *ligamentum arteriosum*. The foramen ovale becomes the *fossa ovalis* and the hypogastric arteries are known as the *obliterated hypogastric arteries* except for the first few centimetres which remain open as the superior vesical arteries.

Respiratory and circulatory changes are not the only ones involved. After birth the baby has to obtain nutrition through the establishment of breast feeding or a breast feeding substitute and to eliminate waste via the kidneys and gastro-intestinal system. In addition, of course, other complex changes take place including the development of communication and the relationship between parents and child (see Ch. 31).

THE FETAL SKULL

The fetal skull contains the delicate brain which may be subjected to great pressure as the head passes through the birth canal. It is large in comparison with the true pelvis and some adaptation between skull and pelvis must take place during labour. The head is the most difficult part to deliver whether it comes first or last.

An understanding of the landmarks and measurements of the fetal skull enables the midwife to recognise normal presentations and positions and to facilitate delivery with the least possible trauma to mother and child. Where malpresentation or disproportion exists she will be able to identify it and alert the medical staff.

Ossification. The bones of the fetal head originate in two different ways. The face is laid down in cartilage and is almost completely ossified at birth, the bones being fused together and firm. The bones of the vault are laid down in membrane and are much flatter and more pliable. They ossify from the centre outwards and this process is incomplete at birth leaving small gaps which form the sutures and fontanelles. The ossification centre on each bone appears as a boss or protuberance.

Bones of the vault

There are five main bones in the vault of the fetal skull.

The occipital bone lies at the back of the head and forms the region of the occiput. Part of it contributes to the base of the skull as it contains the foramen magnum which protects the spinal cord as it leaves the skull. At the centre is the *occipital protuberance*.

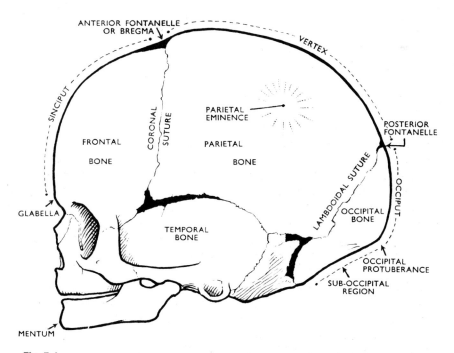

Fig. 5.4
Fetal skull showing regions and landmarks of obstetrical importance.

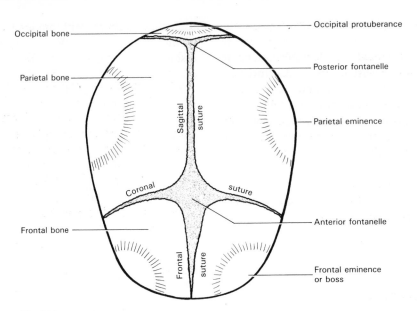

Fig. 5.5
View of fetal head from above (head partly flexed).

The two parietal bones lie on either side of the skull. The ossification centre of each is called the *parietal eminence.*

The two frontal bones form the forehead or *sinciput.* At the centre of each is a frontal boss or frontal eminence. The frontal bones fuse into a single bone by 8 years of age.

In addition to these five the upper part of *the temporal bone* is also flat and forms a small part of the vault.

Sutures and fontanelles

Sutures are cranial joints and are formed where two bones adjoin. Where two or more sutures meet, a fontanelle is formed. There are several sutures and fontanelles in the fetal skull; those of most obstetrical significance are described below.

The lambdoidal suture is shaped like the Greek letter lambda (λ) and separates the occipital bone from the two parietal bones.

The sagittal suture lies between the two parietal bones.

The coronal suture separates the frontal bones from the parietal bones, passing from one temple to the other.

The frontal suture runs between the two halves of the frontal bone. Whereas the frontal suture becomes obliterated in time, the other sutures eventually become fixed joints. Ossification of the skull is not complete until early adulthood.

The posterior fontanelle or lambda is situated at the junction of the lambdoidal and sagittal sutures. It is small, triangular in shape and can be recognised vaginally because a suture leaves from

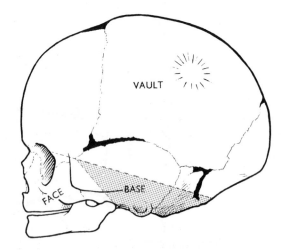

Fig. 5.6
Regions of the skull showing the large, compressible vault and the non-compressible face and base.

each of the three angles. It normally closes by 6 weeks of age.

The anterior fontanelle or bregma is found at the junction of the sagittal, coronal and frontal sutures. It is broad, kite-shaped and recognisable vaginally because a suture leaves from each of the four corners. It measures 3–4 cm long and 1.5–2 cm wide and normally closes by the time the child is 18 months old. Pulsations of cerebral vessels can be felt through it.

The sutures and fontanelles, because they consist of membranous spaces, allow for a degree of overlapping of the skull bones during labour and delivery.

Regions and landmarks of the fetal skull

The skull is divided into the vault, the base and the face. *The vault* is the large, dome-shaped part above an imaginary line drawn between the orbital ridges and the nape of the neck. In the vault the bones are relatively thin and pliable at birth which allows the skull to alter slightly in shape during birth. *The base* is comprised of bones which are firmly united to protect the vital centres in the medulla. *The face* is composed of 14 small bones which are also firmly united and non-compressible. The regions of the skull are described as follows:

The occiput lies between the foramen magnum and the posterior fontanelle. The part below the occipital protuberance is known as the suboccipital region. The protuberance itself can be seen and felt as a prominent point on the posterior aspect of the skull.

The vertex is bounded by the posterior fontanelle, the two parietal eminences and the anterior fontanelle. Of the 96% of the babies born head first, 95% present by the vertex.

The sinciput or brow extends from the anterior fontanelle and the coronal suture to the orbital ridges.

The face is small in the newborn baby. It extends from the orbital ridges and the root of the nose to the junction of the chin and the neck. The point between the eyebrows is known as *the glabella*. The chin is termed *the mentum* and is an important landmark.

Diameters of the fetal skull

The measurements of the skull are important because the midwife needs a practical understanding of the relationship between the fetal head and the mother's pelvis. It will become clear that some diameters are more favourable for easy passage through the pelvic canal and this will depend on the attitude of the head.

There are two transverse diameters:

Biparietal diameter 9.5 cm — between the two parietal eminences.

Bitemporal diameter 8.2 cm — between the furthest points of the coronal suture at the temples.

The remaining diameters described are anteroposterior or longitudinal:

Suboccipitobregmatic 9.5 cm — from below the occipital protuberance to the centre of the anterior fontanelle or bregma.

Suboccipitofrontal 10 cm — from below the occipital protuberance to the centre of the frontal suture.

Occipitofrontal 11.5 cm — from the occipital protuberance to the glabella.

Mentovertical 13.5 cm — from the point of the chin to the highest point on the vertex, slightly nearer to the posterior than to the anterior fontanelle.

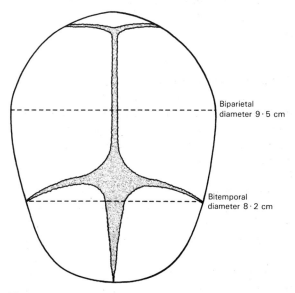

Biparietal
diameter 9·5 cm

Bitemporal
diameter 8·2 cm

Fig. 5.7
Diagram showing the transverse diameters of the fetal skull.

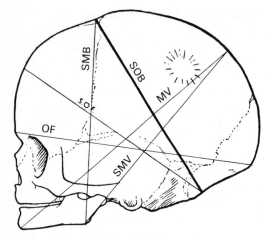

Fig. 5.8
Diagram showing the anteroposterior diameters of the fetal skull.

Diameter			Length
SOB	=	Suboccipitobregmatic	9.5 cm
SOF	=	Suboccipitofrontal	10.0 cm
OF`	=	Occipitofrontal	11.5 cm
MV	=	Mentovertical	13.5 cm
SMV	=	Submentovertical	11.5 cm
SMB	=	Submentobregmatic	9.5 cm

Submentovertical 11.5 cm — from the point where the chin joins the neck to the highest point on the vertex.

Submentobregmatic 9.5 cm — from the point where the chin joins the neck to the centre of the bregma.

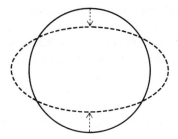

Fig. 5.10
Demonstration of the principle of moulding. The diameter compressed is diminished; the diameter at right-angles to it is elongated.

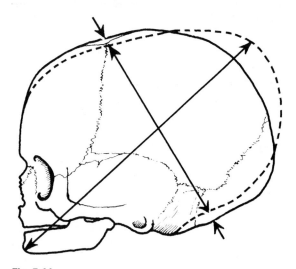

Fig. 5.11
Moulding in a normal vertex presentation with the head well flexed. The suboccipitobregmatic diameter is reduced and the mentovertical elongated.

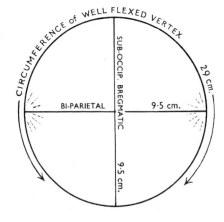

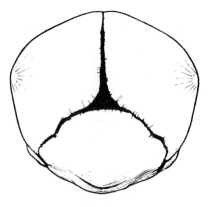

Fig. 5.9
Diagram showing the dimensions presenting when the fetal head is well flexed in a vertex presentation.

Attitude of the fetal head

This term is used to describe the degree of flexion or extension of the head on the neck. The attitude of the head determines which diameters will present in labour and therefore influences the outcome.

Presenting diameters

The diameters of the head which are called the presenting diameters are those which are at right angles to the curve of Carus. There are always two: an anteroposterior or longitudinal diameter and a transverse diameter. The diameters presenting in the individual cephalic or head presentations are as follows:

Vertex presentation. When the head is well flexed, the suboccipitobregmatic diameter and the biparietal diameter present. As these two diameters are the same length, 9.5 cm, the presenting area is circular, which is the most favourable shape for dilating the cervix. The diameter which distends the vaginal orifice is the suboccipitofrontal diameter, 10 cm.

When the head is not flexed but erect, the presenting diameters are the occipitofrontal, 11.5 cm and the biparietal, 9.5 cm. This situation often arises when the occiput is in a posterior position. If it remains so the diameter distending the vaginal orifice will be the occipitofrontal, 11.5 cm.

Brow presentation. When the head is partially extended, the mentovertical diameter, 13.5 cm, and the bitemporal diameter, 8.2 cm, present. If this presentation persists, vaginal delivery is extremely unlikely.

Face presentation. When the head is completely extended, the presenting diameters are the submentobregmatic, 9.5 cm, and the bitemporal, 8.2 cm. The submentovertical diameter, 11.5 cm, will distend the vaginal orifice.

Moulding

This is the term applied to the change in shape of the fetal head that takes place during its passage through the birth canal. Alteration in shape is possible because the bones of the vault allow a

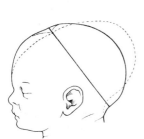

Fig. 5.12 Vertex presentation, head well flexed.

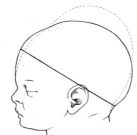

Fig. 5.13 Vertex presentation, head partially flexed.

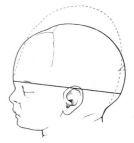

Fig. 5.14 Vertex presentation, head deflexed.

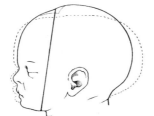

Fig. 5.15 Face presentation.

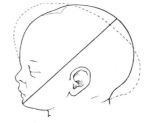

Fig. 5.16 Brow presentation.

Figs 5.12–5.16
Series of diagrams showing moulding when the head presents. Moulding is shown by the dotted line.

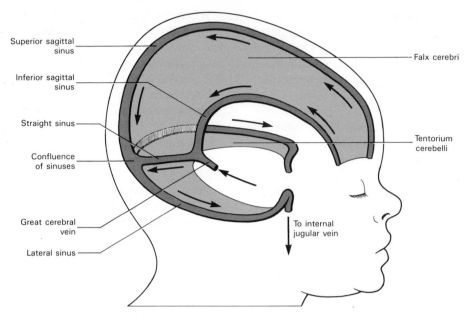

Fig. 5.17
Diagram showing intracranial membranes and venous sinuses. Arrows show direction of blood flow.

slight degree of bending and the skull bones are able to override at the sutures. This overriding allows a considerable reduction in the size of the presenting diameters while the diameter at right angles to them is able to lengthen due to the give of the skull bones.

In a normal vertex presentation with the fetal head in a fully flexed attitude the suboccipito-bregmatic and the biparietal diameters will be reduced and the mentovertical will be lengthened. The shortening may be by as much as 1.25 cm (Figs 5.11–5.16 illustrate moulding in various presentations).

Moulding is a protective mechanism and prevents the fetal brain from being compressed as long as it is not excessive, too rapid or in an un-favourable direction. The skull of the preterm infant, being softer and having wider sutures, may mould excessively; the skull of the postmature infant does not mould well and its greater hard-ness tends to make labour more difficult.

The intracranial membranes and sinuses

The skull contains delicate structures, some of which may be damaged if the head is subjected to abnormal moulding during delivery. Among the most important are the folds of dura mater and the venous sinuses associated with them. These membranes are continuous with the dura mater which lines the cranium.

The falx cerebri is a sickle-shaped fold of mem-brane which dips down between the two cerebral hemispheres and runs beneath the frontal and sagittal sutures, from the root of the nose to the internal occipital protuberance.

The tentorium cerebelli is a horizontal fold of dura mater which lies in the posterior part of the skull at right angles to the falx cerebri. It is shaped like a horseshoe and situated between the cerebrum and the cerebellum over which it forms a sort of tent. The membranes contain large veins or sinuses which drain blood from the brain.

The superior sagittal sinus runs along the upper edge of the falx cerebri from front to back.

The inferior sagittal sinus runs along the lower edge of the falx cerebri in the same direction.

The great cerebral vein of Galen meets the inferior sagittal sinus at the inner end of the junction between the falx and the tentorium.

The straight sinus drains blood from both the great cerebral vein and the inferior sagittal sinus

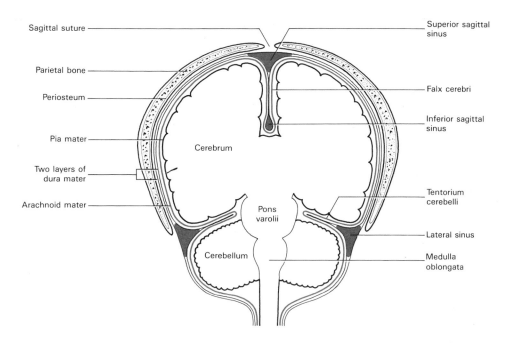

Fig. 5.18
Coronal section through the fetal head to show intracranial membranes and venous sinuses.

along the junction of the falx and the tentorium. The point where it reaches the skull and receives blood from the superior sagittal sinus is known as the *confluence of sinuses*.

The two lateral sinuses pass from the confluence of sinuses along the outer edge of the tentorium cerebelli and carry blood to the internal jugular veins.

The most vulnerable point of these structures is where the falx is attached to the tentorium. The tentorium is liable to tear and there is a danger of bleeding from the great cerebral vein.

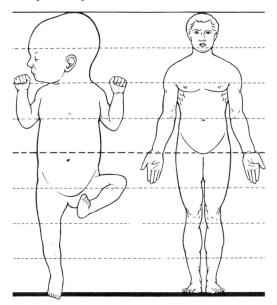

Fig. 5.19
Comparison of a baby's proportions to those of an adult. The baby's head is wider than her shoulders and one-quarter of her length.

Reader Activities

- Examine the head of a baby immediately after birth. From moulding, the position of any caput succedaneum and overlapping of skull bones, calculate the position that the child must have been in during labour. Compare this with the recorded vaginal examinations in labour.
- Take the skull measurements of a newly born baby. (If calipers are available it is possible to take all measurements; if not, use a tape measure to measure the circumferences.) After 3 days take the same measurements and compare the differences.

REFERENCE

Johnson M, Everitt B 1988 Essential reproduction, 3rd edn. Blackwell Scientific, Oxford

FURTHER READING

Burnett C W F 1979 The anatomy and physiology of obstetrics, 6th edn (rev. Anderson M). Faber and Faber, London

Dryden R 1978 Before birth. Heinemann Educational, London

Moore K L 1988 The developing human, 4th edn. Saunders, London

Moore K L 1989 Before we are born, 3rd edn. Saunders, London

Wolpert L 1991 The triumph of the embryo. Oxford University Press, Oxford

6

The female urinary tract

V. RUTH BENNETT   LINDA K. BROWN

The urinary system is chiefly thought of in connection with its elimination function and the production of urine. It also has important functions in connection with the control of water and electrolyte balance and of blood pressure.

In the female it has an importance associated with its proximity to the reproductive organs. When the woman is not pregnant, her uterus lies just behind and partly over the bladder. When she is pregnant the enlarging uterus affects all the parts of the urinary tract at various times and the hormones of pregnancy have an even greater influence than the mechanical effects. The normal, healthy woman may perceive these changes as a minor nuisance created by frequency of micturition and her kidneys continue to function well. A few may experience complications and those who already have diseased kidneys may undergo deterioration in their condition: some women suffer impairment of the function of part of the urinary tract as a direct result of pregnancy. The midwife may have an important part to play in minimising any ill-effect.

The urinary tract begins at the two kidneys which are linked up to the blood supply by the large renal arteries and veins. It continues as a passage for urine in the two ureters, the bladder and the urethra.

THE KIDNEYS

The kidneys are two bean-shaped glands which have both endocrine and exocrine secretions. Their function is to extract soluble wastes from the blood and to excrete such water and minerals as are surplus to the body's requirements. They also prevent substances which are needed by the body from being lost. They have a part to play in red cell production and in maintaining blood pressure.

Position and supports

The kidneys are positioned at the back of the abdominal cavity, high up under the diaphragm. The right kidney is displaced a little downwards by the liver, so the two kidneys are not quite level. They are maintained in position by a generous packing of perinephric fat and by the closeness of neighbouring organs, particularly parts of the gastro-intestinal tract in front and the musculature of the posterior abdominal wall behind (Fig. 6.1).

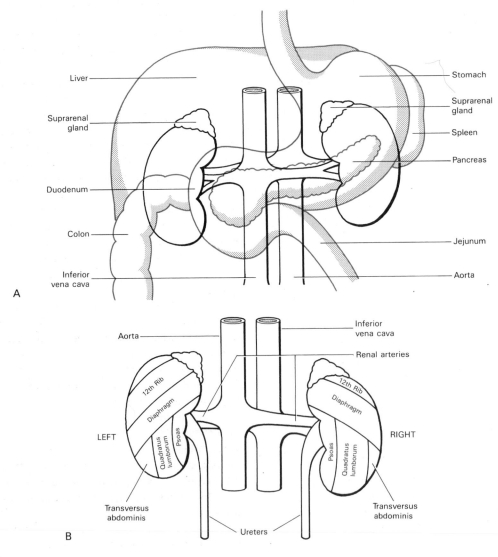

Fig. 6.1
Relations of the kidney: (A) anterior (B) posterior.

Appearance

The gland is recognisable by its dark red appearance and typical shape, so that other similarly shaped objects may be called 'kidney-shaped'. It is about 10 cm long, 6.5 cm wide and 3 cm thick. It weighs around 120 g. It is covered with a tough, fibrous capsule.

The inner border of the organ is indented at the hilum; here the large vessels enter and leave and the ureter is attached by its funnel-shaped upper end to channel the urine away.

Inner structure

The glandular tissue is formed of cortex on the outside and medulla within. The cortex is dark with a rich blood supply while the medulla is paler. A collecting area for urine merges with the upper ureter and is called the pelvis. It is divided into branches or calyces and each calyx cups over a projection from the medulla known as a pyramid. There are some 12 pyramids in all and they contain bundles of tubules leading from the cortex. The tubules create a lined appearance and these are the medullary rays. The base of each pyramid is curved and the cortex arches over it (Fig. 6.2) and projects downwards between the pyramids forming columns of tissue (columns of Bertini).

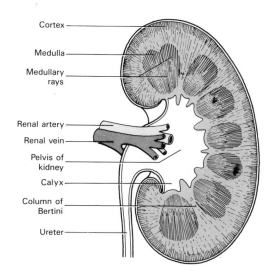

Cortex ——

Medulla ——

Medullary —— rays

Renal artery ——

Renal vein ——

Pelvis of —— kidney

Calyx ——

Column of —— Bertini

Ureter ——

Fig. 6.2
Longitudinal section of the kidney.

The nephrons

When the tissue of the kidney is examined under the microscope, it is found to be formed of about a million nephrons which are its functional units.

The manufacture of urine depends on a constant and generous supply of blood. Each nephron (Fig. 6.3) starts at a knot of capillaries called a *glomerulus*. It is fed by a branch of the renal artery, the *afferent arteriole*, and the blood is collected up again into the *efferent arteriole*. Afferent means 'carrying towards' and efferent, 'carrying away'. This is the only place in the body where an artery collects blood from capillaries. The blood vessel continues alongside the nephron.

Surrounding the glomerulus is a cup known as the *glomerular capsule* into which fluid and solutes are exuded from the blood. The glomerulus and capsule together are the *glomerular body* (Fig. 6.4). The pressure within the glomerulus is raised because the afferent arteriole is of a wider bore than the efferent arteriole and this factor forces the filtrate out of the capillaries and into the capsule. At this stage there is no selection; any substance with a small molecular size will filter out.

The cup of the capsule is attached to a tubule as a wine glass to its stem. The tubule initially winds and twists, then forms a straight loop which dips into the medulla, rising up into the cortex again to wind and turn before joining a *straight collecting tubule* which receives urine from several nephrons. The first twisting portion is the *proximal convoluted tubule*; the loop is termed the *loop of Henle* and the second twisting portion is the *distal convoluted tubule*. The whole nephron is about 3 cm in length. The straight collecting tubule runs from the cortex to a medullary pyramid: it forms a medullary ray (see above) and receives urine from over 4000 nephrons along its length.

Blood supply

The renal arteries are early branches of the descending abdominal aorta and divert about a quarter of the cardiac output into the kidneys. The artery enters at the renal hilum between the ureter behind and the renal vein in front. It sends numerous branches into the cortex and forms a glomerulus for each nephron. Blood is collected up and returned via the renal vein.

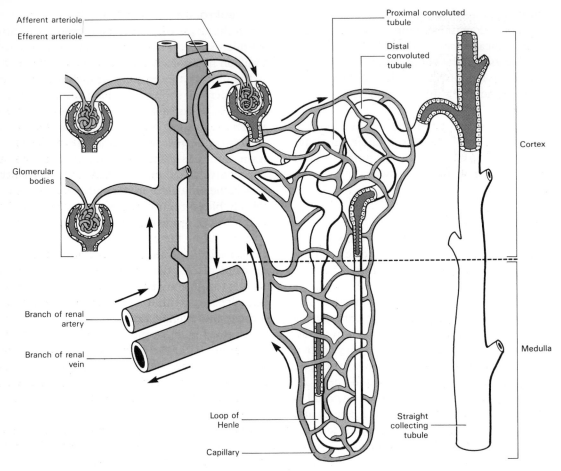

Fig. 6.3
A nephron.

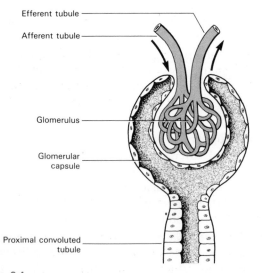

Fig. 6.4
A glomerular body.

Lymphatic drainage

A rich supply of lymph vessels lies under the cortex and around the urine-bearing tubules. It drains into large lymphatic ducts which emerge from the hilum and lead to the aortic lymph glands.

Nerve supply

Nerves enter by the renal hilum and provide a sympathetic and parasympathetic nerve supply.

The making of urine

This takes place in three stages:

- filtration
- reabsorption
- secretion.

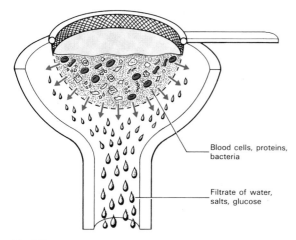

Blood cells, proteins, bacteria

Filtrate of water, salts, glucose

Fig. 6.5
Filtration: larger molecules stay in the sieve (glomerulus) and smaller molecules filter out (into the glomerular capsule).

Filtration is the simple process of water and the substances dissolved in it being passed from the glomerulus into the glomerular capsule as a result of the raised intracapillary pressure. Blood components such as corpuscles and platelets as well as proteins which have a large molecule are kept in the blood vessel; water, salts and glucose escape through the filter as the *filtrate* (Fig. 6.5). A vast amount of fluid passes out in this way, about 2 ml per second or 120 ml per minute. 99% of this must be recovered, or the body would be totally drained of fluid within hours. Filtration is increased in pregnancy as it helps to eliminate the additional wastes created by maternal and fetal metabolism.

Reabsorption. The body selects from the filtrate the substances which it needs: water, salts and glucose.

Normally all the glucose is reabsorbed; only if there is already more than sufficient in the blood, for example after eating sweet, sugary foods, will any be excreted in the urine. The level of blood glucose at which this happens is the *renal threshold* for glucose. In the non-pregnant, the threshold is 10 mmol/ℓ and in the pregnant woman 8.3 mmol/ℓ. It is more likely, therefore, that glucose will appear in the urine during pregnancy.

The water is almost all reabsorbed. If the body has lost fluid by other means, such as sweating,

or if fluid intake has been low, more water is conserved, less urine is passed and the urine appears more concentrated. In the opposite circumstances, when the individual has drunk a lot of water and is sweating little, the urine is more copious and dilute. Note that drinking alcohol does not have this effect. The posterior pituitary gland controls the reabsorption of water by producing antidiuretic hormone (ADH). The more ADH produced, the more water is absorbed. Newborn babies are poorly able to concentrate and dilute their urine and preterm infants even less so. For this reason they are unable to tolerate wide variations in their fluid intake. Pregnant women pass a greater amount of urine than when non-pregnant.

Minerals are selected according to the body's needs. The reabsorption of sodium is controlled by aldosterone which is produced in the cortex of the adrenal gland. The interaction of aldosterone and ADH maintains water and sodium balance. The pH of the blood must be controlled and if it is tending towards acidity, acids will be excreted. This is commonly the case. However, if the opposite pertains, alkaline urine will be produced. Often this is the result of an intake of an alkaline substance.

Secretion. Certain substances, such as creatinine and toxins, are added directly to the urine in the ascending arm of the loop of Henle.

Endocrine activity

The kidney secretes two hormones. One, renin, is produced in the cortex and is secreted when the blood supply to the kidneys is reduced. It combines with hypertensinogen which is present in the blood, to form angiotensin which raises blood pressure.

The second hormone, erythropoietin, stimulates the production of red blood cells.

Summary of functions

The kidney functions may be summarised as follows:

- elimination of wastes, particularly the breakdown products of protein, such as urea, urates, uric acid, creatinine, ammonia and sulphates

- elimination of toxins
- regulation of the water content of the blood and indirectly of the tissues
- regulation of the pH of the blood
- regulation of the osmotic pressure of the blood
- secretion of the hormones renin and erythropoietin.

The urine

Urine is a yellow colour ranging from pale straw colour when very dilute to dark brown if very concentrated. In the newborn baby it is almost clear. It has a recognisable smell which in health is not unpleasant when freshly passed. It should never be cloudy.

An adult passes between 1 and 2 litres of urine daily, depending on fluid intake. Less is produced during the night than in the day. Pregnant women secrete large amounts of urine due to the increased glomerular filtration rate and they often have to rise at night to empty the bladder. In the first day or two postpartum a major diuresis occurs and urine output is copious.

The specific gravity of urine is 1.010–1.030. It is composed of 96% water, 2% urea and 2% other solutes. Urea and uric acid clearance are increased in pregnancy. Urine is usually acid and contains no glucose or ketones, nor should it carry blood cells or bacteria. Women are susceptible to urinary tract infection but this is usually an ascending infection acquired via the urethra. A low count, less than 100 000 per ml, of bacteria in the urine (bacteriuria) is treated as insignificant.

THE URETERS

The tubes which convey the urine from the kidneys to the bladder are the ureters. They assist the passage of the urine by the muscular peristaltic action of their walls. The upper end is funnel-shaped and merges into the pelvis of the kidney where the urine is received from the renal tubules.

Each tube is about 25–30 cm long and runs from the renal hilum to the posterior wall of the bladder (Fig. 6.6). In the abdomen they pass down the posterior wall, remaining outside the peritoneal cavity. On reaching the pelvic brim they descend

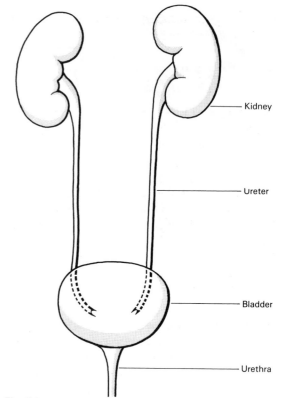

Fig. 6.6
The renal tract.

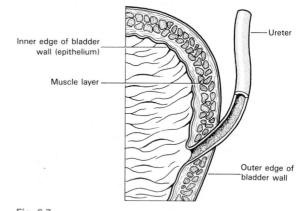

Fig. 6.7
Diagram to show the entry of the ureter into the posterior wall of the bladder.

along the side walls of the pelvis to the level of the ischial spines and then turn forwards to pass beside the uterine cervix and enter the bladder from behind. They pass through the bladder wall at an angle (Fig. 6.7) so that when the bladder contracts to expel urine, the ureters are closed off and reflux is prevented.

Structure
The ureters have three main layers:

The lining is formed of transitional epithelium arranged in longitudinal folds. This type of epithelium consists of several layers of pear-shaped cells and makes an elastic and waterproof inner coat.

The muscular layer is arranged as an inner longitudinal layer, a middle circular layer and an outer longitudinal layer. Waves of peristalsis pass along the ureter towards the bladder.

The outer coat is of fibrous connective tissue which is protective. It is continuous with the fibrous capsule of the kidney.

Blood, lymph and nerve supply
The upper part of the ureter is supplied similarly to the kidney. In its pelvic portion it derives blood from the common iliac and internal iliac arteries and from the uterine and vesical arteries, according to its proximity to the different organs. Venous return is along corresponding veins.

Lymph drains into the internal, external and common iliac lymph nodes.

The nerve supply is sympathetic and parasympathetic.

The ureter in pregnancy

The hormones of pregnancy, particularly progesterone, relax the walls of the ureters and allow dilation and kinking. In some women this is quite marked and it tends to result in a slowing down or stasis of urinary flow, making infection a greater possibility (Fig. 6.8).

THE BLADDER

The bladder is the urinary reservoir which stores the urine until it is convenient for it to be voided. It is described as being pyramidal; its base is triangular. When it is full, however, it becomes

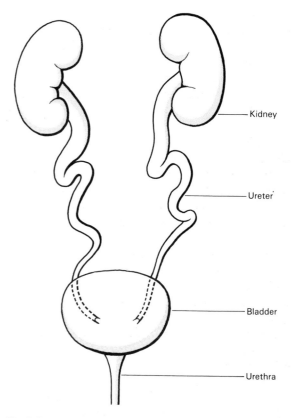

Fig. 6.8
Dilated, kinked ureters in pregnancy.

more globular in shape as its walls are distended. Although it is a pelvic organ it may rise into the abdomen when full, and during labour it is certainly abdominal. It is one of the organs which most greatly concern midwives because of its closeness to the uterus.

Position
In the non-pregnant female, the bladder lies immediately behind the symphysis pubis and in front of the uterus and vagina (Fig. 6.9). In addition the anteverted, anteflexed uterus lies partially over the bladder superiorly. The intestines and peritoneal cavity also lie above. The ureters enter the bladder from behind; the urethra leaves it from below. Underneath the bladder is the muscular diaphragm of the pelvic floor which forms its main support and on which its function partly depends.

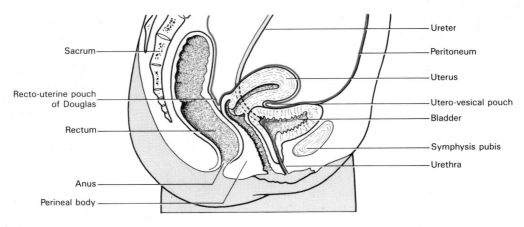

Fig. 6.9
Sagittal section of the pelvis showing the relations of the bladder.

Structure

The base of the bladder is termed the *trigone*. It is situated at the back of the bladder, resting against the vagina. Its three angles are the exit of the urethra below and the two slit-like openings of the ureters above. The apex of the trigone is thus at its lowest point, which is also termed the neck (Fig. 6.10).

The anterior part of the bladder lies close to the pubic symphysis and is termed the apex of the bladder. From it the urachus runs up the anterior abdominal wall to the umbilicus. In fetal life this is the remains of the yolk sac but in the adult is simply a fibrous band.

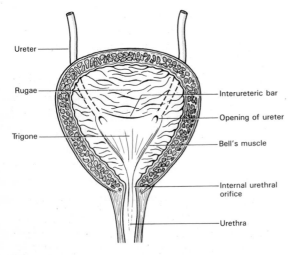

Fig. 6.10
Section through the bladder.

The bladder when empty is of similar size to the uterus but when full of urine it becomes, of course, much larger. Its capacity is around 600 ml but it is capable of holding more, particularly under the influence of pregnancy hormones. The midwife will commonly observe a newly-delivered woman voiding upwards of 1 litre on a single occasion.

Layers

The lining of the bladder, like that of the ureter, is formed of transitional epithelium which helps to allow the distension of the bladder without losing its water-holding effect. The lining, except over the trigone, is thrown into wrinkles or *rugae* which flatten out as the bladder expands and fills.

The mucous membrane lining lies on a submucous layer of areolar tissue which carries blood and lymph vessels and nerves.

The epithelium over the trigone is smooth and firmly attached to the underlying muscle.

The musculature of the bladder consists chiefly of the large detrusor muscle whose function is to expel urine. (To detrude is to thrust down to a lower place.) This muscle has an inner longitudinal, a middle circular and an outer longitudinal layer. Around the neck of the bladder, the circular muscle is thickened to form the *internal urethral sphincter*. It remains constantly contracted except when the individual passes urine.

In the trigone the muscles are somewhat differently arranged. A band of muscle between the ureteric apertures forms the interureteric bar (Mercier's bar). Along the other two sides of the trigone, Bell's muscles run from the entrances of the ureters down through the internal urethral orifice. They are important during voiding of the bladder.

The outer layer of the bladder is formed of visceral pelvic fascia except on its superior surface which is covered with peritoneum (see Fig. 6.9).

Blood, lymph and nerve supplies

The vesical arteries, superior and inferior, are the main suppliers of blood. A few small branches from the uterine and vaginal arteries also bring blood to the bladder. Corresponding veins return used blood.

Lymph drains into the internal iliac glands and into the obturator glands.

The nerve supply is parasympathetic and sympathetic and comes via the important Lee–Frankenhäuser plexus in the pouch of Douglas. The stimulation of sympathetic nerves causes the internal urethral sphincter to contract and the detrusor muscle to relax, while the parasympathetic nerve fibres cause the bladder to empty and the sphincter to relax.

THE URETHRA

The final passage in the urinary tract is the urethra, 4 cm long in the female and consisting of a narrow tube buried in the outer layers of the anterior vaginal wall. It runs from the neck of the bladder and opens into the vestibule of the vulva as the urethral meatus. During labour the urethra becomes elongated as the bladder is drawn up into the abdomen and may become several cm longer.

Structure

The lining. The urethra forms the junction between the urinary tract and the external genitalia. The epithelium of its lining reflects this. The upper half is lined with transitional epithelium while the lower half is lined with squamous epithelium. The lumen is normally closed unless urine is passing down it or a catheter is in situ. When closed, it shows small longitudinal folds. Small blind ducts called urethral crypts open into the urethra of which the two largest are Skene's ducts which open just beside the urethral meatus. Their main significance is in the possibility of infection with an organism such as the gonococcus.

The sub-mucous coat. The epithelium of the urethra lies on a bed of vascular connective tissue.

The musculature. The muscle layers are arranged as an inner longitudinal layer, continuous with the inner muscle fibres of the bladder, and an external circular layer. The inner muscle fibres help to open the internal urethral sphincter during micturition.

The outer layer of the urethra is continuous with the outer layer of the vagina and is formed of connective tissue.

The external sphincter. At the lower end of the urethra, voluntary, striated muscle fibres form the so-called membranous sphincter of the urethra. This is not a true sphincter but it gives some voluntary control to the woman when she desires to resist the urge to urinate. The powerful levator ani muscles which pass on either side of the uterus also assist in controlling continence of urine.

Blood, lymph and nerve supplies

The blood is circulated by the inferior vesical and pudendal arteries and veins. Lymph drains to the internal iliac glands.

The internal urethral sphincter is supplied by sympathetic and parasympathetic nerves but the membranous sphincter is supplied by the pudendal nerve and is under voluntary control.

Micturition

The urge to pass urine is felt when the bladder contains about 200–300 ml of urine but also when psychological stimuli operate such as waking after sleep, arriving or leaving home and from external stimuli such as the sound and feel of water and the feel of the toilet seat. Helpless laughter or paroxysmal coughing may also trigger a desire to empty the bladder.

In newborn babies there is no resistance to the spontaneous prompting of the bladder that it wishes to be emptied. The sphincters relax, the detrusor muscle contracts and urine is passed. After about 2 years a child learns to resist the urge to void and by adulthood it is taken for granted. Many women, particularly the pregnant and parous, experience difficulty in maintaining continence under the stress of coughing, laughing, sneezing and other factors which raise intra-abdominal pressure. Regular muscular exercise such as walking, swimming, running and pelvic floor exercises help to raise the tone of the voluntary muscles.

In summary the bladder fills and then contracts as a reflex response. The internal sphincter opens by the action of Bell's muscles. If the urge is not resisted, the external sphincter relaxes and the bladder empties. The act of emptying may be speeded by raising intra-abdominal pressure either to initiate the process or throughout voiding. The act of micturition can be temporarily postponed but the full bladder becomes progressively more uncomfortable.

FURTHER READING

Beischer N A, Mackay E V 1986 Obstetrics and the newborn, 2nd edn. Baillière Tindall, London
Goodinson S M 1988 Renal function. In: Hinchliff S, Montague S (eds) Physiology for nursing practice. Baillière Tindall, London

3

Pregnancy

7

Preparing for pregnancy

THELMA BAMFIELD

As girls grow up they become aware of their sexuality and the expectation that they will have children. Some will require specialist help before they become pregnant, either for general information about a healthy lifestyle, or for specific advice relating to medical, sexual or fertility problems.

SEXUALITY, LOVE, MARRIAGE AND PARENTHOOD

Sexuality

Sexuality begins to develop at birth. Being born, held and cared for, being suckled at the breast; all are total physical experiences and can bring pleasure and satisfaction or pain and irreversible trauma.

A child's sex education is going on all the time. She is bathed and changed; she begins to explore her own body, to show curiosity about the opposite sex and where babies come from; later she undergoes the changes of puberty and starts to menstruate. Through the way her parents react at every stage she is learning whether her body is something to feel at ease in and derive pleasure from, or something to be embarrassed or ashamed about.

She becomes aware that her parents are sexual beings. From their behaviour she picks up clues which teach her whether sex is about love or power; mutual enjoyment or something a woman must submit to in order to keep the peace.

Sexuality is determined not only by gender but also by social conditioning. Every culture defines the roles which it considers appropriate to males and females, and each individual has to come to terms with these expectations. One of the first questions parents and relatives ask about a baby is whether it is a boy or a girl and the answer defines the way the infant is dressed, brought up, even the way it is nursed. Baby boys in Western society are handled firmly; 'masculine' attributes, such as strong character and wilfulness, are regarded with approval. As they grow they are expected to be adventurous and fearless and play with cars, trucks and guns.

Baby girls are handled more gently; any evidence of strong will is regarded as 'unfeminine'; they are expected to be docile and compliant, behave in a decorous manner and play with dolls.

Although enlightened parents may try to encourage their children to give full expression to every facet of their character, they will have difficulty overcoming the pressures exerted by society, the media and marketing, which still persuasively propound the view that a girl's function in life is to make herself attractive to the opposite sex, marry and have children.

Love

A baby whose needs are fulfilled unstintingly and who is shown unconditional love learns that he or she is worthy of love and can learn to love in return. Without this security, self-esteem is low, the child cannot trust anyone and will be unable to give love. Experiences of being mothered in early life not only affect the well-being of the child but have long-term repercussions on the ability to form relationships as an adult.

As with all basic physiological needs, human societies have always sought to control sexuality and prescribe limits to its gratification. The adolescent has to contend with a newly discovered sexual drive in herself and others and reconcile it with the need to give and receive affection.

The sexuality of adolescent boys tends to be urgent, physical, and tied up with relieving tension and proving their manhood as well as achieving status amongst their peers.

A girl's early encounters may have little to do with her own sexuality. She is expressing romantic love or giving in to a boy's insistence for fear of losing him if she refuses, or else she feels that she is missing out on an experience which all her friends are enjoying.

A girl who feels unloved may permit or even seek out a sexual involvement in her quest for affection and she may well find herself abandoned if she becomes pregnant. She may even deliberately have a baby in order to have someone to love her. She fails to appreciate the demands that a child will make and that a child can only learn to love by example; an example which she will be unable to give because she feels herself intrinsically worthless.

Young people in Western society today receive conflicting messages from parents and peers, school, the media and their culture. On the one hand, sex is seen as a statement of commitment, only appropriate within marriage; on the other they learn that all wants should be instantly gratified and that everyone has the right to sexual fulfilment. One result of this inconsistency is unplanned pregnancy. To use contraception is to admit to premeditation, to acknowledge to another or others, and most importantly to oneself, a deliberate intention to have intercourse. Maintaining the illusion of spontaneity is one way to avoid taking responsibility for one's actions.

Marriage and parenthood

Marriage can provide companionship, a guaranteed sexual outlet, domestic services (for men at any rate) and the opportunity for joint parenthood. Breakdown of marriage is becoming more prevalent: one explanation for this is that individuals nowadays have higher expectations of marriage and are less prepared than their parents to tolerate an unsatisfactory relationship. The high rate of remarriage suggests that the institution itself is as popular as ever and increasing numbers of unmarried couples in stable relationships are having children.

Attitudes to parenthood are largely determined

by experiences in childhood. If they felt loved and secure themselves, young people have a good start towards creating a caring, stable environment for their own children to grow up in. If this early security was denied them or they experienced disruption or violence, they lack a good example on which to model their own parenting.

Before reliable contraception was available, the advent of children within marriage was greeted with a certain fatalism. Now it is more likely that a deliberate choice will be made about when, and indeed whether, to have children.

More women are postponing motherhood until they have established themselves in a career and built up a home. This may mean that by the time they decide to start a family they are past the optimum age for childbearing. Nonetheless, an older couple should try to avoid being rushed into having a baby because they feel that time is running out. They may be mature people but it is impossible to predict how anyone (including oneself) will cope with parenthood.

Young couples should not be in a hurry to begin a pregnancy either. In addition to learning to adjust to each other and allowing their relationship to grow, they need time to mature and develop as individuals.

Preparing for parenthood

However conscientious our antenatal care and attention to health in pregnancy, it does not begin until the most vulnerable stages of embryonic development have passed. After a reproductive disaster a couple will naturally question why it happened and try to prevent the same thing happening again. Hence the interest in health before conception.

Some factors which have an effect on pregnancy are unalterable, such as the parents' relative ages, genetic make-up, intelligence and socio-economic class. Other factors can be influenced, and they too may have a profound effect on pregnancy outcome.

It has been argued that 'it would be premature to make any judgements about prepregnancy advice except to say that on present knowledge its beneficial effects are likely to be extremely modest and it cannot automatically be regarded as harmless' (Lumley & Astbury 1989).

It is true that we know very little about many of the causes of handicap or perinatal death, and it would be both counterproductive and unethical to increase anxiety and apportion blame when things go wrong. Nonetheless, individuals are becoming increasingly aware of the importance of a healthy lifestyle and would welcome constructive advice.

PRE-PREGNANCY CARE

Diet

Gross malnutrition is rare in Western society today but suboptimal nutrition is very common, particularly in areas where unemployment and consequent poverty are increasing.

Much of the food consumed today has been processed by techniques which destroy essential nutrients; in addition it is treated with chemicals, preservatives and artificial colouring and flavouring to increase its shelf life and attractiveness to the customer.

Because of soil depletion, the use of artificial fertilisers and intensive farming, even fresh foods may have low nutritional value and contain harmful substances. Organic farming methods use natural fertilisers and avoid chemical pesticides.

For optimal health, processed and refined foods should be avoided altogether. Items from each of the four main categories should be taken each day.

Bread and cereals
— wholegrain cereals provide carbohydrate, fibre, minerals and vitamins

Fresh fruits and vegetables
— either raw or cooked in such a way as to retain nutritional value:
  - fruits should be stewed in glass or enamel, not aluminium
  - vegetables should be scrubbed, not peeled, then baked or steamed

Protein foods
— meat, fresh and preferably organically raised
— fish

— eggs, preferably free range

— pulses such as dried peas, beans, lentils

Dairy products

— fresh milk contains vitamins and fatty acids which are destroyed by processes such as drying and sterilisation.

A well-balanced diet should contain sufficient vitamins and minerals for daily requirements. Some authorities recommend supplements before pregnancy to correct any deficits.

Allergies to foods and food additives appear to be far more prevalent than was previously thought possible. Symptoms are often non-specific and range from the trivial to the disabling. They include hyperactivity and learning difficulties in children. A susceptible child may be sensitised in utero.

Weight

Pre-pregnancy weight can have an important bearing on pregnancy outcome. Women whose weight falls outside the optimal range have an increased likelihood of amenorrhoea and infertility. If a woman is underweight there is evidence of an association with fetal abnormality and low birth weight. The overweight woman has an increased risk of complications of pregnancy, notably hypertension, in addition to the risk to her own health.

The Quetelet or body-mass index is a method of calculating the ideal pre-pregnancy weight: weight in kilograms divided by height in metres squared.

less than 20 —	underweight
20–24.9 —	desirable
25–29.9 —	moderate obesity
over 30 —	severe obesity.

Advice on diet is given along the lines suggested above. 'Crash dieting' is best avoided as it adversely affects nutritional status. Any woman who does diet rigorously must be strongly advised to use reliable contraception until she is maintaining a desirable weight and a satisfactory intake of nutrients.

Exercise and relaxation

Moderate exercise taken regularly in the fresh air improves health, weight and fitness and aids effective relaxation; yoga exercises are an excellent alternative (see also Ch. 40). The contribution of stress to reproductive disaster is only beginning to be appreciated; it is known to predispose to infertility, spontaneous abortion and preterm labour.

Avoiding hazards

Smoking. The effects of smoking in pregnancy are well documented. There is a higher rate of spontaneous abortion, congenital abnormalities and fetal and neonatal death associated with smoking. Even if the woman gives up during pregnancy the risks are still increased above those for the non-smoker.

Men who smoke have lowered testosterone levels; spermatogenesis, sperm morphology and motility are impaired. Intended pregnancy can therefore provide a good incentive for a couple to give up smoking together.

The effects of smoking are potentiated by caffeine and alcohol.

Alcohol. It is now recognised that alcohol consumed in pregnancy can damage the fetus but the critical dose and time are still not known. Not only the regular drinker, but also the woman who drinks infrequently with the occasional binge may put her fetus at risk at a very early stage. For this reason, women should be advised to reduce or discontinue alcohol consumption before and during pregnancy.

Drugs. Many drugs are known to have an adverse effect on pregnancy but for the most part their influences in the period before conception are simply not known.

As none can be entirely free from suspicion of teratogenicity, medication of any kind should be carefully scrutinised. This includes self-medication such as cold cures, painkillers, antacids and laxatives and the use of psychotropic drugs, prescribed or otherwise.

The oral contraceptive pill lowers blood zinc levels and affects liver function. There is resulting interference with vitamin A metabolism and concentrations which are too high or too low can be teratogenic. The Pill also affects folate and vitamin B_{12} metabolism, and lowers levels of other vitamins of the B complex and of vitamin C.

It is therefore advisable for oral contraceptive use to be discontinued at least 3 and preferably 6 months before a woman tries to become pregnant. In the meantime the couple should use some non-invasive method of contraception, and barrier methods have the best safety record. The safe period may be difficult to calculate while steroid hormones are still circulating. A few couples may be able to use coitus interruptus successfully (see Ch. 17).

Infections. In spite of the publicity about rubella and the policy for immunisation of schoolgirls, between 10 and 25% of women of childbearing age lack rubella antibodies. The vaccination is only 95% effective, therefore any woman planning a pregnancy should have her immune status checked and be given the vaccine if necessary. Stringent contraceptive precautions should of course be taken for 1 to 3 months.

Pregnancy should be avoided following any immunisation. Gamma globulin may be available for protection during an epidemic if pregnancy is a possibility in a susceptible woman.

Any pre-existing infection, for example of the urinary, reproductive, or respiratory tract, or sexually transmitted disease in either partner, should be treated before conception is attempted. The couple should be advised to avoid contact with any infections, particularly viral, as far as possible.

Noxious substances. The reproductive system, the embryo and the fetus are extremely sensitive to insult; they are vulnerable to levels of environmental pollution much lower than those necessary to affect the general health of an adult.

Lead has been most intensively studied, since it is widely encountered, not just in factories but in traffic exhaust fumes, paints, solder and the domestic water supply. The association with mental retardation and hyperactivity in children is well known; evidence also suggests a link with congenital abnormalities and perinatal death. Other heavy metals such as cadmium and mercury may have the same effect.

Industrial processes. There is reliable evidence of toxic effects from chemicals such as gases (including anaesthetic gases), solvents, dusts, pesticides and from ionising radiation. The effect of prolonged exposure to Visual Display Units (VDUs) is still disputed.

Pollutants may affect the gonads of men and women, causing problems ranging from impotence, menstrual disorders and infertility to spontaneous abortion, congenital abnormalities and cancers in the children.

Employers are obliged by law to tell their employees whether they are working with any chemicals or processes known to be hazardous. A couple planning to start a family should seek this information. If there is a danger, they should avoid exposure to the hazard as far as possible. Midwives may be exposed to substances such as nitrous oxide and other gases or to radiation hazards. Unfortunately, although manufacturers are bound by law to research into the effects of their products, few have looked into possible reproductive risks. Statistical proof is indeed hard to collect:

- workers, particularly men, rarely admit to problems related to sexuality unless specifically asked
- doctors investigating fertility problems do not always enquire about work conditions
- the environment is only one of a number of factors which may cause reproductive failure
- experimental work on animals is of limited value, as their susceptibility may be very different from that of humans.

Medical screening

Some couples may seek more specific attention from a general practitioner or preconception clinic before embarking on a pregnancy. The extent of the tests and examinations which the doctor considers appropriate varies greatly.

Basic check-up

Time is allowed for a relaxed discussion covering dietary habits, lifestyle and possible exposure to hazards. A full medical history is taken from both partners and each has a general examination, including measurement of height, weight and blood pressure. The reproductive history of each is taken, and a menstrual history of the woman. A gynaecological examination is performed, including screening for vaginal infection and a cervical smear. The couple are referred for psychosexual counselling or investigation of subfertility if indicated.

Samples will be obtained for a number of tests:

Urinalysis and investigation for urinary tract infection are carried out.

Blood tests will include haemoglobin estimation, rubella immunity, a test for syphilis, estimation of lead levels and any other investigations indicated, for example screening for sickle cell trait.

Hair analysis is organised by some clinics; it reveals concentrations of up to 18 metals. High levels of toxic metals can be reduced by chelating agents, and low levels of essential trace minerals are corrected by appropriate supplements. The use of hair analysis is controversial because it is retrospective.

Stool samples are analysed in order to detect malabsorption or infestation if indicated.

Semen analysis for abnormal sperm should be done in cases of subfertility, high alcohol intake, coeliac disease or recent debilitating illness.

Drinking water samples from the couple's home may be tested, particularly if the water is known to be soft and acid and if the plumbing includes lead pipes and tanks. The finding of high levels of lead, copper, cadmium or aluminium in the water should be referred to the local Water Board.

Individuals with a known medical problem

Drug therapy for any pre-existing medical condition should be reduced to the minimum compatible with stabilisation before pregnancy is attempted. A woman receiving long-term medical treatment should be advised to consult her physician before embarking on pregnancy. Similarly a woman who has undergone major surgery or transplant would be wise to consult her doctor. Women with phenylketonuria should re-introduce dietary therapy.

Epilepsy. Anticonvulsants diminish potency and fertility in men and there is a risk of fetal abnormalities if they are taken by either partner. It is not yet clear to what extent this is due to the fact that they induce folate and vitamin D deficiency; supplements of both should be given before pregnancy is attempted. Anticonvulsants should be withdrawn slowly if there have been no attacks for at least 3 years. Otherwise seizures should be controlled with the single most effective drug. Multiple drugs multiply the risk.

Diabetes. The abnormality rate among babies of diabetic mothers is up to five times higher than among those of non-diabetics; if the condition is poorly controlled, damage occurs to the fetus during organogenesis. Oral hypoglycaemic agents are contra-indicated in pregnancy and insulin is substituted before conception. Women are taught to use self-testing blood glucose kits and educated to achieve the best possible control before attempting to conceive. In severe cases they may be advised against pregnancy.

Genetic counselling

Some couples may seek advice because they or a close relative have already produced a child with some anomaly. If it was due to chance or environmental factors, the prospective parents can be reassured and given advice on how to ensure the best possible outcome for their pregnancy. If hereditary factors were involved they are referred to a geneticist who will take an exhaustive family history and carry out any appropriate investigations. The couple can then be advised about any likelihood of recurrence but they must make their own decision about whether or not to take the risk. It may be possible to offer prenatal diagnosis followed by termination of pregnancy if an anomaly is found. Some couples may opt to avoid pregnancy altogether.

After the birth of an abnormal baby

Any couple who have an abnormal baby should have the cause explained to them as accurately as may be ascertained. If their baby dies the thought of a postmortem is distressing to the parents but they should always be encouraged to give their consent. Determining the exact cause of death may give them peace of mind in the future, even if at the time they cannot imagine ever contemplating another pregnancy. It is the only way that disorders caused by genetic and environmental factors can be distinguished.

Genetically determined disorders

These may be:

- Chromosomal disorders
- Single gene disorders
  - recessive
  - dominant
  - X-linked
- Multifactorial disorders.

Chromosomal disorders

These are usually evident at birth (e.g. trisomies 21, 18 and 13), except in the case of those involving sex chromosomes (e.g. XO [Turner's syndrome], XXY [Klinefelter's syndrome]). Habitual abortion may be due to embryos having a severe chromosomal abnormality incompatible with life. Karyotyping of the parents should be carried out if there is a family history of such disorders, after the birth of an affected baby and in cases of habitual abortion. If one of the parents proves to have a translocated chromosome, it should be possible to predict the likelihood of recurrence.

Single gene disorders

Recessive conditions only occur if each chromosome of a pair carries the affected gene. The disorders are usually severe. In the UK the most common is cystic fibrosis; worldwide, the haemoglobinopathies occur most frequently. Inborn errors of metabolism such as phenylketonuria are also transmitted this way. If the partners are both carriers, their chances of conceiving an affected child are one in four for each pregnancy. The risk of both being carriers is increased in consanguineous marriages, which are common in some cultures.

Dominant conditions occur even if the affected gene is present on only one of a pair of chromosomes. Unless due to a new mutation, one parent will be affected. The disorders tend to be either mild or of late onset: achondroplasia and Huntington's chorea are examples. If a parent is affected there is a one-in-two chance of a child being affected.

X-linked conditions may be carried by girls but usually only appear in boys. Examples are haemophilia and Duchenne muscular dystrophy.

Research is proceeding into detection of single gene disorders but at present only a few can be diagnosed in carriers or prenatally and those only in specialised centres.

Multifactorial disorders

It appears that certain combinations of genes, exposed to certain environmental factors, can produce anomalies such as neural tube defects, cleft lip and palate and congenital heart disease. The risk is enhanced if one parent is affected and increases still further after the birth of an affected child.

PSYCHOSEXUAL COUNSELLING

There are few places where couples with psychosexual difficulties may easily find help. This, together with their understandable reticence about such distressing problems, means that the midwife should always be alert for hints that all is not well within a relationship. Sexual difficulties may be the real reason why a couple or individual asks for advice about preconception care or family planning. Problems grave enough to prevent conception are unusual but comparatively minor difficulties may result in considerable unhappiness. Parenthood brings many stresses of its own, so it is important for the long-term future that the couple's relationship is mutually satisfying before conception is attempted.

Sexual problems are usually caused by emotional factors which are not always consciously recognised. They may result from a traumatic experience in the past or arise from conflicts between particular partners. Untreated, they may manifest themselves in physical or mental illness.

Some difficulties can be alleviated simply by talking them through with an open, caring and accepting listener; others are more deep-seated and need to be referred to an experienced psychosexual counsellor. The aim of treatment is to enable individuals to recognise and overcome the inhibitions which prevent them from trusting and enjoying their own sexuality.

Vaginismus

Spasm of the pelvic floor muscles not only forms a physical barrier to intercourse but is also an emotional barrier to the deeper feelings. The woman may have concluded that she has a rigid hymen, that her vagina is too small or that the penis is too big. It is usually sufficient to demonstrate to her that the muscles are under her own control, describing her anatomy in simple terms and stressing the importance of relaxation and arousal before intercourse is attempted. She may take some time to become comfortable with her own body. Some women need to explore real fears about losing control either to another person or to their own sexual feelings.

'Frigidity'

This imprecise term has been used to cover a whole range of problems, from complete absence of sexual desire to failure to achieve orgasm. The woman may never have found sexual activity pleasurable or satisfying, or the problem may be a feature of a particular relationship, caused by lack of emotional commitment on either side or by poor communication between the partners which results in inadequate stimulation.

A previously responsive woman may lose interest after a stressful life event. It is not uncommon for this to happen following the birth of a baby. Dyspareunia resulting from a sutured perineum may be a factor, as may tiredness, fear of a further pregnancy and anger with the partner. A woman may find it difficult to combine being a mother with being a lover; she finds the baby so absorbing that any other relationship is an intrusion.

Failure to achieve orgasmic release may result in symptoms of mental or physical ill-health. Discussion of technique may help, encouraging the woman to discover what stimulation she needs and to communicate this to her partner. It could be necessary to explore why she is unwilling or unable to give way to her feelings. She may be afraid of emotional commitment or inhibited as a result of a strict upbringing or sexual abuse.

Impotence

It is rare for a man never to have been able to achieve and maintain an erection long enough for intromission to take place but secondary impotence, after previously satisfactory performance, is not unusual. There may be an organic cause, for example endocrine disorders such as diabetes, or it may be induced by alcohol, barbiturates or antihypertensives. Depression, stress and fatigue can all adversely affect sexual function. A man who experiences an episode of impotence may worry about it so much that he fails again. Impotence is sometimes situational, occurring in a particular relationship as a result of conflict or feelings of guilt, while performance elsewhere is unaffected.

Ejaculatory incompetence

Premature ejaculation is only occasionally severe enough to prevent conception but any degree will reduce the likelihood of both partners obtaining satisfaction. It may be learned behaviour from early hurried sexual experiences or an expression of conflicts within the relationship. Well-motivated men can be taught to postpone ejaculation and ensure that their partners reach orgasm; an understanding of the underlying problems could help the couple to achieve emotional as well as physical satisfaction.

A few men are unable to ejaculate intravaginally. This may be the equivalent of orgasmic dysfunction in the woman, an emotional defence mechanism, perhaps after discovery of the partner's infidelity, or it may be a subconscious refusal to become a father.

INFERTILITY

It has been argued that the biological urge to mate does not imply a desire to be a parent; nonetheless, involuntary childlessness can result in considerable distress.

The World Health Organization (WHO) (1988) has defined subfertility as the inability to achieve a pregnancy after 1 year of unprotected intercourse. According to this criterion, 20% of couples are subfertile, though this falls to 10%

after 18 months. The term infertile, strictly speaking, should not be used until it is proved that pregnancy is impossible.

More couples are choosing to start their families later in life but increasing age reduces fertility and the time available for childbearing. Couples over 35 years old should seek help if conception has not occurred within 6 months.

Infertility is said to be *primary* if no conception has ever occurred and *secondary* if there has been a pregnancy, whatever the outcome.

In approximately one-third of cases, male factors are responsible, in another third, female factors; in the remainder, a combination of factors is involved, for instance a low sperm count in association with defective ovulation. It is therefore vitally important that subfertility be investigated as a problem of the couple and not of one partner.

Preliminary investigations

Before any physical investigations are undertaken, time should be allowed for assessing the quality of the relationship and exploring the reasons behind the request for help. The couple are evidently anxious about their apparent infertility but must be encouraged to talk about whether they really want children and if they are both equally committed to that goal. There may be pressure from family or friends, an illusion that a baby would improve a deteriorating relationship, even a concern to obtain better housing. Some may be quite happy to remain childless once they know that they could have children if they wanted to.

It is important to establish whether intercourse is taking place and its frequency and timing. It is occasionally discovered that a relationship has not been consummated.

Infrequent intercourse may be due to lack of interest caused by low sexual appetite or excessive tiredness, or to lack of opportunity. One partner may work away from home for long periods or each may work different shifts. Whatever the reason, the chance of intercourse coinciding with the fertile phase is reduced. Conversely, if ejaculation occurs more than once every other day, sperm count is diminished.

The couple needs to understand the female cycle in order that intercourse may be timed to enhance the possibility of conception. Investigations and attempted treatments of subfertility are stressful and may disrupt the delicate hormonal balance necessary for successful conception. In addition, concentrating exclusively on the potentially fertile period puts great strain on a relationship and may result in the man becoming impotent. For these reasons the couple must be encouraged to maintain as much spontaneity as possible in their lovemaking.

General investigations

A full history is obtained from both partners, including occupation, in case it involves contact with industrial pollutants or radioactive materials. Any medical problems are referred to the appropriate specialist for investigation, treatment or stabilisation. Particular attention is paid to a history of sexually transmitted disease which may have resulted in obstruction of the fallopian or seminal tubes. In the man, orchitis secondary to mumps after puberty may be significant; in the woman, previous pelvic or abdominal surgery raises the possibility of adhesions.

The couple is asked about fertility to date. Each partner should be given the opportunity to elaborate on this individually, as the other may be unaware of a previous pregnancy.

Approximately 20% of women attending infertility clinics have ovulatory dysfunction. Regular menstruation suggests that ovulation is probably occurring; dysmenorrhoea and 'mittelschmerz' (transient mid-cycle pain in the iliac fossa) reinforce this assumption.

Primary amenorrhoea means that a woman has never menstruated; *secondary amenorrhoea* that periods have ceased. If periods are erratic or infrequent (*oligomenorrhoea*) then even if ovulation is occurring, it will be impossible to predict the date.

Both partners are given a complete medical examination which includes the genitalia. In the man this will disclose conditions such as varicocele and hydrocele which affect fertility and may possibly be treatable. In the woman, hirsutism and obesity may be suggestive of endocrine disorders. A bimanual and speculum examination will reveal any gross pelvic pathology and a cervical smear can be obtained.

Male infertility

Causes of male infertility

Defective spermatogenesis
Endocrine disorders
- Dysfunction of:
  - hypothalamus
  - pituitary
  - adrenals
  - thyroid.
- Systemic disease:
  - diabetes mellitus
  - coeliac disease
  - renal failure.
Testicular disorders
- Trauma
- Environmental (high temperature):
  - congenital (hydrocele, undescended testes)
  - occupational (furnaceman, long-distance lorry driver)
  - acquired (varicocele, tight clothing)
- Cancer treatment.

Defective transport
- Obstruction or absence of seminal ducts:
  - infection
  - congenital anomalies
  - trauma.
- Impaired secretions from prostate or seminal vesicles:
  - infection
  - metabolic disorders.

Ineffective delivery
- Psychosexual ⎫ problems (impotence,
- Drug-induced ⎭ ejaculatory dysfunction)
- Physical disability
- Physical anomalies:
  - hypospadias
  - epispadias
  - retrograde ejaculation (into bladder).

Specific investigations of male infertility and significance of findings

Semen analysis
This is the basic test for male infertility. It should be carried out before any further investigations on the couple. Average values are assessed on three samples produced over several weeks, as quality is variable. Specimens are produced by masturbation after 2–3 days' abstinence and examined in the laboratory within 1 hour. If satisfactory, the man is assumed to be potentially fertile.

Normal values (WHO 1988)
Volume: 2–6 ml
Total sperm count: more than 40×10^6 per ml
Motility: more than 60% of the sperm moving forward
Morphology: more than 60% of the sperm should appear normal on examination.

Agglutination of sperm in the semen specimen may be due to:

- *antisperm antibodies*, particularly if the man has had a vasectomy reversal or testicular trauma. Intrauterine insemination with the washed sperm may be successful.
- *infection*, viral or bacterial. If bacterial, it may respond to appropriate treatment.

Azoospermia (absence of spermatozoa in the semen) is usually untreatable but further investigations may give a clue to the cause.

Biopsy of the testes will show whether sperm are actually being produced. If they are, the problem is presumably one of defective transport.

Chromosome studies from blood or buccal smear may reveal Klinefelter's syndrome (XXY) which always results in sterility.

Oligospermia (oligoasthenoteratozoospermia) (total sperm count less than 20×10^6 per ml) may be improved by attention to diet and general health, particularly reducing smoking and alcohol intake. Reducing the ambient temperature of the testicles may encourage sperm development.

Blood tests for hormone levels may suggest possibilities for treatment. If estimation of gonadotrophin levels reveals reduced amounts of follicle-stimulating hormone (FSH), clomiphene therapy may stimulate the pituitary to produce more FSH to act on the testes. Treatment with testosterone appears to have little value. Abnormally high levels of prolactin may respond to bromocriptine.

Post-coital test

A specimen of aspirated cervical mucus from the female partner is examined, at the fertile time of the cycle, within 6 hours of intercourse. The ability of the sperm to penetrate the mucus can be observed, as can the quality of the mucus, and the test gives confirmation that effective intercourse is taking place.

Research into male factor infertility continues, but at present the prognosis is poor. Treatments such as in vitro fertilisation may succeed in circumventing the problem for some couples.

Specific investigations and treatment of female infertility

Ovulation disorders: Tests to establish whether ovulation is occurring:

Cervical mucus becomes clear, copious and stretchy at ovulation and shows a ferning pattern when dried on a glass slide.

Ovulation prediction kits can be purchased at the chemist's; a simple urine test measures luteinising hormone (LH) levels.

Basal body temperature (BBT) drops slightly before ovulation, then rises by about 0.3°C, remaining at the higher level for the rest of the cycle. This method is now considered cumbersome and inaccurate.

Ultrasound scanning can detect a ripening Graafian follicle (follicle tracking) and thickening of the endometrium.

Hormonal assays. A series of blood tests throughout the menstrual cycle should show fluctuations in circulating oestrogens and progesterone, FSH and LH. The results may suggest possibilities for treatment. Other endocrine disturbances, such as thyroid deficiency, and hyperprolactinaemia, should be excluded.

Female infertility

Causes of female infertility

Defective ovulation
Endocrine disorders
- Dysfunction of:
  — hypothalamus
  — pituitary
  — adrenals
  — thyroid.
- Systemic disease:
  — diabetes mellitus
  — coeliac disease
  — renal failure.

Physical disorders
- Obesity
- Anorexia nervosa or strict dieting
- Excessive exercise.

Ovarian disorders
- Hormonal
- Ovarian cysts or tumours
- Polycystic ovary disease
- Ovarian endometriosis.

Defective transport
Ovum
- Tubal obstruction:
  — infection (gonorrhoea, peritonitis, pelvic inflammatory disease)
  — previous tubal surgery.
- Fimbrial adhesions:
  — previous surgery
  — endometriosis.

Sperm
- Vagina:
  — psychosexual problems (vaginismus)
  — infection (causing dyspareunia)
  — congenital anomaly.
- Cervix:
  — cervical trauma or surgery (cone biopsy)
  — infection
  — hormonal (hostile mucus)
  — anti-sperm antibodies in mucus.

Defective implantation
- Hormonal imbalance
- Congenital anomalies
- Fibroids
- Infection.

Stimulation of ovulation

Clomiphene citrate (Clomid) stimulates the hypothalamic-pituitary system permitting FSH production and so inducing ovulation. 50 mg daily are taken in tablet form for 5 days starting within 5 days of the onset of menstruation. Ovulation should occur around day 12–16, and intercourse can be advised on alternate days from days 10–18. Dosage can be increased up to a maximum of 150 mg. Long-term treatment appears to have few benefits.

Human chorionic gonadotrophin (HCG) is identical in action to LH and can be used to trigger ovulation, often in conjunction with clomiphene or some other form of ovulation induction. Intercourse should be advised around the time of administration.

Human menopausal gonadotrophin (HMG) (Pergonal) or pure FSH (Metrodin) may be used if clomiphene has failed or in cases of polycystic ovary disease. It is administered daily by injection from the onset of menstruation until a mature follicle is detected; HCG is then given. Hyperstimulation of the ovaries is a risk. Multiple ovulation can be disastrous if natural conception is intended, though it is necessary for procedures such as in vitro fertilisation (IVF) for which this regime is also used.

Bromocriptine (Parlodel) is used to inhibit synthesis and release of prolactin by the pituitary. Hyperprolactinaemia may result in low oestrogen and progesterone levels and prevent ovulation. It may be caused by stress or the use of drugs such as tranquillisers.

Ovarian disorders may be discovered at laparoscopy. Cysts or tumours may be removed surgically. Endometriosis may be discovered and can be treated by short-term suppression of ovulation with progestogens.

Ovum transport: Investigation of tubal patency

Laparoscopy is carried out under general anaesthetic. Watery dye passed through the cervix can be observed to drip out of the ends of the fallopian tubes if they are patent. Additional information can be obtained such as whether the tubes are mobile and free from adhesions and whether there is evidence of pelvic inflammatory disease or endometriosis. The ovaries are examined for abnormalities and evidence of corpora lutea.

Hysterosalpingography is performed during the first 10 days of the menstrual cycle to avoid possible irradiation of an early pregnancy. Radio-opaque dye is injected through the cervix; an X-ray will reveal whether the tubes are patent and also the shape of the uterine cavity. The procedure can be painful if there is an obstruction, due to build-up of pressure inside the tubes. There is also a risk of chemical or allergic reaction to the dye.

The prognosis for treatment of tubal obstruction is poor. There has been some improvement with the development of microsurgical techniques and argon laser surgery, but even if the damage is repaired there remains a risk of ectopic pregnancy. Increasingly, in vitro fertilisation (IVF), which has the effect of bypassing the blocked fallopian tubes, is being recommended to women with tubal obstruction.

Sperm transport

Psychosexual counselling, antibiotics, surgery or laser treatment are offered as appropriate.

Cervical mucus normally changes from a viscid plug to a copious clear fluid under the influence of progesterone at ovulation in order to facilitate the passage of sperm.

The postcoital test has already been described under investigations for male infertility.

The sperm penetration test demonstrates the behaviour of sperm alongside a sample of mucus taken at the fertile time, on a glass slide. It determines whether sperm function or mucus hostility is the problem.

Crossed hostility tests observe the behaviour of the partner's sperm and fresh donor sperm in the woman's cervical mucus.

If the mucus is hostile, or the woman is producing antisperm antibodies to her partner's sperm, intra-uterine insemination may be successful.

ARTIFICIAL REPRODUCTION

Artificial insemination by husband (AIH)

Indications

- Cervical problems (see above).
- Mechanical problems
  — psychosexual
  — spinal injury
  — other physical disability.
- Antisperm antibodies in the man.
- Mild oligospermia with satisfactory motility.
- Semen stored before commencement of chemo- or radiotherapy.

Procedure

Intra-uterine insemination is mostly used in order to enhance the likelihood of success. There should be no tubal pathology and the woman should be ovulating normally, though mild superovulation may be induced. The sperm are separated from the remainder of the ejaculate in the laboratory and, in 0.2 ml of media solution, are flushed into the uterus via the cervix by means of a fine catheter.

Artificial insemination by donor (AID/DI)

Indications

- Azoospermia or oligospermia in male partner.
- Excessive non-motile and/or abnormal sperm.
- Risk of transmission of a hereditary disease.
- Rhesus iso-immunisation; a Rhesus negative donor may be used.
- Lack of a male partner.

Procedure

A vaginal speculum and syringe are used to bathe the cervix in semen. The woman may be asked to lie still for a few minutes afterwards. It is usually carried out 2–3 days before ovulation and may be repeated a couple of days later. Success rates are comparable to those for normal conception.

Donors are carefully selected. They must be of normal intelligence, fit and healthy, with no personal or family history of disease. Each donation is analysed to ensure satisfactory quality. Tests for sexually transmitted diseases, including human immunodeficiency virus (HIV), are repeated at every visit, and the semen is frozen and stored for at least 3 months before use to be sure that tests were negative. Donors are matched as far as possible to the male partner; skin, hair and eye colouring, height and build, and blood group.

Whether the child is told of his origins is for the parents to decide. If they are encouraged to make love around the time of insemination, there will be a possibility, however remote, that the child's social father will be the genetic father.

Some religious groups oppose DI on the grounds that it profanes the sanctity of marriage. Concern has also been expressed at its use by single women, lesbians and virgins who want a child without being involved with a man.

- All clinics offering DI must be licensed by the Human Fertilisation and Embryology Authority.
- If a man consents to his partner receiving DI, he is legally the father of the child.
- The donor is not considered to be the father of the child.
- The Authority will keep a register of donors and resulting births, in order to limit paternities to 10.

People born as a result of DI will be able to obtain information about their origins, and also whether they are related to an intended partner. Whether this will allow the donor to be identified is not yet clear; nor are the implications for recruitment of donors if confidentiality can no longer be guaranteed.

In vitro fertilisation/embryo transfer (IVF/ET)

Indications

- Tubal damage.
- Oligospermia, poor motility, anti-sperm antibodies.
- Cervical problems.

- Endometriosis.
- 'Unexplained' infertility.

Procedure

Stage 1: Ovulation induction is performed using drugs to stimulate multiple ovulation. Progress is monitored by ultrasound follicle tracking and serum oestradiol levels.

Stage 2: Ovum recovery is planned when four or more follicles reach 20 mm in size. The ova are harvested using vaginal ultrasound guidance under local anaesthetic or laparoscopy under general anaesthetic. Ova and semen are treated separately before being brought together outside the body.

Stage 3: Embryo transfer is performed 2–3 days later when the zygotes have reached the 4- or 8-cell stage. A maximum of three embryos are placed in the uterus via the cervix to increase the chances of success but reduce the risk of higher multiple pregnancy. Any healthy surplus embryos may be frozen for further attempts if necessary.

Gamete intra-fallopian transfer (GIFT)

This may be attempted if there are cervical barriers to conception. At least one fallopian tube must be patent and sperm quality must be good. Ova are harvested as for IVF, aspirated into a catheter with the prepared fresh sperm, and placed in the distal end of the fallopian tube. Fertilisation should then occur in vivo. The procedure is not covered by the new legislation, so a licence is not required in order to offer it, unless donated gametes are used, and there is no restriction on the number of ova which may be transferred.

Zygote intra-fallopian transfer (ZIFT)

Ova are fertilised in vitro, and the embryos are then introduced into the fallopian tube.

Ovum donation

This is the equivalent of DI for the fertile man whose partner is not ovulating but could carry a pregnancy. Most donations are from women undergoing IVF treatment; ova are fertilised in vitro by sperm from the recipient's partner and placed in the recipient's uterus. Timing is crucial, so either the two women's cycles will be synchronised artificially or the embryos may be frozen before use.

The law regarding ovum donation is the same as that for sperm. All potential donors must be offered counselling about the implications, such as their feelings about the potential child, and the possibility of their own childlessness.

Surrogacy

This is the practice whereby one woman carries a child for another with the intention of handing the baby over at birth. It may be seen as the ultimate act of generosity by one woman to another less fortunate than herself, and has probably been going on since time immemorial. However, it arouses considerable public anxiety and following recommendations by the Warnock report (1984) the Surrogacy Arrangements Act became law in 1985. This has since been amended by the Human Fertilisation and Embryology Act 1990.

Surrogacy is legal in the UK as long as no money changes hands (apart from reasonable expenses), but the arrangement is not enforceable in law. The carrying mother is always the legal mother of the child at birth. The commissioning parents, if over 18 years old and married to each other, may apply within 6 months of the birth for a court order making them the legal parents, providing the child was conceived within the law using the gametes of one or both of them and is living with the applicants at the time. The carrying mother cannot agree to the order until 6 weeks after the birth. Both parties are free to change their minds at any time during the pregnancy or until the court order has been made.

Issues raised by artificial reproduction

The birth of the first 'test-tube baby' in July 1978 opened up new possibilities not only in the alleviation of infertility but also for scientific developments. The earliest stages of human development could be observed, raising hopes of detecting and remedying defects along with anxieties about possible experimentation and manipulation.

The Warnock Report (Report of the Committee of Enquiry into Human Fertilisation and Embryology 1984) was commissioned in response to public concern. It made an urgent recommendation for the establishment of a statutory licensing authority to regulate research and infertility services. A Voluntary Licensing Authority was set up by the Medical Research Council and the Royal College of Obstetricians and Gynaecologists; the Human Fertilisation and Embryology Act became statute in 1990.

The Human Fertilisation and Embryology Authority (HFEA) was established by the Act 'to regulate, by means of a licensing system, any research or treatment which involves the creation, keeping and using of human embryos outside the body, or the storage or donation of human eggs and sperm. It must also maintain a Code of Practice giving guidance about the proper conduct of the licenced activities.' (HFEA Code of Practice Consultation Document 1991.)

The legal implications of the reproductive technologies are now somewhat clearer, but the debate surrounding the introduction of the Act raised many practical and ethical issues which remain controversial. For the couple whose infertility is circumvented by assisted reproduction and who achieve a healthy baby, the benefits are clear, but the techniques are very expensive, and success is limited. Writing about IVF/ET, Wagner & St Clair (1989) argue that 'No new technique should become standard until after rigorous evaluation. Until then, it must remain experimental, guided by the principles covering research on human subjects. Evaluation involves assessment of efficacy, safety and costs. . . . IVF/ET and related assisted reproduction technologies have not been scrutinised in this way.' The available evidence is examined regarding the low success rate, the high perinatal mortality and morbidity, the risks to the women, and the financial, psychological and social costs. The authors call for randomised controlled trials to establish the efficacy of treatments, and follow-up studies of the long-term effects. 'With this information, infertile couples can make the best informed choice about their care and countries can make the best informed choice about the appropriate place of IVF/ET in their infertility services.'

Evidently the debate is far from over.

Reader Activities

Identify the health services available to well women of childbearing age in your local community. Talk to staff and users of the services. You might consider health centres, general practitioner surgeries, chemist's shops, occupational health departments, family planning and well-woman clinics, psychosexual counselling and genetic counselling services.

- How accessible are these services (location, hours of opening, 'user-friendliness', ease of referral)?
- Do they make a positive contribution towards encouraging optimum health before conception?
- What provision is there in local schools to educate young people about planning for a healthy pregnancy?
- What services are available for couples concerned about their fertility? What is the pattern of referral for specialist investigation and treatment? How much is available on the National Health Service? What costs might be involved if private treatment is required? How is the money found?

Acknowledgement

The author is grateful to Miss Janice Kerr RGN RM, Clinical Nurse Specialist, Infertility at Birmingham Maternity Hospital, for material submitted for inclusion in this chapter.

Useful addresses

Association to Aid Sexual and Personal Relationships of People with a Disability (SPOD)
286 Camden Road
London N7 OBJ
Tel: 071 607 8851

Birthright
27 Sussex Place
Regent's Park
London NW1 4SP
Tel: 071 262 5337

British Agencies for Adoption and Fostering
11 Southwark Street
London SE1 1RQ
Tel: 071 407 8800

British Diabetic Association
10 Queen Anne Street
London W1M 0BD
Tel: 071 323 1531

British Pregnancy Advisory Service (BPAS)
Austy Manor
Wootton Wawen
Solihull
West Midlands B95 6BX
Tel: 0564 793225

Brook Advisory Centre
153a East Street
London SE17 2SD
Tel: 071 708 1234

CHILD (Infertility, Research, Education, Counselling)
PO Box 154
Hounslow
Middlesex TW3 0EZ
Tel: 081 893 7110

Endometriosis Society
35 Belgrave Square
London SWIX 8QB
Tel: 071 235 4137

Feminist International Network of Resistance to Reproductive and Genetic Engineering (FINRRAGE)
FINRRAGE (Britain)
Box 38
LOP 52 Call Lane
Leeds LS1 6DT
Tel: 0532 681109

Foresight
28 The Paddock
Godalming
Surrey GU7 1XD
Tel: 0483 427839

Genetic Nurses and Social Workers Association
c/o Department of Clinical Genetics

Addenbrookes Hospital
Hills Lane
Cambridge CB2 2QQ
Tel: 0223 216446

ISSUE
St George's Rectory
Tower Street
Birmingham B19 3UY
Tel: 021 359 4887

Pregnancy Advisory Service
11–13 Charlotte Street
London W1P 1HD
Tel: 071 637 8962

Progress
27–35 Mortimer Street
London W1N 7RJ
Tel: 071 436 4528

Women's Health and Reproductive Rights Information Centre (WHRRIC)
52–54 Featherstone Street
London EC1Y 8RT
Tel: 071 251 6580

REFERENCES

Human Fertilisation and Embryology Authority 1991 Code of practice consultation document. HFEA, London

Lumley J, Astbury J 1989 Advice for pregnancy. In: Chalmers I, Enkin M, Keirse M J N C (eds) Effective care in pregnancy and childbirth. Oxford University Press, Oxford, Vol 1, ch 16, p 239

Wagner M G, St Clair P A 1989 Are in-vitro fertilisation and embryo transfer of benefit to all? Lancet 2 (October 28): 1027–1030

World Health Organization 1988 Laboratory recommendations. WHO, Geneva

FURTHER READING

Breen D 1975 The birth of a first child: towards an understanding of femininity. Tavistock Publications, London

Chamberlain G, Lumley J (eds) 1986 Prepregnancy care: a manual for practice. John Wiley, Chichester

Committee of enquiry into human fertilisation and embryology: report, 1984 (Cmnd 9314) (Warnock Report) HMSO, London

Draper K (ed) 1983 Practice of psychosexual medicine. John Libbey, London

Fletcher A C 1985 Reproductive hazards of work. ASTMS/EOC. Equal Opportunities Commission, Manchester

Foresight: The association for the promotion of pre-conceptual care Environmental factors and foetal health — the case for pre-conceptual care; also Guidelines for future parents. Foresight, 28 The Paddock, Godalming, Surrey GU7 1XD

Masters W H, Johnson V E 1980 Human sexual response. Bantam Books, London

Morgan D, Lee R G 1991 Blackstone's guide to the Human Fertilisation and Embryology Act 1990. Blackstone Press, London

Oakley A 1980 Women confined: towards a sociology of childbirth. Martin Robertson, Oxford

Pepperell R J, Hudson B, Wood C (eds) 1980 The infertile couple. Churchill Livingstone, Edinburgh

Pfeffer N, Woollett A 1983 The experience of infertility. Virago Press, London

Snowden R, Mitchell G D, Snowden E M 1983 Artificial reproduction: a social investigation. Allen and Unwin, London

Spallone P 1989 Beyond conception: the new politics of reproduction. Macmillan, London

Tunnadine P 1983 The making of love. Cape, London

Wynn M, Wynn A 1981 The prevention of handicap of early pregnancy origin. Some evidence for the value of good health before conception. Foundation for Education and Research in Childbearing, London

Psychological and physiological changes of pregnancy

VALERIE THOMSON

All changes in a mother's body during pregnancy are due to the effects of specific hormones. These changes enable her to nurture the fetus, prepare her body for labour, develop her breasts and lay down stores of fat to provide calories for production of breast milk during the puerperium. By understanding the normal changes the midwife can detect abnormality.

The woman's psychological state is also affected by hormonal changes. These changes interact with other external factors and influence her transition to motherhood.

It is important to discuss the physical changes that occur so that the midwife may appreciate the psychological effect that they may have on the pregnant woman.

PHYSIOLOGICAL CHANGES IN THE REPRODUCTIVE SYSTEM

The body of the uterus

After conception the uterus develops to provide a nutritive and protective environment in which the fetus will develop and grow.

Decidua

The decidua is the name given to the endometrium during pregnancy.

Progesterone and oestrogen initially produced by the corpus luteum cause the decidua to become thicker, richer and more vascular at the fundus and in the upper body of the uterus. These areas are the usual sites of implantation; the decidua is thinner and less vascular in the lower pole of the uterus. The decidua provides a glycogen-rich environment for the blastocyst until the trophoblastic cells begin to form the placenta (see Ch. 4). Once the placenta has formed, it is able to produce its own hormones and the corpus luteum is no longer maintained by human chorionic gonadotrophin. The corpus luteum then atrophies and becomes the corpus albicans.

Myometrium

Oestrogen is responsible for the growth of uterine muscle. Increase in the size of the muscle fibres is known as *hypertrophy* and the increase in their number is referred to as *hyperplasia*. The uterus continues to grow in this way for the first 20 weeks; after this time it stretches to accommodate its contents.

Increase in weight. From 60 g to 900 g

Increase in size. From 7.5 × 5 × 2.5 cm to 30 × 23 × 20 cm.

The uterus is able to stretch in this way because progesterone encourages relaxation of smooth muscle but even at 8 weeks' gestation the uterus begins to generate small waves of contraction known as *Braxton-Hicks contractions*. These are usually painless although some women do experience pain. Braxton-Hicks contractions last approximately 60 seconds, continue throughout pregnancy and later change in intensity eventually to become the contractions of labour (see Ch. 11).

During pregnancy the muscle layers become more differentiated and organised for their part in expelling the fetus at term (Fig. 8.1).

Muscle layers. The inner circular layer surrounds the cornua, lower uterine segment and cervix. This circular layer is involved in stretching of the lower segment and cervix during labour. The middle oblique layer is involved in the contraction necessary to expel the fetus at the end of pregnancy. This action is also necessary to entrap and enmesh bleeding vessels and ligate them after the placenta is delivered (see Ch. 20).

The outer longitudinal layer muscle fibres contract and retract during labour causing the upper segment to thicken. The thickened upper segment acts as a piston to force the fetus into the receptive, passive lower segment (see Ch. 11).

The perimetrium

This is a layer of peritoneum. It does not totally cover the uterus, being deflected over the bladder anteriorly to form the uterovesical pouch and over the rectum posteriorly to form the pouch of Douglas (see Ch. 2).

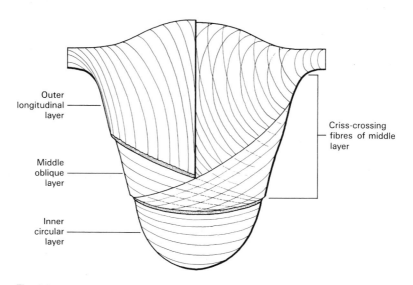

Outer longitudinal layer

Middle oblique layer

Inner circular layer

Criss-crossing fibres of middle layer

Fig. 8.1
Diagrammatic representation of differentiated muscle layers of the uterus in pregnancy.

This arrangement allows for the unrestricted growth of the uterus.

Blood supply

The blood supply to the uterus must increase to keep pace with its growth and also to meet the needs of the functioning placenta.

Oestrogen causes development of new blood vessels. Initially they form a tortuous network through the uterine walls but as the uterus grows and stretches they become straightened, becoming convoluted again in the third stage of labour.

Changes in uterine shape

Healthy growth of the fetus requires adequate space.

After conception the embedded blastocyst demands little space but the upper part of the uterus begins to enlarge due to the effects of oestrogen. The uterus changes to a globular shape in early pregnancy to anticipate fetal growth and also to accommodate increasing amounts of liquor and placental tissue (Fig. 8.2). This causes pressure on other pelvic organs.

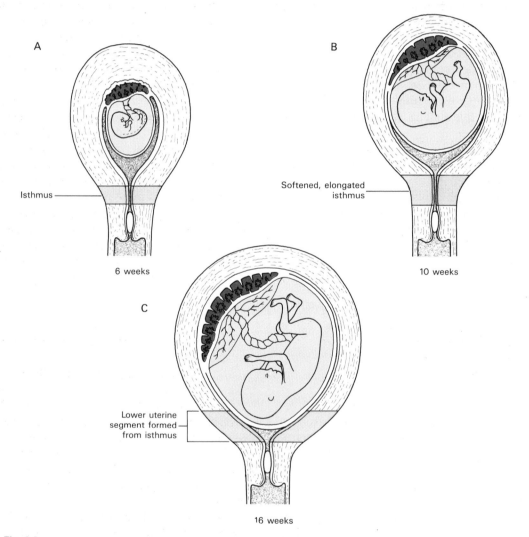

Fig. 8.2
Changes in the uterus between 6 and 16 weeks (not to scale) (A) isthmus 7 mm long, uterine shape ovoid, embryonic sac in upper pole (B) isthmus long and soft, uterus globular, fetal sac in upper pole (C) isthmus open to form lower segment, fetal sac occupies both poles.

The lower part of the uterus consisting of the isthmus, softens and elongates from its original 7 mm until 10 weeks of pregnancy when it measures 25 mm, giving the appearance of a stalk below the globular upper segment. This is the beginning of the differentiation between the upper and lower parts of the uterus which is not completed until the later weeks of pregnancy.

12th week of pregnancy

The uterus is no longer anteverted and anteflexed. It has risen out of the pelvis and become upright although often it inclines and rotates to the right. This is thought to be due to the pressure of the pelvic colon which occupies space in the left part of the pelvis. Further uterine inclination to the right occurs as the pregnancy progresses. This is known as *right obliquity of the uterus.*

The conceptus grows to encroach upon the lower pole of the uterus. The uterus becomes more globular in shape as the isthmus opens out. This area will later become the lower segment and measure approximately one-third of the body of the uterus at term.

At 12 weeks the fundus of the uterus may be palpated abdominally above the symphysis pubis.

20th week

Now restored to its original pear shape, the uterus has a thicker, more rounded fundus. The fallopian tubes appear to issue from a lower level. As the uterus continues to rise in the abdomen the fallopian tubes, being restricted by attachment to the broad ligaments, become progressively more vertical.

30th week

The lower uterine segment can be identified. It is still not complete but can be defined as that portion lying below the reflection of the vesicouterine fold of peritoneum and above the internal os of the cervix.

36th week

The uterus now reaches the level of the xiphisternum. The softening of the tissues of the pelvic floor together with good uterine tone and the formation of the lower uterine segment encourages the fetus to sink into the lower pole of the uterus. This is described as *lightening.* In the primigravida this also encourages the beginning of a gradual descent into the pelvis and the fetal head becomes engaged. In the multiparous woman descent often does not occur until labour aids the process.

The cervix

The cervix acts as an effective barrier against infection; it also retains the pregnancy.

Under the influence of progesterone, endocervical cells secrete mucus which beomes thicker and more viscous during pregnancy. The thickened mucus forms a cervical plug called the *operculum* which provides protection from ascending infection.

The cervix remains 2.5 cm long throughout pregnancy, but the hygroscopic properties of oestrogen cause it to increase in width. This exposes endocervical cells which can give an appearance of erosion. Oestrogen increases cervical vascularity and if viewed through a speculum the cervix looks purple.

In late pregnancy softening of the cervix occurs in response to increasing painless contractions. Prostaglandins released from local tissue are also thought to play a part in cervical softening in readiness for the onset of labour.

The vagina

Oestrogen causes changes in the muscle layer and the epithelium.

The muscle layer hypertrophies. There are also changes in the surrounding connective tissue which allow the vagina to become more elastic. These changes enable it to dilate during the second stage of labour and receive the descending fetal head.

The epithelium has a marked desquamation of the superficial cells which increases the amount of normal white vaginal discharge called *leucorrhoea.*

The epithelial cells also have an increased glycogen content. These cells interact with *Döderlein's bacillus,* a normal commensal of the vagina, and produce a more acid environment. This provides an extra degree of protection against some organisms, but unfortunately an increasing susceptibility to others such as *Candida albicans*.

The vagina is more vascular, appearing reddish-purple in colour.

CHANGES IN THE CARDIOVASCULAR SYSTEM

The heart
Due to an increase in workload the heart may increase in size. It may also be displaced upwards and to the left, rotating anteriorly because of the increasing pressure from the growing uterus.

The cardiac output increases from 5 to 7 litres per minute by late pregnancy. This is effected by:

- increase in resting heart rate of about 15 bpm by the end of pregnancy
- increase in blood volume (see below).

The blood volume
The red cell mass, which is defined as the total volume of red cells in the circulation, increases in response to the extra oxygen requirements made by maternal and placental tissue. There appears to be a constant increase during the pregnancy which results in a total increase of 18% by the end of pregnancy.

The total amount of haemoglobin increases during pregnancy although the mean cell haemoglobin is slightly lower.

Plasma volume increases from the 10th week of pregnancy, reaches its maximum level of approximately 50% above non-pregnant values by the 32nd–34th week and maintains this until term.

A higher circulating volume is required:

- to provide extra blood flow for placental perfusion at the choriodecidual interface
- to counterbalance the effects of increased arterial and venous capacity.

A normal increase in circulating plasma volume is correlated with fetal well-being and good outcome to the pregnancy.

Table 8.1
Summary of changes caused by increased plasma volume

Haemodilution	Increased cardiac output
Physiological anaemia	Heart enlarges
Decrease in concentration of plasma protein	Stroke volume increases
Decrease in concentration of immunoglobulins	

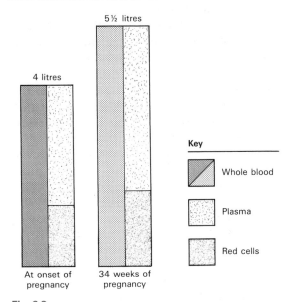

Fig. 8.3
Changes in the blood during pregnancy.
Red cell mass increases steadily throughout; plasma volume peaks at about 34 weeks.

As the plasma increase is much greater than that of the red cell mass there is a haemodilution effect. This is characterised by lowered haemoglobin (Hb) level, haematocrit and red cell count. It occurs in spite of the rise in total circulating haemoglobin. The effect is referred to as *physiological anaemia*. The haemodilution effect is most apparent at 32–34 weeks' gestation (Fig. 8.3).

Most obstetricians would agree that the mean minimum acceptable Hb level in pregnancy is 11–12 g/dl blood.

Iron metabolism
Iron is mobilised from body stores for use by the mother to maintain her circulating haemoglobin level and to supply the fetus.

The fetal need for iron is greatest in the last 4 weeks of pregnancy. Iron absorption from the gut is therefore enhanced in the latter part of pregnancy.

Plasma protein

Plasma proteins increase during pregnancy but the haemodilution effect causes a fall in concentration, particularly of the albumen component. This leads to a decrease in osmotic pressure. In the absence of disease the resultant moderate oedema is seen as physiological and an indicator of a favourable outcome to pregnancy.

Clotting factors

Fibrinogen, factor 7, factor 10, and *platelets* are all increased leading to a change in coagulation time from 12 to 8 minutes. Capacity for clotting is increased, with a resultant higher risk of thrombosis, embolism and, when complications are present, disseminated intravascular coagulation.

White blood cells

Levels in pregnancy are slightly increased reaching levels of $10.0–15.0 \times 10^9/1$. The main change involves an increase in neutrophils which enhances the blood's phagocytic and bactericidal properties: viral resistance is unchanged. Levels of immunoglobulins IgA, IgG and IgM decrease, probably due to the effects of haemodilution and suppression of the immune system (see Ch. 34).

Effects on the blood pressure

The increased cardiac output is balanced by reduced peripheral resistance. Arterial walls relax and dilate as progesterone acts on the smooth muscle. The capacity of veins and venules can increase by a litre.

Blood pressure remains the same or drops slightly in the first trimester, reaches its lowest level in midtrimester, and towards term will return to the level of the first trimester.

During the midtrimester changes in blood pressure may cause fainting. In later pregnancy women should avoid the unsupported supine position as it can cause profound hypotension. The pressure of the gravid uterus compresses the vena cava reducing venous return. Cardiac output is reduced which gives rise to feelings of faintness and paraesthesia of the fingers. Maternal shock ensues which will precipitate fetal heart rate changes.

Blood flow

The majority of increased blood flow is directed to the uterus and, of that, 80% goes to the placenta. In uterine systole the blood is forced into the choriodecidual space and spurts over the chorionic plate allowing exchange of gases, providing nutrition and excretion of waste products from the fetus. Blood flow to the kidney is increased by 30–50%, enhancing excretion. Increased flow to the skin is thought to eliminate extra heat generated by fetal metabolism.

CHANGES IN THE RESPIRATORY SYSTEM

These are necessary in order to maximise maternal oxygen intake and provide efficient carbon dioxide excretion for the mother and through her for the fetus.

In later pregnancy the ribs flare out maintaining the capacity of the thoracic cavity by counteracting the effects of the enlarging uterus which presses upon the diaphragm.

Respiration is made more efficient by:

- progesterone acting on the respiratory centre in the hypothalamus, reducing the threshold for pCO_2 from 5.2 kPa to 4.2 kPa. This is thought to enhance the excretion of CO_2 from the fetus.
- deeper breathing, caused by reduced pCO_2. This increases the oxygen tension from 11.7 kPa to 13.8 kPa.
- decreased residual volume. This means that during respiration there is increased alveolar expansion which enhances gaseous exchange. The tidal volume increases by approximately 40%.

The respiratory rate does not alter but the amount of air exhaled per minute increases from 7 to 11 litres.

Pregnant women often become conscious of a need to breathe. This may be caused by the changes described above.

Nasal congestion occurs during pregnancy and is caused by increased vascularity. Nose bleeds are common.

CHANGES IN THE GASTRO-INTESTINAL SYSTEM

Oestrogen exerts its hygroscopic effect on the gums, which makes them spongy and leads to bleeding during pregnancy. Dental problems occur because of gingivitis rather than from dental caries.

Increased salivation, *ptyalism*, is common. Women often experience changes in their sense of taste, leading to dietary changes and food cravings. Craving for unnatural substances such as coal is termed *pica*.

Effects on digestion

Progesterone relaxes smooth muscle; this has a major influence on the gut. Gastric emptying and peristalsis are slowed in order to maximise the absorption of nutrients. Undesirable effects also result from slow emptying of the stomach and reduced stomach acidity. Heartburn is common and is associated with gastric reflux due to the relaxation of the cardiac sphincter. Constipation is a result of sluggish gut motility. It can exacerbate haemorrhoids which may exist as a result of the relaxing effect of progesterone's action on the smooth muscle of the vein wall.

Nausea and vomiting occur mainly during early pregnancy, possibly due to raised oestrogen or human chorionic gonadotrophin (HCG) levels. In circumstances where hormone levels are further raised, such as multiple pregnancy or hydatidiform mole, vomiting may be excessive.

SKIN CHANGES

Increased activity of the melanin-stimulating hormone causes deeper pigmentation during pregnancy. Women tan more readily. Some develop deeper, patchy colouring on the face which resembles a mask and is known as *chloasma*. Many notice a pigmented line running from the pubis to the umbilicus, and sometimes higher, called the *linea nigra*.

The nipple area is also involved. The deposition of melanin toughens the area in preparation for breast feeding. The perineum darkens in order to enable it to stretch during the birth of the baby.

As maternal size increases, stretching occurs in the collagen layer of the skin particularly over the breasts, abdomen and areas of fat deposition such as the thighs. In some women the areas of maximum stretch become thin and stretch marks, *striae gravidarum*, appear as red stripes during the pregnancy, changing to silvery white lines approximately 6 months after delivery. Stretch marks are also considered to be related to the increase in corticosteroids during pregnancy.

The increased blood supply to the skin leads to sweating. Women often feel hotter in pregnancy. This may be caused by a progesterone-induced rise in temperature of $0.5°C$ together with vasodilatation.

SKELETAL CHANGES

Progesterone and relaxin encourage relaxation of ligaments and muscles, reaching maximum effect during the last weeks of pregnancy. This relaxation allows the pelvis to increase its capacity in readiness to accommodate the fetal presenting part at the end of pregnancy and in labour.

The symphysis pubis softens as do the sacro-iliac joints; the sacrococcygeal joint loosens, allowing the coccyx to be displaced backwards. Unstable pelvic joints result in the rolling gait sometimes seen in pregnant women. In the multigravid woman this is likely to be the cause of backache and ligamental pain.

Posture may alter to compensate for a change in the centre of gravity, particularly if abdominal muscle tone is poor. The gravid uterus pulls the body forward, the woman leans backwards in order to balance and she exaggerates the normal lumbar curve. Chapter 40 gives advice on correct posture.

MATERNAL WEIGHT

Continuing weight increase in pregnancy is considered to be one favourable indicator of maternal adaptation and fetal growth.

Expected increase:

2.0 kg in first 20 weeks
0.5 kg per week until term
12.0 kg approximate total.

Many factors influence weight gain. The degree of maternal oedema, maternal metabolic rate, dietary intake, vomiting or diarrhoea, smoking, amount of amniotic fluid and size of the fetus must all be taken into account. See Figure 8.4 for the distribution of normal increased weight.

CHANGES IN THE ENDOCRINE SYSTEM

Placental hormones
Early effects due to placental hormones are described in Chapter 4. Later effects caused by oestrogen and progesterone have been highlighted throughout the current chapter.

The fetus is dependent on glucose for body and brain growth. In order to ensure that glucose is readily available to the fetus *human placental lactogen* alters maternal metabolism in the following ways:

- The maternal energy needs are met by mobilising free fatty acids. Energy is also conserved by progesterone, reducing muscle tone.
- More insulin is produced centrally but its action is blocked leading to a decreased insulin sensitivity and in consequence a higher circulating blood glucose.

Pituitary hormones
The anterior pituitary gland is enlarged. Adrenocorticotrophic hormone, melanocyte-stimulating hormone and thyrotrophic hormone increase their activities.

Follicle-stimulating hormone and luteinising hormone secretion are inhibited by progesterone and oestrogen. Prolactin secretion increases but is held in abeyance by oestrogen.

The posterior pituitary gland is stimulated to produce increasing amounts of oxytocin during pregnancy although this hormone is not totally effective until the balance between oestrogen and progesterone changes, at a critical point before the onset of labour.

Thyroid function
In normal pregnancy there is a reduced level of plasma iodine, although thyroid activity is not markedly increased. Recent evidence (Rodin et al 1989) suggests that in the absence of iodine deficiency the development of a goitre is unlikely. Raised oestrogen levels in pregnancy cause the liver to produce more thyroxine-binding globulin. As a result T_4 (thyroxine) is mainly bound rather than free in the plasma. A feedback mechanism prompts the thyroid to return the level of free thyroxine to normal (Fig. 8.5). This profile should not be interpreted as hyperthyroidism.

Rising progesterone levels increase the maternal metabolism but also allow fat deposition.

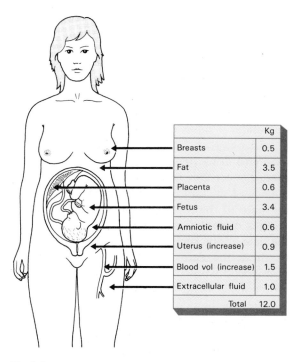

	Kg
Breasts	0.5
Fat	3.5
Placenta	0.6
Fetus	3.4
Amniotic fluid	0.6
Uterus (increase)	0.9
Blood vol (increase)	1.5
Extracellular fluid	1.0
Total	12.0

Fig. 8.4
Disposition of weight gain in pregnancy.

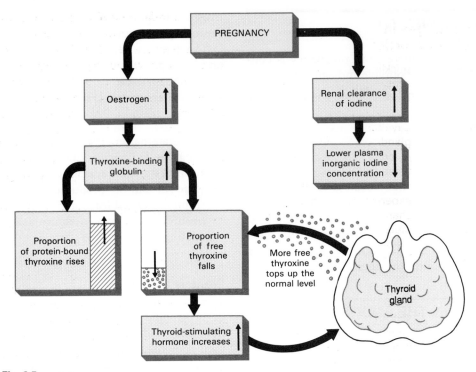

Fig. 8.5
Thyroid function in pregnancy.

The basal metabolic rate is increased in pregnancy due to increased oxygen consumption by the fetus.

Adrenal glands

Corticosteroid production is increased and may be one of the reasons for glycosuria in pregnancy. It is also suggested that hypertension and striae gravidarum are caused by increased secretion.

Excretion of sodium and chloride is increased in the presence of progesterone. Aldosterone, produced in response to the renin–angiotensin mechanism which enhances the reabsorption of sodium, maintains the delicate balance (see Ch. 6).

THE BREASTS

All breast changes are the result of increased hormone activity. Oestrogen develops the duct system and progesterone the glandular tissue. They prepare the nipple for subsequent breast feeding. Prolactin stimulates the production of colostrum.

The breasts enlarge due to increased tissue growth, blood supply and fat deposition.

DIAGNOSIS OF PREGNANCY

Early changes in the breasts often cause a woman to wonder if she is pregnant even before she has missed a period. Feelings of nausea, changes in food and drink preference and an overwhelming tiredness confirm the belief. There may be frequency of micturition and backache. *Quickening*, the date of the first fetal movement felt by the mother, provides an indicator of pregnancy. If the date of quickening is recorded, it can be used to check the date of expected confinement. A primigravid woman feels it at 18–20 weeks, the multigravida at 16–18 weeks.

Other methods of ascertaining pregnancy and estimating early gestational age involve the observation of certain characteristics associated with the physiology of pregnancy.

Hegar's sign. This sign is elicited when a

Breast changes in chronological order

3–4 weeks	prickling, tingling sensation due to increased blood supply particularly around nipple.
6 weeks	developing ducts and glands cause the breasts to be enlarged, painful and tense particularly in women who normally experience pre-menstrual changes.
8 weeks	bluish surface veins are visible.
8–12 weeks	Montgomery's tubercles become more prominent on the areola. These sebaceous glands secrete sebum which keeps the nipple soft and supple. The pigmented area around the nipple darkens and may enlarge slightly. This area is known as the *primary areola.*
16 weeks	Colostrum can be expressed. Further extension of the pigmented area occurs and is often mottled in appearance, *secondary areola.*
late pregnancy	Colostrum may leak from the breasts; progesterone causes the nipple to become more prominent and mobile.

bimanual vaginal examination is performed. Two fingers are inserted into the anterior fornix of the vagina; the other hand is placed behind the uterus abdominally. The fingers of both hands almost meet because of the softness of the elongated isthmus which is marked between the 6th and 12th week of pregnancy. This procedure is seldom employed because of the risk of inducing abortion and has been superseded by ultrasound examination.

Jacquemier's sign. A violet-blue discoloration of the vaginal membrane is observed.

Osiander's sign. This is an increased pulsation felt in the lateral vaginal fornices.

These changes cannot in themselves be considered positive signs of pregnancy as they may all be symptoms of other conditions. Only visualisation of the gestational sac or fetus by ultrasound techniques or X-ray, palpation of the fetus or of fetal movement or auscultation of the fetal heart are positive signs of pregnancy (see Table 8.2).

Once pregnancy has been confirmed, women may experience many different reactions to the news.

Although for most this is a time of great joy and satisfaction, since they have fulfilled a biological function, many experience a period of anxiety about the step they have taken. The first-time mother is likely to undergo the greatest change to her lifestyle. If she was previously financially independent, a reduced income may affect her position in the relationship. If she is unsupported she may envisage financial hardship. Decisions about future work patterns have to be faced and her self-image must change to incorporate motherhood.

The woman will experience changes to her body that are beyond her control. This may be the first time since childhood that she will be both physically and emotionally vulnerable. Concern about loss of independence causes some women to bury themselves in their careers. Similarly, women's partners also experience some anxiety about the future. Even short-term responsibility for mother and child can seem daunting. If these feelings are not resolved the partner may withdraw from the situation both physically and mentally. He may spend greater lengths of time with male friends, playing sports or visiting pubs.

A loving, supportive relationship in which the two partners communicate and discuss their feelings will help resolve these early anxieties.

The first 12–16 weeks are often very uncomfortable and exhausting for the woman. She may feel nauseated. The fetus is growing at such a speed that she often needs to sleep during the day

Table 8.2
Signs of pregnancy

Sign	Time of occurrence (gestational age)	Differential diagnosis
Possible (presumptive) signs		
Early breast changes (unreliable in the multigravida)	3–4 weeks +	Contraceptive pill
Amenorrhoea	4 weeks +	Hormonal imbalance Emotional stress Illness
Morning sickness	4–14 weeks	Gastro-intestinal disorders Pyrexial illness Cerebral irritation etc.
Bladder irritability	6–12 weeks	Urinary tract infection Pelvic tumour
Quickening	16–20 weeks +	Intestinal movement 'Wind'
Probable signs Presence of HCG* in:		
— blood	4–12 weeks	Hydatidiform mole
— urine	6–12 weeks	Choriocarcinoma
Softened isthmus (Hegar's sign)	6–12 weeks	
Blueing of vagina (Jacquemier's sign)	8 weeks +	} Pelvic congestion
Pulsation in fornices (Osiander's sign)	8 weeks +	
Uterine growth	8 weeks +	Tumours
Braxton-Hicks contractions	16 weeks	
Ballottement of fetus	16–28 weeks	
Positive signs Visualisation of fetus by:		
— ultrasound	6 weeks +	
— X-ray	16 weeks +	
Fetal heart sounds by:		
— ultrasound	6 weeks +	No
— fetal stethoscope	20–24 weeks +	alternative diagnosis
Fetal movements:		
— palpable	22 weeks +	
— visible	late pregnancy	
Fetal parts palpated	24 weeks +	

* HCG = human chorionic gonadotrophin
+ = onwards

and retire early. Her body is already changing, breasts are becoming tense and full, her waist is thickening, and frequent and urgent visits to the toilet are necessary due to pressure from an enlarging uterus. All these discomforts occur with no outward signs of pregnancy to compensate! Sometimes women change their posture or wear maternity clothes to declare a pregnancy that seems to them almost a fantasy. Labile emotions are common, due to hormonal changes, and they are often frightening to both partners. Libido is likely to decrease not only because of the discomforts mentioned or the change in body image, but also due to a fear of harming the baby. It is easy to see that this is a time when the woman requires a great deal of support and sensitivity.

Psychologically the woman feels the need to nurture herself and in so doing to nurture the fetus. Some women who have previously suffered miscarriage fear further disappointment and remain detached from the pregnancy until the risk of abortion has passed.

The second trimester confirms the pregnancy to the outside world. The fetus is now moving and is no longer a secret. The woman often feels a unique exclusive closeness with the fetus. Her partner may feel excluded as he is unable to share this experience. Ultrasound techniques reduce these feelings as both partners may now see and hear the fetus. Even so, a man will see the fetus in a different way from his partner. He imagines it as independent of the mother and begins to plan for its future. Decorating the house, re-arranging rooms in preparation for the baby and buying toys are all common responses.

Later in the pregnancy both partners start to change their social contacts, often becoming closer to their own parents, socialising and building links with other couples who have or are expecting children. Childless friends become more distant. A pregnant women evokes many reactions in others which cause her to reflect on the changes to her life.

During the third trimester the mother begins to feel that the fetus could now become independent of her. She feels that it is intruding upon her life. Her normal daily activities become tedious because of her size. She cannot put on her shoes, bending is difficult and getting in and out of the bath may pose problems. She becomes increasingly aware of her new responsibilities and may regret the passing of a more carefree existence. Despite earlier anxieties about labour she now feels ready and impatient to begin her new

experience. Braxton-Hicks contractions become more intense and sometimes painful which makes her wonder if labour has started. Preparations are made well in advance. If her delivery is to be in hospital she will be packed and ready. If a home delivery is anticipated, a room will have been organised and help arranged. Finally the day arrives.

The early signs of labour confirm that the 9 months' preparation is now at an end.

Reader Activities

- Think of a friend or relative who has recently been pregnant and consider if there was any obvious change in her behaviour during pregnancy. If possible, talk to her about the pregnancy and ask her about the changes in her body and the psychological adjustments which she had to make.
- When taking booking histories, ask some of the women to tell you what symptoms first led them to think that they were pregnant.

REFERENCES AND FURTHER READING

Dewhurst C J (ed) 1986 Integrated obstetrics and gynaecology for postgraduates, 4th edn. Blackwell Scientific, Oxford

Hytten F, Chamberlain G (eds) 1991 Clinical physiology in obstetrics, 2nd edn. Blackwell Scientific, Oxford

Llewellyn-Jones D 1986 Fundamentals of obstetrics and gynaecology, vol 1, 4th edn. Faber & Faber, London

Moore M 1983 Realities in childbearing, 2nd edn. Saunders, London

Prince J, Adams M 1987 The psychology of childbirth, 2nd edn. Churchill Livingstone, Edinburgh

Rodin A et al 1989 Thyroid function in normal pregnancy. Journal of Obstetrics and Gynaecology 10(2): 89–94

Sadow J 1980 Human reproduction, an integrated view. Croom Helm, Beckenham

9

Preparing for parenthood: daily life in pregnancy

LEA JAMIESON

Parenthood education can be interpreted in many different ways. At its broadest it describes any interaction between the midwife and the mother or parents when matters related to childbirth and parenting are discussed. This definition covers those occasions, antenatally and postnatally, when a midwife answers queries in personal conversation and builds up a mother's confidence in her ability to carry and mother a new baby. The term more obviously embraces any sessions aimed at giving information or familiarising families with the environment and experience of birth and early parenting. In order to understand parenthood education the midwife needs to understand how people learn and why they learn. This awareness exposes the rich opportunity the midwife has to enhance the couple's experience of pregnancy, childbirth and early parenting.

FACTORS AFFECTING LEARNING

Motivation

Motivation affects learning positively. The reader can apply this personally by examining the reasons for reading this chapter and thus identifying motivation. The student may be about to attend a first parenthood education session and would like to feel prepared or perhaps has an essay to write and feels the need for information! A midwife may have been asked to take on responsibility for more input in parent education than before. Whatever the reasons a motivated reader is in a state of readiness to learn.

Mothers are also in this state. Something very important is happening in their lives. They are hungry to satisfy their need to understand themselves and to gain the knowledge and skills required in order to cope with the coming experiences and responsibilities. Each mother will be wanting to explore her feelings and her thoughts about the amazing reality of a child growing within her. She will need to feel secure about the place of birth and after delivery she will desire to learn very quickly how to care for and nurture her offspring.

Teachers often have students with varying degrees of motivation but the mothers whom a midwife cares for will make eager demands on her which makes sharing her knowledge and expertise very rewarding. Their motivation is very high.

Accurate information

What governs one's choice of textbook? It may be recommended by someone whose judgement is trusted. Perhaps the reader explored parts of it and found that some information confirmed existing knowledge and gave confidence in the accuracy of the remainder. The expertise and professional standing of the editors and writers may appear to guarantee sound midwifery knowledge. Whatever the reasons for choice, the source of information must be trustworthy.

Mothers need to trust the midwife to give accurate, up-to-date information. Insufficient or biased information will not aid their growth and may jeopardise their faith in other midwives. Childbirth has many areas about which individuals need to form opinions after amassing factual, circumstantial and personal information. For example a mother needs to explore the different ways in which her pain can be soothed in labour. If, after considering and discussing the options freely, she chooses to have epidural analgesia it would be inappropriate to request a home delivery. The midwife must help the mother to understand the implications of one choice as it may rule out another. If a mother with a history of back complaints is an unsuitable candidate for epidural anaesthesia, it is unhelpful to explore this form of analgesia in depth with her. These statements may seem obvious but often stock answers and information are given by professionals who fail to give a more individually tailored response.

Presentation

The presentation of information affects learning. If the midwife is able to present relevant information in a way that interests the mothers and their partners, she will enhance their learning both on a one-to-one and a group basis. This may mean being ready to discuss the mother's case notes with her, explaining graphs pertaining to ultrasound or hormone assays, and deciphering and interpreting such abbreviations as *Vx*, *Vert*, *Ceph* and *NAD*. If a midwife who is preparing a session wishes it to be relevant and interesting, this will entail forward planning. She may invite other mothers to share their experiences or breast feed their babies during the discussion. She may use films and slides. The room needs to be welcoming and refreshments should be organised in advance.

Environment

Physical comfort and emotional state affect the attention one can give. If the reader is in a noisy situation, or expects to be disturbed at any moment, is cold or even feeling unhappy or worried about something, study will have less significance and concentration may be lost. The midwife should apply the same principle in parenthood education. Physical needs should usually be attended to first. Discovering the feelings of the mother and determining what she sees as a priority will enable the midwife to begin with that area which is most relevant and important to the mother. For example, if a mother coming to clinic has had her anxieties aroused by an old wives' tale she needs to be assured that it has no relevance before she can grasp information about, say, the alpha fetoprotein blood test. Equally a woman in clinic cannot begin to listen to the midwife explaining how her baby is lying if the surroundings are noisy and her privacy is constantly threatened.

Learning by example

In every interaction with a midwife the mother learns about midwives in general. She identifies midwives' attitudes and skills from the way they communicate with her and she builds up a picture of a 'midwife'. This image will help or hinder her in childbirth and early parenting. The qualities that need to be inherent in the professional approach are gentleness, kindness, understanding and empathy. A mother touched in this way during abdominal examination will be aware of the midwife's respect for her and for her unborn baby. A mother who watches a caring professional will learn by example that it is appropriate to touch and speak to a newborn baby. Whenever a midwife is in contact with mothers, their babies and their families during her working day, she is educating by example, whether consciously or otherwise. Midwives are not alone in their teaching role. All the professionals caring for the mother in pregnancy, childbirth and early parenthood are people with expertise and knowledge. The educative role is shared with colleagues such as the general practitioner and the health visitor. Midwives should be aware of their unique contribution and be professionally secure enough to join with their colleagues in parent education.

SOURCES OF EXISTING KNOWLEDGE

Preconception care

Education is a large part of this aspect of the midwife's role which has been discussed in detail in Chapter 7. The midwife must discover how much understanding the parents have gleaned from previous interaction with professionals.

Childhood role model

Each person has positive and negative experiences within his or her childhood. It is the way in which these are handled and the internal response that affect one's behaviour later. For example Maria, a mother who is described in Michael Deakin's *The Children on the Hill* (1973), had a very sad and restrictive upbringing due to bereavement and an insensitive family and educational environment. Maria's response was to provide for

her children the antithesis to her own experience. Alternatively, another person who has been deeply hurt in childhood may, sadly, pass this abuse on to his or her own children, a fact which is commonly known (Kempe & Kempe 1978). New parents have to be able to perceive how they reacted to the role model set by their own parents. A midwife who seeks to help them to do this must first discover the positive and negative aspects of her own experience during childhood. She must become sensitive to her internal response which may result in strong opinions or definite attitudes that need to be identified and even modified. This journey in self-awareness helps the midwife to aid parents in their own individual growth. This is discussed further later in the chapter.

Family life and school

Schools differ in the amount of teaching which they offer in health care, life skills and related subjects. A survey by Prout (1986) suggests that teenagers gain quite an extensive understanding of antenatal care and that the strategies to enhance knowledge and encourage clinic attendance should take this awareness into account. A midwife is often invited to describe her role to a group of secondary school children or highlight the needs of the unborn baby to primary school children. Professional input which builds on their present knowledge will be valuable and relevant to the children. The relationship with the professional must be open and caring with an atmosphere of mutual trust and respect. This may mean that school groups covering areas such as preconception care, antenatal care and childbirth need to be small and intimate to be effective. This early contact with a midwife will contribute to the children's idea of what a midwife is like.

In parenthood education sessions, awareness of the couple's existing knowledge is vital if the midwife is to build from that point.

EDUCATION DURING PREGNANCY

Much has been written about the time and place for parenthood education. This chapter began by identifying every interaction with a midwife as an opportunity to teach by example. If a midwife chooses, she can make her communication specific and valuable to the individual mother.

Hospital

The booking visit (see Ch. 10) is an excellent opportunity for the midwife to describe the aims of antenatal care and to give the mother an overall concept of what to expect. She can help the mother to become aware of how valuable constant care of herself will be to her unborn baby. If the mother experiences respect she will enjoy her contribution to the growth of a healthy baby. A clinic visit which leaves a mother feeling undervalued as a woman, frustrated and anxious about her pregnancy means that each professional involved has failed to maximise the opportunity to build up the mother and enhance her experience of pregnancy. In the words of Oakley (1980):

Reproduction is not just a handicap and a cause of second-class status; it is an achievement, the authentic achievement of women.

Midwives should be aware of these two attitudes within society and should present the positive view to the mother.

Different stages of pregnancy offer different opportunities for information giving and discussion. For example, nausea and vomiting may be bothersome early in pregnancy and heartburn later. The mother's need for specific advice requires a response from the midwife. Ideally the pace is determined by the mother. The midwife, cognisant that anxieties, embarrassment and lack of trust inhibit communication, will allow time for feelings to be shared and will provide an environment free from interruption. This will enable the mother to go from the clinic emotionally and intellectually satisfied, with her questions answered.

Sometimes major difficulties occur in pregnancy, such as unemployment of a husband, eviction from the home or bereavement. If the midwife has created a caring, listening environment the mother will feel free to seek help. The midwife may need to mobilise other members of the health care team to resolve some of the problems. The clinic should be a point of contact and help.

A clinic visit may provide an opportunity to work through a birth plan in which a mother's personal preferences are noted. This discussion can acknowledge her desires and expectations, inform her of what to expect and help her to adapt her plans in the face of changing circumstances. Ideally the mother should relate to a small number of midwives throughout her pregnancy so that they are all aware of her hopes and aspirations for the birth and able to discuss them sensitively during her visits.

Home

The home provides privacy and an opportunity to meet other important members of the family, such as the husband or a toddler. When a midwife visits at home, delicate topics can be discussed. These may include anxieties about jealousy or the changing relationship within a marriage. In the comfort of a sitting room the midwife acquires an identity which is separate from 'the clinic' and she is more easily seen as a trusted friend. In this setting the mother may feel free to discuss such intimate matters as lovemaking and the relationship with her in-laws. In turn the midwife gains first-hand knowledge of the mother's home situation.

The community or team midwife has the best opportunity for continuity of care and can slowly build up trust. She can evaluate the degree of the mother's understanding and introduce a little more information at each meeting or research to provide specific information requested by a mother.

A midwife can use home visits to provide education on labour and mothering for the single girl or teenager who is too shy or reluctant to attend sessions elsewhere. Sensitivity to needs and future wishes may lead the midwife to visit in everyday clothes rather than in a uniform.

Parenthood education sessions

Effective parenthood education sessions must follow the principles already outlined in this chapter. The midwife explores how she can meet the needs of the mothers in her care. Midwives in different parts of the country will be presented with different problems in terms of the mix of social classes and ethnic groups.

Specialised needs

In considering the special needs of families in a particular area it might be helpful to address the following questions:

* What types of social deprivation may be encountered?
* Is drug or alcohol abuse a possibility?
* Is there a large number of single mothers?
* Is the area one where young families are constantly moving so that little stability is afforded by neighbours and friends?
* Is the area frequented by gypsies or wandering folk who may be difficult to reach and care for?
* Is the area high in unemployment making daytime sessions for both husbands and wives a practicable and valuable proposition?
* Does the area contain immigrant families whose perception of birth and child care differs from that of the potential educators?
* Does the area include Forces families with support but the uncertainty of frequent home changes?

The possible questions are endless but each district has a population with specific needs and the midwife who assesses the demographic picture will at least understand which problems she is likely to face.

Timing

Sessions should be timed in such a way as to meet the needs of the parents as nearly as possible. Some areas may offer preconception sessions which include advice concerning the actual pregnancy. More frequently, the first parenthood education sessions will consist of one or two early meetings in order to discuss topics such as diet, alcohol consumption, smoking, work hazards, fatigue and minor disorders of pregnancy. Meet-

ing other women in this way helps to reduce the feeling of isolation which pregnant women experience.

A longer series of sessions is usually planned for the third trimester when many women have given up work or will shortly be doing so. In the last weeks preparation for labour is the main interest. Multigravid women become more concerned about the baby during the last month and it may be helpful to arrange special sessions for them during this period. If toddlers are brought, they can be included in aspects such as the tour of the hospital and see tiny babies in the post-natal ward, possibly being breast fed. Saving this visit until the later weeks of pregnancy helps to ensure that toddlers will retain the memory until their own brother or sister is born.

If a woman wishes to attend with her partner or has chosen to continue working until late in the pregnancy, evening or weekend sessions will usually be needed. Other sessions should be arranged at times which will suit the clients.

The length of each session depends on accommodation and the needs of the midwife and the mother. Women will not be able to concentrate if they have to get away to collect children from school or playgroup. The attention span is at most 20 minutes before a change of activity is needed. During pregnancy a woman finds it even more difficult to concentrate for long and sessions should allow for frequent breaks and opportunities for discussion and sharing.

Recruitment

The best advertisement for sessions is the satisfied mother in the community! If the sessions are interesting and valuable, mothers will spread the news to one another. The programme, especially new sessions such as toddler tours, couples sessions and single or 'solo' sessions need to be advertised. In society today we are accustomed to professional advertising. In the same way, posters about parenthood sessions need to capture interest, give clear information and be professionally executed. Health Education Departments will often have suitable material. If a midwife has to produce a poster herself, the use of transfer lettering or a stencil can give a professional look. A personal invitation sent to every mother with her booking letter produces good results and makes use of postage already accounted for. A personal word from the midwife at a clinic visit reinforces the information and makes her feel welcome.

Minority groups

The questions addressed under 'Specialised needs' above may have brought to light the needs of single mothers, immigrant families, young families with minimal support, gypsies and families suffering from poor housing, unemployment or eviction. Such situations need specific help and support. Where there is bereavement or chronic illness it might be helpful to put a mother in touch with a self-help group or voluntary organisation.

Pregnancy itself produces minority groups such as:

- the mother having twins or triplets
- the mother who is to have a planned caesarean section
- the mother who has had in vitro fertilisation
- the mother with a drug-induced pregnancy
- the mother who has previously experienced the tragedy of a perinatal death or sudden infant death.

Parents planning to adopt are a minority group often missed by midwife educators. Sessions which teach practical skills and help to develop an awareness of the emotions which *all* new parents experience are helpful to them.

All these groups can benefit from sharing with other mothers and couples who have similar experiences to their own. The initial involvement often leads to very long-standing friendships. People who share their feelings share themselves.

Format of groups

In order to allow exchange within a group and opportunity for every member to participate and learn according to her or his needs, the group should consist of no more than 15 members (Abercrombie 1974). Hospitals and communities which cater for large numbers of deliveries, 2000–5000 per year, need to co-ordinate their services so that there are sufficient groups to keep the numbers small and so that the facilities are fully utilised. A central booking system enables the mothers to attend sessions near their own homes when possible and yet equalises the numbers. This approach has been successfully adopted in some health districts (Zander & Chamberlain 1984). The mothers who book late and the ones who, though invited, choose not to make their arrangements until late in pregnancy are the ones who may not be able to attend the sessions of their choice but can still be accommodated by this method. Figure 9.1 shows a booklet which advertises parent education sessions.

Grouping people with similar needs eases the work of the educator. Mothers having second or third children can meet together to brush up their knowledge and to reflect on their last labours and plan the integration of each new baby into his family. Whereas a second-time mother may be useful in a group of first-time mothers, her needs are different from theirs. It is wisest to invite her specifically to share her experiences and to offer her alternative sessions which meet her differing needs.

The actual schedule of classes offered in any health district must be planned with the location of centres in mind as well as the groups who need to attend. It is valuable if sessions offered by health visitors can be co-ordinated with those run by midwives and this may be the responsibility of a parent education co-ordinator for the district. Varying lengths of courses may be needed. Couples or primigravid mothers attending on their own may need between four and eight sessions, while mothers expecting a second or third baby probably need no more than two or three. 'Solos' often appreciate an open group where attendance is welcome throughout pregnancy and a 'special focus' group for women expecting twins or a caesarean birth may only need a single meeting. Many of the groups which do not cater for the partner as a rule may be able to arrange an evening when the 'dads' can come along.

Content of sessions

The content must match the needs of the mothers. The midwife's own plan should be flexible. She should respond to needs which are stated at the

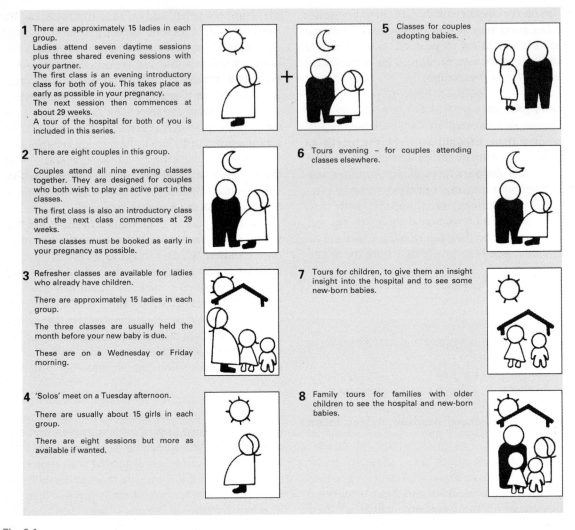

1 There are approximately 15 ladies in each group.
Ladies attend seven daytime sessions plus three shared evening sessions with your partner.
The first class is an evening introductory class for both of you. This takes place as early as possible in your pregnancy.
The next session then commences at about 29 weeks.
A tour of the hospital for both of you is included in this series.

2 There are eight couples in this group.
Couples attend all nine evening classes together. They are designed for couples who both wish to play an active part in the classes.
The first class is also an introductory class and the next class commences at 29 weeks.
These classes must be booked as early in your pregnancy as possible.

3 Refresher classes are available for ladies who already have children.
There are approximately 15 ladies in each group.
The three classes are usually held the month before your new baby is due.
These are on a Wednesday or Friday morning.

4 'Solos' meet on a Tuesday afternoon.
There are usually about 15 girls in each group.
There are eight sessions but more as available if wanted.

5 Classes for couples adopting babies.

6 Tours evening – for couples attending classes elsewhere.

7 Tours for children, to give them an insight into the hospital and to see some new-born babies.

8 Family tours for families with older children to see the hospital and new-born babies.

Fig. 9.1
Leaflet advertising parent education sessions. (Reproduced by permission of the Norwich Health Authority.)

beginning of the sessions and adapt during a session if anxieties and fears become apparent. If the midwife conducting a session discovers, for instance, that a recent television programme on postnatal depression has disturbed the mothers, she should respond by discussing the subject to their satisfaction before continuing. During the introductory session the midwife must offer the mothers an idea of her aims and ask for their suggestions for possible content. The mothers and their partners should be invited to say which areas they hope will be covered in order to satisfy their needs and also to state which additional subjects would interest them. Lists made by parents vary and give the midwife an excellent insight into the perceived needs of the group. Couples might state that both partners would like to see the environment for delivery and to discuss how they might support one another emotionally during labour. The group might ask to learn the practical skill of baby massage. Questions may be asked which seek to evaluate the progressiveness of the unit in which the baby is to be born. Such groups need a confident, competent midwife who can understand their approach and satisfy their particular requests. Another group may be less demanding and almost unable to be clear about what they want but with encouragement will become enthusiastic and enjoy suggesting items for inclusion in their sessions.

It is unwise to prescribe what the content of any programme should be. The following outline suggests a number of questions to which mothers may require to find answers.

A midwife who wishes to build up trust in the group and to help the individuals to grow and change must always accept the other person's perception without being judgemental.

Questions for parents to ask themselves. Besides needing factual answers to their questions, mothers and their partners may be helped to explore their feelings and attitudes to pregnancy and parenthood. The midwife may be able to enhance the mother's perception of herself and build up her self-esteem. She can respond to worries about an unfavourable outcome and broach the subject of emergency intervention and help to prepare for changes in the plans. She can use other people's experiences to help the new parents to imagine how they will deal with their own and to consider ways of coping.

Questions for expectant mothers:
What does antenatal care consist of?
Why is it done?
How will I know that all is well?
Can I choose where to have the baby?
How has pregnancy affected me?
What do I like about being pregnant?
What do I not like about being pregnant?
What is my attitude towards birth?
What do I need to know about the process of labour, physically, emotionally and practically?
What awareness do I have of my own body's ability to give birth?
Do I trust my body?
Who and what may help me at this time?
What makes labours so different?
What are the possible outcomes which I need to understand and anticipate?
What are my attitudes and feelings towards the whole experience?
What will give me confidence at this time in myself, in my partner, my family, my midwife and my attendants?

What skills can I master which will help me to feed and nurture my baby?
Questions for a second or subsequent pregnancy:
Has the care changed since last time?
Will my labour be different?
Will I feel the same afterwards?
Can I avoid jealousy between my present child and the new baby?
How can I ease or help their relationship?
Will I be able to love the baby as much as the first child?
Questions for 'solos':
What will I need if I decide to keep the baby?
How can I budget?
How will I cope with loneliness?
How do other people feel in my position?
How do they cope?
Questions for partners:
What is my attitude towards birth?
What is my experience of birth so far?
How does my life experience contribute?
Do I trust my wife's body to give birth?
What confidence do I have in myself as a supporter?
What strengths do I have?
What will my feelings be towards the baby?

Approaching sessions from the perspective of the mother and her partner enables the midwife to be effective as an educator. A midwife who decides to offer parenthood education needs to develop an awareness of some of her own attitudes, biases and prejudices. She needs to explore the ways in which she can enhance learning and must face her own limitations in order to make appropriate use of others who can help her to cover areas in which she feels insecure. An example is inviting a health visitor to discuss how other children can be helped to accept a new brother or sister or to explain about immunisation. Books which enlarge knowledge of the psychological processes of childbirth include those by Raphael-Leff (1991), Gross (1989), Michaels & Goldberg (1988) and Niven (1992).

The most successful childbirth educator will be someone with sufficient knowledge of childbirth and parenting, an openness to the validity of others' thoughts and ideas, an enthusiasm in planning and conducting the sessions and an honesty and acceptance of the recipients' evaluation. The latter point ensures a response to mothers' changing needs within society in keeping with *The Patient's Charter* (DH 1992).

Session structure

Traditionally, parent education sessions have been approximately 2 hours weekly over a specified period. Workshops covering a day or a half-day can be held. One example is breast-feeding workshops (Jamieson 1990). These workshops which target knowledge, skills and attitudes are very effective in enabling mothers to breast feed successfully. The prolonged time increases the depth of relationship both with professionals and with other mothers. Other subject areas that suit this approach are 'Help yourself to antenatal care — benefits and options', 'Preparing for the birth experience', 'Understanding mothering' and 'Knowledge and skills needed for bottle feeding'.

The workshops allow for a more individualised approach and are well suited to team care.

Part of the sessions can be used for relaxation and focusing on skills which are needed in labour. Ideally an obstetric physiotherapist will lead this part. If the midwife educator is alone, she may be able to integrate the exercises with the rest of the session and make links with attitudes and strengths of the individuals. Opportunities for socialising are vital as friendships formed can give great support in the early months and even years of parenting. Clulow (1982) supports such a view in his book *To Have and To Hold*:

... preparation for parenthood involves more than alerting couples to the likely effects of children upon their marriage. There is a limit to the usefulness of information to parents, although imparting information provides a reason for couples and services to meet. Preparation for the emotional impact of parenthood means establishing relationships which can be called upon later as an aid to integrating experience once that experience has been lived through. The partnership between parents is not alone in requiring preparation. Partnerships between families and the services available to them need to be established before they are required. In addition, the partnerships within the relevant helping agencies will affect the ability of those directly in touch with families to provide an integrated service. In all three contexts, the containing

relationship can serve as midwife to the emerging family unit, enabling those involved both to have and to hold the new life generated by birth. Developing such relationships is a proper objective for preparative and preventive services.

Equally a quotation from a mother's letter to her teacher (Close 1980) helps to show how attitudes are important:

You managed to communicate to me your conviction that it is possible to participate willingly and constructively in the experience of childbirth, through knowledge.

The whole conception of assistance rather than resistance was completely revolutionary to me, apparently my environment had encouraged me to have an irresponsible attitude physically, I simply refused to examine and understand the workings and functions of my body.

The realisation that I could assist the course of my labour, give birth rather than unwillingly allow a child to be dragged from me, created a confidence I had always felt lacking in myself. I do believe that it is a pervasive feeding of inferiority in women that helps to make childbirth the nightmare it undoubtedly is for so many. It was your insistence that we could help ourselves if we wanted to that gave me the courage to attempt it. You really revealed a way of thinking to me, one which I have found myself applying in many other situations besides labour.

Another mother gives insight into structuring the session (Perkins 1980):

I think rather than talk blindly on, they ought to let people ask. You go in, and they give a talk, very helpful really, but they might put you on a subject, or a small item, that will trigger something off and you sit and think 'shall I ask, because I've got that'. At the end they say 'any questions' and they sit looking at one another, and I think that instead of them sitting talking they ought to let you all talk, because it is then that you spill your fears.

Time should be allowed within the session for current anxieties to be broached. Sometimes this will mean shortening the intended input and being prepared to use different methods if time is curtailed by the group.

The midwife as facilitator of the group must be aware of her own attitudes and ideas in the knowledge that example is a powerful teacher. Variety will help each person to come expecting to enjoy the session and to be distracted from the physical discomfort of pregnancy. The midwife may share her own feelings about a recent birth in a way which will help the couples to identify with her as a person and as a midwife. There should always be a break for social exchange and refreshment.

If the session has covered the more disturbing aspects such as forceps delivery and caesarean section or if members of the group have led the discussion into puerperal depression or stillbirth, the session should close on a lighter note. This is possible by looking forward to the next week or by inviting the couples to think about their expected babies. A group should never leave on a sad or anxious note.

The following is a basic framework for couples' sessions. It is not to be copied, simply to be used as an example of content. Each teacher and each group needs to sort out the areas to be covered within the constraints of their own time and facilities. The contents need to be reviewed and altered as the participants experience pregnancy and as the educator grows in skill and perception.

Suggested plan for couples' sessions

Session 1
Introduction
Meeting the babies, listening to their heartbeats
Your expectations and requests
Film — 'Partners in Care'
Session 2
Introduction to labour
Visit to Delivery Suite
Session 3
Labour (continued); skills that help pain relief
Caesarean delivery
Forceps delivery
Relaxation and breathing techniques
Positions for labour
Session 4
Parents sharing their own experience of childbirth and early parenting
Special care nursery
Visit to postnatal ward
Session 5
Film — 'The Amazing Newborn'
Communication with a baby
Bathing a baby
Relaxation exercises

Session 6
Breast feeding
How to help yourself
Relaxation
Session 7
Support networks
Postnatal realities
Parenting: planning a postnatal reunion
Day time (optional)
Baby massage
Limbering up for labour: exercises for ladies.

HEALTH IN PREGNANCY

In her contact with pregnant women, whether in a group or singly, the midwife has ample opportunities to discuss a healthy lifestyle for pregnancy in terms of diet, exercise and personal habits. Sometimes the mother will ask for the midwife's guidance. It is often helpful to link advice to a specific problem which the woman is experiencing, such as a minor disorder of pregnancy, because at such times the woman will be more receptive to health information. Chapter 7 discusses health related to preconception care and most of the information also applies during pregnancy itself.

Diet in pregnancy

Diet is important on three counts: the health of the woman herself, her developing fetus and the alleviation of minor disorders of pregnancy. Some women will not be conversant with the main foods in terms of protein, fat and carbohydrates, fibre, vitamins and minerals, but can readily understand food groups (see Ch. 7). In addition, the midwife may explain that a regular intake of food ensures a regular supply for the unborn baby and should counsel the mother to avoid rushing meals or missing them.

Of particular importance is the intake of protein for the growth of new tissue. Meat, fish and cheese are prime sources, but cheaper sources may be advised such as peas, beans and lentils, milk and eggs. Two minerals are vital in pregnancy: calcium and iron. Milk, cheese and eggs supply the former; soft cheeses such as Brie are best avoided because they have sometimes been found to carry listeriae and eggs must be cooked thoroughly in order to destroy any salmonellae that may be present. Iron is found in red meat and offal but pregnant women are advised to avoid liver and liver products since liver may contain excessive vitamin A. Pâté may also be contaminated with listeriae. Dark green vegetables and red fruits also contain some iron.

Vitamin C helps the absorption of iron, and mothers should be encouraged to eat good quantities of fresh fruit and vegetables — at least half a kilogram per day. These will also contribute to the fibre content of the diet which helps to prevent constipation. Other high fibre foods include wholemeal bread, cereals and pulses. A certain amount of carbohydrate is required to provide energy but mothers should be encouraged to avoid a high sugar intake and to choose instead starches, which are absorbed more slowly.

Some mothers may need specialised advice. Those on low incomes or who are unsupported may need help with budgeting and with making sensible choices. It may have to be pointed out that a filled wholemeal roll is more nourishing and costs less than a fizzy drink and a packet of crisps. New vegetarians may need advice from the dietician to ensure that the range of foods they eat is adequate to supply all their nutritional requirements.

Alcohol

The inadvisability of drinking alcohol whilst pregnant has received much press coverage. Mothers may want to discuss with the midwife the fact that because they did not suspect pregnancy, they have taken alcohol up to the time of missing the first period. Moderate to high levels of alcohol have been found to give rise to fetal problems so a mother who only drinks occasionally may be reassured. No safe level of alcohol consumption has been established, therefore it is wise to stop drinking alcohol prior to conception (see Ch. 7).

Smoking

There is already plenty of literature which discourages the pregnant woman from smoking but the midwife needs to be aware of the social press-

ures and advertising that give a contrary message. Smoking can be a response to stress and it is inappropriate to add to the woman's stress by being over-directive and insensitive to her needs. If she can stop, the outlook for herself and the fetus is improved; if this proves very difficult, she should try to cut down. Smoking is linked with intra-uterine growth retardation, preterm labour and an increase in the perinatal mortality rate. The mother herself is at increased risk of chest infections and thrombo-embolic disorders.

As smoking becomes less acceptable socially it is to be hoped that fewer women will present in pregnancy as smokers; those who do are likely to be those who find it most difficult to give up. Understanding that smoking reduces the baby's oxygen and food supply may motivate a mother to stop but this is not always so. It is helpful if the midwife finds out what triggers the smoking and suggests ways of cutting down. A smoky environment will not be good for the baby in the future and this aspect can be worth discussing.

Tips for giving up smoking
* Leave a longer stub
* Use filter tips
* Keep hands busy
* Only smoke when sitting down
* Do not inhale
* Cut out the first cigarette in the day and the last one at night
* Try chewing gum or sucking peppermints

Sexual intercourse

Sometimes couples fear that sexual intercourse in pregnancy may harm the baby. It is absolutely safe and normal unless special conditions pertain. If the woman is nauseated in early pregnancy she may feel disinclined to have intercourse but the couple can be encouraged to find other ways of being loving. Libido varies throughout pregnancy and the middle trimester is usually the time of most vitality. Towards the end of pregnancy when the abdomen is large, couples sometimes have to adopt different positions.

There are certain situations when caution is advised. If a mother has a history of miscarriages she should avoid intercourse in the early months, especially at the times when her period would usually have started. If any bleeding is seen at any stage the couple should abstain and seek advice.

Some women experience contractions following intercourse due to the prostaglandins in seminal fluid and oxytocin release at orgasm. These will usually pass off with rest. After an episode of pre-term labour which has been successfully averted, abstention should be advised for the same reason.

Exercise and sport

If a mother is used to taking regular exercise such as walking, swimming, riding or cycling, there is no reason why she should not continue for as long as she feels comfortable. Pregnancy is not a time to try out strenuous new sports and the more energetic sports such as squash and wind-surfing will probably need to be discontinued fairly early. A woman could continue to swim quite safely until term and can even do her pregnancy exercises in the water. The mother's own comfort and desire can be used as a guideline. (Exercise is discussed more fully in Chapter 40.)

Travel

Travel is sometimes unavoidable in pregnancy, for example, in Forces families. Airlines ask for a doctor's certificate stating that a pregnant woman is fit to travel and they prefer not to take ladies beyond the 32nd week. Mothers can and do fly safely after this time however. Prior to 32 weeks' gestation a holiday abroad can be very refreshing and of benefit to a couple sharing the experience of looking towards parenting. An important consideration is whether any immunisations are needed because it is not wise to be immunised in pregnancy. The woman should be fastidious about washing fruit and sterilising unsafe drinking water. Sunbathing is often not enjoyed because the mother is already feeling over-warm due to an increase in her basal metabolic rate.

Long, unbroken journeys by whatever transport should be avoided. If travel is essential, taking extra fluids and making definite breaks can ease any discomfort. It is important for the woman to carry up-to-date details of her pregnancy on a co-operation card or similar record, so that

should something unforeseen occur the information needed is readily at hand.

Clothing

This reflects the mother's taste and financial position but loose cool clothing will be the most comfortable. Pinafore dresses and dresses made of ready-gathered material can accommodate the changing shape for longer. Unfortunately, pregnant women often get bored with their maternity dresses, however pretty, because they cannot afford enough to ring the changes. Fashions with loose and flowing lines make it easier for the mother's clothes to accommodate pregnancy in the early months.

Jeans can be made with elastic insets either at the side or at the front to accommodate a growing baby. The feet sometimes spread and shoes need to be comfortable. They should not tip the mother forward. Breasts usually increase in later pregnancy by at least two bra sizes. If the mother intends to breast feed she should buy a suitable bra which opens at the front rather than simply a larger ordinary one. The National Childbirth Trust and main stores often offer a fitting service and advise on size and comfort for the individual mother.

MINOR DISORDERS OF PREGNANCY

Minor disorders are only minor inasmuch as they are not life-threatening. As soon as a midwife becomes pregnant and experiences the fatigue of early pregnancy coupled with nausea and vomiting she realises the inaccuracy of the description. A minor disorder may escalate and become a serious complication of pregnancy. Where sickness develops into hyperemesis gravidarum, a condition which began as a minor disorder has become a life-threatening abnormality. The role of the midwife is to be always alert to any developing complications and refer appropriately. She must, as always, educate: when the changes of pregnancy are understood they are easier to tolerate and unnecessary anxiety is alleviated. She

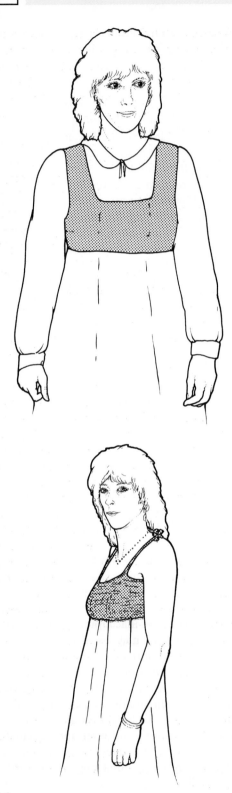

Fig. 9.2
Maternity dresses.

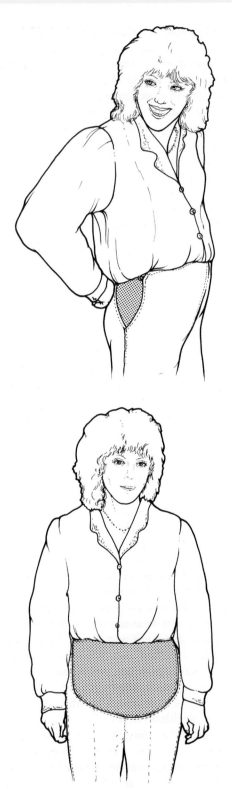

Fig. 9.3
Maternity trousers.

should also provide practical advice to ease the situation as far as is possible and listen attentively to the reality of the experience for the mother.

Causes of minor disorders can be divided into hormonal changes, accommodation changes, metabolic changes and postural changes. Every system of the body adjusts and is affected by pregnancy. In order to make reference easy, the disorders will be dealt with by systems. The mother will only need advice pertinent to some. The skill of the midwife is in anticipating the need for knowledge in the mother in order to equip her to cope with the experience of pregnancy. She also meets the mother's need for specific knowledge when she presents with a discomforting or worrying symptom.

Digestive system

Nausea and vomiting. This presents between 4 and 16 weeks' gestation. Hormonal influences are cited as the most likely cause. Human chorionic gonadotrophin is found in large amounts until the placenta takes over from the corpus luteum at around 12 weeks. Oestrogen and progesterone are also contributors; the transient nausea which may occur when a woman takes the contraceptive pill corroborates this. The sickness is not confined to 'early morning' but can occur at any time in the day. The smell of food cooking will often cause the mother to retch. The midwife can explain the probable reasons and encourage the mother to look positively towards a resolution of the sickness which should occur between 12 and 16 weeks; understanding the cause provides comfort. Mothers often find salads tempting and light snacks more tolerable than full meals. Carbohydrate snacks at bedtime and before rising can prevent hypoglycaemia which is often implicated as a cause of nausea and vomiting. It is always important to remember that other conditions such as appendicitis, unrelated to pregnancy, can present with vomiting so the midwife must be vigilant in her history taking. If vomiting becomes severe, the mother may lose weight and become dehydrated and ketotic. This condition is called hyperemesis gravidarum and warrants specialised care and appropriate referral.

Heartburn. This is a burning sensation in the mediastinal region. Progesterone relaxes the cardiac sphincter of the stomach and allows reflux of gastric contents into the oesophagus. Heartburn is most troublesome at about 30–40 weeks' gestation because at this stage the stomach is under pressure from the growing uterus.

The advice varies according to the severity of the condition. If the heartburn is occasional, the reflux can be prevented by avoiding bending over whilst housekeeping and kneeling to clean the bath or to make the beds. Small meals take up less room in the reduced stomach space and are digested more easily. Sleeping with more pillows than usual and lying on the right side semireclining can sometimes help. For persistent heartburn the doctor may prescribe antacids.

Excessive salivation (ptyalism). This occurs from 8 weeks' gestation and is thought to be caused by the hormones of pregnancy. It may accompany heartburn. Explanation and attentive listening are helpful.

Pica. This is the term used when a mother craves certain foods or unnatural substances such as coal. The cause is unknown but hormones and changes in metabolism are blamed. The midwife needs to be aware that this condition can occur and to seek medical advice if the substance craved is potentially harmful to the unborn baby.

Constipation. Progesterone causes relaxation and decreased peristalsis of the gut, which is also displaced by the growing uterus. It is helpful to increase the intake of water, fresh fruit, vegetables and wholemeal foods in the diet. A glass of warm water in the morning, before tea or breakfast, may activate the gut and help regular bowel movements. Exercise is helpful, especially walking. Aperients are considered only as a last resort: a bulk-increasing agent would be the first choice. Constipation is sometimes associated with the taking of oral iron. The condition can aggravate haemorrhoids and early common-sense advice may avoid much discomfort for the mother. A midwife should be alert to the possibility of constipation if a mother complains of abdominal discomfort and be aware that a full rectum is a cause of non-engagement of the fetal head at term.

Musculoskeletal system

Backache. This is fully discussed in Chapter 40 with advice regarding sitting and posture. The midwife's role is to educate the mother to understand her changing centre of gravity as the fetus grows and which postures to adopt. The hormones sometimes soften the ligaments to such a degree that some support is needed. When the woman appreciates this she is reassured that once birth has occurred the ligaments will return to their pre-pregnant strength. Backache must never be dismissed lightly as it is associated with urinary tract infection and with the onset of labour especially when the fetal occiput is posterior.

Cramp. The cause of leg cramp in pregnancy is unknown. It may be due to ischaemia or result from changes in the pH or electrolyte status. The mother may be advised to dorsiflex the foot (see Ch. 40) and to raise the foot of the bed about 25 cm. It may be helpful to make gentle leg movements whilst in a warm bath prior to settling for the night. This enhances circulation and removes waste products from muscle. Other remedies used are vitamin B complex and calcium.

Genito-urinary system

Frequency of micturition. This occurs in the early weeks of pregnancy when the growing uterus is still situated within the pelvis and competes for space required by the bladder. In the latter weeks the head usually enters the pelvis and reduces the space available. The midwife may reassure the mother, having excluded other causes of bladder irritability such as infection. She may also explain that the problem is resolved when the uterus rises into the abdomen after the 12th week.

Leucorrhoea. This is the term used for the increased white, non-irritant vaginal discharge in pregnancy. If the mother finds the discharge disturbing, it is helpful to offer simple advice concerning personal hygiene. She should wear cotton underwear and avoid tights. Washing with plain water twice a day should be adequate and a mild cream is preferable to talcum powder. The midwife should exclude the possibility of infections such as thrush and trichomonas. Both are dealt with in Chapter 19.

Circulatory system

Fainting. In early pregnancy fainting may be due to the vasodilatation occurring under the influence of progesterone before there has been a compensatory increase in blood volume. Avoiding long periods of standing is helpful and being quick to sit or lie down if she feels slightly faint.

Later in pregnancy a mother may feel faint while lying flat on her back. The weight of the uterine contents presses on the inferior vena cava and slows the return of blood to the heart. Turning the mother quickly onto her side will bring about a rapid recovery. The midwife has to explain to the mother that this occurs in about 10% of pregnant ladies and that she would be wise not to lie on her back except during abdominal examination. Explanation will give the mother confidence to know what to do if she feels faint and will help to ensure her safety.

Varicosities. Progesterone relaxes the smooth muscles of the veins and results in sluggish circulation. The valves of the dilated veins become inefficient and varicosities result. Varicose veins may occur in the legs, anus (haemorrhoids) and vulva. The situation is compounded by pelvic congestion. The midwife must be aware of mothers at risk, for example, those with a family history of varicose veins and those doing work which demands long periods of standing or sitting. Exercising the calf muscles by rising onto the toes or making circling movements with the ankles will help the venous return. In the early days of pregnancy, resting with the legs vertical against the wall for a short time will drain the veins. Support tights increase comfort and should be put on before rising or after resting with the legs elevated.

The avoidance of constipation by fibre in the diet and adequate fluids will reduce exacerbation of haemorrhoids. If appropriate, topical applications should be recommended and medical advice sought.

Vulval varicosities are rare and very painful. A panty-girdle or sanitary pad may give support.

The midwife should listen and offer appropriate advice. She should also be aware of the risk of haemorrhage from a ruptured vein during delivery.

Skin

The mother observes her skin changes closely and will often comment upon the linea nigra and the areola of the breasts. If chloasma occurs, which is a butterfly-shaped area of pigmentation over the face, the mother may be reassured that this will diminish as soon as the baby is born. Sometimes there is generalised itching which often starts over the abdomen. This is thought to have some connection with the liver's response to the hormones in pregnancy and with raised bilirubin levels. It clears as soon as the baby is born and comfort can be gained from local applications. An antihistamine such as Piriton (chlorpheniramine) is often prescribed. If a mother complains of vulval irritation, infection, such as thrush, and glycosuria as a result of diabetes must be excluded before advising on cotton underwear and perhaps washing with unscented soap.

Nervous system

Carpal tunnel syndrome. The mother complains of numbness and 'pins and needles' in her fingers and hands. This usually happens in the morning but it can occur at any time of the day. It is caused by fluid retention which creates oedema and pressure on the median nerve. Wearing a splint at night with the hand resting high on two or three pillows sometimes brings relief. Carpal tunnel syndrome usually resolves spontaneously following delivery. The doctor may prescribe diuretics but the conservative approach is favoured.

Insomnia

This must never be dismissed lightly. There are physical reasons for sleep disturbance such as nocturnal frequency and difficulty in getting comfortable in bed due to the growing fetus. The increased blood supply to the uterus on lying down sometimes causes the baby to move a lot, just as the mother wishes to sleep. This may be overcome by going to bed earlier in the hope that the baby will have an active time earlier and allow the mother to sleep when she wants to.

Remembering the increased anxieties which pregnancy may bring, the midwife may ask the mother what dreams or thoughts she has as she falls asleep. Talking through some of the very common fears of pregnancy may help a mother to come to terms with her own anxieties. It is common to dream of delivering 'monsters' or animals and also to dream that the baby is born dead. Sensitive listening and expressing that the mind is presenting fears through dreams can be helpful. Knowing that it is very common is reassuring.

Later in pregnancy it is wise to recommend that the mother has a lie-in in the morning or has a rest in the afternoon when sleep often comes easily. This may help to prevent the tiredness and some of the depression that can occur in the last trimester of pregnancy. Sharing her feelings can result in a sense of normality and lightness for the mother and can greatly enhance her perception of care and experience of pregnancy.

It is thought that the hormonal changes towards the end of pregnancy also contribute to periods of depression for some women. Self-confidence in pregnancy is also labile and knowing that this is normal can make the experience easier to cope with. It can be frustrating for a woman to feel bouncy and excited one week and the next to feel so insecure that she cannot go into a shop. Explaining such responses helps both the mother and her partner. If a midwife is concerned that the mother's moods are not simply those of normal pregnancy, medical aid should be sought. The minor disorders can provide the midwife with opportunities to advise the mother and help her to achieve the most comfortable and safe pregnancy possible. She will be alert to any need for referral.

Disorders which require immediate action

Most minor disorders can escalate into a more serious complication of pregnancy. Mothers should be encouraged to seek advice if at any time they feel unwell or the signs exceed what they have been led to expect. In addition there are certain incidents which should always be reported to the midwife or doctor. These are:

- vaginal bleeding
- reduced fetal movements
- frontal or recurring headaches
- sudden swelling
- rupture of the membranes
- premature onset of contractions
- maternal anxiety for whatever reason.

The mother can be reassured that her pregnancy is likely to proceed smoothly and without complication. It adds to her security if she knows clearly when she should seek the help of a professional.

Reader Activities

1. Talk to several newly-delivered women. Find out what they wished they had learned in their parent education classes.

Repeat the exercise with a similar number of women whose babies are about 28 days old.

Next ask the same question of a number of women during a subsequent pregnancy.

Compare the findings. How do women's perceived needs change with time and experience?

2. Devise a scheme for evaluating a series of parent education classes. If you have an opportunity carry out such an evaluation. Reflect on your findings and identify the things you would change as a result.

Acknowledgements

I should like to record my thanks to the late Miss Gillian Barnard and all the mothers and fathers who generously shared their experiences with me.

REFERENCES

Abercrombie M L J 1974 Aims and techniques of group teaching. Society for Research in Higher Education, London

Close A 1980 Birth report. NFER Publishing, Windsor

Clulow C F 1982 To have and to hold. University Press, Aberdeen

Deakin M 1973 The children on the hill. Quartet, London, ch 2

Department of Health 1992 The patient's charter. HMSO, London

Gross J 1989 Psychology and parenthood. Open University Press, Milton Keynes

Jamieson L 1990 Breast feeding knowledge and skills shared in a midwife–mother partnership. In: A midwife's love, skill and knowledge. International Congress of Midwives Proceedings, Japan, p 196–197

Kempe R S, Kempe C H 1978 Child abuse. Fontana/Open Books, London, ch 2

Michaels G Y, Goldberg W A (eds) 1988 The transition to parenthood. Current theory and research. Cambridge University Press, Cambridge

Niven C 1992 Psychological care for families before, during and after birth. Butterworth–Heinemann, Oxford

Oakley A 1980 Women confined. Martin Robertson, Oxford

Perkins, E R 1980 Education for childbirth and parenthood. Croom Helm, London

Prout A 1986 Teenage girls' knowledge of antenatal care and its implications for school-based preventive strategies. Health Education Journal 44: 193–197

Raphael-Leff J 1991 Psychological processes of childbearing. Chapman & Hall, London

Zander L, Chamberlain G 1984 Pregnancy care for the 1980s. Royal Society of Medicine and Macmillan Press, London, section V, ch 22

FURTHER READING

Cobb J 1980 Babyshock. Hutchinson, London

Kitzinger S 1977 Education and counselling for childbirth. Baillière Tindall, London

Nichols F, Humenick S 1988 Childbirth education: practice, research and theory. W B Saunders, London

Priest J, Schott J 1991 Leading antenatal classes: a practical guide. Butterworth–Heinemann, Oxford

Scott Peck M 1978 The road less traveled. Simon and Schuster, New York

10

Antenatal care

VALERIE THOMSON

The present pattern of antenatal care has been in existence since the inception of the National Health Service in 1948. Many people are questioning the benefits of routine attendance at hospital antenatal clinics. It is suggested that more flexibility concerning the place of consultation and timing of visits could lead to better attendance and consumer satisfaction. Improvements in maternal health and social conditions, coupled with advances in diagnostic screening techniques, now make it possible to revise current systems and implement new schemes for maximum efficiency (Hall et al 1980).

The Sighthill Project is one such scheme. The Sighthill area of Edinburgh was identified as having a perinatal mortality figure greatly exceeding the national average; associated with this was a poor uptake of hospital antenatal services. A higher than average number of women booked after the 16th week of pregnancy and a higher number of women did not keep their antenatal clinic appointments. A community clinic was set up in the hope that it would encourage attendance. A team approach enabled midwives, general practitioners and health visitors who were already aware of local needs and problems to provide a service that was acceptable to women in the area. All women except those with diabetes or cardiac conditions were seen at the community clinic. A consultant obstetrician visited and was available for consultation at other times as necessary. A protocol was negotiated which would standardise care. If the pregnancy was uncomplicated the woman would be asked to attend much less frequently. Results showed that booking and attendance figures improved. Consumer satisfaction increased and community midwives achieved greater continuity of antenatal and postnatal care. The perinatal mortality figures also improved greatly. Other research (Flint & Poulengeris 1987) has shown that women cared for by a team of midwives known to them seemed to need fewer antenatal admissions.

Aims of antenatal care

* To support and encourage a family's healthy psychological adjustment to childbearing.
* To promote an awareness of the sociological aspects of childbearing and rearing and the influences that these may have on the family.
* To monitor the progress of pregnancy in order to ensure maternal health and normal fetal development.
* To recognise deviation from the normal and provide management or treatment as required.
* To ensure that the woman reaches the end of her pregnancy physically and emotionally prepared for her delivery.
* To help and support the mother in her choice of infant feeding; to promote breast feeding in a sensitive manner and give advice about preparation for lactation when appropriate.
* To offer the family advice on parenthood either in a planned programme or on an individual basis.
* To build up a trusting relationship between the family and their caregivers which will encourage them to participate in and make informed choices about the care they receive.

As demonstrated by the Sighthill project these aims can only be achieved if the service provided is acceptable to women and their families. This has become more apparent in recent years. Women now have more control over their fertility. They are more likely to have planned their pregnancy and if not will have had the opportunity to discontinue it. Many factors have led to a decrease in maternal and perinatal mortality. Women expect a healthy outcome for themselves and their babies and have therefore become less worried about complications and more concerned with the emotional aspects of the experience. Both these factors will influence the type of care that women expect to receive. Education through schools, magazines, television and lay childbirth organisations all emphasise the normality of pregnancy and childbirth. Families are encouraged to participate fully in decision making and to expect emotional satisfaction from the childbearing experience.

In order to respect these views professionals must be approachable and inspire trust and confidence. They must give adequate and unbiased information in order to help families make sensible choices.

For its part the family needs to have realistic expectations of the future and unrealistic demands must be discussed sensitively in the antenatal period. Counselling and discussion must be used to negotiate an acceptable compromise. If this is not attempted there may be confrontation and breakdown in communication when the expectation is not met. This is even more likely when the family is under stress such as during an emergency when the required action is in conflict with the expressed wishes of the family. Ultimately, the woman has the right to refuse treatment for herself and infringement of this could be considered as assault, but the law is less specific when intervention is deemed necessary to protect the fetus.

The midwife requires good communication skills in order to explore a woman's perception of the care she will receive. Together they may use this knowledge to formulate a care or birth plan as a progressive record of the woman's needs and wishes.

BOOKING VISIT

This visit should take place as soon as possible after pregnancy has been confirmed. Advice should be given early because the fetal organs are almost completely formed by the 12th week of pregnancy. Maternal nutrition, infection, smoking, or drug-taking may all have a profound effect on the fetus during this time.

The early few weeks may leave the mother feeling exhausted, nauseous and bewildered about the changes occurring in her body. Unless referral is early she may be denied the midwife's support at this important time. It has been suggested that midwives should be more involved with the confirmation of pregnancy so that an earlier contact would be made. A midwife could then be available for support and counselling should the pregnancy fail. Unfortunately, the risk of early fetal loss often means that booking the place of confinement is postponed until the pregnancy is more established. Inefficient administration also leads to slow referral.

There are many schemes available each with different options for place of antenatal care and confinement and length of stay in hospital. Most entail one consultation with the hospital obstetric team to determine the suitability of the option.

Objectives for the booking visit

* To assess levels of health by taking a detailed history and to employ screening tests as appropriate.
* To ascertain base-line recordings of weight, height, blood pressure and haemoglobin level in order to assess normality. These values are used for comparison as the pregnancy progresses.
* To identify risk factors by taking accurate details of past and present obstetric and medical history.
* To provide an opportunity for the woman and her family to express any concerns they might have regarding this pregnancy or previous obstetric experiences.
* To give advice on general health matters and those pertaining to pregnancy in order to maintain the health of the mother and the healthy development of the fetus.
* To begin building a trusting relationship in which realistic plans of care are discussed.

This is probably the woman's first introduction to the team that is to care for her during pregnancy. First impressions are often lasting and the reception she receives at this interview is likely to colour the rest of her experience. For this reason the midwife must be friendly and approachable. Much of the interview is concerned with exchange of information. Ideally most of it should be conducted in the woman's home, away from the bustle of the busy clinic. This allows the midwife to get to know her in her own environment. The midwife may meet other members of the family and in this way gain a more holistic view of the woman's needs.

If the booking must be done in the hospital it is possible to humanise the process. It is helpful to write to the woman in advance and to advise her of the probable length of the interview, explaining what will happen and who she will see. This will allow her to make preparation for the visit. She may wish to bring a friend or her partner for support. Hospitals can be daunting to those who are not used to them. Two heads are better than one when trying to find the antenatal clinic amongst the many different departments. Children should be welcomed. Involving the toddler in the excitement of early pregnancy paves the way for future trust and lessens his fear of mother going away should she require hospital confinement. Crèche facilities are a great advantage but if not available a well-stocked toy cupboard will provide some distraction and allow mother and midwife to talk. Making the interview room as informal as possible helps to put the woman at ease.

The midwife requires many skills to achieve the aims of this visit and not least of these is her ability to communicate. Listening skills involve showing real interest in the woman as a person, using verbal and non-verbal responses to encourage the woman to talk freely. The midwife must also be able to analyse the information and elicit further details in order to complete the picture. Communication skills also encompass writing accurate, comprehensive yet concise records of information. This is vital when using a team approach to care. Repeated questioning on the same topic not only undermines a woman's confidence in the service but also wastes time that could be used for more important purposes.

The midwife also requires clinical skills in order to carry out the physical examination of the woman which includes screening tests such as cervical smear, high vaginal swab and phlebotomy.

First impressions

A midwife can gain much from observing a woman as she is invited into the interview room. Does she respond to a smile? She may appear nervous or shy. A long wait or the prospect of an interview that she has undergone in other pregnancies may have made her irritable. Perhaps she is distressed at the failure of contraception; unresolved anger may lead to unresponsive behaviour. The most likely response is that of nervous but happy anticipation, as this visit is a further confirmation of a wanted pregnancy. Whatever the response it is essential to acknowledge it, clarify the situation and use the information gained to establish a rapport with the woman and then conduct the interview with sensitivity. It may be that she will need to talk about previous experiences before she can clear her mind and attend to the business in hand. If she is ambivalent about the pregnancy she may value counselling from an abortion agency in order to become aware of her choices before finally accepting the pregnancy; adoption may be an acceptable alternative. Even a woman who has planned and welcomed her pregnancy needs time to discuss her fears and anxieties.

Observation of physical characteristics is also important. Posture and gait can indicate back problems or previous trauma to the pelvis. She may be lethargic which suggests extreme tiredness, malnutrition or depression.

Midwifery history

Although it is very helpful to use a prepared list to ascertain salient information, it is important to resist the temptation to read out a list of questions. It is much more effective to couch questions in conversation leading from one topic to another.

Social history

It is important to assess the response of the whole family to the pregnancy. An additional child may mean overcrowding in the home or even the threat of eviction. A woman may doubt her ability to care for other children during the pregnancy, labour or afterwards; teenage children particularly may be unhappy about their mother being pregnant. The client may herself be a teenager or even younger, still under her parents' care and they may not wish to support her during the pregnancy. Financial problems arise in any family with unemployment being common in some districts. It is not the midwife's responsibility to solve family problems but she must be sympathetic, have a thorough understanding of the financial benefits that are available and be able to refer a family to other professionals as appropriate. Chapter 45 explains the financial benefits.

Environmental factors must be considered when assessing needs during the pregnancy. Studies show that perinatal mortality and morbidity rates are higher in families in social classes 4 and 5 who are more likely to live in poor conditions. Poor housing, lack of hot water, inadequate heating and insufficient money to take a healthy diet or buy items for the baby are all issues that must be addressed. The social worker should be informed if the family wishes, but in deprived inner-city areas the situation is unlikely to improve quickly. The midwife should be aware that women in deprived areas have greater health care needs and should offer realistic advice in order to help them to use all the resources available.

General health

General health should be discussed and good habits reinforced, giving further advice when required.

Exercise is important. Most activities may be continued during pregnancy. The woman's own body is a good indicator of when she should slow down or stop.

The importance of restricting alcohol and nicotine intake is stressed. It may be unrealistic to expect a woman to stop smoking altogether during pregnancy. Exhortations about the effect of smoking on the fetus may exacerbate her fears about the pregnancy so much that she actually increases her intake. Some women even see a bonus in the fact that smoking causes the baby to be smaller. The midwife must give practical advice to help the woman to cut down (see Ch. 9).

Alcohol abuse is less common but can affect the baby (see Ch. 38 for fetal alcohol syndrome). In order to be sure of safety no alcohol at all should be taken during pregnancy, but some suggest that up to one glass of wine per day or the equivalent is acceptable.

Education for parenthood is provided in most areas (see Ch. 9). Sessions should be planned with individual needs in mind, providing for such diverse groups as experienced mothers, first time mothers, teenage mothers, single parents or couples. There may be some women who do not easily fit in to a particular group and it may be possible to meet their needs during antenatal visits. It may be beneficial for a community midwife to visit them at home.

Menstrual history

Determining expected date of delivery (EDD). It is necessary to ascertain the approximate date on which the baby was conceived in order to predict a date of giving birth and calculate gestational age at any point in pregnancy. In this way actual fetal size can be compared with expected size.

The EDD is calculated by adding 9 calendar months and 7 days to the date of the first day of the woman's last menstrual period. This method assumes that:

- conception occurred 14 days after the first day of the last period: this is only true if the woman has a regular 28-day cycle
- the last period of bleeding was true menstruation: implantation of the ovum may cause slight bleeding.

The midwife must enquire about the normal cycle and amount of bleeding in order to assess the reliability of the calculation.

If the woman has taken oral contraceptives within the previous 3 months, this may also confuse estimation of dates because breakthrough bleeding and anovular cycles lead to inaccuracies.

The EDD which is calculated by dates is sometimes confirmed by assessing uterine size vaginally or more commonly by early ultrasound scan. Bimanual examination carries a risk of abortion

and should be avoided particularly for women who have a previous history of spontaneous abortion. Fetal movements are first felt by a multigravid woman at about 16 weeks, and by 20 weeks by a primigravid woman.

Methods of contraception which have been used may affect the pregnancy. Some studies have suggested that the oral contraceptive pill taken in early pregnancy may cause congenital abnormality but this is less likely with modern low-dose pills. Some women become pregnant with an intra-uterine contraceptive device (IUCD) still in place. Although the pregnancy is likely to continue normally, the position of the IUCD should be determined using ultrasound techniques. If it is not evident during delivery the uterus should be explored after labour in order to retrieve it.

Obstetric history

Past childbearing experiences have an important part to play in predicting the likely outcome of the present pregnancy. The way in which a woman will respond to pregnancy, labour and the puerperium cannot be known until she has had at least one child. For this reason the woman who has not been pregnant before, a primigravida, needs closer observation to ensure that all remains normal. Women who have already had one healthy pregnancy are less likely to develop pregnancy-induced hypertension, unless this is the first pregnancy with a new partner. Adequate pelvic capacity can also be assumed if the fetus is of a similar size to previous babies delivered vaginally. Uterine efficiency is better after the first labour (see Ch. 11). If a woman has had more than five previous deliveries, she is considered at high risk particularly of postpartum haemorrhage.

Previous termination of pregnancy must be discussed although it may cause the woman embarrassment or distress. A sympathetic non-judgemental approach is required in order to elicit information and encourage the woman to talk freely about her feelings. Sometimes feelings of guilt or shame are not expressed or resolved at the time of the abortion. This may lead to their suppression which could interfere with emotional adjustment to the present pregnancy. Techniques employed in termination may affect the viability of the pregnancy. Dilatation and curettage could contribute to incompetence of the cervix and cases of later uterine rupture have also been cited (see Ch. 27). Any form of abortion occurring in a Rhesus negative woman requires prophylactic administration of anti-D immunoglobulin.

Repeated spontaneous abortion may indicate such conditions as genetic abnormality, hormonal imbalance or incompetent cervix. Diagnosis of the cause often depends on the time at which the abortion occurred. Screening or treatment may be necessary in the present pregnancy. The woman will also be more anxious about the pregnancy and will be relieved when it progresses past the date of previous abortions. She may be over-anxious, requiring extra time and support. Minor disturbances in pregnancy may cause her undue worry and preoccupation with the pregnancy may lead to difficulties in her home life. She will feel reassured if she hears the fetal heart or sees the image of an ultrasound scan and this may also help her partner. He can assist her to assess the normality of her symptoms and encourage confidence.

In order to give a summary of a woman's childbearing history, the descriptive terms *gravida* and *para* are used.

Gravid means pregnant. Gravida means a pregnant woman; a subsequent number indicates the number of times she has been pregnant regardless of outcome.

Para means having given birth. A woman's parity refers to the number of times that she has given birth to a child, live or still, excluding abortions.

A *grande multigravida* is a woman who has been pregnant five times or more: this tells nothing of outcome.

A *grande multipara* is a woman who has given birth five times or more.

For completeness of the history, reference to old case notes should be made. The woman will not remember everything about past experiences and obstetric or medical detail is usually of least importance to her. The fact that labour was augmented with Syntocinon or that the woman required two injections after the birth of the baby may not be of significance to her but to the midwife such facts will indicate that there may have been inefficient uterine action or a postpartum haemorrhage.

Complications in previous childbearing may be relevant to the present pregnancy. High risk factors listed below will determine the frequency of antenatal visits and alert staff to appropriate screening techniques. The place of antenatal care will be determined by the availability of support services, senior obstetric staff and experienced midwives. Place of birth will also be influenced by these criteria but in all cases the ultimate decision is taken by the mother who must be involved in making the decision.

Medical history

Medical conditions also influence pregnancy. These range from the severe cardiac conditions to the more common but important urinary tract infection (UTI). During pregnancy both the mother and the fetus may be affected.

- Urinary stasis and reflux occur during pregnancy. A UTI can easily develop into pyelonephritis which may lead to premature labour.
- Pregnancy predisposes to deep vein thrombosis and pulmonary embolism.
- Essential hypertension predisposes to pregnancy-induced hypertension (PIH) which results in reduced placental function, fetal intra-uterine growth retardation, fetal compromise and possible antepartum haemorrhage.
- Asthma, epilepsy, infections, psychiatric disorders and so on require drug treatment which may affect early fetal development.

Major medical complications such as diabetes and cardiac conditions require the involvement and support of the medical team (see Ch. 22).

Family history

Certain conditions are genetic in origin, others are familial or racial characteristics and some occur because of the social environment in which the family lives.

Genetic disease in the baby is much more likely to occur if his biological parents are close relatives such as first cousins.

It is known that diabetes, although not genetically inherited, leads to a predisposition in other family

Factors that indicate the need for intensified antenatal care

Booking history

Age less than 18 years or over 35 years
Primigravida over 30 years
Grande multiparity
Vaginal bleeding at any time during pregnancy
Uncertain EDD.

Past obstetric history

Stillbirth or neonatal death
Baby small or large for gestational age
Congenital abnormality
Rhesus iso-immunisation
Pregnancy-induced hypertension
Two or more terminations of pregnancy
Spontaneous abortion twice or more
Premature labour
Previous cervical cerclage
Previous caesarean section
Ante- or postpartum haemorrhage
Precipitate labour.

Maternal health

Previous history of deep vein thrombosis or pulmonary embolism
Chronic illness
Hypertension
History of infertility
Uterine anomaly including fibroids
Smoking more than 10 cigarettes a day
Family history of diabetes.

Booking examination

Blood pressure 140/90 or above
Maternal weight over 85 kg or less than 45 kg
Maternal height less than 5′ (150 cm or less)
Shoe size below 3
Cardiac murmur detected
Other pelvic mass detected
Rhesus negative blood group
Blood disorders.

members particularly if they become pregnant or obese. Hypertension also has a familial component. Multiple pregnancy has a higher incidence in certain families and races.

Examples of conditions which are common in particular races are spina bifida, sickle cell anaemia and thalassaemia.

Tuberculosis is more common in living conditions which are poor and cramped, where it spreads easily. It has been suggested that vitamin deficiency may cause spina bifida. Social factors may also be responsible for abnormalities.

PHYSICAL EXAMINATION

Screening procedures play an important part in ascertaining normality. Clinical observation such as height, weight, shoe size and abdominal examination are enhanced by sophisticated biochemical assessments and ultrasound investigations.

Height of over 160 cm and shoe size above size 3 give an indication of a normal-sized pelvis. Some authorities believe shoe size to be more significant whilst others identify stature as of greater importance (Frame et al 1985, Mahmood et al 1988). Factors which may be thought to affect the fetal size include the genetic contribution of the father but this only has a modest influence: the mother tends to grow a fetus to suit her pelvis.

A woman who is short in stature may come from a small-sized race or family or she may be stunted because of poor nutrition in utero or in childhood. If her nutrition improves subsequently, she may produce a fetus too large for her own pelvis although this is not a common occurrence. This factor is of particular significance in immigrant families. If she continues to be poorly nourished her fetus may be growth-retarded.

At about 36 weeks' gestation when the fetus is almost fully grown the pelvic size is reassessed. The fetal head is an excellent pelvimeter and if it will engage in the pelvic brim there is little cause for concern about cephalopelvic disproportion.

Weight. Obesity can lead to an increased risk of gestational diabetes and PIH.

To be accurate, weight should always be measured using the same scales and the woman asked to wear similar clothing at each visit. Women may record their own weight at home, without clothes, in order to overcome these problems.

Blood pressure is taken in order to ascertain normality and provide a baseline reading for comparison throughout pregnancy. It may be falsely elevated if a woman is nervous or anxious; long waiting times can cause additional stress. If this is the case it is good practice to recheck the blood pressure when the woman is more relaxed, remembering that she should always be in the same position to ensure a comparable reading. Brachial artery pressure is highest when she is sitting and lower when she is in the recumbent position. An adequate blood pressure is required to maintain placental perfusion but systolic blood pressure of 140 mmHg or diastolic pressure of 90 mmHg at booking is indicative of hypertension and could cause damage to the placenta.

The following factors increase accuracy of blood pressure measurement and recording (Bisson et al 1990):

* Using a regularly serviced mercury column sphygmomanometer
* Choosing the correct width cuff
* Initial estimation of the systolic pressure should be by palpation
* Diastolic pressure should be recorded using phase 4 Korotkoff sounds
* Blood pressure should be recorded to the nearest 2 mmHg.

Urinalysis is performed to exclude abnormality. At the first visit a midstream specimen is sent to the laboratory for culture to exclude asymptomatic bacilluria. This condition exists when a culture is grown of a specific bacterium that exceeds 10^5 organisms per ml urine. As it is symptomless the woman is unaware of disease. Pyelonephritis can readily develop because of the changes in the renal tract during pregnancy.

Other possible findings during subsequent routine urinalysis include:

— ketones due to increased maternal metabolism caused by fetal need or due to vomiting
— glucose caused by higher circulating blood levels, reduced renal threshold or disease
— protein due to contamination by vaginal leucorrhoea, or disease such as UTI or PIH.

See Chapter 22 for further information.

Blood tests taken at booking determine *ABO blood group* and *Rhesus (Rh) factor*. Antibody screening is performed followed by titration if present. Normal follow-up of a woman whose blood group is Rh negative will include further blood samples at 28, 32, 36 and 40 weeks, to ensure that the pregnancy is not stimulating antibody activity. If the titration demonstrates a rising antibody response, more frequent assessment will be made in order to plan management (see Ch. 34).

Haemoglobin (Hb) estimations are performed (see Ch. 8 for normal values), and in some areas ferritin levels are also taken in order to assess the adequacy of iron stores. Haemoglobin estimation is repeated at 28 weeks when the physiological effects of haemodilution are becoming more apparent and at 36 weeks to ensure that any anaemia is treated prior to delivery. Iron supplementation is not considered necessary in women who are taking adequate dietary iron and who have a normal Hb at booking although some prefer to give iron in case iron stores, which are not reflected in the Hb level, are low. Supplementation to reproduce pre-pregnancy levels is not desirable (Kassam & Hytten 1989). Iron supplements often have added folic acid (a substance necessary for formation of all new cells) as a precaution against deficiency. Other iron preparations contain vitamin C, which is vital for the optimum uptake of iron. The decision to use supplements should be made on an individual basis and not as a policy decision. Gastro-intestinal upsets are common as a result of oral iron and many women find the tablets unpleasant. If the woman is vegetarian, fasting for cultural reasons, or has an aversion to foods that contain iron, the iron content of the diet should be determined. Frequent conceptions and breast feeding may deplete iron stores and necessitate replacement.

Iron tablets should be taken with meals to reduce gastro-intestinal symptoms. If more than one tablet is necessary, they should be taken separately, one in the morning and one in the evening. In this way maximum absorption will be achieved. The intestinal mucosa have a limited ability to absorb iron and when this is exceeded extra iron is excreted in the stools.

Venereal Disease Research Laboratory (VDRL) test for syphilis is performed although not all positive results indicate active syphilis. Early testing will allow a woman to be treated in order to prevent infection of the fetus (see Ch. 19).

Human Immunodeficiency Virus (HIV) antibodies. Routine screening to detect HIV infection is still controversial. There are many views as to the ethical issues involved in screening and its effectiveness is questioned (see Ch. 19). It is important to gain informed consent for any blood tests undertaken.

Rubella immune status is determined by measuring the rubella antibody titre. Women who are not immune must be advised to avoid contact with anyone suffering from the disease and may be offered termination of pregnancy if they have been exposed. Vaccination is offered during the puerperium and subsequent pregnancy must be avoided for at least 3 months.

Other blood disorders may be sought in members of certain ethnic groups. In some areas testing may be done to screen for sickle cell disease or thalassaemia. If a woman either has or is a carrier of one of these diseases her partner's blood should also be tested. The couple will be given genetic counselling and management during pregnancy will be explained (see Ch. 22).

In some areas authorities also screen for hepatitis. Screening tests for cytomegalovirus and toxoplasmosis are not routinely done in pregnancy. In view of the low prevalence of toxoplasmosis, a health education programme may be more effective in further reducing the incidence (Wang & Smaill 1989).

Alpha fetoprotein screening. Details of this programme are given in Chapter 41.

Midwife's examination

Most of the midwife's examination is performed by exchange of information between the woman and herself rather than physical examination. Communication will be more effective if for most of the time the woman is sitting in a comfortable position feeling that she has the attention of the midwife.

At the booking visit certain aspects of the examination will be more relevant than others but the midwife will explain to the woman what she will be looking for at different stages in the pregnancy.

The midwife's general examination of the woman should follow an orderly direction; for example she may start by looking at the woman's face and then progress downwards to finish with an inspection of her legs and feet. The order should be planned so that after the initial discussion, the woman moves from chair to couch for examination. She should then be invited to return to her chair and asked if she has any final questions.

General appearance. The usual social contact gives the midwife opportunity to look at the woman's face and assess her health. The hair of a healthy woman is shining and glossy, her eyes bright and clear, and her complexion free from blotches. Her general manner will indicate vigour and vitality. Women who are anaemic, depressed, tired or ill appear lethargic, are not interested in their appearance and are likely to be unenthusiastic about the interview.

Lack of energy may be a temporary state. Early pregnancy is particularly tiring as the fetus is growing at its fastest. A woman often feels exhausted and morning or evening sickness may leave her debilitated. Her sleeping patterns should be discussed and advice given as necessary. If she has other young children, they require constant attention and energy and the midwife should help the mother to find ways of sharing the childcare responsibility. Perhaps she could involve a relative or a neighbour or join a playgroup scheme to allow her to rest during the day. Working women are unlikely to be able to rest during the day and many need to sleep as soon as they return home. Most men are now ready to take a greater share in household tasks. The midwife should encourage the mother to accept support from her partner.

Minor disorders of pregnancy may be a nuisance; Chapter 9 discusses these and suggests remedies.

If at any time the midwife notices any sign of ill health she should pass this information on to her medical colleagues.

Breast examination may be linked to the

discussion of infant feeding which will take place at this visit. Breast feeding should be promoted in a sensitive manner and information given about the benefits to both mother and baby. Whether or not a woman wishes to breast feed, the midwife should ask permission to examine the breasts. A woman may feel embarrassed at the prospect and the midwife must be aware of her feelings and gain her co-operation. The breast should be gently palpated with the flat of the hand to feel for any lumps. The nipple should be drawn forward to see if it is protractile: the woman may prefer to do this herself. The midwife will observe the changes due to pregnancy and note the evidence of hormonal activity.

The woman will appreciate information about the changes taking place in her body. Some are distressed by the increase in breast size, others by the obvious large blue veins that are appearing or the increase in areola size. Increasing abdominal size may be an acceptable body change but breast changes may not have been anticipated. For some women breast size and appearance are an important part of their body image (see Ch. 7). Partners may also regret the changes. Unless psychological adjustment is made, the woman may feel that she is no longer attractive which could lead to strain in the relationship. The midwife has a responsibility to counsel the woman who had not realised the extent to which pregnancy would change her body. It may be that she only imagines her partner to be unattracted. Honest discussion between the pair and reassurance that these changes will reverse in the puerperium may help to resolve anxieties. A good relationship in which the couple feel able to share anxieties and fears will minimise the difficulties in making the transition to motherhood.

Elimination should be discussed at every visit. During the booking visit the midwife should ask the woman about her normal bowel habit. Dietary advice may be necessary at this visit or later in the pregnancy when hormonal changes may alter normal function. Oral iron supplementation during pregnancy may cause changes in bowel movement.

Routine urinalysis is carried out at every visit. Frequency of micturition is common in early pregnancy and recurs during late pregnancy. The midwife should always ensure that the woman is free from dysuria.

Vaginal discharge increases in pregnancy. The woman should be asked during the booking visit if she has noticed any increase or changes. Once the woman has identified what is normal she will then be able to report any changes to the midwife during subsequent visits. If the discharge is itchy, causes soreness, is any colour other than creamy-white or has an offensive odour, infection must be suspected and investigated.

Later in pregnancy the woman may report a change from leucorrhoea to a discharge which has the colour and consistency of egg white. It may be tinged with blood. Mucoid loss is evidence of cervical changes and if it occurs before the 37th week of pregnancy should be reported to the obstetrician.

Vaginal bleeding at any time during the pregnancy should be reported to the obstetrician who will investigate its origin. In early pregnancy spotting may occur at the time when menstruation would have been due. Women who have suffered miscarriage in the past will be particularly worried. Early bleeding is not uncommon; the midwife should advise the woman to rest at this time and avoid sexual intercourse until the pregnancy is more stable.

Abdominal examination should be performed at every visit. At the early booking visit the midwife will observe for signs of pregnancy. It is unlikely that the uterus will be palpable abdominally before the 12th week of gestation. If previously it has been retroverted it may not be palpable until the 16th week. See below for a description of the method of examination and an explanation of findings.

Oedema is not likely to be in evidence during the booking visit but occurs as the pregnancy progresses. A degree of oedema is normal and correlates with a healthy outcome to the pregnancy. The midwife must ensure that the observed oedema is physiological and not excessive. This could be associated with pregnancy-induced hypertension. Physiological oedema occurs after rising in the morning and worsens during the day; it is often associated with daily activities or hot weather. At visits later in pregnancy the midwife should ask the woman if she has noticed any swelling. Often the woman has noticed that her rings feel tighter and her ankles are swollen. The midwife should test for pitting oedema in the lower limbs by applying finger-tip pressure for 10 seconds over the tibial bone. If pitting oedema is present a depression will remain when she removes her finger. Pitting oedema that reaches the knee should be reported to the obstetrician.

Varicosities are more likely to occur during pregnancy and are a predisposing cause of deep vein thrombosis. The legs should be examined at every visit and any abnormality discovered must be reported to the doctor. The woman should be asked to remove her tights and footwear to allow the midwife to make a thorough examination of her legs. It is often easier if the woman stands up for this examination because both the back and front of the legs can be visualised. The midwife should inspect the legs for varicosities and record their position and condition. This will enable comparison to be made at future visits. Advice about support hose is given as appropriate. The midwife also observes for reddened areas of the calf which may be caused by phlebitis. Areas that appear white as if deprived of blood could be caused by deep vein thrombosis. The midwife, using the whole of her cupped hand, feels gently along the length of the calf to assess normal warmth of the leg and to exclude irregularity in the shape of the calf. The woman should be asked to report any tenderness that she feels either during the examination or at any time during the pregnancy.

Medical examination

Many doctors see this examination as an opportunity to ascertain health, using screening tests and also to teach women self-examination of the breasts.

Heart and lungs are examined to exclude disease. A soft systolic murmur is heard in 50% of pregnant women but all other abnormality would be referred for the physician's opinion.

A vaginal examination is sometimes performed. A Papanicolaou smear may be taken for cervical cytology, any cervical erosion would be noted, and the examination would also exclude abnormality of the genital tract and pelvic masses.

Some practitioners order ultrasound scans to confirm the gestational age of the fetus.

ABDOMINAL EXAMINATION

Aims of abdominal examination

Women do not always appreciate the importance of attending for regular examination but the skilful midwife will be able to explain that the chief aim is to establish and affirm the normal. The specific aims are:

- to observe signs of pregnancy
- to assess fetal size and growth
- to assess fetal health
- to diagnose the location of fetal parts
- to detect any deviation from normal.

Preparation

The general examination will have been conducted with the mother sitting or standing but during the abdominal examination she must lie on the couch. It is difficult to ask questions while lying in this position and the midwife must explain her findings fully when the woman is sitting up again. The midwife should ensure that the woman has emptied her bladder within 30 minutes before abdominal palpation. Not only will this aid comfort but measurement of fundal height will be more accurate. In a study of black women, Engstrom et al (1989) found fundal height to be significantly larger prior to voiding. It is unnecessary for the woman to undress completely as long as her clothes are loose enough to allow access to the abdomen. Modesty is an important aspect of Islam and women of this faith will wish to keep their arms and legs covered. All women appreciate privacy and respect of their feelings by minimising exposure. The woman should be lying comfortably with her arms by her sides.

Method

Inspection

The size of the uterus is assessed roughly by eye. A distended colon or obesity may give a false impression of size. Multiple pregnancy or polyhydramnios will enlarge both the length and breadth of the uterus whereas a large baby increases only the length.

The shape of the uterus is longer than it is broad when the lie of the fetus is longitudinal as occurs in 99.5% of cases. If the lie of the fetus is transverse the uterus is low and broad.

The multiparous uterus lacks the snug ovoid shape of the primigravid uterus.

Occasionally it is possible to see the shape of the fetal back or limbs. In posterior positions of the occiput a saucer-like depression is seen at or below the umbilicus.

Fetal movement is evidence of fetal life and aids in the diagnosis of position.

Contour of the abdominal wall. A full bladder may be visible and is more obvious in the latter weeks of pregnancy. The umbilicus becomes less dimpled as pregnancy advances and may protrude slightly in later weeks.

When the woman is erect, lightening may be evident.

Lax abdominal muscles in the multiparous woman may allow the uterus to sag forwards: this is known as *pendulous abdomen* or anterior obliquity

of the uterus. In the primigravida it is a serious sign as it may be due to pelvic contraction.

Skin changes. The condition of the skin is noted. Any stretch marks are observed. A linea nigra may be seen. This a dark line of pigmentation running longitudinally in the centre of the abdomen below and sometimes above the umbilicus. Explanation may be needed if the woman is concerned. A line of hair in the same position should alert the midwife to the possibility of an android pelvis.

Scars may indicate previous obstetric or abdominal surgery.

Palpation

The hands should be clean and warm: cold hands do not have the necessary acute sense of touch; they tend to induce contraction of the abdominal and uterine muscles and the mother resents the discomfort of them. Arms and hands should be relaxed and the pads, not the tips, of the fingers used with delicate precision. The hands are moved smoothly over the abdomen in a stroking motion in order to avoid causing contractions.

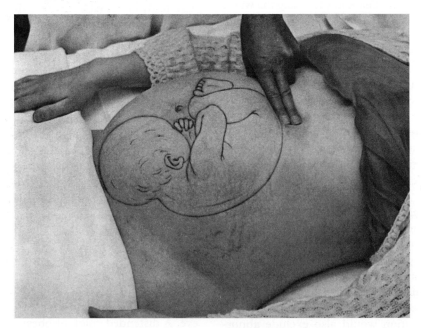

Fig. 10.1
Assessing the fundal height in finger breadths below the xiphisternum.

Estimating the period of gestation. The following method of assessing the period of gestation does not always produce an accurate result because the size and number of fetuses and the amount of amniotic fluid vary. Variations in maternal size and parity may also affect the estimation.

In order to determine the height of the fundus the midwife places her hand just below the xiphisternum. Pressing gently, she moves her hand down the abdomen until the feels the curved upper border of the fundus. She notes the number of finger breadths which can be comfortably accommodated between the two. An alternative and increasingly popular method is to measure the distance of the fundus from the symphysis pubis using a tape measure. This is plotted on a chart which gives average findings for gestational age. The height of the fundus correlates well with gestational age, especially during the earlier weeks of pregnancy (see below).

The overall size of the uterus must be considered along with the height of the fundus. If the uterus is unduly big, the fetus may be large but multiple pregnancy or polyhydramnios may be suspected. When the uterus is smaller than expected, the most likely explanation is that the woman is mistaken in the date of her last menstrual period but retarded intra-uterine growth may be suspected. The experienced midwife will be able to estimate the size of the fetus itself, judging by the size of the head and fetal parts.

Fundal palpation is carried out in order to determine whether it contains the breech or the head. This information will help to diagnose the lie and presentation of the fetus.

Watching the woman's reaction to the procedure, the midwife lays both hands on the sides of the fundus, fingers held close together and curving round the upper border of the uterus. Gentle yet deliberate pressure is applied using the palmar surfaces of the fingers to determine the soft consistency and indefinite outline that denotes the breech. Sometimes the buttocks feel rather firm but they are not as hard, smooth or well-defined as the head. With a gliding movement the fingertips are separated slightly in order to grasp the fetal mass, which may be in the centre or deflected to one side, and to assess its size and mobility. The breech cannot be moved independently of the body as can the head (see Fig. 10.2).

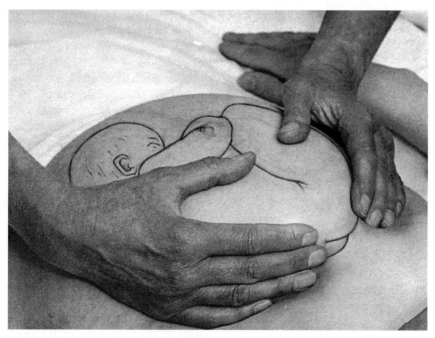

Fig. 10.2
Fundal palpation. Palms of hands on either side of the fundus, fingers held close together palpate the upper pole of the uterus.

The head is much more distinctive in outline, being hard and round; it can be ballotted between the fingertips of the two hands because of the free movement of the neck.

Lateral palpation is used to locate the fetal back in order to determine position. The hands are placed on either side of the uterus at about umbilical level. Gentle pressure is applied with alternate hands in order to detect which side of the uterus offers the greater resistance. More detailed information is obtained by feeling along the length of each side with the fingers. This can be done by sliding the hands down the abdomen while feeling the sides of the uterus alternately. Some midwives prefer to steady the uterus with one hand and, using a rotary movement of the opposite hand, to map out the back as a continuous smooth resistant mass from the breech down to the neck; on the other side the same movement reveals the limbs as small parts that slip about under the examining fingers.

'Walking' the fingertips of both hands over the abdomen from one side to the other is an excellent method of locating the back (see Fig. 10.4). The fingers should be dipped into the abdominal wall fairly deeply. The firm back can be distinguished from the fluctuating amniotic fluid and the

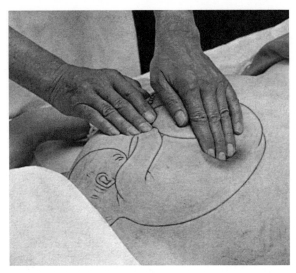

Fig. 10.4
'Walking' the finger tips across the abdomen to locate the position of the fetal back.

receding knobbly small parts. To make the back more prominent fundal pressure can be applied with one hand and the other used to 'walk' over the abdomen.

The anterior shoulder can be located by palpating from the neck upwards and inwards. Its height will vary with the station of the head.

Pelvic palpation. Palpation of the lower pole of the uterus just above the pelvis should not cause discomfort to the woman.

The midwife should ask the woman to bend her knees slightly in order to relax the abdominal muscles and suggest that she breathes steadily through an open mouth. Relaxation may be helped if she sighs out slowly. The sides of the uterus just below umbilical level are grasped snugly between the palms of the hands with the fingers, held close together, pointing downwards and inwards (see Fig. 10.5). If the head is presenting, a hard mass with a distinctive round, smooth surface will be felt. In order to determine if the vertex is presenting, the occipital and sincipital prominences are located. If the head is well flexed the sinciput will be felt on the opposite side from the back and higher than the occiput. If the head is deflexed the prominences are on the same level. If the head is extended as in a face presentation the bulk of the head is felt on the same side as the back. The midwife will also estimate how

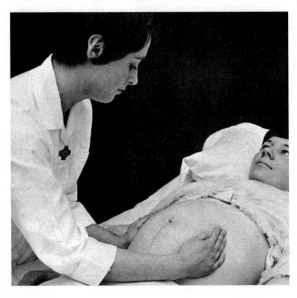

Fig. 10.3
Lateral palpation. Hands placed at umbilical level on either side of the uterus. Pressure is applied alternately with each hand.

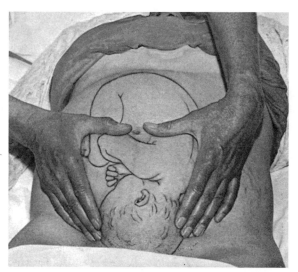

Fig. 10.5
Pelvic palpation. If the hands are in the correct position, the outstretched thumbs will meet at about umbilical level. The fingers are directed inwards and downwards.

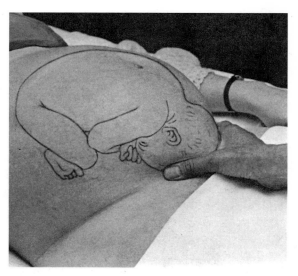

Fig. 10.7
Pawlik's manoeuvre. The lower pole of the uterus is grasped with the right hand, the midwife facing the woman's head.

much of the fetal head is palpable above the pelvic brim.

The two-handed grip is favoured because it is the most comfortable for the woman and gives the most information. *Pawlik's manoeuvre* is sometimes used to judge the size, flexion and mobility

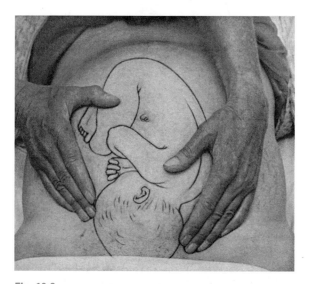

Fig. 10.6
Method of pelvic palpation used to determine position in a vertex presentation. The higher cephalic prominence (the sincipital) will be on the side opposite to the back.

of the head but the midwife must be careful not to apply undue pressure. The midwife grasps the lower pole of the uterus between her fingers and thumb which should be spread wide enough apart to accommodate the fetal head (see Fig. 10.7).

Auscultation
Auscultation must form part of each abdominal examination and must also follow any procedure in order to assess fetal well-being. The sound may be simulated by tapping the fingers together very close to one's ear. Like all heart beats it is a double sound but more rapid than the adult heart. Pinard's fetal stethoscope is commonly used to hear the fetal heart. It is placed on the mother's abdomen and at right angles to it. The ear must be in close, firm contact with the stethoscope but the hand should not touch it while listening because extraneous sounds are produced. The stethoscope should be moved about until the point of maximum intensity is located where the fetal heart is heard most clearly.

Findings

No single piece of information should ever be considered in isolation from other findings. The

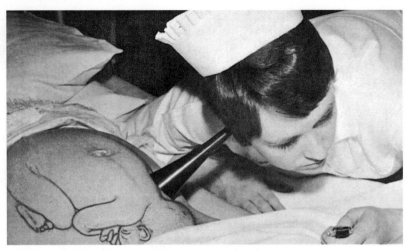

Fig. 10.8
Auscultation of the fetal heart. Vertex left occipito-anterior.

midwife, in making her diagnosis, assesses all the information which she has gathered from inspection, palpation and auscultation and draws the one conclusion which accounts for all of the factors. If one fact does not fit in with the rest she must think again.

Gestational age

During pregnancy the uterus is expected to grow at a predicted rate and in early pregnancy uterine size will usually equate with the gestation estimated by dates (see Fig. 10.9). Later in pregnancy increasing uterine size gives evidence of continuing fetal growth but is less reliable as an indicator of gestational age.

Multiple pregnancy increases the overall uterine size and should be diagnosed by 24 weeks' gestation. In a singleton pregnancy the fundus reaches the umbilicus at 22–24 weeks and the xiphisternum at 36 weeks. In the last month of pregnancy lightening occurs and the fetus sinks down into the lower pole of the uterus. The uterus becomes broader and the fundus lower. In the primigravida strong abdominal muscles encourage the fetal head to enter the brim of the pelvis.

Lie

The lie of the fetus is the relationship between the long axis of the fetus and the long axis of the uterus (see Figs 10.10–10.14). In 99.5% of cases the lie is longitudinal due to the ovoid shape of

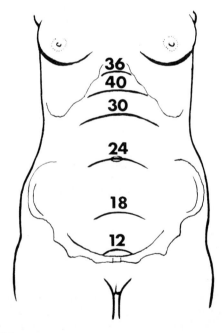

Fig. 10.9
Growth of the uterus, showing the fundal heights at various weeks of pregnancy.

the uterus; the remainder are oblique or transverse. Oblique lie, when the fetus lies diagonally across the long axis of the uterus, must be distinguished from obliquity of the uterus, when the whole uterus is tilted to one side (usually the right) and the fetus lies longitudinally within it. When the lie is transverse the fetus lies at right angles across

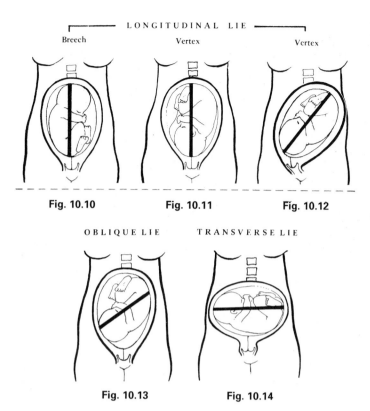

Figs 10.10–10.14
The fetal lie.
Figures 10.10, 10.11 & 10.12 depict the longitudinal lie. Confusion sometimes exists regarding Figure 10.12 which gives the impression of an oblique lie, but the fetus is longitudinal in relation to the uterus and merely moving the uterus abdominally rectifies the presumed obliquity.
Figure 10.13 shows an oblique lie because the long axis of the fetus is oblique in relation to the uterus.
Figure 10.14 shows the true transverse lie with shoulder presentation.

the long axis of the uterus. This is often visible on inspection of the abdomen.

Attitude

Attitude is the relationship of the fetal head and limbs to its trunk. The attitude should be one of flexion. The fetus is curled up with chin on chest and arms and legs flexed, forming a snug, compact mass which accommodates itself to the uterine cavity. Flexion of the fetal head enables the smallest diameters to present to the pelvis and results in an easier labour.

Presentation

Presentation refers to the part of the fetus which lies at the pelvic brim or in the lower pole of the uterus. There are five presentations (see Figs 10.15–10.20). The approximate incidence of each presentation is given below:

- vertex 96.8%
- breech 2.5%
- shoulder 0.4% (1 in 250)
- face 0.2% (1 in 500)
- brow 0.1% (1 in 1000).

Vertex, face and brow are all head or cephalic presentations. When the head is flexed the vertex presents; when it is fully extended the face presents and when partially extended the brow presents (see Figs 10.21–10.24). It is more common for the head to present because the bulky breech finds more space in the fundus which is the widest diameter of the uterus and the head lies in the narrower lower pole. The muscle tone of the

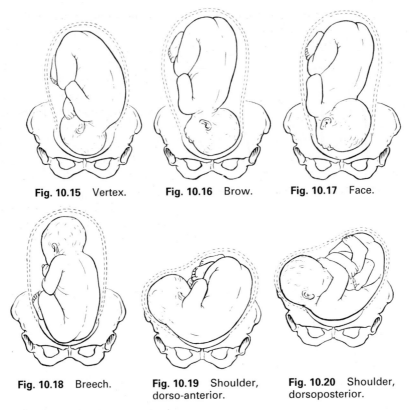

Fig. 10.15 Vertex.   **Fig. 10.16** Brow.   **Fig. 10.17** Face.

Fig. 10.18 Breech.   **Fig. 10.19** Shoulder, dorso-anterior.   **Fig. 10.20** Shoulder, dorsoposterior.

Figs. 10.15–10.20
The five presentations.

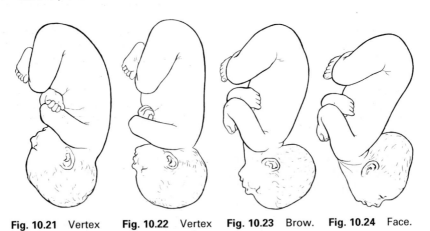

Fig. 10.21 Vertex (well-flexed head).   **Fig. 10.22** Vertex (deflexed head).   **Fig. 10.23** Brow.   **Fig. 10.24** Face.

Figs. 10.21–10.24
Varieties of cephalic or head presentation.

fetus also plays a part in maintaining its flexion and consequently its vertex presentation.

Denominator

Denominate means to give a name to; the

denominator is the name of the part of the presentation which is used when referring to fetal position. Each presentation has a different denominator and these are as follows:

- in the vertex presentation it is the occiput
- in the breech presentation it is the sacrum
- in the face presentation it is the mentum.

Although the shoulder presentation is said to have the acromion process as its denominator, in practice the dorsum is used to describe the position. In the brow presentation no denominator is used.

Position

Position is the relationship between the denominator of the presentation and six points on the pelvic brim (see Fig. 10.25). In addition the denominator may be found in the mid-line either anteriorly or posteriorly, especially late in labour. This position is often transient and is described as direct anterior or direct posterior.

Anterior positions are more favourable than posterior positions because when the fetal back is in front it conforms to the concavity of the mother's abdominal wall and can therefore flex better. When the back is flexed, the head also tends to flex and a smaller diameter presents to the pelvic brim. There is also more room in the anterior part of the pelvic brim for the broad biparietal diameter of the head.

Positions in a vertex presentation

Left occipito-anterior (LOA). The occiput points to the left iliopectineal eminence; the sagittal suture is in the right oblique diameter of the pelvis.

Right occipito-anterior (ROA). The occiput points to the right iliopectineal eminence; the sagittal suture is in the left oblique diameter of the pelvis.

Left occipitolateral (LOL). The occiput points to the left iliopectineal line midway between the iliopectineal eminence and the sacro-iliac joint; the sagittal suture is in the transverse diameter of the pelvis.

Right occipitolateral (ROL). The occiput points to the right iliopectineal line midway between the iliopectineal eminence and the sacro-iliac joint; the sagittal suture is in the transverse diameter of the pelvis.

Left occipitoposterior (LOP). The occiput points to the left sacro-iliac joint; the sagittal suture is in the left oblique diameter of the pelvis.

Right occipitoposterior (ROP). The occiput points to the right sacro-iliac joint; the sagittal suture is in the right oblique diameter of the pelvis.

Direct occipito-anterior (DOA). The occiput points to the symphysis pubis; the sagittal suture is in the anteroposterior diameter of the pelvis.

Direct occipitoposterior (DOP). The occiput points to the sacrum; the sagittal suture is in the anteroposterior diameter of the pelvis.

In breech and face presentations the positions are described in a similar way using the appropriate denominator.

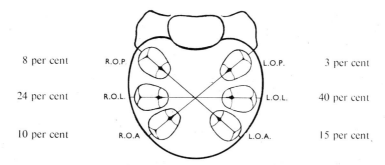

8 per cent   R.O.P.   L.O.P.   3 per cent

24 per cent   R.O.L.   L.O.L.   40 per cent

10 per cent   R.O.A   L.O.A.   15 per cent

Fig. 10.25
Diagrammatic representation of the six vertex positions and their relative frequency.

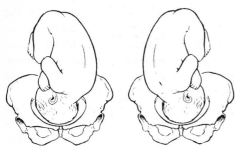

Fig. 10.26
Left occipito-anterior.

Fig. 10.27
Right occipito-anterior.

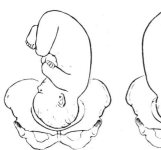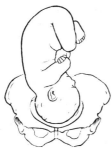

Fig. 10.28
Left occipitolateral.

Fig. 10.29
Right occipitolateral.

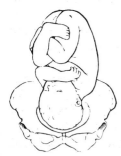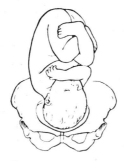

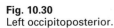

Fig. 10.30
Left occipitoposterior.

Fig. 10.31
Right occipitoposterior.

Figs. 10.26–10.30
Six positions in vertex presentation.

Engagement

Engagement is said to have occurred when the widest presenting transverse diameter has passed through the brim of the pelvis. In head presentations this is the biparietal diameter and in breech presentations the bitrochanteric diameter. Engagement is an important sign that the maternal pelvis is likely to be adequate for the size of the particular fetus and that a vaginal delivery may be expected.

In a primigravid woman the head normally engages between about the 36th and 38th week of pregnancy but in a multipara this may not occur until after the onset of labour. When the vertex presents the following will be evident on clinical examination:

- less than half of the fetal head is palpable above the pelvic brim
- the head is not mobile
- the sinciput is felt less than 5 cm above the brim
- the anterior shoulder is little more than 5 cm above the brim.

On rare occasions the head is not palpable abdominally because it has descended so deeply into the pelvis that the vertex has reached the level of the ischial spines.

If the head is not engaged, the findings are as follows:

- more than half of the head is palpable above the brim
- the head may be high and freely movable but it can also be partly settled in the pelvic brim and consequently *immobile*
- the sinciput may be 7.5 cm above the brim.

If the head remains unengaged in a primigravid woman at 38 weeks, the possibility of cephalopelvic disproportion should be borne in mind. The midwife will refer the woman to the obstetrician who may assess the pelvis clinically, taking the size of the fetal head into account.

Assessment of pelvic capacity

The size of the obstetric conjugate can be estimated by measuring the diagonal conjugate per vaginam.

The diagonal conjugate is measured from the lower border of the symphysis pubis to the centre of the promontory of the sacrum. This is usually 12–13 cm, approximately 2 cm longer than the measurement of the obstetric conjugate. The examination is usually carried out after the 36th week of pregnancy when the vagina and pelvic floor are softer and maximum pelvic joint relax-

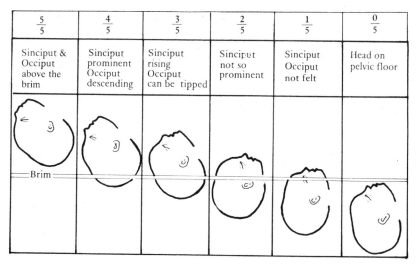

$\frac{5}{5}$	$\frac{4}{5}$	$\frac{3}{5}$	$\frac{2}{5}$	$\frac{1}{5}$	$\frac{0}{5}$
Sinciput & Occiput above the brim	Sinciput prominent Occiput descending	Sinciput rising Occiput can be tipped	Sinciput not so prominent	Sinciput Occiput not felt	Head on pelvic floor

Fig. 10.32
Descent of the fetal head estimated in fifths palpable above the pelvic brim.

ation has occurred, making the procedure less uncomfortable.

Method. The woman should be given the opportunity to empty her bladder. She then lies in the dorsal position with her knees drawn up. Cleanliness is maintained and modesty observed. The first two fingers of the gloved hand are lubricated with obstetric cream and inserted into the vagina. An effort is made to reach the sacral promontory although only the long-fingered will be able to contact it. If bone is encountered the fingers should be directed further upwards. No bone is felt above the promontory because the fifth lumbar vertebra recedes.

The point where the examining hand is in contact with the lower border of the symphysis pubis is marked by the forefinger of the other hand and after withdrawal the distance between that point and the tip of the middle finger is measured with a ruler. On subtracting 2 cm, the measurement of the obstetrical conjugate is obtained.

The cavity and outlet can also be assessed. The ischial spines are palpated to see if they are prominent, which would indicate a reduced bispinous diameter. Two fingers are placed in the greater sciatic notch: this will determine whether it is adequate. The curve of the sacrum is noted. Before removing the fingers the pubic arch is examined to see whether the angle is about 90°. Two fingers can normally be accommodated in the apex of the arch. Finally the distance between the two tuberosities can be gauged by asking the woman to lie on her side and inserting a closed fist between the tuberosities. This is a very rough guide to the anatomical outlet. The amount of maternal tissue and fat will vary as will the size of the individual's fist but one might ascertain whether the outlet is small, average or large.

In the multigravid woman engagement often does not occur until labour has commenced. If, during palpation, it is thought that the present fetus is much larger than previous vaginally delivered babies, further investigations are required (see Ch. 24).

It is usual to avoid diagnosing cephalopelvic disproportion until either X-ray evidence is unequivocal or until after the onset of labour. The reason for this is that the force of labour contractions encourages flexion and moulding of the fetal head and the relaxed ligaments of the pelvis allow the joints to give. This may be suffʳ ᵗo allow engagement and descent. Othʳ non-engaged head at term include:

- occipitoposterior position
- full bladder

- wrongly calculated gestational age
- polyhydramnios
- placenta praevia or other space-occupying lesion
- multiple pregnancy
- pelvic brim inclination of more than 80° as occurs in a high assimilation pelvis.

Presenting part

The presenting part of the fetus is the part which lies over the cervical os during labour and on which the caput succedaneum forms. It should not be confused with presentation.

ONGOING ANTENATAL CARE

It has been stressed that all the information gathered will enable a decision to be made about the subsequent care offered to the pregnant woman and her family.

A woman who has a high number of risk factors identified during the booking or who develops complications during pregnancy will be invited to attend for antenatal care at the hospital unless a scheme exists where consultant obstetricians visit community clinics.

Risk factors arising during pregnancy

Fetal movement pattern changed
Hb lower than 10 g/dl
Poor weight gain, weight loss
Proteinuria, glycosuria, bacilluria
BP systolic above 155, diastolic above 90 mmHg
Uterus large or small for dates
Excess or decreased liquor
Malpresentation
Head not engaged in primigravid woman by 38 weeks
Any vaginal bleeding
Premature labour
Vaginal infection.

The timing and number of visits will depend on the individual. Currently, visits are monthly from booking to 28 weeks, fortnightly to 36 weeks weekly until delivery.

New schemes of antenatal care encourage referral to the midwife much earlier in pregnancy. This would help to make the midwife's support and advice far more effective. Frequency of visiting for those women who are considered at low risk is being reduced. Women are being invited to attend only at key times when a specific reason for examination exists. The frequency of these visits could be decided upon between the woman and her attendant with the option of self-referral if necessary between agreed visits. Should any risk factors develop during pregnancy the woman will be invited to attend more frequently and the place of confinement will be reviewed.

Options for women with few or no risk factors

- Shared care between midwife and GP. Delivery often takes place at home or in a GP unit attached to the hospital.
- Shared care between midwife and GP, with key visits to hospital clinic. Delivery often takes place in hospital.
- Shared care between a hospital midwife and senior obstetrician, delivery in hospital.
- Care by an independent midwife. The woman's GP will have been informed and have agreed to be involved as necessary. The birth will usually be at home.

Purpose of continuing antenatal care

- To continue to observe for maternal health and freedom from infection.
- To assess fetal well-being.
- To ascertain that the fetus has adopted a lie and presentation that will allow vaginal delivery.
- To ensure that the mother and family are confident to decide when labour has commenced and that they have telephone numbers to use if they wish to seek advice.
- To offer an opportunity to express any fears or worries about pregnancy or labour.
- To discuss any views about the conduct of labour and formulate a birth plan if required.

At each visit the midwife will examine the woman, employing the same systematic approach discussed earlier. Some women offer information readily but others will require sensitive questioning.

In order to evaluate the effectiveness of advice or treatment given during a previous visit good record keeping is essential. This is even more important when the care is being shared between practitioners. In some areas women carry their own notes, in others the notes are used only in the hospital but all information is duplicated onto a co-operation card which is carried by the woman.

Indicators of fetal well-being

- Increasing maternal weight in association with increasing uterine size compatible with the gestational age of the fetus.
- Fetal movements which follow a regular pattern throughout pregnancy.
- Fetal heart rate which should be between 110 and 160 beats per minute during auscultation.

Eliciting information about recent fetal movement will reassure the mother. Patterns of fetal movements are a reliable sign of fetal well-being. In order to identify her normal pattern the woman may be asked to complete a fetal kick chart (Grant & Elbourne 1989). Evidence of at least 10 movements a day is considered acceptable. The midwife would, however, expect that these movements had occurred within a 12-hour period. The period of observation usually starts at 9 a.m. but fetal activity is often greatest during the late evening. If this is normal for a particular fetus, then a period of observation should be identified which includes the time during which the fetus is most active. The same time period should be used each day to allow for comparison. The woman should be asked to bring the kick chart with her at each visit for the midwife to assess. If the fetus is taking progressively longer each day to achieve 10 movements, this indicates that the fetus is becoming compromised in utero. It is imperative that the woman is asked to inform the labour ward if the fetus has not moved 10 times in the 12-hour period or if its pattern of activity changes

greatly. She should not wait for the next antenatal appointment or even the next day but ring immediately no matter how late at night. The midwife explains that cardiotocographic monitoring will then be performed to ascertain fetal condition.

Many women believe that it is normal for the fetus to become less active before labour. The midwife can point out that although the type of movements changes because of reduced space, fetal activity should continue throughout pregnancy and labour.

Preparation for labour

During the latter weeks of pregnancy, labour should be discussed. Most hospitals provide a list to remind women what they are likely to need while in hospital. A woman who has decided to deliver at home is visited by her midwife to make final arrangements for the birth (see Ch. 39). In both cases it is important to ensure that women know whom to contact if they are worried or have begun labour.

During the last trimester a birth plan may have been formulated; there should be an opportunity for revision as parents' wishes or original plans may have changed. The midwife should allow time for discussion about the birth plan. She should explain the likely course of labour and the policies adopted by the maternity unit, or any other matters relating to the delivery which she feels need clarification. Most parents are keen to accept change when necessary and are often ready to consider alternatives if the need arises. This is all the more likely if they feel that their needs have been fully considered and that they have been well informed and are involved in decision-making. Parents' wishes should be recorded in the case notes so that they are readily available for labour. Finally the midwife should discuss recognition of the onset of labour, assessing knowledge and adding to it as appropriate. The woman is often psychologically prepared for birth from around 36 weeks. As the pregnancy renders her increasingly encumbered she longs for labour to occur so that she may hold her baby.

Reader Activities

- Look through the case notes of women who have recently booked at the antenatal clinic. Using your own judgement identify one woman who is suitable for midwife care.

  Write down a plan for her future antenatal care. State the key weeks at which you would wish to examine her and list the objectives that you would wish to achieve at each of these visits.

  Discuss your decisions with an experienced midwife.

- Assessment of fetal size is a skill which requires practice. In order to maximise your practice, try to estimate the weight of the fetus when palpating women near the end of their pregnancies. Check your estimation by visiting the mother and baby after delivery.

It is also very helpful to visit the Special Care Baby Unit in order to visualise the size of babies at earlier gestational ages, but remember that not all preterm babies are the birthweight expected for their gestation.

- Compose a letter inviting a woman to attend the antenatal clinic for booking. Assume that she is primigravid and knows nothing about the procedure. Explain in the letter what will happen at this visit and what she should expect. Evaluate the letter by showing it to a woman who has recently attended the booking clinic and ask her how it might be improved upon.

- Consider a room in your hospital in which history taking occurs. List five ways in which it could be made less clinical for the duration of the interview.

REFERENCES

Bisson D L, Golding I, MacGillivray P et al 1990 Blood pressure lability. Contemporary Reviews in Obstetrics and Gynaecology 2: 11–15

Boddy K et al 1981 A schematic approach to prenatal care. Dept. of Obstetrics & Gynaecology, University of Edinburgh

Engstrom J, Osbrenya K, Plass R et al 1989 The effect of maternal bladder volume on fundal height measurements. British Journal of Obstetrics and Gynaecology 96(8): 987–991

Flint C 1986 Sensitive midwifery. Heinemann, London

Flint C, Poulengeris P 1987 The know your midwife report 49 Peckarmans Wood, London

Frame S, Moore J, Peters A et al 1985 Maternal height as a predictor of pelvic disproportion: an assessment. British Journal of Obstetrics and Gynaecology 92: 1239–45

Grant A, Elbourne D 1989 Fetal movement counting to assess fetal wellbeing. In: Chalmers I, Enkin M, Keirse M 1989 Effective care in pregnancy and childbirth. Oxford University Press, Oxford, vol 1, ch 28, p 440–454

Hall M H, Chng P K, MacGillivray I 1980 Is routine antenatal care worthwhile? Lancet I: 78–80

Kassam M, Hytten F 1989 Iron and folate supplementation in pregnancy. In: Chalmers I, Enkin M, Keirse M (eds) Effective care in pregnancy and childbirth, Oxford University Press, Oxford, vol 1, ch 19, p 301–317

Mahmood T A, Campbell D M, Wilson A W 1988 Maternal height, shoe size and outcome of labour in white primigravidas: a prospective study. British Medical Journal 297: 515–517

Maternity Services Advisory Committee 1982 Maternity care in action, Pt. 1 Antenatal care. HMSO, London

Prince J, Adams M 1987 The psychology of childbirth, 2nd edn. Churchill Livingstone, Edinburgh

Staines C 1983 Moving forward in antenatal care: The Sighthill project, Edinburgh. Midwives Chronicle 96(9) supp. p 6–8

Wang E, Smaill F 1989 Infection in pregnancy. In: Chalmers I, Enkin M, Keirse M (eds) Effective care in pregnancy and childbirth, Oxford University Press, Oxford, vol 1, ch 34, p 534–564

Zander L, Chamberlain G 1984 Pregnancy care for the 1980s. Royal Society of Medicine & Macmillan, London

4

Normal labour

11

The first stage of labour: physiology and early care

PATRICIA CASSIDY

The physiological transition from pregnancy to motherhood heralds an enormous change in each woman physically and psychologically. It is a time when every system in the body is affected and the experience represents a major *rite de passage* in the woman's life.

During pregnancy the feto-maternal unit nourishes and protects the growing fetus, the body of the uterus remaining relaxed and the cervix closed. As parturition approaches the non-progressive Braxton-Hicks contractions experienced during pregnancy alter to become the progressive form of labour. The cervix which hitherto was firm and closed becomes soft and dilatable and a life-giving force pervades the woman's body. Accompanying the physical changes are feelings of great intensity varying from excited anticipation to fearful expectancy. The midwife who is the caregiver must exercise great sensitivity at this time in order to meet the needs of the individual woman and her family.

Labour is described as the process by which the fetus, placenta and membranes are expelled through the birth canal.

Normal labour occurs at term and is spontaneous in onset with the fetus presenting by the vertex. The process is completed within 18 hours and no complications arise.

Three stages of labour are described:

The first stage is that of dilatation of the cervix. It begins with regular rhythmic contractions and is complete when the cervix is fully dilated.

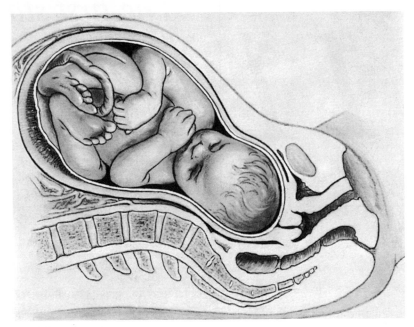

Fig. 11.1
Fetus in utero at the beginning of labour.

The second stage is that of expulsion of the fetus. It begins when the cervix is fully dilated and is complete when the baby is completely born.

The third stage is that of separation and expulsion of placenta and membranes and also involves the control of bleeding. It lasts from the birth of the baby until the placenta and membranes have been expelled.

THE ONSET OF LABOUR

The onset of labour is the most important diagnosis in obstetrics since it is on the basis of this finding that decisions are made which will affect the management of labour (O'Driscoll & Meagher 1966). It is part of the remit of the midwife to ensure women have sufficient information to assist them to recognise the onset of true labour. Contact with the midwife should be made when regular rhythmic uterine contractions are experienced, occurring at 10-minute intervals and perceived as uncomfortable or painful. Contractions will usually be accompanied or preceded by a bloodstained, mucoid 'show'. Occasionally the membranes will

rupture, which should always be reported to the midwife.

Pre-labour (Calder 1985, Gibb 1988) is the term given to the last few weeks of pregnancy during which time a number of changes occur.

Lightening. 2–3 weeks before the onset of labour the lower uterine segment expands and allows the

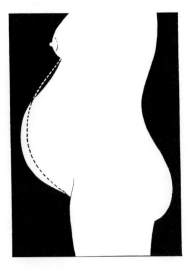

Fig. 11.2
Lightening. The dotted line shows the shape of the uterus prior to lightening.

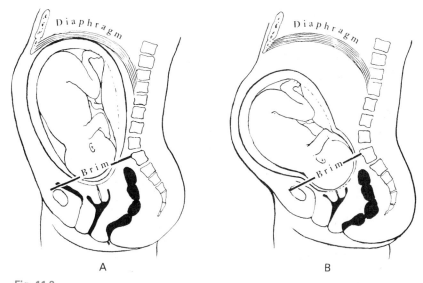

Fig. 11.3
(A) *Prior to lightening*. The fundus crowds the diaphragm. The lower uterine segment is not soft and has not stretched to accommodate the fetal head which therefore remains high. The lower segment is 'V' shaped.
(B) *After lightening*. The fundus sinks below the diaphragm and breathing is easier. The lower segment is 'U' shaped; it has softened and dilated so that the head sinks down into it and may partly enter the pelvic brim.

fetal head to sink lower; it may engage. The fundus no longer crowds the lungs, breathing is easier, the heart and stomach can function more easily and the woman experiences a relief which is known as lightening. The symphysis pubis widens and the pelvic floor becomes more relaxed and soft-ened, allowing the uterus to descend further into the pelvis.

In a primigravid woman the abdominal muscles are in good tone, which braces the uterus into an upright position and helps the head to engage. In the multigravida the abdominal muscles tend to be more lax and, as a result, the abdomen be-comes somewhat pendulous so that the fetal head may not engage.

Walking is more difficult because the sym-physis pubis is more mobile and relaxation of the sacro-iliac joints may give rise to backache.

Relief of pressure at the fundus results in an increase in pressure within the pelvis, which may be accounted for by the presence of the fetal head, venous congestion of the whole area and relaxa-tion of the pelvic joints. Vaginal secretion also becomes more profuse at this time.

Frequency of micturition. Congestion in the pelvis limits the capacity of the bladder, requiring it to be emptied more often. Laxity of the pelvic floor muscles may give rise to poor sphincter con-trol and a degree of stress incontinence.

Spurious labour. Many women experience contractions before the onset of true labour, which may be painful and may even be regular for a time, causing a woman to think that labour has started. The two features of true labour which are absent are retraction, and dilatation of the cervix (see below).

Taking up of the cervix. The cervix is drawn up and gradually merges into the lower uterine segment. In the primigravida this may result in complete effacement but in the multigravida a perceptible canal remains.

During the pre-labour period many women feel cumbersome, ungainly and tired. Mood swings are common and a surge of energy may be expe-rienced. Anxiety can increase the production of adrenaline which inhibits uterine activity and may in turn prolong labour (Seitchik 1987, Wuitchik et al 1989). The attitude of the midwife, the advice

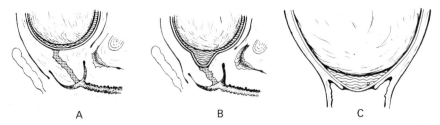

Fig. 11.4
The process of 'taking up' of the cervix by which its canal becomes continuous with the lower uterine segment.

and guidance she gives during pregnancy, influence not only the progress of labour but also the relationship of both partners to each other and to their baby after it is born.

Causes of the onset of labour

The exact cause of the onset of labour remains uncertain but it would appear to be multifactorial in origin, being a combination of hormonal and mechanical factors. Maternal oestrogen reaches optimum levels in the last weeks of pregnancy resulting in the formation of oxytocic receptors in uterine muscle cells and opposing the quiescent action of progesterone. This, coupled with the rise in *prostaglandins* provoked by changes in the decidua and membranes, results in uterine contractions. What is responsible for initiating these changes is unclear but it is thought that fetal factors are involved possibly related to the high levels of *oxytocin* present in the fetal circulation during labour. Emotional and physical stresses operate on the maternal hypothalamus triggering the release of oxytocin. The mutually co-ordinated effects of oxytocin and prostaglandin initiate the rhythmic contractions of true labour.

Uterine activity also results from mechanical stimulation of the uterus and cervix. This may be brought about by overstretching as in the case of a multiple pregnancy or pressure from a presenting part which is well applied to the cervix.

PHYSIOLOGY OF THE FIRST STAGE OF LABOUR

Duration

The length of labour varies widely and is influenced by parity, birth interval, psychological state, presentation and position, pelvic shape and size, and the character of uterine contractions. By far the greater part of labour is taken up by the first stage and it is common to expect the active phase (see below) to be completed within 12 hours. On average the primigravida will take most of this time while the multigravida might expect to reach the second stage within 6 hours or so. In the individual case averages can prove extremely misleading since the onset of labour is a process not an event. It is very difficult to pinpoint exactly when the painless contractions of pre-labour develop into the progressive rhythmic contractions of true labour.

Uterine action

Fundal dominance

Each uterine contraction starts in the fundus near one of the cornua and spreads across and downwards. The contraction lasts longest in the fundus where it is also most intense but the peak is reached simultaneously over the whole uterus and the contraction fades from all parts together. This pattern permits the cervix to dilate and the strongly contracting fundus to expel the fetus.

Polarity

Polarity is the term used to describe the neuromuscular harmony that prevails between the two poles or segments of the uterus throughout labour. During each uterine contraction these two poles act harmoniously. The upper pole contracts strongly and retracts to expel the fetus; the lower pole contracts slightly and dilates to allow expulsion to take place. If polarity is disorganised, the progress of labour is inhibited.

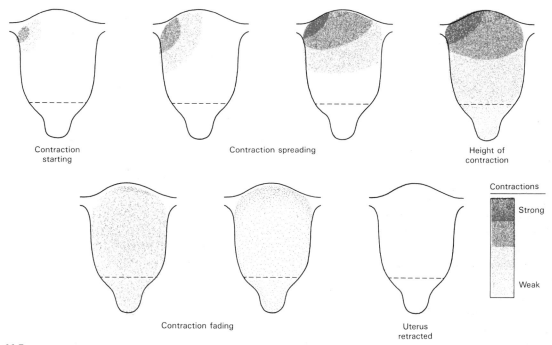

Fig. 11.5
Series of diagrams to show fundal dominance during uterine contractions.

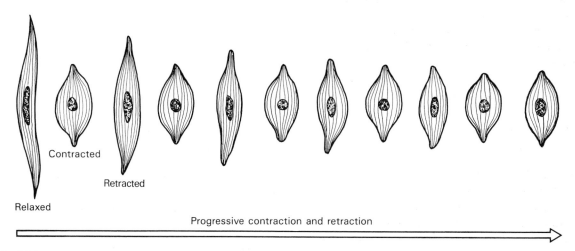

Fig. 11.6
Diagram to show how uterine muscle retains some shortening after each contraction.

Contraction and retraction

Uterine muscle has a unique property. During labour the contraction does not pass off entirely but muscle fibres retain some of the shortening of contraction instead of becoming completely relaxed. This is termed retraction. It assists in the pro-gressive expulsion of the fetus; the upper segment of the uterus becomes gradually shorter and thicker and its cavity diminishes.

In early labour uterine contractions occur every 15–20 minutes and may last for about 30 seconds. They are fairly weak and may even be imper-

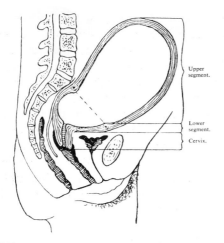

Fig. 11.7
Birth canal before labour begins.

ceptible to the mother. They usually occur with rhythmic regularity and the intervals between them gradually lessen while the length and strength of the contractions gradually increase. By the end of the first stage they occur at 2–3 minute intervals, last for 50–60 seconds and are very powerful.

Formation of upper and lower uterine segments

By the end of pregnancy the body of the uterus has divided into two segments which are anatomically distinct. The upper uterine segment is mainly concerned with contraction and is thick and muscular while the lower segment is prepared for distention and dilatation and is thinner. The lower segment has developed from the isthmus and is about 8–10 cm in length. When labour begins, the retracted longitudinal fibres in the upper segment pull on the lower segment causing it to stretch; this is aided by the force applied by the descending head or breech.

The retraction ring

A ridge forms between the upper and lower uterine segments which is known as the retraction or Bandl's ring. It is customary to use the former term to describe the physiological retraction ring and to reserve the term Bandl's ring for an exaggerated degree of the phenomenon which becomes visible above the symphysis in obstructed labour.

The normal retraction ring gradually rises as the upper uterine segment contracts and retracts and the lower uterine segment thins out to accommodate the descending fetus. Once the cervix is fully dilated and the fetus can leave the uterus, the retraction ring rises no further (see Fig. 11.8).

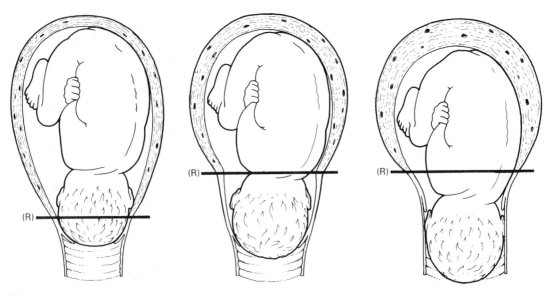

Fig. 11.8
Diagram showing the retraction ring between the upper and lower uterine segments.

Cervical effacement

If the cervix has not already been taken up during the last days of pregnancy, this process will take place in labour. The muscle fibres surrounding the internal os are drawn upwards by the retracted upper segment and the cervix merges into the lower uterine segment. The cervical canal widens at the level of the internal os. In the primigravida the external os remains closed until the cervix is flattened over the presenting part and completely effaced, whereas in the multigravida the external os begins to dilate before effacement is complete. In the highly parous woman the cervix may never be effaced completely.

Cervical dilatation

Dilatation of the cervix is the process of enlargement of the external os from a tightly closed aperture to an opening large enough to permit passage of the fetal head. Dilatation is measured in centimetres and full dilatation at term equates to about 10 cm.

Dilatation occurs as a result of uterine action and the counter-pressure applied by the bag of membranes and the presenting part. A well-flexed fetal head closely applied to the cervix favours efficient dilatation. Pressure applied evenly to the cervix causes the uterine fundus to respond by contraction.

Show. As a result of the dilatation of the cervix, the operculum, which formed the cervical plug during pregnancy, is lost. The woman will see a bloodstained mucoid discharge a few hours before or within a few hours after labour starts. The blood comes from ruptured capillaries in the parietal decidua where the chorion has become detached and from the dilating cervix. There should never be more than bloodstaining; frank bleeding is abnormal.

As the first stage ends, there is often a small loss of bright red blood which heralds the second stage.

Mechanical factors

Formation of the forewaters

As the lower uterine segment stretches, the chorion becomes detached from it and the increased intra-uterine pressure causes this loosened part of the sac of fluid to bulge downwards into the dilating internal os, to the depth of 6–12 mm. The well-flexed head fits snugly into the cervix and cuts off the fluid in front of the head from that which surrounds the body. The former is known as the forewaters and the latter the hindwaters.

The effect of separation of the forewaters is to prevent the pressure applied to the hindwaters during uterine contractions from being applied to the forewaters and keeps the membranes intact during the first stage.

General fluid pressure

While the membranes remain intact, the pressure of the uterine contractions is exerted on the fluid and, as fluid is not compressible, the pressure is equalised throughout the uterus and over the fetal body and is known as general fluid pressure. When the membranes rupture and a quantity of fluid emerges, the placenta is compressed between the uterine wall and the fetus during contractions and the oxygen supply to the fetus is thereby diminished. Preserving the integrity of the membranes, therefore, optimises the oxygen supply to the fetus and it also helps to prevent intra-uterine infection.

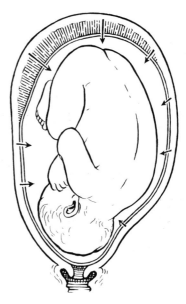

Fig. 11.9
General fluid pressure.

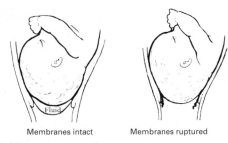

Fig. 11.10
Rupture of the membranes.

Rupture of the membranes

The physiological moment for the membranes to rupture is at the end of the first stage of labour when the cervix becomes fully dilated and no longer supports the bag of forewaters. The uterine contractions are also applying increasing force at this time.

Membranes may sometimes rupture days before labour begins or during the first stage. If for any reason there is a badly fitting presenting part, the forewaters are not cut off effectively and the membranes rupture early but in some cases no reason is apparent. Occasionally the membranes do not rupture even in the second stage and appear at the vulva as a bulging sac covering the fetal head as it is born; this is known as the caul.

Routine amniotomy during the first stage of labour is unjustified and should never be done without the mother's informed consent and a positive indication (Henderson 1990).

Fetal axis pressure

During each contraction the uterus rears forward and the force of the fundal contraction is transmitted to the upper pole of the fetus, down the long axis of the fetus and is applied by the presenting part to the cervix. This is known as fetal axis pressure and becomes much more significant after rupture of the membranes and during the second stage of labour.

RECOGNITION OF THE FIRST STAGE OF LABOUR

Recognition by the mother

It is the woman herself who usually diagnoses the

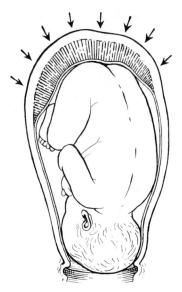

Fig. 11.11
Fetal axis pressure.

onset of labour and many women are apprehensive in case they misdiagnose the beginning of this process. Education during the prenatal period is of paramount importance in order to enable the woman to recognise the beginning of labour and thus avoid expending energy preparing for an occurrence which is not yet about to happen.

- **Show**. It is quite common to lose a jelly-like discharge in late pregnancy but when a pink jelly-like loss is noted, labour is likely to be imminent or under way. It may be lost after a vaginal examination.

- **Contractions**. Braxton-Hicks contractions are more noticeable in late pregnancy and some women experience them as painful. They are irregular or their regularity is not maintained and they often last more than one minute. True labour contractions exhibit a pattern of rhythm and regularity, usually increasing in length, strength and frequency as time goes on. When the woman first feels contractions she may only be aware of backache but if she places a hand on her abdomen she may perceive simultaneous hardening of the uterus. Contractions will be short initially, lasting 30–40 seconds, and may be as much as half an hour apart. The midwife can advise the woman to continue with her normal activities until she feels unable to cope on her own.

• ***Rupture of the membranes***. The woman will have little difficulty in recognising a sudden gush of fluid as rupture of the membranes and she should be instructed to inform the midwife immediately if this happens. It is less easy to recognise a dribble of amniotic fluid and the easiest way to distinguish it from urine is by the smell. If she is certain that it is urine, she need take no action, but if she has any doubt, she should contact the midwife. The midwife may pass a speculum and test the fluid in the vagina with a nitrazine swab. The swab will change from orange to navy blue in the presence of amniotic fluid.

Confirmation by the midwife

The midwife has the opportunity to make an objective assessment of the events recounted by the woman. She will examine the abdomen to evaluate the character of the contractions and, during a vaginal examination, she can assess the state of the cervix and the uterine os. Table 11.1 will help to differentiate between true and spurious labour.

Table 11.1
Differential diagnosis of true and spurious labour

Uterine contractions

True labour	*Spurious labour*
Always present	Not always present
Rarely exceed 60 secs	May last 3–4 minutes
Recur with rhythmic regularity	Are erratic
Are accompanied by abdominal tightening, discomfort or pain	May or may not be painful
Are often accompanied by backache	Not accompanied by backache

The cervix

True labour	*Spurious labour*
The cervix is shortened	The cervix does not shorten progressively
The os is dilating progressively	There is no increase in dilatation
The membranes feel tense during a contraction	The membranes do not become tense
Show is usually present	There is no show

INITIAL EXAMINATION AND CARE

Welcoming the mother and her partner

When she comes to the realisation that labour has started, the woman will experience a mixture of excitement and apprehension. She may be preparing for her first admission to hospital and possibly her first night away from home. Before she arrives at the hospital there will have been a flurry of activity at home making last minute arrangements and informing important members of her family.

When the woman presents at hospital, she should ideally be welcomed by a midwife whom she already knows. Where this is not possible, it is crucial that this first meeting between the midwife and the couple establishes a rapport which sets the scene for the remainder of labour. Skill in inspiring confidence and establishing a trusting relationship with a woman is an integral part of good midwifery care, as is an understanding that each individual couple will respond differently to the onset of labour. The level of anxiety experienced by the woman will be a reflection of cultural expectations, previous experiences, how vulnerable she feels and the degree of knowledge she possesses about the physiological changes occurring within her body. Ideally, a trusting relationship should have been built up during the prenatal period so that when a woman presents in labour peripheral anxieties will be reduced to a minimum. A welcoming attitude and a comfortable environment will encourage the couple to relax and respond positively to the forces of labour.

The midwife must make an immediate assessment of whether delivery is imminent and, if so, admission procedures are curtailed and preparation is made for the birth.

Taking a history

The present labour

Taking the history of labour begins with the woman's telephone call to the midwife. If possible, the midwife should speak to the woman herself rather than to the partner. If the membranes have ruptured or the contractions are strong and frequent, she should advise her to make her way to the hospital. If labour is preterm, admission is always advised (see Ch. 12). Early in the conversation the midwife should ascertain the woman's name, case number, exact location and the number of the telephone from which she is speaking. Providing that there is no complication and labour is not well advanced, the woman can be encouraged to remain at home as long as she feels comfortable and secure.

On arrival a more detailed history should be taken. The midwife will in the meantime have consulted the case notes to obtain information concerning the pregnancy. The woman is asked for an account of events and what made her think that labour had started. The midwife must remember that the woman may not be able to pay attention or respond during a contraction. In addition to ascertaining information about a show, ruptured membranes and contractions, enquiry should be made as to whether the woman has been deprived of sleep and also what food she has taken in the last few hours.

Thought should be given to the social circumstances, particularly the care of other children and whether the partner is available and has been contacted.

Past history

If the woman has booked for a hospital delivery, a full history will have been taken and should be available, either in the case notes or on the co-operation card. Of particular relevance at the onset of labour are:

- parity
- character of previous labours, especially if operative delivery was necessary
- weights of previous babies
- condition of previous babies
- evidence of cephalopelvic disproportion
- age, especially if considered particularly young or old for childbearing
- maternal disease such as pre-eclampsia, anaemia, diabetes or heart disease
- Rhesus iso-immunisation.

Birth plan

Admission of a woman in labour provides the opportunity for the midwife to discuss with each individual and her partner any plans which may have already been prepared by them. An outline may be present in the case notes or the couple may bring the plan with them. Some women will not have prepared a birth plan and, if this is the case, the midwife can encourage the couple to consider any preferences which they may have. A birth plan simply means that a pregnant woman has discussed with her midwife the kind of birth she would like. Frequently the husband or partner is involved in this forward planning which should be a flexible document which can be reviewed and revised during labour. To welcome the woman who is being admitted in labour, to introduce oneself and to ascertain how she would like to be addressed should help establish a trusting relationship. Whether or not they are already identified in a birth plan the midwife should explore the following issues:

- her chosen birth companion
- wearing her own clothes such as an old nightdress or her husband's shirt
- bringing in her own pillow
- games or a radio or cassette player
- ambulation
- pain relief
- episiotomy
- position for delivery
- Syntometrine
- cutting the umbilical cord
- feeding the baby after birth.

An individual plan of labour should then be drawn up based on the woman's wishes and the midwife's observations.

General and abdominal examination of the mother

In order to assess accurately the general condition of the mother and her progress in labour, the midwife must make a thorough examination which begins as the woman enters. Her general demeanour will give an impression of how she is coping with contractions. If she is upright, her build, stature and gait will be evident; height and shoe size should also be noted. The woman will often be flushed with the exertions of labour: pallor or cyanosis give cause for concern.

The woman is asked to empty her bladder and a specimen of the urine is tested for protein, glucose and ketones. The temperature is taken and should be normal. If it is elevated, a cause should be sought. If there is evidence of infection such as gastro-enteritis or upper respiratory tract infection, precautions should be taken to avoid spread to other women or babies. The pulse rate is counted although not during a uterine contraction which increases the heart rate slightly. Blood pressure is recorded and the doctor is notified if it is raised. With the woman lying on the examination couch she is examined for oedema. Slight swelling of the feet and ankles is normal, but pretibial oedema or puffiness of the fingers or face should be reported.

A detailed abdominal examination as described in Chapter 10 should be carried out and recorded. Observations made on admission form a baseline for those carried out throughout labour. The abdominal examination will be repeated at intervals in order to assess descent of the head. This is measured by the number of fifths palpable above the pelvic brim and recorded (see Fig. 10.32).

Vaginal examination

A vaginal examination should always be preceded by an abdominal examination and the woman's bladder must be empty. With the combination of external and internal findings the skilled midwife will have a very detailed picture of the progress of labour.

Indications
- To make a positive diagnosis of labour
- To make a positive identification of presentation
- To determine whether the head is engaged in case of doubt
- To ascertain whether the forewaters have ruptured or to rupture them artificially
- To exclude cord prolapse after rupture of the forewaters, especially if there is an ill-fitting presenting part

- To assess progress or delay in labour
- To apply a fetal scalp electrode
- To confirm full dilatation of the cervix
- In multiple pregnancy to confirm the lie and presentation of the second twin and in order to puncture the second amniotic sac (see Ch. 23).

The midwife should realise that a vaginal examination is not always the only way of obtaining this information and that careful, continuous observation of the labouring mother will enable her to avoid making unnecessary vaginal examinations.

Under no circumstances should a midwife make a vaginal examination if there is any frank bleeding unless the placenta is positively known to be in the upper uterine segment.

Method
A vaginal examination during labour is an aseptic procedure. If it is done carelessly there is a risk of introducing organisms into the vagina. Each institution will have its own vaginal examination pack containing sterile swabs and bowls. Sterile, disposable gloves are also required.

The midwife should first explain the procedure carefully to the woman and give her an opportunity to ask questions. In order to obtain the most information, the woman is usually asked to lie on her back but the technique can be adapted to suit other positions if necessary. During the examination the thighs should be separated and the knees bent but in order to avoid unnecessary exposure the woman can be asked to move and uncover herself when the midwife is ready to begin.

The midwife washes her hands thoroughly and puts on her gloves. The vulva is swabbed using the left hand. The first two fingers of the right hand are dipped into antiseptic cream and gently inserted downwards and backwards into the vagina while the labia are held apart by a thumb and finger of the left hand. The fingers are directed along the anterior vaginal wall and should not be withdrawn until the required information has been obtained. The vagina is gently explored but while turning the hand the thumb must not be brought into contact with the anus where it may be contaminated, nor the clitoris where it may cause great discomfort.

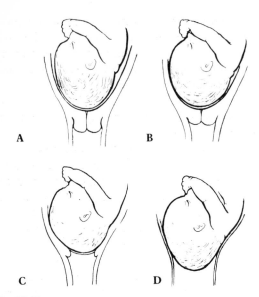

Fig. 11.12
The cervix before and during labour.
(A) Cervix before labour
(B) Cervix partly taken up
(c) Cervix dilating — membranes applied to head
between contractions
(D) Cervix fully dilated — membranes ruptured

Findings

External genitalia. Before cleansing the vulva the midwife should observe the labia for any sign of varicosities, oedema or vulval warts or sores (see Ch. 19). She notes whether the perineum is scarred from a previous tear or episiotomy. Some cultures practise female circumcision (excision of the clitoris and possibly the labia minora) and scarring from this operation would also be evident. She should also note any discharge or bleeding from the vaginal orifice. If the membranes have ruptured the colour and odour of any amniotic fluid are noted. Offensive liquor suggests infection and green fluid indicates the presence of meconium which may be a sign of fetal distress.

Condition of the vagina. The vagina should feel warm and moist. The walls are soft and distensible. A hot, dry vagina is a sign of obstructed labour and should never be found with modern obstetric care. If the woman has a raised temperature the vagina will feel correspondingly hot but should not be dry. If the walls are firm and rigid a longer labour can be anticipated and the presence

of scar tissue from a previous perineal wound may cause delay in the second stage of labour. In a multiparous woman, a cystocele may be found. A loaded rectum may be felt through the posterior vaginal wall.

The cervix. As the examining fingers reach the end of the vagina they are turned so that their sensitive pads face upwards and come into contact with the cervix. Palpate around the fornices and sense the proximity of the presenting part of the fetus to the examining finger. A spongy feeling between the fingers and the presenting part may indicate the possibility of undiagnosed placenta praevia. The os uteri is located by gently sweeping the fingers from side to side. It will normally be situated centrally but sometimes in early labour it will be very posterior. In the rare event of a sacculated retroverted gravid uterus the cervix may be located in an extreme anterior position.

The midwife must assess the length of the cervical canal. A long, tightly closed cervix indicates that labour has not yet started. The cervical canal may be partially or completely obliterated depending on the degree of effacement (see above). In a primigravida the cervix may be completely effaced but still closed; in this case it will be closely applied to the presenting part and can easily be confused with a completely dilated cervix until the small tell-tale depression in the centre is found.

The consistency of the cervix is noted. It should be soft and elastic and applied closely to the presenting part. If it is tight, rigid or unyielding, labour may be prolonged; poor application is associated with an ill-fitting presenting part.

The uterine os. Dilatation of the external os is estimated in centimetres, being the distance across the opening. 10 cm dilatation equates to full dilatation. In preterm labours the smaller fetal head will pass through the os at a smaller diameter. At the point where the maximum diameters of the fetal head have passed through the os, the cervix can no longer be felt.

The midwife should always take care to feel for the cervix in every direction as a lip of cervix frequently remains in one quarter only, usually anteriorly (see also Bishop score, Ch. 25).

The forewaters. Intact membranes can be felt

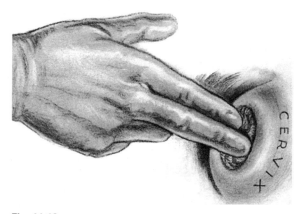

Fig. 11.13
Cervix 4 cm dilated.

through the dilating os. When felt between contractions they are slack but will become tense when the uterus contracts and the fluid behind them is then more readily appreciated. The consistency of the membranes can be likened to cling film. When the forewaters are very shallow it may be difficult to feel the membranes.

If the presenting part does not fit well, some of the fluid from the hindwaters escapes into the forewaters causing the membranes to protrude through the cervix. This will be more exaggerated

in obstructed labour. Bulging membranes are more likely to rupture early and in this case they will not be felt at all. Following rupture of the membranes the midwife needs to satisfy herself that the cord has not prolapsed.

If the forewaters are felt following a leakage of amniotic fluid it may be supposed that the hindwaters have ruptured.

Level or station of the presenting part. The presenting part is defined as the part of the fetus lying over the uterine os during labour. In order to assess the descent of the fetus in labour, the level of the presenting part is estimated in relation to the maternal ischial spines. The distance of the presenting part above or below the ischial spines is expressed in centimetres. As a caput succedaneum may form over the presenting part care must be taken to relate the bony part to the spines and not the oedematous swelling. Moulding of the fetal skull can also result in the presenting part becoming lower without any appreciable advance of the head as a whole. The midwife must bear in mind that the fetus follows the curve of Carus and it is impossible to judge the station precisely. The purpose of making this estimate is to assess progress and it is therefore valuable for

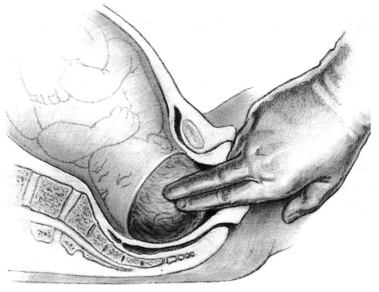

Fig. 11.14
Cervix almost fully dilated.

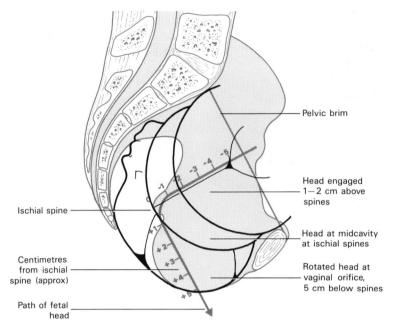

Pelvic brim

Head engaged
1—2 cm above
spines

Head at midcavity
at ischial spines

Rotated head at
vaginal orifice,
5 cm below spines

Ischial spine

Centimetres
from ischial
spine (approx)

Path of fetal
head

Fig. 11.15
Diagram to show stations of the fetal head in relation to the pelvic canal.

the same person to make all the vaginal examinations on any particular mother.

Identity of the presentation. In 96% of cases the vertex presents and is recognised by feeling the hard bones of the vault of the skull and the fontanelles and sutures. For details of the findings in face, brow, breech and shoulder presentations see Chapter 26.

Position. By feeling the features of the presenting part, the position of the presentation can be deduced. The vertex has the fewest diagnostic features but being the most common presentation is the one with which the midwife must become most familiar.

Commonly, the first feature to be felt, even in early labour, is the sagittal suture. Its slope should be noted; most frequently it will be in the right or left oblique diameter of the pelvis, or it may be transverse. Later it rotates into the anteroposterior diameter of the pelvis.

The sagittal suture should be followed with the finger until a fontanelle is reached. If the head is well-flexed, this will be the posterior fontanelle which is recognised because it is small and triangular, with three sutures leaving it. The anterior fontanelle is diamond-shaped, covered with membrane, and four sutures leave it. The location of the fontanelle(s) in relation to the pelvis will give information as to the whereabouts of the occiput.

Moulding (see Ch. 5) can be judged by feeling the amount of overlapping of the skull bones and can also give additional information as to position. The parietal bones override the occipital bone and the anterior parietal bone overrides the posterior.

An understanding of the mechanism of labour (see Ch. 14) will help the midwife to appreciate the significance of flexion, rotation and descent as determinants of progress in labour.

Pelvic capacity. Although the capacity of the pelvis may have been assessed antenatally the midwife should take the opportunity to assure herself of its adequacy as she completes her vaginal examination. She will feel the ischial spines which should be blunt and note the size of the subpubic angle which should be about 90° and accommodate the two examining fingers. Prominent ischial spines and a reduced sub-pubic angle are unfavourable features associated with the android pelvis.

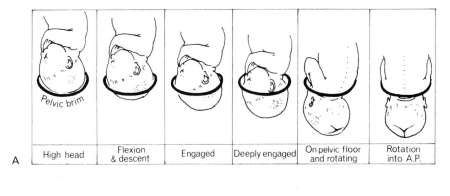

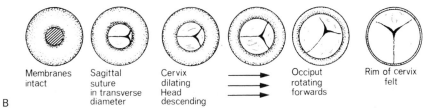

Fig. 11.16
(A) Diagrams showing descent of the fetal head through the pelvic brim
(B) Diagrams showing dilatation of the cervix and rotation of the fetal head as felt on vaginal examination.

Completion of the examination. As the midwife withdraws her fingers from the vagina she should note any blood or amniotic fluid and compare this with the observations made earlier. Finally the midwife should remove her gloves and auscultate the fetal heart prior to assisting the mother to find a comfortable position.

Keeping the woman fully informed of her progress in labour shows sensitivity to her needs and is an integral component of the support provided by the midwife. The midwife records her findings.

CLEANLINESS AND COMFORT

Bowel preparation

If there has been no bowel action for 24 hours or the rectum feels loaded on vaginal examination the woman should be consulted and asked if she would like an enema or suppositories. A small, low volume disposable enema may be administered or two glycerine suppositories. There is no evidence to suggest a full rectum causes delay in the progress of labour (Drayton 1990).

Perineal shave

Research has shown that perineal shaving does not improve infection rates. Most women would prefer to avoid being shaved although a few may request it and others may like long hair clipped. In some cultures all married women keep the vulval area free of hair.

Bath or shower

Immersion in a bath inevitably allows some of the water to enter the vagina. Some see this as opening a potential gate to infection and prefer to advise women with ruptured membranes to take a shower. Others regard this risk as insignificant and consider that the comfort and relaxing effect of a warm bath outweigh the small disadvantage.

In addition to the cleansing of the whole body, soaking in a warm bath may relieve pain and the woman may choose to rest in the bath for a long time. The midwife should invite the mother who is mobile to have a bath or shower whenever she wishes during labour.

Clothing

All hospitals will offer a loose gown to wear but the mother may feel much more comfortable in an old cotton nightdress or a loose shirt. As long as she is aware that the garment may become wet and bloodstained and that she may require more than one, there is no reason to restrict her choice.

RECORDS

The midwife's record of labour is a legal document and must be kept meticulously. Each event must be written down immediately after its occurrence and should be authenticated with the midwife's full signature. An accurate record of the early part of labour provides the basis for management as labour progresses.

The partogram. In recent years the partogram or partograph has been widely accepted as an effective means of recording the progress of labour. It is a chart on which the salient features of labour are entered in a graphic form and therefore provides the opportunity for early identification of deviations from normal. Figure 11.17 shows one example of a partogram but hospitals tend to develop their own to suit their individual requirements. The charts are usually designed to allow for recordings at 15-minute intervals and include:

- fetal heart rate
- maternal temperature
- pulse
- blood pressure
- details of vaginal examinations
- strength of contractions
- frequency of contractions in terms of the number in 10 minutes
- fluid balance
- urine analysis
- drugs administered.

The cervicograph is the diagrammatic representation of the dilatation of the cervix charted against the hours in labour (see Fig. 11.18). Studies have shown (Friedman & Sachtleben 1965, Pearson 1981) that the cervical dilatation time of normal labour has a characteristic sigmoid curve. This curve can be divided into two distinct parts — the latent phase and the active phase.

The latent phase is the period of effacement which begins with the onset of labour and ends when the cervix is 3 cm dilated. In a primigravida this phase lasts from 6–8 hours.

The active phase is the phase of acceleration and is much more rapid. It proceeds at a rate of 1–1.5 cm per hour and a rate of 1 cm an hour in the active phase is commonly accepted as the cut off between normal and abnormal labour. Some centres use a stencil which if superimposed on the cervicograph will identify if the progress of labour lags behind this set rate thus alerting staff to the possibility of prolonged labour.

The disadvantages of using such prescribed parameters of normal is the temptation to make all women fit predetermined criteria for normality. The rate of progress in labour must be considered in the context of the woman's total well-being.

Midwifery record

In some cases the partogram may allow space for a certain amount of comment but usually the midwife will keep a separate written account in which she records her observations of the woman's psychological condition and any other details not included on the graph. If any changes in the birth plan become necessary, the midwife will note down how these were discussed with the woman and her partner and with what outcome. It is relevant to note down what explanations have been given prior to undertaking any procedures and how the woman's consent was obtained.

If it becomes necessary to call a doctor, the midwife records the times and the nature of the message sent including whether the doctor was informed, consulted or summoned to be present. Similarly she will note the doctor's response.

Medical notes

The obstetric record is shared between the midwife and the doctor. The doctor makes notes of his or her findings when he or she visits and any

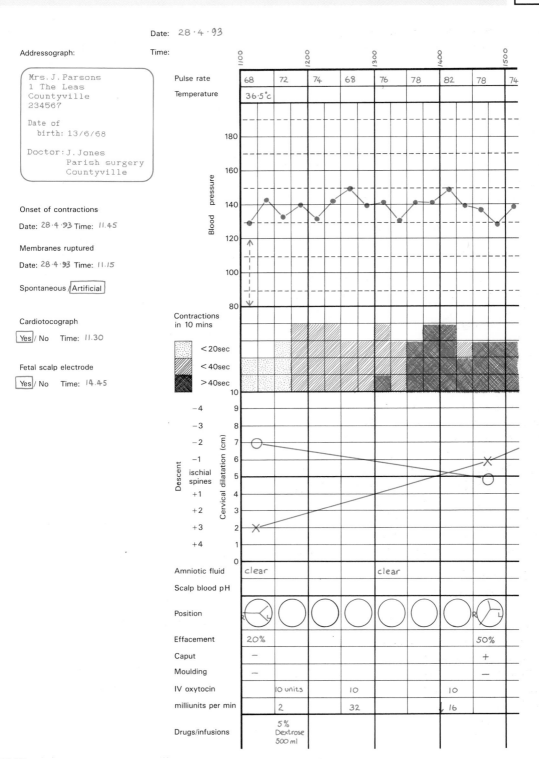

Fig. 11.17
Example of a partogram.

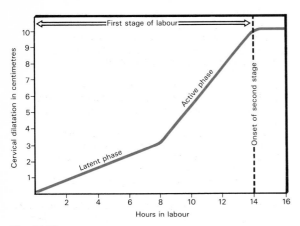

Fig. 11.18
Example of a cervicograph.

prescriptions made. The midwife usually enters the summary of labour and initial details about the baby.

Drug records

As well as being entered on the partogram doses of drugs are recorded on the prescription sheet, in the summary of labour and, in the case of controlled drugs, in the Controlled Drug Register.

INFORMATION TO THE FAMILY

The day on which the baby is born is one of great excitement for the whole family. The partner should be encouraged to act as spokesman and pass on all the news in order to reduce the number of calls to the hospital requesting information.

The person who is the birth companion should be included fully as labour is discussed with the mother and may prove invaluable in interpreting and reinforcing what the midwife wishes to convey to her, as a labouring woman does not always find it easy to concentrate on what she is being told. If the companion is not the partner, the midwife should enquire how he will be kept informed. At all times, priority is given to the closest relatives and the midwife should not divulge information over the telephone unless she is assured that the woman and her partner wish her to do so.

The midwife who communicates with the couple effectively and with sensitivity can enhance their experience and help them to feel secure and supported whatever the circumstances and environment.

Reader Activities

- Establish a relationship with a group of women after 36 weeks of pregnancy.
  — Ask the women to recall information gained from family and friends about the start of labour.
  — Positively reinforce correct information verbalised.
  — Provide information necessary to fill in knowledge gaps to ensure each individual can differentiate between Braxton-Hicks and the regular contractions of true labour.
  — Role play the onset of labour by encouraging each individual to feel her own fundus and time intervals between contractions.

- Select a woman whom you have cared for in labour. Following the normal delivery of her baby invite a student midwife to:
  — examine the baby's head
  — identify caput succedaneum and moulding
  — identify sutures and fontanelles.
  — Using the information obtained encourage the student to determine the position which had been adopted in utero.
  — Explain how this knowledge was obtained on vaginal examination.
  — Discuss the advantages of knowing the position adopted by the fetus in utero.

FURTHER READING

Beazley J M, Lobb M O 1983 Aspects of care in labour. Churchill Livingstone, Edinburgh

Beischer N A, Mackay E V 1986 Obstetrics and the newborn, 2nd edn. Baillière Tindall, London

Bobak I M, Jensen M D, Zalar M K 1989 Maternity and gynecologic care, 4th edn. C V Mosby, St Louis

Bonovich L 1990 Recognizing the onset of labor. Journal of Obstetric Gynecological and Neonatal Nursing 19(2): 141–145

Calder A A 1985 Human labour — an interaction of muscle and gristle. In: The role of prostaglandins in labour. International Congress and Symposium Series Number 92

Cardozo L, Pearce J M 1990 Oxytocin in active-phase abnormalities of labor: a randomized study. Obstetrics and Gynecology 75(2): 152–157

Cunningham F G, MacDonald P C, Grant N F 1989 Williams obstetrics, 18th edn. Prentice-Hall International (UK), London

DHSS 1984 Maternity care in action Part II: Care during childbirth. Chairman: Dame Alison Munro. HMSO, London

Drayton S 1990 Midwifery care in the first stage of labour In: Alexander J, Levy V, Roch S (eds) Intrapartum care: a research based approach. Macmillan, Houndmills

Ferguson J K 1941 A study of the motility of the intact uterus at term. Surgery, Gynecology and Obstetrics 73: 359–366

Flint C 1986 Sensitive midwifery, Heinemann, London

Friedman E A, Sachtleben M R 1965 Station of the fetal presenting part. American Journal of Obstetrics and Gynecology 93(4): 522–529

Gibb D 1988 A practical guide to labour management. Blackwell Scientific, Oxford

Henderson C 1990 Artificial rupture of the membranes In: Alexander J, Levy V, Roch S (eds) Intrapartum care: a research-based approach. Macmillan, Houndmills

Inch S 1982 Birthrights. Hutchinson, London

Llewellyn-Jones D 1990 Fundamentals of obstetrics and gynaecology, 5th edn. Volume one: Obstetrics. Faber, London

Marieb E N 1989 Human anatomy and physiology. Benjamin/Cummings Publishing, California

O'Driscoll K, Meagher D 1986 Active management of labour, 2nd edn. Baillière Tindall, London

Pearson J 1981 Partography. Nursing Mirror (July 8): xxv–xxix

Seitchik J 1987 The management of functional dystocia in the first stage of labour. Clinical Obstetrics and Gynecology 30(1): 42–49

Wuitchik M, Bakal D, Lipshitz J 1989 The clinical significance of pain and cognitive activity in latent labour. Obstetrics and Gynecology 73(1): 25–41

12

Management of the first stage of labour

PATRICIA CASSIDY

Labour, the culmination of pregnancy, is an event with great psychological, social and emotional meaning for the mother and her family. In addition, the woman may experience stress and physical pain and danger may lurk around the corner. The midwife who is the caregiver should display tact and sensitivity, respect the needs of the individual and provide an environment within which each woman can labour and give birth with dignity.

ENVIRONMENT

Physical surroundings should provide protection from harm and be clean and free from the hazards of infection. Facilities should be available for prompt and efficient action in the case of an emergency arising. Soft furnishings, the use of colour and the arrangement of furniture can help to soften a hospital atmosphere with its implications of sickness and institutional rules. The attitude of the staff, however, is much more important than physical surroundings. Anxiety will affect the mother's perception and understanding (Ball 1987) therefore it is essential that the labouring woman is welcomed and encouraged to feel at ease and that the midwife spends time actively listening as the woman recounts the details of the onset of labour. A trusting atmosphere between a woman and her caregivers, a feeling of being among friends and a knowledge of the skills required to cope with the stresses of labour set the scene for a positive childbirth experience (Crowe & von Baeyer 1989, Kitzinger 1985).

EMOTIONAL SUPPORT

The midwife has a traditional role to fulfil, that is being 'with woman' by monitoring the progress of labour and assessing the physical status of mother and fetus. In addition emotional support is provided by exercising skill in imparting confidence, expressing caring and dependability and being an advocate for the childbearing woman. The midwife should display a tolerant non-judgemental attitude, ensuring the woman is accepted whatever her reactions and behaviour may be. Women who feel in control of their own bodies, who retain control of their behaviour and who feel they have an active part in decision-making have a more satisfactory birth experience (Green et al 1990).

Companion in labour
Research has shown that continuous one-to-one support of a woman during labour creates a strong feeling of security and satisfaction (Hodnett & Osborn 1989a and b, Ball 1987) and is associated with a reduction in the length of labour, fewer perinatal complications and a reduced incidence of oxytocin augmentation (Klaus et al 1986). The woman herself is the one who cares most about her baby and therefore she is central to all the decisions made about care during labour. Her chosen companion whether sexual partner, friend or family member should understand this. Ideally he or she would be involved in pre-labour preparation and decision making, have participated in compiling a birth plan and have contingency plans drawn up in the event of everything not remaining straightforward. Admission to hospital is always a traumatic experience and the company of a supportive companion can help reduce anxiety. During labour the companion can keep the woman company, walk with her if she is ambulant in early labour, support her decisions about pain relief and encourage her with breathing techniques.

Providing encouragement and reassurance that labour is progressing is also important, as is helping with physical comfort such as back-rubbing or providing cool cloths or sips of water. The midwife may have to double as the companion since not all women are glad to have a husband or companion present. In some areas a midwife will be assigned to a particular woman and remain with her through her entire labour.

The companion must be encouraged to attend to his (or her) own need for rest and refreshment so that he/she has the necessary stamina to see the labour right through. The midwife should assess events and advise the companion as to the best time to take a break.

The midwife must also appreciate that the companion will have needs. This is particularly evident when a sudden emergency develops. If, for instance, a caesarean section becomes necessary, the midwife must delegate someone to keep the companion fully informed and ensure that he/she is not abandoned and left uncared for.

Explanation
Midwives must also provide support by giving information which encompasses ensuring that the woman understands events, feels free to ask questions and is aware of how labour is progressing. Before performing an examination explanations should be given of what is about to be done and why. Following the procedure the midwife should provide feedback on progress and verbal reinforcement that the woman is capable of managing her own labour and involve both woman and companion if decisions have to be made about care.

Privacy
An unfamiliar setting, the presence of strangers and too many people entering and leaving the room increase stress for the woman, her partner and the midwife. To ensure privacy, individuals should knock before entering, be introduced to all in the room and give an explanation for their presence. Equally the woman has a right to remain alone with her partner if she so wishes and the midwife considers it safe for both mother and fetus.

PREVENTION OF INFECTION

The very nature of the care given during labour may expose both mother and fetus to the risk of infection. The midwife has a responsibility to acquaint herself with the risks, prepare the woman physically during the antenatal period and be scrupulous in her attention to hygiene and asepsis in order to prevent infection occurring.

Mother's well-being during pregnancy

Sound general health is one of the best measures available to resist infection. Antenatal care aims to build up resistance and encourage a healthy lifestyle mainly through education. Information about diet, exercise and hygiene all contribute (see Ch. 9). Socio-economic deprivation is one of the biggest impediments to antenatal health.

Factors affecting resistance

The blood. The haemoglobin level should be adequate and anaemia should be corrected if necessary. White blood cells are needed to fight invading organisms and usually their ability to do so correlates with general health and absence of fatigue.

Nutritional status. In developed countries nutritional status is usually fairly good, although poverty may lead to malnutrition. This may result as much from eating an unwise selection of foods as from being too hard up to buy food. Education in using economical yet nutritious foods, including how to prepare them, may be an invaluable contribution from the midwife.

The skin and membranes. An intact skin provides an excellent barrier to organisms and it is important to protect its integrity. This involves the avoidance of surgical wounds whenever possible, including perineal lacerations and episiotomy. The fetal membranes should also be preserved intact unless there is a positive indication for their rupture which would outweigh the advantage of their protective functions.

Hygiene. A clean body and environment will reduce the organisms which have access to the mother. This implies the need for barrier methods to be used when caring for women with any transmissible infection such as gastro-enteritis, hepatitis or human immunodeficiency virus (HIV) infection.

Rest. A tired, exhausted woman will not be able to combat infection and if the mother has been deprived of sleep and rest prior to admission or during labour, the midwife may need to create an opportunity for sleeping, if necessary by offering a mild sedative drug.

The avoidance of prolonged labour is an important factor in preventing infection.

General hygiene and care of the environment

Hospitals are notorious sources of infection which can be resistant to antibiotic treatment. A modern maternity unit should be constructed so as to limit the spread of such infection. It should be sited at a distance from any source of pathogenic organisms and should be designed for easy and effective cleaning and in a way which will reduce the transfer of airborne organisms. Traffic in and out of a delivery unit should be restricted to people having direct business there and individual rooms should be treated on the same basis. Baths, sinks and toilets should be scrupulously cleaned and disinfected between users as necessary. Beds and rooms are also cleaned thoroughly after use. It is the responsibility of the midwife to ensure that high standards of cleanliness are maintained even if she does not have managerial control over domestic services.

Personal hygiene is important for both mothers and their attendants. The woman should be encouraged to bathe and wash as necessary to maintain personal freshness and the midwife must wash her hands before and after examining the mother and wear gloves when handling used sanitary pads, bloodstained linen or body fluids. The midwife will wish to pay particular attention to her own hygiene as she is in close proximity to the woman and is working in a very warm environment.

Asepsis and antisepsis

A woman's perineal area is bound to be contaminated and procedures such as vaginal examination and delivery itself can never be completely sterile. However the midwife must always use sterile equipment and aseptic technique in order to avoid introducing foreign organisms into the genital tract.

Restriction of invasive techniques

Certain invasive techniques, such as the performance of vaginal examinations, are necessary during labour but the midwife should aim to reduce these to a minimum and ensure that she has a sound reason before embarking on a procedure. Women whose labours are prolonged are at particular risk of infection and are often subjected to a number of invasive procedures including the administration of intravenous fluids. Where progress in labour is slow and it is necessary to involve a doctor, the midwife can avoid a vaginal examination being duplicated by inviting the doctor to do it in the first instance.

POSITION AND MOBILITY

The adoption of the upright position during labour will facilitate efficient uterine contractions, shorten the latent phase and reduce the need for analgesia (Andrews & Chrzanowski 1990, Kakol 1989). Flexibility during labour allows the mother to seek and find the position most suited to her. She may walk about, rock, adopt a kneeling position or squat. The all-fours position may be comfortable if the fetus is in an occipitoposterior position as it relieves the associated backache. Midwives should accommodate the mother's wish to choose her own position remembering that, if a recumbent position is adopted, compression of the inferior vena cava may occur with consequent supine hypotension. Therefore, if the mother wishes to lie down, a lateral position is preferable and this allows the midwife to auscultate the fetal heart and monitor uterine contractions.

Other factors governing choice

Analgesia. If the mother has accepted or requested narcotic analgesia, she will be unable to walk around because she will be unsteady on her feet after receiving the narcotic. A lateral position or supported sitting is suitable.

Epidural analgesia normally demands that a woman should be in bed. She may be sitting up or lying on her side once the anaesthetic has taken effect.

Monitoring. The use of a cardiotocograph may appear to limit the choice of position. A telemetric apparatus allows the woman to walk around freely, provided that she remains within a given range. A conventional cardiotocograph does not necessarily confine the woman to bed but accurate external monitoring of uterine contractions may be difficult if she is very mobile.

Fetal condition. The supine position allows the uterus to compress the inferior vena cava, resulting in maternal hypotension. This not only reduces placental blood flow and thereby fetal oxygenation but also inhibits effective uterine action. More upright positions or a lateral position are to be preferred.

Intravenous infusion. The siting of an intravenous infusion should not in itself prevent mobility as the mother may walk around with a drip stand. The midwife should, however, take account of the reason for the infusion as this may influence the choice of position.

Complications. A woman who has had an antepartum haemorrhage or who has ruptured membranes when the fetal head is still high will be confined to bed.

NUTRITION

Advice prior to admission

The woman's need in labour is for energy and it is carbohydrate that will provide it. Foods such as toast, breakfast cereal, fruit juice, tea, plain biscuits and clear broth are easily digested. Jelly and ice-cream may also be refreshing. Fluids may be taken freely, although fizzy and very sweet drinks may induce vomiting.

Intake in early labour

Opinions are divided and policies vary widely within different hospitals. In some centres all women receive nothing to eat after labour is established and are allowed only ice chips to suck. In others a low residue, low fat diet may be allowed. 'There is widespread concern that eating and drinking during labour will put women at an increased and unacceptable risk of regurgitation and aspiration of gastric contents' (Johnson et al 1990). Aspirated contents from the stomach may contain undigested food and predispose to airway obstruction; if fasting, the strongly acidic gastric juice can cause a chemical pneumonitis if inhaled (Mendelson's syndrome). The cardiac sphincter, rendered inefficient by the effects of progesterone, allows a passive leak of stomach contents into the pharynx when loss of consciousness is induced with general anaesthesia. This, combined with the oedema of the pharynx so often present in pregnancy, makes intubation by the anaesthetist a difficult procedure.

In some centres no food is permitted after labour is established on the basis that an anaesthetic could be needed. In others, because of the relatively low risk of general anaesthesia being required in normal labour, women are allowed light diet and fluids if they want to eat or drink. Different foods and fluids empty from the stomach at different rates and gastric emptying is prolonged following the administration of narcotic analgesia. In an effort to reduce gastric volume and decrease the gastric acidity of the labouring woman, prophylactic antacids may be administered (see Ch. 28).

Glycogenic and fluid requirements

The vigorous muscle contractions of the uterus during labour demand a continuous supply of glucose. If this is not obtained from the diet the body will start to metabolise protein and fat stores in an effort to provide glucose (gluconeogenesis) without which uterine muscle inertia will occur. This relatively inefficient method of producing glucose results in the occurrence of keto-acidosis. If no food is allowed, an intravenous infusion may be sited to correct the homeostatic imbalance by providing glucose and fluids. Care must be taken to assess the individual's needs and to avoid high concentrations of glucose which artificially increase fetal blood glucose levels thereby causing fetal hyperinsulinism.

Comfort

If the woman is permitted to follow her inclinations for drinks she is unlikely to become dehydrated.

Simple measures such as brushing her teeth or using a mouthwash can help relieve the discomfort of a dry and uncomfortable mouth.

BLADDER CARE

The woman should be encouraged to empty her bladder every $1\frac{1}{2}$–2 hours during labour. The midwife should not rely on the mother to request to use the toilet as the sensation of needing to micturate may be reduced and will be absent if there is an effective epidural anaesthetic in progress. If the woman is ambulant she may visit the toilet; the quantity of urine passed should be measured and a specimen obtained for testing. If the woman expresses a desire to defaecate, she may be confusing the sensation with that of imminent delivery.

A full bladder may initially prevent the fetal head from entering the pelvic brim and later impede descent of the fetal head. It will also inhibit effective uterine action. In all cases of delay in labour the midwife should ascertain whether the bladder is full and encourage the woman to empty it. If the bladder remains full, the bladder neck can become nipped between the fetal head and the symphysis pubis. This may give rise to bruising which can slough during the puerperium leaving a vesicovaginal fistula.

Retention of urine. Urinary retention in labour may occur in association with hypotonic uterine action. A woman who is unable to visit the toilet may find it difficult to empty her bladder into a bedpan. The midwife should provide privacy and ensure maximum comfort by placing the bedpan on a stool or chair or letting the woman adopt a squatting position on the bed. The sound or feel of water can also help to trigger the micturition reflex. If the bladder is incompletely emptied or the woman is unable to void for some hours it will become necessary to pass a catheter.

Catheterisation. A plastic disposable catheter is used. If difficulty is encountered while introducing the catheter, the sterile, gloved forefinger of the left hand should be inserted into the vagina and placed along its anterior wall. The tip of the catheter can then be felt and if it is directed parallel with the finger in the vagina, the catheter will enter the bladder without injury to the urethra. If the catheter is obstructed by the fetal head, upward pressure on the head by the finger in the vagina will permit passage of the catheter.

OBSERVATIONS

Mother

Reaction to labour

As with other life events, women vary in their reactions to labour. Some may view the contractions experienced as a positive, motivating, life-giving force. Others may feel them as pain and resist them. One woman may welcome the event with excitement because soon she will see her baby, another may be glad the pregnancy is over and with it the cumbersome ungainliness she experienced. However she views labour, the preparatory phase of pregnancy is at an end and within a relatively short period a baby will be born. There may be feelings of apprehension and fear in case she does not conform to the social expectations of her culture, anxiety in case the experience is painful and concern about her ability to control pain. As labour progresses she may feel less confident in her ability to cope with the relentless nature of the contractions which control her body. The midwife, with her skilful observations, can do much to encourage and help the mother whose expectation is 'to be sustained by another human being, to have relief from pain, to have a safe outcome for self and fetus, to have attitudes and behaviour accepted and to receive bodily care' (Mackey & Lock 1989).

If the midwife concentrates her attention on the woman, she can help to absorb and deflect some of her anxieties. She should give her accurate and easily understood information about her progress and be lavish in praise and encouragement. She will also determine the woman's need for pain relief. The management of pain is discussed in Chapter 13.

Vital signs

Pulse rate. A steady pulse rate is an indication that the woman is in good condition. If the rate increases to more than 100 beats per minute it may be indicative of infection, ketosis or haemorrhage. A rising pulse rate is also a key sign of a ruptured uterus (see Ch. 27).

It is usual to record the pulse rate every 1 or 2 hours during early labour and every 15–30 minutes when labour is more advanced.

Temperature. This should remain within the normal range. Pyrexia is indicative of infection or ketosis. Temperature should be recorded every 4 hours.

Blood pressure is measured every 4 hours unless it is abnormal when more frequent recordings are necessary. The blood pressure must be monitored very closely following the instillation of local anaesthetic into the epidural space (see Ch. 28).

The effect of labour may be to further elevate a raised blood pressure and the midwife must bear this in mind when caring for a woman who has had pre-eclampsia or essential hypertension during pregnancy. Hypotension may be caused by the supine position, shock or as a result of epidural anaesthesia.

Urinalysis

All urine passed during labour must be tested for glucose, ketones and protein. Ketones may occur as a result of starvation or maternal distress when all available energy has been utilised. Unless the mother has recently eaten a large quantity of carbohydrate, glucose is only found in the urine following intravenous administration. A trace of protein may be present following rupture of the membranes but more significant proteinuria may indicate worsening pre-eclampsia.

Fluid balance

A record should be kept of all urine passed to ensure that the bladder is being emptied (see above). If an intravenous infusion is in progress the fluids administered must be recorded accurately. It is particularly important to note how much fluid remains if a bag is changed when only partially used.

Progress

Abdominal examination

An initial abdominal examination is carried out when the midwife first examines the mother. This should be repeated at intervals throughout labour in order to assess the length, strength and frequency of contractions and the descent of the presenting part. The method is described in Chapter 10.

Contractions. The frequency, length and strength of the contractions should be noted. The strength of a contraction cannot be judged by the reaction of the woman but always by laying a hand on the uterus and noting the degree of hardness during a contraction and by timing its length. Some women appear to experience pain and yet the contractions may be neither long nor strong and very little is accomplished; other women appear to suffer very little, yet good progress is made.

When a uterine contraction begins, it is painless for a number of seconds and painless again at the end, so the midwife is aware of the approach of a contraction before the woman feels it and this knowledge can be utilised when giving inhalational analgesia (see Ch. 13). The uterus should always feel softer between contractions. Contractions which are unduly long or very strong and in quick succession give cause for concern as fetal hypoxia may develop.

If a cardiotocograph is in use, the contractions will be recorded electronically. This may be done by means of an external pressure transducer positioned over the uterine fundus and kept in place by an abdominal belt. For effective monitoring the belt must be relatively tight which may cause discomfort to the mother. The midwife must remember that such external monitoring cannot accurately measure the strength of uterine contractions. The size of the peak shown on the tracing is directly related to the ease with which contractions can be felt and not to the intensity of the contraction itself. The thickness of the abdominal wall will affect the reading as will movement of the mother.

If an accurate measurement of the intensity of uterine contractions is required, an internal trans- ducer should be passed into the uterine cavity. A fluid-filled catheter is frequently used but this has the disadvantage that it may become blocked with vernix, meconium or blood clot. A transducer-tipped catheter avoids this problem and is easier to place.

Descent of the presenting part. During the first stage of labour, descent can be followed almost entirely by abdominal palpation. It is usual to describe the level in terms of the fifths of the head which can still be felt above the brim (see Figs 10.32 and 11.16).

In the primigravida the fetal head is usually engaged before labour begins. If this is not the case, the level of the head must be estimated frequently by abdominal palpation in order to observe whether the head will pass through the brim with the aid of good contractions.

When the head is engaged, the occipital pro-tuberance can only be felt with difficulty from above but the sinciput may still be palpable, due to increased flexion of the head, until the occiput reaches the pelvic floor and rotates forwards.

Vaginal examination

While it is not essential to examine the woman vaginally at frequent intervals, it may be useful to do so when progress is in doubt or another indication arises (see Ch. 11). The features which are indicative of progress are effacement and dilatation of the cervix, and descent, flexion and rotation of the fetal head.

Effacement and dilatation of the cervix. In normal labour the primigravid cervix effaces before dilating, whereas in the multigravida these two events occur simultaneously. In many centres, dilatation of the cervix up to 3 cm is discounted when calculating the length of labour because of the difficulty of deciding prospectively whether a small amount of dilatation indicates that true labour has begun. (See also latent and active phases of labour, Ch. 11.)

Progressive dilatation is monitored as labour continues and if active management is practised (see below) it will be compared with the cervico-graph (Fig. 11.18).

Descent. When assessed vaginally, the level or station of the presenting part is estimated in relation to the ischial spines which are fixed points at the outlet of the bony pelvis. During normal labour the head descends progressively (see Fig. 11.15). The midwife must be aware, while estimating whether the head is lower than previously, that marked moulding or a large caput will give a false impression of the level of the fetal head.

Flexion. In vertex presentations, progress depends on increased flexion. The spine is attached nearer to the back of the skull than the front. When the head is driven down onto the pelvic floor it encounters resistance: a lever principle causes the anterior part of the head to flex because there is less counter-pressure on it from above. The midwife assesses flexion by the position of the sutures and fontanelles. If the head is fully flexed, the posterior fontanelle becomes almost central; if the head is deflexed, both anterior and posterior fontanelles are palpable.

Rotation is assessed by noting changes in the position of the fetus between one examination and the next. The sutures and fontanelles are palpated in order to determine position. If insufficient information is gained to make a definitive diagnosis, a record is made of what *is* felt and the findings will be evaluated with the abdominal findings at the time and compared with the findings of earlier or later vaginal examinations.

The fetus

Fetal condition during labour can be assessed by obtaining information about the fetal heart rate and patterns, the pH of the fetal blood and the amniotic fluid.

The fetal heart

The fetal heart may be assessed intermittently or continuously.

Intermittent recording. This term is used when the fetal heart is auscultated at intervals using a monaural fetal stethoscope (Pinard's) or a Doppler ultrasound apparatus (Doptone or Sonicaid). The following assessments of the fetal heart can be made:

Rate. This should be counted over a complete minute in order to allow for variations. The rate should be between 120 and 160 beats per minute (bpm). The Doppler apparatus can be used throughout a contraction but listening during a contraction with a monaural stethoscope is uncomfortable for the woman and the fetal heart sounds may be inaudible. Normally the rate is maintained during a contraction and immediately after it. Episodes of fetal bradycardia may suggest hypoxia (see below).

Rhythm. The normal fetal heart has a coupled beat which should remain steady. Any noticeable irregularity in the rhythm may give cause for concern.

Continuous recording. This depends on the use of electronic apparatus in the form of a fetal heart monitor. Continuous recording usually combines a fetal cardiograph and a maternal tocograph in a cardiotocograph apparatus (CTG). This presents a graphic record of the response of the fetal heart to uterine activity as well as information about its rate and rhythm. The CTG can be applied for periods of about 20 minutes (periodic cardiotocography) or be used for the whole of labour (continuous cardiotocography).

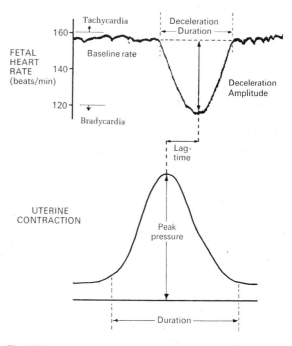

Fig. 12.1
Terms used in describing continuous fetal heart traces.

Method. An ultrasound transducer may be strapped to the abdomen at the point where the fetal heart is heard at maximum intensity. This method is non-invasive and does not require rupture of the membranes. The quality of the fetal heart recording may be affected by the thickness of the abdominal wall, fetal position, maternal or fetal movement and uterine contractions.

A better quality recording may be obtained by applying an electrode to the fetal scalp over a bone. In order to achieve this the membranes must be ruptured and the cervix be at least 2–3 cm dilated. The electrode is connected to the CTG by electrical wiring. A small scalp wound is inevitable but this rarely causes problems.

Internal cardiography may be used in conjunction with telemetry to monitor the fetal heart when the mother wishes to move away from the machine. A portable battery-operated transmitter is carried about by the ambulant woman. The scalp electrode transmits the fetal heart recording by radio to the cardiotocograph where it is recorded on the strip chart. It is impossible to obtain a recording of uterine activity when the mother is walking about but if she depresses a hand-held button at the onset of each contraction the strip chart will be marked accordingly.

Findings. The cardiotocograph provides information on:

- baseline fetal heart rate
- baseline variability
- response of the fetal heart to uterine contractions.

Baseline fetal heart rate. This is the fetal heart rate between uterine contractions. A rate more rapid than 160 bpm is termed *baseline tachycardia*; a rate slower than 120 bpm is *baseline bradycardia*. Either may be indicative of hypoxia but fetal tachycardia may be associated with maternal ketosis and in some fetuses the baseline rate is constant at between 110 and 120 bpm. Continuous compression of the umbilical cord, as in cord prolapse, will result in a prolonged, severe bradycardia.

Baseline variability. Electrical activity in the fetal heart results in minute variations in the length of each beat. This causes the tracing to appear as a jagged, rather than a smooth, line. The baseline rate should vary by at least 5 beats over a period of 1 minute. Loss of this variability may indicate fetal hypoxia but may also be noted for a short period after the administration of maternal pethidine which depresses the cardiac reflex centre in the fetal brain. Periods of 'fetal sleep' also cause a reduction in variability and commonly last for 20–30 minutes even in advanced labour (Gibb 1988).

PROLONGED ACCELERATION PATTERN

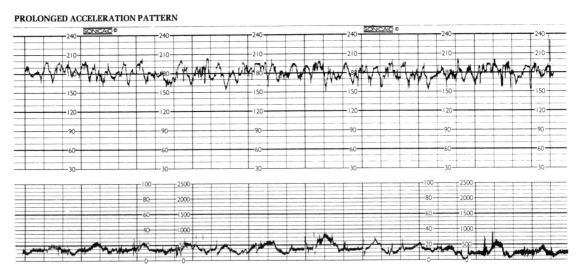

Fig. 12.2
Baseline tachycardia.

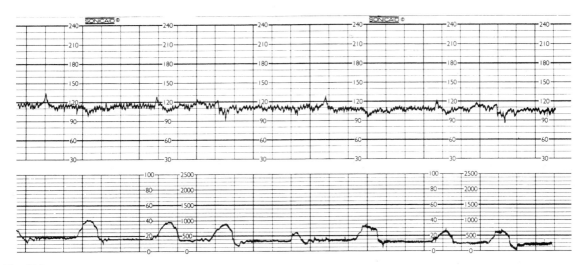

Fig. 12.3
Baseline bradycardia — normal.

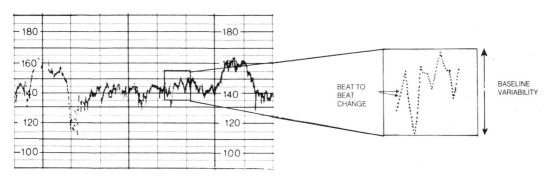

Fig. 12.4
Baseline variability.

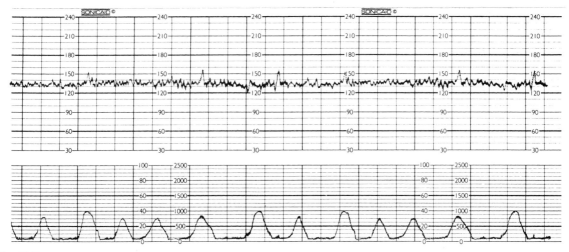

Fig. 12.5
Baseline variability: normal baseline rate.

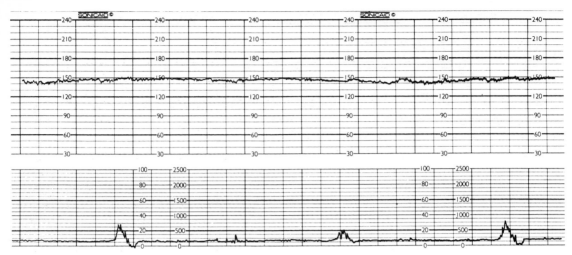

Fig. 12.6
Uncomplicated loss of baseline variability: normal rate, no decelerations.

Response of the fetal heart to uterine contractions. The fetal heart rate will normally remain steady or accelerate during uterine contractions. In order to assess the significance of fetal heart rate decelerations accurately, their exact relationship to uterine contractions must be noted. An *early deceleration* begins at or after the onset of a contraction, reaches its lowest point at the peak of the contraction and returns to the baseline rate by the time the contraction has finished. On the graph it produces a mirror image of the contraction. An early deceleration is commonly associated with compression of the fetal head, for example as it engages, but may indicate early fetal hypoxia.

A *late deceleration* begins during or after a contraction, reaches its nadir after the peak of the contraction and has not recovered by the time that the contraction has ended. Sometimes the deceleration has barely recovered by the onset of the next contraction. The *time lag* between the peak of the contraction and the nadir of the deceleration is more significant of severity than the drop in the fetal heart rate. If this occurs

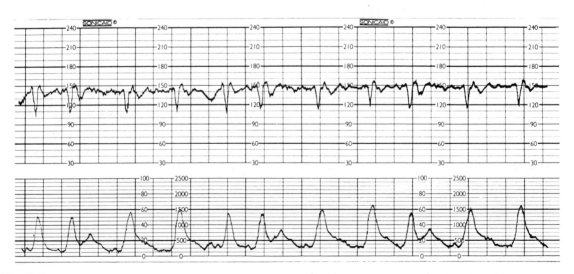

Fig. 12.7
Early decelerations.

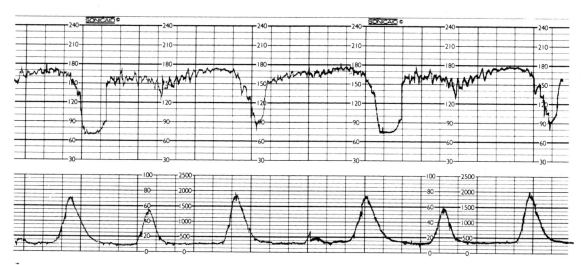

Fig. 12.8
Late decelerations.

the doctor must be informed as it always indicates fetal hypoxia. A vaginal examination should be performed to exclude prolapse of the cord as late decelerations are suggestive of cord compression.

Interpretation of recordings. If contact is lost, artifacts may appear on the tracing which can be confused with abnormal fetal heart patterns especially decelerations. However, the midwife is cautioned against disregarding abnormalities of the tracing on the assumption that the machine is 'playing up'. An attempt should be made to improve the quality of the recording and the fetal heart rate should be checked using a monaural stethoscope or Doppler apparatus.

Some mothers will request avoidance of electronic monitoring. This request should be respected as research has not confirmed a need for continuous monitoring in normal labour (Pello et al 1988). The mother will not usually object to the use of a hand-held Doppler to monitor the fetal heart; her concern is commonly that she wishes to be free to move around. Some units will suggest a 20-minute period of monitoring on admission with or without additional periods throughout labour.

Fetal blood sampling

The fetus who has become hypoxic will also become acidotic as the pH of its blood is lowered.

The normal pH of fetal blood is 7.35 or above. If it falls below 7.25 in the first stage of labour, action must be taken: in the second stage of labour a level of 7.2 is acceptable if delivery is imminent. Cardiotocograph recording of the fetal heart may suggest hypoxia but acidosis can only be confirmed by fetal blood sampling.

An amnioscope is passed through the cervix to provide access to the fetal scalp. A small blade is used to puncture the skin and 0.5 ml of blood is collected in a heparinised capillary tube. The

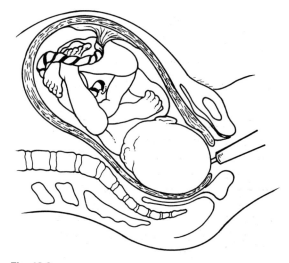

Fig. 12.9
Fetal blood sampling. Access to fetal scalp via amnioscope passed through the cervix.

specimen must be analysed immediately. While it is in transit to the blood gas analyser, care must be taken to ensure that the blood is not allowed to clot and does not come into contact with atmospheric oxygen. To prevent clotting an iron filing is added to the tube and moved backwards and forwards with a magnet to mix the heparin with the blood. The ends of the capillary tube are sealed with wax to prevent spillage and exclude air during transit.

Amniotic fluid

Following rupture of the membranes amniotic fluid escapes from the uterus continuously and may provide information about the condition of the fetus. This fluid should normally remain clear. If the fetus becomes hypoxic, he may pass meconium, as hypoxia causes relaxation of the anal sphincter. The amniotic fluid becomes green as a result of meconium staining. Amniotic fluid which is a muddy yellow colour or which is only slightly green may signify previous distress from which the fetus has recovered.

If the breech is presenting and is compacted in the pelvis, the fetus may pass meconium due to the compression of the abdomen; a fetus presenting by the breech is also prone to fetal distress and may pass meconium as a result of hypoxia.

In the rare case of a fetus who is severely affected by Rhesus iso-immunisation the amniotic fluid may be golden-yellow due to an excess of bilirubin.

Bleeding which is of sudden onset at the time of rupture of the membranes may be the result of a ruptured vasa praevia and is an acute emergency (see Ch. 27).

Fetal distress

Fetal distress occurs when the fetus suffers oxygen deprivation and becomes hypoxic. Severe hypoxia may result in the baby being stillborn or he may be asphyxiated at birth and suffer brain damage.

Signs of fetal distress. Any or all of the following may be present:

- fetal tachycardia which is an early sign of oxygen deprivation

- fetal bradycardia or fetal heart rate decelerations related to uterine contractions
- passage of meconium-stained amniotic fluid.

Management of fetal distress. When signs of fetal distress occur the midwife must call a doctor. If Syntocinon is being administered, it must be stopped and the woman placed in a favourable position, usually on her left side. In cases of maternal oxygen lack, such as eclampsia or shock due to antepartum haemorrhage, oxygen may be given via a face mask. The doctor may wish to take a sample of fetal blood for testing and arrangements should be made for this.

If fetal distress is more than transient, delivery will be expedited. In the first stage of labour this will necessitate caesarean section. In the second stage of labour an episiotomy may be sufficient to effect delivery but failing this a forceps delivery or ventouse extraction may be performed. In all cases of delivery following fetal distress a paediatrician is summoned to be present.

PRETERM LABOUR

Preterm labour (for causes, see Ch. 35) is defined as labour occurring before the 37th completed week of pregnancy, and judging whether it has started or not is just as difficult regardless of the period of gestation. Of all women who present for help because of preterm uterine contractions, between 30 and 50% will have spontaneous cessation of contractions and pregnancy will continue (Pearce 1985). Increased perinatal survival attributed to increased neonatal facilities and appropriately trained personnel has altered policies towards management of the woman in preterm labour. If the labouring woman is not in an area where there is a special care unit and resident neonatal staff she should be transferred there as quickly as possible. Betamimetic drugs to suppress uterine contractions (tocolysis) may be administered until the woman has been transferred to such a centre. Ritodrine hydrochloride (Yutopar) and salbutamol (Ventolin) are commonly used betamimetic drugs. Side-effects include maternal tachycardia, palpitations and hypotension and fetal tachycardia. The main contra-indications are hypertension, haemorrhage, rupture of the membranes and drug incompatibilities.

Ritodrine is administered by intravenous infusion commencing with a low dose which is increased at 10-minute intervals until contractions cease. The infusion is maintained at the same rate for 24 hours. Oral ritodrine is commenced half an hour before the intravenous infusion is completed and continued for 14 days or more.

Management of preterm labour

No attempt should be made to arrest labour if pregnancy has advanced to 34 weeks gestation and the fetus is estimated to have grown to 2500 g (Pearce 1985). Generally speaking the more preterm the fetus the greater the risks from labour and delivery. Skilled care is required for the woman and the fetus during labour. The mother is faced with an unexpected emotional crisis because of the interruption of the normal progress of pregnancy. The high perinatal mortality rate means the woman and her partner have to face the possibility of the death or disability of their baby. The fetus is at risk of hypoxia and therefore continuous electronic heart rate monitoring is advisable. To reduce the risk of intraventricular haemorrhage an episiotomy should be performed unless there is a very relaxed vaginal outlet. Caesarean section may be undertaken if there is an abnormal presentation or the infant is expected to be of very low birth weight. If the mother requires analgesia during labour, narcotics which cross the placental barrier and depress the fetal respiratory centre should be avoided. The presence of a paediatrician at delivery will ensure that skilled resuscitation is carried out promptly. For management of the baby see Chapter 35.

ACTIVE MANAGEMENT OF LABOUR

The term *active management of labour* is used to describe a range of policies which aim to prevent prolonged labour. It implies a commitment to attaining delivery within a fixed time span, usually 12–18 hours. The use of artificial rupture of the membranes and Syntocinon augmentation of contractions is favoured. Many obstetricians will be guided by the cervicograph; if the curve of actual dilatation is 2 hours later than the guide curve which is being followed, intervention is considered to be justified.

Principles

The policy of active management has been developed in the search for greater fetal and maternal safety during labour. Obstetricians strive to lower the perinatal mortality rate and to avoid the maternal exhaustion and despondency which accompany a long and tedious labour.

Close observation of maternal and fetal condition is essential to this type of management and vaginal examination will be performed at regular intervals, for example 2- or 4-hourly. Cardiotocography will often be carried out on a continuous basis. Membranes are usually ruptured at an early stage, by artificial means if necessary. If dilatation of the cervix is slow or lags behind the cervicograph guide curve, Syntocinon infusion will be commenced in order to augment contractions (see Ch. 25).

Disadvantages

Whereas some women are pleased to be guaranteed delivery within a specified time, others are more interested in achieving delivery by natural means and dislike the suggestion of intervention. Maternal preference must be taken into account when offering active management of labour.

In active management the membranes are artificially ruptured in order to shorten the labour but this is at the cost of the advantages of intact membranes. Some would also question the advantage of speed for its own sake. If the membranes are intact, hydrostatic pressure is applied evenly to the placental surface and to the fetus and the amniotic sac prevents the entry of pathogenic organisms.

It is less easy to take advantage of an upright position if active management is practised. However, the midwife may still be able to assist a mother to use positions which favour uterine action, such as the left lateral or a kneeling position, if necessary by putting a mattress on the floor.

Contractions augmented by Syntocinon may be experienced as more painful than those of spontaneous labour. This may in turn necessitate the use of pain-relieving drugs which may disappoint the woman who had hoped to manage without them.

The midwife's role

If a policy of active management is practised, it is the midwife's responsibility to inform the mother fully of what procedures to expect and to help her to make a decision on the basis of that information. Whatever the mother's preferences, the midwife will give supportive care and endeavour to achieve an outcome in keeping with that choice.

RECORDS

Throughout the first stage of labour the midwife must keep meticulous records of all events and of the woman's physical and psychological condition and the condition of her fetus (see Ch. 11). While observing the progress of labour she should be alert for signs of the second stage (see Ch. 14).

An individualised approach to care will attempt to follow the plan which was devised in pregnancy. If the woman changes her mind as her labour progresses adjustments can be made. Whether or not a formal birth plan has been prepared the midwife who is caring for the woman should communicate effectively with her, evaluate whether the labour is proceeding as expected and listen to her requests. A comprehensive record of the discussions which take place about changes in plan or about proposed measures which the midwife may suggest will ensure that the closest possible attention is paid to achieving the outcome that the parents are hoping for and also provide an excellent documented history of the labour.

Acknowledgement

Figures 12.1–12.8 are reproduced from *Fetal heart rate patterns and their clinical interpretation* (Sonicaid Obstetrics) by kind permission of Sonicaid Limited, Chichester, West Sussex.

Reader Activity

After caring for a particular woman through the whole of her labour attempt to measure the quality of care which has been provided.

Select the appropriate case notes and examine records for nursing observations. Then review with the mother the events of her childbirth experience. Show an interest in finding out how the mother feels about her labour. Initiate dialogue by asking questions, such as:

- 'Tell me about . . .'
- 'Can you tell me how you felt about . . .?'

These require more than a yes or no answer and by describing a situation the woman should understand it better herself.

Allow the mother to express any feelings of anger or embarrassment or pride in her achievement. In this way emotional support is provided by the midwife as the woman talks through her feelings and compares what she expected to happen with the actual event.

Re-examine the case notes following the interview with the mother to identify areas where care could have been improved.

USEFUL ADDRESSES

Association for Improvements in the
Maternity Services (AIMS)
40 Kingswood Avenue
London NW6 6LS

International Active Birth Centre
55 Dartmouth Park Road
London NW5 1SL

Maternity Alliance
15 Britannia Street
London WC1X 9JP

National Birthday Trust Fund
27 Sussex Place
Regents Park
London NW1 4RG

National Childbirth Trust
Alexandra House
Oldham Terrace
Acton
London W3 6NH

REFERENCES

Andrews C M, Chrzanowski M 1990 Maternal position, labor, and comfort. Applied Nursing Research 3(1): 7–13

Ball J A 1987 Reactions to motherhood. Cambridge University Press, Cambridge

Crowe K, von Baeyer C 1989 Predictors of a positive childbirth experience. Birth 16(2): 59–63

Gibb D 1988 A practical guide to labour management. Blackwell Scientific Publications, Oxford

Green J M, Coupland V A, Kitzinger J V 1990 Expectations, experiences and psychological outcomes of childbirth: A prospective study of 825 women. Birth 17(1): 15–24

Hibbard B 1987 The aetiology of preterm labour. British Medical Journal 294: 59–60

Hodnett E D, Osborn R W 1989a Effects of continuous intrapartum professional support on childbirth outcomes. Research in Nursing and Health 12: 289–297

Hodnett E D, Osborn R W 1989b A randomized trial of the effects of montrice support during labor: Mother's views two to four weeks postpartum. Birth 16(4): 177–183

Johnson C et al 1989 Nutrition and hydration in labour. In: Chalmers I, Enkin M, Keirse M J N C (eds) Effective care in pregnancy and childbirth, Vol. 2 Oxford University Press, Oxford, pp 827–832

Kakol K 1989 Position in labour — does mother know best? The Professional Nurse 4 (July): 481–484

Kitzinger S 1985 What do women want? In: Studd J (ed) The management of labour. Blackwell Scientific Publications, Oxford

Klaus M H, Kennell J, Robertson S, Sosa R 1986 Effects of social support during parturition on maternal and infant morbidity. British Medical Journal 293: 585–587

Mackey M C, Lock S E 1989 Women's expectations of the labor and delivery nurse. Journal of Obstetric Gynecological and Neonatal Nursing 18 (November/December): 505–512

Pearce M J 1985 The management of pre-term labour. In: Studd J (ed) The management of labour. Blackwell Scientific Publications, Oxford

Pello L C, Dawes G S, Smith J, Redman C 1988 Screening of the fetal heart rate in early labour. British Journal of Obstetrics and Gynaecology 95: 1128–1136

Taylor K, Copstick S 1985 Psychological care in labour. Nursing Mirror 161(4): 42–43

Thomas E A 1987 Pre-operative fasting — a question of routine? Nursing Times 83(7): 46–47

FURTHER READING

Alexander J, Levy V, Roch S (eds) 1990 Intrapartum care — a research-based approach. Macmillan Education, Houndmills

Balaskas J 1983 Active birth. Unwin Paperbacks, London

Ball J A 1987 Reactions to motherhood. Cambridge University Press, Cambridge

Beischer N A, Mackay E V 1986 Obstetrics and the newborn, 2nd edn. Baillière Tindall, London

Flint C 1986 Sensitive midwifery. Heinemann, London

Inch S 1982 Birthrights. Hutchinson, London

Llewellyn-Jones D 1990 Fundamentals of obstetrics and gynaecology, 5th edn. Volume one: Obstetrics. Faber, London

Maternity Services Advisory Committee 1984 Maternity care in action Part II: Care during childbirth. Chairman: Dame Alison Munro. HMSO, London

Oakley A 1980 Women confined. Martin Robertson, Oxford

O'Driscoll K, Meagher D 1986 Active management of labour, 2nd edn. W B Saunders, Philadelphia

Reading A 1983 Psychological aspects of pregnancy. Longman, London

13

Pain relief and comfort in labour

RUTH BEVIS

In the late twentieth century women are wanting to take control of their bodies, make informed choices and to be treated as individuals. Labour is one of the major life-events a woman will experience. Its memory will remain with her; negative impressions may give rise to psychological sequelae with implications for the whole family. This chapter explores the variety of ways in which midwives use their skills to achieve for each woman and her partner in labour an experience which they regard as positive.

PERCEPTION OF PAIN

The way in which an individual perceives and reacts to pain is affected by many different factors.

Fear and anxiety will heighten the individual's response to pain. Fear of the unknown, fear of being left alone to cope with an experience such as labour and fear of failing to cope well will increase anxiety. A previous bad experience will also increase anxiety.

Personality plays a part and the woman who is naturally tense and anxious will cope less well with stress than one who is relaxed and confident.

Fatigue. The woman who is already fatigued by several hours of labour, perhaps preceded by a period when sleep was disturbed by the discomforts of late pregnancy, will be less able to tolerate pain.

Cultural and social factors also play a part. Some cultures expect stoicism while others encourage expression of feeling. The perception of pain may be altered if the woman has experienced pain and hardship previously.

Expectations colour the experience. The woman who is realistic in her expectations of labour and about her likely response to it is probably the best equipped, as long as she feels confident that she will receive the help and support she needs and is assured that she will receive appropriate analgesia.

PHYSIOLOGY OF PAIN

Pain pathways

The *pain pathway* or ascending sensory tract originates in the sensory nerve endings at the site of trauma. The impulse travels along the sensory nerves to the dorsal root ganglion of the relevant spinal nerve and into the posterior horn of the spinal cord. This is known as the *first neurone*.

The *second neurone* arises in the posterior horn, crosses over within the spinal cord (the sensory decussation) and transmits the impulse via the

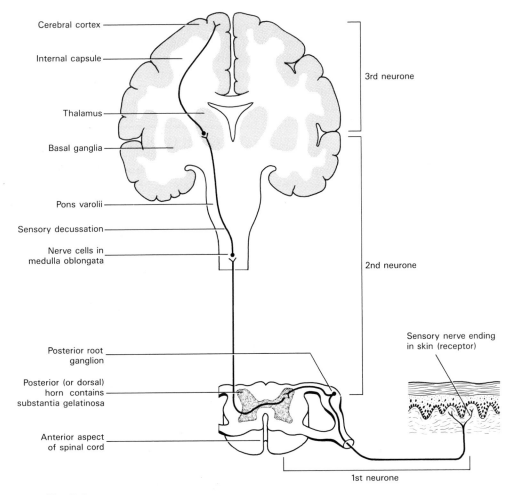

Fig. 13.1
The sensory pathway showing the structures involved in the appreciation of pain. (Reproduced from Bevis (1984) by courtesy of Baillière Tindall.)

medulla oblongata, pons varolii and the midbrain to the thalamus.

From here it travels along the *third neurone* to the sensory cortex.

Acute pain. Such sensations are transmitted along *A delta fibres*, which are large diameter nerve fibres, dealing with acute pain. This type of pain is perceived as pricking pain which is readily localised by the sufferer.

Chronic pain. The pathway for chronic pain is slightly different; the nerve fibres involved are of smaller diameter and are called *C fibres*. Chronic pain is often described as burning pain, which is difficult to localise.

Neurotransmitters. Transmission of nervous stimuli is effected or inhibited by substances called neurotransmitters. These may be excitatory or inhibitory. They interact to maintain equilibrium of pain appreciation. An example of an *excitatory neurotransmitter* is acetylcholine, and one of the *inhibitory neurotransmitters* is enkephalin. Local anaesthetic solutions act by competing for the acetylcholine receptors on the neurone and blocking the action.

Inhibitory mechanisms. The thalamus, hypothalamus and parts of the cerebral cortex are known collectively as the *limbic system*. This system links the endocrine and autonomic nervous systems and regulates certain visceral functions. Some emotions arise in the limbic system and it has a part to play in inhibition of the pain response.

There is a substance in the dorsal roots of the spinal cord called *substantia gelatinosa*. If a pain stimulus is not sufficiently strong, or if it is superseded by a different stimulus, the substantia gelatinosa may inhibit its passage. In the *gate control theory* the substantia gelatinosa is likened to a gate. Pain impulses must be sufficiently strong to open the gate in order to ascend the sensory tract any further. The gate may be closed by a competing stimulus such as local application of heat or cold.

Endogenous opiates play an important part in pain inhibition. Opiate receptors are found at various points in the central nervous system and the body produces opiate-like substances which give natural analgesia. The two main classifications are the *endorphins* and the *enkephalins*. It is thought that transcutaneous electrical nerve stimulation (TNS or TENS) and acupuncture stimulate the production of endogenous opiates; the gate control system is also involved.

Pain in labour

The pain experienced by the woman in labour is caused by the uterine contractions, the dilatation of the cervix and, in the late first stage and the second stage, by the stretching of the vagina and pelvic floor to accommodate the presenting part. These painful stimuli are transmitted by thoracic, lumbar and sacral nerves.

The nerve supply of the uterus passes to the last two thoracic nerves, T11 and T12, via the paracervical plexus. These nerves transmit the pain caused by cervical dilatation. In the later first stage T10 and the first lumbar nerve, L1, are also involved. The pudendal nerve relays the pain impulses from the stretching of the pelvic floor to sacral nerves S2, S3 and S4.

PSYCHOLOGICAL SUPPORT

Preparation for labour

At some stage in her pregnancy every woman will realise the inevitability of the delivery of her baby. Not every woman will experience labour but the mother who delivers by planned caesarean section will also have fears and anxieties and will wonder just how she will cope with the experience.

Giving information. Ideally every pregnant woman should have the opportunity to form a relationship with one particular midwife so that advice may be given consistently and the woman become relaxed and feel able to ask for information freely. In this way each woman is able to obtain as much information as she wishes. Some will state that they do not wish to be told too many details, while others feel reassured if they know exactly what they may expect.

Discovering what level of information is required and meeting the individual woman's needs presents the midwife with a challenge. It is best done in an informal, relaxed setting and on a one-to-one basis.

It is more difficult to give information to a group of women, since some are likely to become anxious

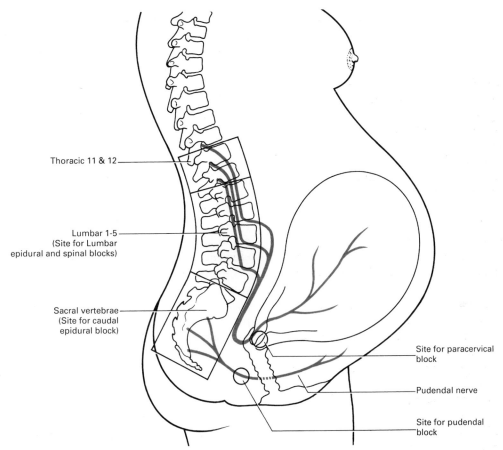

Thoracic 11 & 12

Lumbar 1-5
(Site for Lumbar
epidural and spinal blocks)

Sacral vertebrae
(Site for caudal
epidural block)

Site for paracervical
block

Pudendal nerve

Site for pudendal
block

Fig. 13.2
Pain pathways in labour, showing the sites at which pain may be intercepted by local anaesthetic technique. (Reproduced from Bevis (1984) by courtesy of Baillière Tindall.)

if too much information is given. The best approach when talking to a group of women is probably to attempt to meet the perceived needs of the majority and to offer an opportunity for further discussion with those who would like it.

The giving of information is supplemented by handing out leaflets and recommending books to read. Many women will wish to attend additional classes such as those run by the National Childbirth Trust (NCT).

Reassuring women that they will be given appropriate analgesia and telling them what is available are very important parts of the information given.

Allaying anxiety. While every woman is likely to be apprehensive about some aspect of pregnancy or labour, many fears will be unfounded. Some women may be anxious at the thought of being given an episiotomy, for example, and if this is no longer routine practice in the local maternity unit a needless fear may be allayed.

Many old wives' tales are still in circulation and a discussion of these may be useful. The pregnant woman is often the recipient of such misinformation just when she is especially vulnerable. Some women seem unable to resist the temptation to recount their own horrific experiences to the innocent primigravida. This is not to say that other women may not be a great source of support and constructive advice.

Participation in planning. Entering hospital for any reason is often seen as a dehumanising experience. The person becomes a 'patient' as he or she enters the building and assumes the sick role. Personal clothing is removed, an identity band is attached to the wrist and the person begins to feel helpless.

Women having babies have been no less prone to these experiences and during the last decade many have complained that they had no control over what was done to them. A normal physiological process had become medicalised. Giving back to the woman as much control as possible reduces her feeling of helplessness and increases her ability to tolerate the sensations of labour. This may begin by encouraging her to consider her particular needs and wishes and to discuss these with the midwife.

The birth plan is becoming common (see Ch. 11). This is a document, which the woman compiles together with the midwife, on which she states her preferences for care during and after labour. Completing this document provides a useful opportunity for discussion of pain relief and the exchange of information between the woman and her midwife.

Couples who are able to participate in planning their care in this way will feel that they matter to the professionals and are likely to be less apprehensive about the whole experience of entering hospital. The midwife should remember that for many young couples a hospital is an alien, unfamiliar environment associated with sickness and death and that they may have had no personal experience of it.

Meeting staff. Meeting the staff of the labour ward and seeing the environment will be very helpful to many women. If the use of equipment is explained it will seem less clinical and fearsome. The team approach to care is designed to offer continuity of care and of caregiver to each woman so that she has the reassuring experience of meeting familiar people throughout her contact with the maternity service. The woman is allocated to a team of 6–12 midwives and will get to know them during her pregnancy: hopefully the midwife giving care in labour is therefore not a stranger.

Support during labour

The environment. A relaxed, homely atmosphere will help the woman and her partner feel at ease more quickly. The attitude of the staff is very important, perhaps more so than the physical details of the environment.

The labour room must be furnished in such a way that an emergency may be dealt with swiftly and efficiently and for this reason the clinical aspect can never be removed. However, wallpaper and curtains in attractive, restful colours and the use of screens to hide equipment soften the clinical appearance of the room. Furniture now includes less formal items and rocking chairs, reclining chairs and bean bags are in widespread use.

Lighting should be versatile. Many women prefer subdued lighting or semi-darkness while they are in labour but it may be necessary to direct an efficient light onto the working area.

Piped music may be a source of irritation, but women may be encouraged to bring cassette players with tapes of their own choice and possibly personal headphones.

A television set may be a useful distraction for the woman in early labour and a pleasant sitting room with a variety of comfortable chairs is a desirable provision.

The midwife should endeavour to ensure that there are as few intrusions into the labour room as possible and should aim to maintain an unhurried, peaceful atmosphere.

A supportive companion. Some men are unwilling companions during labour and couples should be encouraged to be honest about this. A supportive companion is a great source of strength to the woman in labour and provides the continuity which the staff cannot promise (see Ch. 11).

Midwife means 'with woman' and she should also aim to be a supportive companion, working with the woman and her partner. The skilful, sensitive midwife works to develop a rapport with the woman and with her chosen supporter.

Mobility. If the woman can be encouraged to be upright and mobile, labour is likely to progress more quickly and the woman will feel more in control, especially if she is encouraged to change position from time to time in order to become as comfortable as possible.

Giving information. The couple should be kept fully informed of progress and all developments during the course of labour. Any treatment or intervention, imminent or probable, should be anticipated and explained. The prospective parents should be involved in the decision-making.

Relaxation techniques. If the woman has been taught relaxation techniques she should be reminded of them and supported as she puts her knowledge into practice. The midwife should be careful to discover just how the woman has been taught and should follow the same method.

If the woman has not attended classes the midwife will aim to give her very simple instructions in breathing techniques and to encourage the use of these (see Ch. 40).

Conversation. When a woman is in labour there are times to talk and times to be silent. A companionable, sympathetic silence is infinitely preferred by most women in advanced labour. At this stage a woman is becoming tired and each contraction requires her complete concentration and all the physical and emotional reserves she can muster. She may close her eyes and become rather distant at this stage. If she is very aware of what is going on in her body, she is concentrating on the baby's progress and her own response and inconsequential conversation is inappropriate. Conversation over the woman is even more inappropriate; attention should be focused on her and her needs throughout the labour.

When silence seems appropriate, touch and facial expressions become more important.

Encouragement. The midwife should aim to encourage the woman throughout her labour. Most women will reach a stage when they feel they cannot continue any longer and will despair. Just a few quiet words of praise after each contraction or some non-verbal encouragement will often suffice. The woman who is made to feel she is coping and progressing very well will usually respond by continuing to do so. The midwife whose communication skills are well developed and who responds with warmth and enthusiasm will usually achieve this.

PHYSICAL CARE

The details of physical care are covered in Chapter 11 but the following points relate particularly to comfort.

Hygiene and comfort

The woman in labour will become very hot and will perspire profusely so that she will appreciate the opportunity to have a bath or shower if she feels able. A warm bath may be very comforting for the woman with backache and she may enjoy soaking herself in deep warm water.

If the woman is not able to get up she will appreciate frequent sponging, particularly of her face and neck, with cold water.

A clean, cool gown will be appreciated and a fan will be comforting.

The mouth may be refreshed by cleaning the teeth or using a mouthwash. The woman may like to have some ice to suck.

Position

The woman may need help to find a position which is comfortable. Leaning forward with the arms resting on a convenient windowsill, table or shelf during a contraction may help the woman to cope with backache. She may prefer to sit astride or kneel on a chair, leaning on the back of it. The midwife should make use of wedges, bean bags and pillows. A rocking chair provides a soothing, rhythmic distraction during contractions and the motion probably encourages release of endogenous opiates; most rocking chairs give good support to the back. A reclining chair also gives good support.

Birthing beds and chairs are designed specifically for women in labour and most are very versatile. Ideally they are used for delivery only and the woman is encouraged to walk about and use alternative positions during the first stage of labour.

An alternative position may be described as any position other than recumbent, semi-recumbent or sitting on the bed; the woman follows her natural instincts and finds a position which feels right, making use of gravity to assist descent of the presenting part. Women wishing to have an active birth will certainly want to make full use of alternative positions but any woman in normal labour may benefit from freer mobility.

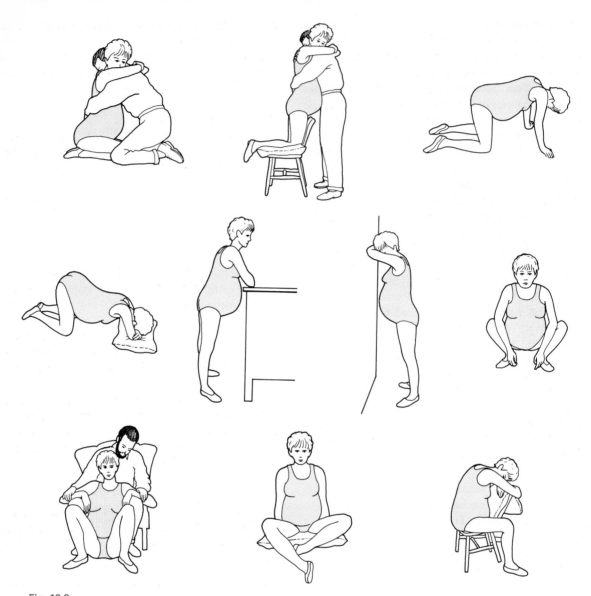

Fig. 13.3
Some of the alternative positions women may find helpful during labour.

Immersion in warm water may be a useful aid to relaxation and comfort for women. An ordinary bath may be used but greater use of alternative positions is possible in the larger 'birthing pools' available in some centres (Milner 1988).

In *active birth* the woman participates fully in her labour, is very aware of all that is going on within her body and aims to respond to these events naturally. She will have prepared herself during her pregnancy by exercising in order to be aware of her pelvic floor and to control these muscles. She may also practise squatting. She will not wish to have any form of medical intervention if this can be avoided. She may use any position she finds comfortable, such as squatting, kneeling on all fours or kneeling upright. Most women prefer such positions if they have the confidence to try them and they find that they can cope with the contractions better than when sitting on the bed.

Physical contact

The woman may not wish to talk but she may find physical contact comforting. Her partner should be encouraged to hold her hand, rub her back, sponge her face or just cuddle her. Some couples may wish to practise *effleurage*, where the partner strokes the woman's abdomen and thighs, or similar techniques. Those who are wanting an active birth may wish to try nipple or clitoral stimulation to encourage the release of oxytocin from the pituitary gland and so stimulate uterine contractions in a natural way. This will also stimulate the production of endogenous opiates, giving some natural analgesia. The midwife should be sensitive to each couple's wishes and should respect them. It may be appropriate at times to leave the couple alone together, if that is what they prefer.

The woman's partner may support her in her chosen alternative position, although this becomes a physical endurance test after a time and the midwife may have to suggest practical alternatives.

Some women become very irritable as labour progresses and find any touch annoying and intrusive.

The midwife should not be afraid to make sensitive use of physical contact herself but should learn to recognise when this becomes intrusive.

Massage

The woman who is suffering from backache or pain during her labour may find appropriate massage very soothing. The midwife or partner may perform circular massage over the lumbosacral area, reducing friction with the use of talcum powder or body lotion.

Deep massage is given by applying pressure with the heel of the hand, the knuckles or an object such as a tennis ball.

Some women may find it comforting to have abdominal massage; light circular strokes over the whole abdomen may be soothing, using both hands and passing the fingertips lightly up from the symphysis pubis, across the fundus of the uterus and down either side of the abdomen. Some may prefer a similar two-handed technique across the lower abdomen, where the pain of uterine contractions is usually felt. Women may like to do this for themselves.

If the woman finds it difficult to relax any part of herself, such as her face, she may benefit from sensitive use of massage in that area.

Care of bladder and bowels

This is discussed more fully in Chapter 12 but care of the bladder and bowels is an important aspect of the mother's comfort.

PSYCHOPHYSICAL METHODS OF COPING WITH PAIN

History

In the 1930s Grantly Dick-Read postulated that fear of the unknown led to muscular tension thus increasing the pain of labour. He maintained that in order to break this vicious circle, it was necessary to give women more information and then to teach them specific methods of relaxing. The relaxation techniques were also intended to serve as a distraction.

Lamaze was a proponent of psychoprophylaxis.

Michel Odent advocates a natural approach, allowing women to feel in control of their bodies and what happens to them and encouraging them to respond instinctively to labour.

Principles

The principles in psychophysical methods of pain relief are to allay anxiety, encourage relaxation, provide distraction and to encourage a positive attitude.

SEDATIVES AND ANALGESICS

Until recent years sedatives were widely used for women in early labour, to encourage sleep and rest. The sedatives given were usually the chloral derivatives. Welldorm, commonly used until 1991, is now contra-indicated because of a change in composition.

Analgesics which are used in early labour are in the mild to moderate analgesic range, for example paracetamol.

Such drugs are usually included in the standing orders which allow a midwife to administer specified drugs in certain situations at her own discretion.

NARCOTICS

A narcotic is a strong analgesic drug with some sedative properties. Narcotic drugs include the opiates.

Pethidine

Pethidine has been used as an analgesic for women in labour since the 1940s. Although other drugs have been introduced from time to time, none shows any distinct advantage over pethidine.

Pethidine, given by intramuscular injection, appears to give satisfactory analgesia to some individuals but not to others. Some women afterwards claim that they felt unpleasantly drowsy and detached in labour but did not have adequate pain relief. They may complain of nausea or may vomit following the administration of pethidine.

Infants of mothers who received pethidine during labour may be slow to establish spontaneous respirations at birth because the respiratory centre is depressed. As alternative methods of analgesia such as epidural are available, it should not be necessary to give large doses. The baby is less likely to be affected if pethidine is not given between 2 and 4 hours before delivery. The baby whose mother received pethidine during labour is also likely to be affected in more subtle ways. Detailed neurobehavioural studies show that these babies tend to be slightly less alert, suck less frequently and demonstrate reduced peak sucking pressures when feeding. They show a slightly slower response to light and sound, a less brisk Moro reflex and tend to be less cuddly and consolable. These very subtle effects are said to last for up to 48 hours but some authorities state that these babies are affected for much longer periods, possibly several months.

Parents have often read about these effects on the baby in the popular medical press and may be unduly anxious. They need careful advice to enable them to make an informed decision regarding pain relief in labour.

In obstetric units where active management of labour is practised an initial dose of 50 mg of pethidine may be given. This may be repeated after 30 minutes if it is not effective.

In other units the Cardiff palliator may be used. This device is designed to administer an intravenous dose of 25 mg of pethidine on demand from the mother. In-built safety mechanisms include a time limit so that the dose may not be repeated too frequently.

It is easy to give a standard dose of pethidine to women in labour without considering variations in body weight. Thus a large lady would receive the same amount of analgesic as a small, slim woman, when it would be appropriate to give her a considerably larger amount. This may account in part for the apparent inadequacy of opiate analgesia in labour.

Pethidine is often given together with a tranquilliser such as promazine or promethazine. These drugs make the woman feel relaxed and potentiate the analgesic effect.

An anti-emetic drug may be prescribed, to be given with the pethidine if necessary. Some drugs possess both anti-emetic and tranquillising qualities.

Other opiate drugs

Diamorphine or morphine may be used instead of pethidine. All these drugs have similar disadvantages. Some authorities feel that diamorphine offers better analgesia; it certainly gives the woman a pleasant feeling of detachment and well-being. Those who do not favour its use fear the possibility of addiction and it is more likely than pethidine to cause respiratory depression in the neonate.

Opiate antagonist. The action of the opiate drugs may be reversed by the use of the opiate antagonist naloxone (Narcan). Naloxone will reverse any respiratory depression caused by the opiate but will also reverse the analgesic effect. It acts by competing for the opiate receptors and blocking them, so that the opiate is rendered ineffective. Very occasionally the naloxone may become ineffective before the opiate has been excreted. The opiate may then become effective again.

The most common use of naloxone in obstetrics is in its paediatric form. This is given to the baby who is born with respiratory depression due to the administration of an opiate to the mother.

Pentazocine

Pentazocine (Fortral) has not enjoyed great popularity. Its analgesic effect is said to be equivalent to that of pethidine and it does cause less nausea and vomiting. It is also less likely to cause respiratory depression in the infant but if this effect is seen naloxone is effective in reversing it. Some women who have received pentazocine have complained of unpleasant dreams and of feeling hot and sweaty and they have disliked it for these reasons.

Meptazinol

Meptazinol (Meptid) has been introduced in the mid-1980s, and may well have advantages over pethidine as the side-effects, although similar, are less marked. It is claimed to give rise to less respiratory depression.

INHALATIONAL ANALGESIA

With the advent of epidural analgesia inhalational methods of analgesia have become less widely used but they do still have their uses.

They offer effective pain relief for the majority of women, with the advantage that all their effects are short-lived and they do not give rise to any complications in the neonate.

One approved inhalational analgesic agent is available for use by the midwife in the UK without medical supervision, provided she has been trained in its use. This agent is Entonox.

Entonox

Entonox is the trade name used to describe an equal mixture of oxygen and nitrous oxide. Nitrous oxide is used in higher concentrations as a general anaesthetic.

Physical qualities. Entonox is colourless and odourless; women may complain of a smell associated with its use but this arises from the black rubber tubing and not from the gas itself.

Equipment. In major obstetric units Entonox is usually piped to each labour room. Alternatively a medium-sized cylinder on a wheeled stand may be used and is easily moved from room to room. The community midwife may obtain Entonox in a small cylinder which is fairly easy to transport; the apparatus is compact but quite heavy.

Piped Entonox comes from a bank of large cylinders situated at a central point. These must be checked and maintained so that there is always a good supply of full cylinders.

Cylinders should always be stored on their sides rather than upright. Nitrous oxide is heavier than oxygen and the two gases may separate in extreme cold (below −7°C). If the cylinder is kept on its side the two gases may be remixed more effectively before use. The temperature of the storage site should be kept above 10°C. If the cylinders have been subjected to freezing conditions they should be kept in a temperature of at least 10°C for 2 hours prior to use, or placed for 5 minutes in a bath of warm water (no hotter than 35°C), keeping the part of the cylinder above the neck dry. Afterwards the cylinder is inverted at least three times to mix the contents.

Entonox apparatus. This is manufactured by the British Oxygen Company (BOC) and is probably the most commonly used device for delivering nitrous oxide and oxygen in midwifery practice in the UK. The apparatus and the cylinder are made so that neither will fit any other equipment. They fit together by means of matching pins and holes (the pin index system). The cylinder is blue with a blue and white quartered shoulder. The apparatus has a demand valve which opens on inspiration by the user and the mask has an expiratory valve which prevents exhaled gas from being re-breathed. A cylinder pressure gauge indicates when the cylinder is becoming empty.

When Entonox is provided to the labour room from a piped supply the demand valve and non-return expiratory valve are still incorporated. In some units *scavenging equipment* to extract expired gases from the room may be fitted.

Principles involved. It is important that the

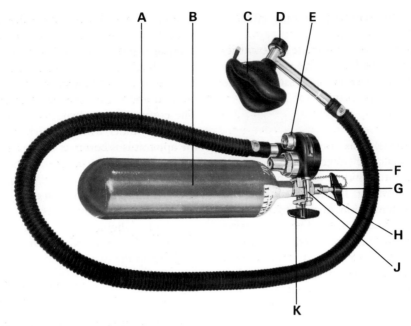

Fig. 13.4
Entonox analgesic apparatus, intended for use in the home.
(A) corrugated rubber tubing; (B) 500 litre cylinder; (C) face mask; (D) expiratory valve; (E) cylinder pressure gauge; (F) demand regulator; (G) cylinder valve key; (H) pin-index valve; (J) cylinder yoke; (K) cylinder yoke key. (Reproduced by courtesy of British Oxygen Company Ltd.)

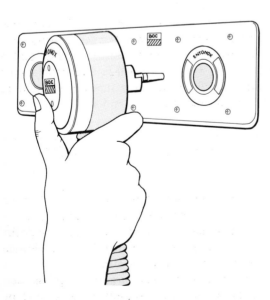

Fig. 13.5
Entonox apparatus; pipeline model. (Reproduced by courtesy of British Oxygen Company Ltd.)

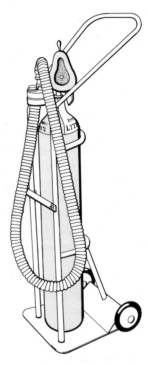

Fig. 13.6
Entonox apparatus; hospital cylinder model. (Reproduced by courtesy of British Oxygen Company Ltd.)

mother be instructed correctly if she is to obtain maximum benefit from inhalational analgesia.

Entonox does not flow continuously from the cylinder but must be obtained by the woman's own inspiratory efforts. She must therefore be instructed to fit the mask firmly over her nose and mouth and take a steady breath in. Care must be taken to avoid hyperventilation; if this occurs the woman will complain of dizziness and numbness of the face and hands. She exhales into the mask which has an expiratory valve.

Analgesia is obtained from Entonox within about 20 seconds and the maximum effect is felt after about 45–60 seconds. The mother is instructed to start using the Entonox as soon as the uterus begins to harden and to continue until the peak of the contraction has passed. The midwife needs to help the woman to recognise when a contraction is starting as there will be no pain at first.

The mother should be persuaded, for her own safety, to hold the mask herself, since part of the principle of self-administration is that she will drop the mask if she takes too much of the gas.

If a woman fears feeling claustrophobic when using the face mask, or in practice dislikes the sensation, she may be offered a mouth piece. She closes her lips firmly around this, and proceeds as already described.

Use with narcotics. For most primigravid women Entonox does not provide adequate analgesia alone and is often used in conjunction with pethidine. Ideally it is not used for long periods of time, although it is excreted quickly and therefore does not have any residual effects.

Effects on the fetus. Because Entonox is excreted quickly from the mother via her lungs it is not thought to have any residual effect on the fetus. It will cross the placenta following the *concentration gradient*; this means that if levels are higher in the mother Entonox will pass from her to the fetus and vice versa, so that the situation is one of continual change.

The midwife's responsibilities

In the UK the United Kingdom Central Council for Nursing, Midwifery and Health Visiting (UKCC) lays down both rules and guidelines governing the midwife's practice (see Ch. 48).

Training and supervision. The midwife who is involved in the administration of inhalational analgesia is only permitted to do this if she has been trained and supervised in the use of both the agent and the apparatus concerned. Although her employer has a responsibility in this, the midwife herself is expected to seek further help and training if she does not feel confident in this area.

There are four types of apparatus approved for use by midwives on their own responsibility. These are:

- the original BOC Entonox apparatus described above
- the PneuPac apparatus
- the SOS Nitronox—midwifery model
- the Peacemaker (approved in 1990).

Care of equipment. The equipment used must be serviced and maintained at the prescribed intervals. The community or independent midwife takes the responsibility for this herself, while in hospital practice it may be delegated to the appropriate service department or a midwifery manager. However, the individual midwife still has a responsibility to check equipment before use, and not to use it if there is any question at all as to its safety.

Selection of women. The use of inhalational analgesia is rarely contra-indicated. The midwife must check the woman's medical history and if she has any reason to consider that inhalational analgesia may be an unwise choice, she should seek a medical opinion.

TRANSCUTANEOUS ELECTRICAL NERVE STIMULATION (TNS OR TENS)

This is a recently introduced method of pain relief in labour. It has been welcomed by many because it is non-pharmacological and not surgically invasive. It does not appear to have any residual effect on the fetus or the mother.

It is thought to work by interrupting pain transmission along the sensory pathway and by stimulating production of endogenous opiates.

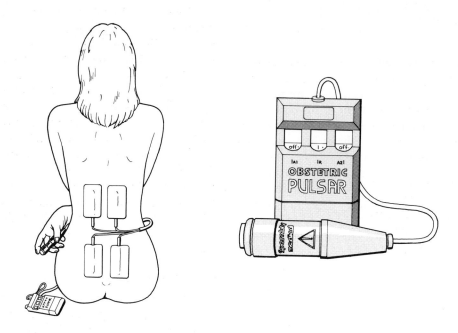

Fig. 13.7
TENS equipment in use, showing the electrodes in position on the back. (Reproduced by courtesy of Spembly Medical Company Ltd.)

Electrodes are attached to the woman's back on the skin areas, known as *dermatomes*, overlying the nerve endings of thoracic and lumbar nerves T10 to L1, and over those of sacral nerves S2 to S4. Electrodes may also be placed on the woman's abdomen. It is important that these are accurately placed if the woman is to receive maximum benefit. The equipment is operated by the mother and this adds to its acceptability by women. Ideally the mother should become familiar with the equipment during pregnancy. The apparatus is activated by pressing a small button which causes a small electric current to pass through the electrodes. The electric current may be low frequency and intermittent (*pulsed*) or high frequency and continuous. Low frequency TENS stimulates the release of endogenous opiates while high frequency current closes the pain gate. As the pain of labour intensifies the woman increases the intensity of the electric current and graduates from low frequency to high frequency current. She may feel this as tingling, or as a sharper elec-

tric shock sensation. Some women will not tolerate this and for some it will not provide adequate analgesia when used alone. It is most effective when started in early labour. Because there are no residual effects the woman may receive some other form of analgesia whenever she feels the need.

Many women will be keen to persevere with its use because they do not want drugs or invasive techniques such as epidural or spinal anaesthesia.

Some anaesthetists and obstetricians are sceptical as to its efficacy but many midwives feel that if it is safe and acceptable to women, many of whom express great satisfaction, then it is a welcome adjunct to the other methods of pain relief in labour.

It is probably most useful for the multigravid woman, who may expect a shorter labour, though many primigravidae will also find it beneficial. It will be most helpful for the woman who is highly motivated to use it and who is confident that it will be effective.

In 1991 the UKCC approved TENS for use by midwives on their own responsibility provided that:

- they have received adequate and appropriate instruction; this is to be determined by local policy
- safety standards should conform to those laid down by the Department of Health Medical Devices Directorate or the equivalent body in Scotland, Wales or Northern Ireland.

TENS may interfere with certain electronic fetal monitors. If this is suspected TENS apparatus should be switched off to obtain an accurate trace from the monitor. A different fetal monitor may be satisfactory.

ALTERNATIVE METHODS OF PAIN RELIEF

Many mothers are anxious to avoid pharmacological or invasive methods of pain relief in labour and this contributes to the popularity of alternative methods of analgesia which are coming into more common use.

Acupuncture. The mode of action of this ancient practice is still not understood. It may be related to stimulating the release of endogenous opiates as well as interruption of the transmission of pain stimuli.

Women may wish to employ this method of pain relief. They may have difficulty in finding a practitioner who is willing to be available whenever they commence labour. The presence of the acupuncturist would need to be negotiated.

Hypnosis. A few medical practitioners offer hypnosis as a pain-relieving technique. Women are usually taught self-hypnosis and in suitable subjects it may be successful.

Homeopathy and aromatherapy. Homeopathic remedies include raspberry leaf tea to encourage cervical dilatation and caullophyllum to stimulate uterine contractions. Aromatherapy involves the use of aromatic oils.

Biofeedback. An individual receives a visual or auditory signal indicating the satisfactory performance of an autonomic body function. It is thought that, by conditioning, a person may be able to control that function. The use of biofeedback has been well documented in the control of chronic pain and it has been suggested that it could be helpful in labour. Electromyography (EMG) feedback may be used to reduce voluntary muscle tension. Women could be taught to focus on relaxing the abdominal muscles when feeling pain or uterine contractions (St James-Roberts et al 1983).

Midwives who are interested in alternative forms of pain relief should be prepared to make a thorough study of the remedies available, their uses and mode of action and the possible side-effects.

Acknowledgement

Figures 13.1 and 13.2 are reproduced from Bevis R 1984 Anaesthesia in midwifery. Baillière Tindall, London with permission of the publishers.

Reader Activities

- Devise a study designed to find out how newly delivered women's expectations of labour differed from the reality.
- Aim to elicit how they felt they could have been better prepared in the antenatal period, and also try to evaluate the support they received from their carers during labour.
- Run a pilot study to test the format, but discuss the procedure with a mentor first.

- Select some case notes of recently delivered women in your care, including some with one or more complications.
- Discuss the care and support these women received with a group of colleagues. Attempt to evaluate their care.
- Consider what kind of support you would wish to have if you were in these circumstances.

FURTHER READING

Bevis R 1984 Anaesthesia in midwifery. Baillière Tindall, London

British National Formulary 1986 British Medical Association and Pharmaceutical Press, London

Flint C 1986 Sensitive midwifery, Heinemann, London

Green J H 1974 An introduction to human physiology, 3rd edn. Oxford University Press, London

McFarlane A 1977 Psychology of childbirth. Fontana, London

Melzack R, Wall P D 1982 The challenge of pain. Penguin, Harmondsworth

Milner I 1988 Water baths for pain relief in labour. Nursing Times 84 (Jan 6): 1

Moir D D 1986 Obstetric anaesthesia and analgesia, 5th edn. Baillière Tindall, London

Polden M 1985 Transcutaneous nerve stimulation in labour and post-caesarean section. Physiotherapy 71(8)

St James-Roberts I, Hutchinson C, Haran F et al 1983 Biofeedback as an aid to childbirth British Journal of Obstetrics and Gynaecology 90(1): 56–60

UKCC 1991 Handbook of midwives rules. UKCC, London

Williams M, Booth D 1985 Antenatal education, 3rd edn. Churchill Livingstone, Edinburgh

14

Physiology and management of the second stage of labour

JENNIFER SLEEP

Physiological changes

The mechanism of normal labour

Midwifery care

Perineal repair

The second stage of labour is a time when the whole tempo of activity changes. The mother's passive control during the long hours of the first stage is replaced by intense physical effort and exertion for a comparatively short period. Both parents require stamina, courage and confidence in the skill of the attendant midwife. Excitement and expectation mount as the birth becomes imminent. A happy outcome will depend upon a successful partnership between professionals and parents. A mother will never forget the midwife who delivered her baby.

PHYSIOLOGICAL CHANGES

The second stage of labour begins when the cervix is fully dilated and ends with the baby's birth. A knowledge of the physiological processes and of the actual mechanism of delivery forms the basis for determining midwifery care.

The physiological changes result from a continuation of the same forces which have been at work during the first stage of labour but activity is accelerated once the cervix has become fully dilated. This acceleration, however, does not occur abruptly. There may be a lull before the woman experiences the full expulsive nature of the second stage contractions.

Uterine action

Contractions become stronger and longer but may be less frequent, affording mother and fetus a recovery period during the resting phase. There is continued, progressive contraction and retraction of the upper uterine segment while the lower segment and cervix passively dilate and thin. The membranes often rupture spontaneously at the onset of the second stage. The consequent drainage of liquor allows the hard, round fetal head to be directly applied to the vaginal tissues and aid distension. Fetal axis pressure increases flexion of the head which results in smaller presenting diameters, more rapid progress and less trauma to both mother and fetus.

The nature of the contractions changes. They become more expulsive as pressure is exerted on the rectum and the pelvic floor. The mother feels a compelling urge to push. This reflex may initially be controlled to a limited extent but becomes increasingly compulsive, overwhelming and involuntary during each contraction. The mother's response is to employ her secondary powers of expulsion by contracting her abdominal muscles and diaphragm.

Soft tissue displacement

As the hard fetal head descends, the soft tissues of the pelvis become displaced. Anteriorly, the bladder is pushed upwards into the abdomen where it is at less risk of injury during fetal descent. This results in the stretching and thinning of the urethra so that its lumen is reduced. Posteriorly, the rectum becomes flattened into the sacral curve and the pressure of the advancing head expels any residual faecal matter. The levator ani muscles dilate, thin out and are displaced laterally and the perineal body is flattened, stretched and thinned. The fetal head becomes visible at the vulva, advancing with each contraction and receding during the resting phase until crowning takes place and the head is born. The shoulders and body follow with the next contraction, accompanied by a gush of amniotic fluid. The second stage culminates in the birth of the baby.

Recognition of the commencement of the second stage of labour

The transition from the first to the second stage is not always clinically apparent. Several of the signs are presumptive and not a reliable index that this stage has been reached. Nevertheless the midwife should be able to diagnose the onset of the second stage of labour. The purpose is not to impose a time limit on its duration but to conserve maternal energy and minimise the avoidable soft tissue trauma caused by premature pushing.

Presumptive signs and differential diagnoses

Expulsive uterine contractions. It is possible for a woman to feel a strong desire to push before the cervix is fully dilated, especially if the fetus is in an occipitoposterior position, the rectum is full or the woman is highly parous.

Rupture of the forewaters. This may occur at any time during labour.

Dilatation and gaping of the anus. Deep engagement of the presenting part and premature maternal effort may produce this sign during the latter part of the first stage.

Appearance of the presenting part. Excessive moulding may result in the formation of a large caput succedaneum which can protrude through the cervix prior to full dilatation. Similarly a breech presentation may be visible when the cervix is only 7–8 cm dilated.

Show. This must be distinguished from bleeding due to partial separation of the placenta or that caused by ruptured vasa praevia.

Congestion of the vulva. Enthusiastic premature pushing may also cause this.

The appearance of several presumptive signs may indicate that the second stage of labour has been reached.

Confirmatory evidence

This is only available when no cervical rim can be felt on vaginal examination. Although the midwife should be reluctant to perform repeated vaginal examinations she should conduct the delivery on the basis of accurate observation and assessment of progress.

THE MECHANISM OF NORMAL LABOUR

As the fetus descends soft tissue and bony structures exert pressures which force him to negotiate the birth canal by a series of passive movements. Collectively, these movements are called the mechanism of labour. Knowledge and recognition of the normal mechanism enable the midwife to anticipate the next step in the process of descent which in turn will dictate her conduct of the delivery. Her understanding and constant monitoring of these movements ensure that normal progress is recognised, the delivery safely completed and early assistance sought should any delay occur. During vaginal delivery the fetal presentation and position will govern the exact mechanism as the fetus responds to external pressures. Principles common to all mechanisms are:

- descent takes place throughout
- whichever part leads and first meets the resistance of the pelvic floor will rotate forwards until it comes under the symphysis pubis
- whatever emerges from the pelvis will pivot around the pubic bone.

During the mechanism of normal labour the fetus turns slightly to take advantage of the widest available space in each plane of the pelvis. The widest diameter of the pelvic brim is the transverse: at the pelvic outlet the greatest space lies in the anteroposterior diameter.

At the onset of labour the way that the fetus is situated may be described as follows:

- the lie is longitudinal
- the presentation is cephalic
- the position is right or left occipito-anterior
- the attitude is one of good flexion
- the denominator is the occiput
- the presenting part is the posterior part of the anterior parietal bone. (See Ch. 10 for definitions of these terms.)

Main movements

Descent. Descent of the fetal head into the pelvis often begins before the onset of labour. In primigravidae it occurs during the latter weeks of pregnancy when engagement of the head provides confirmation that vaginal delivery is probable. In multigravidae muscle tone is lax and therefore engagement may not occur until labour actually begins. Throughout the first stage of labour the forces of contraction and retraction aid descent. Following rupture of the forewaters and full dilatation of the cervix, maternal effort speeds progress.

Flexion. This increases throughout labour. The fetal spine is attached nearer the posterior part of the skull; pressure exerted down the fetal axis will be more forcibly transmitted to the occiput than the sinciput. The effect is to increase flexion which results in smaller presenting diameters which will negotiate the pelvis more easily. At the onset of labour the suboccipitofrontal diameter, 10 cm, is presenting; with greater flexion the suboccipitobregmatic diameter, 9.5 cm, presents. The occiput becomes the *leading part.*

Internal rotation of the head. During a contraction the leading part is driven downwards onto the pelvic floor. The resistance of this muscular diaphragm brings about rotation. As the contraction fades, the pelvic floor rebounds causing the occiput to glide forwards. Resistance is therefore an important determinant of rotation. (This explains why rotation is often delayed following epidural anaesthesia which causes relaxation of pelvic floor muscles.) The slope of the pelvic floor determines the direction of rotation. The muscles are gutter-shaped and slope down anteriorly so whichever part of the fetus first meets the lateral half of this slope will be directed forwards and towards the centre. In a well-flexed vertex presentation the occiput leads and meets the pelvic floor first and rotates anteriorly through one-eighth of a circle. This causes a slight twist in the neck of the fetus as the head is no longer in direct alignment with the shoulders. The anteroposterior diameter of the head now lies in the widest (anteroposterior) diameter of the pelvic outlet, facilitating an easy escape (Fig. 14.1). The occiput slips beneath the sub-pubic arch and crowning occurs when the head no longer recedes between contractions and the widest transverse diameter (biparietal) is born. If flexion is maintained, the suboccipitobregmatic diameter, 9.5 cm, distends the vaginal orifice.

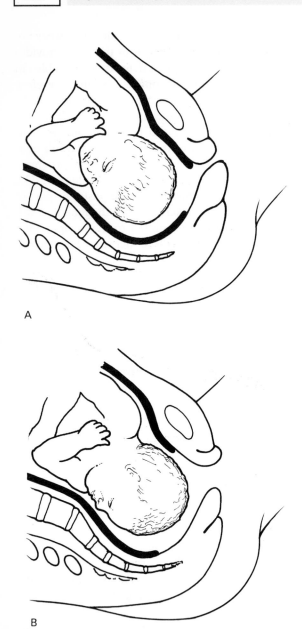

A

B

Fig. 14.1
(A) Internal rotation of the head begins. (B) Upon completion, the occiput lies under the symphysis pubis.

Extension of the head. Once crowning has occurred the fetal head can extend, pivoting on the suboccipital region around the pubic bone. This releases the sinciput, face and chin which sweep the perineum and are born by a movement of extension. The suboccipitofrontal diameter, 10 cm, distends the vaginal outlet.

Restitution. The twist in the neck of the fetus which resulted from internal rotation is now corrected by a slight untwisting movement. The occiput moves one-eighth of a circle towards the side from which it started (Fig. 14.2).

Internal rotation of the shoulders. The shoulders undergo a similar rotation to that of the head to lie in the widest diameter of the pelvic outlet, namely anteroposterior. The anterior shoulder is the first to reach the levator ani muscle and therefore rotates anteriorly to lie under the symphysis pubis. This movement can be clearly seen as the head turns at the same time (*external rotation of the head*) (Fig. 14.2). It occurs in the same direction as restitution and the occiput of the fetal head now lies laterally.

Lateral flexion. The shoulders are born sequentially, usually the anterior shoulder first. The anterior shoulder slips beneath the sub-pubic arch and the posterior shoulder passes over the perineum. This enables a smaller diameter to distend the vaginal orifice than if both shoulders were born simultaneously. The remainder of the body is born by lateral flexion as the spine bends sideways through the curved birth canal.

Duration of the second stage

Once the onset of the second stage has been confirmed a woman should not be left without a midwife in attendance, especially if she is to be delivered at home. Accurate observation of progress is vital, for the unexpected can always happen. The duration of the second stage is difficult to predict with any degree of certainty. In multigravidae it may last as little as 5 minutes; in primigravidae the process may take 2 hours. More important than the time factor is the evidence of progressive descent and the condition of mother and fetus. There is no good evidence to suggest that the imposition of an upper time limit for duration of second stage improves the outcome for mother or baby (Sleep et al 1989). Two phases in progress may be recognised, the latent phase followed by the active phase.

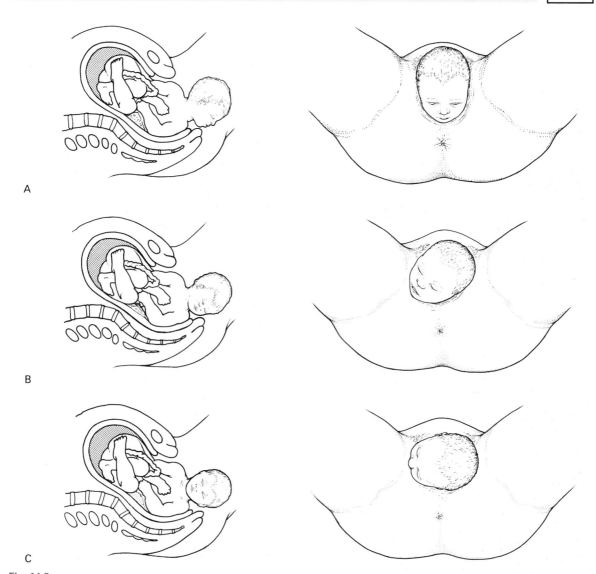

Fig. 14.2
(A) Delivery of the head. (B) Restitution. (C) External rotation.

The latent phase

This begins at full cervical dilatation although the presenting part may not yet have reached the pelvic outlet. The soft tissues of the vagina and pelvic floor gradually stretch and thin under the pressure of the advancing fetal head. The woman may experience little expulsive urge until the head has descended sufficiently to exert pressure on the rectum and perineal tissues. The head will then become visible.

There is scant evidence that active pushing during the latent phase achieves much, apart from exhausting and discouraging the mother. On the contrary, uterine supports and vaginal and perineal muscle may become strained and damaged as a result of the woman's efforts to push before these tissues have been able to stretch gradually (Benyon 1957). This same study showed that spontaneous delivery was not speeded by maternal effort at this stage. Passive descent of the fetus should be allowed to continue until the head is visible at the vulva.

Active phase

Once the fetal head is visible the woman will probably experience a compulsive urge to push. In the absence of this reflex, the midwife's instruction and encouragement may enable the mother to use her contractions effectively to expedite delivery but such intervention is rarely needed.

The recognition of the two phases of descent is particularly important if an effective epidural is in progress as there is little benefit in allowing the analgesia to wear off until the active phase has been reached.

The time taken to complete the second stage will vary considerably between mothers; clearly it should not be allowed to continue for many hours. However, in the presence of regular contractions, good maternal and fetal condition and progressive descent, considerable flexibility in duration should be allowed.

MIDWIFERY CARE

Care of the parents

The couple will now realise that the birth of their baby is imminent. They may feel excited and elated but at the same time anxious and frightened by the dramatic change in pace. The midwife's calm approach and information about what is happening can safeguard a co-operative partnership. This is critical at a time when a woman may feel a lack of control over events which can result in a sensation of panic. This is especially true when a supportive companion is not present. In this situation the midwife's role is even more important. The relationship of trust which she is able to build up during the earlier stages of labour will help to establish the mother's confidence in her skills. In order to achieve this, it is eminently preferable that the same midwife should look after the couple throughout labour. It may not always be possible but continuity of care is advantageous for both parents and professional. The father's wishes about being present at the actual birth should have been fully discussed with the couple and documented prior to the start of labour.

In practice even the most reluctant of partners may decide to change his mind and witness the birth. He is then able to offer his continued support and the couple can share the climactic moment when their baby is born. If, however, the father chooses not to be present, his wishes should be respected. In this case the mother should be given the opportunity to select another companion of her choice.

Throughout the second stage of labour the parents need explanations of events; the midwife should praise and congratulate the mother on her hard work, regardless of apparent progress, so that she is encouraged to participate actively.

Observations during the second stage of labour

Four factors determine whether the second stage may safely continue and these must be carefully monitored:

- uterine contractions
- descent of the presenting part
- fetal condition
- maternal condition.

Uterine contractions. The strength, length and frequency of contractions should be assessed continuously. They are usually stronger and longer than during the first stage of labour, lasting up to 1 minute with a longer resting phase between. The posture and position adopted by the mother may influence the contractions. The left lateral or the upright position may improve their effectiveness.

The progress of descent. Progress is observed by noting the descent of the fetal head as it advances during contractions and recedes afterwards. This becomes apparent during the active phase. Initially, descent occurs slowly, especially in primigravidae, but it accelerates during the active phase. It may occur very rapidly in multigravidae. If descent is progressive it should not be necessary for the midwife to make a further vaginal examination. If, however, there is a delay in progress of more than half an hour, a vaginal examination should be performed. This will confirm whether or not internal rotation of the head has taken place, the station of the presenting part and whether a caput succedaneum has formed. If the occiput has rotated anteriorly, the head is well flexed and caput succedaneum is not excessive it is likely that progress will continue.

If there is anxiety about either fetal or maternal condition, a doctor must be notified. In these circumstances vaginal assessment may be delayed until his arrival.

Fetal condition. The liquor amnii is observed for signs of meconium staining. As the fetus descends, fetal oxygenation may be less efficient due to either cord or head compression or to reduced perfusion at the placental site. The midwife should learn to recognise the normal changes in fetal heart rate patterns during the second stage, so that assistance may be sought at the earliest indication of fetal distress whilst avoiding the risk of unwarranted interference (see Ch. 12).

Maternal condition. The midwife's observation includes an appraisal of the mother's ability to cope emotionally as well as an assessment of her physical well-being. Maternal pulse rate is usually recorded quarter-hourly and blood pressure hourly, provided that these are within normal limits.

Pushing

The urge to push may come before the vertex is visible. In order to conserve maternal effort and allow the vaginal tissues to stretch passively, the mother should be helped to avoid active pushing at this stage. She may lie on her left side in order to relieve pressure on the rectum and improve placental blood flow. The breathing exercises learned during pregnancy may help her to control this urge (see Ch. 40). Once the head becomes visible each mother should be encouraged to follow her own inclinations in relation to expulsive effort. Few women need formalised instruction on how to push; the desire is so overwhelming that the response becomes involuntary and compelling. Her pushing effort will be regulated in response to the varying intensity of her contractions. Most women fall into their own rhythm after the first few exertions. Attempts to override spontaneous efforts by encouraging sustained pushing accompanied by prolonged breath-holding

(the Valsalva manoeuvre) may result in potentially adverse haemodynamic consequences (McKay & Roberts 1985). The mother is therefore the best judge of when and how to push. This concept is endorsed by Inch (1982) who advocates that mothers should be allowed 'to follow their physiological inclinations'. This results in maximum pressure being exerted at the height of a contraction which is beneficial. Delaying active pushing in this way allows the vaginal muscles to become taut and prevents bladder supports and the transverse cervical ligaments from being pushed down in front of the baby's head. This may help to prevent prolapse and urinary incontinence in later life (Benyon 1957). Some mothers may become frightened by the overwhelming urge and cry out. This may help a woman to cope with the contractions and she should feel free to express herself in this way. If, however, these sounds are an embarrassment to the mother or cause distress to other couples, the woman may wish to use the Entonox mask to inhale the analgesia or simply to help to muffle the sound. The midwife's gentle reassurance and praise will help to boost confidence enabling the mother to assert her control over events. The atmosphere should be calm and the pace unhurried.

Maternal comfort and hygiene

As a result of her exertions the woman usually feels very hot and sticky and she will find it soothing to have her face and neck sponged with a cool flannel. Her mouth and lips may become very dry. Sips of iced water are refreshing and a moisturising cream can be applied to her lips. Her partner may help with these tasks as a positive contribution to ease her discomfort. Pain relief remains important but this is discussed further in Chapter 13.

Bladder care

As the fetus descends into the pelvis the bladder is particularly vulnerable to damage from the pressure of the advancing head. The bladder base may become compressed between the pelvic brim and the fetal head. The risk of trauma is greatly increased if the bladder is distended. The woman should be encouraged to pass urine at the beginning of the second stage unless she has recently done so. Small amounts of urine may dribble during contractions.

Position

General considerations

The position the mother may choose to adopt is dictated by several factors:

- *Maternal and fetal condition.* If there is any concern about the well-being of either the woman or her baby then a need for frequent or continuous monitoring may limit the choices available to her.
- The *mother's personal preference* should always be a primary consideration.
- *The environment.* For reasons of safety and privacy it may not be possible to consider all the alternative positions.
- The *midwife's confidence* in her own skills to supervise the delivery when the mother prefers to adopt a posture with which she has little or no experience. However, a real understanding of the mechanism of labour should enable the midwife to adapt to any position that the woman wishes to adopt.

A full discussion of these issues should take place during pregnancy and the woman's preference should be ascertained and documented. The physiotherapist and midwife in partnership may advise about preparatory exercises which may be necessary to enable a particular position such as squatting to be sustained. Practicalities such as physical support and protection of furnishings and carpets should also be discussed.

The semi-recumbent or supported sitting position, with the thighs abducted, is the posture most commonly encouraged in Western cultures. There is evidence to suggest that if the mother lies flat on her back, vena caval compression is increased resulting in hypotension and this can lead to reduced placental perfusion and diminished fetal oxygenation (Humphrey et al 1974, Kurz et al 1982). The efficiency of uterine contractions may also be reduced. Unless she is well supported, it may be difficult for a mother to direct her pushing efficiently and if she is semi-

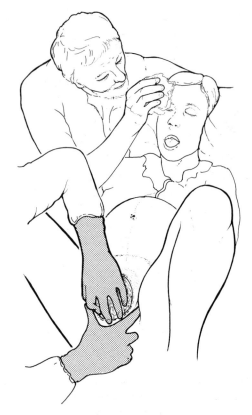

Fig. 14.3
Supported sitting position.

recumbent, her weight is on her sacrum, which directs the coccyx forwards and reduces the pelvic outlet. Dorsal positions afford the midwife good access and a clear view of the perineum (Fig. 14.3).

Squatting, kneeling or standing. In Western countries these positions have been encouraged only in recent years. In primitive cultures where women follow their own inclinations, the majority choose to adopt a variation or combination of these postures (Russell 1982). Science supports their choice. Radiological evidence demonstrates an increase of 1 cm in the transverse diameter and 2 cm in the anteroposterior diameter of the pelvic outlet when the squatting position is adopted. This produces a 28% increase in the overall area of the outlet when comparing the supine with the squatting position, resulting in obvious benefit to the progress and ease of delivery (Russell 1969).

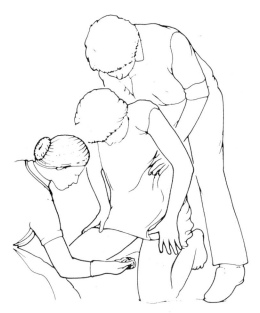

Fig. 14.4
Squatting/kneeling position with father lending support.

The birthing chair is an attempt to reconcile the advantages of an upright posture with ease of access to the perineum. Women using birthing chairs are, however, at increased risk of postpartum haemorrhage (Stewart et al 1983, Turner et al 1986). This may arise as a consequence of perineal trauma exacerbated by obstructed venous return which is reflected in the excessive perineal oedema and haemorrhoids reported in women who spend long periods of time in birthing chairs (Cottrell & Shannahan 1986). This tendency to postpartum haemorrhage is unlikely to be due to increased risk of bleeding from the placental site.

Left lateral position. This is not widely used in current practice. The perineum can be clearly viewed and uterine action is effective but an assistant may be required to support the right thigh. It provides an alternative for women who find it difficult to abduct their hips. The mother usually turns back into the dorsal position for delivery of the placenta. During this manoeuvre she should keep her knees together to prevent the uterus from filling with air; the contracted fundus should be supported by the midwife's hand.

Overall there is no evidence that posture during the second stage of labour affects the incidence of operative delivery, perineal trauma or episiotomy.

Whichever position the mother chooses, she is most likely to trust a midwife who allows her freedom of choice and active participation in her labour. Flexibility is the keynote. Positive and dramatic effects can be achieved by encouraging the mother to change and adapt her position in response to the way her body feels (Fig. 14.5).

Leg cramp is a common occurrence whichever posture is adopted. It can be relieved by massaging the calf muscle, extending the leg and dorsiflexing the foot.

Preparation for delivery

Once the onset of the second stage has been confirmed the midwife should make preliminary preparations for delivery. There is usually little urgency if the woman is primigravid but multigravidae may progress very rapidly.

The room in which the delivery is to take place should be warm with a spotlight available so that the perineum can be easily observed. The woman may wish other family members to witness the birth, especially if delivery is taking place at home. A clean area should be prepared to receive the baby and waterproof covers provided to protect the bed and floor. A sterile delivery pack which includes cord clamps, a midwife's gown and rubber gloves are placed to hand. An oxytocic agent (usually Syntometrine 1 ml) is prepared in readiness for the active management of the third stage or for use during an emergency and is checked by a second person. It must be kept separate from any neonatal drugs to avoid risk of error.

A warm cot and clothes should be prepared for the baby. In hospital a heated mattress may be used; at home, a *warm* water bottle (as opposed to a hot water bottle) can be placed in the cot.

Neonatal resuscitation equipment must be thoroughly checked and readily accessible and should include portable oxygen equipment for home deliveries.

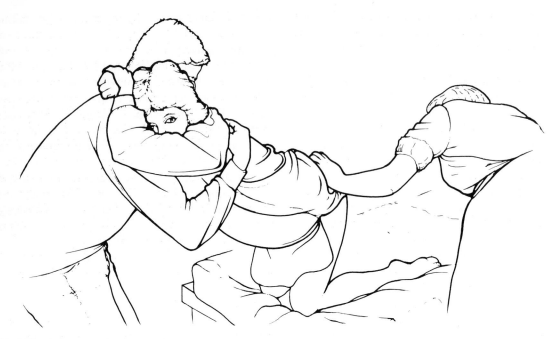

Fig. 14.5
A change of position can sometimes speed progress.

Conducting the delivery

The midwife's skill and judgement are crucial factors in minimising maternal trauma and ensuring a safe delivery for the baby. These qualities are acquired by experience but certain basic principles should be applied whatever the expertise of the accoucheuse. They are:

- observation of progress
- prevention of infection
- emotional and physical comfort of the mother
- anticipation of normal events
- recognition of abnormal developments.

Asepsis

During delivery both mother and baby are particularly vulnerable to infection. Care must be taken to observe meticulous aseptic technique when preparing sterile equipment. Sterilised surgical gloves must be worn during the delivery for the protection of both mother and midwife.

The time at which the midwife decides to scrub up will vary. If the mother is multigravid it is wise to prepare as soon as the fetal head becomes visible: in primigravidae the head usually takes a little longer to advance over the perineum. Once she has put on her gown and gloves the midwife prepares her sterile equipment. This includes the following main items:

- warm antiseptic solution
- cotton wool and pads
- cord scissors and clamps.

Delivery of the head

Throughout these preparations the midwife must not be distracted from monitoring the descent of the fetus. She must either watch the advance of the fetal head or control it with her hand or both. Quick action may be necessary if advance is rapid.

The perineum is swabbed, the delivery area draped with sterile towels and a pad used to cover the anus. There is currently no evidence to show whether or not the practice either of guarding or of massaging the perineum is effective in minimising spontaneous trauma. With each contraction the head descends. As it does so the superficial muscles of the pelvic floor can be seen to stretch, especially the transverse perineal muscles. The head recedes during the resting phase, which allows these muscles to thin gradually. The skill of the midwife in ensuring that the active phase is unhurried helps to safeguard the perineum from trauma.

The midwife places her fingers on the advancing head to monitor descent and prevent expulsive crowning which may result in perineal laceration. As the perineum distends, the decision is made as to whether an episiotomy is necessary. Light pressure on the head is maintained so that its birth is controlled. For her part, the mother can achieve control by gently blowing or 'sighing' out each breath in order to avoid pushing. The midwife will have prepared her to listen for instructions and the partner can be very supportive in relaying these. Delivery of the head in this way may take two or three contractions but delicate control will avoid unnecessary maternal trauma (Fig. 14.6).

Once crowned, the head is born by extension as the face appears at the perineum. During the resting phase before the next contraction the midwife has time to check that the cord is not around the baby's neck. If found, it should, if possible, be slackened to form a loop through which the shoulders may pass. If tightly applied,

it may still be possible to deliver the baby without cutting the cord by keeping the head near the perineum as the shoulders deliver, rather than attempting to place the baby on the mother's abdomen. If, however, the cord is very tightly wound around the neck, two artery forceps are applied 3 cm apart and the cord is severed between the two clamps. Great care must be taken that in this confined space other tissues are not clamped in error. When cutting the turgid cord it is always a wise precaution to hold a swab over the area as it is incised. This will reduce the risk of the attendants being sprayed with blood during the procedure. Once severed the cord may be unwound from around the neck.

The mother may now be able to see and touch her baby's head and assist in delivery of the trunk.

Delivery of the shoulders

Restitution and external rotation of the head must occur in order to deliver the shoulders safely and to avoid perineal laceration. External rotation shows that the shoulders are rotating into the anteroposterior diameter of the pelvic outlet which is the largest space. The midwife proceeds to deliver

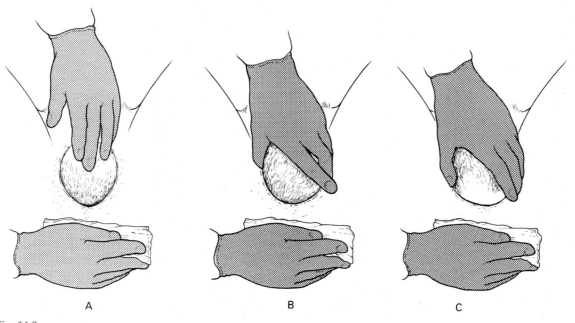

A B C

Fig. 14.6
Delivering the head: (A) Preventing too rapid extension; (B) Controlling the crowning; (C) Easing the perineum to release the face.

one shoulder at a time to avoid overstretching the perineum. A hand is placed on each side of the baby's head, over the ears, and downward traction is applied. This allows the anterior shoulder to slip beneath the symphysis pubis while the posterior shoulder remains in the vagina. If the third stage is to be actively managed the assistant is instructed to give intramuscular Syntometrine 1 ml. When the axillary crease is seen, the head and trunk are guided in an upward curve to allow the posterior shoulder to escape over the perineum (Fig. 14.7). The midwife or mother may now grasp the baby around the chest to aid the birth of the trunk and lift the baby towards the mother's abdomen. This not only allows the mother immediate sighting of her baby and close skin contact with him but removes the baby from the gush of liquor which accompanies release of the body. The time of delivery is noted.

The cord is severed at whatever time is considered appropriate (see Ch. 31). The baby is dried

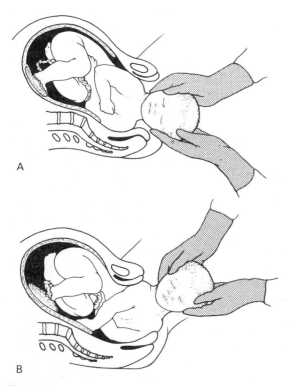

Fig. 14.7
(A) Downward traction releases anterior shoulder. (B) An upward curve allows the posterior shoulder to escape.

and warmly wrapped to prevent cooling. Swabbing of the eyes and aspiration of mucus during and immediately following delivery are not considered to be necessary providing the baby's condition is satisfactory. Oral mucus extractors should not be used because of the risks of mucus which is contaminated with a virus such as the hepatitis virus or human immunodeficiency virus (HIV) entering the operator's mouth.

The moment of birth is both joyous and beautiful. The midwife is privileged to share this unique and intimate experience with the parents.

Episiotomy

This is an incision through the perineal tissues which is designed to enlarge the vulval outlet during delivery. The UKCC sanctions its use by midwives, advocating prior infiltration of the perineum. As this is a surgical incision it is essential that the mother gives consent prior to the procedure. A detailed discussion should take place during pregnancy so that each woman is aware of the indications for and implications of the intervention. She should be assured that its use is selective and discretional. The mother's personal wishes for her own care should be clearly documented and respected.

The risks and benefits of episiotomy have been well reviewed (Banta & Thacker 1982, Hofmeyr & Sonnendecker 1987). The rationale for its use depends largely on the need to minimise the risk of severe, spontaneous, maternal trauma and to expedite the birth when there is evidence of fetal distress. During a normal delivery the indications for its use are few and the midwife should adopt a restrictive policy.

Justifiable indications
- To speed delivery if there is fetal distress.
- Prior to an assisted delivery such as forceps or ventouse extraction.
- To minimise the risk of intracranial damage during preterm and breech delivery.

Dubious indications
- To prevent overstretching of the perineal muscles with the intention of preventing the longer term problem of prolapse and stress incontinence.

• To reduce the risk of spontaneous 'explosive' trauma where the midwife has intuitive concern.

Recent evidence generated by randomised, controlled trials has provided sound scientific evidence on which practice may be based. Sleep and colleagues (1984) demonstrated that the liberal (51%) use of episiotomy during normal deliveries resulted in few advantages for mothers in terms of healing and comfort, either at 10 days or at 3 months postpartum, when compared with a restrictive (10%) episiotomy policy. On the contrary, the liberal use of episiotomy is associated with higher rates of perineal trauma (Harrison et al 1984), although it does seem to protect against anterior trauma around the labia and urethra. This, however, appears not to influence the incidences of pain on intercourse and of urinary incontinence either in the short or longer term (Sleep & Grant 1987). The midwife should use her skills to avoid this intervention if at all possible.

The timing of the incision

An episiotomy involves incision of the fourchette, the superficial muscles and skin of the perineum and the posterior vaginal wall. It can therefore successfully speed delivery only when the presenting part is directly applied to these tissues. If the episiotomy is performed too early it will fail to release the presenting part and haemorrhage from cut vessels may ensue. In addition, the levator ani muscles will not have had time to be displaced laterally and may be incised as well. If performed too late there will not be enough time to infiltrate with a local anaesthetic. There is also little reason for superimposing an episiotomy if a tear has already begun.

Types of incision

There are two main directions of incision:

Mediolateral. This begins at the mid-point of the fourchette and is directed at a 45° angle to the midline towards a point midway between the ischial tuberosity and the anus. This line avoids the danger of damage to both the anal sphincter and Bartholin's gland but it is the more difficult to repair. This is the incision largely used by midwives in the UK.

Median. This is a mid-line incision which follows the natural line of insertion of the perineal muscles. It is associated with reduced blood loss but a higher incidence of damage to the anal sphincter. It is the easier to repair and results in less pain and dyspareunia. This incision is favoured in the USA.

Infiltration of the perineum

The perineum should be adequately anaesthetised prior to the incision. Lignocaine is commonly used, 0.5% 10 ml or 1% 5 ml. The advantage of the more concentrated solution is that a smaller volume is needed. Lignocaine takes 3–4 minutes to take effect and, if possible, two or three contractions should be allowed to occur between infiltration and incision. The timing is not always easy to calculate but it is better to infiltrate and not perform an episiotomy than to incise the perineum without an effective local anaesthetic.

Method of infiltration. The perineum is cleansed with antiseptic solution. Two fingers are inserted into the vagina along the line of the proposed incision in order to protect the fetal head. The needle is inserted beneath the skin for 4–5 cm following the same line. The piston of the syringe should be withdrawn prior to injection to check whether the needle is in a blood vessel. If blood is aspirated the needle should be repositioned and the procedure repeated until no blood is withdrawn. Lignocaine is continuously injected as the needle is slowly withdrawn. Some practitioners inject the whole amount in one operation. Anaesthesia is, however, more effective if about one-third of the amount is used at first and two further injections are made, one either side of the incision line (Fig. 14.8). The needle must be redirected just before the tip is withdrawn.

The incision. A straight-bladed, blunt-ended pair of Mayo scissors is usually used. The blades should be sharp to ensure a clean incision. (Some doctors prefer to use a scalpel for this reason.) Two fingers are inserted into the vagina as before and the open blades are positioned (see Fig. 14.8). The incision is best made during a contraction when the tissues are stretched so that there is a clear view of the area and bleeding is less likely to be severe. A single, deliberate cut 4–5 cm long is

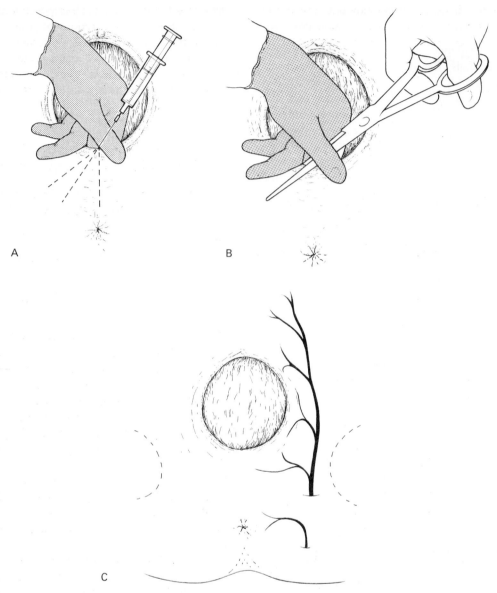

Fig. 14.8
(A) Infiltrating the perineum. (B) Performing an episiotomy. (C) Innervation of the vulval area and perineum.

made at the correct angle. Delivery of the head should follow immediately and its advance must be immediately controlled in order to avoid extension of the episiotomy. If there is any delay before the head emerges, pressure should be applied to the episiotomy site between contractions in order to minimise bleeding. Postpartum haemorrhage can occur from an episiotomy site unless bleeding points are compressed.

PERINEAL REPAIR

Midwives who have had instruction and supervised practice in suturing the perineum and are judged to be proficient may carry out the procedure. Trauma is best repaired as soon as possible after delivery in order to secure haemostasis and before oedema forms. It is also much kinder to the mother to complete this aspect of her care without undue delay and while the tissues are still anaesthetised. Prior to commencement the mother must be made as warm and comfortable as possible. The lithotomy position is usually chosen as it affords a clear view of the area. Other positions may be more appropriate in the home setting. A good, directional light is essential and the operator should be seated comfortably during the procedure.

The trolley, set with the appropriate instruments, antiseptic solution, suture materials and local anaesthetic, should be prepared before the mother's legs are placed in the stirrups. This minimises the time spent in this uncomfortable, undignified position and reduces the risks of complications such as deep vein thrombosis. The midwife scrubs and puts on sterile gown and gloves. The perineum is cleaned with warm antiseptic solution. Blood oozing from the uterus may obscure the field of vision, so a taped vaginal tampon may be inserted into the vault of the vagina. The tape is secured to the towelling drapes by a pair of forceps as a reminder that it must be removed upon completion of the procedure. Both insertion and removal should be recorded. The full extent of the trauma is assessed and explained to the mother. The procedure for repair should also be outlined so that she is aware of what is happening.

Spontaneous trauma may be of the labia anteriorly, the perineum posteriorly or both. A gentle, thorough examination must be carried out to assess the extent of the trauma accurately and to determine whether a doctor should carry out the repair, if it is extensive.

Anterior labial tears. It is debatable whether or not these should be sutured. Much depends upon the control of bleeding as the labia are very vascular. A suture may be necessary to secure haemostasis.

Posterior perineal trauma. Spontaneous tears are usually classified in degrees which are related to the anatomical structures which have been traumatised. This classification only serves as a guideline because it is often difficult to identify the structures precisely.

- *1° tear* involves the fourchette only.
- *2° tear* involves the fourchette and the superficial perineal muscles, namely the bulbo-

cavernosus and the transverse perineal muscles and in some cases the pubococcygeus.
- *3° tear.* In addition to the above structures there is damage to the anal sphincter.
- *4° tear.* This classification is sometimes used to describe trauma which extends into the rectal mucosa.

Third and fourth degree tears should be repaired by a senior obstetrician. A general anaesthetic or effective epidural or spinal anaesthetic is necessary.

Prior to the commencement of repair infiltration of the wound with local anaesthetic will be required. It is unlikely that any perineal infiltration carried out before delivery will be sufficient to ensure the mother's comfort during the procedure. Lignocaine 1% is used and time must be allowed for it to take effect before repair begins. If an epidural block is in progress, a 'top up' should be given.

The apex of the vaginal incision is identified and the posterior vaginal wall repaired from the apex downwards. A continuous suture affords better haemostasis. The suture material most commonly used is 2/0 chromic catgut. The thread should not be pulled too tightly as oedema will develop during the first 24–48 hours (Fig. 14.9). Care must be taken to identify other vaginal lacerations which should also be repaired. The deeper interrupted sutures are then inserted to repair the perineal muscles. Good approximation of tissue is important. The subsequent strength of the pelvic floor will depend largely upon adequate repair of this layer.

The best choice of method and materials for repair is debated. Grant (1986) highlights the lack of controlled trials to evaluate the different techniques and suture threads in terms of improved maternal comfort and reduced morbidity. This is likely to be of greatest significance in the choice for skin closure. A tear is usually repaired using interrupted sutures (with or without buried knots); for an episiotomy a continuous subcuticular stitch may be used (see Fig. 14.9). There is little substantiated evidence from recipient mothers as to which is preferable in terms of reduced pain, ease of sitting and comfortable sexual intercourse. Suture material may be absorbable (e.g. chromic

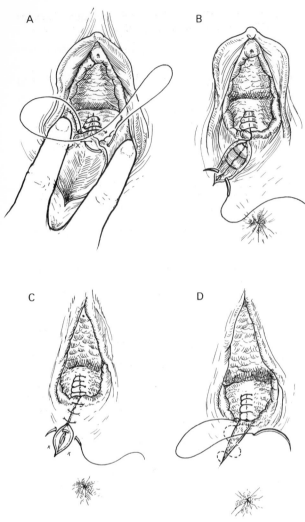

Fig. 14.9
Perineal repair: (A) A continuous suture is used to repair the vaginal wall. (B) Three or four interrupted sutures repair the fascia and muscle of the perineum. (C) Interrupted sutures to the skin. (D) Subcuticular skin suture.

catgut, Dexon) or non-absorbable (e.g. black silk). A continuous, subcuticular stitch using an absorbable thread appears to produce fewest maternal problems (Grant 1989).

Whatever the choice of material or type of suture, repair of the skin edges should begin at the fourchette so that the vaginal opening is properly aligned. When the wound has been closed, any further vulval lacerations should be repaired. Anterior labial tears occur more frequently when

episiotomy has been avoided. This trauma does not appear to cause additional maternal discomfort 10 days after delivery (Sleep et al 1984).

The sutured areas should be inspected in order to confirm haemostasis before the vaginal pack is removed. A vaginal examination is made to ensure that the introitus has not been narrowed. Upon completion a rectal examination is made in order to ensure that no sutures have penetrated the rectal mucosa. Any such sutures must be removed to prevent fistula formation. It is essential to warn the mother before this examination is performed.

The area is cleaned and a sterile sanitary pad positioned over the vulva and perineum. The mother's legs are then gently and simultaneously removed from lithotomy support and she is made comfortable. The nature of the trauma and repair should be explained to her and information given on whether or not sutures will need to be removed. If the midwife suspects damage to the upper vagina, cervix, anal sphincter or rectal mucosa, a senior obstetrician should be notified as this repair will be outside her province. A general anaesthetic is occasionally necessary if the trauma is extensive.

Records

It is the responsibility of the midwife conducting the delivery to complete the labour record. This should include details of any drugs administered, of the duration and progress of labour, of the reason for performing an episiotomy and of perineal repair. This information is recorded on the mother's notes and may be duplicated on her co-operation card and domiciliary record as well as in the birth register. Details of the baby's condition including Apgar score are also recorded.

The birth notification must be completed within 36 hours of delivery. This may be undertaken by anyone present at the birth but is usually carried out by the midwife. The notification is sent to the medical officer in the health district in which the baby was born.

The development of computerised records has minimised the need for duplication of information and has also reduced the time spent by midwives in completing several sets of documents. Computerised data are subject to the Data Protection Act.

Reader Activities

1. What information is given to women who attend parentcraft classes in your area of practice in relation to perineal management at delivery and perineal care postpartum? It may prove enlightening to replicate part of Lyn Cater's study (1984).

Following childbirth, women were invited to draw on a prepared diagram the direction and extent of perineal damage they believed they had sustained during delivery. The results highlighted how ill-prepared and poorly informed most women were; such findings have important implications for practice.

2. In the unit in which you work search for documents which influence or dictate any aspect of practice related to second stage management, for example, the imposition of an upper limit of duration or an episiotomy policy. These documents may be guidelines for practice, defined standards of care or policy statements. When were these documents compiled and by whom? Are any of the recommendations supported by research evidence? What can you do to change, improve or remove such limitations on practice?

REFERENCES

Banta D, Thacker S B 1982 The risks and benefits of episiotomy. Birth 9 (1 Spring): 25–30

Benyon C 1957 The normal second stage of labour. Journal of Obstetrics and Gynaecology, British Empire 64: 6.1

Cater L 1984 A little knowledge... Nursing Mirror 159 (11): ii–viii

Cottrell B H, Shannahan M D 1986 Effect of the birth chair on duration of second stage labor and maternal outcome. Nursing Research 35: 364–367

Grant A 1986 Repair of episiotomies and perineal tears. British Journal of Obstetrics and Gynaecology 93: 176–178

Grant A 1989 Repair of perineal trauma after childbirth. In: Chalmers I, Enkin M, Keirse M J N C (eds) Effective care in pregnancy and childbirth. Oxford University Press, Oxford, p 1170–1181

Harrison R F, Brennan M, North P M, Reed J V, Wickham E A 1984 Is routine episiotomy necessary? British Medical Journal 288: 1971–1975

Hofmeyr G J, Sonnendecker E W W 1987 Elective episiotomy in perspective. South African Medical Journal 71: 357–359

Humphrey M D, Chang A, Wood E C, Morgan S, Hounslow D 1974 A decrease in fetal pH during the second stage of labour when conducted in the dorsal position. Journal of Obstetrics and Gynaecology, British Commonwealth 81: 600–602

Inch S 1982 The second stage. Birthrights. Hutchinson, London, p 117–144

Kurz C S, Schneider H, Hutch R, Hutch A 1982 The influence of maternal position on the fetal transcutaneous oxygen pressure. Journal of Perinatal Medicine 10 (Suppl. 2): 74–75

McKay S, Roberts J 1985 Second stage of labour: what is normal? Journal of Obstetric, Gynaecologic and Neonatal Nursing 14: 101–106

Mendez-Bauer C et al 1976 Effects of different maternal positions during labour. In: 5th European Congress of Perinatal Medicine, (9–12 June, Stockholm) Uppsala, Sweden

Ohel G 1978 Fetal heart rate in the second stage of labour and fetal outcome. South African Medical Journal 54: 1130–1131

Russell J G B 1969 Moulding of the pelvic outlet. Journal of Obstetrics and Gynaecology 76: 817–820

Russell J G B 1982 The rationale of primitive delivery positions. British Journal of Obstetrics and Gynaecology 89 (September): 712–715

Sleep J, Grant A 1987 West Berkshire perineal trial: three-year follow up. British Medical Journal 295: 749–751

Sleep J, Grant A, Garcia J, Elbourne D, Spencer J, Chalmers I 1984 West Berkshire perineal management trial. British Medical Journal 289: 587–590

Sleep J, Roberts J, Chalmers I 1989 Care during the second stage of labour. In: Chalmers I, Enkin M, Keirse M J N C (eds) Effective care in pregnancy and childbirth. Oxford University Press, Oxford, p 1129–1144

Stewart P, Hillan E, Calder A A 1983 A randomised trial to evaluate the use of a birth chair for delivery. Lancet i (June 11): 1296–98

Turner M J, Romney M L, Webb J B, Gordon H 1986 The birthing chair: an obstetric hazard? Journal of Obstetrics and Gynaecology 6: 232–235

FURTHER READING

Johnstone F D, Aboelmagd M S, Harouni A K 1987 Maternal posture in the second stage and fetal acid base status. British Journal of Obstetrics and Gynaecology 94: 753–757

Knauth D G, Haloburdo E P 1986 Effect of pushing techniques in birthing chair on length of second stage of labour. Nursing Research 35: 49–51

Roberts J 1980 Alternative positions for child birth. Part II. Journal of Nurse-Midwifery 25(5): 13–19

Roberts J E, Goldstein S A, Gruener J S, Maggio M, Mendez-Bauer C 1987 A descriptive analysis of involuntary bearing down efforts during the expulsive phase of labour. Journal of Obstetric, Gynecologic and Neonatal Nursing 16: 48–55

Stewart K S 1984 The second stage. In: Studd J (ed) Progress in obstetrics and gynaecology, vol 4. Churchill Livingstone, Edinburgh, p 197–216

15

Physiology and management of the third stage of labour

JENNIFER SLEEP

This is a time when the activity and excitement accompanying the birth of the baby are replaced by the parents' quiet and wondrous contemplation of their offspring. The focus shifts from the mother's concentrated exertions to the miracle of the newborn. There is a sense of emotional and physical relief. Yet for the mother this is the most dangerous stage of labour when the skill and expertise of the midwife will be crucial factors in ensuring her safety.

PHYSIOLOGICAL PROCESSES

These are a continuation of the processes and forces at work during the earlier stages of labour. It is an understanding of these changes which dictates the midwife's care. During the third stage separation and expulsion of the placenta and membranes occur as the result of an interplay of mechanical and haemostatic factors. The time at which the placenta actually separates from the uterine wall may vary. It may shear off during the final expulsive contractions accompanying the birth of the baby or remain adherent for some considerable time. The third stage usually lasts between 5 and 15 minutes but any period up to 1 hour may be considered normal.

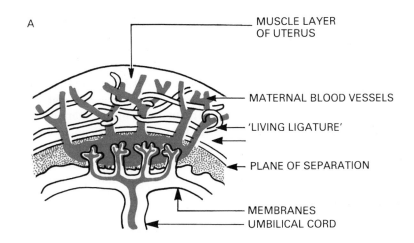

A

MUSCLE LAYER
OF UTERUS

MATERNAL BLOOD VESSELS

'LIVING LIGATURE'

PLANE OF SEPARATION

MEMBRANES
UMBILICAL CORD

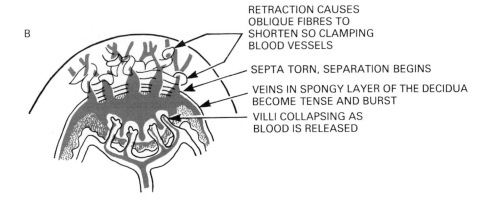

B

RETRACTION CAUSES
OBLIQUE FIBRES TO
SHORTEN SO CLAMPING
BLOOD VESSELS

SEPTA TORN, SEPARATION BEGINS

VEINS IN SPONGY LAYER OF THE DECIDUA
BECOME TENSE AND BURST

VILLI COLLAPSING AS
BLOOD IS RELEASED

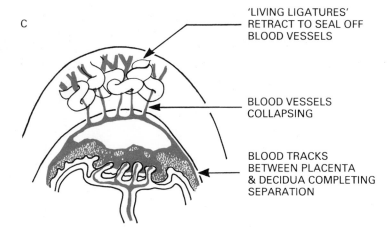

C

'LIVING LIGATURES'
RETRACT TO SEAL OFF
BLOOD VESSELS

BLOOD VESSELS
COLLAPSING

BLOOD TRACKS
BETWEEN PLACENTA
& DECIDUA COMPLETING
SEPARATION

Fig. 15.1
The placental site during separation. (A) Diagram of uterus and placenta before separation. (B) Separation begins. (C) Separation almost complete.

Separation and descent of the placenta

Mechanical factors

The unique characteristic of uterine muscle lies in the power of retraction. During the second stage of labour the uterine cavity progressively empties so enabling the retraction process to accelerate. Thus by the beginning of the third stage the placental site has already begun to diminish in size. As this occurs the placenta itself becomes squeezed and the blood in the intervillous spaces is forced back into the spongy layer of the decidua. Retraction of the oblique uterine muscle fibres exerts pressure on the blood vessels so that blood does not drain back into the maternal system. The vessels thus become tense and congested. With the next contraction the turgid veins burst and a small amount of blood seeps between the thin septa of the spongy layer and the placental surface stripping it from its attachment (Fig. 15.1). In addition, as the surface area for placental attachment reduces, the non-elastic placenta begins to detach from the shrinking uterine wall.

Separation usually begins centrally so that a retroplacental clot is formed (Fig. 15.2). This may further aid separation by exerting pressure at the mid-point of placental attachment so that the increased weight helps to strip the adherent lateral borders. This increased weight also helps to peel the membranes off the uterine wall so that the clot, thus formed, becomes enclosed in a membranous bag as the placenta descends, fetal surface first. This process of separation (first described by Schultze) is associated with more complete shearing of both placenta and membranes and less attendant fluid blood loss. Alternatively, the placenta may begin to detach asymmetrically at one of its lateral borders. The blood escapes so that separation is unaided by the formation of a retroplacental clot. The placenta descends, slipping sideways, maternal surface first. This process (first described by Matthews and Duncan) takes longer and is associated with ragged, incomplete expulsion of the membranes and a higher fluid blood loss.

Once separation has occurred, the uterus contracts strongly, forcing placenta and membranes to fall into the lower uterine segment and thence into the vagina.

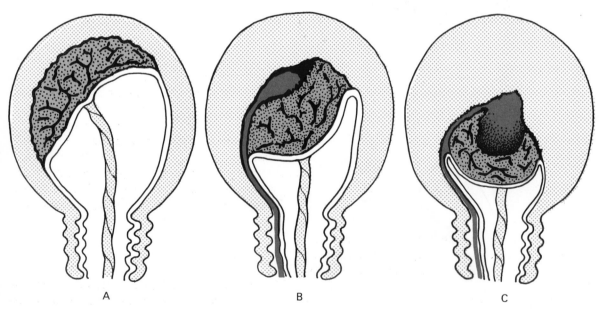

A   B   C

Fig. 15.2
The mechanism of placental separation: (A) Uterine wall partially retracted but not sufficiently to cause placental separation. (B) Further contraction and retraction thicken uterine wall, reduce placental site and aid placental separation. (C) Complete separation and formation of retroplacental clot.
Note. The thin lower segment has collapsed like a concertina following the birth of the baby.

1. The tortuous uterine blood vessels are woven between the oblique muscle fibres present in the upper uterine segment. As these fibres retract, their resultant thickening exerts pressure on the torn vessels acting as clamps, so securing a ligature action. This is shown in Figure 15.1. It is the absence of oblique fibres in the lower uterine segment which explains the greatly increased blood loss which usually accompanies placental separation in placenta praevia.

2. Following separation a vigorous uterine contraction brings the walls into apposition so that further pressure is exerted on the placental site.

3. There is evidence to suggest that there is a transitory activation of the coagulation and fibrinolytic systems during, and immediately following, placental separation (Bonnar et al 1970). It is believed that this protective response is especially active at the placental site so that clot formation in the torn vessels is intensified. Following separation the placental site is rapidly covered by a fibrin mesh utilising 5–10% of the circulating fibrinogen. This secures haemostasis.

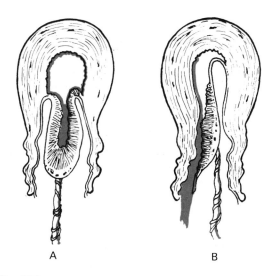

Fig. 15.3
Expulsion of the placenta: (A) Schultze method.
(B) Matthews Duncan method.

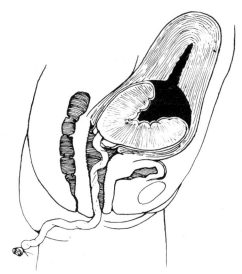

Fig. 15.4
Third stage. Placenta in lower uterine segment.

Haemostasis

The normal volume of blood flow through the placental site is 500–800 ml per minute. At placental separation this has to be staunched within seconds or serious haemorrhage will occur. The normal physiological processes which control bleeding are critical factors in minimising this blood loss and safeguarding maternal condition, indeed the mother's life. The interplay of three factors is involved:

MANAGEMENT OF THE THIRD STAGE

The midwife's care of the mother should be based on an understanding of the normal physiological processes at work. Her actions can help to reduce the very real risks of haemorrhage, infection, retained placenta and shock, any of which may increase maternal morbidity and even threaten life. A mother's ability to withstand these complications depends, to a large degree, upon her general condition and the avoidance of debilitating, predisposing problems, e.g. anaemia, ketosis, exhaustion and hypotonic uterine action.

Position of the mother

This may vary according to the mother's personal preference, the normality of progress and the experience and confidence of the attendant midwife, and may be influenced by the need for the midwife to monitor closely factors such as uterine contraction and blood loss.

Dorsal position

This position enables the parents to cuddle and inspect their new baby in safety, and it is essential if the third stage is to be actively managed as it allows easy palpation of the uterine fundus. However, blood is more likely to pool in the uterus and vagina, thus disguising the true blood loss.

Upright/kneeling/squatting position

One of these positions should be recommended when the third stage is to be passively managed except when the mother has had an epidural block during labour. Gravity and intra-abdominal pressure may now aid and speed the process. Blood loss can be more easily observed as fluids will drain out of the vagina. However, the mother will need support while she cuddles her baby (Fig. 15.5).

Whichever position is adopted the use of wedges, pillows and physical support from the father will help to ensure the mother's comfort and safety. Some women feel cold and shivery at this time especially if labour has progressed rapidly. This is usually transient and not abnormal. Additional warmth provided by clean, dry linen, a woollen bed

jacket, an extra blanket and bed socks help to remedy the situation.

Asepsis

The need for asepsis is even greater now than in the preceding stages of labour. Laceration and bruising of the cervix, vagina, perineum and vulva provide a route for the entry of micro-organisms. At the placental site a raw wound provides an ideal medium for infection. Strict attention to the prevention of sepsis is therefore vital.

Cutting the umbilical cord

This may have been carried out during delivery of the baby if the cord was tightly around the neck. However, opinions vary as to the most beneficial time for clamping the cord during the third stage of labour (Inch 1985). Early clamping is carried out in the first 1–3 minutes immediately after birth and before cord pulsation ceases. This enables freedom of movement for either parent to hold their baby or for the midwife to take resuscitative measures if necessary. It has been suggested that this practice:

- reduces the time to placental separation (Botha 1968).
- may reduce the volume of blood returning to the fetus by as much as 75–125 ml, especially if clamping occurs within the first minute (Montgomery 1960). This in turn may reduce neonatal haemoglobin levels in the short term but, in the only published study to assess longer term outcomes, by 6 weeks after birth the haemoglobin levels in these babies had been restored (Pau-Chen & Tsu-Shan 1960).
- may prematurely interrupt the respiratory function of the placenta in maintaining O_2 levels and combating acidosis in the early moments of life. This may be of particular importance in the baby who is slow to breathe.
- results in lower neonatal bilirubin levels but the effect on the incidence of clinical jaundice is unclear (Prendiville & Elbourne 1989).
- increases the likelihood of fetomaternal transfusion as a larger volume of blood remains in the placenta. Venous pressure is further

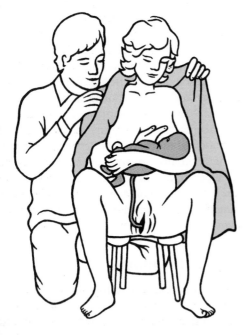

Fig. 15.5
Mother sitting up, supported by her partner. The cord remains unclamped.

increased as retraction continues and may be sufficiently high to rupture surface placental vessels thus facilitating the transfer of fetal cells into the maternal system. This may be a critical factor where the mother's blood group is Rhesus negative (Ladipo 1972).

- results in the truncated umbilical vessels containing a quantity of clotted blood which provides an ideal medium for bacterial growth.

The proponents of late clamping suggest that no action be taken until pulsation ceases or until the placenta has been completely delivered, thus allowing the physiological processes to take place without intervention. Postulated advantages include:

1. The route to the low-resistance placental circulation remains patent which provides the newborn with a safety valve for any raised systemic blood pressure. This may be critical when the baby is preterm or asphyxiated, as raised pulmonary and central venous pressures may exacerbate the difficulties in initiating respiration and accompanying circulatory adaptation (Dunn 1985).

2. The reduction in the length of time for the cord to separate postnatally.

3. The transfusion of the full quota of placental blood to the newborn. This may constitute as much as 40% of the circulating volume depending on when the cord is clamped and at what level the baby is held prior to clamping (Yao & Lind 1974) and therefore may be important in maintaining haematocrit levels.

Another factor which may influence the amount of placental transfusion is the use of an oxytocic agent prior to the completion of labour. This may precipitate a strong uterine contraction with resultant over-transfusion of the baby.

It would seem therefore that the timing of the clamping of the cord may be of considerable significance to both mother and baby. There is, however, no evidence to suggest that it influences the incidence of postpartum haemorrhage. The most common current practice is to clamp and cut the cord some time before delivery of the placenta. This is necessary if controlled cord traction is to be used to complete the third stage. Care should be taken to apply the clamp nearest the baby 3–4 cm clear of the abdominal wall to avoid

pinching the skin or clamping a portion of gut which, in rare instances, may be in the cord. A greater length of cord is left when umbilical vessels are needed for transfusion, e.g. in preterm babies and cases of Rhesus haemolytic disease. Holding a swab over the cord as it is cut will help to reduce the risk of the midwife being sprayed with blood as the congested umbilical vessels are incised.

Oxytocic agents

These are drugs which stimulate the uterus to contract. They may be administered at crowning of the head, at delivery of the anterior shoulder, at the end of the second stage of labour or following the delivery of the placenta to ensure effective uterine contractions, thereby minimising blood loss and promoting rapid separation and descent of the placenta. They do, however, carry the risk of side-effects such as maternal hypertension.

During the antenatal period it is important to discuss these drugs with each mother, explaining their use in relation to the events of labour and the method of placental delivery. Prophylactic oxytocics may be specifically indicated where ineffective or hypotonic uterine action has arisen during the first or second stages of labour but they are commonly used routinely. Emergency use is usually in the event of haemorrhage. If the mother specifically requests that these drugs be withheld from routine use the midwife should clarify the circumstances in which this decision may be reversed. If an oxytocic drug is *not* to be used, the third stage must be *passively* managed and the mother's preference for the care recorded in her notes. Some would wish the record to be signed by the mother. It would be expedient for the midwife to notify her supervisor of such a request if it is contrary to local guidelines. In practice one of the following oxytocic drugs is usually used:

Syntometrine
1 ml contains 5 units of Syntocinon and 0.5 mg ergometrine and is administered by intramuscular injection. The Syntocinon acts within $2\frac{1}{2}$ minutes, and the ergometrine within 6–7 minutes (Fig. 15.6). Their combined action results in a rapid uterine

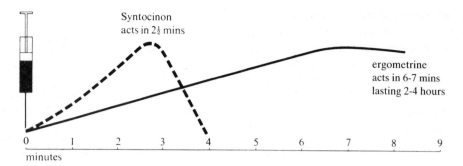

Fig. 15.6
Showing the rapid action of Syntocinon in comparison with ergometrine.

contraction enhanced by a stronger, more sustained contraction lasting several hours. It is usually administered as the anterior shoulder of the baby is delivered thus stimulating good uterine action at the beginning of the third stage. It is important, however, that the placenta should be delivered before the ergometrine component acts, otherwise it may be retained. The evidence to date suggests that this is the oxytocic of choice in the management of the third stage of labour where reducing the risk of haemorrhage is the primary consideration, for example in women who have a previous history of postpartum haemorrhage.

Syntocinon

If the mother is hypertensive, it may be considered expedient to give Syntocinon in order to reduce the risks of hypertension and increased vomiting associated with the administration of ergometrine. Questions remain about the most appropriate dose. Current evidence suggests 5–10 units administered intramuscularly or given intravenously in emergency situations (Elbourne 1992).

Intramuscular ergometrine 0.5 mg

Because of the 6- to 7-minute time delay between administration and action of this drug it is usually given at an earlier stage of delivery, namely crowning of the head. Its use is not widely advocated as it carries a greater risk of prolonged third stage and retained placenta (Prendiville & Elbourne 1989). Furthermore in the event of subsequent shoulder dystocia there is an increased risk of fetal anoxia and of uterine rupture.

Intravenous ergometrine 0.25 mg

This acts within 45 seconds; therefore it is particularly useful in securing a rapid contraction where hypotonic uterine action results in haemorrhage. If a doctor is not present in such an emergency, the injection may be given by a midwife.

CAUTION. No more than 2 doses of ergometrine 0.5 mg should be given as it can cause headache, nausea and hypertension. Great caution is therefore required where a hypertensive state already presents and its use may be contra-indicated.

Chapter 42 deals with the procedures concerning administration of drugs.

DELIVERY OF THE PLACENTA AND MEMBRANES

Active management by controlled cord traction

This method is in widespread use as it is believed to reduce blood loss, shorten the third stage of labour and therefore minimise the time during which the mother is at risk from haemorrhage. It is designed to enhance the normal physiological process. Successful results depend upon understanding the action of Syntometrine, timing the procedure properly and being alert to the possibility of a second twin in the uterus. Intramuscular Syntometrine 1 ml may be given as the head is crowned or more commonly with the delivery of the anterior shoulder. This allows time for completion of the second stage and preliminary care of the baby before the Syntocinon component causes a strong uterine contraction.

The abdomen is draped with a sterile towel and a hand placed lightly on the fundus to monitor progress. It is important not to manipulate the uterus in any way as this may precipitate incoordinate action. No further step should be taken until a strong contraction is palpable. If tension is applied to the umbilical cord without this contraction, then uterine inversion may occur. Consequentially, a joyous, normal delivery may rapidly change to an acute obstetric emergency with life-threatening implications for the mother.

A sterile receiver should be placed against the perineum to collect blood loss and receive the placenta. If artery forceps are used to clamp the cord it is useful if they are moved and re-applied near the vulva so that they can be used to provide a handhold when applying cord traction. If a clamp is not applied, the cord is best held firmly by winding it around the hand so that tension can be applied without losing grasp of the slippery surface.

There is debate about whether controlled cord traction (CCT) should be applied before or after the signs of placental separation have been noted. Levy & Moore (1985) observed that blood loss was reduced when CCT was delayed until lengthening of the cord and a trickle of fresh blood loss had been observed. There are, however, four checks to be made before applying traction to the cord:

- that an oxytocic drug has been administered
- that it has been given time to act
- that the uterus is well contracted
- that counter-traction is applied.

When the uterus palpably contracts, one hand is placed above the level of the symphysis pubis with the palm facing towards the umbilicus exerting pressure in an upwards direction. This is counter-traction. The other hand, firmly grasping the cord, applies traction in a downward and backward direction following the line of the birth canal (Fig. 15.7). Some resistance may be felt but it is important to apply steady tension by pulling the cord firmly and maintaining the pressure. Jerky movements and force should be avoided. The aim is to complete the action as one continuous, smooth, controlled movement. However, it is only possible to exert this tension for 1 or 2 minutes as it may

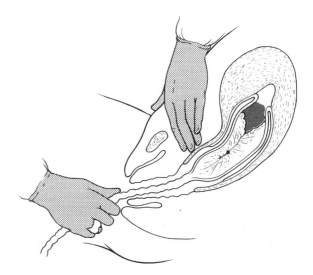

Fig. 15.7
Controlled cord traction.

be an uncomfortable procedure for the mother and the midwife's hand will tire.

Downward traction on the cord must be released *before* uterine counter-traction is relaxed. If the manoeuvre is not immediately successful there should be a pause before the uterine contraction is again checked and a further attempt is made. Should the uterus relax, tension is temporarily released until a good contraction is again palpable. Once the placenta is visible it may be cupped in the hands to ease pressure on the friable membranes. A gentle upward and downward movement or twisting action will help to coax out the membranes and increase the chances of delivering them intact. Artery forceps may be applied to gradually ease them out of the vagina. This process should not be hurried; great care must be taken to avoid tearing them.

Recent evidence suggests that active management of the third stage of labour shortens it and results in less blood loss, fewer blood transfusions and a reduced need for therapeutic oxytocics. The neonatal effects associated with increased placental transfusion include higher mean birth weight and higher neonatal haematocrit accompanied by an increase in the incidence of jaundice (Prendiville et al 1988). Its present and continued use in midwifery practice would therefore appear to be justified.

Breaking of the cord

This is not an unusual occurrence during this procedure. Before further action, it is crucial to check that the uterus remains firmly contracted. If the placenta remains adherent, no further action should be taken before a doctor is notified. It is possible that manual removal may be indicated (Ch. 29). Should placental separation have occurred (see passive physiological management), maternal effort is likely to secure expulsion. If there is any doubt, the midwife applies fresh sterile gloves before performing a vaginal examination to ascertain whether the placenta is palpable per vaginam. If so, it is probable that separation has occurred and when the uterus is well contracted maternal effort may be encouraged. As a last resort, if the mother is unable to push effectively, fundal pressure may be used. An oxytocic must have been given. Great care is exercised to ensure that placental separation has already occurred, and the uterus is well contracted. The mother should be relaxed as the midwife exerts downward and backward pressure on the firmly contracted fundus. This method can cause considerable pain and distress to the mother and result in the stretching and bruising of supportive uterine ligaments. If it is performed without good uterine contraction, acute inversion may ensue. This is an extremely dangerous procedure in unskilled hands and is not advocated in everyday practice when alternative, safer methods may be employed.

Passive physiological management

This allows the physiological changes to take their natural course with minimal intervention and normally excludes the administration of oxytocic drugs. The processes of placental separation and expulsion are quite distinct from one another and the signs of separation and descent must be evident before maternal effort can be used to expedite expulsion. If the mother is sitting or squatting at this stage, gravity will aid expulsion.

Signs of placental separation and descent

At the beginning of the third stage, a strong uterine contraction results in the fundus being palpable below the umbilicus. It feels broad as the placenta is still in the upper segment. As the placenta separates and falls into the lower uterine segment:

— there is a small fresh blood loss
— the cord lengthens

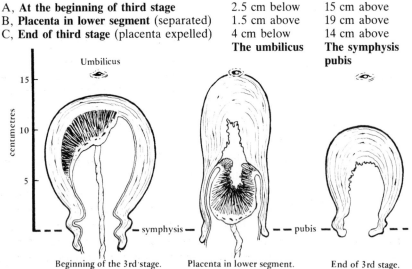

SUMMARY OF FUNDAL HEIGHTS DURING THIRD STAGE

		The umbilicus	The symphysis pubis
A,	**At the beginning of third stage**	2.5 cm below	15 cm above
B,	**Placenta in lower segment** (separated)	1.5 cm above	19 cm above
C,	**End of third stage** (placenta expelled)	4 cm below	14 cm above

Umbilicus

Symphysis pubis

centimetres

15

10

5

— symphysis —   — — pubis —

Beginning of the 3rd stage.   Placenta in lower segment.   End of 3rd stage.

Fig. 15.8
Fundal height relative to the umbilicus and symphysis pubis.

— the fundus becomes rounder and smaller; it rises in the abdomen and becomes more mobile as it is perched on top of the placenta.

If good uterine contractions are sustained, maternal effort will usually bring about expulsion. The mother simply pushes as during the second stage of labour. Encouragement is important as by now she may be exhausted and the contractions will feel weaker and less expulsive than those during the second stage of labour. Providing that fresh blood loss is not excessive and the mother's condition remains good and her pulse rate normal, there need be no anxiety. This spontaneous process can take from 20 minutes to an hour to complete. It is important that the midwife monitors uterine action by placing a hand lightly on the fundus. She can thus palpate the contraction whilst checking that relaxation does not result in the uterus filling with blood. Vigilance is crucial as it should be remembered that the longer the placenta remains undelivered, the greater the risk of bleeding as the uterus cannot contract down fully whilst the bulky placenta is still in it. Great patience, calm and confidence are required on the part of the midwife to secure a successful conclusion. An oxytocic agent need not be given unless uterine tone is poor.

These physiological changes may be enhanced by encouraging the mother to suckle the baby. This will result in the reflex release of oxytocin from the posterior lobe of the pituitary gland, which helps to secure good uterine action.

Cord blood sampling
This may be required for a variety of conditions:

— when the mother's blood group is Rhesus negative or as a precautionary measure if the mother's Rhesus type is unknown.
— when atypical maternal antibodies have been found during an antenatal screening test.
— where a haemoglobinopathy is suspected, e.g. sickle-cell disease.

Using a syringe and needle, the sample should be taken from the fetal surface of the placenta where the blood vessels are congested and easily visible. This must be done before the blood clots, but is a quick procedure if preparation has been made.

If the cord has not been clamped prior to placental delivery the fetal vessels will not be congested, but a sample of sufficient volume may still be easily obtained. The appropriate containers should be used for the investigations requested. These may include the baby's blood group, Rhesus type, haemoglobin estimation, serum bilirubin level, Coombs' test or electrophoresis. Maternal blood for Kleihauer testing can be taken upon completion of the third stage.

COMPLETION OF THE THIRD STAGE

The midwife must first check that the uterus is well contracted and fresh blood loss is minimal. Careful inspection of the perineum and lower vagina is important. A strong light is directed onto the perineum in order to assess trauma accurately prior to instigating repair. This should be carried out as gently as possible as the tissues are often bruised and oedematous. Slight lacerations such as damage to the fourchette may be repaired immediately. However, if repair of a more extensive wound such as an episiotomy or a 2° tear is necessary, the mother should be made comfortable by changing soiled bed linen or placing a clean, waterproof-backed pad beneath her buttocks and back whilst the necessary preparations are made (see Ch. 14).

The vulva and perineum are gently cleansed using warm water or an appropriate antiseptic solution, softly dried and a clean pad placed in position. Maternal pulse, blood pressure and temperature are recorded. Once the mother is comfortable, examination of the placenta and membranes is the next priority.

Examination of placenta and membranes
This should be performed as soon after delivery as possible so that if there is doubt about their completeness, further action may be taken before the mother leaves the labour ward or the midwife prepares to leave the home. Meticulous inspection must be carried out in order to make sure that no part of the placenta or membranes has been retained. The membranes are the most difficult to examine as they become torn during delivery

and may be ragged. Every attempt should be made to piece them together to give an overall picture of completeness. This is easier to see if the placenta is held by the cord, allowing the membranes to hang. The hole through which the baby was delivered can then usually be identified and a hand spread out inside the membranes to aid inspection (Fig. 15.9). The placenta should then be laid on a flat surface and both placental surfaces minutely examined in a good light. The amnion should be peeled from the chorion right up to the umbilical cord, which allows the chorion to be fully viewed.

Any clots on the maternal surface need to be removed and kept for measuring. Broken fragments of cotyledon must be carefully replaced before an accurate assessment is possible.

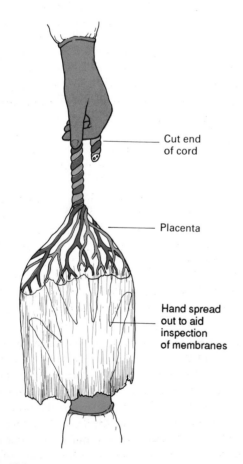

Cut end of cord

Placenta

Hand spread out to aid inspection of membranes

Fig. 15.9
Examination of the membranes.

Recent infarctions are bright red, old infarctions form grey patches whereas localised calcification can be seen as flattened white plaques feeling gritty to the touch. (None of these is of great significance at this stage, but may provide retrospective evidence of an intra-uterine problem.) The lobes of a complete placenta fit neatly together without any gaps, the edges forming a uniform circle. Blood vessels should not radiate beyond the placental edge; if they do this denotes a succenturiate lobe which has developed separately from the main placenta (see Ch. 4). When such a lobe is visible there is no cause for concern, but if the tissue has been retained the vessels will end abruptly at a hole in the membrane. On the fetal surface the position of insertion of the cord is noted. This is most commonly central but may be lateral (for abnormal insertion, see Ch. 4). Two umbilical arteries and one vein should be present. The absence of one artery may be associated with congenital abnormality, particularly renal agenesis: the paediatrician should be informed. In some units the placental weight may be recorded. This will vary according to the time of clamping of the cord. Delayed clamping produces a placenta weighing approximately one-sixth of the baby's birth weight, whereas early clamping results in an additional volume of contained blood which increases the weight to nearer one-fifth of the birth weight. The cord length averages 50 cm.

Disposal of placenta
It is important to remember that the placenta is the property of the mother and her wishes regarding its disposal must be solicited and respected. The majority of women will rely on the midwife to undertake this task. It then becomes her responsibility to do so with maximum safety. This does not pose a problem in hospital where incinerators are available; where delivery has taken place in the home, the midwife is best advised to take the placenta to the nearest hospital for incineration. Home delivery packs usually include a plastic bag for this purpose. Disposal by burial is not recommended because of the risk of preying animals.

If there is any suspicion that the placenta or membranes are incomplete, they must be kept for inspection and a doctor informed immediately. Blood loss should be estimated as accurately as possible although Newton et al (1961) and Levy & Moore (1985) have demonstrated that the average normal recorded loss of between 150 and 300 ml represents a gross underestimate. Account must be taken of blood which has soaked into linen and swabs as well as measurable fluid loss and clot formation.

Upon completion of the examination the midwife should return her attention to the mother. The empty uterus should be firmly contracted. If the fundus has risen in the abdomen a blood clot may be present. This should be expelled while the uterus is in a state of contraction by pressing the fundus gently in a downward and backward direction — with due regard to the risk of inversion and acute discomfort to the mother. Force should *never* be used.

Immediate care

It is advisable for mother and baby to remain in the midwife's care for at least an hour after delivery, whether in the home or in a labour ward. Much of this time will be spent in clearing up and completion of records but careful observation of mother and baby is very important. If an epidural cannula is in situ it is usually removed and checked at this time.

Most mothers appreciate a wash although a bath or shower may be preferred especially if the mother is at home. The father is the ideal person to help. A fresh nightie, hair brush, the use of a deodorant, talcum powder or perfume do much to restore comfort and increase a sense of well-being. Cleaning the teeth and the application of lip salve or cream can help relieve the discomfort of a dry mouth and sore lips, especially if inhalational analgesia has been used during labour. The mother should be encouraged to pass urine because a full bladder may impede uterine contraction. She may not actually feel an urge to do so especially if she has passed urine immediately prior to delivery or an effective epidural has been in progress but she should be asked to try. Following use of the bedpan or toilet, the vulva should be douched, dried and a clean pad applied.

Uterine contraction and blood loss should be checked on several occasions throughout this first hour. The mother is left warm and resting comfortably with good pillow support and in a dry bed. A hot drink is usually welcomed by both parents. If the mother is hungry there is no reason why she should not enjoy a light snack such as toast, but in practice this can often precipitate vomiting especially if pethidine has been given during labour. The choice can be left to her discretion.

Throughout this same period the midwife should pay regard to the baby's general well-being. She should check the security of the cord clamp and observe general skin colour, respirations and temperature. A baby will quickly chill in the comparative cool following birth. She or he needs to be thoroughly dried and then wrapped in a clean, dry towel so that body heat is retained. In many labour wards, electrically warmed cot mattresses and perspex heat shields are used, but the warmest place for a baby is cuddled close to his mother. At an early stage a full examination of the baby is made in the presence of his parents (see Ch. 32).

Most mothers intending to breast feed will wish to put their babies to the breast during these early moments of contact. This is especially advantageous as babies are usually very alert at this time and their sucking reflex particularly strong. There is also evidence to suggest that women who breast feed soon after delivery successfully breast feed for a longer period of time (Salariya et al 1979). An additional benefit lies in the reflex release of oxytocin from the posterior lobe of the pituitary gland which stimulates the uterus to contract. This may result in the mother experiencing a sudden fresh blood loss as the uterus empties and she should be reassured. The desire to feed a newborn baby is a warm, loving and instinctive response and a bottle feed should be available for those who do not wish to breast feed. This may contain water, dextrose solution or artificial milk according to the unit policy. It may be appropriate for the father to give part of a bottle feed.

It is important that the midwife allows the new parents a quiet, private time together to admire and inspect their new offspring (Fig. 15.10). She should remain unobtrusively in attendance and this affords the ideal time to complete the labour record.

Records

A complete and accurate account of the labour including the documentation of all drugs and observations is the midwife's responsibility. This should also include details of examination of the placenta, membranes and cord with attention drawn to any abnormalities. The volume of blood loss is particularly important. This record not only provides information which may be critical in the future care of both mother and baby but is a legal document which may be used as evidence of the care given. Signatures are therefore essential with co-signatories where necessary. Many mothers now carry their own notes or are supplied with a co-operation card. The completed records are a vital communication link between the midwife responsible for delivery and other caregivers, including the community midwife.

It is usually the midwife who completes the birth notification form. This must be sent within 36 hours to the medical officer of the health district in which the baby was born.

Transfer from the labour ward

The midwife is responsible for seeing that all observations are made and recorded (as specified above) prior to transfer of mother and baby to the postnatal ward or before the midwife leaves the home following the birth.

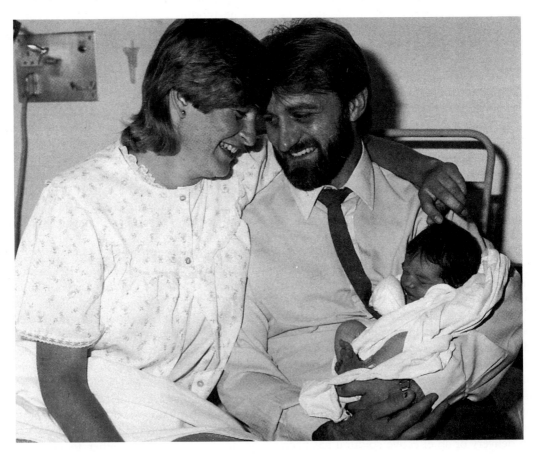

Fig. 15.10
The joy of parenthood.

The postnatal ward midwife should verify these details prior to transfer of mother and baby. Following a domiciliary delivery the midwife should leave details of a telephone number where she may be contacted should the parents feel any cause for concern.

Reader Activities

1. One simple and effective means of demonstrating the inaccuracy of estimating blood loss to colleagues is to replicate part of the Levy & Moore study (1985).

Four units of expired blood were obtained from the haematology laboratory. These were divided into measured amounts: to each was added citrate to prevent clotting plus 200 ml of normal saline to mimic a moderate quantity of amniotic fluid. The calculated volumes were poured over sets of drapes and pads laid out on trolleys. Staff were then invited to estimate the blood loss, which served to demonstrate gross under-estimation.

2. In the unit in which you work search for documents which influence or dictate any aspect of practice related to third stage management. This may include policy statements, guidelines for practice or defined standards of care. When were these documents compiled and by whom? Are any of the recommendations supported by cited research evidence? What can you do to change or improve such statements?

REFERENCES

Bonnar J, McNicol G P, Douglas A S 1970 Coagulation and fibrinolytic mechanisms during and after normal childbirth. British Medical Journal 25 April: 200–203

Botha M G 1968 The management of the umbilical cord in labour. South African Journal of Obstetrics and Gynaecology 6(2): 30–33

Dunn P M 1985 Management of childbirth in normal women: The third stage and fetal adaptation. In: Perinatal medicine. Proceedings of the IX European Congress Perinatal Medicine, Dublin, September 1984. MTP Press, Lancaster, ch 7, p 47–54

Elbourne D 1992 Prophylactic syntometrine vs oxytocin in third stage of labour: an overview of the evidence from controlled trials. In: Chalmers I (ed) Oxford data base of perinatal trials. Version 1.2 Disc Issue 7, Spring, Record 2999

Inch S 1985 Management of the third stage of labour — Another cascade of intervention. Midwifery 1: 114–122

Ladipo O A 1972 Management of third stage of labour, with particular reference to reduction of feto-maternal transfusion. British Medical Journal 1: 721–723

Levy V, Moore J 1985 The midwife's management of the third stage of labour. Nursing Times 81(5): 47–50

Montgomery T L 1960 The umbilical cord. Clinical Obstetrics and Gynaecology 3: 900–910

Newton M, Mosey L M, Egli G E, Gifford W B, Hull C T 1961 Blood loss during and immediately after delivery. Obstetrics and Gynaecology 17: 9–18

Pau-Chen W, Tsu-Shan K 1960 Early clamping of the umbilical cord: a study of its effect on the infant. Chinese Medical Journal 80: 351–355

Prendiville W, Elbourne D 1989 Care during the third stage of labour. In: Chalmers I, Enkin M, Keirse M J N C (eds) Effective care in pregnancy and childbirth. Oxford University Press, Oxford, p 1145–1169

Prendiville W J, Harding J E, Elbourne D, Stirrat G 1988 The Bristol third stage trial: 'active' versus 'physiological' management of the third stage. British Medical Journal 297: 1295–1300

Salariya E, Easton P, Cater J 1979 Early and often for best results. Nursing Mirror 148: 15–17

Yao A C, Lind J 1974 Placental transfusion. American Journal of Diseases of Children 127: 128–141

FURTHER READING

Prendiville W, Elbourne D, Chalmers I 1988 The effects of routine oxytocic administration in the management of the third stage of labour: an overview of the evidence from controlled trials. British Journal of Obstetrics and Gynaecology 95: 3–16

5

The Normal Puerperium

16

Physiology, psychology and management of the puerperium

JEAN A. BALL

The puerperium is a time of great change which spans a period of transition from the pinnacle experience of birth to the assumption of the joys and responsibilities of family life.

Well-integrated postnatal care has an important role to play in assisting this transition and launching the family on their new life together.

The puerperium is a period of 6 weeks which begins as soon as the placenta is expelled. During this time a number of physiological and psychological changes take place:

- the reproductive organs return to the non-pregnant state
- other physiological changes which occurred during pregnancy are reversed
- lactation is established
- the foundations of the relationship between the infant and his parents are laid
- the mother recovers from the stresses of pregnancy and delivery, and assumes responsibility for the care and nurture of her infant.

The care which mothers and babies require during the puerperium should be based upon three main principles:

- promoting the physical well-being of the mother and baby
- encouraging sound methods of infant feeding and promoting the development of good maternal–child relationships

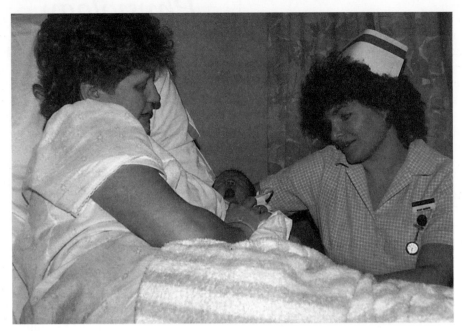

Fig. 16.1
Building a trusting relationship is vital.

● supporting and strengthening the mother's
  confidence in herself, and enabling her to fulfil
  her mothering role within her particular
  personal family and cultural situation.

PHYSIOLOGY OF THE PUERPERIUM

Changes in endocrine activity

Oxytocin

Oxytocin is secreted by the posterior pituitary
gland and acts upon uterine muscle and upon
breast tissue. During the third stage of labour the
action of oxytocin brings about the separation of
the placenta. It then continues to act upon the
uterine muscle fibres maintaining their contraction,
reducing the placental site and preventing haemorrhage. In women who choose to breast feed their
babies, the suckling of the infant stimulates further
secretion of oxytocin and this aids the continuing
involution of the uterus and expulsion of milk.

After the placenta is expelled, the circulating
levels of human chorionic gonadotrophin, human
placental lactogen, oestrogen and progesterone

fall rapidly, and this brings about a number of
physiological changes.

Prolactin

The fall in oestrogen allows prolactin, which is
secreted by the anterior pituitary gland, to act upon
the alveoli of the breast to stimulate the production
of milk. In women who breast feed, the levels of
prolactin remain high and the resumption of follicle
stimulation in the ovary is suppressed. In women
who do not breast feed, the levels of circulating
prolactin fall within 14–21 days of the birth and
this fall allows the follicle-stimulating hormone
secreted by the anterior pituitary gland to act upon
the ovary, leading to the resumption of normal
patterns of oestrogen and progesterone production,
follicle growth, ovulation and menstruation.

Other changes

The fall in oestrogen and progesterone brings
about several other physiological changes.

During pregnancy normal blood volume is
considerably increased. Although the mechanism

is not fully understood, it is thought that the high levels of circulating oestrogen augment the anti-diuretic hormone which allows the blood volume to be increased. In addition, progesterone acts upon smooth muscle fibres reducing their excitability and increasing their vascularity. This affects the ureters and the pelves of the kidneys, the gut and abdominal wall, the ligaments of the uterus, the muscle fibres in the walls of the veins, the pelvic floor, perineum, vagina and vulva.

Pelvic floor, perineum, vagina, vulva and bowel

The fall in circulating progesterone allows its effects upon the smooth muscle fibres of the pelvic floor, perineum, vagina and bowel to be reversed. This process aids the recovery of normal muscle tone in these areas and in the ligaments of the uterus. This is a gradual process which is aided by early ambulation of the mother, by postnatal exercises, and by the avoidance of constipation. Progesterone also increases the vascularity of the vagina and vulva during pregnancy and delivery of the baby frequently causes some degree of bruising and oedema in these tissues and in the perineum. The excess fluid in these tissues is usually re-absorbed by the 3rd or 4th day of the puerperium.

Bladder, urethra and ureters

The pelves of the kidneys and the ureters have also been affected by progesterone leading to dilatation and stasis of urine and this is associated with the increased risk of urinary tract infection during pregnancy. The effect of progesterone diminishes after delivery of the placenta but many women remain prone to urinary tract infection during the first weeks of the puerperium. During labour the bladder is displaced into the abdomen, stretching the urethra to a considerable degree and this frequently leads to bruising of the urethra and loss of muscle tone in the bladder. The bruising of the urethra makes micturition painful and the bladder may easily become overdistended. Retention of urine is a frequent occurrence and if unchecked, retention with overflow may result. The increased renal flow during the first 48 hours of the puerperium adds to the ease with which overdistension may occur. Where retention with overflow does occur it leads to continuing loss of muscle tone, back pressure on the ureters and pelves of the kidneys and increased likelihood of urinary tract infection. This situation is prevented by frequent micturition and by ensuring that the bladder completely empties on each occasion. In some women it may be necessary to relieve retention of urine by catheterisation but this should be avoided if possible because of the increased risk of infection which is associated with catheterisation.

The cardiovascular system

During pregnancy the normal blood volume increases to accommodate the increased blood flow needed by the placenta and uterine blood vessels. The withdrawal of oestrogen allows a diuresis to take place, rapidly reducing the plasma volume to normal proportions. This action takes place within the first 24–48 hours following the birth of the baby. During this time mothers pass copious amounts of urine. The loss of progesterone helps to reduce the fluid retention inherent in increased vascularity of the tissues during pregnancy, together with that due to trauma during delivery of the baby.

The kidneys

Renal action is increased in the early part of the puerperium because of the reduction of blood volume and the excretion of the waste products of autolysis. The peak of this activity occurs within the first 7 days of the puerperium.

The breasts

The rise in circulating prolactin acts upon the alveoli of the breasts and stimulates milk production. During the first 3–4 days of the puerperium the breasts become heavy and engorged. They are tender and must be handled gently and supported well. Engorgement is reduced as the baby begins to suckle. In women who do not breast feed engorgement is gradually reduced by the fall in prolactin which occurs when its secretion is no longer stimulated by suckling. Fuller details of the physiology of breast changes are given in Chapter 33.

The involution of the uterus

At the completion of labour the uterus weighs approximately 1 kg. By the end of the puerperium it has returned to its non-pregnant weight of 60 g. This represents a reduction of 16 times the weight and size of the uterus immediately after the delivery of the placenta. This physiological phenomenon is brought about by the process known as autolysis, during which proteolytic enzymes digest the muscle fibres which have increased during pregnancy to 10 times their normal length and 5 times their normal thickness. The end products of autolysis are removed by the phagocytic action of polymorphs and macrophages in the blood and lymphatic systems. This process is further assisted by the contraction and retraction of the uterine muscles under the influence of oxytocin, and this results in compressing the blood vessels and reducing the uterine blood supply. Breast feeding stimulates the continuing secretion of oxytocin thus assisting involution. The contraction and retraction of the uterine muscles reduce the size of the placental site and prevent excessive bleeding, and the site is gradually covered, first by granular tissue and then by endometrium.

The most marked reduction in size of the uterus takes place during the first 10 days of the puerperium, but involution is not complete until 6 weeks later. Immediately after delivery the fundus of the contracted uterus is found at or just below the mother's umbilicus. One week after delivery it is palpable just above the symphysis pubis, and by the 10th or 12th day it is no longer palpable.

The cervix is soft and vascular immediately after delivery and may be seen protruding into the vagina. It loses its vascularity rapidly and normally regains its usual hard consistency within 2 or 3 days of the delivery. The cervical os also reduces in size and measures 1 cm wide 10 days after delivery. The process of normal involution is a gradual one. The list given below in Table 16.1 is a guide to the usual progression of change in the uterus.

Table 16.1
Progression of change in the uterus after delivery

	Weight of uterus	Diameter of placental site	Cervix
End of labour	900 g	12.5 cm	Soft, flabby
End of 1 week	450 g	7.5 cm	2 cm
End of 2 weeks	200 g	5.0 cm	1 cm
End of 6 weeks	60 g	2.5 cm	A slit

The lochia

Lochia is the term used to describe the discharges from the uterus during the puerperium and the term is plural. Lochia have an alkaline reaction in which organisms can flourish more rapidly than in the normally acid secretions of the vagina. The odour of the lochia is heavy but not offensive, and the amount varies in different women.

The lochia undergo sequential changes as involution progresses:

Red lochia (lochia rubra). This is the name given to the lochia during the first 3–4 days of the puerperium. As the name implies they are usually red in colour and consist of blood from the placental site and debris arising from the decidua and chorion.

Serous lochia (lochia serosa). These are pink in colour and discharged during the next 5–9 days. The lochia now have less blood and more serum and contain leucocytes from the placental site.

White lochia (lochia alba). The discharges are paler, creamy-brown in colour, and contain leucocytes, cervical mucus and debris from healing tissues. Some evidence of blood may continue to be seen for a further 2 or 3 weeks.

The quantity, colour and odour of the lochia are significant. An increase in the amount lost and in the blood content may be seen when the mother becomes more active. Scanty lochia may suggest infection. The presence of small blood clots may be normal during the first 24 hours, especially in multiparae, but if this continues or is accompanied by pain, it suggests that products of conception may not have been fully expelled. Offensive lochia may indicate poor vulval hygiene and contamination by faecal debris; if, however, this situation persists in spite of improvement in vulval hygiene, then it is indicative of infection of the genital tract, possibly of the uterus itself.

PSYCHOLOGY OF THE PUERPERIUM

In addition to the rapid and wide-ranging physiological changes of the puerperium, this is also a time of major psychological change and adjustment.

The birth of a baby is an eagerly anticipated event, surrounded by high expectations and some trepidation. The care required by a small infant brings considerable changes into the life of his mother and father and to the other members of the family. Social life is restricted and there may be financial problems to be faced.

It is important to realise that psychological adjustment to motherhood is a varied and gradual process which takes time. Parenting is a complex experience, affected by expectation of the family and society and by the expectations of the parents themselves. It is accompanied by a number of conflicting reactions and feelings, some of which may be surprising to the parents. The mother must learn to care for her new baby during the time in which she is still recovering from the physical stress of pregnancy, labour and delivery. Older children in the family must learn to share the love and attention of their parents with this newcomer, and this may not be easy to accept.

The puerperium is a time of transition during which both parents but especially the mother adjust their patterns of living to meet the needs of a small infant. Many women have little or no experience of caring for a newborn infant and may feel overwhelmed by the responsibility. They will be very sensitive to any suggestion that they are not coping as well as they ought, and easily confused and distressed by conflicting or ill-considered advice. The patterns of mothering which develop will depend partly upon the mother's degree of experience in caring for babies, but much more upon her expectations, her emotional reactions and upon the sensitivity of the help she receives from her husband, family and friends. There is no set pattern by which a mother may be expected to take complete responsibility for the care of her baby. This will depend upon her confidence in herself, and in the natural degree of anxiety in her personality. The more anxious a mother is, the more difficult it may be for her to respond to instructions. It is important that a mother's self-esteem is not impaired by criticism or by any suggestion that she is not being a 'good mother'. This is particularly true of feeding the infant. When a mother is feeding her baby either by breast or bottle, she is doing far more than providing him with nourishment, she is communicating her love and care to him, and is rewarded by his satisfaction with the feed. This is of much greater significance than the degree of skill displayed and midwives must recognise that it is the mother who is the most important person in her baby's life. This relationship must not be impaired by the skilled midwife usurping the mother's role. The midwife should provide help, encouragement and advice, and should praise the mother for her prowess both in the act of giving birth and in mothering her infant. The role of the midwife is to nurture the mother and her self-confidence in order that she can give to her baby. In this way, the maternal–child relationship is built up and enriched.

Maternal–child relationships

The maternal–child relationship begins during pregnancy as the mother becomes aware of the fetal movements and activity. This relationship develops rapidly following the birth of the baby. The time immediately following the delivery of the baby is a most important time for the fostering of good parent–child relationships. The mother and father should be left in peace with their baby to rejoice in his birth and delight in his perfection. Touch and eye contact between parents and infant are particularly important and parents should be encouraged to hold their baby as soon as possible after birth. Whenever possible the mother should give the baby a feed soon after birth either at the breast or by bottle.

Close contact

Close physical and eye contact should be en-

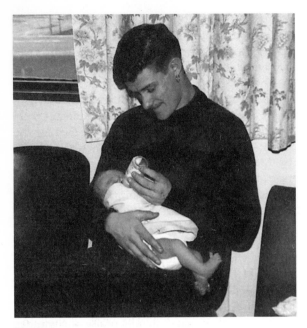

Fig. 16.2
Fathers enjoy feeding too.

couraged throughout the puerperium. Eye contact between mother and baby is achieved when the baby is held in the en-face position in her arms. This can be easily achieved when the baby is suckling at the breast or when held to be bottle fed. A mother should be encouraged to look into her baby's eyes and to smile and talk to him. She should also be encouraged to handle, cuddle and enjoy her baby as much as possible. The father of the baby must not be forgotten and he should also be encouraged to hold his baby when he visits. Parents delight in examining the baby's body and both should be able to share in bathing the baby.

Feelings

It is important that mothers are assured that maternal feelings vary in their development. Many women feel an immediate and overwhelming rush of affection for the baby as soon as he is born but others take several days or even weeks before these feelings are fully experienced. They should be reassured that this delay is not unusual and the midwife should ensure that close and intimate

contact between the mother and her baby is not being restricted or prevented.

Mood changes in the early puerperium

With rapid physiological and psychological change taking place during the first week of the puerperium it is not surprising to find that many women experience emotional lability and changes of mood in the first 3 or 4 days. The natural anxiety of pregnancy, and fear of labour, the physical efforts of labour and delivery together with the peak experience of giving birth all contribute to a mixture of emotional reactions.

Many women experience some degree of mood change during the first few days of the puerperium, and one in three experience a transient period of tearfulness, anxiety and irritability which is usually called the '3rd day or baby blues'. Its incidence is increased by fatigue and any undue stress or anxiety arising from family tensions or insensitive handling by those responsible for caring for the mother. Anxiety about her ability to cope with the demands of the baby may also add to the mother's transient distress. For some women, however, this distress may last longer than usual and may indicate that the mother needs more support and care than she is at present receiving. It may also lead to a more prolonged period of emotional distress or depression.

The role of the midwife

The role of the midwife is to provide the kind of consistent, kindly and relevant support which each individual mother requires in order to recover from physical stress of labour and to grow in confidence in caring for her baby.

Mothers vary in their needs, expectations and attitudes and babies vary in their developing patterns of feeding and sleeping. No routine approach to care will meet these varying needs. The midwife must be non-judgemental in her approach and see her function as that of adviser and counsellor. It is not her role to make decisions on behalf of the mother nor should she convey disapproval of a mother's decisions.

The process of adjustment to motherhood continues throughout the puerperium and beyond it. Many women may take several months before becoming really confident in their mothering role. Midwives working in hospital and in the community have a unique opportunity to assist this adjustment process by their competence, skill and sensitivity to the needs and expectations of individual mothers and their families.

MANAGEMENT OF POSTNATAL CARE

The management of care begins in the delivery suite and extends throughout the postnatal period and should be directed to achieve the following objectives:

- ensuring that postnatal care is related to the needs of each individual mother rather than to any routine pattern
- promoting a relaxed environment in which the mother can be certain of adequate rest and freedom from unnecessary stress
- identifying potential problems in physical or emotional well-being as early as possible and ensuring prompt and appropriate help and treatment
- ensuring good communications between all the people providing care for the mother and baby
- enabling parents to become confident in the necessary skills of caring for an infant by providing opportunities for learning and discussion.

The Midwife's responsibilities during the postnatal period

The Midwives' Rules (UKCC 1991) define the postnatal period as a period of not less than 10 days and not more than 28 days after the end of labour during which the continued attendance of a midwife on the mother and baby is requisite.

During this period the midwife will normally visit the mother and baby daily. Rather than adhere to a rigid routine, it may be more effective to miss out a day when all is going well and arrange an extra visit later on when the mother has been managing the baby herself for a while.

The midwife must endeavour to promote breast feeding whenever possible. If the mother decides to use artificial feeding the midwife must give advice and guidance on the preparation of artificial feeds.

The midwife must, with the permission of the mother, carry out routine screening tests on the baby. She must take steps to ensure that sufficient heating is available so that the baby is nursed in the correct temperature by day and night.

Registration of infant birth

It is primarily the duty of the father or mother of the child to report the birth to the Registrar of Births and Deaths within 42 days whether the baby was live or stillborn. The midwife must inform the parents of their responsibility and if they default in this duty, anyone present at the birth, including the midwife, may be called upon to register the birth (see Ch. 43).

Planning postnatal care

Continuity of care
Ideally the midwife who provides postnatal care will have been caring for the mother throughout her pregnancy, labour and delivery and will already be familiar with the mother's needs and her obstetric and family history. Midwives have, in many areas, devised schemes which aim to increase continuity of care and of carer, inspired by the Know Your Midwife study (Flint & Poulengeris 1987). The Winterton Report (House of Commons 1992) stresses the importance of continuity in postnatal care. Whether or not team midwifery is in operation locally, midwives need to co-operate in providing consistency of advice and continuity of personal contact.

Welcome to the ward
As soon as the postnatal ward is notified that a newly delivered mother and her baby are to be transferred to the ward, the midwife should arrange for a bed to be prepared in a single room or in a

quiet area of the ward so that the mother will be able to sleep following her efforts during delivery. The midwife should then be ready to greet the mother by name when she arrives. The midwife ensures that the uterus is contracted, the lochia are not excessive and that the bladder is empty. She must ascertain whether the mother, father and baby have been able to spend some time alone together in the delivery suite, and whether the baby has been put to the breast or been bottle fed by his mother. If this has not taken place, then the parents should be left quietly alone together to enjoy their baby and rejoice in his birth. The mother should then be encouraged to rest.

History

Whilst the mother is resting, the midwife should familiarise herself with the obstetric and family details of the mother, taking particular note of the following:

- age and parity
- blood group and Rhesus factor
- the result of the most recent estimation of maternal haemoglobin
- the events of labour and delivery, including the amount of blood loss
- the baby's condition at birth and his birth weight
- the mother's chosen method of infant feeding
- the mother's social and family needs and the observations of the community midwife
- the mother's wishes about the length of time she spends in the postnatal care of the hospital.

The midwife should ascertain what examinations and tests have already been carried out and plan for those which must be done during the next few days.

Screening

The baby is examined at birth by the midwife responsible for the delivery to ascertain if any congenital abnormalities are present. This examination is repeated by a paediatrician or general practitioner during the first few days of the puerperium (see Ch. 32).

Prevention of Rhesus iso-immunisation in the mother. A series of tests is undertaken on the fetal and maternal blood samples taken at birth from women with Rhesus negative blood. It is the responsibility of the midwife to ensure that these tests have been carried out, to ascertain their results and to ensure that anti-D immunoglobulin is given as necessary (see Ch. 34).

Identification of metabolic and endocrine disorders. On the 6th postnatal day a blood sample is taken from the baby by heel stab in order to screen it for phenylketonuria, hypothyroidism and occasionally other disorders (see Chs 32 and 38).

Recording the date and time of the tests. The date and time of screening tests and the results of examinations must be recorded and the information passed on to the community midwife and health visitor.

Prevention of anaemia

Women are prone to develop iron deficiency anaemia during pregnancy and a further haemo-globin estimation is undertaken early in the puerperium to identify any mother who may be in need of treatment to alleviate or prevent the development of anaemia. The postnatal blood sample should not be taken less than 24 hours after completion of the delivery as the effect of any blood loss upon the volume of haemoglobin will not be seen if the test is performed earlier.

Discussing and agreeing the care plan with the mother

Once the mother has rested from the immediate effects of labour and delivery she and the midwife should discuss her needs and expectations for postnatal care. A care plan should then be agreed between them. This plan will be tailored to the individual needs of each mother and baby and recorded in such a way that all who provide care for the mother and baby can have easy access to relevant information.

The care plan should note the following:

- The mother's choice of feeding, her degree of experience in the care of a newborn baby and her feelings of confidence.

- Care required as a result of problems identified during pregnancy, e.g. anaemia or hypertension, and that required as a result of trauma sustained during the delivery of the baby, e.g. a perineal wound, bruising of the perineum during forceps delivery, postpartum blood loss.
- Any special needs of unsupported mothers, those whose babies are to be adopted or those with more than normal anxiety about the baby, for instance who have had a previous stillbirth or cot death.
- The day on which screening tests are expected to be carried out.
- The provisional arrangements made for returning home to the care of the community midwife.
- The needs of the family such as the husband's need to take time off work or the care of other children.

Following discussion of the mother's needs, her wishes and the various options about post-natal care at home or in the hospital, a provisional care plan is agreed and details are noted in such a way as to avoid conflicting advice and ensure continuity of care. This care plan can then be re-assessed in the light of each day's progress or any change in the mother's wishes. The information it contains should be made available to the community midwife when she takes over the care of the mother and baby.

Daily assessment of needs

Each day the midwife should carry out an examination of the mother, observing her general health and noting her physical and emotional well-being. This daily assessment provides an opportunity for the midwife and mother to discuss the mother's needs and the needs of the baby and should become the basis of postnatal care decisions. A physical examination should be carried out for at least 10 days after the birth, and for as long afterwards as the mother's condition requires. It should be repeated before the midwife finally discharges the mother from care.

Daily examination

General well-being

The mother should be greeted and asked how she is feeling. The midwife should take particular note if the mother complains of feeling unduly tired. Any woman who is developing an infection or who is anaemic will not feel well.

Temperature, pulse and blood pressure

The temperature may be labile during the first few days following delivery as a result of breast activity and may rise as a result of engorgement of the breasts but such elevation should be transient and the temperature should not exceed 37.3°C. It is not now considered necessary to take the temperature routinely unless indicated.

The pulse rate is normally at or below 80 beats per minute. Any rise in the pulse rate may be indicative of excessive bleeding or of a developing puerperal infection. A rising pulse rate which is due to excessive bleeding will be accompanied by a fall in the blood pressure and the midwife must check the state of the uterus and lochia in order to identify postpartum haemorrhage. Excessive blood loss or heavy lochia would alert the midwife to take the pulse.

The blood pressure is checked during the first 24 hours following a normal delivery and for a longer period of time if there has been any history of bleeding, hypertension during pregnancy or if the mother has had a caesarean section or has required any other surgical intervention.

Tiredness and fatigue

Many women feel tired following delivery but they do not feel unwell. Undue fatigue may result from sleep disturbance because of the baby's needs and may be relieved by arranging a quiet period and place where the woman can gain extra sleep. If necessary a mild sedative may be offered. Many women will recover rapidly after only a few hours of extra and undisturbed rest. A mother who complains of tiredness in spite of adequate opportunity to sleep may be showing early signs of depression and should be given an opportunity to discuss her feelings and provided with extra help with the baby until she feels more able to cope. A further cause of feeling tired may be the presence of anaemia and care should be taken to check the last estimation of haemoglobin level and the amount of blood lost at delivery.

The breasts

A complete breast examination should be carried out on each occasion. The technique for this and possible findings are discussed in Chapter 33.

The uterus

The abdomen should be palpated daily until the uterine fundus is no longer palpable above the symphysis pubis. Although the rate of reduction in size varies in different women, involution should follow a progressive pattern. It is usually more rapid in women who breast feed and in primigravidae. The uterus should be well con-tracted and not painful. Sub-involution is identified if the uterus remains the same size for several days. A bulky uterus may indicate the presence of blood clots or of retained products of conception. Tenderness of the uterus suggests infection. The midwife must report such findings to the doctor. A bulky uterus may also be due to a full rectum. A correct impression of size will not be gained if the bladder is full and the uterus may be displaced to one side, commonly the right.

The lochia

The character and amount of the lochia are noted and the midwife should expect to see a gradual change in the colour and amount of the lochia as the puerperium progresses (see above). An increase in the volume of lochia is normal when the mother first becomes ambulant.

Continuity of observation

Observation of changes in the uterus and in the lochia is more likely to detect deviation from normal physiology if the same midwife examines the woman on successive occasions. Abnormal changes are discussed in Chapter 30.

After-pains

Multiparae frequently suffer from 'after-pains' in the first 2 or 3 days after the birth of the baby. These are caused by mild contractions of the uterus which is more flaccid than that of a primipara. A degree of discomfort can be relieved by 500 mg of paracetamol but the midwife should palpate the uterus and examine the lochia to ensure that the contractions are not caused by the uterus attempting to expel clots or retained products.

Micturition

The woman should be encouraged to pass urine as soon as possible after delivery and preferably within 12 hours. She will produce large quantities of urine in the postpartum diuresis within 24–48 hours of giving birth. Most women are fit enough to visit the lavatory where they can enjoy privacy and a more normal position than seated on a bedpan in bed. It is common to measure urine passed for about 24 hours in order to monitor voiding of the bladder. If a woman has difficulty in emptying her bladder, the reason must be sought. It may be due to bruising or lacerations, however small, to oedema of the urethra, to fear or to inhibition. If the problem is not resolved early, retention of urine may occur. Remedies which may be tried include the sound of running water or sitting in the bath. Catheterisation should be regarded as a last resort when all else has failed. Strict asepsis is mandatory. Once mic-turition has been achieved it usually proceeds normally thereafter but the midwife should ensure that it continues to be pain free, that the bladder is not palpable and that adequate amounts of urine are being passed.

The perineum, vulva and anus

The perineum, anus and vulva should be inspected to ensure that any trauma is healing satisfactorily. The midwife should ensure that vulval pads are being changed frequently and that the perineum is free from stale lochia which could be a source of infection. Any perineal wound should be inspected daily to exclude any signs of infection. The bowels should be opened daily and a mild aperient given if necessary.

The legs

The mother's legs should be examined for any tenderness which might suggest thrombosis of the superficial veins or of the deep veins. Thrombophlebitis of the superficial veins is characterised by swelling, hardness and redness of the affected vein.

Deep vein thrombosis which may predispose to pulmonary embolism should be suspected if there is any tenderness on walking or when the deep veins in the calf of the leg are pressed. Either condition should be reported to the doctor.

PROMOTING PHYSICAL AND EMOTIONAL WELL-BEING

Prevention of infection

Puerperal infection is still a cause of maternal death although its incidence is infrequent in the developed countries. It must be prevented by strict cleanliness. The uterus provides an ideal environment for the multiplication of organisms. Any degree of trauma will increase the tendency for development of infection.

Possible foci of puerperal infection are:

— breast infection (see Ch. 33)
— infection of the genital tract
— infection of the urinary tract
— upper respiratory tract infection.

Genital tract infection is most likely to occur in women who have suffered tears or abrasions to the vulva, vagina and perineum. Bruising reduces the tissues' resistance to infection and there is danger that ascending infection may involve the uterus and the placental site.

It can be prevented by careful attention to the mother's hygiene, encouragement of drainage of lochia by early ambulation and by the prevention of cross-infection.

The mother's hygiene should be maintained by a bath or shower at least once a day, frequent use of the bidet and careful vulval toilet. Vulval pads should be changed frequently and the mother should be warned not to let the pad rub between the anus and vulva when removing it as this may transmit organisms from the anus, contaminating the perineum and vulva. Vulval cleanliness promotes the healing of trauma and prevents urinary tract infection.

In many centres the midwife wears disposable gloves when handling vulval pads and she must maintain aseptic technique when applying any treatment or removing sutures.

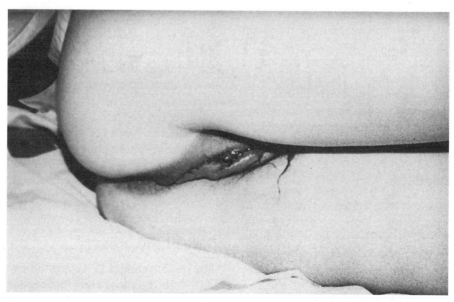

Fig. 16.3
Bruising and oedema of the vulva and perineum in a primipara 3 days after a forceps delivery.

Urinary tract infection affects a number of women during pregnancy and may recur in the puerperium. It may be caused by lack of vulval hygiene and is more likely to occur if there is retention of urine or stasis due to poor fluid intake or lack of exercise. Constipation must be avoided.

Upper respiratory tract infection may occur to any person at any time. Midwives suffering from colds should not work in the wards during the most acute phase of the condition, and should wear a face mask when attending to the mother or baby.

Ambulation and exercise

Ambulation increases muscle tone and venous return from the legs and lower abdomen. It also increases the drainage of the lochia and the voiding of urine. Ambulation should be encouraged as soon as possible after delivery and most women are able to walk to the bathroom with help approximately 6 hours after delivery. Those mothers who had a forceps delivery or suffered marked bruising of the perineum may find walking difficult at first but should be encouraged to persevere , the increase in venous return helps to red e oedema and bruising.

Increas g amounts of exercise should be taken each d and it is important that mothers are enco aged to walk about and not just sit by th edside as this will help them to feel better otionally and physically.

Postnatal exercises help to increase muscle tone and are usually commenced during the first 3 days after delivery. Further information will be found in Chapter 40.

Rest and sleep

Ensuring adequate rest and sleep is a vital part of postnatal care and should form an important part of care planning. The healing of trauma is aided by physical rest; emotional well-being can be eroded when a mother has insufficient sleep or time for personal refreshment (Ball 1989).

However, achieving adequate rest for mothers is not easy. Caring for a small baby brings busy days and broken nights. Hospital wards are full of bustle and eager visitors, and staff members may not always appreciate the mother's need for peace and quiet.

These difficulties can be overcome by a number of stratagems.

1. It should be a cardinal rule in all hospitals that a sleeping mother is not woken for any reason. Mothers should not be woken at a set time in the morning to fit in with hospital regimens nor for breakfast. A mother often falls into a deep sleep in the early hours after feeding her baby and should be allowed to sleep on. A buffet breakfast should be made available when required. The use of 'do not disturb' signs should be encouraged.

2. The practice of 'rooming-in' during the night, should not be allowed to create a situation where mothers are repeatedly disturbed by crying babies. The mother's permission should be sought, so that a baby who does not settle after being fed could be taken out of the ward.

3. Each ward should have a number of side rooms or a section of the ward which is ear-marked for the use of women who have just given birth or who have had a particularly trying night with a hungry baby. This area of the ward should be kept as quiet as possible. Many women benefit from the opportunity of a few hours uninterrupted sleep during the daytime and sedation may be offered to assist this if necessary.

4. It is helpful for a particular period of each day to be set aside as a rest period, when busyness in the ward is kept to a minimum and visitors discouraged.

When the mother returns home, the need for adequate rest should be emphasised and the family encouraged to take over the care of the baby for a period of time each day to allow the mother to continue her pattern of resting at least once during the day.

Care of the breasts

The breasts should be supported by a well-fitting bra worn by day and if necessary by night. Engorgement is usually most marked in women who do not breast feed and may cause considerable discomfort for a few days. This can be relieved by frequent bathing with warm, but not hot, water when some milk will flow into the bath. Engorgement may be relieved by expressing small quantities of milk. Excessive expression will stimulate the production of oxytocin and prolactin thus increasing the engorgement and delaying suppression of breast milk. If milk production is high, the mother may sometimes be persuaded to breast feed her baby after all. Discomfort may be relieved by the use of paracetamol and by providing firm support. If engorgement makes it impossible for a normal bra to be worn, a comfortable support may be made out of a length of sheeting approximately 4 feet long and 18 inches wide. The mother lies down and the sheeting is placed under her with its lower edge at her waist level. The sheeting is then brought forward, kept taut, and pinned together with large safety pins above waist level. One end is then folded over each breast, brought over the mother's shoulder and pinned to the sheeting at the back. The sheeting should be kept taut in order to provide firm but not constricted support. When the pieces are securely fastened, a tuck can be made in each piece just below the armpit and pinned into place. Further care of the breasts is covered in Chapter 33.

Nutrition

The diet of a puerperal woman should be nourishing, varied and balanced. It should include adequate protein to aid tissue renewal and milk production, iron and vitamins to counteract anaemia, fibre to aid excretion and improve muscle tone, and plenty of fluids.

Prevention of anaemia

Pregnant women are prone to develop iron deficiency anaemia and this is most commonly due to lack of iron in the diet or malabsorption of iron from the intestine. In developed countries anaemia is judged to be present when the concentration of haemoglobin is less than 10.5 g per 100 ml.

Even a moderate blood loss at delivery may reduce the haemoglobin to less than 10.5 g, if the concentration before delivery was assessed at 11–12 g per 100 ml. Any degree of anaemia will reduce the body's resistance to infection and its capacity for healing. It is important therefore that any degree of anaemia is identified and reported to the doctor for treatment.

Methods of treating anaemia are identical to those used in pregnancy (see Ch. 22). Most cases can be corrected with a course of oral iron.

Emotional needs

Major changes. It is not surprising that giving birth is an emotional experience as it is the culmination of many hopes and fears and the beginning of a new human life and family relationship. Mothers need to be supported as they adjust to this experience and the secret of providing emotional support is to have an encouraging attitude, showing confidence in the mother's ability and preventing her from being made to feel a failure in any way. Much of what is written in the popular press or portrayed in television advertising suggests that every mother must also be a perfect wife, companion and housekeeper. The reality is that caring for a newborn infant is a demanding 24-hour-a-day commitment which leaves little time for anything else. The household routine is changed and both husband and wife have major adjustments to make.

Many primiparae have unreal expectations of mothering and this unreal image may also be fostered in some of the health education material used in parentcraft classes and by the attitude of the midwife who may have an image of the kind of 'mothering model' she expects or approves.

Taking on new responsibilities. A mother needs to be helped to cope with caring for the baby and the needs of her family by a gradual process which is related to her particular ability and physical and emotional condition. Taking increasing responsibility for the care of the baby should be staged and the mother enabled to build upon the successful completion of one aspect of care before being expected to master another. Thus one mother may feel ready and eager to bath her baby on the 3rd or 4th day after his birth while another may not feel sufficiently confident that she can handle him safely until he is a week old.

Rest and relaxation. The mother also needs to have time for rest and relaxation and should be encouraged to spend some time each day on herself.

No comparisons. It is important that comparisons are not drawn between the competence of different mothers, and midwives should discourage a woman from comparing her prowess in infant care with that of other mothers in her ward. There should not be a routine pattern of care which expects that each mother will follow an unvarying sequence of increasing responsibility for the care needed by her baby.

Praise and encouragement. Some mothers will be highly competent and irritated by receiving too much advice and help, while others may feel foolish if they cannot cope as well as they feel they should. In developing happy relationships between a mother and her baby, nothing succeeds like success and the mother should be praised and encouraged in the things she does well, advised and supported in the things she cannot yet master and she should not be criticised or made to feel inadequate.

Consistent advice. Conflicting advice is a potent cause of discouragement and mothers experiencing emotional distress and those most vulnerable to emotional distress tend to blame themselves for being unable to understand what the midwife is advising them to do. Anxious mothers need to have instructions repeated on a number of occasions before they can take the information in fully; conflicting information is confusing and ineffective.

All advice or instructions that are given should be clearly recorded in the care plan so that any other midwife or doctor may provide continuity of care and advice.

Mothers' self-esteem

It cannot be emphasised too strongly that midwives must endeavour to maintain and enhance the self-esteem of the mothers for whom they care. Each mother should be helped to realise her unique and inestimable worth in providing for the welfare of her baby and the attitudes of midwives and doctors should convey their respect for her. The mother's role as a woman must also

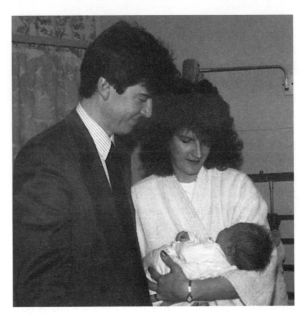

Fig. 16.4
Family group.

be recognised; she is not only a mother but she is a person of worth in her own right. She should be encouraged to take time for herself and to resume some social contacts.

It can be helpful to suggest to the husband that he arranges to take his wife out for an evening as soon as possible after the mother and baby have returned home or even before. Some maternity units will offer to 'baby-sit'. Couples should be assured that a carefully chosen helper could take care of the baby for a short period of time in order to enable his parents to spend a little time together.

When the mother returns home the midwife should ensure that the family and friends understand the mother's needs and offer help readily. The family should take care that the mother still has a time to rest and that the family do not make unreasonable demands upon her.

Promoting good maternal–child relationships

There is a natural empathy between a mother and her baby and this grows into a strong and mutually enriching relationship as the two spend time with each other. Mothers who are well cared for are able to enjoy caring for the baby. The midwife should seek to foster the growth of a strong relationship by building the mother's confidence, preventing or alleviating physical discomfort and ensuring that the mother is protected from unnecessary stress and anxiety.

It has been demonstrated that close contact between a mother and her baby enriches the developing relationship between them (Klaus & Kennell 1982). Every effort should be made to enable the mother and baby to be together as much as possible. The baby should be nursed close to his mother and in her direct line of vision. The mother should be encouraged to handle and talk to her baby as much as she wishes and the rest of the family should be encouraged to cuddle the baby. In the past, fear of infection led midwives and doctors to discourage family members from handling the baby when they visited the ward but this fear has proved groundless.

Rooming-in. The baby should remain by his mother's bedside throughout the day and possibly at night or at least be brought to her for feeding during the night. This approach to care is known as 'rooming-in' and provides the mother with ample opportunity to become familiar with her baby and to develop confidence in caring for him before she returns home. However, this approach must be practised with care and rooming-in at night should not be allowed to conflict with the mother's need for adequate rest and sleep. Sleeping in the strange environment of a hospital ward is not easy and if a ward is continually disturbed by the crying of babies in the night it is not possible for mothers to enjoy the kind of deep sleep which they need. If a mother wishes to care for her own baby throughout the night but he continues to cry after feeding, she may agree to take him out of the ward.

Building confidence

The midwife can build up the mother's confidence by giving clear and careful instructions and by providing opportunities for the mother to ask questions and to discuss any anxieties. It may be necessary to repeat explanations on a number of occasions and the midwife must be patient in teaching and encouraging those mothers who are particularly anxious. The midwife should plan for a number of sessions of teaching which should include:

- advice about baby's feeding
- how to bring up the baby's wind
- sterilisation of feeding bottles, teats and comforters (for mothers who are bottle feeding)
- bathing the baby, dealing with sore buttocks, skin rashes, etc.
- coping with crying spells
- the emotional needs of parents
- the needs of the family
- the role of the health visitor
- the mother and baby clinic
- the postnatal examination
- family planning advice (see Ch. 17).

These sessions should be spread over a period of time and it is usual that some will be undertaken by the midwife in hospital and others by the community midwife. Whenever possible, the father and other members of the family should be included.

CARE OF SPECIAL GROUPS

Caesarean section

In addition to normal postnatal care, women delivered by caesarean section will require the degree of nursing care needed by any patient who has undergone major surgery. Those who have had an emergency caesarean section may be debilitated because the stress of surgery has been added to that of a difficult labour or anxiety over danger to the baby.

Women delivered by caesarean section have an increased risk of developing thrombophlebitis or deep vein thrombosis and there may be some risk of haemorrhage from the placental site during the first 48 hours after delivery. Prophylactic antibiotic therapy is commonly used to reduce or prevent infection (Enkin et al 1989).

During the first 24 hours the major needs are for adequate relief of pain and for maintenance of fluid intake. The first is achieved by giving the prescribed postoperative drug, usually pethidine

100 mg or papaveretum 10–20 mg intramuscularly as required. Fluid intake is normally maintained by intravenous infusion and by encouraging the mother to take some oral fluids. Once consciousness has been regained, the mother should be given the opportunity to see and touch her baby and she may be able to feed him if she is helped into a comfortable position.

On the day following the operation, the mother should be assisted to sit in a chair for a short time, to do deep breathing exercises and to do leg exercises. If she is able, she should be helped to walk to the bathroom and lavatory. Many women experience considerable discomfort from distension of the gut during the first 48 hours and this may be relieved by passing a flatus tube or giving a suppository. Sitting on the lavatory seat also helps in the expulsion of flatus. After 48 hours the mother should be encouraged to move around more and to undertake as much of the care of her baby as she feels able. It must be remembered that lifting a baby is painful for a woman with an abdominal wound and a mother who has had a caesarean section should not be left to cope on her own until she feels fully able to do so.

Sick and preterm babies

The mother of a preterm or sick baby will feel anxious, disappointed and may be very distressed. She will be anxious about her baby's health and prognosis and distressed at being unable to feed and care for him herself. It is important that she is allowed to express her fears, and that she is enabled to have as much contact with her baby as possible. It has been found that it is helpful for the mother to have a photograph of the baby to keep at her bedside and the midwife should use this to initiate conversation about the baby and encourage the mother to talk about him. Close and frequent contact between the mother and her baby in the special care baby unit should be encouraged and the mother should be taken to visit her baby if necessary in a wheelchair.

The parents should visit the baby together every day and arrangements should be made for the mother to feed the baby herself as soon as it is possible for her to do so. If the condition of the baby is causing particular anxiety, both parents should be enabled to stay as close to him as possible. Many units now have facilities for mothers

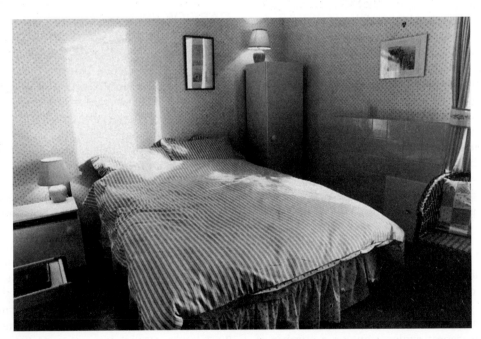

Fig. 16.5
Double bedroom for the use of parents of stillborn or sick infants.

to stay and sleep in the special care unit itself. Some hospitals also provide rooms with double beds to enable a couple to stay near their sick infant together thus providing each other with comfort and support.

Stillbirth or neonatal death

Recent years have seen the development of increased understanding of the needs of bereaved parents (Oglethorpe 1989). A couple who have lost a baby should be given privacy in which to grieve together.

The provision of a double room where husband and wife can stay together is especially helpful. Arrangements should be made for the mother to return home as soon as she is sufficiently recovered from the birth.

The midwife should ensure that the father or other responsible relative has understood the need to register the stillbirth or the birth and death of the baby (see Ch. 43) and that some arrangements have been made for the burial or cremation of the baby's body. It must be remembered that distressed people do not easily take in or retain information and care should be taken that no further distress is caused because the necessary procedures are not understood. Most hospitals provide very clear guidelines for staff and a set of written instructions for the family. (See Chapter 49 for a much fuller discussion of the needs of bereaved parents.)

Continuity of care between hospital and community midwives

The bulk of postnatal care in the UK is undertaken in the mother's own home by the community midwifery service. The role of the hospital midwife is to provide immediate postnatal care and to ensure that her community colleague has the necessary information which will enable her to continue the care of the mother and baby. This will include:

- relevant details of labour and delivery, including details of any trauma which has been sustained

- the condition of the baby at birth and results of his physical examination
- the results of any screening tests which have been undertaken and the dates when any further tests are required
- the current physical and emotional status of the mother
- any known problems or needs in the immediate family
- the current condition of the infant, and his method of feeding
- the mother's competence in feeding and care for her baby and details of advice that has been given.

If possible, a full copy of the hospital midwife's care plan and nursing records should be sent to the community midwife. It is important that the community midwife is informed of the mother's transfer to her care in sufficient time for her to make proper arrangements for the care of the mother and baby. The family will also need to have time to prepare for the mother and baby to come home.

Postnatal examination

It is important that the mother's full recovery from the effects of pregnancy, labour and delivery is confirmed by a postnatal examination when the baby is 6 weeks old. In the majority of cases this examination is carried out by the general practitioner although mothers who have experienced a difficult labour or had a caesarean section may receive their postnatal examination from the hospital consultant.

At this examination the mother's general physical and emotional health is checked and particular attention is paid to any symptoms of anaemia, urinary tract infection or of emotional distress or depression.

A physical examination is carried out of the breasts, abdomen and pelvis to ensure that involution is complete and any trauma which was sustained during delivery is fully healed. The integrity of the pelvic floor should be assessed and the woman asked directly if she has any dribbling or stress incontinence. She is asked whether she has any dyspareunia. A cervical smear is usually taken for cytology and the blood pressure is recorded. When the breasts are examined the woman is instructed in self-examination. Any problems which are found may then be treated promptly in order to ensure the mother's physical and emotional well-being. Advice about family planning and the continuing care of the baby is also given during this examination.

The midwife and the health visitor should advise each mother to attend for her postnatal examination. Ideally any woman who does not attend as arranged should be visited at home. Those who miss their postnatal examination either do so because they feel fit and do not see any point in it or because they are having difficulty coping and may be apathetic or depressed. For this reason defaulters should be followed up.

The midwife's role in caring for the mother and baby normally comes to an end with the transfer of care to the health visitor. The midwife may have the opportunity to meet mother and baby again when they attend the general practitioner's surgery for the postnatal visit. She may also have arranged a postnatal reunion group for mothers who attended the same set of parentcraft classes in order that they may share experiences and provide mutual support. Midwives and health visitors often share these sessions to provide a link between past and future care.

Acknowledgements

The help of the following is gratefully acknowledged: Miss P. Preston and midwives at the Dukeries Centre, Kings Mill Hospital, Sutton in Ashfield, Notts; Mrs Curry, Miss Hanson and midwives of Lincoln County Hospital.

REFERENCES

Ball J A 1989 Postnatal care and adjustment to motherhood. In: Robinson S, Thomson A M (eds) Midwives, research and childbirth, Vol 1. Chapman & Hall, London

Enkin M, Enkin E, Chalmers I, Hemminki E 1989 Prophylactic antibiotics in association with caesarean section. In: Chalmers I, Enkin M, Keirse M J N C (eds) Effective care in pregnancy and childbirth. Oxford University Press, Oxford

Flint C, Poulengeris P 1987 The 'know your midwife' report. Flint 49 Peckarmans Wood, Sydenham Hill, London SE26 6RZ

Reader Activities

1. Write out an interview schedule which could be used as the basis for discussing and planning postnatal care with:

- a woman who has just given birth normally to her first baby and who intends to breast feed
- a mother who has been delivered of her third child by caesarean section in the last few hours.

What facts would you need to know in order to make judgements about needs?

What choices and patterns of care would you wish to offer?

2. What arrangements are made in your hospital to ensure that mothers get adequate rest?

Check whether there are any guidelines on the care of:

- newly-delivered women
- waking mothers for meals
- dealing with fractious babies at night
- work of domestic staff.

House of Commons 1992 Health Committee 2nd report: Maternity services. HMSO, London

Klaus M H, Kennell J H 1982 Parent–infant bonding. Mosby, St Louis

Oglethorpe R J L 1989 Parenting after perinatal bereavement — a review of the literature. Journal of Reproductive and Infant Psychology 7: 227–244

United Kingdom Central Council 1991 Midwives rules. UKCC, London

FURTHER READING

Alexander J, Levy V, Roch S (eds) 1990 Postnatal care: a research-based approach. Macmillan, Basingstoke

Amiel G J 1981 Essential obstetric practice. MTP Press, Lancaster

Ball J A 1986 Reactions to motherhood: The role of postnatal care. Cambridge University Press, Cambridge

Ball J A 1988 Mothers need nurturing too. Nursing Times 84: 17

Boyd C, Sellers L 1982 The British way of birth. Pan, London

Maternity Services Advisory Committee 1985 Maternity care in action Part 3 Postnatal and neonatal care. HMSO, London

Prince J, Adams M E 1987 The psychology of childbirth, 2nd edn. Churchill Livingstone, Edinburgh

17

Family planning

JO ALEXANDER

Family planning is considered today as a basic human right. It is an important component both of primary health care and maternal and child health. It is the means of planning families that are wanted, spaced according to choice and timed to fit in with life decisions such as marriage or a break in career. Since stillbirth and infant mortality rates have dropped and epidemics and famine are better controlled, contraception has become a key element in population policy. The problem of overpopulation is now acute as every 10 seconds the world population increases by 30 individuals and is likely to double over the next 40 years.

On a personal level, unplanned pregnancy can be catastrophic and in a recent survey of live births (Fleissig 1991) it was found that 31.3% had been unintended pregnancies; those mothers whose pregnancies had not been planned were mainly single, young, had left school under the age of 18 or already had two or more children. This seems tragic.

This chapter will review the family planning methods available and the midwife's role in relation to contraception.

History of family planning services

Dr Marie Stopes set up the first birth control clinic in London in 1921 and following this, independent societies were formed and opened clinics in other parts of the country. 'Children by choice, not chance' was their declared intent with the aim of increasing marital happiness, and these societies were later to become the Family Planning Association (FPA). In 1930 the first real governmental recognition came when the Ministry of Health allowed Local Health Authorities to provide family planning advice for women who for health reasons should avoid further pregnancies. Gradually interest in the subject of fertility and relationships broadened and in 1943 a centre investigating male sub-fertility was opened in London, and sessions for helping those with marital difficulties were started in 1946. In the same year some formal training for doctors and nurses was established.

There were nearly 300 FPA clinics by 1958 and a Church of England conference accepted the statement that birth control is a 'right and important factor in Christian family life'. Oral contraceptives and intra-uterine contraceptive devices were approved for use in FPA clinics in 1961 and 1965 respectively, and in 1967 the Local Health Authorities in England and Wales were allowed to provide family planning advice without regard to marital status and on social as well as medical grounds.

Following the 1973 National Health Service (NHS) Reorganisation Act, the FPA clinics and domiciliary services were gradually handed over to the NHS; family planning advice and supplies were made available free of charge and irrespective of age and marital status. In 1975 general practitioners began to provide family planning services under the NHS and in 1977 the FPA and Health Education Council jointly set up the Family Planning Information Service (FPIS). This provides both the public and professionals with information about family planning, sexuality and related subjects. A survey in 1982 found the NHS family planning services to be cost effective.

The work of the International Planned Parenthood Federation is noteworthy in promoting population and family planning activities throughout the world.

SERVICES AVAILABLE

Today *Family Planning Clinics* are run by District Health Authorities in England and Wales, Health and Social Services Boards in Northern Ireland and Health Boards in Scotland. Self-referral is normal practice. The doctors and nurses have usually undergone specialist post-registration training. All the National Boards for Nursing, Midwifery and Health Visiting run courses in family planning. These consist of both theoretical instruction and experience at clinics. Family planning clinic addresses are available at public libraries, post offices, child health clinics and in telephone directories. Many women prefer the relative anonymity of these clinics and confidentiality is complete. It is however usual to ask a woman who is being prescribed the contraceptive pill if her general practitioner may be informed.

A list of *general practitioners* offering these services (some with post-registration training) is compiled by Family Health Service Authorities (Health Boards in Scotland) and available at post offices and public libraries. Clients may choose a doctor other than their own general practitioner, the doctor being paid on an item of service basis.

In heavily populated areas the District Health Authority may provide *Domiciliary Family Planning* services for those unable or unwilling to attend clinics. This service is unfortunately becoming increasingly rare.

Private services and some run by *charitable organisations* also exist. Addresses are available from the FPIS and telephone directories.

All services should offer routine screening for cervical cancer, but for an apprehensive client vaginal examination is better not carried out at a first visit. Some authorities also advocate routine screening by palpation for breast cancer and the teaching of breast awareness. Pregnancy testing should be available for anyone concerned about a delayed period.

Young people under 16 years of age should always be encouraged to involve their parents or guardians. In England and Wales, however, it is legal for contraceptive or abortion advice or treatment to be given without parental consent provided the client understands the nature and consequences of the treatment. The practitioner should also be of the opinion that if contraception was withheld, sexual intercourse would still be likely to take place and that to withhold treatment would damage the young person's physical or mental health. In Scotland this applies to girls over 12 years of age but in Northern Ireland the situation is unclear.

The role of the midwife in family planning is acknowledged by the World Health Organization, International Confederation of Midwives, International Federation of Gynaecologists and Obstetricians and the EC Midwives Directives. She must be able to provide reliable and up-to-date information. Her counselling skills (Ch. 49) are of paramount importance and she must be careful never to make moral judgements. Knowledge of colloquial names for contraceptive methods and parts of the body is desirable. Some clients may need advice about the risks associated with their sexual lifestyle.

When a midwife is giving *pre-conception advice* she may suggest that oral contraceptives are discontinued 3 months prior to conception. A balanced diet should rectify any vitamin deficiencies which may have resulted (see below). In the case of combined pills this gap allows the woman's own menstrual cycle to become re-established. Calculation of gestation is then more accurate. A barrier method is probably the best alternative over this period. There is, however, no need for a woman to worry if she conceives immediately after discontinuing oral contraceptives.

After rubella vaccination the use of contraception for 1 month is advised.

A woman may wish to discuss family planning *antenatally* and it may be suitable for her partner to be involved. *Postnatally* the midwife should consider discussion of this topic to be an integral part of her care. Talking with a mother about pelvic floor exercises often leads on quite naturally to the subject of intercourse. This allows practical information to be given about the various methods and also enables the midwife to indicate that intercourse may be resumed as soon as the couple desire. Laryea (1980) has shown that whilst primiparae would have welcomed discussion concerning resumption of intercourse, they waited for the midwives to initiate it. Midwives thought that for them to broach the subject was an intrusion into the mother's private relationship and an impasse arose.

Another study (Sleep et al 1984) has shown that 32% of women resume intercourse during the first postnatal month. It is not uncommon for either partner to experience diminished libido and it may help to discuss this. This problem is said to be more common amongst breast-feeding women and they may also appreciate being forewarned that milk ejection can occur with orgasm. Alternative positions may lessen perineal discomfort and help to prevent painful pressure on the breasts. Lack of vaginal lubrication is a common problem postnatally and proprietary jellies (e.g. K–Y) may be of use.

The midwife needs to be aware that *factors governing an individual's choice of method* vary enormously and can include religious and cultural considerations, the stability of the relationship, frequency of intercourse, and lifestyle. The ability of the client to understand any method must also be considered and the FPIS produces user-friendly pamphlets in English and ethnic minority languages. (Where relevant, postnatal factors are discussed under the method concerned.)

The motivation of clients to use their chosen method will be governed by the strength of their desire to prevent pregnancy. A couple with a family history of a genetically inherited disorder may be highly motivated, whereas a girl receiving little attention from her parents or a woman attempting to cement a failing relationship may be less so. Age may also influence choice but although a woman's fertility is reduced by the age of 45, contraception is still advised for 2 years after her last period if a woman is under 50 and 1 year if she is older.

It is not yet within a midwife's practice in Britain to insert intra-uterine contraceptive devices or to prescribe family planning supplies other than sheaths. However, because of her work, she is in an ideal position to provide advice concerning all aspects of sexual medicine. If her knowledge and experience are inadequate to help the couple, she should refer them to a practitioner with specialist training.

The *ideal contraceptive* would be 100% effective, perfectly safe, and painlessly reversible. There would be no interruption of spontaneity, no mess and no unpleasant odour or taste. It would be easy to use, cheap, not reliant on the user's memory and independent of the medical professions. Needless to say it will never exist, but if she is aware of the person's preferences the midwife may be able to advise the most suitable option.

For each contraceptive method discussed below the failure rate is stated per 100 woman years (HWY) of use. This is the number who would become pregnant if 100 women used the method for 1 year. It is slightly misleading as it does not reflect the fact that fertility varies with age and that the success of a method is partially dependent on motivation and the teaching received. When counselling clients it is perhaps more helpful to talk in terms of success rates and to calculate for them the likelihood of a pregnancy occurring during a certain period of usage. It is important to remember that unprotected intercourse for young women results in 80–90 pregnancies per HWY, and not 100.

NATURAL METHODS

Interest in these methods is increasing. Just as many women, given the opportunity, express a strong preference for natural childbirth, so a similar attitude is being taken about family planning.

Natural methods are particularly attractive to people who hold certain moral convictions and also to women who on medical advice are seeking an alternative to hormonal contraception and intra-uterine contraceptive devices.

Methods involving abstention

The following methods involve *abstention* from intercourse around the time of ovulation. Their use involves individual preparatory instruction, careful observation of changes in the body and self-control by both partners. The communication between a couple which is necessary for these methods to work may enhance the quality of their relationship and they may find ways of expressing affection apart from intercourse. Adequate instruction is beyond the scope of most midwives and family planning clinics but can be obtained via the Natural Family Planning Service (Catholic Marriage Advisory Council, Clitherow House, 1 Blythe Mews, Blythe Road, London W14 0NW)

and the Natural Family Planning Centre (Queen Elizabeth Medical Centre, Edgbaston, Birmingham B15 2TG). It is advisable for several indicators of fertility to be used.

Observation of cervical mucus

Following menstruation thick mucus blocks the cervical canal and acts as a barrier to spermatozoa. The woman is aware of dryness at the vulva. As oestrogen levels rise, the mucus absorbs water and nutrients, softens and begins to flow. This mucus is opaque, white or creamy and gives a sensation of stickiness.

Around the time of ovulation the mucus becomes transparent, slippery and capable of considerable stretching between finger and thumb. This latter property is called spinnbarkeit and occurs as the molecules become parallel to one another to facilitate the passage of spermatozoa. This 'fertile' mucus looks like raw egg white. Progesterone subsequently causes the mucus to thicken and the sensations of stickiness and then dryness return.

Observations of mucus are made throughout the day. The fertile phase begins when mucus is first noticed and ends four days after the last day of 'fertile' mucus. Semen can make interpretation difficult and in the pre-ovulatory infertile phase it is recommended that alternate nights only are used for intercourse. Some suggest that there must be abstinence from intercourse during menstruation because if any mucus were to be produced it might not be noticed.

If these observations alone are relied on, the failure rate is between 6 and 11 per HWY. After cessation of lochia postnatally mucus patterns can be interpreted with expert help but much abstinence may be required because oestrogen surges result in mucus flow.

In couples trying to conceive, observation of cervical mucus will help them to determine their most fertile time. The characteristics of this mucus may also be of clinical value when sub-fertility is being investigated.

Observation of body temperature

The temperature is taken immediately on waking every day (special large scale thermometers and charts are available from family planning clinics). Progesterone production following ovulation causes body temperature to rise by 0.2°C (0.4°F). Thus once three consecutive readings are higher than the previous six, it is unlikely that intercourse during the remainder of the cycle will result in pregnancy. (After getting up during the night, the woman must be resting in bed for at least 2 hours before taking her temperature.) Factors such as stress or a late night may affect temperature and considerable care needs to be taken when interpreting these charts.

Palpation of the cervix

Around the time of ovulation the cervix shortens, softens and dilates slightly. This is an oestrogenic effect and some women are able to detect these changes. 12 weeks after delivery they may again be interpreted with expert help.

Calendar or rhythm method

This is used to calculate the period during which intercourse is most likely to result in pregnancy. The remainder of the cycle used to be called the 'safe period'.

This method assumes, wrongly, that ova remain capable of being fertilised for up to 48 hours after ovulation, and that spermatozoa are viable within the female for 72 hours during the fertile phase. (In fact ova survive for 12–24 hours.) The woman records the length of six menstrual cycles. Her first fertile day is calculated by subtracting 20 days from the length of her shortest cycle and her last fertile day by subtracting 10 days from the length of her longest cycle. Thus if her cycles varied between 25 and 31 days, she would be fertile between days 5 and 21.

Amongst advocates of natural family planning, calendar calculation on its own is rarely used. The menopause and the postnatal period pose special problems.

Symptothermal method (Fig. 17.1)

The symptothermal method combines temperature charting with observation of cervical mucus and use of the calendar formula to identify the beginning of the fertile phase. Other cyclical symptoms such as ovulation pain, breast tenderness and cervical changes may be recorded. The failure rate is 1–4 per HWY.

Couples aiming to prevent rather than delay pregnancy should be advised to rely on the post-ovulatory phase of the cycle only.

A urine-testing kit which responds to the luteinising hormone surge and changes colour shortly before ovulation is now available and useful for women wishing to conceive. It does not give sufficient warning of the approach of ovulation to be useful for contraceptive purposes.

The contraceptive effect of breast feeding

In some cultures abstention is practised during lactation, but even taking this into consideration it has been estimated that in developing countries breast feeding prevents more pregnancies than the combined effects of all other methods of artificial contraception put together.

The precise contraceptive effect of breast feeding is uncertain. It has been shown that whilst blood prolactin levels are raised and those of oestradiol and progesterone lowered, gonadotrophins are either at, or just below, normal levels.

Howie et al (1982) have shown that the return of ovulation postnatally is significantly delayed in breast-feeding women. Ovulation may still occur prior to the first postnatal menstruation but often only if supplementary feeds have been introduced. The lack of a night feed may be important. The results of one small study (McNeilly et al 1983) have suggested that, if a woman wishes to rely on the contraceptive action of breast feeding, the baby must be completely breast fed and suckle at least five times and for more than a total of 65 minutes daily. Women wanting to use natural methods at this time will be taught to watch for the return of mucus symptoms and for changes in the temperature chart, and to palpate the cervix.

Large scale introduction of artificial feeding into a developing country is likely to result in a rapid rise in population growth which could only be controlled by a very substantial increase in contraceptive usage.

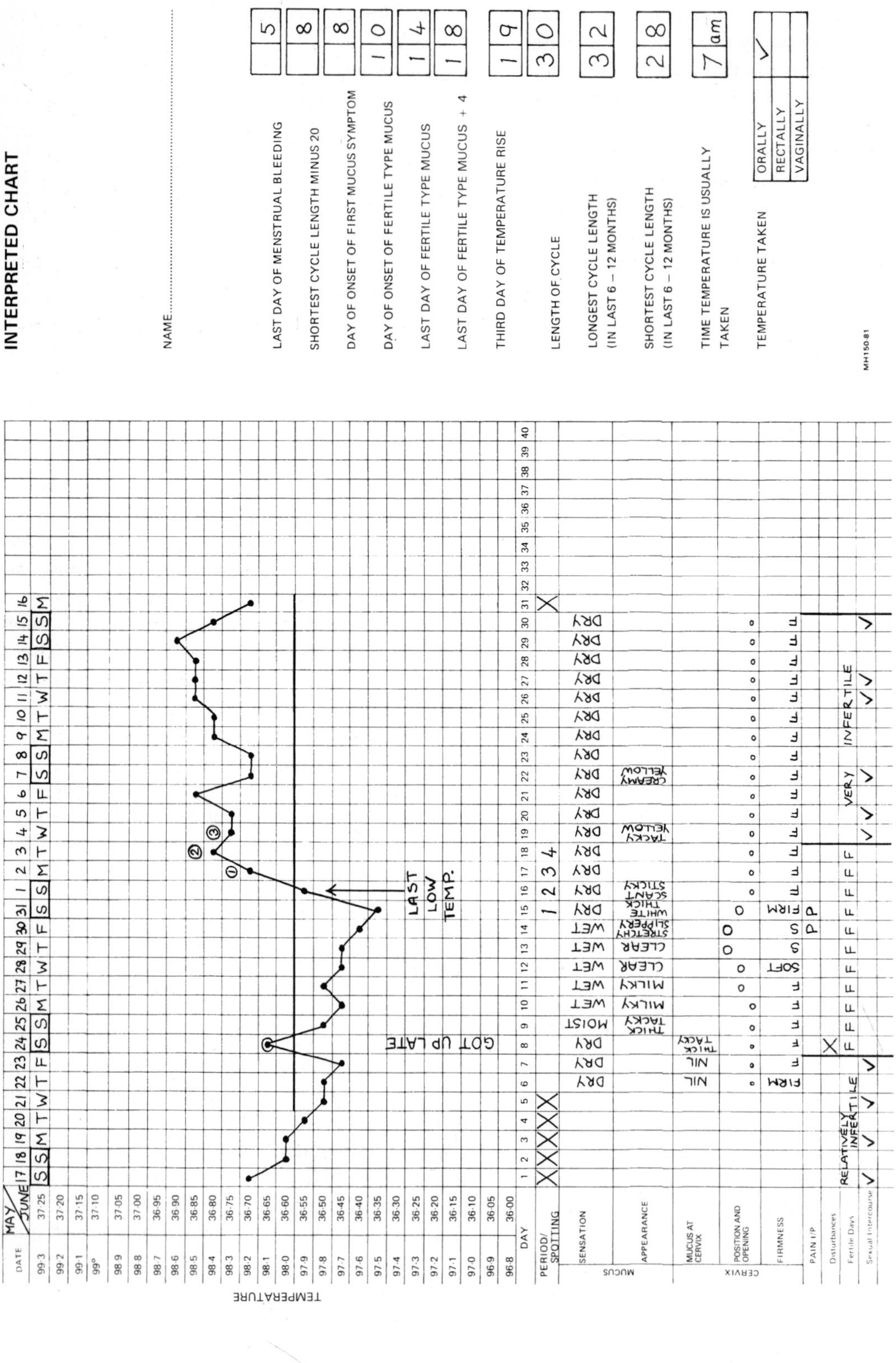

INTERPRETED CHART

NAME.........................

LAST DAY OF MENSTRUAL BLEEDING	5
SHORTEST CYCLE LENGTH MINUS 20	8
DAY OF ONSET OF FIRST MUCUS SYMPTOM	8
DAY OF ONSET OF FERTILE TYPE MUCUS	10
LAST DAY OF FERTILE TYPE MUCUS	14
LAST DAY OF FERTILE TYPE MUCUS + 4	18
THIRD DAY OF TEMPERATURE RISE	19
LENGTH OF CYCLE	30
LONGEST CYCLE LENGTH (IN LAST 6 – 12 MONTHS)	32
SHORTEST CYCLE LENGTH (IN LAST 6 – 12 MONTHS)	28
TIME TEMPERATURE IS USUALLY TAKEN	7 am
TEMPERATURE TAKEN	ORALLY ✓
	RECTALLY
	VAGINALLY

MH150-81

Fig. 17.1
Symptothermal fertility chart.

Coitus interruptus

This involves withdrawal of the penis prior to ejaculation and necessitates tremendous self-control. It is often referred to as 'being careful' or 'taking care' and both partners may find this interruption of intercourse frustrating. The method is widely practised but the failure rate may be as high as 25 per HWY as semen leakage can occur prior to ejaculation. It is, however, much more effective than using no contraception at all.

Vaginal douching

Douching after intercourse will not prevent pregnancy as spermatozoa can reach the internal cervical os within 90 seconds of ejaculation.

BARRIER METHODS

Sheath or condom

This tube of thin rubber is rolled on to the erect penis. It must be applied before any genital contact takes place because some semen often escapes prior to ejaculation. About 1/2" of air-free space must be left at the tip to accommodate the ejaculate, otherwise the sheath may burst. Some designs incorporate a teat end for this purpose. The sheath may slip off unless it is held in place during withdrawal of the still erect penis. Sheaths can tear and need to be handled carefully.

Spermicides (see below) increase the efficacy of the sheath, some of which are already impregnated with them. The lubrication they afford may reduce the risk of tearing associated with poor vaginal lubrication which is not uncommon postnatally. Vaseline should not be used as it damages rubber.

Failure rate: 2–15 per HWY.

Considerations in relation to use

If the packet bears the British Standards KiteMark, the sheaths have been batch-tested for strength. Many different colours are available and special sheaths are made for those allergic to rubber. Each sheath should be used once only and not after the expiry date. Although available at family planning clinics, chemists, some super-markets and by mail order, sheaths cannot be obtained on prescription. It has been shown that they afford some protection against sexually transmitted diseases and also cervical cancer.

A female condom consisting of a lubricated, loose-fitting polyurethane pouch for insertion into the vagina is now available. An inner ring (which is part of the closed end of the pouch) should be situated in the fornices; an outer ring lies flat against the vulva.

The failure rate is expected to be similar to that of the male condom. They are used once only and are available from family planning clinics and retail outlets.

Diaphragm

This thin rubber dome forms a barrier in the vagina between the semen and the cervix (see Fig. 17.2). It has a circumference of soft metal to help maintain its shape. The woman is individually fitted. The rim should lie closely against the vaginal walls and rest in the posterior vaginal fornix and against the back of the symphysis pubis. Before its insertion spermicidal cream or jelly should be applied to the upper surface (some authorities say to the lower surface also) but not around the rim. After insertion the woman must check that her cervix is covered. She may need to be shown the diaphragm's position on a model and reassured that it cannot wander round the body. The im-

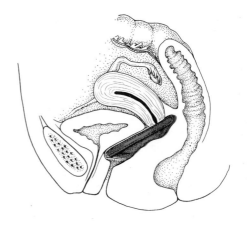

Fig. 17.2
The diaphragm in place.

portance placed on the use of spermicides and the close fit of the diaphragm is currently being questioned, as considerable dilatation of the upper portion of the vagina takes place during arousal.

Failure rate: 2–15 per HWY.

Important considerations in relation to use

In order to preserve spontaneity the woman may decide to insert her diaphragm every night as a matter of routine but if intercourse is anticipated more than 3 hours after its insertion a spermicidal pessary is needed (see below). The diaphragm must be left in situ for 6 hours following intercourse, but not for more than 24. The woman should not bathe for 3 hours after intercourse. On removal the diaphragm should be washed with a mild soap and inspected for holes. The diaphragm appears to predispose to vaginal candidiasis, especially in diabetic women. Nystatin (or rather its base) may rot the rubber and it is best if the sheath is used instead during treatment. Clotrimazole does not appear to have the same effect.

Postnatally the woman should not rely on her previous diaphragm but have its size checked 5–6 weeks after delivery when the vagina and pelvic floor muscles will have regained some of their tone. A 3 kg (7 lb) alteration in weight also necessitates refitting as fat is stored in the vaginal walls and pelvic connective tissue. A new diaphragm should be fitted annually. It is likely that the diaphragm affords some protection against sexually transmitted diseases and cervical cancer. Some women may not find it acceptable to handle their external genitalia to the extent that this method requires. Water for cleaning the diaphragm must be readily available.

Contra-indications include rubber allergy or uterine prolapse.

Recurrent cystitis may be aggravated and physically handicapped or arthritic women may have difficulty in inserting the diaphragm.

Cervical and vault caps cover only the cervix, adhering to it by suction. Their use is similar to that of the diaphragm, but they are uncommon.

Work was done on caps moulded to fit the cervix of the individual concerned. They could be worn continuously for about a year as they contained a one-way valve to allow for menstrual flow. Unfortunately they had a very high failure rate.

Vaginal sponge

This synthetic sponge is impregnated with spermicide. After moistening with water and insertion high into the vagina it remains effective for 24 hours. The woman needs to check that her cervix is covered, but even if intercourse is repeated no additional spermicides are required. It must remain in situ for at least 6 hours after intercourse and the type currently available is not re-usable. A bath can be taken with the sponge in situ, but it should not be used during menstruation.

Failure rate. This is claimed by the manufacturers to be 9–11 per HWY when used according to instructions, but in one British study of its use by young, highly motivated and well educated women (Bounds & Guillebaud 1984) the failure rate was approximately 25 per HWY. Despite this, and the fact that it is expensive, it may prove to be popular as no contact with professionals is needed. The sponge may prove to be suitable for women whose fertility is lowered (for example those over the age of 40 or who are breast feeding), but quite unsuitable for those to whom it is vital to avoid pregnancy. Contra-indications include existing vaginal infection, allergy and previous toxic shock syndrome.

Spermicidal pessaries, creams, jellies, foaming tablets and aerosols

These preparations kill spermatozoa, but as there are usually several hundred million spermatozoa per ejaculate, they are not usually recommended for use on their own. They must be applied immediately before or, in the case of pessaries, 10 minutes before intercourse. Allergy can occur. Concern has been expressed about possible teratogenicity if spermicides are used around the time of conception, but most studies are very reassuring. Spermicides may afford some protection against human immunodeficiency virus (HIV), gonorrhoea and syphilis.

Failure rate (when used alone): 14–25 per HWY.

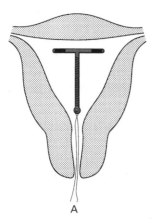 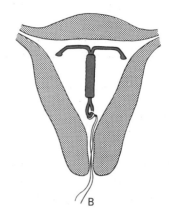

Fig. 17.3
Intra-uterine contraceptive devices; (both are radio-opaque). After insertion through the cervix, the device assumes the shape shown; the threads attached to it protrude into the vagina. (A) Copper-carrying device. (B) Hormone-carrying device — available in some countries.

INTRA-UTERINE CONTRACEPTIVE DEVICES (IUCD)

There are several types (see Fig. 17.3).

Mode of action
This is not fully understood. When an IUCD has been in position long term, its main effect appears to be to block fertilisation by action on the sperm. The IUCD also increases tubal motility, making it likely that any conceptus will pass through the uterine cavity before it is ready to implant.

It renders the endometrium less suitable for implantation; the mechanism is uncertain but the endometrium has been found to contain more leucocytes.

It may increase prostaglandin production making expulsion of any conceptus more likely.

The larger the surface area of the device the less likely is conception, but the greater the chance of expulsion or menstrual problems. Copper-carrying devices are more efficient, possibly because they increase inflammatory response in the endometrium.

Failure rate: 0.3–4 per HWY.

Important considerations in relation to use
The device may be inserted at any time of the cycle, but expulsion is more likely if it is performed during heavy menstrual flow. The best time is probably around ovulation when the cervix is slightly dilated, or during the first half of the cycle. Aseptic technique must be scrupulous. Insertion usually causes some pain but prior explanation significantly reduces this.

The length and volume of the menstrual loss may increase; prospective users should be warned of this and those with menorrhagia or chronic anaemia may be considered unsuitable. It may also prove a problem for the physically or mentally handicapped. Dysmenorrhoea is likely to increase and inter-menstrual bleeding may occur.

The expulsion rate is between 5 and 15% per annum and depends on many factors including parity, type of device and the experience of the fitter. The woman is usually taught to check for the presence of the threads at the end of each period. If her partner is aware of the device during intercourse this may be because it is being expelled or the threads need shortening.

Yearly check-ups are advised. Manufacturers recommend that copper-carrying devices are changed every 2–5 years. If a woman in her forties has a device inserted, it may remain in situ until the menopause.

Other possible side-effects
An increase in pelvic inflammatory disease may be related to the easier access that spermatozoa have to the uterus and uterine tubes. It is possible that

concurrent use of spermicides may reduce both this and the failure rate. Current pelvic inflammatory disease is a contra-indication to insertion and it may be considered that the risk of salpingitis and infertility makes the device unsuitable for nulliparae. Structural cardiac abnormality is a contra-indication because of the risk of bacterial endocarditis.

IUCDs are associated with an increase in ectopic pregnancies. This may be a result of tubal damage caused by salpingitis. However it is possible that these ectopics were destined to occur anyway, for whereas other methods of contraception prevent fertilisation this device probably prevents intra-uterine pregnancies much more effectively than tubal ones.

Should pregnancy occur, there is an increased incidence of spontaneous abortion. If pregnancy continues most obstetricians advise removal of the device to reduce the risk of septic incomplete abortion which can be fatal. There is also an increased incidence of premature labour and antepartum haemorrhage. There is no evidence of teratogenicity.

To reduce the chances of perforation of a softened uterus, insertion is usually delayed until 6 weeks after vaginal delivery and for 6–8 weeks after caesarean section. The uterine contractions caused by breast feeding do not increase the expulsion rate but uterine perforation is more likely.

Some argue that insertion immediately following spontaneous or therapeutic abortion can increase the risk of sepsis (although this is probably only likely if there is retained tissue) and that women after therapeutic abortion may be persuaded to accept a device against their better judgement. Others feel that a delay following termination may result in another genuinely unwanted pregnancy.

Following hydatidiform mole an IUCD can be inserted after 6–8 weeks provided the serum HCG level has returned to normal. If the level remains high the IUCD might precipitate malignant spread to the circulation. If intermenstrual bleeding occurs this must not be blamed on the device until the HCG level has been shown to be normal.

Work is progressing on hormone-carrying devices. These often cause amenorrhoea which the users seem to like provided that they have been counselled in advance.

HORMONAL METHODS

Combined oral contraceptive pill (containing oestrogen and a synthetic form of progesterone, a progestogen)

Mode of action

Oestrogen and progestogen suppress follicle-stimulating hormone and luteinising hormone production, so that ovarian follicles do not mature and ovulation does not usually take place.

Progestogen also causes thickening of the cervical mucus, making penetration by spermatozoa difficult. It renders the endometrium unsuitable for implantation. It also slows uterine tube motility making the blastocyst less likely to reach the uterus at the optimum time for implantation.

One pill is usually taken daily for 21 days and vaginal bleeding due to hormone withdrawal should occur during the 7 pill-free days before the next packet is started. The woman's own cycle is suppressed, periods are regular and often lighter due to poor endometrial development. Dysmenorrhoea and premenstrual tension are usually reduced.

Failure rate: 0.1–7 per HWY.

Important considerations in relation to use

Contraceptive pills of all types are currently designed to be taken orally by the woman concerned; it has been known for them to be taken by the partner and for surprise to be expressed when pregnancy occurred.

If a tablet is forgotten it should be taken late. If it is more than 12 hours late, additional contraceptive measures must be used for 7 days (if these 7 days run beyond the end of the packet, the new packet should be started as soon as the old one is finished). No more than two tablets should be taken at one time.

If vomiting or severe diarrhoea occur within 3 hours of taking a pill additional measures are needed as above. If other medications are taken the doctor should be consulted about possible interactions: broad spectrum antibiotics may impair intestinal absorption, most anti-convulsants increase liver enzyme production and hence drug breakdown, large doses of vitamin C increase oestrogen absorption. Absorption of oestrogen and progestogen varies between women as much as ten-fold.

There may initially be 'minor' side-effects which usually resolve spontaneously. These include breast tenderness, nausea, weight increase, mild depression, diminished libido, amenorrhoea and intermenstrual bleeding. If the latter continues, a pill containing a higher dose of hormones may be required.

Possible major side-effects

Over recent years the hormone dosage of all oral contraceptives has been greatly reduced in order to reduce these effects.

Arterial or venous thrombosis. (Clotting factors, platelet aggregation and serum lipids are increased.) Consequences can be serious and include deep vein thrombosis, pulmonary embolus and cerebral ischaemia. This does not appear to be a problem with the progestogen-only pill.

Hypertension. This is thought to be an oestrogenic effect but can be potentiated by progestogen.

(Women who smoke and are over 35 are at considerably increased risk from both thrombosis and hypertension.)

Predisposition to impaired glucose tolerance, pyridoxine deficiency and depression; the latter two may be linked. Blood levels of riboflavin, folacin, vitamin B_{12}, ascorbic acid and zinc are lowered and those of vitamin K, iron and copper are raised. The clinical significance of these is uncertain.

There *may* be a link between *breast cancer* occurring under the age of 35 and the long-term use of pills before the age of 25.

Evidence linking the combined pill with *cervical carcinoma* is controversial. This carcinoma is not hormonally dependent, but it is probably relevant that this method affords the cervix no protection from contact with semen. Cigarette smokers and partners of men who smoke are at an increased risk of cervical carcinoma. The combined pill however offers valuable protection against cancer of the ovary and endometrium.

Women discontinuing the pill take, on average, 3 months longer to conceive than women discontinuing other methods.

Contra-indications

These include the following:

— History of thrombo-embolic problems or known abnormal clotting factors
— Hypertension
— Familial hyperlipidaemia
— Valvular heart disease
— Diabetes mellitus with complications (e.g. retinopathy)
— Oestrogen-dependent malignancy
— Gross obesity
— Smokers over 35
— Current liver disease
— Idiopathic jaundice of pregnancy
— Hydatidiform mole (until serum HCG is no longer detectable; see Ch. 18)
— Pregnancy (evidence that conception whilst taking the pill predisposes to limb reduction deformities has not been confirmed by large scale studies)
— Puerperal psychosis
— Lactation. Oestrogen suppresses prolactin production and hence diminishes milk production and the duration of lactation.

This pill is not usually prescribed during the 3 weeks following delivery as postnatal women are already at an increased risk of thrombo-embolism. Women who have had severe pre-eclampsia or a caesarean section should probably wait longer (Guillebaud 1989) but the pill can be prescribed immediately following spontaneous or therapeutic abortion.

Similarly it should not be taken for 4 weeks before and for 2 weeks following full mobilisation after a major operation. This is because of the risks of thrombo-embolic complications but some authorities feel that this is unnecessary.

Fit, non-obese women who do not smoke may continue using low-dose pills until the menopause.

Clients taking any form of oral contraceptive are seen every 3–6 months when the blood pressure and weight are noted.

Biphasic and triphasic oral contraceptive pills

The dosage of oestrogen and progestogen alters two or three times during the 21 days that these pills are taken and, provided the pills are taken in the correct sequence, normal monthly hormonal blood levels will be imitated. The overall hormone dosage is lower than in traditional combined pills and there is less alteration of blood chemistry. The failure rate is comparable with traditional combined oral contraceptives.

Progestogen-only pill

Mode of action — see above. In about 50% of cycles ovulation is not suppressed.

Important considerations in relation to use

The effect on cervical mucus is at its maximum between 4 and 22 hours after this pill has been taken; there are no pill-free days. It is best taken about 4 hours before the usual time of intercourse and it should be taken at the same time every day. If forgotten for more than 3 hours, additional contraceptive methods will be needed for 48 hours (some would say 7 days) and the late pill should be taken as soon as possible. Following vomiting or severe diarrhoea additional contraceptive methods will be needed until 48 hours (some say 7 days) after the illness ceases.

Antibiotics do not adversely affect the progestogen-only pill, but the woman should consult a doctor about possible interactions with other drugs.

Menstruation is not due to artificial hormone withdrawal; amenorrhoea or irregular light periods are common.

As with the combined pill the emphasis on time may prove difficult for women of some cultures.

Failure rate: 0.5–7 per HWY.

Possible side-effects

- Impaired glucose tolerance (minimal effect)
- Ectopic pregnancy is increased in incidence (note the action of progesterone on uterine tubes)
- Functional ovarian cysts.

Contra-indications

- Current pregnancy
- History of ectopic pregnancy
- Recent hydatidiform mole (until the serum HCG has disappeared)

- Heavy, frequent or irregular periods (because they tend to be exacerbated)
- Severe arterial disease.

The physician may not consider the contra-indications listed for the combined pill as absolute in relation to the progestogen-only pill. As thrombosis is not a problem, the remarks concerning operations do not apply and this pill may be prescribed immediately following spontaneous or induced abortion and 1 week following delivery. Puerperal break-through bleeding, however, tends to be less if the pill is not started for 3–4 weeks.

Some progestogen crosses in breast milk but does not diminish supply and is thought to be harmless.

This form of contraception may be prescribed for women with diabetes mellitus, a previous history of thrombo-embolism or who have developed hypertension with the combined pill.

Intramuscular long-acting progestogen

Mode of action

As with the progestogen-only pill but ovulation is much more likely to be suppressed.

Contraceptive action lasts for 2–3 months depending on dosage but so do any adverse effects. Periods can be lighter, irregular or nonexistent. Irregular, heavy and prolonged bleeding is more common if the injection is given in the puerperium.

Currently the Licensing Authority and Minister of Health only sanction the long-term use of this injection when other methods are contra-indicated, have caused unacceptable side-effects or are otherwise unsatisfactory. Informed consent must be given.

Links with breast cancer and congenital abnormalities have not been confirmed, but there may be some delay in the return of fertility. The same contra-indications apply as for the progestogen-only pill. For breast-feeding mothers it is suggested that administration is delayed until 4–6 weeks after delivery when the baby's enzyme system is more fully developed. This delay may also reduce the risk of heavy and prolonged periods which can be confused with secondary postpartum haemorrhage.

The use of this drug for mentally handicapped women has been the subject of hot debate, as has its wide use in certain developing countries where other contraceptive methods are not as easily available as perhaps they should be.

Failure rate: 0–1 per HWY.

Future methods of carrying long-acting progestogens

Work is progressing with the implantation of small silastic tubes beneath the skin of the upper arm; these may be effective for 6 or 7 years, unless removed earlier. A silastic ring has also been developed which when placed in the vaginal vault remains effective for 3 months; slightly increased vaginal discharge has been a problem.

Emergency contraception

This is reserved for use when no contraception was used or contraception failed or was used incorrectly.

An *IUCD* is the most effective method. If it is inserted within 5 days, implantation can be avoided and it can be left in situ if desired.

Alternatively, two *combined pills* each containing 50 μg of ethinyloestradiol and 250 μg of levonorgestrel can be taken within 72 hours of intercourse and an identical further dose 12 hours later; nausea is a problem. The next period often starts later than expected. Follow-up is essential as in 1% of cases this fails and there is then an increased risk of ectopic pregnancy. The risk of teratogenicity is extremely small but must be discussed.

Large oral doses of *progestogen* may have the same effect.

Work is progressing on a pill (RU 486) which, if taken in the days before the next period is due, blocks the action of progesterone so that menstruation occurs early, carrying with it the fertilized ovum.

MALE AND FEMALE STERILISATION

Sterilisation should be viewed as a permanent move and couples need to consider carefully what their feelings might be if any existing children or one partner died, or if their relationship ended. Although consent of a spouse is not legally required joint counselling is desirable. The operation is available for both sexes under the NHS, but the waiting list for male sterilisation (vasectomy) may be especially long.

With the commonly used techniques neither male nor female sterilisation results in any hormonal changes. Diminished libido may result for psychological reasons, but some find the freedom from fear of pregnancy very liberating.

Female sterilisation

The passage of ova from ovary to uterus is interrupted by occluding the uterine tube by division and suturing or by clip application. Modern methods aim at minimal tissue destruction and the isthmus is chosen (for here the tube is of static diameter) so as to increase the chance of a reversal being successful. The operation may be carried out via laparotomy, laparoscopy or more rarely by entry into the Pouch of Douglas via the posterior vaginal fornix.

Attempts are being made to develop a method using removable silicone plugs.

Failure rate of tubal clips applied abdominally: 2 per 1000 cases.

Important considerations

Unless carried out at caesarean section, delay until at least 6 weeks after delivery is usually considered advisable because of the increased risk of thromboembolic problems over this period and the time it allows for assessment of the baby's health. If carried out earlier, the operation is more difficult because of the upward displacement of the tubes and their wider diameter. The argument advanced in favour of its being performed during the postnatal stay is that of convenience, but more women regret the operation if it is carried out at this time. The incidence of regret is also high if sterilisation is performed at the time of abortion or on women aged less than 30.

In women with menstrual problems or prolapse, a hysterectomy might be more suitable.

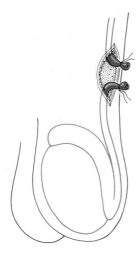

Fig. 17.4
A vas deferens divided.

Female sterilisation is immediately effective but admission to hospital and general anaesthetic are usually required; local anaesthetic is, however, becoming increasingly popular. Postoperative complications are commoner than after vasectomy and longer convalescence is needed. Following reversal of the operation or the rare event of spontaneous recanalisation there is an increased risk of ectopic pregnancy.

Male sterilisation by vasectomy

A small incision is made on both sides of the scrotum, each vas deferens having its cut ends sutured (see Fig. 17.4).

Contraception must be used until two sperm counts have been negative; a sample of semen is usually examined at 3 and 4 months postoperatively. Frequent ejaculation may expel spermatozoa proximal to the occlusion more rapidly.

The man usually undergoes the operation under local anaesthetic as an outpatient.

Haematoma and infection are the commonest complications but continuous local support for 2 weeks will reduce bruising.

After vasectomy the spermatozoa produced are destroyed by phagocytosis and although some men produce antibodies these do not appear to be detrimental to health. They may however lead to persistent infertility following vasectomy reversal. Thus although the operation is easier to reverse than female sterilisation, the subsequent pregnancy rates are lower. The volume of ejaculate is not reduced and this may be important for morale.

Work is progressing on injecting the vasa with a synthetic polymer which then solidifies. This plug can subsequently be removed if desired.

Failure rate: 0–0.2 per HWY.

POSSIBLE FUTURE DEVELOPMENTS

The search for a *male pill* is proving difficult as diminished libido often accompanies any reduction in testicular activity. As mature spermatozoa take 3 months to be produced it takes a long time for any treatment to cause azoospermia and equally long for fertility to return. Gossypol (an extract from cotton-seed oil) upsets potassium balance and sometimes permanently impairs fertility.

It has been found that if the *combined pill* is inserted into the vagina, rather than taken orally, absorption may be satisfactory and medical complications fewer. Progestogen vaginal rings are, however, better.

A nasal spray of *gonadotrophin-releasing hormone* (GnRH), which is not a steroid, appears to block natural secretion of GnRH so that ovulation does not take place. Dosage is critical as oestrogen suppression can result in menopausal symptoms.

Immunising men and women against spermatozoa or follicle-stimulating hormone, or women against the outer covering of the oocyte or so that they will reject a pregnancy, are methods which are being researched.

Acknowledgements
The author wishes to acknowledge the help of the following in the writing of this chapter: Dr E. Cooper; Mr J. Guillebaud and the staff of the Margaret Pyke Centre; and Dr E. Clubb.

Reader Activities

- It may be useful to role play the following and then to discuss the feelings elicited from those playing the various roles (it is important to be very careful to leave the role behind once you have finished):
  — you have been asked by a couple for preconception advice (cover family planning in particular)
  — you have been asked by an antenatal woman for advice concerning intercourse during pregnancy
  — you have been asked for family planning advice by a recently-delivered woman.
- Find out from an experienced midwife how she discusses with a mother the subject of the resumption of sexual intercourse. Ask how she broaches the subject before the mother is transferred home and the information she gives.

USEFUL ADDRESSES

International Planned Parenthood Federation
Regent's College
Regent's Park
London

Family Planning Information Services
27–35 Mortimer Street
London W1N 7RJ

REFERENCES

Bounds W, Guillebaud J 1984 Randomised comparison of the use-effectiveness and patient acceptability of the Collatex (Today™) contraceptive sponge and the diaphragm. British Journal of Family Planning 10: 69–75

Fleissig A 1991 Unintended pregnancies and the use of contraception: changes from 1984 to 1989. British Medical Journal 302: 147

Guillebaud J 1989 Contraception and sterilisation. In: Turnbull A, Chamberlain G (eds) Obstetrics. Churchill Livingstone, Edinburgh, ch 79: 1135–1152

Howie P W, McNeilly A S, Houston M J, Cook A, Boyle H 1982 Fertility after childbirth: post-partum ovulation and menstruation in bottle and breast feeding mothers. Clinical Endocrinology 17: 323–332

Laryea M G G 1980 The midwife's role in the postnatal care of primiparae and their infants in the first 28 days following childbirth. Unpublished M.Phil thesis for Newcastle upon Tyne Polytechnic

McNeilly A S, Glasier A F, Howie P W, Houston M J, Cook A, Boyle H 1983 Fertility after childbirth: pregnancy associated with breast feeding. Clinical Endocrinology 18: 167–173

Sleep J, Grant A, Garcia J, Elbourne D, Spencer J, Chalmers I 1984 West Berkshire perineal management trial. British Medical Journal 289: 587–590

FURTHER READING

Bromwich P, Parsons T 1990 Contraception — the facts, 2nd edn. Oxford University Press, Oxford

Clubb E, Knight J 1987 Fertility: a comprehensive guide to natural family planning. David & Charles, Newton Abbott

Family Planning Association 1992 Contraceptive handbook. FPA, London

Family Planning Information Services fact sheets and information leaflets; send SAE to F.P.I.S., 27–35 Mortimer Street, London W1N 7RJ

Guillebaud J 1989 Contraception — your questions answered. Revised reprint. Churchill Livingstone, Edinburgh

Loudon N (ed) 1991 Handbook of family planning, 2nd edn. Churchill Livingstone, Edinburgh

Phillips A, Rakusen J (eds) 1989 The new our bodies ourselves: a health book by and for women. Penguin, London

VIDEO

Clubb E, Knight J 1989 Fertility — a guide to natural family planning. Available from Dept of medical illustration, John Radcliffe Hospital, Oxford OX3 9DU

6

Abnormalities of Pregnancy, Labour and the Puerperium

Abnormalities of early pregnancy

SARAH KELLY

BLEEDING IN PREGNANCY

The midwife's role

Vaginal bleeding in pregnancy is a cause for concern to most mothers, particularly any mother who has had a previous experience of vaginal bleeding which resulted in fetal loss. Any mother who has had an unsuccessful outcome to pregnancy, for whatever reason, is likely to enter any subsequent pregnancy with some degree of anxiety which will be compounded if vaginal bleeding occurs. The midwife must be aware of the mother's emotional situation when caring for her during the antepartum period. Whatever the mother's age and parity, the successful outcome to pregnancy is a live, healthy baby. When the midwife takes the initial health history she must ensure that the mother is aware of the need to report any blood loss per vaginam either to her midwife or to her doctor as timely intervention may save the pregnancy.

It is not unusual for some mothers to have an episode of vaginal bleeding which is a past event by the time she presents for pregnancy diagnosis and health history. This should be recorded by the midwife in the mother's notes as the episode may recur.

Vaginal bleeding occurs in 16% of all pregnant women during the first trimester, which is the period extending from conception to 12 weeks.

The exact aetiology of bleeding in early pregnancy is not always known but there are identifiable reasons in most instances. Any episode of vaginal bleeding, however slight, could place the mother and baby at high risk and ideally all mothers who bleed from the genital tract should be referred to the care of a consultant obstetrician.

Assessing the mother's condition

The midwife must view seriously any report of vaginal bleeding by the mother. With the mother's help the midwife should establish the gestation, when the episode occurred and identify, if possible, whether the commencement of bleeding was associated with any particular activity.

A history of recent illness or episodes of headaches, nausea or vomiting may assist in making a differential diagnosis regarding the cause of the bleeding.

An attempt should be made to quantify the amount of blood lost and whether it is red or dark brown in colour. It is also important to enquire of the mother whether she is experiencing any pain, its locality and whether it is intermittent or continuous in nature.

The midwife needs to assess the general appearance of the mother. She notes her colour and whether the skin is dry, suggesting dehydration, or moist, which in conjunction with other signs may denote shock.

Respirations should be observed and the temperature and pulse should be taken.

Assessing the fetal condition

Assessment of the fetal condition will depend upon the gestational age. As early as the sixth week of gestation the embryonic sac can be identified by ultrasound and crown–rump length can be measured; heart movements can be seen by the seventh week of pregnancy. Now that ultrasound is widely used in antenatal clinics, a mother may have seen her baby long before she experiences other signs that he is alive. In the second trimester the fetal heart sounds may be elicited using a Sonicaid or a cardiotocograph machine. The presence of fetal heart sounds will be very comforting to the mother.

It may be possible to obtain a history of the presence or cessation of fetal movements if the duration of pregnancy is beyond the 16th week.

All observations of the mother and fetus should be carefully recorded. An accurate history and examination will enable the midwife to give the doctor a concise appraisal of the maternal and fetal conditions so that swift and appropriate action can be instituted. In community practice it may be necessary for the midwife to call to her assistance the emergency obstetric team when bleeding is excessive, so that resuscitation can begin prior to the mother's admission to hospital.

Any further assessments, investigations and plan of care become the responsibility of a registered medical practitioner.

Aims of care

The general aims of care are to establish the cause of the bleeding, to preserve the life of the mother and maintain the life of the baby where possible.

The role of the midwife in caring for a woman with vaginal bleeding is to assess the maternal and fetal conditions, to provide emotional support for the mother and family and to carry out treatment prescribed by a medical practitioner relative to the mother's situation.

Mothers with Rhesus negative blood may develop Rhesus antibodies following placental-site bleeding with a leak of fetal cells into the maternal circulation. A Kleihauer test should be performed and anti-D immunoglobin administered as necessary (see Ch. 34).

MISCELLANEOUS CAUSES OF VAGINAL BLEEDING

Implantation bleeding

This occurs about the 7th day after fertilisation, when the syncytial layer of the primary trophoblast, which has invasive properties, erodes

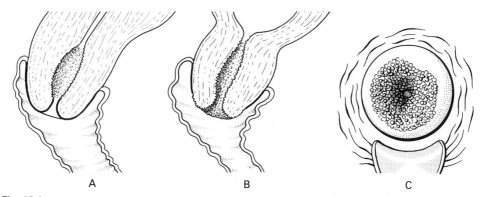

Fig. 18.1
(A) Nulliparous cervix. (B) Pregnant cervix with eversion of the columnar epithelium. (C) Eversion as seen on speculum examination.

the uterine epithelium, stroma and blood vessels to form a ragged implantation cavity. It is sometimes referred to as implantation haemorrhage and may be difficult to distinguish from a threatened abortion, although the former is usually slight in amount and the colour bright red. The bleeding settles quickly within 3–4 days when the blastocyst is completely embedded and covered by endometrial (decidual) cells.

The mother may confuse this type of bleeding with a menstrual period and think nothing of it until she is aware of other bodily changes suggestive of pregnancy. This episode of bleeding can ultimately lead to some confusion regarding the period of gestation as the mother may date her pregnancy from the missed period following this episode.

Confirming gestation later by ultrasonic scan easily remedies any uncertainty.

Cervical lesions

Eversion

Eversion occurs when the endocervical columnar epithelium pouts through the external cervical os. This is due to increased levels of oestrogen and progesterone which produce swelling and softening of the cervical tissues.

The columnar epithelium proliferates more rapidly than the squamous epithelium which results in ectopy. This condition is commonly called an erosion. As columnar epithelium secretes mucin, the pregnant woman may present with a history of profuse vaginal discharge. This may be

bloodstained due to rupture of the capillaries of the endocervical epithelium. Bleeding frequently occurs following sexual intercourse.

There may also be a history of low backache, dysmenorrhoea, menorrhagia and dyspareunia. The condition is unpleasant for the mother who may be reluctant to divulge her situation unless directly questioned in respect of vaginal bleeding and discharge. Cervical ectopy is not uncommon in women, and can be remedied by cauterisation postnatally using diathermy or cryosurgery.

Although complications of cervical diathermy are rare, they include cervical stricture, haemorrhage and infertility arising from destruction of the mucus-producing glands. Infection is also a risk and should be treated in order to bring relief to the mother.

Polyps

Polyps are small, bright red, fleshy, pedunculated, benign growths which may cause bleeding. Usually originating in the cervical canal they often accompany eversion. They are removed by torsion and sent for microscopic examination. Polyps and erosions are diagnosed on speculum examination often during the initial examination made by the doctor when assessing the woman's health in the early weeks of pregnancy or as part of the investigation for a local cause of vaginal bleeding.

Physiologically the blood supply to the cervical area increases during pregnancy which is why polyps tend to bleed at this time but they may already have been present for some while.

Carcinoma of the cervix

Cervical cytology performed routinely in the antenatal period has demonstrated that approximately 1 in 200 mothers have abnormal cell changes. When cervical intra-epithelial neoplasia (CIN) is suspected, a repeat papanicolau smear is indicated followed by colposcopic assessment. This procedure must be undertaken by a medical practitioner experienced in carrying out colposcopic examinations. The examination will identify the extent of the lesion. If the lesion is limited, no treatment is indicated other than careful observation. When the lesion is found to be invasive the mother will need to be admitted for wedge or cone biopsy under general anaesthesia. Bleeding may be excessive due to the increased vascularity in pregnancy and suturing may be required. Haemorrhage may be delayed and careful postoperative observation is essential. Biopsy carried out in the first trimester does not necessarily precipitate abortion, whereas the incidence of abortion following mid-trimester cone biopsy is substantial and cervical cerclage is advisable.

The pregnancy usually continues and vaginal delivery at term is the norm. The mother is examined again 3 months after delivery when the cervical oedema occasioned by childbirth has subsided.

Carcinoma of the cervix occurs in approximately 1 in 5000 women of childbearing years and it is a serious complication of pregnancy.

There is no evidence to suggest that cervical tumours become more rapidly invasive during pregnancy therefore treatment is prescribed on an individual basis in consultation with the mother and her partner. They face the appalling dilemma of opting to terminate pregnancy and possibly losing a healthy baby or of allowing a pregnancy to continue with the risk of shortening the mother's life.

Any decisions made are influenced by the degree of invasion and the duration of the pregnancy at the time of diagnosis. With the aid of ultrasonic scans the extent of the growth may be identified and the development of the baby assessed. Continuation of the pregnancy will culminate in caesarean section followed by radical hysterectomy and excision of pelvic lymph nodes. This is usually followed by irradiation of the surrounding viscera.

Blood transfusion will be required to replace the increased loss from the vascular genital tract and to counteract shock due to major surgery. The mother will require high-dependency physical care and the whole family will need empathy, support and information in order to cope with this traumatic situation. The delivery of a stillborn, preterm or sick baby will be an added stress at this time.

ABORTION

Abortion can be defined as the death or expulsion of the fetus either spontaneously or by induction, before the 24th week of pregnancy. This was changed under the Still-Birth (Definition) Act 1992 which brought the definition of stillbirth down to 24 weeks. The prognosis for survival of very small infants has so greatly improved that it had become incongruous to continue to include babies of between 24 and 28 weeks' gestation as 'abortions'.

Between 10 and 15% of all pregnancies terminate as spontaneous abortions, and a further 10–60% are terminated by an induced (either legal or criminal) abortion (Llewellyn-Jones 1990).

The majority of spontaneous abortions occur between the 8th and 12th weeks of pregnancy when the level of progesterone secreted by the corpus luteum falls and the placental hormone has not reached a sufficiently high level to sustain the conceptus.

Fetal causes

Chromosomal abnormality or disease of the fertilised ovum may account for 60% of spontaneous, first trimester abortions. Malformation of the trophoblast and poor implantation of the blastocyst may result in placental separation with consequent hypoxia and impaired embryonic development.

Maternal causes

General conditions

Diseases acquired during pregnancy such as rubella or influenza, especially if they are accompanied by acute fever, interfere with transplacental oxygenation and may precipitate abortion. Chronic disorders, for example renal disease accompanied by hypertension, may have a similar effect.

Drugs. Large doses of any drug are poisonous and should be avoided; anaesthetic gases and medication prescribed for malignancy and diseases of the immune system result in an increased incidence of abortion. Women who are or are intending to become pregnant should not be employed in industries where toxic substances are utilised or manufactured: some would extend this to intending fathers. The midwife will need to obtain employment information within the context of the social history. It is advisable to assess the blood concentration of toxic substances when pregnancy has occurred.

ABO incompatibility between mother and embryo may result in abortion.

Psychological factors such as stress and anxiety can adversely affect the functioning of the hypothalamic region of the brain and the pituitary gland. Alteration in the level of pituitary hormones affects uterine activity and may lead to abortion. It is important for the midwife to assess the mother's emotional state on every encounter and to be aware of any changes in the mother's life which may occasion stress. Recording of such information is an important element in the management of the pregnancy.

Local disorders of the genital tract

A retroverted uterus which is unable to rise out of the pelvis may occasionally predispose to abortion. Early diagnosis of retroversion by pelvic examination or ultrasonic scan allows for correction of this anomaly.

Developmental defects such as bicornuate uterus and myomas which distort the uterine cavity and inhibit uterine enlargement may cause midtrimester abortion.

Cervical incompetence may be present due to congenital weakness, trauma resulting from previous dilatation and curettage or lacerations sustained during past childbearing. As the pregnancy progresses and intra-uterine pressure increases, cervical dilatation occurs resulting in abortion. An accurate surgical and obstetric history may indicate a pregnancy at risk from possible cervical incompetence.

Approximately 20% of mothers who have a history of recurrent abortion are found to have an incompetent cervix although this may be an overestimate (Grant 1989). This is usually diagnosed by direct examination early in pregnancy or by serial ultrasonic scanning when a gradual painless dilatation of the cervix is detected. The usual treatment for this is cervical cerclage provided that the membranes are intact.

Cervical cerclage. A purse-string suture of strong non-absorbable material is inserted beneath the cervicovaginal mucosa to encircle the cervix at the level of the internal os and then tied. This is sometimes called a Shirodkar suture. Following the procedure the mother needs to rest in bed for 3–5 days. Occasionally uterine activity is stimulated and abortion may become inevitable in which case the suture must be removed. If no adverse sequelae occur the mother can go home, although adequate rest throughout the remainder of the pregnancy is essential.

Midwives should be aware that the cervical suture must be removed between the 38th and 39th week of pregnancy or sooner if the woman goes into premature labour, otherwise severe damage will be inflicted on the dilating cervix.

Types of abortion

Spontaneous abortion

Signs and symptoms. Many mothers will speak of a period of uneasiness prior to the onset of specific signs and symptoms.

Vaginal bleeding is generally the earliest sign of an impending abortion. The bleeding may consist of a bloodstained discharge, brown spotting or a bright red loss which may be variable in amount.

Pain is usually felt in a central position, low in the abdomen, and is intermittent in character due to uterine contractions. This may be accompanied by backache.

Dilatation of the cervix is present when an abortion becomes inevitable.

Missed abortion

This is the term applied to the fetus which has died and is retained with its placenta in the uterus. Early ultrasonic scan may identify missed abortion before the mother experiences any symptoms. Pain and bleeding may cease but the mother may experience a residual brown vaginal discharge. This has been described by some women as having an odour of decaying matter and it can be offensive and distressing. All other physiological signs of pregnancy will regress, uterine enlargement will cease and a pregnancy test will prove negative. Some obstetricians prefer not to treat a missed abortion actively as the dead conceptus will be expelled eventually. This decision can aggravate the mother's distress. Alternatively prostaglandin E_2 may be given to induce expulsion in conjunction with i.v. oxytocin or a vacuum aspiration of the uterine contents may be performed.

Blood coagulation disorders may develop in cases of missed abortion which persist for over 6–8 weeks. It is advisable that plasma fibrinogen estimations be made at weekly intervals and that fresh compatible blood is available if several weeks have elapsed between death and expulsion of the conceptus.

Blood mole

Occasionally a missed abortion will progress to form a blood mole. This is a smooth brownish-red mass which is completely surrounded by the capsular decidua. Within the capsular decidua

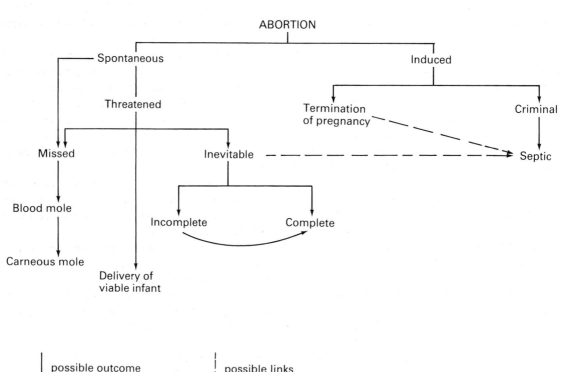

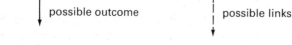

Fig. 18.2
Classification of abortion.

the fetus and placenta are surrounded by clotted blood. The mole usually forms before the 12th week and if it is retained in utero for a period of months, the fluid is extracted from the blood and the fleshy, firm, hard mass remaining is known as a *carneous mole*. On histological examination following expulsion the embryo may be found in the centre of the mass.

Treatment. Prostaglandin E_2 pessaries will be inserted into the vagina to soften the collagen fibres of the cervix and aid dilatation. This will be followed by an intravenous oxytocin infusion administered via a calibrated pump. The dosage is adjusted according to uterine activity.

Analgesia will be required to relieve the pain of induced contractions and the mother will require close observation throughout the whole procedure.

Threatened abortion

It is presumed that a pregnancy is threatening to abort when vaginal bleeding occurs before the 24th week. The bleeding is not usually severe and when a gentle speculum examination is performed after the cessation of bleeding the cervical os is found to be closed. Backache may be present and occasionally lower abdominal pain but the membranes remain intact.

Treatment of threatened abortion. The mother will be extremely agitated at the possibility of losing her baby and understanding, empathy and tranquil surroundings will help her to relax as much as possible. It is essential that the mother is encouraged to rest in bed with the minimum of disturbance. A mild sedative may be prescribed to aid relaxation and analgesia may be given for pain.

All loss per vaginam should be observed and recorded.

Vulval swabbing should be performed at least twice daily while the discharge persists in order to minimise discomfort.

Temperature and pulse should be taken twice daily or 4-hourly if a pyrexia is present. Between 24 and 48 hours after the bleeding a speculum examination is performed to exclude local lesions and to note the state of the cervical os.

48 hours after the bleeding ceases the mother can commence gentle ambulation and, if in

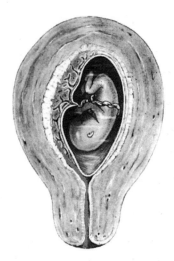

Fig. 18.3
Threatened abortion: slight placental separation, slight bleeding, membranes intact, os closed.

hospital, she may return home. If the mother is working she may be advised to stop work and to rest as much as possible. Should the bleeding recur, the woman should go to bed and contact her midwife or doctor.

Subsequent pregnancy care includes advice regarding a high fibre diet to prevent constipation and specific tests for placental function later in pregnancy. Abdominal examinations will determine uterine growth rate and the onset and degree of fetal movement should be noted. Serial scans to observe fetal growth and development are usually prescribed.

The presence of a threatened abortion places both mother and baby in a high-risk category. Subsequent care is usually carried out by the obstetrician and his team.

70–80% of all mothers diagnosed as having a threatened abortion in the first trimester will continue with their pregnancies to term.

If the contractions fail to subside and if the bleeding becomes bright red and increases in amount abortion is usually *inevitable*.

Inevitable abortion

This term is applied when it is impossible for the pregnancy to continue. Vaginal bleeding is free which suggests that a large section of the placenta has separated from the uterine wall.

The abdominal pain becomes more acute and rhythmic in character. The membranes may have ruptured and amniotic fluid will be seen. Alternatively the fetal sac and its contents, and possibly the placenta, will protrude through the dilating cervical os. The mother will become extremely distressed with the pain and the knowledge that she is about to lose her baby.

The midwife should continue to care for the mother by offering emotional support and maintaining observations. The pain of the contractions is equal to that of labour and adequate pain relief is essential.

Bleeding and uterine contractions will continue and all or part of the conceptus will be expelled vaginally.

Complete abortion

A complete abortion is more likely to occur prior to the 8th week of pregnancy and constitutes the expulsion of the embryo, placenta and intact membranes.

An ultrasonic scan can confirm that the uterus is empty of any placental tissue and avert a general anaesthetic and surgical procedure.

Incomplete abortion

This usually occurs in the second trimester. The fetus is expelled from the uterus but all or part of

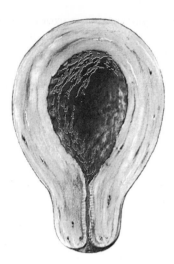

Fig. 18.5
Complete abortion: fetus and placenta expelled, bleeding scanty, os closed.

the placenta is retained. Bleeding is profuse but the abdominal pain and backache may cease. The cervix will be soft and purplish in colour and will be partly closed.

Placental tissue must be removed otherwise the bleeding will continue and the uterus will remain bulky.

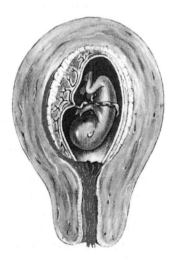

Fig. 18.4
Inevitable abortion: placental separation, moderate bleeding, membranes ruptured, os dilated.

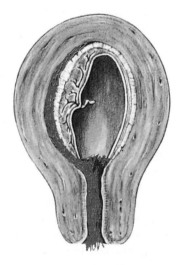

Fig. 18.6
Incomplete abortion: fetus expelled, placenta partially separated, free bleeding, os dilated.

The fetus and blood-soaked garments and pads should be kept for inspection so that the amount of blood to be replaced can be estimated.

Treatment. Once diagnosis is confirmed the midwife should carry out the treatment prescribed by the medical practitioner. She should make herself available to listen to the fears and anxieties of the mother which will aid her through her grief.

Specific treatment prior to the 12th week will include the administration of ergometrine 500 mcg (0.5 mg) i.m. to expel the uterine contents and reduce bleeding from the placental site, followed by evacuation of any tissue retained. The latter procedure is carried out under general anaesthesia and midwives should remain aware of anaesthetic complications such as Mendelson's syndrome. After the 12th week an oxytocin infusion will be administered using a pump.

A dose of ergometrine will be given on completion of surgery but if this is within 30 minutes of any previous dose the mother may vomit. This is due to the action of ergometrine upon the plain muscle fibres of the stomach. Suction apparatus to clear the airway should be readily available if the mother is still unconscious.

Uterine aspiration is commonly used but where this is not available the uterus will be evacuated digitally or by dilatation and curettage.

Digital evacuation. The equipment required for this procedure is as for a vaginal examination in labour.

The vulva is cleansed; antiseptic cream is applied to the gloved right hand. The left hand is placed upon the abdomen and the uterus is anteverted and pressed downward. Simultaneously the index finger of the right hand is inserted into the vagina and through the cervical os: the placenta and other tissue is removed.

If severe haemorrhage occurs and medical assistance is not available, the midwife may need to perform digital evacuation of the uterus.

Dilatation and curettage. This is a potentially hazardous procedure as the uterine texture softens during pregnancy. Following expulsion of the fetus the uterus remains bulky due to retained placental tissue and the muscular tone of the uterine body and cervix is poor. The procedure calls for gentle and gradual dilatation of the cervix to prevent splitting of the tissues. It is important that the length of the uterine cavity is determined before the ovum forceps or curette are inserted so that uterine perforation does not occur. Damage sustained at this time could require major surgery. Cervical incompetence which predisposes to recurrent abortion and pelvic inflammatory disease with infertility are possible sequelae.

Prior to the procedure a full blood count is performed and at least 2 units of blood should be cross-matched. An intravenous infusion is always commenced before admission to the operating theatre.

Recurrent abortion (habitual)

This term is applied when a mother has had at least two consecutive spontaneous abortions. The risk of further abortion increases with each successive aborted pregnancy.

The majority of mothers who encounter this problem will lose their babies in the early weeks or pregnancy. If a pregnancy continues following a mid-trimester threatened abortion there is a greater risk of preterm labour. The midwife should let parents know of this possibility so that their future plans may be made realistically.

Women who suffer recurrent abortion will require future pre-pregnancy counselling (see Ch. 7).

Induced abortion

Termination of pregnancy

In the United Kingdom, legal termination of pregnancy is a therapeutic procedure carried out under the terms of the 1967 Abortion Act. It is important to provide adequate counselling and support prior to and following the operation. Many mothers do not make the decision to have a pregnancy terminated without some inner conflict. There are religious, psychological, social and cultural factors which affect the woman's decision. Important considerations are her economic and marital status, the health and well-being of existing children in the family and the presence of an abnormal fetus. Some mothers will consult their general practitioners having clearly thought through their reasons for wishing to have a pregnancy terminated. Others may require to be taken through a process of careful counselling before they can make an appropriate decision. A few may be advised on health grounds to discontinue the pregnancy.

The 1967 Abortion Act made the following provisions: Two registered medical practitioners should be of the opinion that the pregnancy should be terminated if:

- the continuance of the pregnancy would involve a risk to the life of the pregnant woman or of injury to her physical or mental health
- the continuance of the pregnancy would be detrimental to the health and well-being of the existing children in the family
- there is a substantial risk that the child when born would suffer from such physical or mental abnormalities as to be seriously handicapped.

The termination must be reported to the Chief Medical Officer, Department of Health (Eng.) or the Home and Health Department (Scot.). Therapeutic abortions may be carried out in National Health Service hospitals or registered private hospitals and nursing homes.

Before the 12th week of pregnancy vacuum aspiration is the chosen method of terminating a pregnancy as there is less blood loss. Alternatively dilatation and curettage may be performed. Pelvic infection is a common complication of abortion by curettage and selective prophylactic administration of antibiotics may be used in some units although this is a controversial issue.

After the 12th week a prostaglandin preparation will be used either intra- or extra-amniotically to produce abortion within 48 hours. Prostaglandin may cause nausea, vomiting and diarrhoea. Therapeutic abortion is a painful procedure and adequate pain relief is essential.

If pregnancy must be terminated after 20 weeks for reason of serious maternal illness, hysterotomy is the method of choice. After 24 weeks the baby may be able to survive with intensive neonatal care.

All terminations performed after 8 weeks' gestation should be carried out in hospital where resuscitation facilities are available. In all instances ergometrine or Syntometrine will be administered intravenously to prevent haemorrhage.

Any midwife involved with caring for mothers postoperatively must make careful observations and record and report any abnormality of the lochia, temperature, pulse, blood pressure or urine output.

Many mothers experience feelings of guilt or regret following termination and this may be manifest in sleep disturbance and marital disharmony. Occasionally severe depression, mania and psychosis occur. There may be signs of anguish and disturbance in the early postoperative period and these too should be reported, although it is usually the general practitioner and community services who will encounter such sequelae.

Attention has been drawn to the need for post-termination care as for any postnatal mother but no conclusive decision has been made.

Criminal abortion

A criminal abortion is one performed in contravention of the 1967 Abortion Act. Such procedures are illegal and are punishable by imprisonment.

The abortion is attempted by an unqualified, inexpert person. The operation has often been hurried and lacking in asepsis; consequently placental tissue is left inside the uterus resulting in haemorrhage.

Injuries to the birth canal and pelvic organs can occur if implements are inserted. The insertion into the uterus of abortifacients such as soap solutions or pastes may result in sudden death from air embolism or shock. Haemolysis and renal damage may also occur.

A midwife should not give advice or information which could result in illegal abortion; neither should she assist anyone to perform an illegal abortion.

It is usually the subsequent bleeding which causes a mother to seek professional help and care should be given as for a threatened abortion until medical assistance arrives. The mother will be nervous because of the action which she has taken and may fear for her life. The woman must be accepted without criticism and her physical needs attended to.

While she needs reassurance, counselling in depth should be delayed until the mother is well.

Septic abortion

Infection may occur following any abortion.

It may be associated with incomplete abortion but is more commonly found after an induced abortion. In countries where legislation permits termination of pregnancy, septic abortion has become rarer but has not been eradicated. Good aseptic techniques are essential for all procedures which require intra-uterine exploration.

The infection may be limited to the decidual lining of the uterus but virulent organisms may cause the infection to spread and involve the myometrium, fallopian tubes and pelvic organs.

Symptoms and signs. The mother will complain of feeling unwell and may have a headache and nausea accompanied by sweating and shivering.

On examination she will look flushed, her skin will be hot to the touch and it may be clammy. There will be a spiking pyrexia in excess of 38°C and a steadily rising pulse, both of which will worsen if the infection becomes extensive. After the 12th week of pregnancy abdominal examination will identify tenderness of the uterus which will be bulky and soft in texture. The vaginal discharge will have an offensive odour and may be pinkish in colour, but this may not be very marked if the infection has spread to the inner tissues. Specific investigations will include high vaginal and cervical swabs, full blood culture and haematological investigations.

Midwifery care is related to the mother's condition and may be of high or low dependency.

In all instances 4-hourly recording of the temperature, pulse and blood pressure will be necessary. Urinalysis will be carried out at least daily and urine output must be measured accurately. Isolation may be required which will have the advantage of giving the mother a tranquil, restful atmosphere.

Treatment. Amoxycillin 500 mg three times daily and metronidazole 200 mg 6-hourly is the treatment of choice until bacteriological results are obtained, after which the antibiotic treatment will be more appropriately prescribed.

Dilatation and curettage will be performed preferably after the acute infection subsides.

Bacteraemic shock (endotoxic or septic shock)
Despite the availability of good antimicrobial drugs, septicaemia still occurs and is a major cause of death associated with septic abortion. Fever is persistent, yet the extremities are cold and cyanosed. Rigors, nausea, vomiting and diarrhoea will be accompanied by oliguria and hypotension. Confusion will progress to delirium, coma and death if the condition remains untreated. Disseminated intravascular coagulation may also develop resulting in persistent bleeding from the uterus and venepuncture sites. Bacteraemic shock may occur postnatally in cases of puerperal sepsis.

Treatment. The aims of the treatment are to cure the infection and to restore the blood volume, the haematological status and the electrolyte concentrations to normal.

Whenever a mother develops a pyrexia following abortion or childbirth, diligent observations by the midwife may help to diagnose infection and prevent bacteraemic shock.

ECTOPIC PREGNANCY

If the fertilised ovum embeds outside the uterus, the condition is known as an ectopic or extra-uterine pregnancy. Most commonly this occurs in the fallopian tube, but it may occasionally be abdominal or rarely ovarian. The incidence of ectopic pregnancy is 1 in 150 conceptions and this may be due to the prevalence of pelvic inflammatory disease as a result of early and indiscriminate sexual activity.

Tubal pregnancy

The main cause is damage and distortion of the fallopian tubes. Implantation can occur at any point along the fallopian tube.

Signs and symptoms. The mother will complain of mild lower abdominal discomfort

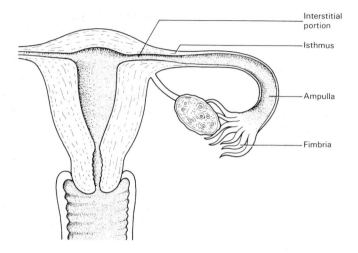

Fig. 18.7
Diagram showing the sites of implantation in tubal pregnancy.

with an occasional attack of sharp, stabbing pain accompanied by nausea. This may be sufficiently severe for the mother to seek medical advice. Unless it is established that the mother has experienced amenorrhoea, other conditions such as ovarian cysts, salpingitis, appendicitis or urinary tract infection may be suspected. Other physiological signs of pregnancy may not be present and the mother may have a slight brown vaginal discharge.

Ultrasonic scan may assist diagnosis. In many instances the mother may present with acute abdominal pain accompanied by shock, in which case urgent treatment is needed.

Outcomes of the pregnancy
The endometrium thickens and the uterus enlarges under the influence of hormones from the corpus luteum. The muscle layers of the fallopian tube also thicken and the ovarian, arcuate and uterine arteries and veins become more tortuous.

The trophoblast enlarges and erodes into the tissues of the fallopian tube causing repeated episodes of bleeding. The developing trophoblast may become separated from the wall of the tube by a layer of blood clot resulting in the development of a *tubal mole*. If this occurs near the distal end of the tube the mole may be extruded into

the peritoneal cavity resulting in a *tubal abortion* which will usually regress and be absorbed.

The closer to the uterus that the trophoblast embeds, the less room there will be for expansion. Eventually the tube ruptures. The ovarian artery and vein may be torn. Severe haemorrhage into the broad ligament or peritoneal cavity will cause sudden collapse of the mother.

In the case of a ruptured ectopic tubal pregnancy the mother will be transferred to hospital where resuscitation will commence prior to salpingectomy.

Abdominal pregnancy

Abdominal pregnancy is rare but it occurs when the placenta develops in the distal end of the tube or is attached to the ovary and abdominal organs or the outside of the uterus. The fetus usually dies and calcifies but a few abdominal pregnancies go to term.

If the pregnancy continues, ultrasonic scans provide a valuable diagnostic tool. On abdominal examination the irregular enlargement may be mistaken for large uterine fibroids but near term fetal movement is evident very close to the surface. Delivery is by laparotomy when the baby may be born alive but often has compression deformities. It is usual to leave the placenta in situ to avoid uncontrollable haemorrhage.

chorionic villi proliferate and become avascular. The villi are filled with fluid so that collectively they take on the appearance of a bunch of grapes. The choriodecidual spaces become obliterated and maternal blood cannot circulate. The absence of maternal blood and intervillous circulation gives the whole structure a creamy-white appearance. Oxygen and nutrition cannot reach the fetus which dies and becomes absorbed. The villi continue to multiply so that uterine enlargement occurs, usually out of proportion to the duration of the pregnancy.

In the developed countries of the Western world the incidence of vesicular mole is approximately 1 in 2000 pregnancies, but this does not imply that it is specific to any ethnic group. In England and Wales where cases of hydatidiform mole have to be registered annually, the incidence doubled between 1973 and 1983 to reach a level of 1.54 per 1000 live births. The mothers at greatest risk of developing vesicular mole are those under 15 and over 50 years of age. Women who have a hydatidiform mole may, if untreated, develop malignant choriocarcinoma and are regarded as being in a high-risk group.

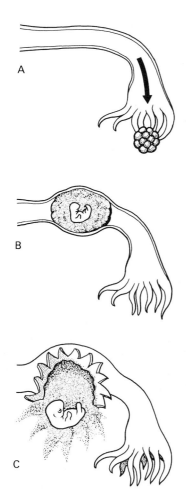

Fig. 18.8
Possible outcomes of a tubal pregnancy. (A) Tubal abortion. (B) Tubal mole. (C) Ruptured tubal pregnancy.

Ectopic pregnancy accounted for 11 maternal deaths in the triennium 1985–87 in the UK (DH et al 1991). The majority were due to tubal rupture but two were abdominal pregnancies. The most important feature was failure to diagnose the ectopic pregnancy.

VESICULAR (HYDATIDIFORM) MOLE

Hydatidiform mole is the term applied to a gross malformation of the trophoblast in which the

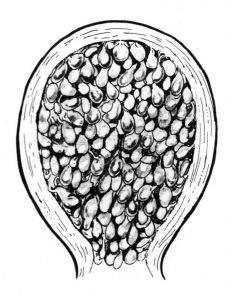

Fig. 18.9
Uterus with hydatidiform mole in situ.

Signs and symptoms

Clinically the first sign of hydatidiform mole is vaginal bleeding similar to that found in threatened abortion. The mother may have a history of nausea and vomiting which can become excessive and be accompanied by other symptoms of hyperemesis gravidarum. Alternatively signs and symptoms of pre-eclampsia may develop (see Ch. 20).

On examination the midwife may find that the uterine size far exceeds that expected for the period of gestation. Alternatively if the mole becomes detached from the uterine wall it may cease to grow and the uterus may be normal in size.

The midwife will not be able to palpate fetal parts nor hear the fetal heart and the mother will not have experienced fetal movements. In normal circumstances the level of human chorionic gonadotrophin falls after the 12th week of pregnancy. The large surface area of the vesicles causes the gonadotrophin level to continue to rise. There will be increased levels in the woman's urine and blood. Hydatidiform mole may be diagnosed earlier in pregnancy if ultrasonic scanning is available, although diagnosis is often not made until vesicles are passed per vaginam.

Treatment

The mother will be admitted to hospital and care will be as for threatened abortion until a conclusive diagnosis is made. The mole may be removed by vacuum aspiration or dilatation and curettage. An intravenous infusion of Syntocinon will be administered during, and for several hours after, the operative procedure in order to prevent sudden haemorrhage. Occasionally the mole will be removed by hysterotomy. In the older mother a hysterectomy will be performed with the mole in situ.

Trophoblastic tissue left inside the uterus may become highly malignant and form a *choriocarcinoma*.

Every mother who has had a vesicular mole will be screened postoperatively to identify the serum human chorionic gonadotrophin level. In the majority of mothers the gonadotrophin level does not return to normal until 8 weeks after surgery.

In the presence of choriocarcinoma the levels will rise. Tests are carried out every month for 1 year, then 3-monthly for the second year. If choriocarcinoma is suspected a dilatation and curettage will be performed and the curettings will be sent for histopathological examination. In most instances cytotoxic chemotherapy will eliminate the tumour but occasionally hysterectomy has to be performed in order to prevent death of the mother. It is important that the mother receives contraceptive counselling in order to prevent a pregnancy occurring for at least 2 years.

Midwives should note that hydatidiform mole may recur in subsequent pregnancies in a small proportion of mothers.

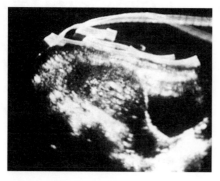 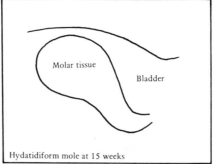

Hydatidiform mole at 15 weeks

Fig. 18.10
Ultrasonogram of hydatidiform mole: white speckled area indicates the mole.

Reader Activities

- Consider what supplementary questions you, as a midwife, would ask a woman whom you were booking at 10 weeks' gestation and who informs you that she had already had a loss of blood during this pregnancy.

- Similarly, what questions would you ask if a woman told you at booking that she had had three miscarriages in the past? What health education may be appropriate for this woman?

REFERENCES

Department of Health, Welsh Office, Scottish Home and Health Department and Department of Health and Social Services, Northern Ireland 1991 Report on confidential enquiries into maternal deaths in the United Kingdom 1985–87. HMSO, London

Grant A 1989 Cervical cerclage to prolong pregnancy. In: Chalmers I, Enkin M, Keirse M J N C Effective care in pregnancy and childbirth. Oxford University Press, Oxford, p 633–646

Llewellyn-Jones D 1990 Fundamentals of obstetrics and gynaecology. Vol 1 Obstetrics, 4th edn. Faber & Faber, London

FURTHER READING

Atkinson D 1987 Life and death: moral choices at the beginning and end of life. Oxford University Press, Oxford

Bagshawe K D, Dent J, Webb J 1986 Hydatidiform mole in England and Wales 1973–1983. Lancet i: 637–677

Bigrigg A, Bourne T, Read M D 1990 A comparison of the efficacy of gameprost vaginal pessaries and extra-amniotic prostaglandin E_2 gel in the induction of middle trimester abortion. Journal of Obstetrics and Gynaecology 10: 304–305

Farrer H 1987 Gynaecological care, 2nd edn. Churchill Livingstone, Edinburgh

Frater A, Wright C 1986 Coping with abortion W R Chambers, Edinburgh

Gibbons M 1984 Psychiatric sequelae of induced abortion. Journal of the Royal College of General Practitioners 34: 146–150

Guillebaud J 1990 Medical termination of pregnancy combined with prostaglandin RU486 is effective. British Medical Journal 301: 18–25

Kenney A 1985 Cancer of the cervix in young women. In: Studd J (ed) Progress in obstetrics and gynaecology, vol 5. Churchill Livingstone, Edinburgh

Lee R, Morgan D 1989 Birthrights: law and ethics at the beginnings of life. Routledge, London

Levallois P, Rioux J E 1988 Prophylactic antibiotics for suction curettage abortion: results of a clinical controlled trial. American Journal of Obstetrics and Gynecology 158(1): 101–105

Panting G 1990 The Abortion Act 1967. Update (June): 1192–1197

Pipes M 1986 Understanding abortion. The Women's Press, London

Sutton A 1990 Arguments for abortion of abnormal fetuses and the moral status of the developing embryo. Ethics and Medicine 6(1)

Urquhart D R et al 1990 The efficacy and tolerance of mifepristone and prostaglandin in first trimester termination of pregnancy: UK multicentre trial. British Journal of Obstetrics and Gynaecology 97: 480–486

Ylikorkala O et al 1989 Outpatient therapeutic abortion with mifepristone. Journal of Obstetrics and Gynaecology 74(4)

Genital and sexually transmissible infections in pregnancy

CAROLYN ROTH

The relevance of sexually transmissible infection for women of childbearing age

Local infection of the vagina and vulva

Bacterial infections

Viral infections

The range of sexually transmitted diseases (STDs) and genital infections, their social and health consequences and their significance during pregnancy are areas of growing importance and understanding.

This chapter reviews issues relating to a number of infections that are important in relation to pregnancy. The title highlights the facts that:

- not all genital infections are sexually acquired
- infections acquired by other means may also be sexually transmitted
- many sexually transmissible infections do not produce genital symptoms or disease.

Since the focus of the chapter is pregnancy, other sources of information should be consulted for consideration of the broader issues involved in the presentation, diagnosis and treatment of genital and sexually transmissible infection such as that offered by Adler (1990).

The initial sections of the chapter consider the general significance to midwives of this group of infections in pregnancy. This is followed by a consideration of those infections which give rise to local symptoms in the vagina and vulva. Finally, other infections, some of which have a more generalised impact on the pregnant woman and newborn baby are discussed, including infection with human immunodeficiency virus (HIV).

Referral of a woman to a clinic for genito-urinary medicine (GUM) which specialises in the diagnosis and treatment of many of the infections discussed here will often be most appropriate. Clinics have at their disposal a range of diagnostic facilities as well as personnel who are familiar with relevant social, psychological and physical issues and can offer counselling and facilitate contact tracing when required. Midwives should familiarise themselves with local provision so that liaison and referral between the two services are facilitated.

The range of genital and sexually transmissible infections

A variety of organisms are capable of being transmitted sexually; in the case of some, for example group B streptococcus (GBS) and *Candida albicans*, sexual transmission is an incidental feature, whereas in the case of others, such as *Neisseria gonorrhoeae* and *Treponema pallidum*, sexual contact is the primary mode of transmission. There are other organisms, such as human immunodeficiency virus (HIV) and hepatitis B virus (HBV), whose presence in blood and other body fluids, including semen and cervical secretions, facilitates their spread by sexual contact.

THE RELEVANCE OF SEXUALLY TRANSMISSIBLE INFECTION FOR WOMEN OF CHILDBEARING AGE

- A number of sexually transmitted organisms (e.g. *N. gonorrhoeae* and *Chlamydia trachomatis*) cause salpingitis, which may lead to chronic pelvic inflammation and permanent damage to the fallopian tubes, resulting in reduced fertility and ectopic pregnancy.
- The mechanisms that enable the sexual spread of infection that is the presence of an organism within or around the genitalia, or its presence in the blood and sexual secretions, also facilitate vertical (perinatal) transmission of infection, from mother to fetus or newborn baby.
- Some perinatally acquired infections have serious and prolonged consequences for the fetus or neonate.
- Pregnancy may have an impact on the presentation and course of infection giving rise to

difficulties in diagnosis or management. Some infections, such as human papillomaviruses (HPV), become more virulent; some, such as GBS, are asymptomatic in the woman but may produce serious neonatal disease.
- Some infections, such as HIV and HBV, are incurable and have serious, lifelong implications for the health and infectivity status of those infected.
- The diagnosis of a sexually transmitted infection may have stressful or destructive consequences for the relationship between the woman and her partner, which may be particularly difficult to manage during pregnancy.
- Women may experience high levels of anxiety and guilt about the implications for their baby of a perinatally transmissible infection.

Educational issues

The advent of the HIV epidemic in the 1980s stimulated educational efforts to heighten awareness about sexually transmissible infection and the necessity for people to avoid this serious, incurable infection by changing their sexual behaviour and practising 'safer sex'. However, research carried out in late 1990 suggests that a significant proportion of people remain ignorant of the risks to women of contracting HIV infection (International Nursing Review 1991).

Suggestions on how to reduce the risk of contracting a sexually transmissible infection can be easily listed. These include using a condom during sexual intercourse, avoidance of multiple sexual partners and partners with other partners, avoidance of sexual contact with a partner experiencing symptoms of infection or genital lesions and avoidance of genital contact with oral 'cold sores'. Anyone at risk should have regular medical examinations (Adler 1990). Translation of these 'principles' into accessible and usable information both for pregnant women as a group and for individual women is a challenge for midwives. Barriers of language and social attitudes are two issues that need to be addressed in meeting the challenge successfully.

Social issues

For many women the balance of power in sexual

relationships is such that their capacity to insist on safer sexual practices may be limited. In addition, the condom, which is the most effective barrier method to protect from STDs, is a method under the control of the man, and in this respect, a woman's power to control her situation is constrained (Stein 1990). Female condoms, however, have now been introduced. Pregnancy, customarily, is a time during which use of barrier contraceptives has not been considered necessary, yet a woman's exposure to a sexually transmissible infection is as liable to occur during pregnancy as at other times of unprotected intercourse. Anatomical and immunological changes of pregnancy may increase susceptibility to some infections (Brunham et al 1990) and the consequences of sexually transmitted infection are liable to be greater during pregnancy than at other times: preterm delivery is associated with infection of the membranes and amniotic fluid and there is risk of fetal exposure and puerperal maternal illness.

Midwives should seek to maximise the opportunity for women to ask questions and express concerns about their sexual health. Women need access during pregnancy, as well as postnatally, to information and supplies of condoms.

A legacy of stigma, misinformation and guilt surrounding the issue of sexually transmissible infection has consequences for women seeking and receiving care in relation to this problem. A woman may be reluctant to report symptoms or exposure to infection because she fears judgemental attitudes from her caregivers or is worried about the risk of the confidence being disclosed to others. There is some evidence that women are less likely than men to report symptoms of genital infection (Harris 1975). Many women find a speculum examination of the vagina, especially when conducted by a man, a disturbing experience; midwives and doctors should be sensitive to this distress and provide care which is acceptable to the woman. Midwives may appropriately be taught to conduct such examinations.

When infection is diagnosed during pregnancy, midwives should use the opportunity to offer education and counselling which may enable the woman to prevent future infection. It is important that women receive a constructive response to their expression of feelings of guilt or fear. Midwives may need to spend some time considering their own attitudes around issues of sexuality, in addition to building up knowledge of sexually transmissible infection. Provision of appropriate information will also require understanding and sensitivity to the particular circumstances of a woman's life, her sense of self-esteem and her attitudes about her sexuality.

Confidentiality

Ensuring the security of information which women share with their caregivers and the results of investigations carried out is essential to creating an environment in which clients feel safe to seek advice about symptoms and to discuss their concerns, and this may be particularly true in the sensitive area of sexually transmissible infection.

It is important for midwives to address the general issue of how, where and whether sensitive information is to be documented in notes. It is inappropriate to document certain information in the notes that women carry, although there may be a need to share information with other caregivers, the GP for example. Women should be consulted about how information should be documented and should, where possible, be enabled to be responsible for relaying relevant information to other professionals involved in their care.

Protection of confidentiality and establishment of a sound relationship of trust between the pregnant woman and her caregiver is best facilitated by a system of continuity of care and carer. In such a scheme, information about a woman's health status is contained amongst the small number of people who are actually engaged in giving her care reducing the likelihood of an inadvertent breach of trust.

As a registered . . . midwife . . . you are personally accountable for your practice and, in the exercise of your professional accountability, must: . . .
10. protect all confidential information concerning patients and clients obtained in the course of professional practice and make disclosures only with consent . . . (United Kingdom Central Council, 1992).

Screening

Syphilis is the only sexually transmitted infection for which there is presently a policy of routine screening during pregnancy.

Other sexually transmissible infections do not lend themselves as easily to routine screening, since many require culture and analysis of the infecting organism rather than serological diagnosis and the tests are therefore more labour-intensive and costly to perform.

It may be that the simplicity of serological testing for syphilis and the rarity of a positive diagnosis have contributed to a fairly cavalier approach to the conduct of the test. The blood specimen is usually taken as one of several during the booking visit, often without adequate explanation of the test to be performed. The result, if negative, may be recorded without further discussion with the woman (personal observation). Clearly, these practices breach the principle of informed consent and are a poor basis for establishing an effective exchange of information between a woman and her attendants. Equally, an opportunity is lost of raising the awareness and knowledge of women about the risks and prevention of sexually transmissible infections.

Where screening is carried out, it is essential that midwives have sufficient knowledge of the condition, its significance for the woman and her baby, the treatment available should the diagnosis be positive, the time it will take for a diagnostic result to be available and other relevant details.

In addition, time must be available for sufficient discussion and to answer any questions which the woman might want to pose. An offer of screening should always be used to better inform women about their sexual health as well as to diagnose particular infection. (See below for discussion of HIV testing in pregnancy.)

LOCAL INFECTION OF THE VAGINA AND VULVA

The vagina, far from constituting a sterile environment, is host to a rich variety of micro-organisms. These are subject to dynamic alteration in quantity and composition, reflecting at any given time a woman's current physiological state, her immunological defence mechanisms and her past exposure. Transfer and sharing of micro-organisms between partners occurs during sexual intercourse, and may include the exchange of infective organisms.

There is, however, a distinction between the presence of an infective agent in the vagina and the existence of infection. Clinical disease may occur because of the introduction of organisms that are new to the woman or because of a redistribution of existing microbiological flora due, for example, to the physiological changes of pregnancy or the action of antibiotics. Changes may occur in a woman's susceptibility to, or the pathogenicity of, previously encountered organisms.

Fungal infections

The most common of these is *Candida albicans* (thrush), which accounts for the vast majority of fungal vulvovaginal infections, with a minority caused by organisms such as *Torulopsis glabrata* and *Candida tropicalis* (Lossick 1986).

Candida is a common inhabitant of the mouth, large intestine and vagina in 25–50% of healthy individuals, and isolation of the organism does not correlate strongly with the presence of clinical disease. Colonisation of the vagina and vulva may originate from contamination of the peri-anal region; many women are colonised by the same organism and phenotype in different sites.

The particular environmental and biological factors that give rise to clinical infection by *C. albicans* are not understood, but some women may be more susceptible; predisposition to infection is associated with diabetes, pregnancy and the administration of antibiotics, particularly those, like penicillin, that are effective against vaginal lactobacilli.

Resistance to fungal infection depends on cell-mediated immunity, and therefore compromise of this by disease, such as HIV infection, or immunosuppressive therapy increases infection risk. Some individuals develop candida-specific reduced cell immunity.

The role of sexual transmission in candida infection is not clear; although the organism is often shared by sexual partners, it is unlikely that just the deposition of the organism gives rise to infection (Lossick 1986). Tight clothes and mild skin abrasions may contribute to clinical presentation of infection.

Presentation and diagnosis

A woman may complain of vulval pruritus (itchiness) and on examination there may be evidence of vulvovaginitis and/or vulval, vaginal and cervical erythema. Dyspareunia (pain during intercourse) is a common complaint.

A vaginal discharge is common but not universal, and may be scant, or thick and white with a curd-like consistency. In less than 20% of cases white thrush patches may be present on the vulva or walls of the vagina (Lossick 1986).

Half of the babies born to infected women will be infected by *Candida* (Lossick 1986), generally involving oral or gastro-intestinal infection. Such infection is usually mild, but treatment of the mother prior to delivery is clearly desirable.

Diagnosis of *C. albicans* is by detection of spores and mycelia by microscopy from a swab sent for culture (see Table 19.1).

Treatment

Vaginal infection is treated by the insertion of vaginal pessaries at night to maximise the time for local action, with cream provided for application to the vulval and peri-anal area.

A number of antifungal treatments are available, including:

- Clotrimazole pessaries — 100 mg for 6 nights **or** 200 mg for 3 nights
  with
  Clotrimazole cream (1%) — applied to the vulva two or three times daily
- Miconazole pessaries — 150 mg for 3 nights
- Nystatin pessaries — 100 000 i.u. × 2 for 14 nights
  with
  Nystatin gel for external use. — 100 000 i.u./g

Signs of clinical infection in a man, usually small red spots or plaques on the glans penis, should be treated with cream applied to the infected area.

Generally it is advised that sexual intercourse be avoided until after treatment is complete, perhaps to avoid local irritation which might provoke re-infection. Advice may be offered about maintaining cleanliness of the peri-anal area, the importance of wiping in the direction of the anus after defaecation, the advantages of cotton underwear, and the avoidance of tights and clothing which is tight or constricting in the crotch.

Table 19.1
Transport media for swabs prior to culture

Infection suspected	Type of medium	Comments
Candidiasis or gonorrhoea	Stuart's	a. White and opalescent — as oxygen content rises it becomes bluish and unsuitable for use b. Stored refrigerated. It must be at room temperature when the swab is inserted and not refrigerated again if the organism is to survive Gonococcus should be cultured within 6 hours
Group B streptococcus	Stuart's	See above
Trichomoniasis	Special medium containing a broad-spectrum antibiotic (this prevents swamping of the organism by fungal or bacterial growth)	As point (b) above Stuart's may be used if the special medium is not available
Herpes simplex or Cytomegalovirus	Viral transport medium (contains antibiotics as above)	Stored frozen; liquefied prior to insertion of swab Refrigerated if there is delay in transport
Chlamydia trachomatis	Special medium containing antibiotics and sucrose to protect the organism	As for herpes simplex but should ideally reach the laboratory within 1 hour

Protozoal infection

The protozoon, *Trichomonas vaginalis*, is an anaerobic organism which is highly pathogenic to the epithelium in the vagina. Its prevalence varies considerably in different populations, but it is estimated on the basis of serological screening that about one-third of American women have been exposed to it (Lossick 1986).

The major mode of transmission is sexual intercourse. 80% of women whose partners are infected with *T. vaginalis* themselves become infected, although the rate of female-to-male transmission is lower than this (Lossick 1986).

T. vaginalis is significant because of the severe vaginitis experienced by some infected women and also because of its common association with other sexually transmitted infections, particularly *Neisseria gonorrhoeae* and *Chlamydia trachomatis*. Infection of the neonate seems to be uncommon.

Presentation and diagnosis
About half to two-thirds of infected women will complain of symptoms. In addition to the pruritus and burning of vaginitis, these include an increase in vaginal discharge, which may range from normal to copious, greyish in colour and somewhat bubbly in character. The green, frothy discharge and friable erythematous cervix, which are the 'classic' presenting feature of infection, are rarely seen (Lossick 1986). Urethritis may also be a feature.

Asymptomatic infection may sometimes be detected on a Papanicolaou smear.

A wet swab examined immediately under a microscope will demonstrate the presence of the pear-shaped protozoon, with 3–5 flagellae and an undulating membrane.

Alternatively, a swab may be sent for culture in special medium (see Table 19.1).

Because of the high co-incidence of *Trichomonas* with other infections, swabs should be taken to exclude the presence of gonococcal and chlamydial infection.

Treatment
A single oral dose of metronidazole 2 g or a 5-day course of 400 mg twice daily is the treatment of choice. Although there is no evidence of a tera-togenic effect in human pregnancy, metronidazole has been found to be carcinogenic to rodents and mutagenic for some bacteria, and is generally avoided in the first trimester of pregnancy. Clotrimazole (see above) may be used as local treatment in early pregnancy.

A woman's partner should also be prescribed treatment with metronidazole.

Metronidazole interacts with alcohol, causing sickness, and therefore alcohol should be avoided while taking it. It may also potentiate the action of anticonvulsants and warfarin. Because of its excretion in breast milk, it is contra-indicated for breast-feeding mothers.

Conventional advice suggests the avoidance of intercourse until treatment is complete.

BACTERIAL INFECTIONS

Bacterial vaginosis

Bacterial vaginosis is a term applied to vaginal discharge associated with a variety of anaerobic organisms including *Gardnerella vaginalis* and *Bacteroides spp*. It has been associated with postpartum pyrexia, amniotic fluid infection, preterm labour and pelvic inflammatory disease (Lossick 1986).

Presentation, diagnosis and treatment
The infection presents with a grey or white, fishy smelling discharge, which may be adherent or of normal consistency and may be more profuse than normal.

Diagnostic clues are the distinctive fishy odour of the discharge and a vaginal pH of >4.5.

Treatment is with metronidazole 400 mg twice daily for 5 days.

Chlamydial infection

Chlamydia trachomatis is one of a group of intracellular parasites, closely related to Gram-negative bacteria. The organism is responsible for a number of human disorders including trachoma, inclusion conjunctivitis, non-gonococcal urethritis, salpingitis, cervicitis and neonatal pneumonitis. Its prevalence in pregnant women varies widely with estimates ranging from 2–37%, with higher rates among young women, unmarried women, women from lower socio-economic groups and those attending inner-city antenatal clinics (Wang & Smaill 1989).

C. trachomatis is the major cause of salpingitis and pelvic inflammatory disease (PID) with their sequelae of ectopic pregnancy and infertility, and postpartum and postabortal infection. Chlamydial infection has been associated with increased risk of low birthweight, preterm rupture of membranes (Alger et al 1988) and a shorter gestation (Brunham et al 1990). It is currently the most common cause of neonatal conjunctivitis and it is estimated that from 3 to 18% of infants born to infected mothers will develop chlamydial pneumonia (Abel & von Unwerth 1988).

Presentation and diagnosis

The condition is often asymptomatic in the woman, although a mucopurulent cervicitis may be detected clinically, or she may present with salpingitis or the urethral syndrome (Wang & Smaill 1989).

Screening for chlamydia. In the light of its association with maternal and neonatal morbidity, detection of chlamydial infection during pregnancy could offer significant benefits, but until recently isolation of *C. trachomatis* involved extremely labour-intensive and expensive techniques. Recently developed antigen detection systems may allow for cost-effective screening to be undertaken; Schachter & Grossman (1981) suggest that if the prevalence of maternal infection in the antenatal population exceeds 6%, it will be cost-effective to use the new techniques to identify and treat chlamydial infection in all pregnant women.

The United States' Centers for Disease Control (CDC) recommend that pregnant women satisfying the following criteria should have at least one prenatal culture for *C. trachomatis*:

- age less than 20 years
- unmarried
- history of other sexually transmitted disease
- multiple sexual partners
- a partner with multiple partners (Bell & Grayson 1986).

If such a strategy is adopted, it is essential for midwives to consider how to discuss this information with women and offer screening in a non-judgemental, non-discriminatory and sensitive way.

Treatment

Erythromycin, 400 mg four times a day for 7 days, is the antibiotic of choice during pregnancy.

Group B streptococcus

Group B streptococcus (GBS, *Streptococcus agalactiae*) is part of the vaginal flora of 5–25% of women. One-third or more pregnant women may be vaginal carriers of GBS at any time during pregnancy and intermittent colonisation may occur.

This asymptomatic maternal infection is significant in pregnancy as the most frequent cause of overwhelming sepsis in neonates, estimated to occur in 0.6–3.7 cases per 1000 live births (Wang & Smaill 1989). The mortality rate of neonatal GBS in the US is 50% (Brunham et al 1990).

In addition, GBS has been associated with early spontaneous rupture of membranes and with a threefold increase in preterm delivery at less than 32 weeks' gestation (Brunham et al 1990).

Of the neonates of women with GBS colonisation, 65–75% will be colonised with the organism, although only 1–2% of exposed neonates will develop invasive disease (Brunham et al 1990).

Management and treatment of GBS colonisation in pregnancy

The efficacy of routine antenatal screening and treatment of GBS is limited because of the intermittent nature of maternal infection and the tendency for recurrence after treatment.

Minkoff & Mead (1986) propose the treatment of women with preterm rupture of membranes or preterm labour with ampicillin until culture results are available. The use of a rapid screening test which can identify heavy vaginal GBS colonisation within 5 hours in women with preterm rupture of membranes would facilitate this strategy (Wang & Smaill 1989).

The recommended treatment is intravenous administration of ampicillin (or erythromycin if the woman is allergic to penicillin), which should be continued if the result is positive or unavailable (Wang & Smaill 1989).

Gonococcal infection

Gonorrhoea is caused by *Neisseria gonorrhoeae*, a Gram-negative diplococcus, which has an affinity for columnar epithelial tissue. In women infection occurs in the urethra or cervix. The vagina in women of childbearing age, composed of transitional and stratified squamous epithelium, is protected from being a site of infection, although resistance may be lowered in prepubertal and postmenopausal women. Colonisation of pharyngeal tissue also occurs, as a result of oral sexual contact with an infected partner, as does infection of the rectum due to anogenital contact.

Incidence of maternal infection varies greatly between populations, ranging from 1 to 5% (Wang & Smaill 1989). The rate of asymptomatic infection is high, and as many as 50% of women diagnosed in STD clinics are asymptomatic (Adler 1985).

Effect of gonococcal infection in pregnancy

Gonorrhoea may give rise to local or systemic infection, and pregnancy appears to increase the likelihood of infection presenting as arthritis or systemic disease. This apparent increase may be attributable to better follow-up during this period (Wang & Smaill 1989) or may be associated with the higher rate of pharyngeal infection in pregnancy that has been noted in some US studies and the greater risk of dissemination associated with pharyngeal colonisation (Brunham et al 1990).

Among non-pregnant women with endocervical infection, about 10–20% have clinical evidence of pelvic inflammatory disease (PID) and up to 50% of those with recent infection develop PID. Acute PID is rare in pregnancy, although positive *N. gonorrhoeae* cultures are sometimes associated with fever and pain.

The signs and symptoms which may charac-terise local gonococcal infection in pregnant women are:

- dysuria–sterile pyuria syndrome (urethral infection)
- cervicitis (endocervical infection)
- proctitis (rectal infection)
- conjunctivitis (ophthalmic infection).

Less common manifestations include acute inflammation of Bartholin's glands (bartholinitis), endometritis and salpingitis (Wang and Smaill 1989).

Arthritis is the most common manifestation of disseminated infection. Infection usually presents with fever and rigors and there may be a characteristic purpuric-petechial rash (Wang & Smaill 1989).

Impact of gonococcal infection on pregnancy

Pregnancy complicated by endocervical gonococcal infection is associated with prelabour rupture of membranes, chorio-amnionitis, preterm rupture of membranes and preterm delivery. The effect of gonococcal infection on early pregnancy is not well studied but early infection is associated with septic abortion and chorio-amnionitis (Brunham et al 1990, Wang & Smaill 1989).

Intrapartum infection is associated with postpartum endometritis and upper genital tract infection (Brunham et al 1990).

Infection in the neonate

Neonatal infection most commonly presents as conjunctivitis, but infection at other body sites can occur and may be associated with a higher risk of disseminated infection (Brunham et al 1990).

Diagnosis

Because of the presence of other Gram-negative diplococci in the female genital tract, Gram staining is not adequate for diagnosis of gonococcal infection in women, and culture of the organism is required.

Swabs should be taken from the cervix and the urethral meatus. If culture is being conducted because of known contact with an infected partner, other sites of exposure such as the throat and anus should be swabbed.

Screening

Screening all women for gonococcal infection in pregnancy has been advocated by a number of authors, on the grounds of its serious effects on pregnancy and the risks of neonatal and puerperal infection (Brunham et al 1990, Wang & Smaill 1989) and the fact that a high proportion of infection in women is asymptomatic. Repeat cultures in the last trimester are suggested for women with a previous history of gonorrhoea or other sexually transmitted infection.

Treatment

Penicillin is the drug of choice, intramuscularly with probenecid 1 g orally, or ampicillin may be prescribed in a single dose orally with probenecid 1 g orally (Adler 1990). In cases of disseminated disease penicillin should be administered either intravenously or intramuscularly, with an initial dose of 10 mega-units per day and continued at a reduced dose for 10–14 days. If arthritis is a feature of infection, a longer therapy is indicated (Wang & Smaill 1989).

Repeat swabs should be cultured because of the rising incidence of penicillin-resistant strains of gonococcus.

Conclusions

Prevention of complications of pregnancy and neonatal disease associated with *N. gonorrhoeae* depends on early detection and treatment of infection, which it has been argued (Wang & Smaill 1989) would be best accomplished by screening of all pregnant women.

If routine screening is introduced or when testing is undertaken on an individual basis, it should be accompanied by information about how gonorrhoea is transmitted, the need for the woman's sexual partner also to be diagnosed and treated, and the use of barrier protection during sexual intercourse to reduce transmission of gonorrhoea and other infections.

Syphilis

Syphilis is an infection caused by *Treponema pallidum*, one of a family of three spirochaetes associated with human disease. In pregnancy its particular significance is the devastating effect it has on fetal well-being.

The natural course of adult infection is divided into stages:

- Early infectious
  - primary: 9–60 days after exposure
  - secondary: 6 weeks to 6 months after exposure (4–6 weeks after appearance of primary lesion)
  - early latent: 2 years after exposure
- Late non-infectious
  - late latent more than 2 years after exposure
  - neurosyphilis, cardiovascular syphilis or gummatous syphilis (Adler 1990).

Most pregnant women diagnosed will be in the primary or secondary stages and untreated infection will affect almost all fetuses. About 20% of infants will deliver preterm and 20% of pregnancies result in miscarriage or perinatal death. 20% of surviving infants will present with subclinical infection and 40% with congenital syphilis with resulting disability (Wang & Smaill 1989). Untreated early latent syphilis results in a 40% rate of prematurity or perinatal death, while about 10% of infants of mothers with untreated late syphilis will show signs of congenital syphilis with a 10 times increased perinatal death rate (Brunham et al 1990). Whereas sexual transmission of untreated infection does not usually occur after 2 years, women may remain infectious for their fetuses for much longer (Brunham et al 1990).

Prenatal diagnosis and treatment through routine serological testing in early pregnancy has been the key to the prevention of congenital syphilis in the United Kingdom. It has also contributed to the general decline in the incidence of syphilis to the extent that it functions as an indirect population screening programme, facilitating referral of women to GUM clinics where contact tracing and treatment of infected partners can be initiated (Clay 1989).

In spite of the rarity of syphilis amongst women of childbearing age in England and Wales, there is evidence that there may be pockets of increase (Horner et al 1989) and calculations have demonstrated a benefit to cost ratio of 30:1 in favour of continuing screening (Williams 1985).

O'Mahony & Holland (1989) have argued in favour of performing a second screening test in late pregnancy or the introduction universally of the more sensitive *Treponema pallidum* haemagglutination test (TPHA), in addition to the Venereal Diseases Research Laboratory (VDRL) test for detection of infection. They report experience of a number of infants presenting with congenital syphilis although their mothers had had negative serology in early pregnancy.

Treatment

Penicillin is the drug of choice and the dosage depends on the stage of the woman's infection. If it is 2 years or less since the time of infection, she should receive aqueous procaine penicillin 600 000 units intramuscularly daily for 10 days. In late latent infection (more than 2 years since infection) the dosage is 900 000 units/day for 21 days.

If the woman is allergic to penicillin, erythromycin 500 mg 6-hourly for 15 days in early infection or 30 days in latent infection will be required. The baby should then be treated with penicillin at birth, because of less efficient placental transfer of erythromycin.

Ideally, case identification and treatment should be initiated in early pregnancy. Problems of third trimester diagnosis include treatment failure due to inadequate dosage of penicillin. In addition, treatment may give rise to a Jarisch–Herxheimer reaction, which may provoke uterine contractions and fetal distress (Horner et al 1989). The Jarisch-Herxheimer reaction, common in the treatment of primary and secondary syphilis, is characterised by fever and flu-like symptoms, which may occur 3–12 hours after the first injection of penicillin (Adler 1990).

The baby should be examined and have serological tests done to exclude infection, even if the mother has been treated early with penicillin. Passively transmitted maternal antibodies may persist for up to 6 weeks, and therefore serological tests should be done at 6 weeks and 3 months of age.

Treatment of a woman in subsequent pregnancies is advocated by some, because of the possibility of persistent treponemes after treatment. Adler (1990) suggests that if the woman has already been followed up for 2 years and discharged as cured, an alternative to re-treating the mother is to carry out serology on the infant at 3 months of age to exclude infection. It is important that the woman is informed of this necessity so that she can arrange for follow-up of the baby.

Congenital syphilis

Incidence — 2 per 10 000 live births.

The diagnosis rests on the same factors as for adults. Blood tests can be confusing, some babies having specific IgM present whilst in others all serology is negative. A 3-month follow-up is needed to exclude any possibility of the disease. Physical characteristics of the placenta are no longer considered a useful guide to diagnosis.

Early signs may be present at birth or develop within the first 2 years but primary syphilis is not found as the treponemes have been blood borne. Highly contagious vesicles ('syphilitic pemphigus') on the palms, soles and possibly other areas burst and leave their dull red, raised bases exposed. Aborted and stillborn babies may have similar lesions. Ulcers can occur on the lips and mouth, and if on the larynx the cry can be thin or soundless. Ulcers of the nasal periosteum cause a purulent, bloodstained or watery nasal discharge teeming with treponemes. Poor feeding and weight loss can result.

Periostitis produces swelling of the long bones and the pain may cause the baby to behave as if he has a fracture. There may be patchy alopecia, hepatosplenomegaly and mild jaundice. Surprisingly the prognosis is excellent if the early hazards are survived.

Late signs may develop any time from the 2nd to the 30th year of life even if none of the early ones were exhibited. Corneal scarring can cause impaired vision or blindness; meningitis can result in convulsions, blindness and mental retardation. Gummata in the nasal septum can leave deformity and there may be eighth nerve deafness. Rarely neurosyphilis may develop. The prognosis depends on the damage which exists prior to treatment.

Scars and deformities resulting from the infection are known as *stigmata* and, although characteristic, are not always present. There may be a *'saddleback' depression of the nasal bridge* or linear scars resulting from ulcers around the mouth, nares and anus; these are known as *rhagades*. The permanent incisors may be widely spaced and have sides which converge to resemble the end of a screwdriver, the cutting edge being notched (*Hutchinson's teeth*).

Management. In the presence of contagious lesions the baby must be barrier nursed until antibiotics have been given for 48 hours. He may be very ill. Intramuscular procaine penicillin 50 000 i.u. per kg body weight is given in divided doses over 10 days.

Some advocate routine lumbar puncture to look for treponemes. Follow-up is prolonged and the parents will need investigation.

Prior to May 1984 it was legally required in England and Wales that a child for adoption (or his mother) should be screened for syphilis 6 weeks after delivery. Now, under the Adoption Agencies Regulations of 1983, all examinations and tests are at the discretion of the adoption agency's medical adviser. Some form of screening is usual.

VIRAL INFECTIONS

Herpes simplex virus

Herpes simplex is one of a family of herpes viruses, which includes varicella-zoster, cytomegalovirus (CMV) and Epstein–Barr virus. All within the family share the ability to establish lifelong, persistent infection in their host and to undergo periodic reactivation. Reactivated infection may have characteristics different from the primary episode.

Infections of the mouth and lips caused by herpes simplex virus were recognised by the ancient Greeks; genital infections were described by an 18th century French physician, Astruc. Neonatal herpes infections were first documented 50 years ago (Stagno & Whitley 1990).

It was only in the mid-1960s that two herpes simplex viruses (HSV), type 1, associated with infections of the lip and oropharynx, and type 2,

associated with genital infection, were demonstrated. The recognition that neonatal infection was most often associated with HSV type 2 and that maternal viral excretion could be present at the time of delivery, suggested transmission by exposure to genital secretions at delivery. However, postnatal infection of the newborn baby with HSV type 1 from maternal or non-maternal sources, such as staff and visitors, has also been documented.

For transmission to occur the HSV virus must come into contact with mucosal surfaces or abraded skin. Viral replication occurs at the site of infection and then the virus or particles of it are transmitted by neurons to the ganglia where they remain dormant until there is an alteration in the host environment that gives rise to recurrence of active infection.

Presentation of infection with HSV

Primary infection of HSV type 1 in young children is usually asymptomatic, though may present with gingivostomatitis. In young adults, primary infection is associated with pharyngitis and mononucleosis-like illness.

Primary infection with HSV type 2 usually presents with painful genital ulcers after an incubation period of less than 7 days. Skin lesions begin with erythema, progress to vesicles and then ulcers and finish with crusting. Local lesions with viral shedding may last about 12 days, with complete healing taking another week (Adler 1990). Both the vulva and cervix are involved in most primary attacks in women, but single sites may be affected.

Recurrent infection involves reactivation of the virus at the same site, rather than re-infection. Patients may experience prodromal symptoms of local tingling or numbness at the site of the lesions about 24–48 hours prior to onset of lesions. There may be fewer lesions, milder symptoms and a shorter duration in recurrent attacks.

Both primary and recurrent infection may be asymptomatic; this presents a particular problem in the case of primary infection in pregnancy, which is the situation in which the fetus is at greatest risk.

Effect of HSV infection in pregnancy

The main concerns about HSV during pregnancy are the association of primary infection with an increased risk of spontaneous abortion, prematurity and the acquisition of serious infection by the neonate (Nahmias et al 1971). Transmission of virus to the fetus or neonate is thought to occur at delivery and only rarely transplacentally (Brunham 1990). In primary maternal infection the rate of transmission has been estimated to be as high as 50% (Nahmias et al 1971); in recurrent maternal infection, however, the rate is low, with estimations of between 3 and 8% (Prober et al 1987). The difference in infection rate between the two groups of babies is attributed to the presence of a high titre of passively acquired maternal antibodies to HSV in the babies of mothers with recurrent infection (Prober et al 1987, Anon 1988).

Neonatal infection with HSV can present in localised or disseminated form. Localised infection may occur in the central nervous system, the eyes, the skin and mouth. Multiple organs are affected in disseminated infection including the brain, lungs, stomach, kidneys, liver and others. Neonatal HSV infection is associated with an overall mortality rate of about 60%, although rates vary with the site of infection.

Management of HSV in pregnancy

Recommendations for the management of late pregnancy and delivery of women with a history of genital HSV have evolved in the light of the accumulating evidence about perinatal transmission, although there have been no randomised trials to evaluate clinical policy and the evidence for recommended policy remains weak (Wang & Smaill 1989).

Recommended policy is summarised by Wang and Smaill (1989):

- All women with prodromal symptoms or visible herpetic lesions at the outset of labour should have samples taken and examined by electron microscopy for the presence of herpes virus.
- If no virus is detected, vaginal delivery should be allowed to proceed.

- If the results are not available at the time of delivery and membranes have been ruptured for less than 4–6 hours, the presence of virus should be assumed and a caesarean section performed.
- If membranes have been ruptured for longer than 4–6 hours, caesarean section is not thought to confer any advantage, because of the possibility of ascending infection, and vaginal delivery should proceed.

The use of fetal scalp electrodes and fetal blood sampling should be avoided if there is a risk of viral shedding.

Swabs should be taken from the eyes, nasopharynx, umbilicus and skin abrasions of the baby exposed to viral shedding during labour, to exclude colonisation and infection.

Women who experience recurrent HSV infection during pregnancy should be reassured that the transmission rate is very low and that antiviral therapy is available if infection of the baby occurs. There is some evidence that administration of acyclovir during the late antenatal period to women with recurrent genital herpes may be a successful strategy for preventing transmission to the neonate at delivery (Stray-Pederson 1990).

Cytomegalovirus (CMV)

This virus is a member of the herpes group and can be excreted in saliva, urine, breast milk, semen and cervical secretions. Infection in adults usually occurs by contact between mucous membranes (e.g. on kissing) and may be sexual. The primary infection may occasionally result in manifestations similar to glandular fever or influenza with headache, sore throat and anorexia. There may be hepatitis with prolonged pyrexia. Subsequently the virus may remain dormant but be subject to reactivation and be excreted for many years.

Diagnosis is confirmed on culture of specimens of urine, blood or saliva, or of a swab from the cervix (see Table 19.1). Serology is performed for antibody levels.

Infection in pregnancy

There is increasing evidence that at any stage of

pregnancy both primary infections and reactivation can result in transplacental infection, although the results are probably most serious in the former case. Abortion, stillbirth, growth retardation and premature labour may result. The incidence of infected babies in Britain is estimated to be 4 per 1000 live births. 2% of these develop serious problems (for example micro- or hydrocephaly, spastic quadriplegia, psychomotor retardation and deafness). 8% have minor problems (e.g. hepatosplenomegaly and thrombocytopenia). 90% are symptom free at birth but some will not attain their expected intellectual potential or will become deaf in later childhood.

If *transplacental infection* is suspected, cord blood is examined for specific IgM and a urine sample and nasopharyngeal swab are sent for culture. Treatment is supportive only and infection of other babies and members of staff (especially those who are pregnant) must be avoided. The virus may be shed for a prolonged period.

Babies may be infected by breast milk, but this does not cause serious disease. Transfusion of infected blood may result in pneumonitis, especially in preterm babies and in some centres only blood free of CMV antibodies is given.

Whilst it is estimated that 50% of women of childbearing age have been infected by cytomegalovirus, only about 1% of their infants will become infected.

Routine screening in pregnancy is not thought desirable as it is difficult to know what advice to give parents and, as attacks are often sub-clinical, repeated screening would be needed.

Cytomegalovirus is an increasing problem and work on the development of a vaccine has been slow. It has been suggested that in countries where rubella vaccination levels are high, cytomegalovirus is now the more important cause of congenital abnormalities.

Hepatitis B or serum hepatitis

This virus is present in the blood of those who have been infected. Particles of it are also present in all their body fluids, for example vaginal secretions, menstrual blood, semen, saliva, sweat,

urine and faeces. Sexual activity, blood and blood products appear to be the main modes of transmission. Drug addicts or those tattooed with dirty needles are at especial risk. It should be noted that in adults with syphilis or gonorrhoea, hepatitis B is also often present.

This infection can lead to chronic liver disease or to an asymptomatic carrier state. Pregnant women have an increased risk of a severe attack because of their slightly immunosuppressed state.

Antenatal screening of all pregnant women is recommended, so that the need to treat the baby prophylactically can be determined and staff can exercise suitable precautions in relation to venepuncture, delivery and postnatal care. If hepatitis B surface antigen (HBs Ag — formerly known as the Australia antigen) is present, then the serum is also examined for 'e' antigen (HBe Ag) which indicates that the disease is at a highly infectious stage. (If there is delay in transport of this blood, it must be stored at 4°C.)

An acute attack in a pregnant woman may result in abortion or premature labour and it is recommended that specific immunoglobulin should be offered to sexual contacts of men who develop the acute disease. Transplacental infection probably does not occur in carriers as maternal antibodies also cross the placenta.

Intrapartum infection may occur, the virus entering eye mucosa, gastro-intestinal tract or through breached skin. It is rare in babies of carrier mothers, but prophylaxis is recommended for the babies of those who develop acute hepatitis B in the last trimester or who are HBe Ag positive. (Cord blood is not a reliable indicator of which babies need treatment.) The first dose of hepatitis B vaccine (consisting of highly purified surface antigen) must be given within 24 hours of delivery and is repeated at 1 and 6 months of age. This protects the baby from becoming a carrier and from the long-term dangers of chronic hepatitis, cirrhosis and hepatocellular carcinoma. Acute hepatitis B in the neonate is rare, serious and may have a poor prognosis. In order to prevent it several doses of specific immunoglobulin are given during the first 6 months of life, the first at the same time as the vaccine.

In Britain 0.1% of the population are carriers

but the rate may be as high as 10% in some parts of Africa and Asia.

Breast feeding is probably not a significant mode of transmission to babies of carrier mothers. However, if a woman is highly infectious following an acute attack it should not be started until her baby has a good level of passive immunity.

Babies who have not been vaccinated may contract the infection later in childhood from their parents or siblings.

The following specific recommendations are modified from Goodall et al (1987) and reproduced with the permission of the Royal College of Nursing.

Delivery and postnatal care of women suspected or infected with Hepatitis B (acute or chronic)

1. It is advisable that all staff present at the delivery should be vaccinated and in any case the team should be kept to essential staff who are aware of the hazards.

2. Delivery should be performed aseptically.

3. **Protective clothing.** During delivery the following must be worn:

   a. A plastic apron under a sterile water-repellant disposable gown
   b. Gloves (these must also be worn at all times when handling bloodstained materials)
   c. Mask and goggles or visor.

Disposable bed sheets should be used with a plastic liner underneath.

4. **Spillages of blood or body fluids** should be dealt with promptly. Wearing strong rubber gloves and a plastic apron they should be absorbed into disposable towels and 1% sodium hypochlorite (10 000 p.p.m. available chlorine) poured onto them. This should be left for 30 minutes if possible (but at least 15). The towels should then be discarded into the appropriate colour-coded bags and secured prior to incineration. The area should finally be thoroughly washed with detergent and water and then dried.

5. **Mishaps.** All accidents must be reported immediately. In order to reduce needlestick injuries needles should never be re-sheathed.

   a. An accidental puncture wound should be encouraged to bleed by gentle squeezing *not* sucking and then washed with soap and warm water or other skin wash.
   b. Any contamination of the skin by blood or other body fluids should be cleaned with soap and warm water.
   c. Splashes in the eye should be well rinsed with water or sterile saline.

Unless the injured person was previously vaccinated and shown to have immunity, it is likely that they will be given hepatitis B immunoglobulin and a course of vaccine.

6. During the puerperium a plastic apron and gloves should be worn when attending the mother or baby if there is likely to be contact with blood or other body fluids. After the procedure the gloves should be removed and the hands washed thoroughly.

7. The mother should be instructed to dispose of soiled sanitary material into the appropriate colour-coded bag before washing her hands.

8. Arrangements must be made for strict sanitisation of lavatory seats immediately after use.

Specific guidance is also given in the above-mentioned publication in relation to collection and transport of specimens, cleaning of equipment, care during and after surgery and disposal of waste and sharps.

Genital warts

Genital warts are caused by the human papillomavirus (HPV) and are nearly always transmitted by sexual contact although, rarely, a baby may acquire a laryngeal papilloma as a result of exposure at the time of delivery.

The special significance of warts in pregnancy is that they occasionally increase very dramatically in size, which may be extremely distressing for the woman and may infrequently jeopardise the possibility of a vaginal delivery.

The preferred first line of treatment for genital warts is 10–25% podophyllin, but as this is contra-indicated during pregnancy because of its toxicity, the recommendation is not to treat warts at this time. Other treatments that may be attempted in pregnancy are trichloroethanoic acid, cryotherapy or electrocautery (Adler 1990).

It is suggested that women presenting with genital warts should have full investigations to exclude other sexually transmitted infections. In addition, the cervix should be examined by colposcopy to exclude flat warts on the cervix, which may be associated with malignant changes. Because of the possible association between HPV and cervical intra-epithelial neoplasia (CIN), cytological screening is recommended for women with vulval or vaginal warts or those whose partners have penile warts (Adler 1990).

Human immunodeficiency virus (HIV)

HIV is a retrovirus which may be transmitted in three ways:

- in blood
- during sexual intercourse
- from mother to fetus in utero, at delivery or via breast feeding.

It is recognised that there are at least two varieties of HIV, designated as HIV-1 and HIV-2. So far, in the UK, HIV-1 is the predominant form and the following discussion relates to HIV-1 unless otherwise stated.

For a full discussion of the pathophysiology of HIV and HIV-associated illness see Pratt (1991).

HIV infection in pregnancy

Because of the alterations in the immune system that occur in pregnancy, there are grounds for a theoretical concern that the interaction of pregnancy with HIV might provoke acceleration of the infection (Schoenbaum et al 1988).

A number of prospective studies have failed to demonstrate marked advance of HIV illness during pregnancy in women with asymptomatic infection (Schoenbaum et al 1988, MacCallum et al 1988) in spite of early suggestions that this might have been the case. There may, however, be some evidence for an acceleration of immune compromise during pregnancy (Schaefer et al 1988, Biggar et al 1989). In addition, a recent study demonstrates the vulnerability to serious infection during pregnancy of those HIV-positive women who have become immune-compromised (Minkoff et al 1990).

Further research charting the natural course of infection in women, both pregnant and not, is required (Minkoff & DeHovitz 1990). Until additional data are available, it has to be acknowledged that pregnancy may confer additional risks for the HIV-positive woman, but the evidence for acceleration of HIV-related disease is not strong. Decision making about continuation of the pregnancy and its management will require full physical and immunological assessment of the individual woman.

With regard to the impact of HIV infection on pregnancy, there is no evidence of marked differences in the outcome of comparable pregnancies of HIV-positive and HIV-negative women (Johnstone et al 1988, Selwyn et al 1989).

However, the perinatal outcome of a group of infants born to HIV-positive mothers in Zaire, amongst whom the rate of AIDS was 18%, demonstrated higher rates of prematurity, lower birthweights and higher neonatal death rates than in a comparable group of HIV-negative mothers (Ryder et al 1989). Many of the neonatal deaths are likely to have been associated with prematurity and low birthweight, possibly due to symptomatic maternal illness rather than HIV infection per se.

The risks of perinatal transmission

On the basis of the most recent figures from an ongoing multi-centred European prospective study (European Collaborative Study 1991) the rate of mother-to-child transmission has been estimated to be about 13%. Higher rates have been reported in other studies, which may be a result of study designs in which children are retrospectively included. In addition, factors such as the length of time that the infection is present in a population, the prevalence of immune compromise within the maternal population and other as yet unidentified factors may influence the rate of transmission.

As data accumulate, analysis is beginning of the factors that are associated with transmission from mother to child (European Collaborative Study 1992). Improved understanding of the mechanism will provide more accurate information on which to base decisions about continuation of and management of pregnancy, as well as practices that may be adopted to minimise the risks of neonatal HIV acquisition.

There is evidence that HIV infection may be transmitted by breast feeding and that the risk of infection is greater to the breast-fed baby (Dunn et al 1992). Where safe alternatives to breast feeding are available, HIV-infected women should be discouraged from breast feeding (Dunn et al 1992). However, where there are high rates of infant infection and high rates of malnutrition and infant mortality, breast feeding should continue to be encouraged, regardless of HIV infection status (Global Programme on AIDS, 1992).

Diagnosis of HIV infection

The diagnosis of asymptomatic HIV infection is made on the basis of the presence in serum of antibodies to the virus. The identification of anti-HIV antibodies represents merely a marker for the presence of infection, as they do not have a neutralising effect on it. Most individuals will produce antibodies (seroconvert) within 3 months of infection with the virus. If an HIV antibody test is carried out less than 3 months after the most recent possible exposure, during the so-called 'window of infectivity', a negative result will require a repeat test in order to take account of the possibility of late seroconversion.

All serum for HIV antibody testing in the UK will be subject to two tests. The ELISA (enzyme linked immunosorbent assay) test is highly sensitive to the presence of antibodies. Its sensitivity increases the possibility of false positive results and thus a Western Blot test, which has a greater specificity for HIV is always used to confirm the presence of the antibodies. Often a second specimen of blood will be tested to confirm the result.

HIV antibody testing in pregnancy

The discovery by an individual that she is infected with HIV will have profound effects on her psychologically, socially and economically. For complex social reasons, it is also a uniquely stig-

matised infection. Decision-making about HIV testing is likely to be more complex during pregnancy, because the woman will need to consider the implications not only for herself but also for her unborn baby and the impact that the diagnosis might have on her social and family relationships at this vulnerable time. Given the implications of a positive result, it is crucial that any woman who is tested for the virus has had an opportunity to consider the impact of a positive result on her, both in the short and the long term.

Such consideration requires information about the nature of the infection, the meaning of the test results, the choices and options available for surveillance and management of the infection and available support networks.

For these reasons, the implementation of a policy of routinely testing for HIV unless a woman 'opts out' (Boyd 1990) may confer a risk that some women will receive a positive HIV test result without having been adequately prepared to understand and to deal with it. In addition, many women will be tested and found negative, but the individual may not gain any knowledge about the infection and how she might protect herself from exposure in future.

On the other hand, there may be strong reasons for a woman deciding to be tested for HIV during her pregnancy (Brierley & Roth 1991).

It is essential that midwives and other caregivers are able to provide the time, information and support needed for a woman to make a choice about HIV testing in an informed and knowledgeable way. Caregivers must also be able to facilitate access to whatever medical and supportive resources a woman may require in the event of a positive test result.

The notion of risk in relation to HIV

The prevalence of HIV in different communities and under different circumstances varies enormously, and a notion of 'high risk groups' has evolved as a way of identifying individuals thought more likely to have come into contact with the virus.

It is, however, more useful and accurate to identify 'risk activity', because infection with the virus is linked not to who or what a person is but rather to what she does that might expose her to infection. This change in perspective may also guard against the tendency to apply the notion of 'high risk group' in a way that is perceived by women to be discriminatory or threatening.

The activities that put individuals at risk are:

• Unprotected sexual intercourse with an infected partner. Because it is impossible with any certainty to distinguish an infected partner from an uninfected one, unprotected intercourse with anyone who has had unprotected intercourse with anyone else or who has shared injecting equipment with anyone else can be considered to be an infection risk.
• Injecting drugs using needles and syringes that have been used by someone else.
• Being transfused with blood or other blood products that have not been screened for HIV infection.

If health education and availability of testing is to serve the interests of the client, it is essential that women acquire information which will empower them to protect themselves more effectively against HIV in future, whether they decide to be tested or not.

Issues of infection control

Because it is impossible to know the HIV status of all individuals or indeed to exclude the presence of other blood-borne infections that might constitute a transmission risk, the principle of 'universal precautions' has been proposed (Centers for Disease Control 1988) as a basis for infection control policy. This recommends that there be the application, in the care of *all* clients, of measures to protect staff and others from accidental exposure to potentially infectious body fluids. In the midwifery context such fluids include blood, liquor, cervical secretions, cerebrospinal fluid and any bloodstained fluid.

Special considerations for care of women in relation to HIV

In the following section some of the issues likely to arise in relation to the care of the HIV-positive pregnant woman are highlighted. Throughout

Practical application of universal precautions

• When exposure to body fluids is anticipated, protective clothing should be worn.
• Contaminated surfaces should be disinfected and mopped up using a hypochlorite solution 1:100 or 1:10.
• Skin accidentally exposed should be washed thoroughly with soap and water.
• Care should be exercised in handling sharps; injuries should be encouraged to bleed and washed thoroughly, the accident should be reported and agreed local policy followed.

the discussion reference is made to 'the woman', although where appropriate this should be taken to include her partner or other support persons. The circumstances of women are so variable that it is difficult to find a phrase that applies equally well to all women.

Breaking the news

A diagnosis of HIV will give rise to shock and extreme emotion, and this is likely to be intensified in pregnancy. A woman should be told, at the time her blood specimen is taken, when to expect the result to be available and from whom she will receive it. She should be encouraged to involve her partner or a reliable close friend who might accompany her, but because of the stigma and prejudice which marks reactions to HIV infection she may need to guard herself against disclosure which may be detrimental to her.

Midwives must be prepared to offer the woman immediate access to a support network and formal counselling should she want it.

A further appointment with the doctor and midwife should be offered in the next few days to discuss her care and answer the questions which she will have, and she should be given a phone number she can ring to make contact before that.

Termination of pregnancy?

Counselling should be offered to enable the woman to consider her plans for this pregnancy in the light of her diagnosis. The counsellor should be able to discuss the most recent information available about the impact of HIV on the mother's and baby's health in order to facilitate an informed decision.

The stage of the pregnancy, the woman's immune status, her desire for a child and her attitude towards termination will all be important factors in the discussion of this issue.

Continuity of care

Throughout the pregnancy of this woman the midwife has an essential contribution to make in co-ordinating appropriate care and providing an accessible source of information and support.

Early and regular surveillance of the woman's general health and immune status should be organised with the appropriate specialist physician. Co-ordination of care with other agencies, such as the Drug Dependency Unit (DDU) should be ensured.

Early reporting, investigation and treatment of signs of HIV-related and other infections should be encouraged, with particular attention to non-specific signs such as weight loss, oral thrush and diarrhoea. The woman may experience recurrence of HSV lesions; evidence of this should be sought and investigations initiated if delivery is imminent. Because of the increased risk of CIN in the HIV-infected woman (Minkoff & DeHovitz 1990), colposcopy or cytology may be indicated.

Opportunity should be provided for the woman to meet the paediatrician who will care for the baby, and to discuss the pattern of follow-up and treatment that may be undertaken if the baby is infected.

The midwife should encourage the woman to talk about her plans for feeding. If she had hoped to breast feed it is important to discuss with her the additional risk to the baby. She can be helped to achieve the physical closeness of breast feeding even if she decides to use formula milk.

A decision not to breast feed may be an additional source of disappointment which she may want to talk about.

Discussion should also be initiated about self-care at the onset of labour such as how she should manage spilled liquor.

Care in labour

Care by a midwife already known to the woman is desirable. This ensures that confidentiality will continue to be protected and allows care to be given within an established, supportive relationship.

Postnatal care

The midwife should discuss with the woman whether she has preference for a single room; if not, a separate room and toilet or bath facilities are unnecessary. There should be adequate facilities for the safe disposal of sanitary towels and the woman should be aware of the need for immediate attention to the disinfection and cleaning of any spilled blood.

The stress and adjustment of the postnatal period are likely to be intensified for the woman who is HIV-positive and complicated by anxiety about her baby's health and her own, uncertainty about the future and the long-term well-being and care of her baby. She may also lack confidence in

---

Care in labour: suggestions for minimising infection risks to staff

- Wear waterproof protective gowns and gloves when exposure to body fluids is expected.
- Leave membranes intact to avoid unnecessary contamination with liquor.
- Avoid the use of fetal scalp electrodes and fetal blood sampling to minimise unnecessary exposure of the baby.
- Protect against splashes to the eye by wearing British Standard approved safety glasses if directly involved in care where a splash might occur, e.g. at delivery, cutting the cord. Masks should also be available.
- Use mechanically operated suction in preference to a mouth-operated device, if mucus extraction is required.
- Bath the baby as soon as possible after delivery, in water at 37.5°C, provided he or she is well and body temperature is 36.5°C or above. Rubber gloves and plastic apron should be worn; gloves should be worn when handling the baby until the bath is done.

her skills as a new mother and experience the sense of inadequacy that accompanies this. Continued care by a known midwife, familiar with the woman and her circumstances and confident to respond to her questions and doubts, is especially important at this time. The midwife should be alert to the woman's sense of isolation, loneliness and guilt and should offer support or referral to a counsellor or social worker, or contact with a self-help group as appropriate.

The midwife's daily examination should specifically elicit signs or symptoms suggestive of physical illness and emotional distress. Gloves need only be worn if exposure to blood is anticipated, for instance when examining the perineum, lochia or an abdominal wound.

The mother should be encouraged to manage the baby's care herself with the support of the midwife. Gloves need only be worn by the midwife if she is carrying out cord care or nappy changing in the presence of bleeding or for invasive procedures, such as the collection of a capillary sample of blood from a heel stab, when contamination of the operator's hands is difficult to avoid.

Plans for follow-up care of the mother and baby should be reviewed prior to discharge, and the woman should be encouraged to consider the roles that might be played by the community midwife, GP and health visitor. The decision to inform these caregivers of her HIV status should rest with the woman herself and she should understand that they will not be informed without her consent.

Discussion of contraception should be offered before her transfer home and she should be advised to use condoms as well as another method for birth control. Even if both partners are HIV positive, condoms should be used in order to prevent possible exposure to other STDs. Evidence for a preferred additional method of contraception is lacking. An intra-uterine contraceptive device (IUCD) may not be ideal because of increased risk of pelvic inflammatory disease; oral contraceptives may alter the metabolism of other drugs used in the treatment of HIV-infected women (Minkoff & DeHovitz 1990).

Some women will not have confided their HIV status to their partner, and discussion of contraception might offer an opportunity to explore this difficult problem. Further formal counselling may assist a woman to find a way of discussing her infection with her partner.

Appointments should be arranged for follow-up cervical smear or colposcopy as well as for general assessment by the physician. She should be given appointments for the baby's follow-up assessments and should be given a contact number should any problems arise about which she needs advice.

Care and follow-up of the baby

All babies who are born to HIV-positive women will have passively acquired maternal antibodies to HIV and these may persist for as long as 18 months. Therefore diagnosis of HIV cannot be achieved by antibody testing and confirmation of the infant's infection status may not occur for some time. The uncertainty and doubt which parents may experience is an additional stress.

Data from the European Collaborative Study (1991) has allowed a picture of the natural history of infection to be described.

There were no differences identified in birthweight, gestation, head circumference or gestation-adjusted birthweight between infected and uninfected babies.

It was found to be possible to use immunological and clinical signs as predictors of HIV infection in children less than 18 months of age, and it is estimated that the monitoring of immunoglobins and other indices of immune function together with clinical signs could identify 48% of infected children by 6 months of age.

A number of signs and symptoms were identified as being strongly associated with HIV infection. These are:

- oral candidiasis on two consecutive examinations at least 2 months apart
- a combination of two of the following persisting for 2 months: lymphadenopathy, hepatomegaly, splenomegaly (LHS)
- abnormal immunological findings.

Of children within the study, 83% of those infected showed laboratory or clinical features by 6 months of age. By 12 months, 26% of infected children had AIDS and 17% had died of HIV-related disease. The remainder seemed to remain stable and some improved during the second year (European Collaborative Study 1991).

Treatment

It is beyond the scope of this chapter to discuss the complex issue of the treatment of women and babies with HIV disease and the opportunist infections associated with it. The treatment of HIV-infected women, and in particular pregnant women, is a very under-researched area. Current literature should be consulted for on-going trials and case reports.

Conclusion. The woman whose pregnancy is complicated by HIV infection will face a multitude of complex physical, social and emotional challenges during her pregnancy and after. It is essential that the care she is offered acknowledges those complex needs and attempts to respond to them.

This will be best achieved by continuity of care provided by a midwife who is sensitive to the woman's needs, well informed about HIV infection and who can contribute to and co-ordinate the appropriate medical and supportive services.

Reader Activities

1. Imagine that a woman in your local antenatal clinic wants to confide her worries about having been exposed to, or having symptoms of, a sexually-transmitted disease.

With a colleague, take the parts of woman and midwife, talking as if you were the real people, for about 10 minutes. You might like to make a tape recording of the conversation. At the end, debrief by saying, 'I am not X, Y, or Z (this woman or midwife). I am (your own name) and I am in (the place where you are).'

Then, play back the recording and discuss how it went. You might address:

- which aspects of the conversation were difficult and which worked well for the 'midwife'
- which were difficult and which worked well for the 'client'
- did the 'midwife' feel comfortable and confident of her knowledge and the advice she offered?

Try to explore with each other:

- why the midwife responded the way she did

- why she asked the questions she did
- why she offered information in the way she did
- whether the client found the interventions useful.

Each of you might choose to conduct the role play with another colleague, or again with one another, taking the opposite role.

2. Prepare a leaflet about safer sex.

Talking with women about sex and enabling them to express their concerns about sexual issues can be difficult, especially during pregnancy.

With a colleague or friend with whom you feel comfortable, try brainstorming about what it is that makes such discussion difficult. This might range from problems of language or assumptions about women and their sexual interests to the environment of the clinic.

Attempt to translate the results or insights of your brainstorming into a leaflet for women which might be a way of opening the possibility of discussion for them. The theme might be on 'safe sex' or another theme that you think is relevant to pregnant women.

REFERENCES

Abel E, von Unwerth L 1988 Asymptomatic chlamydia during pregnancy. Research in Nursing and Health, 11(6): 359–365

Adler M 1985 Sexually transmitted diseases. In: Holland W W, Detels R, Knox G (eds) Oxford textbook of public health. Oxford University Press, Oxford, vol 3(31)

Adler M W 1990 The ABC of sexually transmitted diseases, 2nd edn. British Medical Journal, London

Alger L S, Lovchik J C, Hebel J R et al 1988 The association of *Chlamydia trachomatis, Neisseria gonorrhoeae*, and group B streptococci with preterm rupture of the membrane and pregnancy outcome. American Journal of Obstetrics and Gynecology 159(2): 397–404

Anonymous 1988 Virological screening for herpes simplex virus during pregnancy. Lancet 24 September: 722–723

Bell T A, Grayson J T 1986 Centers for Disease Control: guidelines for prevention and control of *Chlamydia trachomatis* infections. Annals of Internal Medicine 104: 524–526

Biggar R J, Pahwa S, Minkoff H et al 1989 Immunosuppression in pregnant women infected with human immunodeficiency virus. American Journal of Obstetrics and Gynecology 161: 1239–1244

Boyd K M 1990 Institute of Medical Ethics: working party report: HIV infection: the ethics of anonymised testing and of testing pregnant women. Journal of Medical Ethics 16: 173–178

Brierley J, Roth C 1991 Pregnancy, childbirth and HIV infection. In: Claxton R, Harrison T (eds) Caring for children with HIV and AIDS. Edward Arnold, London

Brunham R C, Holmes K K, Embree J E 1990 Sexually transmitted diseases in pregnancy. In: Holmes K K, Mardh P A, Sparling P F et al (eds) Sexually transmitted diseases, 2nd edn. McGraw-Hill, New York

Centers for Disease Control 1988 Universal precautions for prevention of transmission of human immunodeficiency virus, hepatitis B virus and other blood borne pathogens in health care settings. Morbidity and Mortality Weekly Report 37: 377–388

Clay J C 1989 Antenatal screening for syphilis must continue. British Medical Journal 299: 409–410

Dunn D T, Newell M L, Ades, A E, Peckham C S 1992 Risk of human immunodeficiency virus type 1 transmission through breastfeeding. Lancet 340: 585–588

European Collaborative Study 1991 Children born to women with HIV-1 infection: natural history and risk of transmission. Lancet 337: 253–60

European Collaborative Study 1992 Risk factors for mother-to-child transmission of HIV-1. Lancet 339: 1007–1012

Global Programme on AIDS 1992 Consensus statement from the WHO/UNICEF constitution on HIV infection and breast-feeding. Weekly Epidemiological Record; 67: 177–184

Goodall B et al 1987 Introduction to Hepatitis B and nursing guidelines for infection control. Royal College of Nursing, London

Harris J R W 1975 Epidemiological and social aspects of candidiasis. In: Morton R S, Harris J R W (eds) Recent advances in sexually transmitted disease. Churchill Livingstone, Edinburgh, p 231–234

Horner P J, Goldmeier D, Byrne M, Hay P E 1989 Antenatal screening for syphilis (letter). British Medical Journal 299:859

International Nursing Review 1991 The UK women are complacent about AIDS. 38(1):5

Johnstone F, MacCallum L, Brettle R et al 1988 Does infection with HIV affect the outcome of pregnancy? British Medical Journal 496: 467

Lossick J G 1986 Sexually transmitted vaginitis. Seminars in Adolescent Medicine 2(2): 131–142

MacCallum L R, France A J, Jones M E 1988 The effects of pregnancy on the progression of HIV infection. IV International Conference on AIDS Stockholm, Abstract 4032

Minkoff H, Mead P 1986 An obstetric approach to the prevention of early onset group B beta-hemolytic streptococcal sepsis. American Journal of Obstetrics and Gynecology 154:973–977

Minkoff H L, Willoughby A, Mendez H et al 1990 Serious infections during pregnancy among women with advanced immunodeficiency virus infection. American Journal of Obstetrics and Gynecology 162(1): 30–34

Minkoff H L, DeHovitz J A 1990 Care of women infected with the human immunodeficiency virus. Journal of the American Medical Association 266(16): 2253–2258

Nahmias A J et al 1971 Perinatal risk associated with maternal genital herpes simplex virus infection. American Journal of Obstetrics and Gynecology 100: 825–833

O'Mahoney C, Holland N 1989 Antenatal screening for syphilis (letter). British Medical Journal 299:859

Pratt R J 1991 AIDS: a strategy for nursing care, 3rd edn. Edward Arnold, London

Prober C G et al 1987 Low risk of herpes simplex virus infections in neonates exposed to the virus at the time of vaginal delivery to mothers with recurrent genital herpes infections. New England Journal of Medicine 316: 240–244

Ryder R W, Nsa W, Hassig S E et al 1989 Perinatal transmission of the human immunodeficiency virus type 1 to infants of seropositive women in Zaire. New England Journal of Medicine 320: 1638–1642

Schachter J, Grossman M 1981 Chlamydial infections. Annual Review of Medicine 3: 45–61

Schaefer A, Grosch-Woerner I, Friedmann W et al 1988 The effects of pregnancy on the natural course of HIV infection. IV International Conference on AIDS Stockholm, Abstract 4039

Schoenbaum E E, Davenny K, Selwyn P A 1988 The impact of pregnancy on HIV-related disease. In: Hudson C N, Sharp F (eds) AIDS and obstetrics and gynaecology. Royal College of Obstetricians and Gynaecologists, London

Selwyn P A, Schoenbaum E E, Davenny K et al 1989 Prospective study of human immunodeficiency virus infection and pregnancy outcomes in intravenous drug users. Journal of the American Medical Association 261: 1289–1294

Stagno S, Whitley R J 1990 Herpesvirus infection in the neonate and children. In: Holmes K K, Mardh P A, Sparling P F et al (eds) Sexually transmitted diseases, 2nd edn. McGraw-Hill, New York

Stein Z A 1990 HIV prevention: the need for methods women can use. American Journal of Public Health 80(4): 460–462

Stray-Pederson B 1990 Acyclovir in late pregnancy to prevent neonatal herpes simplex. Lancet 336: 756

United Kingdom Central Council 1992 Code of Professional Conduct. UKCC, London

Wang E, Smaill F 1989 Infection in pregnancy. In: Chalmers I, Enkin M, Keirse M J N C (eds) Effective care in pregnancy and childbirth. Oxford University Press, Oxford

Williams K 1985 Screening for syphilis in pregnancy: an assessment of costs and benefits. Community Medicine 7: 37–42

FURTHER READING

Claxton R, Harrison T (eds) 1991 Caring for children with HIV and AIDS. Edward Arnold, London

Gordon P, Mitchell L 1988 Safer sex: a new look at sexual pleasure. Faber, London

Richardson D 1989 Women and the AIDS crisis, 2nd edn. Pandora Press, London

Vance C S (ed) 1984 Pleasure and danger: exploring female sexuality. Routledge Kegan Paul, London

CHAPTER

20

Disorders caused by pregnancy

SARAH KELLY

Many of the disorders associated with pregnancy are rarely seen today in their most severe forms. This is mainly due to improvements in the general health of the population, improved social conditions and lower parity. Regular antenatal health checks beginning in early pregnancy have contributed to the early diagnosis of such conditions and immediate and appropriate treatment has greatly influenced the reduction in maternal and fetal mortality resulting from them.

The midwife's role

The midwife's role in relation to the disorders specific to pregnancy is clear. At initial and subsequent encounters with the pregnant woman it is essential that an accurate health history is obtained. General and specific physical examinations must be carried out and the results meticulously recorded. The examination and recordings give direction towards future referral and management. Whilst the elements of antenatal care are routine for the midwife they will be very individual for the mother in her charge.

Where a complication of pregnancy is diagnosed the midwife must refer the mother to the appropriate registered medical practitioner.

VOMITING IN PREGNANCY

Vomiting is a common symptom in pregnancy and it is usually engendered by the pregnancy.

The less serious manifestation is that of morning sickness which occurs in 50% of women as a result of rising pregnancy hormones. It usually improves after 12–14 weeks' gestation without recurrence unless other factors producing increased pregnancy hormones are present, for example, hydatidiform mole, acute polyhydramnios and monozygotic twins (see Ch. 9).

It is important for the midwife to be aware that in some instances the usually innocuous morning sickness can persist throughout the day and inhibit any desire of the mother to eat and drink with the result that dehydration and ketosis develop. Whilst anti-emetic preparations would improve the situation they should only be administered on prescription as the chemical content of some preparations is known to induce malformations of the developing embryo. The mother will feel extremely miserable if the condition persists.

Hyperemesis gravidarum

Excessive vomiting in pregnancy is a rare condition found in approximately 1 in 500 pregnancies. Nausea and vomiting persist and dehydration and keto-acidosis escalate with the result that the serum electrolyte balance is disrupted. The liver and kidney tissues necrose and malfunction, polyneuritis and encephalopathy may result due to lack of vitamin B, and sodium and potassium imbalance affects the activity of the heart musculature.

Vomiting over an extended period affects the availability of the intrinsic factor essential for the absorption of vitamin B_{12}. The vitamin C and folic acid levels fall and the whole results in anaemia.

The aetiology of hyperemesis gravidarum is unclear but it is known to be associated with multiple pregnancy, hydatidiform mole and a history of unsuccessful pregnancies. A proportion of women who experience this condition will have a recurrence in subsequent pregnancies.

Assessing the mother's condition

An accurate history regarding previous pregnancy experiences is essential. Evidence of vomiting in previous pregnancies will alert the midwife to a possible recurrence.

The midwife should enquire of all women who attend for early antenatal care whether they are experiencing nausea or vomiting and the answer should be recorded. On subsequent encounters with the mother the midwife should ask if the symptoms have improved and whether normal diet has been resumed and tolerated. It is also important to identify any events producing stress or anxiety as these may exacerbate any vomiting. The midwife should ascertain whether the nausea and vomiting are accompanied by pain; the location of any pain should be elicited. This information is essential if the correct cause of the vomiting is to be diagnosed.

The mother's appearance should be observed and dryness or inelasticity of the skin should be noted. Where the condition has become serious, jaundice may be apparent which signifies liver damage. The mother's breath will smell of acetone; her tongue and oral mucosa will be dry and pale if anaemia is present. Her eyes will appear dry and sunken and she may complain of blurred vision. The mother's weight will be less than expected for gestation. She may even have lost weight since the beginning of the pregnancy. Lack of food and persistent vomiting will result in anaemia.

The pulse rate will be weak and rapid and the blood pressure will be low. The urine will smell of acetone, be scant and dark in colour and should be tested for specific gravity, acetone, bile, protein and sugar. A midstream specimen should be obtained for laboratory examination, especially if protein is found, so that urinary tract infection may be excluded as a cause for the vomiting.

Where vomiting has persisted into the second trimester the midwife should perform an abdominal examination and note and record any deviation from the normal. Multiple pregnancy or hydatidiform mole may be suspected if the uterus is larger than expected for gestation. Absence of fetal movements after the 18th week in a multigravida or after the 20th week in a primigravida may be suggestive of a hydatidiform mole.

Having completed her examination the midwife should carefully record her findings and contact a medical practitioner, giving a concise appraisal of the situation so that swift and appropriate action may be instituted.

It is usual for a mother suffering from hyperemesis gravidarum to be admitted to hospital. This enables the obstetrician to undertake further examinations and monitor the progress of the disorder once treatment has commenced. It has the added advantage of enabling the mother to have adequate rest, especially if she has small children at home who demand her attention.

The midwife should be sensitive to the effects on the family when the mother is removed from the home environment. She may need to inform the social worker or health visitor of the family's need.

Aims of care

The general aims of care are:

- to identify the cause of the vomiting
- to give treatment which will stop the vomiting and reverse the effects of starvation and dehydration
- to provide a tranquil atmosphere in which the mother can return to good health.

The role of the midwife is to provide emotional support for the mother and her family, to make regular assessments of the maternal condition and carry out treatment prescribed by a medical practitioner.

Treatment

The midwife should receive the mother with an awareness of her psychological needs. She may be fearful of losing the pregnancy or feel guilty that her body is reacting abnormally and almost certainly feels a loss of control. Calm reassurance and sensitive information-giving should be accompanied by competent attention to physical needs.

On arrival in hospital blood will be taken to determine the plasma electrolytes. The potassium and sodium levels will be corrected by intravenous therapy, and dehydration and ketosis will be corrected with an infusion of dextrose 5%. Similarly the serum electrolyte levels will be corrected by the administration of Hartmann's solution. The infusion will be continued until hydration and electrolytes return to normal. Vitamins B_{12} and C, folic acid and iron will be required to correct the anaemia if it is present. Promethazine 25 mg may be given if the vomiting persists and a sedative may be prescribed to produce rest. The mother should not be given food or fluid whilst the vomiting persists, although small quantities of ice to suck may keep the mouth moist.

It will be necessary for the midwife to observe the blood pressure, pulse rate and temperature at least 4-hourly and to test the urine twice daily for specific gravity, acetone, sugar, protein and bile. The intake and output of fluids, including vomitus, will need assiduous monitoring and recording.

A marked improvement in the mother's general condition will be apparent in response to treatment. Once vomiting has ceased for a period of 24 hours, oral fluids may be commenced and if these are tolerated a light diet may follow. Normal food is gradually introduced and intravenous therapy discontinued.

The mother should be made as comfortable as possible throughout these ministrations.

Regular oral and general hygiene should be carried out. Vomitus must be removed from the vicinity of the mother as the odour may precipitate further vomiting.

The mother may feel cold due to general debility and the environment should be maintained at a suitable temperature. Bed linen should be changed for comfort, particularly if it becomes soiled.

Once the mother's health is stable and she feels well enough to return home she will be able to do so. The midwife may visit regularly for a short time until the mother settles into her home routine.

Very occasionally the disorder fails to improve with the treatment outlined above and the mother will subside into a coma and be in danger of dying. Termination of pregnancy is indicated to save the mother's life. The method will depend upon the length of the pregnancy (see Ch. 18).

This will be an added distress for the mother and her family and they will require emotional support from all members of the team involved with the care.

Vomiting at any time is extremely debilitating for the sufferer. Even when transient it will predispose to depression. Great sensitivity on the part of the midwife and other members of the team will be required if vomiting is prolonged. It is important to advise the mother's family that a restful home environment will contribute to her recovery and prevent a recurrence of the symptoms. Help may be required in the home for a short period after the mother's discharge from hospital and if there are no relatives to assist, the midwife may ask the social services for a home help.

Other causes of vomiting

Whilst vomiting may be pregnancy-induced the midwife should not lose sight of the fact that a pregnant woman is susceptible to illnesses and disorders which cause vomiting. The history relative to the onset of vomiting in conjunction with the presenting signs and symptoms will assist in making a differential diagnosis.

Urinary tract infection

Infections in the urinary tract often cause vomiting and the mother may present with a history of frequency of micturition, dysuria and possibly loin pain before vomiting occurs. There may be a history of previous or recurrent urinary tract infection and a urine test will identify protein; acetone, bile and sugar will not be found. An odour of stale fish may be noticed. The infection will be accompanied by a marked pyrexia (up to 40°C) and rigors may be a feature.

In contrast to hyperemesis gravidarum, the onset of symptoms is sudden and the mother rarely presents with signs of starvation. Whilst anaemia may be present the underlying cause is renal impairment causing a reduction in erythropoietin which results in the production of immature red cells (see Ch. 22).

Appendicitis

During pregnancy the appendix is displaced in an upward direction by the enlarging uterus which makes the diagnosis of appendicitis difficult. Pain and tenderness may be mistaken for a threatened abortion in the early weeks of pregnancy; there wil be no vaginal blood loss. Later in pregnancy as the appendix is further displaced, urinary tract infection may be suspected. With appendicitis, however, pain will be acute and will be in the abdomen rather than the loin and back.

There will be no protein, bile or sugar in the urine. The temperature is generally lower with appendicitis than with a urinary tract infection but the pulse rate may be higher.

Vomiting may also occur with the following disorders:

- acute polyhydramnios
- pre-eclampsia
- acute hepatic failure
- gastro-enteritis
- acute intestinal obstruction
- torsion of an ovarian cyst
- cerebral tumour.

ABDOMINAL PAIN IN PREGNANCY

Abdominal pain is quite common during pregnancy and it may be due to a variety of causes.

During the early weeks it may be occasioned by abortion or ectopic pregnancy (see Ch. 18). Occasionally pain is due to the presence of fibroids and these may be palpable during pregnancy as they enlarge when the muscle fibres hypertrophy.

Red degeneration of a fibroid

As the muscle fibres hypertrophy the fibroid (myoma) enlarges. Large fibroids situated within the myometrium may receive a diminished blood supply and occasionally the central core necroses. The cells of the capillaries supplying the area undergo haemolysis and aseptic inflammation occurs. The affected area is tender on palpation and there may be a low-grade pyrexia present.

The pain usually subsides with rest and analgesia and the pregnancy will progress to term. Occasionally enlargement of the fibroid may impede the progress of labour. Rupture of the uterus at the affected site is a possibility which should always be considered when caring for the mother in labour (see Ch. 27).

In the presence of a breech presentation an enlarged fibroid can impede the descent of the head. Manipulative procedures constitute a particular hazard to the integrity of the myometrium when fibroids are present.

Other causes of abdominal pain are given in Chapter 21.

PREGNANCY-INDUCED HYPERTENSION AND PRE-ECLAMPSIA

These terms are often used interchangeably but may be differentiated as follows:

Pregnancy-induced hypertension is a condition specific to pregnancy occurring mainly after the 28th week. It disappears following delivery.

Pre-eclampsia is similar but more severe and is also associated with proteinuria. As its name implies it may lead on to *eclampsia*.

Eclampsia is a very serious state in which generalised convulsions occur. The triennial report of maternal deaths in the United Kingdom 1985–1987 (DH et al 1991) identified that hypertensive disorders of pregnancy were the second most common cause of maternal death with 6.7 deaths per million (10^6) births from pre-eclampsia and 5.4 deaths/10^6 from eclampsia; cerebral haemorrhage and adult respiratory distress syndrome were the sequelae which resulted in most of these deaths.

Incidence

Between 5 and 8% of all pregnancies are complicated by hypertension and of these pre-eclampsia accounts for 80% (Llewellyn-Jones 1990). It occurs more frequently in young primigravidae, first pregnancies from a new partner and in mothers over 35 years of age. With the latter pre-eclampsia may be superimposed upon an already existing hypertension. It is known to be associated with hydatidiform mole, multiple pregnancy and diabetes and this is believed to be related to the greater mass of placental tissue. It is also more common in obese mothers and women from low socio-economic groups who may have inadequate antenatal care.

Careful observation of this disease worldwide has identified that the incidence varies with geographical location and race.

Aetiology

Much study has been devoted to the aetiology of pre-eclampsia but it still remains obscure. It has been referred to as a 'disease of theories' but MacGillivray (1983) suggested that it would be more appropriate to refer to pre-eclampsia as the 'disease of cascades' as there are so many systems involved and all interact one with another to form a type of cascade similar to that responsible for blood coagulation.

Pathological changes

Whilst cardiac output appears to decrease as pre-eclampsia worsens, generalised vasoconstriction occurs which affects much of the physiological activity of the tissues within the body. Capillary permeability increases and the fluid which escapes contributes to the oedema within the tissues. The presence of excess fluid within the cells impedes oxygenation and tissue hypoxia occurs which may cause tissue necrosis of the vital organs.

In the kidney vasospasm of the afferent arterioles results in a decreased renal blood flow which produces hypoxia and oedema of the endothelial cells of the glomerular capillaries. Fibrinoid deposits are laid down in the glomerular basement membrane as the condition worsens. Permeability increases and serum albumin filters through into the urine. This alters the plasma osmotic pressure resulting in tissue fluid retention producing generalised oedema. The circulating plasma volume is reduced resulting in haemoconcentration.

Disseminated intravascular coagulation (DIC) results and as the process progresses fibrin and platelet deposits occur in many organs including the brain and liver.

The uterus is also affected, particularly the vessels supplying the placental bed. Vasoconstriction and DIC reduce the uterine blood flow and vascular lesions occur in the placental bed. Placental abruption can be the result. Reduction in blood flow to the choriodecidual spaces diminishes the oxygen which diffuses through the cells of the syncytiotrophoblast and cytotrophoblast into the fetal circulation within the placenta. The result is that the placental tissue becomes ischaemic, the capillaries in the chorionic villi thrombose and infarctions occur. Hormonal output is impaired with reduced placental function. This has serious implications for the survival of the fetus. In their research into Doppler umbilical and uterine flow wave forms in severe pregnancy hypertension, Trudinger & Cook (1989) concluded that an abnormal Doppler flow velocity wave form correlated with adverse fetal outcome. They also suggested that the associated placental lesion may precede the maternal hypertension.

The liver is affected in severe cases where intracapsular haemorrhages and necrosis occur. Oedema of the liver cells produces epigastric pain and impaired liver function may result in jaundice.

The brain becomes oedematous and this, in conjunction with DIC, can produce thrombosis and necrosis of the blood vessel walls resulting in cerebrovascular accident. DIC was identified in 12 women out of 27 who died as a result of pre-eclampsia or eclampsia in the triennium 1985–87 (DH et al 1991). Sheehan identified that cerebral venous thrombosis could account for eclampsia occurring in the postpartum period (cited in MacGillivray 1983).

The lungs become congested with fluid in severe cases; oxygenation is impaired and cyanosis occurs.

Diagnosis of pre-eclampsia

Symptoms are rarely experienced by the mother until the disease has arrived at an advanced state. It is possible to identify the onset by the following which are known as the *cardinal signs*:

- **Blood pressure.** A rise of 15–20 mmHg above the mother's normal *diastolic* pressure or an increase above 90 mmHg on two occasions elicited at least 6 hours apart when the mother has been at rest signifies that cardiovascular changes have taken place. A diastolic increase is significant because the diastolic pressure is not affected by excitement. A marked increase in the systolic pressure above that expected for the mother's age, for example 140–170 mmHg is also important to note.

In order to detect an incipient increase the midwife should take the mother's blood pressure early in pregnancy and compare this with all subsequent recordings, taking into account the normal pattern in pregnancy. The pressure identified at the muffling stage is a more accurate measurement of the diastolic pressure and should be the one recorded.

- **Proteinuria** in the absence of urinary tract infection is indicative of renal damage.

If the midwife identifies protein in a midstream specimen of urine, laboratory investigation is essential. The amount of protein in the urine is frequently taken as an index of the severity of pre-eclampsia.

- **Oedema** of the ankles in late pregnancy is a common occurrence and may be found in 40% of pregnant mothers. It is of a dependent nature, usually disappears overnight and is not significant in the absence of raised blood pressure and proteinuria. Oedema affects approximately 85% of women with pre-eclampsia. It may appear rather suddenly and be associated with a rapid rate of weight gain (Wallenburg 1989). Generalised oedema is significant and may be classified as occult or clinical.

Occult oedema may be suspected if there is a marked increase in weight but this may be due to causes other than fluid retention.

At each encounter with the mother when antenatal screening is carried out the midwife should obtain and record the mother's weight. If the weight is in excess of that anticipated for gestation, the midwife will see the mother more frequently and notify the mother's medical practitioner of her findings.

Clinical oedema may be mild or severe in nature and the severity is related to the worsening of the pre-eclampsia. The oedema pits on pressure and may be found in the following anatomical areas:

- Feet, ankles and pre-tibial region.

• The hands. It may be noticed that the mother's rings are tight. It is advisable to ask her to remove them temporarily and the midwife may suggest that the mother wear them on a chain round her neck. The mother may be reluctant to remove her rings but should be encouraged to do so to prevent circulatory impairment should the oedema worsen.

• The lower abdomen. In the first instance the midwife will probably identify abdominal oedema by the circular indentation caused when using Pinard's stethoscope when listening to the fetal heart sounds.

• The vulva. This is an uncomfortable and distressing occurrence for the mother and fortunately it rarely occurs.

• Sacral oedema generally occurs when the mother is confined to bed.

• Facial oedema may be mild resulting in puffiness of the eyelids. The mother may have observed that her face feels tight in the mornings.

The midwife should remember that excessive tissue fluid responds to gravitational pull and should examine the most appropriate anatomical site in order to identify the presence of oedema.

In the presence of two of the three cardinal signs a provisional diagnosis of pre-eclampsia may be made. Proteinuria is considered to be the most serious manifestation and a significant increase in proteinuria coupled with diminished urinary output indicates serious renal impairment.

Classification

Mild pregnancy-induced hypertension is diagnosed when, after resting, the mother's diastolic blood pressure rises 15–20 mmHg above the basal blood pressure recorded in early pregnancy or when the diastolic blood pressure rises above 90 mmHg. Oedema of the feet, ankles and pretibial region may be present.

Moderate pre-eclampsia is usually diagnosed when there is a marked rise in the systolic and diastolic pressure, when proteinuria is present in the absence of a urinary tract infection and when there is evidence of a more generalised oedema.

Severe pre-eclampsia is diagnosed when the blood pressure exceeds 170/110 mmHg, when there is an increase in the proteinuria and where oedema is marked. The mother may complain of frontal headaches and visual disturbance.

Effects on the mother

• The condition may worsen and eclampsia may occur (see below).

• Placental abruption may occur with all the complications stated in Chapter 21.

• Haematological disturbance can occur and the kidneys, lungs, heart and liver may be seriously damaged.

• The capillaries within the fundus of the eye may be irreparably damaged and blindness can occur.

Effects on the fetus

• Reduced placental function can result in low birth weight. This will be further aggravated if the mother smokes.

• There is an increased incidence of hypoxia in both the antenatal and intranatal periods.

• Placental abruption, if minor, will contribute to fetal hypoxia; if major, intra-uterine death will occur.

• Early delivery if the disease worsens, or if abruption occurs, will produce a preterm baby requiring resuscitation.

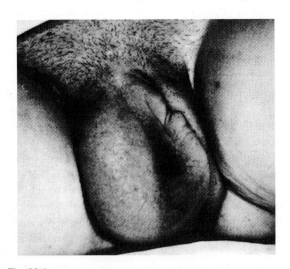

Fig. 20.1
Oedema of the vulva.

The midwife's role in detection

Whilst it is unlikely that pregnancy-induced hypertension can be prevented, early detection and appropriate management can minimise the severity of the disease. A high standard of antenatal care will contribute to the maintenance of good health. The midwife is in a unique position to identify those mothers with a predisposition to pre-eclampsia. She will start at their first meeting by taking a careful history, particularly noting the following:

— adverse social circumstances or poverty which could prevent her from attending for regular antenatal care
— a familial tendency towards hypertension
— the mother's age and parity
— any history of renal disease
— any new partnership
— a past history of pre-eclampsia.

On subsequent visits the midwife must take note of any further predisposing factors such as multiple pregnancy. The mother's weight, urine and blood pressure are monitored carefully.

If the midwife identifies any abnormality the mother should be referred to a registered medical practitioner so that appropriate care can be commenced. The mother may be admitted directly from the antenatal clinic to a maternity unit for care and treatment.

A mother who has mild pregnancy-induced hypertension may be advised to return home and go to bed where she will be visited by the midwife or doctor once or twice weekly or on a daily basis until the condition improves. Where there are children at home, relatives may be called upon to help; otherwise Social Services can be asked to provide a home help.

If the mother is in her own home when the diagnosis is made, the midwife should advise the mother to rest in bed.

The mother may feel very well and energetic with mild or moderate pre-eclampsia and both she and her husband may be surprised when bed rest is advised. A clear but simple explanation of the situation should be given and the need for rest reinforced without aggravating their anxiety.

Occasionally a community midwife may encounter a mother with severe pre-eclampsia. This may be in a mother who has not received antenatal care, either due to default or because the pregnancy has been concealed.

A medical practitioner should be informed or there may be a need to call out the emergency obstetric team. The midwife should remain with the mother and commence the examinations and recordings which are given later in this chapter.

The midwife will need to be sensitive to the needs of the family when the mother is admitted to hospital. Visiting may be limited to her immediate family: if the mother's condition permits, her own children should be encouraged to visit. The mother will be anxious about the well-being of her other children, especially if she feels well enough to be at home, and their visits will allay many of her fears. The mother and her partner will be very anxious about the progress of the current pregnancy, and sensitive counselling, emotional support and encouragement will be required of the midwife.

The aims of care

The aims of care are to provide rest and a tranquil environment, to monitor the disease and to prevent it worsening by giving appropriate care and treatment. The ultimate aim is to prolong the pregnancy until the baby is sufficiently mature to survive while safeguarding the mother's life.

Management of pregnancy-induced hypertension

Depending upon the severity of the disease a mother may be admitted to a multi-bedded ward or to a single room. Treatment is symptomatic because the cause of pre-eclampsia is unknown.

Bed rest. The mother should be nursed in bed and will be encouraged to adopt a sitting position or to lie on her side in order to encourage uterine blood flow. A supine position predisposes to aortocaval compression. Bed rest has the added advantage of reducing oedema by improving the renal circulation, facilitating kidney filtration and producing a diuresis. There is usually a reduction in blood pressure with bed rest. Except in severe cases the mother may get up for toilet facilities. Where pre-eclampsia is severe high dependency care should be instituted.

Diet. There is little evidence to support dietary intervention for preventing or restricting the advance of pre-eclampsia. As for any pregnant woman a diet rich in protein, fibre and vitamins may be recommended. There is no reason to support attempts at weight restriction or low-salt diets (Green 1989). Fluids should be encouraged. In very severe pre-eclampsia intravenous therapy will be used but oral fluids may still be given.

Weight should be estimated and recorded twice weekly if the mother is ambulant and *oedema* should be observed daily.

Urine should be tested for protein and ketones twice daily and specimens should be sent to the laboratory as ordered so that the levels of protein can be estimated. The level of protein indicates the degree of vascular damage. It also signifies the degree to which the fetus is at risk. 24-hour urine samples may be obtained three times a week in order to estimate the oestriol levels as an indication of placental function.

Fluid intake and output should be conscientiously measured. Adequate urine output signifies good renal function; oliguria or urinary suppression may occur if the disease becomes severe.

Blood pressure is ascertained 4-hourly in moderate pre-eclampsia but will be taken 2-hourly or more frequently if the mother is severely affected.

Abdominal examination will be carried out at least twice daily. Any discomfort, tenderness or pain experienced by the mother should be recorded and reported immediately to the doctor.

The fetal heart rate should be elicited when the abdominal examination is performed. A cardiotocograph machine used for 20 minutes twice daily will indicate uterine activity in addition to supplying further details about the fetal heart including its response to uterine contraction and fetal movement.

Kick charts are maintained to monitor the degree of fetal movement and serial *ultrasonic scans* are undertaken to assess fetal growth.

Aspirin treatment may be in use in some maternity units to prevent pre-eclampsia and intra-uterine growth retardation. Low doses of 60–75 mg may be started after 12–14 weeks' gestation when embryonic development is complete. A collaborative trial of low-dose aspirin in pregnancy (CLASP) is in progress at the time of writing (McParland et al 1990).

Sedation may be prescribed if the mother needs to be encouraged to rest and sleep. Sedatives do not improve the pre-eclampsia directly.

Hypotensive agents are prescribed where there is a marked increase in the blood pressure. An example of such medication is methyldopa 250 mg three times daily. The treatment is instituted to prevent cerebrovascular accidents.

Anticonvulsant therapy may be used where the condition is severe, for example diazepam 10–20 mg orally or intramuscularly.

The duration of the care and treatment will depend upon the severity of the pregnancy-induced hypertension, the response to treatment and the period of gestation.

When the pregnancy-induced hypertension remains mild, labour will be induced at term if it has not begun spontaneously prior to this.

If the serum urate levels rise or the urinary and plasma oestriol levels are below the normal levels for gestation, delivery will be expedited either by caesarean section or by induction of labour.

Management of labour

The midwife should remain with the mother throughout the course of labour. Pre-eclampsia can suddenly worsen at any time and it is essential to document the presence of oedema, the blood pressure, urinary output and the result of urinalysis at the outset so that any marked deviation will be noted and medical assistance sought. The mother should be made as comfortable as possible which will necessitate attention to oral and bodily hygiene at regular intervals. The bed linen should be changed frequently as amniotic fluid usually drains throughout. Positioning the mother on her side will prevent supine hypotension. *Epidural analgesia* may procure the best pain relief, reduce the blood pressure and facilitate rapid caesarean section should the need arise. The midwife should encourage the mother to move her legs. If she is unable to do so, passive leg exercises will stimulate the circulatory return to the heart.

Care of the bladder is essential and the mother should be encouraged to void urine regularly. All specimens should be tested for protein, ketones and glucose and the results recorded. If intravenous dextrose is being administered it is unusual for ketones to be present in the urine. If the mother does develop keto-acidosis, the fetus is at great risk. Maternal acid–base balance must be returned to normal immediately.

The blood pressure and pulse rate should be elicited half-hourly. *Respirations* may need to be observed hourly if there is pulmonary oedema and the *temperature* should be taken 4-hourly.

Abdominal examination should be performed on transfer to the delivery suite and at regular intervals in order to assess the progress of labour.

The fetal heart should be recorded at least half-hourly if a Pinard's stethoscope is used. A cardiotocograph will permit observation of the heart rate throughout a contraction which is advantageous. The midwife should conscientiously record all her findings and summon medical assistance if any deviation from the normal is observed.

When the second stage commences the obstetrician and paediatrician should be notified. The latter will be present at the delivery in case the baby requires resuscitation. The midwife will continue her care of the mother throughout the second stage and will usually deliver the baby. Occasionally a short second stage is prescribed and in this instance the obstetrician will perform a forceps delivery.

Care after delivery

The blood pressure will be recorded after delivery and at least 4-hourly for 24 hours. If proteinuria has been present the urine should be tested once or twice daily until it is clear and urinary output should be recorded. Any other treatment prescribed should be carried out. Postnatal care will be as normal.

Signs of impending eclampsia

The midwife must be vigilant in monitoring the maternal condition and be alert to the following signs and symptoms which signal the onset of eclampsia:

- A sharp rise in blood pressure
- Diminished urinary output which is due to acute vasospasm
- Increase in proteinuria caused by decreased glomerular filtration
- Headache which is usually severe, persistent and frontal or occipital in location
- Drowsiness or confusion due to cerebral oedema
- Visual disturbances such as blurring of vision or flashing lights due to retinal oedema
- Nausea and vomiting
- Epigastric pain which denotes liver oedema and impairment of liver function. The mother may interpret this pain as indigestion.

The midwife who observes any one of these signs in a woman with pre-eclampsia must make a full examination in order to establish if others are present. Meanwhile she must summon a registrar or consultant immediately and remain with the mother. Assistance will be required to prepare necessary equipment and medication.

The aims of care at this time are to control hypertension, prevent convulsions and coma and to prevent death of the mother and fetus. Treatment is intensified to this end and delivery will be expedited either by induction or by caesarean section. In some instances eclampsia will occur before medical assistance arrives. This constitutes an emergency situation. A midwife must be able to preserve the mother's life until help arrives.

ECLAMPSIA

Eclampsia is rarely seen today especially if there are good facilities for antenatal care. Usually pregnancy-induced hypertension is diagnosed and treatment instituted in order to prevent eclampsia. Occasionally pre-eclampsia is so rapid in onset and progress that eclampsia ensues before any action can be taken. In this situation pre-eclampsia is termed *fulminating*.

The incidence of eclampsia is approximately 1 in 1500 pregnancies and of these about 20% occur in the antenatal period, 25% occur intrapartum and 35% within the first few hours after delivery. Eclampsia is characterised by convulsions and coma and the progress of the convulsion is usually described in four stages.

The stages of an eclamptic fit

Premonitory stage (lasts 10–20 seconds). The mother is restless and rapid eye movements can be noted. The head may be drawn to one side and twitching of the facial muscles may occur. The mother has no perception of the impending fit and shows altered awareness.

Tonic stage (lasts 10–20 seconds). The muscles of the mother's body go into spasm and become rigid and her back may become arched. Her teeth will become tightly clenched and her eyes staring. As the diaphragm is in spasm, *the mother's respiration is checked and cyanosis ensues*.

The clonic stage (lasts 60–90 seconds). Violent contraction and intermittent relaxation of the mother's muscles produces convulsive movements and these may be very severe. Salivation increases and foaming at the mouth occurs. This will be bloodstained if the mother bites her tongue during this episode.

The mother's face becomes congested and bloated and the features become distorted. She is unconscious, her breathing stertorous and her pulse full and bounding. Gradually the convulsion subsides.

Stage of coma. Stertorous breathing continues and coma may persist for minutes or hours. Further convulsions may occur before the mother regains consciousness.

Care of a mother with eclampsia

The aims of immediate care are to:

- clear and maintain the mother's airway. This may be achieved by the insertion of an airway as soon as the premonitory stage is observed, by placing the mother in a semi-prone position in order to facilitate the drainage of saliva and vomitus and by aspirating if suction facilities are available
- administer oxygen and prevent severe hypoxia
- prevent the mother from being injured during the clonic stage.

The midwife must remain with the mother constantly. She will assist the doctor who arrives in answer to her summons. In the first instance all effort is devoted to the preservation of the mother's life and the well-being of the baby is secondary. This may seem arbitrary but if the mother dies fetal death is inevitable.

Treatment may be given as follows:

- Intravenous therapy will be commenced to maintain adequate hydration. The regimen will be prescribed according to the mother's needs and keto-acidosis must be prevented. Dextrose 5% will be used for intravenous drug administration.
- Intravenous diazepam 10 mg is usually administered as a bolus injection, followed by 40 mg in 500 ml of dextrose 5% at 60 drops per minute or via a titration pump. This will prevent convulsions and produce relaxation in the mother. A suitable alternative to diazepam may be prescribed and the regimen for administration stipulated.
- Where the hypertension is severe and requires rapid reduction, intravenous hydrallazine 10 mg may be given. When administered via the intravenous route it is given very slowly and the blood pressure will be estimated at 5-minute intervals until the diastolic pressure reaches a sufficiently low and safe level. Once the blood pressure is reduced it can be maintained at a satisfactory level by the continued administration of hydrallazine.

   The midwife should be aware that hydrallazine can precipitate headache, vomiting and muscle tremors.
- When prolonged intravenous therapy is necessary it is usual to establish a central venous pressure line.
- The volume of urine and the albuminuria need to be monitored 4-hourly and to this end a self-retaining catheter is inserted into the bladder. This may be left on continuous

drainage or spigotted and released at regular intervals. It is important that specimens collected for testing are fresh and that they are not removed from the drainage container.

- Blood specimens will be obtained for cross-matching and haemoglobin estimation so that blood is available for transfusion should haemorrhage occur at delivery. The blood samples may also be used for other biochemical tests.

The role of the midwife

The mother will require intensive care as she may remain comatose for a time or may be heavily sedated.

Recordings should be carried out as previously mentioned for severe pre-eclampsia. The midwife must observe for periodic restlessness associated with uterine contraction, which indicates that labour has commenced.

If he is not present the mother's partner should be informed as soon as possible. The midwife will need to give him emotional support through this unexpected and anxious time.

It is usual to expedite delivery of the baby as soon as possible when eclampsia occurs. In this instance caesarean section is the usual mode of delivery. The next of kin is usually required to give consent for surgery.

As soon as the baby is delivered the partner should be encouraged to hold the baby and accompany him to the neonatal intensive care unit where he is to be cared for. It is important that the partner has early interaction with the baby so that he can give the mother an account of the baby's progress from the time of birth. A photograph is taken of the baby so that the mother can see it as soon as she recovers from the anaesthetic.

Intensive care will be continued when the mother returns from theatre and this is usually maintained for 24–48 hours. Convulsions rarely occur after this time. It is important to note that there is an increased risk of pulmonary embolism following caesarean section for fulminating pre-eclampsia (DH 1989).

All the usual postpartum care is given and as soon as the mother's condition permits she should be taken in her bed or a chair to see her baby.

Alternatively if the baby's condition is good he may be returned to his mother.

Complications of eclampsia

Cerebral: haemorrhage, thrombosis and mental confusion.
Renal: acute renal failure.
Hepatic: liver necrosis.
Cardiac: myocardial failure.
Respiratory: asphyxia, pulmonary oedema, bronchopneumonia.
Visual: temporary blindness.
Injuries: bitten tongue, fractures.
Fetal: hypoxia and stillbirth.

Future management

There is no indication that pregnancy-induced hypertension causes later hypertensive disease but it can bring to the fore an inherent disposition towards hypertension.

Usually the blood pressure returns to normal within several weeks but the protein may persist for a longer period. 6 months after delivery the mother is examined by the obstetrician and if all is well she will be discharged and advised to seek advice as soon as a subsequent pregnancy occurs.

The mother may have very little recollection of the birth and the events surrounding it if she was unconscious or heavily sedated at the time. It is essential that the midwife enquire further if a mother gives no clear history of a previous delivery or if she says that she was ill. It is advisable to obtain the previous case notes where possible. In this way good care can be provided and prophylactic management established where indicated.

PELVIC ARTHROPATHY

Pelvic arthropathy is characterised by abnormal relaxation of the ligaments supporting the pubic joint. This is brought about by high levels of pregnancy hormones. The result of the relaxation is increased mobility of the joint; the pubic bones move up and down alternately as the mother walks. Strain on the sacro-iliac joints may also occur. This is more common in grande multiparae.

Symptoms and signs

The mother will complain of pain in the pubic region and of backache. Pain may be experienced in the abdominal muscles due to an attempt to stabilise the bones by muscular action.

On examination the mother will complain of tenderness over the pubic symphysis.

Care of the mother

The midwife should note whether there is any history of pelvic fractures which may be aggravated by the pregnancy. Otherwise the midwife should explain to the mother the cause of this anomaly and advise her to rest as much as possible especially as the pregnancy advances and abdominal distension increases. The mother should be advised to wear a supportive panty-girdle when she is up and about.

The midwife should notify the doctor of this condition and of the advice which she has given. In severe cases, bed rest may be necessary. A fracture board will be required.

The ligaments should slowly return to normal following delivery. Physiotherapy will aid the strengthening and stabilisation of the joint.

JAUNDICE IN PREGNANCY

The metabolic changes in pregnancy influence hepatic function. These changes are brought about by the increased hormone levels.

Pregnancy may worsen an already existing liver disease or the mother may become infected with viral hepatitis. Jaundice may accompany severe pre-eclampsia and severe hyperemesis gravidarum. Occasionally a mother may have jaundice associated with obstruction of the common bile duct due to gallstones.

The midwife should refer the mother to a medical practitioner immediately if jaundice is observed.

Very rarely, *acute yellow atrophy of the liver* occurs. This is associated with vomiting, haematemesis and abdominal pain in the third trimester and is a severe complication of pregnancy which may result in maternal death. It may be associated with the administration of large doses of drugs in pregnancy.

SKIN DISORDERS

Herpes gestationis is a disease specific to pregnancy which usually occurs in the mid-trimester and persists into the postnatal period.

Signs and symptoms

The mother complains of generalised itching of the skin and a burning sensation. An erythematous rash appears. This is initially over the abdomen and it spreads to involve the remainder of the trunk and limbs. Blisters develop which may become infected and purulent, especially if the mother scratches.

Management

The midwife should refer the mother to a medical practitioner and be supportive to the mother throughout her care.

The lesions should be kept clean and may be covered to prevent the mother scratching. A diet high in vitamins should be encouraged.

The mother will usually have her labour induced at about the 37th week of pregnancy. The baby may have a rash when born and will need paediatric examination and treatment.

Prognosis

The condition may recur in subsequent pregnancies.

Reader Activities

- Take the blood pressure in the right arm of a pregnant woman who is lying on her left side. Take it again in the same arm when the woman has turned so that her brachial artery is level with the left atrium of her heart. You should be listening for the fourth Korotkoff sound which is when the sound becomes muffled. What difference did you notice? For a discussion of the significance of your findings see Wallenburg (1989).
- Talk to a woman who has been admitted to hospital for rest in pregnancy because she has hypertension. Find out how this has affected her and her family socially and psychologically.

REFERENCES

Department of Health, Welsh Office, Scottish Home and Health Department, Department of Health and Social Services, Northern Ireland 1991 Report on confidential enquiries into maternal deaths in the United Kingdom 1985–87. HMSO, London

Department of Health 1989 Report on confidential enquiries into maternal deaths in England and Wales 1982–84. HMSO, London

Green J 1989 Diet and the prevention of pre-eclampsia. In: Chalmers I, Enkin M, Keirse M J N C Effective care in pregnancy and childbirth. Oxford University Press, Oxford

Llewellyn-Jones D 1990 Fundamentals of obstetrics and gynaecology. Vol 1 Obstetrics, 5th edn. Faber & Faber, London

MacGillivray I 1983 Pre-eclampsia, the hypertensive disease of pregnancy. W B Saunders, London

McParland P, Pearce J M, Chamberlain G V P 1990 Doppler ultrasound and aspirin in recognition and prevention of pregnancy-induced hypertension. Lancet 335(June): 1552–1555

Trudinger B J, Cook C M 1990 Doppler umbilical and uterine flow wave forms in severe pregnancy hypertension. British Journal of Obstetrics and Gynaecology 97(2): 142–148

Wallenburg H C S 1989 Detecting hypertensive disorders of pregnancy. In: Chalmers I, Enkin M, Keirse M J N C Effective care in pregnancy and childbirth. Oxford University Press, Oxford

FURTHER READING

Davey D A, MacGillivray I 1988 The classification and definition of the hypertensive disorders of pregnancy. American Journal of Obstetrics and Gynecology 158(4): 892–898

de Swiet M 1990 The use of aspirin in pregnancy. Journal of Obstetrics and Gynaecology 10(6): 467–482

Perry I J et al 1991 Conflicting views on the measurement of blood pressure in pregnancy. British Journal of Obstetrics and Gynaecology 98(3): 241–243

Pickles C J, Symonds E M, Broughton Pipkin F 1989 The fetal outcome in a randomised double-blind controlled trial of labetalol versus placebo in pregnancy-induced hypertension. British Journal of Obstetrics and Gynaecology 96(1): 38–43

Pickles C 1987 Pregnancy-induced hypertension. Midwife, Health Visitor and Community Nurse 438–442

Plouin P F et al 1990 A randomised comparison of early with conservative use of antihypertensive drugs in the management of pregnancy-induced hypertension. British Journal of Obstetrics and Gynaecology 97(2): 134–141

Steel S A et al 1990 Early Doppler ultrasound screening in prediction of hypertensive disorders of pregnancy. Lancet 335(June): 1548–1551

Studd J 1985 Progress in obstetrics and gynaecology, vol 5. Churchill Livingstone, Edinburgh

Weigel M M, Weigel R M 1989 Nausea and vomiting of early pregnancy and pregnancy outcome: an epidemiological study. British Journal of Obstetrics and Gynaecology 96(11): 1312–1318

21

Disorders of the pregnancy

SARAH RANKIN

Antepartum haemorrhage

Blood coagulation failure

Disorders of the amniotic fluid

Maternal mortality due to severe haemorrhage continues to decline in the industrialised world but maternal morbidity remains a consistent feature. The situation is different in some parts of the developing world where Burke & Duigin (1991) describe the maternal mortality rates as 'appalling'.

Midwives need to be alert for the possibility of bleeding in late pregnancy. The effects of hypovolaemia and reduced haemostasis are features of moderate to severe haemorrhage and continue to place the life of the mother and unborn child at risk. Pre-eclampsia frequently co-exists with placental abruption which further compounds a potentially life-threatening situation.

ANTEPARTUM HAEMORRHAGE

Definition

Bleeding from the genital tract in late pregnancy, after the 28th week of gestation and before the onset of labour, is referred to as antepartum haemorrhage.

Effect on the fetus

Fetal mortality and morbidity are increased as a result of severe vaginal bleeding in pregnancy. Stillbirth or perinatal or neonatal death may occur. Premature placental separation and consequent hypoxia may result in the birth of a child who is mentally and physically handicapped.

Effect on the mother

If bleeding is severe, it may be accompanied by shock, disseminated intravascular coagulation and renal failure. The mother may die or be left with permanent ill-health.

These events are infrequently seen by practitioners in the UK.

Types of antepartum haemorrhage

If bleeding from local lesions of the genital tract (*incidental causes*) is excluded, vaginal bleeding in late pregnancy is confined to placental separation due to *placenta praevia* or *placental abruption*.

Initial appraisal of a woman with antepartum haemorrhage

When a woman first loses blood per vaginam during pregnancy, she has little idea of the cause and will find the episode frightening and disturbing. She may call the midwife or present herself at hospital. Her first need is for a feeling that someone capable is in control of the situation. She will fear that she is losing her baby; the partner may fear for the life of both mother and child. The midwife's role at this stage is to be supportive and to ascertain as much detail as possible of the history and the circumstances surrounding the blood loss. These will assist both in assessing the woman's condition and in making a diagnosis.

Assessment of physical condition

Maternal condition. The first priority is the well-being of the mother. The midwife will look for any pallor or breathlessness which may indicate shock. She will weigh up the woman's emotional state as she greets her and begins to ask for a history of events. She must generate the trust of both partners and remain calm.

Observation of pulse rate, respiratory rate, blood pressure and temperature will be made and recorded. The midwife must assess the amount of blood lost in order to ensure adequate fluid replacement. She will discuss with the couple how much has been lost earlier and should ask to see all soiled articles, retaining them for the doctor's inspection.

An abdominal examination is made, observing for signs that the woman is going into labour. *On no account must any vaginal or rectal examination be made* nor may an enema or suppository be given to a woman suffering from an antepartum haemorrhage.

Fetal condition. The mother should be asked if the baby has been moving as much as normal. The midwife must attempt to ausculate the fetal heart and may use ultrasound apparatus to obtain the information.

Factors to aid differential diagnosis

The location of the placenta is perhaps the most critical piece of information which will be needed in order to make a correct diagnosis; initially the midwife will not usually have this fact at her disposal. The following questions will help to arrive at a provisional diagnosis:

Pain. Did pain precede bleeding and is it continuous or intermittent?

Onset of bleeding. Was this associated with any event such as coitus?

Amount of visible blood loss. Is there any reason to suspect that some blood has been retained in utero?

Colour of the blood. Is it bright red or darker in colour?

Degree of shock. Is this commensurate with the amount of blood visible or more severe?

Consistency of the abdomen. Is it soft or tense and board-like?

Tenderness of the abdomen. Does the mother resent abdominal palpation?

Lie, presentation and engagement. Are any of these abnormal when taking account of parity and gestation?

Audibility of the fetal heart. Is the fetal heart heard?

Ultrasound scan. Does a scan suggest that the placenta is in the lower uterine segment?

Supportive treatment

After emotional reassurance the first need is for restoration of physical condition. This will necessitate fluid replacement, initially with a plasma expander and later with whole blood. If the mother is in severe pain she must have strong analgesia to help counteract shock. If the midwife is in attendance at home she must summon the emergency obstetric unit. The obstetric registrar will institute these measures before transfer of the woman to hospital.

Subsequent management depends on the definitive diagnosis.

Placenta praevia

The placenta is partially or wholly implanted in the lower uterine segment on either the anterior or posterior wall. The anterior location is less serious than the posterior.

The lower uterine segment grows and stretches progressively after the 12th week of pregnancy. In later weeks this may cause the placenta to separate and severe bleeding can occur. Bleeding is caused by shearing stress between the placental trophoblast and maternal venous blood sinuses. In some instances bleeding may be precipitated by coitus.

Placenta praevia places the mother and fetus at high risk and it constitutes an obstetric emergency. Medical assistance is vital if the lives of the mother and fetus are to be saved. Mothers with suspected placenta praevia should be transferred to a consultant obstetric unit either at the request of the general practitioner or via the obstetric emergency service.

Degrees of placenta praevia

Type 1 placenta praevia. The majority of the placenta is in the upper uterine segment. Vaginal delivery is possible. Blood loss is usually mild and the mother and fetus remain in good condition.

Type 2 placenta praevia. The placenta is partially located in the lower uterine segment near the internal cervical os (marginal placenta praevia). Vaginal delivery is possible particularly if the placenta is anterior. Blood loss is usually moderate, although the conditions of the mother

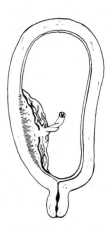 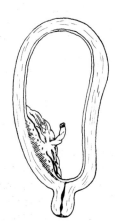 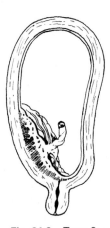 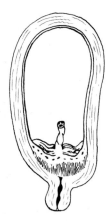

Fig. 21.1 Type 1.   **Fig. 21.2** Type 2.   **Fig. 21.3** Type 3.   **Fig. 21.4** Type 4.

Figs 21.1–21.4
Types of placenta praevia.

   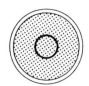

Fig. 21.5 Type 1.   **Fig. 21.6** Type 2.   **Fig. 21.7** Type 3.   **Fig. 21.8** Type 4.

Figs 21.5–21.8
Relationship of placenta praevia to cervical os.

and fetus can vary. Fetal hypoxia is more likely to be present than maternal shock.

Type 3 placenta praevia. The placenta is located over the internal cervical os but not centrally. Bleeding is likely to be severe particularly when the lower segment stretches and the cervix begins to efface and dilate in late pregnancy. Vaginal delivery is inappropriate because the placenta precedes the fetus.

Type 4 placenta praevia. The placenta is located centrally over the internal cervical os and torrential haemorrhage is very likely. Vaginal delivery should not be considered. Caesarean section is essential in order to save the life of the mother and fetus.

Indications of placenta praevia

Bleeding per vaginam is the only sign and it is painless. The uterus is not tender or tense. The presence of placenta praevia should be suspected when:

- the fetal head remains unengaged in a primigravida
- there is malpresentation, especially breech
- the lie is oblique or transverse
- the lie is unstable, usually in a multigravida.

Localisation of placenta using ultrasonic scanning will confirm the existence of placenta praevia and establish its degree.

Assessing the mother's condition

The amount of vaginal bleeding is variable. Some mothers may have a history of a small repeated blood loss at intervals throughout pregnancy. Others may have a sudden single episode of vaginal bleeding after the 20th week but severe haemorrhage occurs most frequently after the 34th week of pregnancy.

The haemorrhage may be mild, moderate or severe, is often not associated with any particular type of activity and may occur at rest.

The colour of the blood is bright red, denoting fresh bleeding. The low placental location allows all of the lost blood to escape unimpeded and a retroplacental clot is not formed. For this reason pain is not a feature of placenta praevia.

General examination. If the haemorrhage is slight the mother's blood pressure, respiratory rate and pulse rate may be normal.

In severe haemorrhage the blood pressure will be low and the pulse rate raised due to shock. The degree of shock correlates with the amount of blood lost per vaginam. Respirations are also rapid and the mother may have air hunger due to a reduction in the number of red blood cells in the circulation available for the uptake of oxygen. The mother's colour will be pale and her skin cold and moist. The temperature is usually normal as haemorrhage from a placenta praevia is not associated with infection.

Abdominal examination. The midwife may find that the lie of the fetus is oblique or transverse and the fetal head may be high in a primigravida near term. The uterine consistency is normal and there is no pain experienced by the mother when her abdomen is palpated.

The midwife *should not attempt to do a vaginal examination* as this could precipitate a torrential haemorrhage and worsen the situation.

An attempt should be made to quantify the amount of blood lost and all blood-soaked material used by the mother should be saved. Although this will not provide an accurate estimation of the quantity, it may be helpful.

Assessing the fetal condition

The mother should be asked whether fetal activity has been normal. She may be aware of diminution or cessation of fetal movements which may occur if fetal hypoxia is severe. In some instances she may report that her fetal movements have been excessive which is another indication of severe fetal hypoxia.

The midwife should assess the fetal condition using an electronic fetal monitor such as a cardiotocograph or Sonicaid machine. A Pinard fetal stethoscope may be used if these are not available. Fetal oxygenation depends upon the proportion of the placenta remaining attached. Fetal hypoxia is an emergency and medical assistance should be called urgently.

Management of placenta praevia

The management of placenta praevia depends on:

- the amount of bleeding
- the conditions of mother and fetus
- the location of the placenta
- the stage of the pregnancy.

Conservative management is appropriate if bleeding is slight and the mother and fetus are well. The woman will be kept in hospital at rest until bleeding has stopped. A speculum examination will have ruled out incidental causes. Further bleeding is inevitable if the placenta encroaches into the lower segment and therefore it is usual to require the woman to remain in hospital for the rest of the pregnancy. Placental function is monitored by means of fetal kick charts, antenatal cardiotocography and possibly hormonal assays. Ultrasound scans are repeated at intervals in order to observe the position of the placenta in relation to the cervical os as the lower segment grows. Fetal growth is also monitored.

A woman who is asked to stay in hospital for many weeks will have particular psychological and social needs. If she has other children, she will be anxious to know that good arrangements have been made for their care and they must be allowed to visit her frequently. She should be given parenthood education and sometimes may be able to continue with the group which she has been attending. Occupational therapy should be arranged.

If heavy bleeding should occur or when the fetus is mature, an examination per vaginam will be carried out under general anaesthetic. The theatre and personnel are in readiness for immediate caesarean section. The doctor will perform a gentle palpation through the vaginal fornices. If the placenta is felt, caesarean section will be performed without delay. If the placenta does not appear to be covering the os, a finger will be inserted through the cervix to explore the margins. If no placenta is felt, the membranes will be ruptured and labour induced with an oxytocin infusion.

Vaginal delivery is usual with Type 1 placenta praevia and possible with Type 2 unless the placenta is situated immediately above the sacral promontory where it is vulnerable to pressure from an advancing fetal head and may impede descent. The degrees of placenta praevia which are amenable to vaginal delivery may be termed *minor*.

The midwife should be aware that even if vaginal delivery is achieved, there remains a danger of postpartum haemorrhage because the placenta has been situated in the lower segment where there is paucity of oblique muscle fibres and therefore the living ligature action will be poor.

Active management. Severe vaginal bleeding will necessitate immediate delivery by caesarean section. This should take place in a unit with facilities for special care of the newborn especially if the baby will be preterm.

An intravenous infusion will be in progress and several units of blood must be cross-matched. In emergency it may be necessary to give Group O blood, if possible of the same Rhesus group as the mother.

During the assessment and preparation for theatre the mother will be extremely anxious and the midwife must comfort and encourage her, giving her as much information as possible. The partner will also need to be supported, especially if he has to wait outside the theatre during the operation.

If the placenta is situated anteriorly in the uterus, this may complicate the surgical approach as it underlies the site of the normal incision.

In major degrees of placenta praevia (types 3 and 4) caesarean section is required even if the fetus has died in utero. This will prevent torrential haemorrhage and possible maternal death.

Placenta accreta is now being encountered more frequently following previous caesarean section. Clark et al (1985) cited the incidence as being 'as high as 24% among patients with placenta praevia who had only one previous caesarean section'.

Incidence

Placenta praevia occurs in 0.5% of all pregnancies. It is more than twice as common in multigravidae, with an incidence of 1 in 90 deliveries. In primigravidae the incidence is 1 in 250 deliveries. Burke & Duigin (1991) found that 'placenta praevia remains one of the commonest causes of massive obstetric haemorrhage'.

Complications

Postpartum haemorrhage is the most probable complication following delivery. Oxytocic drugs should be given as the baby is delivered. Occasionally uncontrolled haemorrhage may continue and a caesarean hysterectomy may be required.

Other complications:

- maternal shock may result from blood loss and hypovolaemia
- maternal death occasionally ensues — the rate is between 0.1 and 3%
- fetal hypoxia due to placental separation
- fetal death — mortality is from 5 to 15%.

Placental abruption

Premature separation of a normally situated placenta occurring after the 28th week of pregnancy is known as a placental abruption.

The aetiology of this type of haemorrhage is not always clear, but it is often associated with pregnancy-induced hypertension or with a sudden reduction in uterine size. Rarely, direct trauma to the abdomen may partially dislodge the placenta.

Unlike inevitable haemorrhage which is due to placenta praevia, placental abruption is an accidental occurrence of haemorrhage in 2% of all pregnancies. Accidental in this context does not denote trauma.

Partial separation of the placenta causes bleeding from the maternal venous sinuses in the placental bed. Further bleeding continues to separate the placenta to a greater or lesser degree.

If blood escapes from the placental site it separates the membranes from the uterine wall and drains through the vagina.

Blood which is retained behind the placenta may be forced into the myometrium and it infiltrates between the muscle fibres of the uterus. This extravasation can cause marked damage. The uterus appears bruised and oedematous. This is termed *Couvelaire uterus* or *uterine apoplexy*. There is no vaginal bleeding. The mother will have all the signs and symptoms of hypovolaemic shock. This is caused by *concealed* bleeding into the muscle of the uterus. The concealed haemor-rhage causes uterine enlargement and extreme pain.

A combination of these two situations where some of the blood drains via the vagina and some is retained behind the placenta is known as a *mixed haemorrhage*.

Types of placental abruption

The blood loss from a placental abruption may be defined as revealed, concealed or mixed haemorrhage as described above. An alternative classification, based on the degree of separation and therefore related to the condition of mother and baby, is of mild, moderate and severe haemorrhage. The midwife cannot rely on visible blood loss as a guide to the severity of the haemorrhage; on the contrary, the most severe haemorrhage is that which is totally concealed.

Assessing the mother's condition

There may be a history of pregnancy-induced hypertension. A recent history of headaches, nausea, vomiting, epigastric pain and visual disturbances may be a feature. Road traffic accidents are probably the most likely cause of trauma to the abdomen. External cephalic version injudiciously performed may result in placental separation. The midwife should be aware of the possibility of placental separation after the birth of a first twin or loss of copious amounts of amniotic fluid.

The mildest degrees of placental abruption are relatively pain-free, although the mother may experience a slight localised pain. The blood loss is revealed. More severe degrees are associated with abdominal pain and the midwife should enquire as to the time of onset and whether the bleeding (if any) began simultaneously or later.

General examination. The mother is likely to be anxious, experiencing abdominal pain and her skin will be pale and moist if she is shocked. On clinical examination the mother may have obvious oedema of the face, fingers and pretibial area of the lower limbs.

The blood pressure and pulse should be taken immediately. A low blood pressure and raised pulse rate are signs of shock; if the mother has pregnancy-induced hypertension the blood pressure may be within normal limits, having been raised prior to the haemorrhage. The respirations may be normal or rapid and reduced oxygenation may lead to air hunger. The temperature will usually be normal but as placental abruption may be caused by severe infection, it should be taken.

The amount of any visible blood loss should be estimated. Its colour is noted. Freshly lost blood is bright red; blood that has been retained in utero for any length of time changes to a brown colour.

Abdominal examination. Concealed haemorrhage may lead to uterine enlargement in excess of gestation. The uterus has a hard consistency and there is guarding on palpation of the abdomen. Palpation may be difficult and should not be attempted if the uterus is rigid and excessively painful. Fetal parts may not be palpable. In less severe cases palpation should be kept to a minimum in order to avoid further damage. The location and nature of the pain should be established.

The fetal heart is unlikely to be heard with a fetal stethoscope if there has been any concealed haemorrhage; a Sonicaid apparatus should be used. If the haemorrhage is severe, fetal death is probable.

Assessing the fetal condition

Retroplacental haemorrhage is a major threat to fetal survival with the perinatal mortality rate rarely less than 300 per 1000 of which more than half will have died before the mother reaches hospital (Fraser & Watson 1989).

The mother may be aware of a cessation of fetal movements. It is said that excessive fetal movements may also occur as a result of profound hypoxia. A cardiotocograph recording will give more complete information about fetal condition. Failure to elicit heart sounds with a Pinard fetal stethoscope is not confirmation of fetal death but in cases of severe haemorrhage this is unfortunately the usual outcome.

The midwife should take care how she conveys information about the fetus to the mother. If the heart is inaudible on first examination, she should explain that a fetal monitor is needed to establish the condition of her baby. If fetal heart sound can be detected with ultrasonic apparatus, this will be of great comfort to the mother.

Management

Any woman with a history suggestive of placental abruption needs urgent medical attention. She should be transferred speedily to a consultant obstetric unit, preferably by the emergency obstetric service. The general practitioner may be called to the home in the first instance.

On arrival at the hospital the woman is admitted to the delivery suite and the registrar or consultant obstetrician is informed. The midwife should offer the mother comfort and encouragement by attending to her physical and emotional needs, including her need for information.

Pain. Pain exacerbates shock and must be alleviated. As it may be extreme, a suitable analgesic would be morphine 15 mg or pethidine 100–150 mg. If the mother has had a narcotic drug prior to admission, the midwife must alert those in attendance to the fact that analgesia has been given.

The acute pain of concealed haemorrhage from placental abruption is due to the extravasation of blood between the muscle fibres of the uterus. This must be differentiated from the pain of uterine contraction due to the onset of labour and from subcapsular liver haemorrhage as a result of pre-eclampsia. The nature of the pain should be discussed because labour may supervene following placental abruption.

Shock may be due to hypovolaemia, to extravasation and consequent pain or to consumptive coagulopathy. The latter is due to tissue damage and the liberation of thromboplastins into the circulation with resulting disseminated intravascular coagulation. This is discussed later in this chapter.

Whole blood is traditionally used to restore the blood volume. Letsky (1985) suggests the infusion of 1 unit of fresh frozen plasma for every 4–6 units of bank blood to replenish the clotting factors.

If blood is not available for immediate transfusion, hypovolaemia may be reduced by administering a suitable plasma expander. Letsky (1985) favours the use of Haemaccel which does not interfere with platelet function or subsequent blood grouping and cross-matching of blood. It helps to improve renal function. This is only a temporary palliative, however, and blood transfusion must follow as quickly as possible.

The mother should rest on her side in order to prevent vena caval occlusion and aortic compression by the gravid uterus. The legs may be raised but the body must remain horizontal. Elevating the foot of the bed will cause pooling of blood in the vagina and is unlikely to reduce shock.

Observations. The mother's blood pressure and pulse rate should be taken at frequent intervals, which would depend on the severity of her condition. If a pyrexia is present the temperature may be recorded every 1 or 2 hours; if the mother is not feverish a 4-hourly recording is adequate. A central venous line is usually inserted in order to monitor the central venous pressure 2-hourly or more frequently as necessary (see Ch. 29).

Urinary output is accurately assessed by the insertion of an indwelling catheter. Oliguria or anuria indicates suppression of renal function which may persist until a postpartum diuresis occurs. The urine should be tested for the presence of protein, which may also be linked to pregnancy-induced hypertension.

Fluid intake must also be recorded accurately and fluid balance assessed with the aid of the central venous pressure recordings.

Fundal height and abdominal girth are measured hourly. An increase indicates continued bleeding behind the placenta.

If the fetus is alive, the fetal heart rate should be monitored continuously with the aid of a cardiotocograph.

Any deterioration in the maternal or fetal condition must be immediately reported to the obstetrician.

Investigations. In concealed haemorrhage, because of the possibility of coagulation defects, clotting studies may be carried out. Blood samples may be needed at intervals in order to monitor the progress of the condition.

Management of different degrees of placental abruption

Mild separation of the placenta. In this case the placental separation and the haemorrhage are slight. Mother and fetus are in a stable condition. There is no indication of maternal shock and the fetus is alive and the heart sounds are normal. The consistency of the uterus is normal and there is no tenderness on abdominal palpation. It may be difficult to differentiate this condition from placenta praevia and from an incidental cause of vaginal bleeding.

Ultrasonic scan can determine the placental location and identify any degree of concealed bleeding. Fetal condition should be continuously assessed while bleeding persists, using an electronic fetal monitor. Subsequently electronic monitoring should be carried out once or twice daily because any degree of abruption by definition involves partial separation of the placenta.

If the mother is not in labour and the gestation is less than 37 weeks she may be cared for in an antenatal area for a few days. She may then be allowed home if there is no further bleeding and the placenta has been found to be in the upper uterine segment. Mothers who have passed the 37th week of pregnancy will have an amniotomy to induce labour. Further bleeding or evidence of fetal distress may indicate that a caesarean section is necessary.

Moderate separation of the placenta. This describes placental separation of about one-quarter. Up to 1000 ml of blood may be lost, some of which will escape per vaginam and some be retained behind the placenta as retroplacental clot or extravasation into the uterine muscle. The mother will be shocked, with a raised pulse rate and a lowered blood pressure. There will be a degree of uterine tenderness and abdominal guarding. The fetus may be alive although hypoxic; intra-uterine death is a probability.

The immediate aims of care are to reduce shock and to replace blood loss. Fluid replacement should be monitored with the aid of a central venous pressure line (see above). The fetal condition should be assessed with an electronic fetal monitor and if the fetus is alive, immediate caesarean section may be indicated.

If the fetus is in good condition or has already died, vaginal delivery may be contemplated. Delivery is advantageous because it enables the uterus to contract and control the bleeding. Amniotomy is usually sufficient to induce labour but oxytocin may be used if necessary. Delivery is often quite sudden after a short labour.

Moderate separation of the placenta may on occasion deteriorate into a more serious degree of separation.

Severe separation of the placenta. This is an acute obstetric emergency; at least two-thirds of the placenta has become detached and 2000 ml of blood or more are lost from the circulation. Most or all of the blood will be concealed behind the placenta. The mother will be severely shocked to a degree far beyond what might be expected from the amount of visible blood loss. The blood pressure will be lowered; the reading may lie within the normal range due to a preceding hypertension. The fetus is almost certainly dead. The woman will have very severe abdominal pain with excruciating tenderness; the uterus has a boardlike consistency.

Features associated with severe haemorrhage are coagulation defects, renal failure and pituitary failure.

Treatment is the same as for moderate haemorrhage. 1500 ml of whole blood should be transfused rapidly and subsequent amounts calculated in accordance with the woman's central venous pressure. Labour may begin spontaneously in advance of amniotomy and the midwife should be alert for signs of uterine contraction causing periodic intensifying of the abdominal pain.

Care of the baby

Preparation should be made for an asphyxiated baby. The paediatrician must be present at the birth to resuscitate the infant. The baby may need neonatal intensive care following delivery and the staff of the neonatal unit will have been alerted. In addition to the insult of the haemorrhage the baby may suffer from the effects of preterm delivery and his stay in the neonatal unit may be prolonged.

A baby who is born in good condition will of course require minimal resuscitation and may be transferred to the postnatal area with his mother.

Psychological care

When a woman has a placental abruption she and her partner must be kept fully informed of what is happening at all times. The doctor should have a full and frank discussion with them about the events and the prognosis. The midwife should ensure that the partner is offered support and adequate explanation if the woman requires emergency surgery or if her condition deteriorates suddenly. Whenever possible he should continue to be present and he may need another member of the family to share the burden.

If the fetus is alive, a midwife from the neonatal unit should visit the couple in order to introduce herself and explain where the baby will be cared for after delivery. The partner should be encouraged to visit the unit.

When the baby is born, if it is at all possible, his parents should be given a chance to see and handle him before he is transferred to the neonatal unit. It is most helpful to have a photograph taken which the mother can keep beside her and the father should visit the baby at the earliest opportunity. Later the mother will be taken to see the baby, if necessary in her bed or in a wheelchair. As her condition improves she will be encouraged to participate in caring for him.

At a suitable time following her recovery, the woman must be invited to discuss the events and the prognosis for her baby. She may ask about the possibility of haemorrhage occurring in future pregnancies and can usually be reassured.

Complications

- Disseminated intravascular coagulation is a complication of moderate to severe placental abruption.
- Postpartum haemorrhage may occur as a result of the Couvelaire uterus and disseminated intravascular coagulation or both. Intravenous ergometrine 0.5 mg is given at delivery as a prophylactic measure.

- Renal failure may occur as a result of hypovolaemia and consequent poor perfusion of the kidneys.
- Pituitary necrosis is another possible consequence of prolonged and severe hypotension.

BLOOD COAGULATION FAILURE

Normal blood coagulation

Haemostasis means the arrest of bleeding. Its function is to prevent loss of blood from the blood vessels. It depends on the mechanism of coagulation. This is counterbalanced by fibrinolysis which ensures that the blood vessels are reopened in order to maintain the patency of the circulation.

Blood clotting occurs in three main stages:

- When tissues are damaged and platelets break down, *thromboplastin* is released
- In the presence of *calcium* ions thromboplastin leads to the conversion of *prothrombin* into *thrombin*
- Thrombin is a proteolytic (protein-splitting) enzyme which converts *fibrinogen* into *fibrin*.

Fibrin forms a network of long, sticky strands which entrap blood cells to establish a clot. The coagulated material contracts and exudes serum which is plasma depleted of its clotting factors.

This is the final part of a complex cascade of coagulation involving a large number of different clotting factors. These factors have been assigned numbers in order of their discovery and a summary of the process is shown in Figure 21.9.

It is equally important for a healthy person to maintain the blood as a fluid in order that it can circulate freely. The coagulation mechanism is normally held at bay by the presence of heparin which is produced in the liver.

Fibrinolysis is the breakdown of fibrin and occurs as a response to the presence of clotted blood. Unless fibrinolysis takes place, coagulation will continue. It is achieved by the activation of a series of enzymes culminating in the proteolytic enzyme *plasmin*. This breaks down the fibrin in the clot and produces *fibrin degradation products* (FDPs).

Disseminated intravascular coagulation (DIC)

This is a situation of inappropriate coagulation within the blood vessels which leads to the consumption of clotting factors. As a result clotting fails to occur at the bleeding site.

Aetiology. DIC begins with an event which triggers widespread clotting with the formation of microthrombi throughout the circulation. Clotting factors are used up. The DIC triggers fibrinolysis and the production of FDPs. FDPs reduce the efficiency of normal clotting.

When DIC occurs during or after delivery, the reduced level of clotting factors and the presence of FDPs prevent normal haemostasis at the placental site. FDPs inhibit myometrial action and prevent the uterine muscle from constricting the blood vessels in the normal way. Torrential haemorrhage may be the outcome. Visible blood loss may be observed to remain uncoagulated for several minutes and, even when clotting does occur, the clot is unstable.

Microthrombi may cause circulatory obstruction in the small blood vessels. The effects of this vary from cyanosis of fingers and toes to cerebrovascular accidents and failure of organs such as the liver and kidneys.

Events which trigger DIC

There are a number of obstetric events which may precipitate DIC:

- placental abruption
- intra-uterine fetal death including missed abortion
- amniotic fluid embolism
- intra-uterine infection including septic abortion
- pre-eclampsia and eclampsia.

Each of the conditions is dealt with in the appropriate chapter and only those aspects relating to DIC are discussed here.

Placental abruption. Due to the damage of tissue at the placental site large quantities of thromboplastin are released into the circulation and may cause DIC. If the placenta is delivered as soon as possible after the abruption the risk of DIC is reduced.

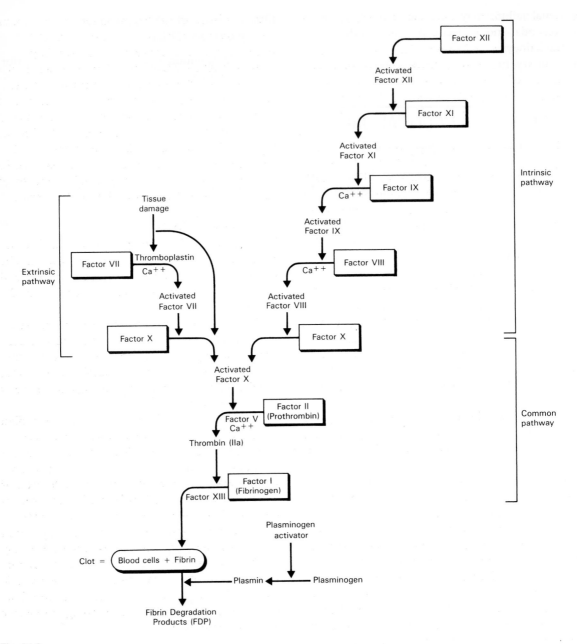

Fig. 21.9
The coagulation cascade.

Intra-uterine fetal death. If a dead fetus is retained in utero for more than 3 or 4 weeks thromboplastins are released from the dead fetal tissues. These enter the maternal circulation and deplete her clotting factors. If labour does not follow fetal death spontaneously, it should be induced.

Amniotic fluid embolism. If death does not occur from pulmonary embolism and maternal collapse, DIC may develop. Thromboplastin in the amniotic fluid is responsible for setting off the cascade of clotting.

Intra-uterine infection. The causes of this include septic abortion, hydatidiform mole, placenta accreta and endometrial infection before or after delivery. DIC is caused by endotoxins entering the circulation and damaging the blood vessels.

Pre-eclampsia and eclampsia. The exact aetiology of pregnancy-induced hypertension is unknown and the factors which precipitate DIC as a complication of this condition are unclear. FDPs are increased in the serum and urine which indicates that fibrinolysis is taking place.

Management

The midwife should be aware of the conditions which may cause DIC. She should be alert for signs that clotting is abnormal and the assessment of the nature of the clot should be part of her routine observation during the third stage of labour. Oozing from a venepuncture site or bleeding from the mucous membrane of the mother's mouth and nose must be noted and reported.

The doctor will carry out clotting studies such as prothrombin time and clotting time; the levels of platelets, fibrinogen and FDPs will be estimated.

Treatment involves the replacement of blood cells and clotting factors in order to restore equilibrium. This is usually done by the administration of fresh frozen plasma and platelet concentrates. Banked red cells will be transfused subsequently. The use of fresh whole blood is not now common because the screening processes undertaken in the modern transfusion service take up to 24 hours and the components are best given separately. In situations where the transfusion service is not so sophisticated, whole blood will be used.

In some instances there are specific considerations in the choice of treatment.

Intra-uterine fetal death. When the fetus is known to have died some time previously, clotting studies should be undertaken before any attempt is made to induce labour. If DIC is diagnosed, heparin is given to prevent further clotting.

This is discontinued before induction of labour and fresh frozen plasma should be available as postpartum haemorrhage is still a possibility.

Intra-uterine infection. When infection is the cause of DIC the infection itself must be treated aggressively with antibiotic therapy. If there is a haemolytic septicaemia any blood administered may be destroyed by the bacteria in the bloodstream. The baby may also need treatment following delivery if the infection is antepartum. In postpartum infection, any retained products of conception must be evacuated from the uterus.

Care by the midwife

DIC causes a frightening situation which demands speed of recognition and of action. The midwife has to maintain her own calmness and clarity of thinking as well as reassuring the couple.

Frequent and accurate observations must be maintained in order to monitor the woman's condition. Blood pressure, pulse rate and temperature are recorded. The general condition is noted. Fluid balance is monitored with vigilance for any sign of renal failure.

The father in particular is likely to be baffled by a sudden turn in events when previously all seemed to be going well. The midwife must make sure that someone is giving him appropriate attention and he will need to be kept informed of what is happening and be excluded as little as possible. The carers need to be aware that he may find it impossible to absorb all that he is told and may require repeated explanations. He may be the best person to help the woman to understand. The death of the mother is a real possibility and this may be one of the rare situations when the midwife finds herself needing to minister to a grieving partner.

DISORDERS OF THE AMNIOTIC FLUID

Normal amniotic fluid increases in amount throughout pregnancy from a few millilitres until 38 weeks when there is about a litre. After this it diminishes to approximately 800 ml at term. Amniotic fluid is not static; the water of which it is largely composed is changed every hour and the solutes are changed about every 3 hours.

There are two chief abnormalities of amniotic fluid, *polyhydramnios* and *oligohydramnios*.

Polyhydramnios

Polyhydramnios is defined as being a quantity of amniotic fluid which exceeds 1500 ml. It may not be clinically apparent until it reaches 3000 ml. It occurs in 1 in 250 pregnancies.

Causes

- Oesophageal atresia
- Open neural tube defect
- Multiple pregnancy, especially in the case of monozygotic twins
- Maternal diabetes mellitus
- Rarely, Rhesus iso-immunisation is associated with polyhydramnios
- Chorioangioma, a rare tumour of the placenta.

Types

Chronic polyhydramnios is gradual in onset, usually from about the 30th week of pregnancy. It is the most common type.

Acute polyhydramnios is very rare. It occurs at about 20 weeks and comes on very suddenly. The uterus reaches the xiphisternum in about 3 or 4 days. It is frequently associated with monozygotic twins or severe fetal abnormality.

Recognition

The mother may complain of breathlessness and discomfort. If the polyhydramnios is acute in onset, she may have severe abdominal pain. The condition may cause exacerbation of symptoms associated with pregnancy such as indigestion, heartburn and constipation. Oedema and varicosities of the vulva and lower limbs may be present.

Abdominal examination. On inspection, the uterus is larger than expected for the period of gestation and is globular in shape. The abdominal skin appears stretched and shiny with marked striae gravidarum and obvious superficial blood vessels.

On palpation the uterus feels tense and it is difficult to feel the fetal parts but the fetus may be balloted between the two hands. A *fluid thrill* may be elicited by placing a hand on one side of the abdomen and tapping the other side with the fingers. A wave of fluid will move across from the side which is tapped and is felt by the opposite examining hand. It may be helpful to measure

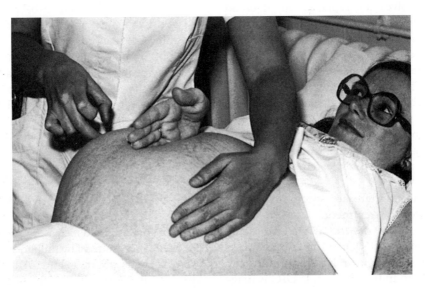

Fig. 21.10
Eliciting a fluid thrill in polyhydramnios.

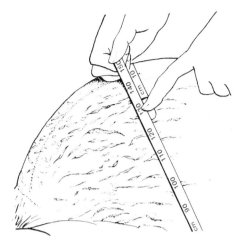

Fig. 21.11
Measuring abdominal girth in a case of polyhydramnios.

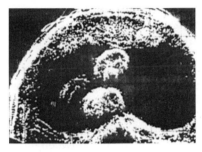

Fig. 21.12
Polyhydramnios. Ultrasonogram.

the abdominal girth, particularly in cases of acute polyhydramnios, in order to observe the rate of increase.

Auscultation of the fetal heart is difficult because the quantity of fluid allows the fetus to move away from the stethoscope.

Ultrasonic scan may be used to confirm the diagnosis of polyhydramnios and may reveal a multiple pregnancy or fetal abnormality. X-ray examination is not often performed and the images are usually hazy if there is a large quantity of amniotic fluid.

Complications

- Increased fetal mobility leading to unstable lie and malpresentation
- Cord presentation and cord prolapse
- Premature rupture of the membranes
- Placental abruption when the membranes rupture
- Premature labour
- Postpartum haemorrhage.

Management

The cause of the condition should be determined if possible. The mother will usually be admitted to a consultant obstetric unit. Subsequent care will depend on the mother's condition, the cause of the polyhydramnios and the stage of pregnancy. Diabetes mellitus will be managed as an entity; the polyhydramnios is managed much as in other cases. The presence of fetal abnormality will be taken into consideration in choosing the mode and timing of delivery. If gross abnormality is present, labour may be induced; if the fetus is suffering from an operable condition such as oesophageal atresia, it may be appropriate to arrange transfer to a neonatal surgical unit.

The mother should rest in bed. An upright position will help to relieve any dyspnoea and she may be given antacids to relieve heartburn and nausea. If the discomfort from the swollen abdomen is severe, abdominal amniocentesis may be considered. This is not without risk, as infection may be introduced or the onset of labour provoked. No more than 500 ml should be withdrawn at any one time. It is at best a temporary relief as the fluid will rapidly accumulate again and the procedure may need to be repeated.

Acute polyhydramnios is managed by amniocentesis but the outlook is very poor. The usual course of events is that the fluid continues to increase at an alarming rate, the membranes rupture spontaneously and the fetus or fetuses are washed out in a river of amniotic fluid. As this generally occurs prior to 24 weeks the babies are unlikely to survive.

The mother may need to have labour induced in late pregnancy if the symptoms become worse. The lie must be corrected if it is not longitudinal and the membranes will be ruptured cautiously, allowing the amniotic fluid to drain out slowly in order to avoid altering the lie and to prevent cord prolapse. Placental abruption is also a hazard if the uterus suddenly diminishes in size.

Labour is usually normal but the midwife should be prepared for the possibility of postpartum haemorrhage. The baby should be carefully examined for abnormalities and a tube must be passed in order to confirm the patency of the oesophagus.

Oligohydramnios

Oligohydramnios is an abnormally small amount of amniotic fluid. At term it may be 300–500 ml but amounts vary and it may be much less. It is associated with renal agenesis (absence of kidneys) or Potter's syndrome in which the baby also has pulmonary hypoplasia. The lack of amniotic fluid reduces the intra-uterine space and causes compression deformities. The baby has a squashed-looking face, flattening of the nose, micrognathia and talipes. The skin is dry and leathery in appearance.

Recognition

On inspection, the uterus appears smaller than expected for the period of gestation. The mother who has had a previous normal pregnancy may have noticed a reduction in fetal movements. When the abdomen is palpated the uterus is small and compact and fetal parts are easily felt. Breech presentation is possible. Auscultation is normal.

Ultrasonic scan will enable differentiation from intra-uterine growth retardation. Renal abnormality may be visible on the scan.

Management

The woman should be admitted for investigations which will include placental function tests. If there is no fetal abnormality the pregnancy will be allowed to continue.

Labour may begin early or may be induced because of the possibility of placental insufficiency. Epidural analgesia may be indicated because uterine contractions may be very painful. Impairment of placental circulation may result in fetal hypoxia. Constriction rings are a possibility due to the small amount of amniotic fluid. In rare cases the membranes may adhere to the fetus.

The paediatrician should be present to resuscitate the baby who will be examined carefully for abnormality.

Reader Activities

- Outline the midwife's assessment and care plan for a woman with vaginal bleeding in late pregnancy caused by a placental abruption. What criteria would you utilise to evaluate the care of:
  a. the mother?
  b. the unborn child?
- How would you recognise acute polyhydramnios? What are the dangers of this condition to:
  a. the mother?
  b. the fetus?
- A woman in late pregnancy calls her community midwife to the home because she is bleeding severely from the vagina. What emergency treatment would be needed? How would the midwife make a differential diagnosis between the possible causes?

REFERENCES

Burke G, Duigin N M 1991 Massive obstetric haemorrhage. In: Studd J (ed) Progress in obstetrics and gynaecology — 7. Churchill Livingstone, Edinburgh, p 114–116

Clark S L, Koonings P P, Phelan J P 1985 Placenta praevia/accreta and prior caesarean section. Journal of Obstetrics and Gynaecology 66: 89–92

Fraser R, Watson R 1989 Bleeding during the latter half of pregnancy. In: Chalmers I, Enkin M, Keirse M J N C Effective care in pregnancy and childbirth. Oxford University Press, Oxford, ch 37, p 594–611

Letsky E A 1985 Coagulation problems during pregnancy. Churchill Livingstone, Edinburgh

Llewellyn-Jones D 1986 Fundamentals of obstetrics and gynaecology. Vol 1 Obstetrics, 4th edn. Faber & Faber, London

Thorne T 1984 Disseminated intravascular coagulation. Nursing Times 80: 41

22

Diseases associated with pregnancy

CARMEL LLOYD   VICKY LEWIS

Infection

Cardiac disease

The anaemias

Hypertension

Renal problems

Diabetes mellitus

Epilepsy

Diseases which predate pregnancy are important because of the way that pregnancy affects them, and because of the way in which the disease, or the treatment, affects the pregnancy; they are also important for their social and psychological consequences. For example a woman with anaemia not only has a medical problem but may become tired and depressed, she may find herself unable to cope with existing children and she may have to take time off from her employment. If she is admitted to hospital for a prolonged period her family may suffer and she can become bored and frustrated as well as physically weak through lack of exercise. Her ideals about the place of confinement and the conduct of her labour may be compromised and the added anxiety of her medical condition may increase her need for pain-relieving drugs; anxiety has even been shown to decrease uterine efficiency in some species. Postnatally, the woman's lactation may suffer and her ability to enjoy her baby may be inhibited which may predispose her to postnatal psychological problems. It can be seen that the woman's physical, social and psychological conditions are inseparable.

When the midwife is assessing the needs of the woman and her family and planning their care, this interplay of social, psychological and physical factors is important.

If the medical problem is one that is likely to continue into the next pregnancy, the midwife can use the postnatal period to begin preconception care and advice. If the midwife can make the experience of this pregnancy a positive one, the woman will be encouraged to seek contact with the maternity services early in subsequent pregnancies or even before.

INFECTION

Pregnancy produces a degree of altered immuno-responsiveness which helps to prevent fetal rejection but predisposes the woman to infection. The physiological events of childbearing also predispose her to genito-urinary infection and if she is already the mother of small children the likelihood of exposure to the viral diseases of childhood is increased.

Midwives taking a detailed medical history from the pregnant woman should note any infections that she has had while pregnant and during the previous 3 months. Infection in pregnancy will affect the fetus as well as the mother. Maternal pyrexia produces fetal tachycardia and severe febrile illness can lead to abortion or premature labour.

Transmission of infection to the fetus can occur as follows:

— via the transplacental route, for example the human immunodeficiency virus (HIV) and rubella
— by ascending via the vagina after rupture of the membranes, for example faecal bacteria
— as the baby passes through the birth canal, for example herpes simplex and hepatitis B.

(Infection of the neonate after delivery is dealt with in Chapter 34.)

Viral infections are commonly transmitted via the placenta; some bacteria, such as the *Treponema pallidum* of syphilis and *Listeria monocytogenes*, and protozoa, such as *Toxoplasma gondii*, are also transferred. The effect on the fetus is very variable and includes abortion, fetal death and stillbirth, major or minor morphological abnormality, apparent normality at birth with an abnormality such as deafness becoming apparent later and no effect at all. The earlier the fetus is infected the more severe the problem.

Most of these infections gain access to the fetus via the placenta. The degree to which the fetus is affected is generally dependent on:

- the virulence of the infecting organism
- the mother's resistance to disease
- the stage of fetal development.

Immunisation

If the woman is planning to go abroad during or shortly after pregnancy she may wish to discuss vaccination.

Immunisation in pregnancy with a killed vaccine is generally considered safe. Some vaccines, however, such as cholera and typhoid, are contra-indicated because they can produce pyrexia which can cause spontaneous abortion or premature birth. Live vaccines such as rubella can damage the fetus and therefore must not be used during pregnancy. Polio vaccine is only advocated if the woman is travelling to a country where the disease is endemic and then a killed vaccine is used in preference to the live oral type.

Care of the woman with an infection

If the woman contracts an infection she should be cared for in isolation from other pregnant women.

Investigations of the cause of infection include blood culture and culture of a high vaginal swab, a throat swab and a urine sample as appropriate. Blood samples for blood count, antibody titres and immunoglobin M (IgM) determination may also be required.

Treatment

Antimicrobial therapy is undertaken with care. Overuse of broad-spectrum antibiotics has produced resistant organisms and some antibiotics are contra-indicated in pregnancy because of their effect on the fetus. Sulphonamides, when given close to the time of delivery, can produce neonatal jaundice. Co-trimoxazole, which is prescribed for urinary tract infection, is a folate antagonist and is therefore avoided in the first trimester of pregnancy. Later it can be given in conjunction with folic acid supplements and the midwife can discuss with the woman ways of increasing her dietary intake of folic acid. The aminoglycosides such as streptomycin cause fetal auditory nerve damage, while tetracycline stains the child's deciduous teeth.

Viral infections

According to Best and Banatvala (1990) the list of viruses that may cause congenital infections is growing. These include rubella virus, cytomegalovirus, varicella zoster virus, the human immunodeficiency viruses (HIV I and HIV II) and human parvovirus B19.

Congenital rubella is usually the result of a primary maternal infection. A secondary attack which produces clinical illness in the mother is not thought to put the fetus at risk. If the mother contracts rubella during the first 10 weeks of pregnancy there is a 90% risk that the fetus will be affected. Between 12 and 16 weeks the fetal infection rate is about 50% and the risk of defects is 25%. Although infection may occur after 16 weeks defects do not necessarily follow. Defects not identified at birth may become evident later. Up to 20% of apparently normal newborn infants develop defects later on. Careful follow-up of potentially infected babies is therefore necessary.

All women have their rubella antibody titre assessed during the antenatal period. If they are shown to be susceptible to the disease they are advised to avoid contact with anyone who may be infectious. They will be offered the vaccination during the postnatal period and advised to take precautions to avoid becoming pregnant for 3 months. Should a non-immune woman contract rubella during a critical period of fetal development she may be offered a termination of pregnancy.

The rubella vaccination programme has substantially reduced the susceptibility among women of childbearing age and the introduction of the measles, mumps and rubella vaccine in October 1988 for children aged 1–2 years should reduce the circulation of the virus in the community.

Cytomegalovirus (CMV) is a herpes virus which becomes latent after primary infection and may be reactivated later. Primary CMV infection usually causes a subclinical illness and therefore makes diagnosis difficult. Approximately 50% of women are susceptible to primary CMV, 1% of whom will be infected during pregnancy. Unlike the rubella virus, CMV can damage the fetus if maternal infection occurs at any stage of the pregnancy and 10% of fetuses will be severely damaged (Morgan-Capner 1991). Recurrent CMV infection only very rarely causes congenital anomalies. Screening pregnant women for primary CMV infection is of little value due to the asymptomatic nature of the disease. In addition, no treatment is available and as yet a safe, effective vaccine for those found to be susceptible has not been identified.

Varicella zoster virus (chickenpox) presents a risk both in early pregnancy and at term. Morgan-Capner (1991) states that 'there have been a number of reports of infants with characteristic abnormalities, such as microcephaly and skin scarring, after maternal varicella in the first 20 weeks of pregnancy'. Equally the risk to the neonate is substantial if maternal infection occurs near or soon after delivery. Because of these risks, hyperimmune varicella zoster immune globulin (VZIG) can be offered to susceptible mothers in contact with chickenpox or shingles. In addition Sills et al (1987) recommended the use of prophylactic acyclovir for those babies at risk. Best and Banatvala (1990) recommend the use of ultrasonography to monitor women who have acquired varicella in the first 20 weeks of pregnancy, 'as it is the only method for detecting defects induced by varicella such as severe scarring and limb deformities'.

Human immunodeficiency virus (HIV). Recent studies have shown that increasing numbers of women of childbearing age are infected with HIV, 30–40% of whom will transmit the infection to their infants in utero or during the perinatal period. There is no known cure at present and for pregnant women with acquired immune deficiency syndrome (AIDS) there are poor maternal and perinatal outcomes. 25–40% of infected infants will die before their second birthday.

Those at risk of developing AIDS are sexual partners of men with AIDS, intravenous drug abusers, recipients of blood transfusions (particularly pre-1985 as blood was not then screened for the AIDS virus) and women from parts of tropical Africa and Asia. It is recommended that these women are screened in pregnancy and, if found to be seropositive, an abortion before 12 weeks is advisable. If a pregnancy is carried to term, long-term follow-up studies on mother and child are needed as antiviral treatment may be beneficial if started in infancy (Katz & Wilfert 1989).

Human parvovirus B19 infection in adults may be asymptomatic or produce a rubella-like rash and arthralgia. In children it is the cause of erythema infectiosum (fifth disease) which is characterised by a widespread lacy erythematous rash with malar flushing.

A study done by the Public Health Laboratory Service Working Party on Fifth Disease (1990) showed that when infection occurs in pregnancy 84% of mothers had a normal outcome. Transplacental transmission of the virus occurs in approximately 10% of cases and results in abortion or stillbirth associated with hydrops fetalis. The risk of fetal loss is greatest in the second trimester.

Pregnant women may be monitored by ultrasonography for evidence of hydrops fetalis induced by B19. As the condition is relatively rare there is no role for routine antenatal screening, and infection in pregnancy is not an indication for therapeutic termination. Information about B19 virus should be added to that of other infections in pregnancy for expectant parents.

Bacterial infections

With the advent and increasing use of convenience foods, pregnant women are becoming more susceptible to food-borne organisms and to developing subsequent infections such as listeriosis. This may be responsible for abortion, fetal disease or death depending upon the severity of the infection and the duration of pregnancy.

The bacterium which is the cause of listeriosis, *Listeria monocytogenes*, is widespread in the environment. It can be found in soil, dust, mud, vegetation, silage, sewage and most of the animals that have been tested. Thus access to the human food chain is easily gained. Foods implicated in the outbreaks of listeriosis are raw vegetables, coleslaw, milk, soft cheeses and meat paté. Cook–chill catering is also a hazard as the organism has the unusual characteristic of being able to grow, albeit slowly, at temperatures as low as 6°C.

Infection in pregnancy may vary from a mild 'flu-like' to a severe illness. This may precipitate premature birth or abortion and cause meningitis in neonates or adults whose immunity to infection is impaired. When intra-uterine infection is present, amniotic fluid may be heavily contaminated and, at birth, attendant staff's hands, clothing and equipment will also become contaminated.

The diagnosis is made by culturing the organism from blood and/or cerebrospinal fluid. In the event of infection the mother and child are treated with large doses of penicillin or erythromycin.

It is important that the midwife and other health professionals that the mother comes into contact with give simple, but comprehensive, education on personal, environmental and food hygiene. This is in order to reduce the risk of fetal morbidity and mortality.

Protozoal infections

Toxoplasmosis, a multisystem disease caused by the protozoon *Toxoplasma gondii* causes spontaneous abortion, preterm labour, stillbirth and congenital malformations.

The parasite is endemic in Europe and less common in the UK. It is capable of infecting all mammals but is most commonly found in cats. These domestic pets hunt rodents harbouring the parasite and subsequently excrete infective oocytes in the faeces. Human infection follows hand to mouth contact after disposal of cat litter or ingestion of undercooked meat from cattle or sheep grazed in contaminated fields.

Parasitaemia can result in fetal infection acquired transplacentally; the fetal bloodstream is invaded by parasites. If the primary infection of the mother occurs in the first or second trimester the damage to the fetus is high. The principal locus of the infection is the central nervous system leading to developmental and neurological damage;

10–15% of babies born with congenital toxoplasmosis will die.

The disease can only occur in the fetus when there is acute maternal infection, hence those mothers who have antibodies before conception are safe. Those mothers who have no antibodies must be advised to eat only well-cooked meat during their pregnancy and to avoid handling cat litter.

In today's society pregnant women have become more likely to travel abroad and may be exposed to certain endemic diseases such as malaria and tuberculosis. Equally, the rising immigrant population within the UK may carry these diseases.

Malaria is a parasitic infection, the most common causative organism being *Plasmodium falciparum* which is carried by mosquitoes. It may cause infertility and complicates pregnancy. Intrauterine growth retardation, spontaneous abortion, stillbirth and neonatal death are typical. Exacerbation or relapse of malaria is particularly common during pregnancy, for unknown reasons. Each attack may precipitate abortion or the onset of preterm labour. Approximately 10% of infants born of women with plasmodial infection will have plasmodia in cord blood samples.

Severe complications of malaria include cerebral malaria, massive haemolysis and acute renal failure, this is more commonly found with the *P. malariae* type of infection.

The prevention and treatment of malaria during pregnancy is complicated by the increasing resistance of *P. falciparum* to chloroquine. In addition, no antimalarial drug is completely safe for use during pregnancy. If a pregnant woman must be treated for malaria it is recommended that advice be sought from experts such as the National Hospital for Tropical Diseases.

Pregnant women planning to travel in hot countries should be advised to avoid geographical areas where chloroquine-resistant malaria is endemic.

The parasite is not thought to be transmitted in milk, but breast feeding should be discouraged in women with clinical evidence of malaria. Women receiving any anti-malarial agent who are breast feeding should be told that their infants are not protected against malaria.

Pulmonary tuberculosis

The prevalence of pulmonary tuberculosis in Great Britain is between 0.5 and 1% although its incidence is much higher amongst certain sections of the Asian population.

Effects on the woman

The onset of primary tuberculosis is often insidious producing night sweats, weight loss, anorexia, purulent sputum, haemoptysis (as the blood vessels in the lung are eroded), low grade fever and general malaise. The overall effect is to debilitate the woman, making her less able to cope with pregnancy and her existing family. Although pregnancy makes extra demands on her respiratory system dyspnoea may not be the principal problem.

Transplacental infection of the fetus is rare but possible and there is a suggestion that the risk of abortion may be increased. The woman's poor state of health may affect fetal growth.

Management

The woman will be under the care of an obstetrician and a chest physician during her pregnancy.

If there are clinical signs of tuberculosis or the woman is known to have been in contact with tuberculosis, a chest X-ray is performed during the third month, at term and 6 months after delivery. A full-size plate is used as this involves a lower dose of radiation. The fetus is protected by a lead apron. Sputum specimens are taken and any pleural effusions may be aspirated to help identify the organism.

Most treatment is given on an outpatient basis although the woman may be admitted to an isolation unit if her sputum test is positive as the disease is communicated by droplet infection. The rest of her household will also be referred for investigation. The treatment for tuberculosis includes rest (physical and emotional), hospitalisation if the disease is moderate or advanced, and chemotherapy.

None of the drugs available for treating tuberculosis is ideal. Table 22.1 gives those used, their doses and reported side-effects. Treatment is usually with isoniazid and ethambutol during the first trimester; rifampicin may be used after

Table 22.1
Drugs used in the treatment of tuberculosis

Drug	Dose	Reported side-effects
Isoniazid	5 mg/kg/day	Abnormalities seen in animals. Interferes with pyridoxine metabolism. Supplements are needed. Found in significant amounts in breast milk.
Ethambutol hydrochloride	15–20 mg/kg/day	No effects on fetus apparent.
Rifampicin	6–12 mg/kg/day	Increased incidence of neural tube defects: not usually given in first trimester.
Streptomycin sulphate	1 g/day i.m.	Fetal auditory and vestibular nerve damage.

that. If treatment is begun soon enough the sputum test will be negative by the time the baby is born, although drug therapy is likely to continue for 9 months. Some women are admitted for rest during the last 2 weeks of pregnancy.

Part of the midwife's role is to consider the woman's social and domestic situation. If she has financial difficulties or poor housing the help of a social worker will be needed. She may welcome information about other people or organisations who could care for existing children during the day while she rests. An examination of her eating habits and subsequent dietary counselling may help to improve her nutritional status.

Intrapartum care

If the mother is infectious she should be allocated a single room during her stay in hospital.

Problems in labour stem from fatigue and reduced lung function and the midwife should seek advice before offering the woman nitrous oxide and oxygen. Episiotomy and forceps delivery may be advocated to reduce the strain of the second stage. Unnecessary blood loss can be avoided by careful management of the third stage.

The interaction between her regular medication and the drugs given in labour may be important, e.g. streptomycin potentiates the effect of muscle-relaxing drugs.

Postnatal care

Separation of the baby from his family is not always necessary. The baby can be vaccinated with an isoniazid-resistant BCG (bacille Calmette–Guerin) whilst being protected from the disease by the prophylactic use of isoniazid syrup 25 mg/

kg/day. The vaccine becomes effective in 3–6 weeks as shown by a positive Mantoux test. Without vaccination the child has a 50% chance of catching the disease. If any of the baby's family are infected with an isoniazid-resistant organism, separation will be advised until the baby is Mantoux positive.

Breast feeding is contra-indicated if the woman has an active infection. Women who breast feed whilst still undergoing treatment may need their medication altered.

Caring for a child at home makes great demands on the woman. If it is possible for her to have extra help in the home this could be arranged in advance of her return. Friends, relatives or the home help service could be contacted. Midwives should explain that poor nutrition, stress and over-tiredness will encourage a recurrence of active disease.

Family planning advice is an integral part of postnatal and preconception care as it is advisable for the woman to avoid further pregnancies until the disease has been quiescent for at least 2 years. When choosing her method of family planning, the woman needs to be aware that rifampicin reduces the effectiveness of oral contraception.

Follow-up. Long-term medical and social follow-up is necessary in order to monitor the disease and its treatment and to provide help for the socially and economically disadvantaged.

CARDIAC DISEASE

Trends in cardiac disease

The overall incidence of cardiac disease in pregnancy is falling in Europe and North America, largely due to the lower incidence of rheumatic heart disease (less than 1% in the UK). However, the number of women with congenital cardiac defects who survive to childbearing age is increasing as medical and surgical care improves. Coronary artery disease is also increasing.

In the developing world rheumatic heart disease is still the most common cardiac problem. In parts of Africa, cardiomyopathy is often seen during pregnancy or the puerperium although it is rare in the UK.

> To manage pregnancy effectively in a patient with heart disease the normal compensatory changes in the cardiovascular system that occur during pregnancy must be understood. These normal responses are only detrimental to the mother and fetus if heart disease is present. (Nolan 1990)

Changes in cardiovascular dynamics during pregnancy

In normal pregnancy the cardiovascular dynamics alter in order to meet the increased demands of the feto-placental unit. This increases the work load of the heart quite significantly.

The major cardiac changes to occur are:

- an increase in cardiac output by 40%
- an increase in blood volume by 35%
- a decrease in total peripheral resistance.

These changes commence in early pregnancy and gradually reach a maximum at the 30th week, where they are maintained until term. Oestrogens and prostaglandins are thought to be the mediators of the alterations in haemodynamics during pregnancy. These changes are associated with several clinical signs:

- The increased cardiac output may produce a physiological systolic flow in one-third of pregnant women.
- The heart dilates and a third heart sound is common.
- As the uterus enlarges, the heart may be displaced upwards by the growing uterus.
- During the third stage of labour 300–400 ml of blood is added to the circulating volume by the contracting uterus.

Classification

The New York Heart Association classification based on exercise tolerance is useful for describing the extent of the immediate problem but has little predictive value:

1. No symptoms during ordinary physical activity
2. Symptoms during ordinary physical activity
3. Symptoms during mild physical activity
4. Symptoms at rest.

It used to be said that women would deteriorate by one grade in pregnancy, but it is now thought more useful to consider the prognosis for each specific problem. For example, valvular incompetence may improve during pregnancy as peripheral resistance drops and more blood flows in the right direction, whereas the woman with mitral stenosis may deteriorate three grades in a matter of hours.

Rheumatic heart disease

Valvular lesions predominate in rheumatic heart disease.

Mitral and aortic valve incompetence. Pregnancy can be helpful in this case as it lowers the pressure in the arterial system, encouraging blood to flow the right way through the valves. There is, however, a risk of endocarditis.

Mitral stenosis. A non-pregnant woman with this condition already requires an increase in left atrial pressure in order to push blood through the mitral valve. As the demand for cardiac output rises in pregnancy, pressure in the left atrium rises still further. This may lead to back pressure in the pulmonary system and pulmonary oedema. The left atrium, unable to cope with the demands made upon it, begins to fibrillate and heart failure may occur.

Congenital heart disease

The most common congenital defects which may remain uncorrected during the childbearing years are:

— atrial septal defect
— patent ductus arteriosus
— ventricular septal defect.

All of these are openings which allow communication between the right and left sides of the heart or, in the case of patent ductus arteriosus, between the pulmonary artery and the aorta.

The main determinant of the woman's well-being during pregnancy and the early puerperium is the amount of blood flowing in the right direction. Blood flows easily from a high-pressure area to a low-pressure area. For this reason, blood is more likely to flow from the left side of the heart into the aorta, where the pressure is low, rather than through a septal defect into the right side of the heart. Similarly, blood flows easily from the right heart into the low-pressure pulmonary circulation which reduces the chance of shunting from right to left via a defect.

Problems arise when pulmonary vascular resistance rises, as it does in pre-eclampsia, and blood flows from the right side to the left instead of passing through the lungs, leading to cyanosis. This may also happen in the third stage of labour when there is a sudden return of blood to the heart.

Other, less common defects produce permanent cyanosis. Fallot's tetralogy (pulmonary stenosis, ventricular septal defect, an aorta which overrides the septum and right ventricular hypertrophy) and Eisenmenger's syndrome (the occurrence of pulmonary hypertension due to vascular changes induced in the lungs by a large left-to-right shunt leading to shunt-reversal cyanosis (Nolan 1990)) produce cyanosis and blood flows from the right ventricle into the aorta. Eisenmenger's syndrome is associated with a high maternal mortality.

Any structural defect, whether congenital or acquired, predisposes the woman to bacterial endocarditis and thrombo-emboli.

Risk to mother and fetus

In rheumatic heart disease (RHD) the maternal mortality can now be very low and pregnancy does not affect long-term survival. The fetal outcome in RHD is usually good and little different from that in patients who do not have heart disease (de Swiet 1989).

Maternal mortality is most likely in those conditions where pulmonary blood flow cannot be increased as, for example, in Eisenmenger's syndrome (DH 1991).

During pregnancy, the babies are generally growth-retarded and fetal loss may be high. However, there is no increase in the perinatal mortality rate (PMR) although there is an increased incidence of congenital heart disease (CHD) in children born to mothers who have CHD themselves (Nolan 1990).

Preconception care and advice

A woman who knows that she has cardiac disease would be wise to seek advice from both a cardiologist and an obstetrician before becoming pregnant so that the risks of her condition can be discussed. In some cases, preconception surgery such as mitral valvotomy may be advised.

The woman should be helped to control obesity, cut down smoking and choose a diet which will prevent anaemia in order to minimise risk.

It is advisable that family size should be limited, as the risks increase with each pregnancy. Contraceptive advice is therefore an important aspect of management.

Antenatal care

Diagnosis of cardiac disease in some women may only be made during antenatal visits. The midwife may detect a problem when taking the woman's history. Breathlessness, fatigue, swollen ankles and palpitations may all be attributable to the normal changes associated with pregnancy but if they were present before the pregnancy began they may indicate something more sinister and the woman must be referred to a cardiologist. Diagnosis will be made with the aid of the clinical picture, radiography, ECG and echocardiography.

Assessment of the problem and its prognosis can be made at a combined cardiac and obstetric clinic where the couple can discuss the options open to them. Where there is no evidence of a cardiac lesion, no further follow-up will be required. Some may have a mild lesion with no haemodynamic effect in which case pregnancy may not be affected, although prophylactic antibiotic cover in labour is recommended. For those with a significant lesion with real or potential haemodynamic implications, the future of the pregnancy needs to be considered and careful counselling given. First trimester termination of pregnancy is preferable, as termination after 16 weeks gestation is no safer than later delivery.

Management. All pregnant women with heart disease should be managed in a combined obstetric/cardiac clinic by one obstetrician and one cardiologist. In this way most pregnancies in women with heart disease will be successful. The aim of management is to maintain or improve the physical and psychological well-being of mother and fetus. This involves keeping a steady haemodynamic state and preventing complications. The major maternal complications are:

— bacterial endocarditis
— thrombo-emboli
— cyanosis
— heart failure.

The risk factors for heart failure include:

— infections, particularly urinary tract infection (UTI)
— hypertension
— anaemia
— multiple pregnancy
— obesity
— smoking.

Physical care

Depending on the woman's condition, antenatal clinic visits may be more frequent than usual. Women with cardiac disease will require the same health and dietary advice as other pregnant women, although each mother must be considered individually. An important aspect of care is that of dental treatment and antibiotic cover to eliminate sources of sepsis and reduce the risk of endocarditis.

In late pregnancy it may be advisable to restrict activity or admit the woman to hospital for rest and close monitoring.

Obstetric management in pregnancy includes early ultrasound examination of the fetus to confirm gestational age and detect congenital abnormality. Following this the fetus should be monitored to assess fetal well-being. This may be done by:

- assessment of fetal growth and amniotic fluid volume both clinically and by ultrasound
- monitoring the fetal heart rate by cardiotocography
- measurement of fetal and maternal placental blood flow indices by Doppler.

Social care

With more frequent antenatal visits the midwife may need to give advice about assistance with fares or transport to the hospital.

If the mother is required to reduce her physical activity and leave work earlier than she had planned, the midwife may need to give advice regarding the Employment Protection Act and any DSS benefit to which she may be entitled (see Ch. 45). If the problem is complex, referral to a social worker will be appropriate.

A woman who finds it necessary to restrict her activities in the home could be put in contact with the home help service.

Psychological care

Psychological support by the midwife is important during pregnancy particularly at times when there are intercurrent problems which may require admission to hospital. Consideration must particularly be given to the emotional stress caused by a woman being separated from her other children.

Intrapartum care

The first stage of labour

The least stressful labour for a woman with cardiac disease will be spontaneous in onset and result in a vaginal delivery. The midwife should inform the anaesthetist and cardiologist of her admission. Blood may be cross-matched in case of need. Oxygen and resuscitation equipment should be available and functioning.

Observations of pulse and respiratory rate should be made every 15 minutes. The heart may be monitored by ECG. Deviations from the normal, such as breathlessness and tachycardia, should be reported immediately. Blood pressure and fetal condition should be carefully monitored and recorded.

As these women are at an increased risk from endocarditis it would seem prudent to administer antibiotic prophylaxis in labour (de Swiet 1989).

Positioning. The mother will need encouragement to adopt a position in which she is comfortable. It is important to remember that women with heart disease are particularly sensitive to aortocaval compression by the gravid uterus in the supine position. This results in marked hypotension and maternal and fetal distress. Positions such as the lithotomy position in which the feet are higher than the trunk are best avoided because of the risk of acute heart failure resulting from the sudden increase of venous return to the heart.

Fluid balance. Women with significant heart disease require care concerning fluid balance in labour. Indiscriminate use of intravenous crystalloid fluids will lead to an increase in circulating blood volume, which women with heart disease will find difficult to cope with and they may easily develop pulmonary oedema.

Pain relief. Women with heart disease usually have quite rapid, uncomplicated labours. The midwife should help the woman to use the techniques that she has learned for coping with stress, as she and her labour companion are likely to be very anxious.

In the majority, an epidural would be the analgesia of choice, inserted by a skilled anaesthetist. It is effective analgesia which decreases cardiac output and heart rate. It causes peripheral vasodilation and decreases venous return which alleviates pulmonary congestion.

Nitrous oxide and oxygen (Entonox) and pethidine are usually considered safe but it is wise to consult a doctor before administering any form of pain-relieving drug.

Preterm labour. If the woman should labour prematurely beta-sympathomimetic drugs such as salbutamol, widely used for the treatment of premature labours, are not recommended. The vasodilatory side-effects cause tachycardia and an increase in circulatory blood volume which may lead to the development of pulmonary oedema and heart failure. In addition these drugs have metabolic effects which may further impair myocardial function.

Induction is only considered safe if the benefits outweigh the disadvantages. A failed induction leads to caesarean section and a risk of sepsis which is especially dangerous for a damaged heart.

Labour is not usually induced for uncomplicated heart disease. If it is necessary to induce labour the use of prostaglandin pessaries is advocated. Oxytocin by intravenous infusion causes a degree of fluid retention and it is important for the midwife to keep a careful record of fluid balance if this is used.

The second stage of labour

The second stage should be short and without undue exertion on the part of the mother. Prolonged pushing with held breath such as the Valsalva manoeuvre, which is undesirable for healthy women, may be dangerous for a woman with heart disease. It raises the intrathoracic pressure, pushes blood out of the thorax and impedes venous return, with the result that cardiac output falls. When a breath is taken, blood rushes back to the right side of the heart and to the lungs, and a beat or two later to the left side of the heart. This alteration in haemodynamics can have a serious effect on a heart which relies on a steady flow.

Midwives may need to suggest to the woman that she avoids holding her breath and follows her natural desire to push, giving several short pushes during each contraction. In this way she will also avoid facial petechiae and subconjunctival haemorrhages.

Some doctors perform a forceps delivery electively, while others see no reason for this if the woman is expected to deliver quickly and easily. Some midwives and doctors advocate delivery in the left lateral position.

The third stage of labour

Views on the management of the third stage vary. Syntometrine (ergometrine 0.5 mg and Syntocinon 5 units) causes a tonic contraction which returns 300–500 ml of blood to the venous system. Syntocinon may be used in order to prevent haemorrhage as it has less effect on blood vessels than ergometrine. If the woman is in heart failure, oxytocics should be avoided. In the case of actual haemorrhage Syntocinon can be given by infusion accompanied by intravenous frusemide to prevent pulmonary oedema.

Postnatal care

During the first 48 hours following delivery the heart must cope with the extra blood from the uterine circulation and it is important to monitor the woman's condition closely during this time. A 4-hourly record of her temperature will help in the early detection of infection.

The baby is examined very carefully for any sign of hereditary heart disease. Breast feeding is not contra-indicated unless the woman is in heart failure. Her drugs may be transmitted through breast milk and she may need advice on any possible effect on the baby. Antibiotic cover may continue for up to 2 weeks after the birth.

When the woman has discussed the implications of future pregnancies on her condition with the cardiologist and obstetrician, she may need help to choose a suitable method of family spacing. The intra-uterine contraceptive device has been associated with an increased risk of infection which may lead to endocarditis. The combined pill increases the risk of thrombo-embolism and hypertension but the progesterone-only pill and barrier methods with spermicides are suitable alternatives. Sterilisation, if chosen, is usually delayed for 2–3 months after delivery.

On her return home the woman may benefit from extra help in the house. Friends and relatives often fulfil this need but the home help service could be approached.

Major complications of heart disease

Cardiac failure and pulmonary oedema
The risk of cardiac failure increases throughout pregnancy, reaching a peak in the early puerperium. Signs and symptoms include tachycardia, tachypnoea, cyanosis, oedema and liver distension.

Pulmonary oedema may accompany cardiac failure or it may have an acute onset in conditions like mitral stenosis. Signs and symptoms include acute dyspnoea, frothy sputum and haemoptysis; pulmonary congestion may be seen on X-ray.

Management of acute heart failure and pulmonary oedema in pregnancy is similar to that in a non-pregnant woman. The woman's anxiety is likely to be increased through concern for her baby; an honest but supportive approach by medical personnel will help to increase her confidence.

Drug therapy includes analgesia to reduce anxiety and pain and to aid vasodilation. Morphine 15–20 mg i.v. may be used but this can produce neonatal respiratory depression if given in labour. A diuretic such as frusemide will relieve oedema. A bronchodilator such as aminophylline will relieve dyspnoea but it has been known to produce neonatal irritability. Digoxin counteracts dysrhythmias. Oxygen and prophylactic antibiotics may also be given.

The woman is nursed upright in a supported sitting position, with suction apparatus and resuscitation equipment close at hand. Intermittent positive pressure ventilation may be needed and sometimes venesection is used to reduce venous congestion and the pressure on the right side of the heart.

Cardiac failure and pulmonary oedema must be brought under control before caesarean section or induction of labour is attempted.

Management of chronic cardiac failure. The woman with chronic cardiac failure will be admitted for bed rest. Leg exercises should be taught to help to avoid deep venous thrombosis. Fluid balance and apex beat are recorded and digoxin, diuretics and potassium are likely to be prescribed. Salt and fluid intake may be restricted.

Thrombo-emboli
Women with artificial heart valves run a risk of developing thrombo-emboli unless anticoagulants are given. There is debate about the choice of drug. The oral anticoagulant warfarin crosses the placenta and is known to be teratogenic in the first 13 weeks of pregnancy; it also predisposes to fetal and neonatal haemorrhage. Heparin is not passed to the fetus but it is thought by some

doctors to be less effective in reducing thrombo-emboli. Some doctors prescribe subcutaneous heparin throughout pregnancy; others prescribe heparin in early pregnancy then warfarin until 36 weeks, reverting to subcutaneous heparin which is given until the day of delivery. Heparin and war-farin are given again after delivery. Warfarin appears in breast milk but there is no evidence that it harms the baby although some doctors prefer not to prescribe it. Whilst the mother is taking warfarin the prothrombin time is moni-tored.

THE ANAEMIAS

Anaemia is a reduction in the oxygen-carrying capacity of the blood which may be due to:

- a reduced number of red blood cells
- a low concentration of haemoglobin or
- a combination of both.

Physiological haemodilution of pregnancy

During pregnancy the blood volume increases. The increase in plasma volume is greater than the increase in the red cell mass. This has the following effects:

- there are fewer red cells in each litre of blood which means that the haemoglobin (Hb) con-centration is reduced
- the blood becomes less viscous which may help to reduce cardiac workload and make perfusion of the placental bed easier.

These changes result in an apparent anaemia but as this represents a normal pregnancy state they should not be regarded as pathological.

The criteria used for diagnosing true anaemia in pregnancy vary. In 1972 the World Health Organization definition was an Hb level of less than 11g/dl but many doctors only begin to investigate and treat anaemia when the Hb falls below 10.5 g/dl. Studies in the developing world have demonstrated that many women show no ill effects with an Hb of 10 g/dl.

The effects of anaemia

Mother
- Reduced enjoyment of pregnancy and motherhood due to fatigue
- Reduced resistance to infection caused by impaired cell-mediated immunity
- Predisposition to postpartum haemorrhage
- Problems caused by treatment
- Potential threat to life

Fetus/baby
- Increased risk of intra-uterine hypoxia and growth retardation
- Higher perinatal morbidity and mortality if maternal Hb is less than 6 g/dl

Signs and symptoms
- Pallor of mucous membranes
- Dyspnoea
- Fainting
- Fatigue
- Tachycardia and palpitations.

Routine screening for anaemia

Physiologic and pathologic changes in the mother during pregnancy make the determination of anaemia difficult. Not only do blood values during pregnancy differ from those in the non-pregnant patient, but these factors also vary with the course of pregnancy. (Benson 1983)

The examination of the red cell indices gives a guide to the diagnosis of anaemia in pregnancy. The size of the red cell (MCV), its haemoglobin content (MCH) and Hb concentration (MCHC) can be calculated from red blood count (RBC) and packed cell volume (PCV).

Pregnant women are usually screened at their first antenatal visit and thereafter at monthly intervals from the 28th week.

Normal blood changes in pregnancy

— Red blood count (RBC). The number of red blood cells falls from $4.2 \times 10^{12}/l$ to $3.8 \times 10^{12}/l$.
— Mean cell volume (MCV). The average volume of a red cell fluctuates within the non-pregnant range 77–93 femtolitres (a thousand million millionth of a litre).
— Mean cell haemoglobin (MCH). The average amount of Hb in a red cell falls within the non-pregnant range 26–32 picograms (see Ch. 42).
— Mean cell Hb concentration (MCHC) indicates how well filled with Hb the cells are. This remains within the non-pregnant range 32–36 g/dl.
— Packed cell volume (PCV) or haematocrit (Hct) may fall from 0.45–0.33 l/l.

Anaemia in the developing world

In developed countries it is estimated that approximately 2% of women are anaemic; in the developing world this figure may be as high as 50% and this contributes to the high rate of maternal mortality. Iron, folic acid and vitamin B_{12} deficiencies are more common; the unavailability of correct food, food taboos and eating and cooking customs all play a part. In order to help prevent anaemia, midwives must not only understand the medical problem but also any social circumstances that give rise to it.

Other contributory causes to the high incidence of anaemia include infections such as amoebic dysentery, malaria (particularly *Plasmodium falciparum)* and *Clostridium welchii*, which cause increased haemolysis. Hookworm, which is a parasite found in the tropics, lives in the duodenum and gains its nutrition from the host's blood, causing anaemia. The ova of the worm may be found in the woman's stools. The haemoglobinopathies are discussed later.

Iron deficiency anaemia

Iron deficiency in women is usually due to blood loss resulting from excessive menses, postpartum haemorrhage or iron deprivation from previous pregnancies. About 95% of pregnant women with anaemia have the iron deficiency type (Benson 1983). During pregnancy approximately 1400 mg iron is needed for:

- the increase in the number of red blood cells
- the fetus and placenta
- replacement of daily loss (about 1 mg/day) through stools, urine and skin
- replacement of blood lost at delivery
- lactation.

Absorption of iron is increased in pregnancy but this does not adequately meet the extra demand. In addition a well-nourished woman has sufficient stores of iron on which to draw. These stores are usually about 1000 mg in women in Britain.

Causes

- Reduced intake or absorption of iron or protein or both. (Iron is stored in combination with ferritin which is a protein.)

Examples include dietary deficiency and gastrointestinal disturbance such as morning sickness.
- Excess demand such as multiple pregnancy, frequent or numerous pregnancies or chronic inflammation, particularly of the urinary tract.
- Blood loss, for example from menorrhagia before conception, bleeding haemorrhoids, antepartum or postpartum haemorrhage or hookworm.

Prevention

The midwife can help to identify the woman at risk of anaemia by taking an accurate medical, obstetric and social history. This may reveal a pre-existing problem or a woman whose racial origin or lifestyle puts her at risk of anaemia. It may also suggest that the woman is suffering from the effects of anaemia.

Advice and explanations which are appropriate to the particular woman can be given, taking into account health, religious and cultural preferences.

Women need to be taught about the sources of iron and ways in which absorption can be increased. Iron is most easily absorbed in the form found in red meat. It is also found in wholegrain products such as wholemeal bread. Egg yolks contain iron but it is less well absorbed. Absorption of iron is inhibited by tea and coffee but increased by ascorbic acid which is present in orange juice and fresh fruit.

Some doctors prescribe iron supplements for all pregnant women although there is little evidence to support this practice; some give it to those at risk of anaemia while some only use iron to treat anaemia if it occurs. Many doctors avoid giving iron during the first trimester of pregnancy due to the gastro-intestinal side-effects. It may be more appropriate to administer prophylactic iron therapy in the third trimester of pregnancy. During this time the maternal iron stores become depleted due to the increasing fetal demand. Indications for prophylactic iron therapy include:

- previous anaemia
- dietary conditions
- chronic blood loss
- low haemoglobin on booking
- close family spacing.

Oral iron preparations given prophylactically consist of one of the iron salts, either alone or in combination with folic acid. Pregaday contains ferrous fumarate 304 mg (this has 100 mg iron) and folic acid 350 μg. Iron may also be combined with ascorbic acid or other vitamins.

Investigation

A low Hb concentration only indicates that the woman is anaemic; it does not reveal the cause. Iron deficiency is *microcytic*, that is, it produces small red cells; the MCV falls first, followed by the MCH, Hct and Hb. By the time the Hb falls, the iron stores will already be depleted. Lack of iron is demonstrated by measuring the serum iron level which will be reduced (normal range 11–30 μmol/l) and the serum iron-binding capacity which will be raised (normal range 54–75 μmol/l). Serum ferritin levels show changes before the Hb falls and correspond well with iron stores but the test is expensive.

A mid-stream specimen of urine should be taken to exclude urinary tract infection.

Management

The midwife's role lies in helping the woman to understand the condition, its cause and treatment. The dietary advice already discussed will help her to increase her iron intake. Fatigue may be lessened if other family members can share the work load. It is sometimes appropriate to arrange day care for other children.

Oral iron. The daily dose of iron for treating anaemia is between 120 and 180 mg in divided doses. Two examples are:

- ferrous sulphate: 200 mg tablets contain 60 mg iron
- ferrous gluconate: 300 mg tablets contain 35 mg iron.

Side-effects of oral iron. The woman should be warned that her stools may turn black but that this does not mean that iron is not being absorbed. Other side-effects are dose-related and include nausea and epigastric pain and diarrhoea or constipation. These discomforts may be reduced by taking iron after meals. Some women find one form of iron salts more tolerable than another.

Parenteral iron. If iron is given intramuscularly or intravenously it bypasses the gastro-intestinal tract. This is not a common method of treatment due to its unpleasant side-effects, although it is an advantage for women who are unable to take, tolerate or absorb oral iron but the Hb level will only rise at the same rate. Women receiving parenteral iron do not require any further iron therapy during pregnancy. Parenteral iron is contra-indicated for women who have liver or renal disorders.

Intramuscular iron is given in the form of iron sorbitol 50 mg/ml. The dose is 1.5 mg iron/kg body weight daily or weekly. Injections should not be given in conjunction with oral iron as this enhances toxic effects such as headache, dizziness, nausea and vomiting. The injection should be given deep into the muscle to prevent staining of the skin, formation of abscesses and fat necrosis.

Total dose iron infusion is given as iron dextran 50 mg/ml in a slow intravenous infusion of normal saline. The dosage is calculated by taking account of body weight and the Hb concentration deficit. Side-effects include allergic reaction which may take the form of severe anaphylactic shock; joint pain, occurring within 24 hours of the infusion, is not uncommon. A test dose must be given and the woman's condition monitored strictly during and immediately following the infusion according to local procedure. Women who are prone to allergies should not receive this form of iron.

Blood transfusion is used rarely to treat severe iron deficiency anaemia. It may be used to raise the Hb level quickly if delivery is imminent.

Folic acid deficiency anaemia

Folic acid is needed for the increased cell growth of both mother and fetus but there is a physiological decrease in serum folate levels in pregnancy. Folic acid is found in leafy green vegetables such as broccoli and spinach but is destroyed easily by prolonged boiling or steaming and by the addition of alkalis such as bicarbonate of soda. It is also found in avocado pears and in mushrooms but these are expensive sources.

Anaemia is more likely to be found towards the end of pregnancy when the fetus is growing rapidly. It is also more common during winter when folic acid is more difficult to obtain and in areas of social, economic and nutritional deprivation.

Causes
• Reduced dietary intake, for example as a result of overcooking vegetables.
• Reduced absorption, for instance in coeliac disease and tropical sprue.
• Interference with utilisation. Drugs such as anticonvulsants, sulphonamides and alcohol are folate antagonists.
• Excessive demand and loss. In haemolytic anaemia there is an increased demand for production of new red cells and consequently for folic acid. Multiple pregnancy also results in an increased demand.

Prevention
The risk of folic acid deficiency can be reduced by advising pregnant women on correct selection and preparation of foods which are high in folic acid.

Folic acid may be prescribed prophylactically in the following conditions:

— folate deficiency
— malabsorption syndrome
— haemoglobinopathies
— anticonvulsant treatment
— multiparity
— multiple pregnancy
— adolescence.

The dose is 300–500 µg daily.

Signs and symptoms
These are pallor, lassitude, progressive anorexia, mental depression, nausea and vomiting, glossitis, gingivitis and diarrhoea. There are no abnormal neurological findings.

Investigation
In folic acid deficiency the red cells are reduced in number but enlarged in size. It is termed *macrocytic* or *megaloblastic* anaemia. The MCV rises; the MCH may remain the same but as there are fewer cells the Hb level falls.

Management
Folic acid is available in oral and intramuscular forms, the usual daily dose being between 5 and 15 mg in divided doses. Side-effects are rare. Folic acid should not be given in cases of vitamin B_{12} deficiency as it can hasten subacute degeneration of the spinal cord.

Complications of folic acid deficiency in pregnancy
These include infection, placental separation, bleeding and possible congenital abnormalities such as neural tube defects.

Vitamin B_{12} deficiency anaemia

Deficiency of vitamin B_{12} also produces a megaloblastic anaemia. Vitamin B_{12} levels fall during pregnancy but anaemia is rare because the body draws on its stores. Deficiency is most likely in vegans, who eat no animal products at all, and in some Asians.

Haemolytic anaemia

Haemoglobin consists of a group of four molecules, each of which has a haem unit which is made up of an iron porphyrin complex, and a protein chain. The position of the amino-acids in the protein chains determines the type of haemoglobin produced. Adult Hb (HbA) has 2 alpha and 2 beta chains while fetal Hb (HbF) has 2 alpha and 2 gamma chains. By 6 months of age 96% of a baby's Hb is HbA. The type of protein chain is genetically determined. Defective genes lead to the formation of abnormal Hb and a more fragile red cell.

Haemoglobinopathies

This term describes conditions where haemoglobin is abnormal. They prevail in certain geographical areas and racial groups. Screening of parents may be carried out by electrophoresis which detects different types of Hb. From 7 weeks onwards fetal blood obtained by cordocentesis can be examined for abnormalities, making early diagnosis possible using genetic probes. Chorionic villus sampling may also be done in the first trimester.

Many decisions about investigations or treatment are made by balancing risks against benefits as some of these investigations carry a risk of miscarriage. Prospective parents who are known to have (or carry genes for) abnormal Hb need genetic counselling in order to help them make an informed decision before embarking on a pregnancy.

Thalassaemia. This condition is most commonly found in people of Mediterranean, African, Middle and Far Eastern origin. The basic defect is a reduced rate of globin chain synthesis resulting in either alpha or beta chains being missing. This leads to ineffective erythropoiesis and to haemolysis and a resultant inadequate haemoglobin content. The severity of the condition depends on whether the child has inherited abnormal genes from one parent or from both. Figure 22.1 shows the possible offspring from a couple who both carry one faulty gene and Table 22.2 shows the number of abnormal genes in each type of thalassaemia.

Thalassaemia intermedia and minor produce an anaemia which is similar to iron deficiency in that the Hb, the MCV and the MCH are all lowered. A deficiency in iron is not, however, usually a problem because red cells are broken down more rapidly than normal and the iron is stored for future use. Iron therapy is inappropriate but the woman should be given folic acid supplements.

The incidence of thalassaemia minor in the UK is in the region of 1 in 10 000.

Thalassaemia major. The child inherits abnormal genes from both parents. Rapid red cell breakdown produces a severe anaemia. In the worst form (alpha thalassaemia major) this condition is incompatible with extra-uterine life. Beta thalassaemia major may result in cardiac failure and death in early childhood although the use of frequent blood transfusion increases the possibility of survival to childbearing age. The constant breakdown of red cells from donated blood results in an accumulation of iron in the body which must be removed by the chelating agent desferrioxamine.

A pregnant woman with thalassaemia major should have shared care from an obstetrician and a haematologist. It may be preferable for her to be referred to a specialist centre where members of staff giving care are experienced in managing this condition. The mother will need to increase her dietary intake of folic acid and to take folic acid supplements throughout pregnancy. Repeated blood transfusions may be required. The midwife has a role to play in supporting the woman and in maintaining links with other departments such as haematology, social work and voluntary bodies, for example, the thalassaemia society.

Sickle cell anaemia. In this condition defective genes produce abnormal haemoglobin beta chains; the resulting Hb is called HbS. In *sickle cell disease* (HbSS) abnormal genes have been inherited from both parents while in *sickle cell trait* (HbAS) only one abnormal gene has been inherited.

When subjected to low oxygen tension, HbS

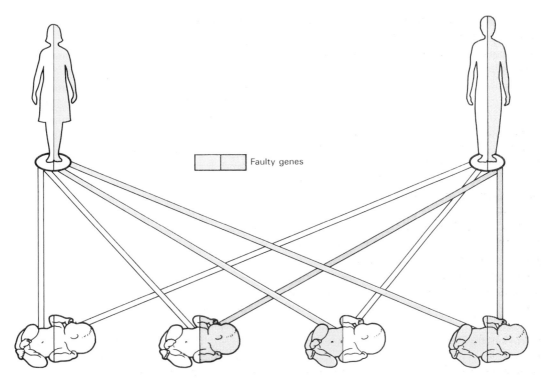

Fig. 22.1
The inheritance of thalassaemia when both parents are heterozygous.

contracts, damaging the cell and causing it to assume a sickle shape. Damaged cells block capillaries in the kidney, brain or placental bed and cause ischaemia and pain. The cells are haemolysed and anaemia develops.

Sickle cell anaemia is found most commonly in people of African or West Indian origin.

Table 22.2
Types of thalassaemia and their inheritance

Alpha chains are formed by 2 genes from each parent
Beta chains are formed by 1 gene from each parent

Therefore:
Alpha thalassaemia major = 4 defective alpha genes
Beta thalassaemia major = 2 defective beta genes

Alpha thalassaemia intermedia = 3 defective alpha genes

Alpha thalassaemia minor = 2 or 1 defective alpha genes
Beta thalassaemia minor = 1 defective beta gene

Sickle cell trait is usually asymptomatic. The blood appears normal, although the sickle screening test is positive. There is no anaemia even under the additional stress of pregnancy.

Sickle cell anaemia. Women with sickle cell anaemia may be subfertile but those who do become pregnant may already have organ damage. This occurs as a result of sickling crises which may occur whenever oxygen concentration is low, for instance during anaesthesia, illness, cold, at high altitude or during pregnancy. The red cells sickle and clump together, blocking small blood vessels. The resulting infarction leads to pain, affecting particularly the bones, joints and abdominal organs. Emboli may be thrown off into the circulation, which may threaten life. Sickle cells have an increased fragility and shortened life span of 17 days. This results in chronic haemolytic anaemia.

Antenatal care. Women in groups at risk are screened. Those who are diagnosed as having sickle cell anaemia will be referred to a specialist centre.

Monitoring of pregnancy is performed at regular intervals under the joint supervision of obstetricians and haematologists with back-up from the laboratory and a sickle cell centre and with the support of trained haemoglobinopathy counsellors. This role is both supportive and educational to the sufferers, families and health care workers. In addition they provide a counselling service for the at-risk community in the screening programme before, during and after pregnancy.

During pregnancy it is important that women with sickle cell anaemia avoid situations which may precipitate a crisis such as cold, stress, dehydration, hypoxia and infection.

Regular monitoring of the Hb concentration is required throughout pregnancy. Treatment may include a 3–4 unit blood transfusion every 6 weeks to maintain an adequate Hb level. Alternatively an exchange transfusion may be needed in an emergency.

Possible complications which may occur include pre-eclampsia, urinary tract infection, pneumonia, spontaneous abortion, preterm labour and intra-uterine growth retardation. Both fetal and maternal mortality rates are increased.

The midwife's role is to identify preventative measures as well as to provide social and psychological support.

Intrapartum care. During labour the midwife must ensure that the woman is kept well hydrated with intravenous fluids, given prophylactic antibiotics and effective analgesia, preferably epidural, and oxygen therapy if needed.

The fetus should be monitored closely for signs of distress. Neonatal testing of all babies at risk must be undertaken by obtaining a cord blood sample at delivery.

The sickle cell test does not yield positive results until the age of 3–4 months as fetal haemoglobin (HbF) recedes. A positive test does not distinguish between sickle cell trait and sickle cell anaemia, therefore all children showing positive results should be investigated and followed up by the haematologist.

In order to prevent the high incidence of infant mortality from sickle cell anaemia, early prophy-laxis with antibiotics is recommended in the early months.

Postnatal care. Prevention of puerperal sepsis is paramount, therefore antibiotic cover is continued throughout the postnatal period.

Combinations of abnormal haemoglobins. Sickle cell haemoglobin C anaemia (HbSC) is a mild variant of HbSS more commonly found in Ghanaians. It presents with normal or near-normal levels of Hb. Owing to its mildness, neither the woman nor the obstetrician is aware of its presence or its complications. Women with HbSC may have mild sickling episodes, therefore close supervision is required to avoid any stimulus to a crisis such as hypoxia, dehydration or trauma. This particularly applies immediately after delivery. These women should be managed during labour in the same way as those with HbSS.

Sickle cell disease may be combined with beta thalassaemia.

Other rare inherited abnormalities

Glucose-6 phosphate dehydrogenase (G6PD) deficiency is found in Africa, Asia and Mediterranean countries. It is inherited through an X-linked gene and is therefore seen predominantly in males. G6PD is an enzyme necessary for the survival of the red cell. When it is deficient red blood cells are destroyed in the presence of certain substances. These include fava beans, sulphonamides, vitamin K analogues, salicylates and camphor (found in products such as Vick). Clinically G6PD deficiency takes two forms:

- Jaundice in the neonatal period, usually occurring on the second or third day of life, reaching a maximum by the sixth day and subsiding by the end of the first week.
- Acute self-limiting haemolysis precipitated by contact with the substances listed above. This may be indirect contact via the placenta or breast milk. Death from haemolysis is rare.

Spherocytosis is found in Northern Europe. In this condition the red cells are spherical instead of biconcave and are easily destroyed. In this disease the abnormal gene is dominant. It may cause a haemolytic jaundice in the neonate.

HYPERTENSION

Hypertension is the term used to describe a blood pressure deemed to be higher than average (de Swiet 1989). Hypertension in pregnancy has three possible causes:

- It may be a long-term problem, present before the beginning of the pregnancy, for example essential hypertension which accounts for 5% of the cases of hypertension in pregnancy.
- It may be caused by the pregnancy itself. This is known as pregnancy-induced hypertension and is discussed in Chapter 20.
- It may be secondary to existing medical problems such as:
  — renal disease
  — systemic lupus erythematosus
  — coarctation of the aorta
  — Cushing's syndrome
  — phaeochromocytoma, which is a rare but dangerous tumour of the adrenal medulla.

Investigation

When taking a history the midwife may identify potential or existing problems which may include a known medical condition. Women with essential hypertension tend to be older, parous and have a family or personal history of hypertension. The midwife can enquire about the woman's social background and investigate her psychological needs, offering her support as necessary.

Consistent blood pressure recordings of 140/90 mmHg or more during the first 20 weeks of pregnancy suggest that the hypertension is a chronic problem and unrelated to pregnancy. Hypertension which is essential or secondary is most easily detected during the first trimester because of the physiological fall in blood pressure which occurs in pregnancy.

Accurate readings are important and the midwife should bear in mind points such as avoidance of postural hypotension, placing the cuff at the level of the left atrium and using a cuff large enough for the arm. Consistency between observers is improved by agreeing, for example, that the diastolic reading is at the point where the sound becomes muffled, i.e. Korotkoff sound IV. Several blood pressure recordings should be made in order to determine the true pattern as even normotensive women show occasional peaks (see also Ch. 10).

The doctor's physical examination of the woman may reveal the long-term effects of hypertension such as retinopathy, ischaemic heart disease and renal damage. Weak femoral pulses indicate coarctation of the aorta. Renal function tests may be performed; however, it is important to realise the extent to which the alterations in the physiological norms may affect clinical interpretation in pregnancy (Davison 1989). Blood urate levels may help to differentiate between essential hypertension and pre-eclampsia (Ch. 20); they do not rise in the former as they do in the latter.

Admission to hospital or a day unit for initial assessment may be necessary.

Complications

Women with essential or secondary hypertension have a predisposition to a superimposed pre-eclampsia. Other complications are independent of pregnancy and include renal failure and cerebral haemorrhage.

The perinatal outcome in essential hypertension is good unless the blood pressure exceeds 200/130 mmHg for a prolonged period. If essential hypertension is complicated by pre-eclampsia, however, there may be severe fetal compromise (Ch. 20).

Phaeochromocytoma has a 50–60% maternal mortality rate if untreated.

Management

Mild essential hypertension

This is defined as a blood pressure of between 140/90 and 150/95 mmHg. The woman is unlikely to need antenatal admission to hospital and may be cared for by the community midwife and the general practitioner. The woman's condition should be carefully monitored in order to identify any pre-eclampsia which develops.

Severe essential hypertension

The blood pressure is above 150/95 mmHg. Ideally

the woman will be cared for by the obstetric team in conjunction with the physician and may need to visit the hospital more frequently than normal.

Antihypertensive drug therapy is used in order to prevent maternal complications but has no proven benefit for the fetus nor to the prognosis of the pre-eclamptic process. The most commonly used agent is methyldopa 1–4 g/day in divided doses. It has a sedative effect lasting 2–3 days and can also cause urine to darken. Other drugs in common usage include labetalol, atenalol and oral hydralazine.

Sedative drugs may be given to reduce anxiety and help the woman to rest. The midwife may do much to settle anxiety by the use of counselling skills and by mobilising resources to meet social needs if required. Diuretics are rarely used in pregnancy.

In the rare event of a phaeochromocytoma being present the blood pressure will be treated with appropriate antihypertensive drugs during pregnancy and the tumour resected postnatally.

Monitoring of fetal well-being and of placental function will be carried out assiduously because of the risk of fetal compromise. This would include using serial growth scans and placental blood flow studies by Doppler ultrasound (see Ch. 41). If maternal or fetal condition deteriorates, the woman will be admitted to hospital. The timing of the delivery is planned according to the needs of mother and fetus. If early delivery is deemed necessary, induction of labour is preferred to caesarean section (see also Ch. 20).

Renal function should be reassessed postnatally and the woman should be seen by the physician with a view to long-term management of persistent hypertension. The midwife who is advising the woman on family planning should be aware of the hypertensive effect of the combined oral contraceptive pill.

RENAL PROBLEMS

A knowledge of the effects of pregnancy on the urinary tract and on renal function will assist the midwife to understand the impact of pregnancy on existing urinary tract disease and the predis-position pregnant women have to develop urinary tract infection (see Ch. 6).

Tests of renal function

Creatinine is a product of muscle breakdown and is excreted by the kidney at a regular rate; for this reason it is a useful indicator of renal function. The glomerular filtration rate rises by 50% during pregnancy leading to a greater clearance of creatinine; the plasma creatinine level falls but rises again during the third trimester. *Plasma urea* levels follow a similar pattern:

	Plasma creatinine	Plasma urea
Normal non-pregnant values	70–130 μmol/l	2.5–6.6 mmol/l
Pregnancy upper limit	75 μmol/l	4.5 mmol/l

Plasma urates fall during mid-trimester and rise again to almost non-pregnant levels at term.

	Plasma urates
Normal non-pregnant values	0.12–0.42 mmol/l
Mid-trimester values	0.12–0.24 mmol/l
Values towards term	0.24–0.36 mmol/l

Pyelonephritis

Pyelonephritis occurs in 1–2% of all pregnancies. The causative organism is often *Escherichia coli*. Bacteriuria in early pregnancy is a predisposing factor. Intra-uterine growth retardation and pre-term labour are associated with pyelonephritis and there is a suggestion that there may be an increase in congenital abnormality.

The mother feels extremely unwell and usually has a marked pyrexia which may reach 40°C. Rigors may occur. Maternal and fetal heart rates are accelerated. The mother may be nauseated and vomit to the point of dehydration.

Pain and tenderness over the loins may be accompanied by muscle guarding. The pain follows the path of the ureters and radiates down to the suprapubic region. The mother may complain of scalding on micturition and a desire to pass urine even when her bladder is empty.

Examination of the urine shows it to be cloudy. If the infecting organism is *E. coli* the urine will usually be acid but with other organisms may be acid or alkaline.

Management of acute pyelonephritis

If the mother exhibits any of the above symptoms the midwife must refer to a doctor immediately. Admission to hospital is usual and the midwife should help the mother to arrange for care of any other children.

A mid-stream specimen of urine (MSU) should be sent to the laboratory for culture and sensitivity. An appropriate antibiotic will be prescribed; this will be given intravenously at first and orally as the condition improves. In some centres antibiotics may be continued for as long as 6 weeks and nitrofurantoin given until 2 weeks after delivery. A further MSU may be required 48 hours after commencement of treatment and this should be repeated at intervals after resolution of the infection in order to ensure that there is no recurrence.

Intravenous fluids may also be required to correct dehydration and an accurate record of fluid balance must be kept.

During the early stages of the illness the woman will be confined to bed and the midwife should take steps to prevent complications of immobility such as deep vein thrombosis and constipation.

The midwife must monitor uterine activity as there is a risk of labour commencing when the temperature rises. It may be necessary to reduce the temperature by the use of tepid sponging and antipyretics prescribed by the doctor. The temperature and pulse should be recorded at least 4 hourly.

The mother may be in considerable pain which may be eased by a heat pad applied to her back. Buscopan 20 mg may be used to relieve pain and anti-emetics given to counteract nausea.

Follow-up excretion urography is often carried out 3 months postnatally as persistent or recurrent infection, with or without symptoms, may be associated with an abnormality of the renal tract.

Chronic renal disease

The chances of a woman becoming pregnant decrease with declining renal function; pregnancy is rare if the kidneys are functioning at less than 50% efficiency. A pregnant woman with pre-existing renal disease is considered to be at high risk of pre-eclampsia; intra-uterine growth retardation, preterm birth and perinatal mortality are increased. The woman's own condition is likely to deteriorate. Hospital delivery is essential.

Disagreement exists over whether it is pregnancy or pregnancy complications which cause deterioration in renal condition. It is argued that the physiological increase in glomerular filtration can shorten the life of a damaged kidney (Brenner et al 1982).

During pregnancy proteinuria tends to increase. A loss of more than 30% of protein in 24 hours leads to oedema. Damage to the kidney tubules causes an activation of the renin–angiotensin system, leading to salt and water retention and a consequent rise in blood pressure. Production of erythropoietin may be reduced, leading to anaemia. The presence of chronic infection predisposes the mother to superimposed acute infection.

The outcome of pregnancy depends on the degree of renal dysfunction, the blood pressure and episodes of infection. Termination of pregnancy or early induction of labour may be offered if the renal condition deteriorates severely.

Examples of pre-existing renal disease are:

- polycystic kidney disease
- glomerular nephritis
- chronic pyelonephritis
- renal calculi
- nephrotic syndrome.

The implications for mother and baby and the management vary according to the condition.

Management

Apart from routine monitoring of the pregnancy (see Ch. 10), the aim of management is to prevent deterioration in renal function. This will necessitate more frequent attendance for antenatal care and the midwife may need to help the mother make the necessary arrangements (see Ch. 45).

Renal function tests are performed at intervals throughout the pregnancy. The emergence and severity of hypertension and pre-eclampsia are monitored by recording blood pressure and estimating urea and uric acid levels (see Ch. 20).

Admission to hospital is advised if there is evidence of fetal compromise, if renal function deteriorates and proteinuria increases or if the blood pressure rises. In severe cases it may be necessary to transfer the woman to a renal unit for dialysis.

If pregnancy remains uncomplicated, some doctors suggest induction of labour at 38 weeks while others hope for spontaneous labour and delivery at term.

Renal transplant

The fertility of women who have had successful transplants is greater than that of women on haemodialysis. There is an increase in ectopic pregnancy as a result of pelvic adhesions but pregnancy does not affect the acceptance of the graft or the survival of the recipient.

Women are advised to wait 2 years after the transplant before attempting to become pregnant as this allows time for the success of the graft to be evaluated. Preconception advice is particularly important as the woman must be in optimal health before embarking on a pregnancy. The choice of contraceptive must be made with care because the combined pill may raise the woman's blood pressure and the intra-uterine contraceptive device may predispose her to infection.

Davison (1987) suggests the following indicators for successful pregnancy and delivery:

- good health for 2 years following transplant
- stature compatible with good obstetric outcome
- no proteinuria
- no significant hypertension
- no evidence of graft rejection
- no evidence of distension of the renal pelvis and calyces on a recent excretory urogram
- plasma creatinine of 180 μmol/l or less
- limited drug therapy, for example prednisolone 15 mg/day or less and azothioprine 2 mg/kg/day or less.

Immunosuppressive therapy is continued during pregnancy which makes the woman more vulnerable to infections such as cytomegalovirus. Hypertension, proteinuria, urinary tract infection, anaemia, intra-uterine growth retardation and premature delivery are all more common. The midwife must be aware of these possible deviations.

During pregnancy the woman should be seen by both the obstetrician and a nephrologist. Clinic visits will be more frequent. Fetal well-being, renal function, blood pressure, haemoglobin and the status of the graft will all be assessed.

During labour steroid therapy may be increased and antibiotics may be prescribed. Special care should be taken to prevent infection and monitor fluid balance.

The baby will be more prone to infection as the mother's immunosuppressive therapy reduces the number of antibodies crossing the placental barrier. The midwife should discuss with the parents ways in which the risk of infection can be minimised. The baby's adrenal function may also be depressed. Long-term follow-up of mother and baby is usually undertaken.

Acute renal failure

Acute renal failure is said to have occurred if urinary output falls below 400 ml in 24 hours. It is characterised by a reduced glomerular filtration rate which causes a rise in blood urea and creatinine.

Causes of renal failure can be classified according to the site of the problem. Reduced blood flow is *pre-renal*, obstruction of the renal capillaries as in disseminated intravascular coagulation is *intrinsic* and obstruction of the urinary tract as in renal calculi is *postrenal*.

Consideration of the mother's history may reveal one of the following:

- haemorrhage
- reduction in blood volume, as in hyperemesis gravidarum
- shock
- septic shock
- coagulopathy

— severe pre-eclampsia
— acute pyelonephritis
— acute fatty liver of pregnancy.

Occasionally acute renal failure occurs for no apparent reason 3–6 weeks after the birth.

Investigations

Blood samples will be taken for estimation of urea, electrolytes and plasma proteins. Dehydration can be assessed by estimating the haematocrit and osmolality of the blood and blood culture or liver function tests may help to reveal the cause of the failure.

Urine samples will be sent to the laboratory for culture and sensitivity, osmolality, specific gravity and protein estimation.

Termination of pregnancy may be advised in the case of acute fatty liver; haemodialysis or peritoneal dialysis may be used to reduce blood urea.

Management

The aims of medical management of acute renal failure are to reverse oliguria or anuria and to treat the cause.

The midwife will be involved in careful assessment of fluid intake and urinary output which may necessitate catheterisation of the bladder. She may also be requested to monitor the woman's central venous pressure. If possible the woman should be weighed daily in order to help monitor fluid retention or loss. Fluid replacement is calculated according to the volume lost in the previous 24 hours. An extra 500 ml is given in order to replace insensible fluid loss; in the presence of pyrexia a further 200 ml is added for every degree Celsius that the temperature exceeds the normal. When the circulating volume is reduced a plasma expander such as Haemaccel will be given; mannitol is both a volume expander and an osmotic diuretic.

A dietician may be consulted to advise on nutrition. The woman needs a high calorie, low protein, low salt and low potassium diet which will need adjustment as renal function improves.

Prognosis depends on the degree of renal failure. Women with acute tubular necrosis will even-

tually recover full renal function while those with complete cortical necrosis require haemodialysis and a subsequent kidney transplant.

Midwives can provide continuity and support for a woman who is transferred to a renal unit for treatment as they retain a responsibility for midwifery care.

DIABETES MELLITUS

Carbohydrate metabolism in pregnancy

The fetus obtains glucose from its mother via the placenta by a process of facilitated diffusion. From the 10th week of pregnancy there is a progressive fall in the maternal fasting glucose level from 4 mmol/l in early pregnancy to 3.6 mmol/l at term. During the third trimester the mother begins to utilise fat stores which were laid down during the first two trimesters. This results in a rise in free fatty acids and glycerol in the bloodstream and the woman will become ketotic more easily.

The fetoplacental unit alters the mother's carbohydrate metabolism in order to make glucose more readily available. The placenta manufactures human placental lactogen (HPL) which produces a resistance to insulin in the maternal tissues. This results in blood glucose levels which are higher after meals and remain raised for longer than in the non-pregnant state. Oestrogen and progesterone contribute to these changes and at the end of pregnancy cortisol levels rise which also leads to a rise in blood glucose. More insulin is produced, sometimes two or three times as much as in the non-pregnant state.

The extra demands on the pancreatic beta cells can precipitate glucose intolerance or overt diabetes in women whose capacity for producing insulin was only just adequate prior to pregnancy. If a mother was already diabetic before pregnancy, her insulin needs will be increased.

Glycosuria in pregnancy

Glucose is more liable to appear in the urine of a pregnant woman for the following reasons:

- In a non-diabetic the blood glucose remains within normal limits but the glomerular filtration rate rises. Glucose passes through the proximal convoluted tubule faster than it can be reabsorbed.

- In the diabetic, the rise in blood glucose leads to more glucose in the glomerular filtrate due to the lowering of the renal threshold for glucose.
- Renal tubular damage interferes with glucose reabsorption and may be revealed for the first time during pregnancy.

Glycosuria in pregnancy is not diagnostic of diabetes nor can it be used as a monitor of diabetes in the pregnant woman. Two episodes, however, are regarded as an indication for a glucose tolerance test.

Gestational diabetes

Certain women are at special risk of developing diabetes during pregnancy and may be identified when the history reveals one or more of the following:

- diabetes in a first degree relative
- recurrent abortion
- unexplained stillbirth
- congenital abnormality
- a baby whose birthweight was greater than the 97th centile for gestational age, for example a baby weighing more than 4360 g at 40 weeks
- previous gestational diabetes or impaired glucose tolerance
- persistent glycosuria.

In addition the woman may exceed the normal weight range by more than 20%.

The progressive increase in insulin demand during pregnancy can make latent diabetes appear. This may resolve after the pregnancy. Some women show a slightly impaired glucose tolerance during pregnancy which returns to normal after delivery.

Detection of diabetes in pregnancy

Women considered to be at risk of gestational diabetes undergo a glucose tolerance test. This will indicate whether they have normal or im-

paired glucose tolerance or have developed diabetes. The criteria for carrying out this test vary but would include the presence of the risk factors listed above and also heavy or repeated glycosuria.

When testing for the presence of glucose in urine it should be remembered that while most reagent *strips* are specific for glucose, reagent *tablets* will give a positive reaction in the presence of other sugars such as lactose which is not abnormal in the urine of pregnant women.

Before proceeding to a full glucose tolerance test a fasting blood sample may be examined for glucose.

Glucose tolerance tests vary slightly but the aim is always to assess the body's response to a glucose load. The woman is asked to fast for a period of time. The fasting blood glucose level is estimated and the woman is given a measured amount of glucose in the form of a drink such as Lucozade 353 ml which provides 75 g glucose. Blood samples are obtained at intervals for glucose estimation and the results compared with a normal range. The blood glucose level will rise initially but should return to normal within a given length of time. This time will vary with the amount of glucose administered. It would be considered abnormal if, between 28 and 34 weeks of pregnancy, glucose levels in two out of four venous samples exceeded the following:

- Fasting   8.0 mmol/l
- 1 hour after ingestion of   11.0 mmol/l 75 g glucose
- 2 hours after ingestion of   9.0 mmol/l 75 g glucose
- 3 hours after ingestion of   7.0 mmol/l 75 g glucose

(WHO 1980).

The effect of pregnancy on diabetes

In the early stages of pregnancy diabetic control may be complicated by nausea and vomiting. Throughout pregnancy there is a tendency to lose glucose in the urine. As the fetus grows the mother needs more carbohydrate and ketosis is induced more easily, particularly in the latter stages of pregnancy. The diabetic who is controlled by diet may become dependent on insulin.

Blood sugar must be kept within narrow limits in order to avoid exacerbating the effects of the diabetes. Women who have had diabetes since childhood and already have nephropathy or retinopathy can progress to kidney failure and blindness.

The effect of diabetes on pregnancy

When diabetes is well controlled its effect on pregnancy may be minimal. If the control is inadequate there may be complications. Maternal haemoglobin (Hb) can become irreversibly bound to glucose; this is termed glycosylated Hb and it normally constitutes 4–8% of the woman's total Hb, increasing during hyperglycaemia.

Fertility is reduced and should conception occur there is an increased risk of spontaneous abortion, stillbirth and fetal abnormality. The perinatal mortality rate is 2 or 3 times higher for diabetic mothers.

Diabetic women are more prone to urinary tract infection and they have a greater susceptibility to *Candida albicans*. The incidence of pre-eclampsia and of polyhydramnios is increased.

Effects on the fetus. The effect of uncontrolled diabetes on the fetus is partially due to disturbed maternal metabolism. Fetal blood glucose is similar to that of the mother and it is thought that congenital abnormality is caused by fetal hyperglycaemia during the first trimester of pregnancy. Even if glucose control is optimal preconceptionally and in the first trimester the incidence of congenital abnormality is increased. Severe maternal ketosis can cause intra-uterine death.

No particular congenital abnormality is typical but the rare combination of sacral agenesis and neurological defects is most often seen in babies of diabetic mothers. Neural tube defects are twice as common amongst babies of diabetic mothers and defects in the kidney and heart are also seen.

Glycosylated Hb releases oxygen poorly to the fetus and this may lead to intra-uterine growth retardation. A compensatory fetal polycythaemia develops and will result in neonatal jaundice when the excess red cells are broken down. This is exacerbated by relative immaturity of liver enzymes in these babies.

Babies of mothers with poorly controlled diabetes may be large (macrosomic) rather than small. The fetus responds to the extra glucose by producing more insulin which can increase its body fat and muscle mass. Birthweight and body length are both greater and the kidneys and adrenal cortex are larger. The head circumference and brain size are normal, however.

Pre-pregnancy care of the known diabetic

As pregnancy complications are reduced if diabetes is well controlled, a diabetic woman should consult her physician for preconception care and advice. Pregnancy may lead to a deterioration of the diabetes; for this reason she must be carefully examined for the presence of renal, cardiovascular or retinal changes before becoming pregnant. A woman with severe nephropathy might be advised to await transplant, a woman with ischaemic heart disease and shortened life expectancy might like to reconsider the advisability of pregnancy and a woman with proliferative retinopathy might be offered laser treatment.

The woman will need to continue using some form of contraception while improving control of her diabetes. She may be advised to use the progesterone-only pill or barrier methods. This reduces the risk of arterial changes associated with the combined oral contraceptive pill and the possibility of intra-uterine infection caused by an intra-uterine contraceptive device.

The midwife will offer advice on giving up smoking and weight control. She will also remind women of the importance of early antenatal care because of the effects of pregnancy on insulin requirements. All women with diabetes should be told by those who care for them how essential it is to ensure that their diabetes is well controlled before considering a pregnancy.

Antenatal care

A diabetic woman should be advised to book to

have her baby in a hospital with a Neonatal Intensive Care Unit. She should be seen at a combined antenatal and diabetic clinic. The woman is seen as often as is required in order to maintain good diabetic control; this may entail fortnightly visits until 28 weeks' gestation and then weekly until term.

The midwife should remember the woman's predisposition to genito-urinary infection and her need to pay particular attention to hygiene; she should alert her to signs and symptoms so that she will seek treatment as soon as possible.

It is necessary to assess the progress of the pregnancy in the normal way and to detect any complications. Alpha fetoprotein screening results must be interpreted in the light of the fact that open neural tube defects have been found at lower levels in diabetic mothers. Fetal growth and detailed anomaly scans must be observed carefully because of the risk of either growth retardation, macrosomia or fetal abnormality. Examination of maternal weight and of the abdomen will help the midwife to detect polyhydramnios. In addition the woman must be examined for any sign of diabetic complications. In severe cases such complications may provide sufficient grounds for termination of the pregnancy.

Control of diabetes in pregnancy

The aims of diabetic control in pregnancy are to avoid hypoglycaemia, to maintain the preprandial blood glucose between 4.0 and 5.5 mmol/l and to ensure that the postprandial peak does not exceed 7.2 mmol/l.

The dietician should be consulted and will advise the woman on her nutritional requirements. Special attention will be paid to such problems as nausea and vomiting and the woman might need advice on the importance of maintaining an adequate calorie intake. A diet which is high in fibre produces a more constant blood glucose because the carbohydrate is released for absorption more slowly. The need for carbohydrate increases as the fetus grows and the diet must be reviewed frequently. 24-hour urine samples can be taken to estimate glucose loss.

Subcutaneous insulin provides the best method of control for most women. A combination of a short- and an intermediate-acting insulin is usually given twice daily. The dose must be adjusted during pregnancy as insulin requirements increase.

In the case of a newly diagnosed diabetic the midwife's role will include teaching the woman how to give herself injections. Insulin is absorbed most quickly from the upper arm, then from the abdomen and more slowly from the thigh. The same area should be used at the same time each day so that the rate of absorption is predictable. The midwife will also ensure that the woman understands her dietary requirements and is able to complete any records accurately. The woman is usually given a kit containing glucagon which can be administered subcutaneously in the event of severe hypoglycaemia. The woman and members of her family should be taught how and when to use it.

Some women are able to alter their insulin dose once they are familiar with the variations in their own glucose pattern. Some centres have a doctor on call 24 hours a day to advise women on any concerns they may have.

Diabetic women may be admitted to hospital due to poor diabetic control, a destabilising illness or obstetric complications.

Monitoring diabetic control. As far as possible the woman monitors her own diabetes at home. The purpose of these home blood glucose measurements is:

- to detect hyperglycaemia and hypoglycaemia
- to measure changes of blood glucose during a 24-hour period
- to assess blood glucose control in times of special need so that insulin dosage can be readjusted accordingly
- to obtain a full blood glucose profile; samples should be taken at the following times:

  — before the morning injection
  — 1–2 hours after breakfast
  — before lunch
  — 1–2 hours after lunch
  — before the evening injection
  — 1–2 hours after the evening meal
  — before bedtime
  — at some point during the night.

The woman should try to do two home profiles before visiting the diabetic clinic; this will give a clearer picture of what is happening (Knopfler 1989). She may need to be taught how to take capillary blood samples and test them using a reflectance meter. Some women also test their urine but a reliable estimation cannot be obtained during pregnancy (see section on glycosuria in pregnancy).

At the clinic random blood glucose estimations may be carried out in order to check the woman's self-monitoring. Blood samples for estimation of glycosylated haemoglobin (HbA_1) are often taken throughout pregnancy in order to gain a retrospective picture of the blood glucose levels over a 6-week period. The HbA_1 levels reflect overall control and correlate with the blood glucose profiles. In a non-diabetic person the HbA_1 level averages 6 mmol/l throughout pregnancy. In a diabetic pregnancy, levels of 5–8.5 mmol/l should be aimed for. A rise in HbA_1 during the first trimester is associated with an increase in fetal abnormality.

Management of labour and delivery

If diabetes has been well controlled, the risk of stillbirth is small. The former practice of routine delivery between 35 and 37 weeks of pregnancy is unnecessary.

Fetal lungs mature more slowly when the mother is diabetic and it is important to take this into account if induction of labour is being considered. Ideally labour should be allowed to commence spontaneously at term but poor diabetic control or a deterioration in maternal or fetal condition may necessitate earlier, planned delivery.

If labour begins prematurely beta sympathomimetics such as ritodrine hydrochloride or salbutamol may be used to relax the uterus in order to allow the lungs more time to mature. These drugs increase insulin requirements and blood glucose must be monitored frequently while they are being administered. Steroids such as dexamethasone which may be used to aid lung maturation also increase insulin requirements. Some doctors prefer not to attempt inhibition of preterm labour in diabetic women.

Control of diabetes in labour. Although regimens for diabetic control vary, the aim is to maintain blood glucose between 4 and 5 mmol/l. Maternal hyperglycaemia leads to an increase in fetal insulin production which will cause neonatal hypoglycaemia. See Figure 22.2 for an example of a regimen for diabetic control in labour. If labour is induced some women will be allowed a light breakfast while others will receive nil orally and the insulin dose will be adjusted accordingly.

The midwife should monitor fetal condition continually throughout labour using electronic fetal monitoring. A paediatrician should be present during delivery especially if labour has been induced as a baby with immature lungs may require resuscitation.

Polyhydramnios increases the risk of malpresentation, cord prolapse and uterine inertia during labour. Birth asphyxia is more common in both the macrosomic and the growth-retarded baby. The large baby is prone to birth injuries. Shoulder dystocia is a possible hazard to which the midwife must be alert during delivery. Caesarean section is not indicated for diabetes alone and should be reserved for obstetric indications.

Postnatal care

Mother

Carbohydrate metabolism returns to normal very quickly after delivery of the placenta and insulin requirements will fall rapidly. The woman can resume her pre-pregnancy regimen.

A diabetic mother who is breast feeding may need to increase her carbohydrate intake by 50 g a day and may need to adjust her insulin requirements according to a preprandial blood glucose estimation. Poor diabetic control will interfere with lactation. Although small amounts of insulin may enter breast milk these are destroyed in the baby's stomach.

The diabetic woman is more prone to infection and delayed healing. The midwife may need to advise her to change her pads frequently in order to keep any wound clean and dry.

Gestational diabetes. A woman with gestational diabetes requiring insulin will stop this

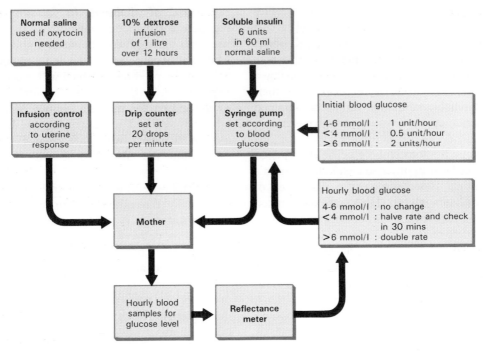

Fig. 22.2
The management of diabetes during labour.

immediately after delivery. A postpartum glucose tolerance test should be performed approximately 3 months after delivery. If this is normal the woman should be warned that the condition may recur in a subsequent pregnancy.

All women who have had gestational diabetes, particularly those who are overweight, are encouraged to keep to their diet for the rest of their lives, regardless of whether their glucose tolerance test is normal (Knopfler 1989).

Baby

Asphyxia is common in both macrosomic and growth-retarded babies. The former are also prone to birth injuries because of their size. The baby must be examined carefully at birth as there is an increased risk of congenital abnormality.

After birth the baby continues to produce more insulin than he needs. As he is no longer receiving high levels of glucose from his mother, hypoglycaemia may occur. To prevent this complication the baby should be fed soon after

delivery. Monitoring of neonatal blood glucose is often undertaken on the postnatal ward. If the baby's blood glucose is unstable he may be admitted to a neonatal unit for monitoring (see also Ch. 35).

Fetal hyperinsulinism results in polycythaemia. The destruction of many red cells and the relative immaturity of the liver in the newborn predispose the baby to jaundice.

EPILEPSY

The prevalence of epilepsy in the general population is 1:200 and it affects 0.3–0.5% of pregnant women. Between 1985 and 1987 three women died as a result of status epilepticus during pregnancy (DH 1991).

These days many women with epilepsy have children and it is important that midwives are aware of the implications in order to improve their care and reduce the risk of maternal death.

Antenatal care

In general, women whose epilepsy is well controlled have few problems from their condition in pregnancy. Most of the complications to pregnancy are increased when the epilepsy is poorly controlled (Saunders 1989). Care should be shared between the neurologist, the obstetrician and the midwife, preferably at a combined clinic as this maximises professional surveillance of the woman's condition without the added stress of multiple hospital appointments (Lindsay 1990).

The physiological changes of pregnancy produce a haemodilution and an increased metabolism of anticonvulsant drugs which lead to a fall in the plasma concentration. This results in difficulties with controlling seizures as pregnancy progresses. The pregnant mother should be advised to continue her anticonvulsant therapy at a dose that maintains therapeutic levels.

Complications of anticonvulsant therapy

Most of these drugs act as folic acid antagonists and may produce anaemia. Additionally long-term phenytoin treatment produces vitamin D deficiency and therefore women affected should receive supplementary vitamin D throughout pregnancy. Some anticonvulsant drugs have been associated with birth defects (Saunders 1989). Many different malformations have been reported, the most common being oro-facial clefts and congenital heart defects. Abnormalities are more common if anticonvulsant drugs are prescribed in high concentration and particularly if more than one is used. In spite of these potential problems most babies are unaffected and 90% are born normal.

Carbamazepine is not a folate antagonist and appears to be relatively safe in terms of teratogenicity. Nowadays it is considered to be the drug of choice in pregnancy. Preconception advice is important as it allows time for changes in medication and stabilising the condition prior to pregnancy. The antenatal care should include a detailed anomaly scan, which will detect any fetal abnormalities and allow the option of terminating the pregnancy.

Intrapartum and postnatal care

Care during labour and delivery is not likely to be any different from that of other mothers. Seizures are more likely to occur in conditions such as sleep deprivation, hypoglycaemia, anaemia, stress or hyperventilation. This holds implications for the care of the mother during labour and the early postnatal period where careful observation by the midwife is required (RCM 1989a & b).

Effect on fetus and neonate

According to Donaldson (1989), when status epilepticus occurs, one third of mothers and half of the fetuses do not survive. A single seizure may cause fetal morbidity from hypoxia or placental abruption.

Anticonvulsants cross the placenta freely and decrease production of vitamin K producing the risk of haemorrhagic disease. This can be prevented by routine administration of vitamin K to the mother from 36 weeks' gestation and to the baby shortly after birth (Brodie 1990).

The rate of clearance of anticonvulsant drugs varies according to the drug. Newborn infants may therefore suffer harmful effects from the anticonvulsant level and, as a group, tend to be less efficient at feeding and gain weight more slowly. A minority will suffer withdrawal symptoms such as tremor, excitability and convulsions. Anticonvulsants pass into the breast milk in relatively small quantities. Breast feeding is not contraindicated and helps to initiate a good mother and baby relationship.

Acknowledgements

The chapter authors are grateful for the help and advice of Ms K. Morton, Consultant Obstetrician, The Royal Surrey County Hospital, Guildford and Ms J. Wilson, Senior Registrar, Queen Charlotte's Hospital, London.

Reader Activities

- Bearing in mind the risk of food-borne infections to the pregnant woman and fetus, outline the dietary advice which you would give to a pregnant woman on her first and subsequent visits to the antenatal clinic.
- Highlight the specific problems associated with caring for a woman with cardiac disease during labour. As a midwife, how can you ensure that this labour will have a satisfactory outcome for mother and baby?
- Arrange a visit to the haematology laboratory and ask to be shown microscopic slides showing different forms of anaemia.
- Explore the literature on the use of iron therapy during pregnancy and clarify for yourself the advice that midwives should give concerning this controversial issue.
- Discuss the value and cost-effectiveness of routinely carrying out urinalysis, weighing and blood pressure measurement during pregnancy.
- Devise a care plan covering the first 24 hours after delivery for a woman who has epilepsy. Refer to the RCM booklets, *The care of mothers with epilepsy* and *Guidelines for mothers with epilepsy* (RCM 1989a & b) to assist you in this.

REFERENCES

Benson B 1983 Handbook of obstetrics and gynaecology. Lange Medical Publications, California

Best R, Banatvala J E 1990 Congenital virus infections. British Medical Journal 300 (5 May): 1151–1152

Brenner B M et al 1982 Dietary protein intake and the progressive nature of kidney disease. The role of hemodynamically medicated glomerula-injury in the pathogenesis of progressive glomerular sclerosis in ageing, renal ablation and intrinsic renal disease. New England Journal of Medicine 307: 652-659

Brodie M J 1990 Management of epilepsy during pregnancy and lactation. Lancet 336(8712): 426–427

Davison J M 1987 Pregnancy in renal allograft recipients: prognosis and management. Clinical Obstetrics and Gynaecology 1(4): 1027–1045

Davison J 1989 Renal disease. In: de Swiet M (ed) Medical disorders in obstetric practice. Blackwell Scientific Publications, Oxford

Department of Health et al 1991 Report on confidential enquiries into maternal deaths in the United Kingdom 1985–1987. HMSO, London, p 95–102

de Swiet M (ed) 1989 Medical disorders in obstetric practice. Blackwell Scientific Publications, Oxford

Donaldson J 1989 Neurology of pregnancy. W B Saunders, London

Katz S L, Wilfert C M 1989 Human immunodeficiency virus infection of newborns. New England Journal of Medicine 320: 1687–1689

Knopfler A 1989 Diabetes in pregnancy. Positive health guide. Macdonald, London, p 35

Lindsay P 1990 Epilepsy in pregnancy. Nursing Times 86(24): 36–38

Morgan-Capner P 1991 Viral infections in pregnancy. British Journal of Hospital Medicine 45 (March): 150–157

Nolan J 1990 Heart disease in pregnancy. Maternal and Child Health 15(3): 94–96

Public Health Laboratory Service Working Party on Fifth Disease 1990 Prospective study of human parvovirus B19 infection in pregnancy. British Medical Journal 300 (5 May): 1166–1170

Royal College of Midwives 1989a The care of mothers with epilepsy. RCM, London

Royal College of Midwives 1989b Guidelines for mothers with epilepsy. RCM, London

Saunders M 1989 Epilepsy in women of childbearing age. British Medical Journal 299: 581

Sills J A et al 1987 Acyclovir prophylaxis and perinatal varicella. Lancet i: 161

WHO 1980 World Health Organization Expert Committee: Diabetes mellitus technical report issues. WHO, Geneva, p 646

23

Multiple pregnancy

BEATRICE GRANT

The term 'multiple pregnancy' is used to describe the development of more than one fetus in utero.

Twin pregnancy occurs approximately once in every 100 pregnancies in the United Kingdom but in other parts of the world the incidence is different: in West Africa it is much higher and in Japan much lower. Triplets occur once in every 8000–9000 pregnancies and quadruplets once in every 700 000. Naturally occurring quintuplets are rare but because of an increased use of drugs like clomiphene to stimulate ovulation the consequent superovulation has led to an increase in pregnancies where quintuplets, sextuplets and septuplets have been conceived. Survival rates in such pregnancies, however, are poor.

Recent research suggests that the incidence of triplets and higher order multiples in England and Wales has increased since 1970 (Botting et al 1990).

TWIN PREGNANCY

Types of twin pregnancy

Twins may be monozygotic or dizygotic. *Monozygotic or uniovular twins* develop from one ovum and one spermatozoon. These twins have two amniotic sacs, one placenta and, usually, one chorion, although occasionally two chorions are found. There is a connection between the fetal circulations. These twins are always of the same sex and have similar palm and finger prints.

There is a high incidence of errors in development and malformations which give rise to abnormal fetuses. There may be a connection with the fact that complete division of the fertilised ovum is in itself abnormal. Conjoined or Siamese twins are monozygotic in origin.

Perinatal mortality rates for twins are higher than for singleton fetuses and are higher in monozygotic twins than in dizygotic (Botting et al 1990).

Dizygotic or binovular twins develop from two ova and two spermatozoa and are more common than monozygotic twins. These twins have two placentae which may be fused to form one, two amniotic sacs, two chorions and no connection between fetal circulations. These twins may be of the same sex, but are often of different sexes. There is a well-known familial tendency. The genetic factor which causes double ovulation is carried by the mother and passed on by the females in the family. Dizygotic twinning is a sign of fertility.

Table of comparison

Monozygotic or uniovular	Dizygotic or binovular
one ovum	two ova
one spermatozoon	two spermatozoa
one placenta	two placentae (may be fused)
one chorion (rarely two)	two chorions
two amnions (rarely one)	two amnions
same sex	different sexes or same sex

One fetus may die in utero and become a fetus papyraceous which is expelled with the placenta at delivery.

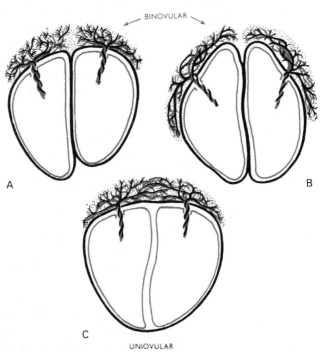

DIZYGOTIC OR BINOVULAR

BINOVULAR

A

B

C

UNIOVULAR

MONOZYGOTIC OR UNIOVULAR

Fig. 23.1
Twin placentae (A and B). Dizygotic twins have two placentae and two chorions.
(A) Placentae fused together. (B) Placentae separate. (C) Monozygotic twins have one shared placenta, one chorion and two amnions.

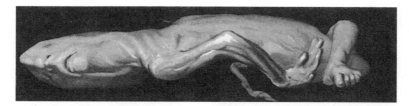

Fig. 23.2
Fetus papyraceous.

At delivery an apparently single placenta may be the result of the fusion of two separate placentae. On examination the presence of two chorions and two amnions should make the diagnosis of dizygotic twins obvious even if they are of the same sex (see Fig. 23.1).

The babies may be small and are often preterm but larger babies may be delivered. One twin may be considerably larger than the other and there may be a marked discrepancy in weights.

Diagnosis of twin pregnancy

Diagnosis of twin pregnancy may be difficult, although a family history of twins should alert the midwife to the possibility.

Ultrasound

Ultrasound can be used to detect the presence of more than one fetal sac from as early as 8 weeks' gestation but the presence of two fetuses may not be detected until 15 weeks when the outline of the heads will be noted. Only one twin may survive beyond 28 weeks' gestation. The expression 'vanishing twin' is sometimes used to describe the disappearance, in early pregnancy, of the other twin who can no longer be seen on the scan of the uterus.

Abdominal examination

On abdominal examination the following may be found:

Inspection. On inspection the size of the uterus may be larger than expected for the period of gestation, particularly after the 20th week. The uterus may look broad or round and fetal movement may be seen over a wide area, although this is not diagnostic. Fresh striae gravidarum may be apparent. Up to twice the amount of amniotic fluid may be expected but polyhydramnios may co-exist with twin pregnancy, particularly monozygotic twins.

Palpation. On palpation the fundal height may be greater than expected for the period of gestation. The presence of two fetal poles (head or breech) in the fundus of the uterus may be revealed on palpation and multiple fetal limbs may also be palpable. The size of the head in relation to the size of the uterus may lead one to suspect that the fetus is small and that there may be more than one in utero. Lateral palpation may reveal two fetal backs or limbs on both sides. Pelvic palpation may give findings similar to those on fundal palpation although one fetus may lie behind the other and make palpation difficult. Location of three poles in total is diagnostic of at least two fetuses.

Combinations of presentations in descending order of frequency

First twin		Second twin	
Vertex	:	Vertex	40–45%
Vertex	:	Breech	30–40% (³⁄₄)
Breech	:	Vertex	(¹⁄₄)
Breech	:	Breech	
Vertex	:	Shoulder	
Breech	:	Shoulder	

Auscultation. Hearing two fetal hearts is not diagnostic as one can often be heard over a wide area in a singleton pregnancy. If simultaneous comparison of the heart rates reveals a difference of at least 10 beats per minute, it may be assumed that two hearts are being heard.

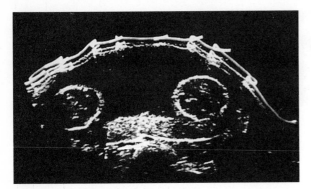

Fig. 23.3
Ultrasound picture of twins at 21.5 weeks' gestation.
Both heads are seen in oblique section. The placenta is
the speckled area near the bottom of the picture.

Effects on pregnancy

Exacerbation of minor disorders

The presence of more than one fetus in utero and
the higher levels of circulating hormones lead to
an exacerbation of the minor disorders of pregnancy. Morning sickness, nausea and heartburn
may be more persistent and more troublesome
than in a singleton pregnancy.

Anaemia

Iron deficiency and folic acid deficiency anaemias
are common in twin pregnancies. Early growth
and development of the uterus and its contents
make greater demands on maternal iron stores
and in later pregnancy (after the 28th week) fetal
demands for iron deplete those stores further. Poor
response to iron therapy may lead the midwife to
suspect folic acid deficiency.

Pregnancy-induced hypertension

This is more common in twin pregnancies and
may be associated with the larger placental site or
the increased hormonal output. The incidence
tends to be greater in monozygotic twin pregnancies.

Polyhydramnios

This is also common and is particularly associated
with monozygotic twins and with fetal abnormality.
If acute polyhydramnios occurs it tends to lead to
abortion. Polyhydramnios will add to any discomfort which the woman experiences.

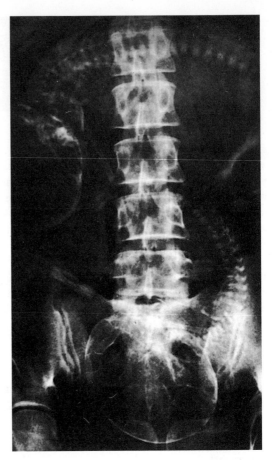

Fig. 23.4
X-ray picture of twins in utero. One is presenting by the
vertex, the other is lying transversely in the fundus.

Pressure symptoms

The increased weight and size of the uterus and
its contents may be troublesome. Impaired venous
return from the lower limbs increases the tendency
to varicose veins and oedema of the legs. Backache may be common and the increased uterine
size may also lead to marked dyspnoea and to
indigestion.

Management of pregnancy

Early diagnosis of twin pregnancy is important in
order to anticipate or prevent problems. Once the
diagnosis has been made, prevention of anaemia
is essential and haemoglobin estimations should
be carried out at regular intervals. Dietary advice

and the prescription of iron, folic acid and vitamins should help the woman to keep her haemoglobin at an acceptable level. Foods rich in iron, folic acid, vitamins and calcium should be advised and an adequate protein intake is essential. The obstetrician will wish to supervise this pregnancy closely and he should explain the reasons to the mother.

The detection of pregnancy-induced hypertension may necessitate more frequent visits to the clinic and, if necessary, admission to hospital for rest and observation may be arranged.

For relief of discomfort in later pregnancy it may be helpful for the woman to wear a light-weight support girdle or support tights. She may also require extra pillows at night either to prop her up in bed or to support the weight of the uterus.

The midwife should help the parents to prepare for twins by ensuring that they are given the opportunity to discuss any problems or worries which they may have about the prospect of caring for two babies. It can be a considerable shock to discover that two babies are on the way. The parents should be encouraged to ask questions and be informed about preparation for parenthood groups. Other parents who have had twins may be invited to come and talk to the prospective parents.

Admission to hospital will be necessary if complications arise and some women may be admitted to hospital around 30–32 weeks' gestation for a period of rest and observation.

Two babies will add considerably to the financial burdens of the family. The midwife should gently probe in order to find out the family circumstances in case they need to be referred to the social worker.

LABOUR AND DELIVERY

Effects on labour

Labour often occurs spontaneously before term due to the overstretching of the uterus or may be induced early if complications arise. In addition to being preterm the babies may be light for dates and prone to the associated complications of both.

If spontaneous labour begins at a time when the ability of the babies to survive outside the uterus is in doubt, ritodrine hydrochloride may be given in an attempt to suppress uterine activity.

It is unusual for a twin pregnancy to last more than 40 weeks and induction of labour will be considered if pregnancy continues beyond term.

Malpresentations are common and in the small number where the first twin presents by the breech, this may have an adverse effect on the length of the labour.

Management of labour

The woman may adopt whichever position she finds most comfortable. The use of a foam rubber wedge under the side of the mattress will help to prevent supine hypotensive syndrome by giving a lateral tilt. It may be preferable for her to adopt a semi-prone position, well supported with pillows or a bean-bag. A birthing chair or a reclining chair, if available, may be more comfortable than a delivery bed.

Analgesia is given as required and in view of the possibility of operative delivery epidural analgesia may be the first choice. Use of the Entonox apparatus may be helpful, particularly in the late first stage and during second stage of labour. Intramuscular pethidine 100 or 150 mg may be given in early labour but because of the depressant effect on fetal respiratory centres this drug is usually avoided if possible.

The woman should be encouraged to use whatever form of relaxation she finds helpful. If she expresses a wish to use drugs only after other methods have been tried and found inadequate, her wishes should be respected. The midwife should explain that if complications arise, intervention and the use of drugs may be necessary. This should be discussed prior to the onset of labour.

Both fetuses should be monitored continuously if possible. Initially two external transducers may be used but once the first sac of membranes is ruptured a scalp electrode may be applied to the first fetal head and the external transducer used to monitor the second fetal heart. Uterine activity will be monitored simultaneously.

If cardiotocography is not available, use of the Doptone or Sonicaid may give more accurate recordings of the fetal heart rates than a fetal stethoscope. If the latter has to be used, two people should auscultate simultaneously so that both fetal heart rates are counted over the same minute.

If fetal distress occurs during labour, delivery will need to be expedited, often by caesarean section. Action may also need to be taken if the maternal condition gives cause for concern.

If the uterine activity is poor, the use of intravenous Syntocinon may be required once the membranes are ruptured. Artificial rupture of the membranes may be sufficient in itself to stimulate good uterine activity but may be used in conjunction with intravenous Syntocinon. The cardiotocograph will give a good indication of the pattern of uterine activity, whether the labour is induced or spontaneous. The response of the fetal hearts to uterine contractions can be observed on the graph paper.

If the babies are expected to be of low birth weight, the neonatal unit should be informed that the woman is in labour so that they can make preparations. When delivery is imminent, the paediatric team should be summoned so that they may be present to receive the infants when they are born.

Throughout labour the general physical and psychological state of the mother must be considered. She requires support from the midwife and may be apprehensive about the outcome of her labour. The presence of her partner or companion will be helpful to her and the midwife should encourage her to ask questions and express her feelings.

Management of delivery

The onset of the second stage of labour should be confirmed by making a vaginal examination. The obstetrician, paediatrician and obstetric anaesthetist should be present for the delivery because of the risk of complications.

If epidural analgesia has been used it may be 'topped-up' prior to delivery, either by the anaesthetist or by the midwife if this is within her sphere of competence. The possibility of emergency caesarean section is ever present and the operating theatre should be in a state of readiness to receive the mother at short notice.

Monitoring of both fetal hearts should continue until delivery. Provided that the first twin is presenting by the vertex, the delivery can be expected to proceed normally, as with a singleton pregnancy (see Ch. 14). An elective episiotomy may be considered if there are complications. When the first twin is born the time of delivery and the sex are noted. This baby must be labelled as 'twin one' immediately. The identity bracelets should be completed and the midwife must check them with the mother before they are applied to the infant's ankle and wrist. The mother may wish to hold her baby and if he is in good condition this should be encouraged. He may be put to the breast because suckling stimulates uterine contraction. If he requires active resuscitation, the paediatric team will place him on the resuscitaire to facilitate this.

After delivery of the first twin, an abdominal examination is made to ascertain the lie, presentation and position of the second fetus and to auscultate the fetal heart. If the lie is not longitudinal an attempt is made to correct it by external cephalic version. If it is longitudinal, a vaginal examination is made to confirm the presentation. If the presentation is not engaged it should be pushed into the pelvis by fundal pressure before the second sac of membranes is ruptured. The fetal heart should be auscultated again and a scalp electrode may be applied once the membranes are ruptured. If uterine activity does not recommence, intravenous Syntocinon may be used to stimulate it.

When the presenting part becomes visible, the mother is encouraged to push with contractions to deliver the second twin. The midwife should be aware that, owing to the reduced size of the placental site following the birth of the first twin, the second fetus is somewhat deprived of oxygen. Delivery will proceed as normal if the presentation is vertex but if the fetus presents by the breech, the midwife may need to hand over to the doctor. An oxytocic drug is usually given intramuscularly or intravenously, depending on local policy.

This baby is labelled as 'twin two'. A note of the time of delivery and the sex of the child is made. The risk of asphyxia is greater for the second twin and the paediatric team may need to resuscitate this infant actively. He may need to be transferred to the neonatal unit immediately after delivery. He should, however, be shown to his mother prior to transfer and if possible she should be allowed to cuddle him. Some units make a point of keeping twins together which may result in the transfer of a healthy twin to the neonatal unit.

After both babies have been delivered, the midwife prepares to deliver the placentae. Once the oxytocic drug has taken effect, controlled cord traction is applied to both cords simultaneously and delivery of the placentae should be effected without delay. Emptying the uterus enables the control of bleeding and the prevention of postpartum haemorrhage.

The placenta(e) should be examined and the number of amniotic sacs, chorions and placentae noted (see Fig. 23.1). If the babies are of different sexes, the twins are dizygotic but if they are of the same sex it may be more difficult to determine whether they are monozygotic or dizygotic. The presence of one chorion and two amnions is indicative of monozygotic twins but two chorions and two amnions may indicate either dizygotic or monozygotic twins. Pathological examination of the placenta and membranes will confirm the diagnosis. The umbilical cords should be examined and the number of cord vessels and the presence of any abnormalities noted.

COMPLICATIONS ASSOCIATED WITH MULTIPLE PREGNANCY

Abortion

Abortion is more common in association with multiple pregnancy. If abnormality is present, the pregnancy may end in abortion quite early on. Over-distension of the uterus may lead to late abortion. In some cases one twin is lost at an early stage and the remaining fetus continues to develop normally.

Polyhydramnios

Acute polyhydramnios may occur at around 26–30 weeks and may be associated with fetal abnormality. It is found in association with monozygotic twins and the outcome is usually abortion. It is rare. Chronic polyhydramios is also a possibility. It may occur in one or both sacs (see also Ch. 21).

Fetal abnormality

This is particularly associated with monozygotic twins.

Malpresentations

Although the uterus is large and distended, the fetuses are less mobile than may be supposed. They can restrict each other's movements, which may result in malpresentation, particularly of the second twin. After delivery of the first twin, the presentation of the second twin may have changed.

Premature rupture of the membranes

Malpresentations or polyhydramnios may predispose to premature rupture of the membranes.

Prolapse of the cord

This, too, is associated with malpresentations and polyhydramnios and is more likely if there is a poorly fitting presenting part. The second twin is at particular risk of prolapse of the cord.

Prolonged labour

Malpresentations are a poor stimulus to good uterine action and a distended uterus is likely to lead to poor uterine activity and consequent prolonged labour.

Locked twins

This is a rare but serious complication of twin pregnancy. There are two varieties. One occurs when the first twin presents by the breech and the second by the vertex, the other when both are vertex presentations. In both instances the second twin prevents the continued descent of the first by the position of its head (see Fig. 23.5).

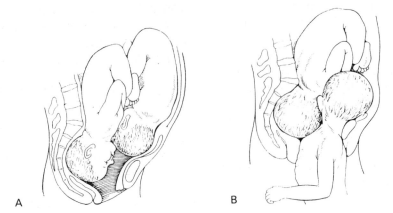

Fig. 23.5
Two varieties of locked twins. (A) Both twins presenting by the vertex. (B) Twin one — breech presentation. Twin two — vertex presentation.

Conjoined twins

If obstruction occurs during a twin delivery, the possibility of conjoined twins should be considered. Caesarean section is necessary and separation is sometimes possible.

Delay in the birth of the second twin

After delivery of the first twin uterine activity should recommence within 5 minutes. The second twin should be delivered within 15–20 minutes at the most. Poor uterine action as a result of malpresentation may be the cause of delay. The risks of such delay are intra-uterine hypoxia, birth asphyxia following premature separation of the placenta and sepsis as a result of ascending infection from the first umbilical cord which lies outside the vulva. After delivery of the first twin the lower uterine segment begins to re-form and the cervical canal may have to dilate again to full dilatation. The midwife may need to rub up a contraction and to put the first twin to the breast to stimulate uterine activity. If there appears to be obstruction, medical aid is summoned and caesarean section may be necessary. If there is no obstruction, Syntocinon infusion may be commenced or forceps delivery considered.

Premature expulsion of the placenta

The placenta may be expelled before delivery of the second twin. In dizygotic twins where the placentae are not fused, one placenta may be delivered separately; in monozygotic twins the shared placenta may be delivered. The risks of severe asphyxia and death of the second twin are high. Haemorrhage is also likely if one twin is retained in utero as this prevents adequate retraction of the placental site.

Postpartum haemorrhage

Poor uterine tone as a result of overdistension or hypotonic activity is likely to lead to postpartum haemorrhage. The placental site is also large and may encroach on the lower segment (see also Ch. 29).

Undiagnosed twins

The possibility of undiagnosed twins should be considered if the uterus appears larger than expected after delivery of the baby, or if the baby is smaller than expected. If an oxytocic drug has been given after delivery of the anterior shoulder of the first baby, the second baby is in grave danger and delivery should be expedited. He will require active resuscitation because of severe asphyxia.

The midwife should break the news of undiagnosed twins gently to the parents. These parents will require special support and guidance during the postnatal period.

THE POSTNATAL PERIOD

Care of the babies

Immediate care at delivery will involve ensuring that both babies have a clear airway. Maintenance of body temperature is vital, particularly if the infants are small, and use of an overhead heater on the resuscitaire will help to prevent heat loss. The infants should not be over-exposed and gentle handling is important. Identification of the infants should be clear and the parents are given the opportunity to check the identity bracelets and handle their babies. The infants may be admitted directly to the neonatal unit from the labour ward or they may be transferred to the postnatal ward if they are in good condition.

Temperature control

Maintenance of a thermoneutral environment is essential, particularly for infants in the neonatal unit. They may need to be nursed in incubators. One infant may be in the neonatal unit and one in the postnatal ward if he is of normal weight but some prefer to keep the babies together. Clothing should be light but warm and allow air to circulate. The babies' temperatures should be checked regularly and recorded. If they are below normal range, rewarming is required.

Nutrition

Both babies may be breast fed simultaneously or serially or they may be artificially fed. The mother may elect to breast feed one and artificially feed the other, although it is preferable to use the same method for both. The milk supply may appear insufficient for two babies, in which case they may alternate between breast and bottle feeds. The midwife should bear in mind that lactation responds to the demands made upon the breast and should encourage the mother to attempt total breast feeding. The mother should be shown how to hold the babies so that she can feed them simultaneously.

As the babies are likely to be preterm or light for dates or both, their ability to co-ordinate the sucking and swallowing reflexes may be poor. If so, they must be fed by nasogastric tube, naso-jejunal tube or intravenously depending on their size and general condition. The mother should be encouraged to participate whatever method is used. Careful monitoring of weight gain is required. Hypoglycaemia may occur and capillary blood glucose estimation should be made regularly.

Prevention of infection

The principles of hygiene should be re-inforced as prevention of infection is a priority. If the infants are of low birth weight they are more susceptible to infection. The mother should be encouraged to wash her hands before handling her babies.

Mother–baby relationships

It may be difficult for the mother to relate equally to each child. For example, if the babies are of markedly different sizes, she may favour one or the other or if one infant is in the neonatal unit and the other with her in the postnatal area she may have a preference for the one that she sees more of. If she has had an operative delivery she may find it difficult to care for two babies and extreme tiredness or anaemia will exacerbate the situation. The midwife should be alert for such circumstances and help the mother to divide her attention between both.

Care of the mother

Involution of the uterus will be slow because of its increased bulk. 'After pains' may be troublesome and analgesia should be offered. Some mothers may benefit from a night sedative and all need rest. A good diet is essential and if the mother is breast feeding she requires a high protein, high calorie intake. Hunger between meals may be appeased by snacks of the mother's choosing kept in her locker. A dietitian may be able to offer help.

The midwife must give the mother of twins support and help in caring for her babies as initially she may be frightened or feel inadequate about coping on her own. Her confidence may be built up by teaching her simple parenting skills and encouraging her to carry them out with increasing assurance.

The mother may feel very 'left out' in the postnatal period when all the care and attention seems to be centred on the babies. She may find it difficult to come to terms with the fact that she has two infants to care for. If one infant is very ill or dies she will experience additional psychological problems.

Postnatal exercises should be encouraged. They help to improve the muscle tone of the abdomen and pelvic floor and also bladder and bowel function.

The mother may be discharged home without the babies if both are in the neonatal unit or she may take one child with her and leave the other. Great demands are placed on the mother if she is required to care for one child at home and visit the other in hospital. If both babies are discharged home with the mother she will probably require help until she becomes familiar with handling and caring for the babies. A home help may be organised or a relative or friend may stay. The community midwife will visit until the 10th postnatal day and beyond if she feels it is necessary. She will reinforce the mother's knowledge and give help and advice where necessary. Once the mother goes home she must have adequate rest and sleep in order to recover from the effects of pregnancy and delivery and be able to care for her family adequately. It might be more helpful to the mother if visitors are discouraged in the first week at home while she adjusts to the new circumstances. The father should be encouraged to help as much as possible.

Voluntary groups provide support and practical help. The Twins and Multiple Births Association may have a local group. It can be helpful to meet other parents who have had twins and who have faced the same kind of problems that new parents of twins are experiencing. Practical help may involve hiring or selling second-hand prams, cots or clothes and some clubs use this as a means of fund raising.

Parents of twins should be encouraged to think of their children as individuals. Ways to emphasise their individuality include choosing names which do not rhyme or sound similar and using dress and hair styles which are different, particularly if the twins are of the same sex. Children should be addressed by name, not 'twin', and when it comes to birthdays, separate cards and different presents help to retain individuality. Parents should also be alerted to the feelings of any older children who may suffer a particularly acute loss of attention with the arrival of twins.

HIGHER MULTIPLES

The incidence of higher multiples has increased with greater use of drugs which stimulate ovulation such as clomiphene or Pergonal.

Considerations during pregnancy
Triplets, quadruplets or quintuplets are prone to the same complications as twins but are even more likely to deliver before term. Perinatal mortality rates are higher than in twins or singletons.

The mother may have difficulty in coming to terms with the idea of three, four or five fetuses in utero and if, at the end of labour, none of the fetuses survives, she will have considerable problems adjusting to this loss. It can be helpful to contact other parents with similar problems. The Twins & Multiple Births Association (TAMBA) Twinline is a useful resource. (See also Ch. 49.)

Mode of delivery
The mode of delivery is chosen with regard to maternal and fetal well-being. Complications may necessitate delivery being effected early, often by caesarean section. The midwives must be prepared to receive several very small babies within a very short time-span. It is essential to have the paediatric team present as expert care is required.

Special dangers
Asphyxia, intracranial injury and perinatal death are all much more likely in higher multiples.

Publicity
If the babies are born alive the parents may have to contend with media coverage and this requires careful handling. Staff must be careful to maintain confidentiality. Baby food manufacturers and other interested parties may wish to supply the new family with their products in return for

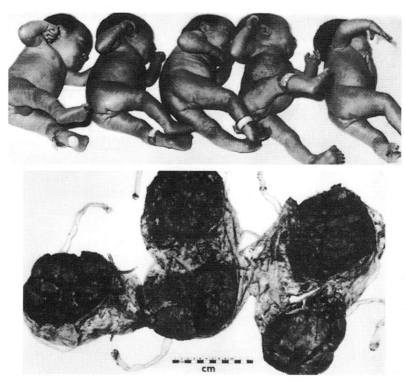

Fig. 23.6
Quintuplets born in 1972. Weights: 1470 g, 1250 g, 1490 g, 1596 g and 1250 g. Placentae: total weight 1780 g.

advertising rights. The midwife should be ready to discuss such matters with the parents if they wish and to refer them to a suitable adviser.

Reader Activities

Find out if there is a branch of TAMBA in your area. If possible visit the group and listen to the parents and the children.
Decide how you could use the information gained:

- to help other parents in similar circumstances
- to increase your own understanding.

USEFUL ADDRESSES

Twins and Multiple Births Association (TAMBA)
360 Woodham Lane
Newham
Weybridge
Surrey

Scottish contacts:
Mrs Ruth Campbell-Smith
72 Craigton Drive
Newton Mearns
Glasgow

Mrs Dorothy Lynch
2 Glebe Grove
Corstorphine
Edinburgh

Multiple Births Foundation
Queen Charlotte's & Chelsea Hospital
Goldhawk Road
London W6 0XG

REFERENCES

Botting B, Macfarlane A J, Prince F V 1990 Three, four and more: a study of triplet and higher order births. HMSO, London
Bryan E 1983 The nature and nurture of twins. Baillière Tindall, London
Linney J 1983 Multiple births. H M and M, London
Moore K L 1983 Before we are born: basic embryology and birth defects, 2nd edn. W B Saunders, Eastbourne
Willocks J B (ed) 1986 Essentials of obstetrics and gynaecology, 3rd edn. Churchill Livingstone, Edinburgh

FURTHER READING

Atkinson R L, Atkinson R C, Smith E E, Bem D J Hilgard
E R 1990 Introduction to psychology, 10th edn. Harcourt
Brace, Jovanovich, San Diego

Clay M M 1989 Quadruplets and higher multiple births.
MacKeith, Oxford

Leigh G 1989 All about twins — a handbook for parents.
Routledge, London

Patel N, Campbell D, Barrie N, Howat R, Melrose E,
Redford D, McIlwaine G, Smalls M 1983 Scottish twin
study. University of Glasgow Social and Paediatric
Research Unit, Glasgow

24

Structural abnormalities affecting pregnancy

JOHNANNA T. MATTHEW

For pregnancy and labour to be achieved with minimal difficulty, a woman must have normal reproductive anatomy. When structural abnormality of the pelvic organs or of the bony pelvis exists, problems arise which can place an extra burden on mother and fetus. The possible effects of such abnormalities are explored in this chapter.

UTERINE MALFORMATIONS

Embryological development of the uterus

The female genital tract is formed in early embryonic life when a pair of ducts develop. These paramesonephric or Müllerian ducts come together in the midline and fuse into a Y-shaped canal. The open upper ends of this structure open into the peritoneal cavity and the unfused portions become the uterine tubes. The fused lower portion forms the uterovaginal area which further develops into the uterus and vagina.

Types of uterine malformation

Various types of structural abnormality can result from failure of fusion of the Müllerian ducts. Three of these abnormalities can be seen in Figure 24.1. A double uterus with an associated double vagina will develop where there has been complete failure of fusion. Partial fusion results in various degrees of duplication. A single vagina with a

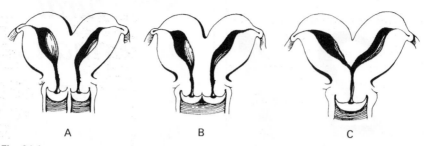

Fig. 24.1
(A) Double uterus with duplication of body of uterus, cervix and vagina. (B) Duplication of uterus and cervix with single vagina. (C) Duplication of uterus with single cervix and vagina.

double uterus is the result of fusion at the lower end of the ducts only. A bicornuate uterus (one with two horns) is the result of incomplete fusion at the upper portion of the uterovaginal area. In rare cases, one Müllerian duct regresses and the end result is a uterus with one horn — termed a unicornuate uterus.

Effect of abnormality on pregnancy

When pregnancy occurs in the woman with an abnormal uterus, the outcome depends on the ability of the uterus to accommodate the growing fetus. A problem only exists if the tissue is insufficient to allow the uterus to enlarge for a full-term fetus lying longitudinally.

If there is insufficient hypertrophy, the possible difficulties are abortion, premature labour and abnormal lie of the fetus. In labour, poor uterine function may be experienced.

Minor defects of structure cause little problem and might pass unnoticed with the woman having a normal outcome to her pregnancy. Occasionally problems arise when a fetus is accommodated in one horn of a double uterus and the empty horn has filled the pelvic cavity. In this situation, the empty horn has grown due to the hormonal influences of the pregnancy, and its size and position will cause obstruction during labour. Caesarean section would be the method of delivery.

DISPLACEMENT OF THE PREGNANT UTERUS

Retroversion of the gravid uterus

Definition

When the long axis of the uterus is directed backwards during pregnancy, the uterus is said to be retroverted.

Causes

- Congenital
- Poor uterine tone
- Overdistended ligaments
- Adhesions
- Fibroid on anterior uterine wall.

Diagnosis

Retroversion should be suspected if the woman complains of low back pain in the early weeks of pregnancy. Confirmation is made on vaginal examination. In a significant number of women, there are no symptoms and the condition will only be found on vaginal examination.

Possible outcomes

In most cases the retroversion corrects itself spontaneously when the uterus rises above the pelvic brim at 12 weeks' gestation. For this reason, a retroverted uterus diagnosed in early pregnancy is not treated. At 12 weeks' gestation the obstetrician will check that correction has occurred. If spontaneous anteversion has not taken place, the position will be corrected by bimanual manipulation.

Incarceration of the gravid uterus is a rare complication of retroversion. The retroverted gravid uterus becomes imprisoned in the pelvic cavity with the fundus trapped in the sacral hollow and it cannot rise above the pelvic brim. This occurs between the 12th and 14th week of pregnancy.

Signs and symptoms. The woman complains of frequency of micturition with dysuria and paradoxical incontinence (retention of urine with overflow). Low abdominal pain is present because of the associated retention of urine. Difficulty in micturition and retention are caused by pressure of the cervix on the bladder.

Management. The midwife must send for medical aid. Bladder catheterisation is carried out but may prove difficult as the urethra is elongated and the external meatus slit-like and difficult to locate. Once the bladder has been emptied, manual correction of the retroversion will be attempted. An impacted bowel will make the procedure difficult, therefore an enema will be given prior to manipulation. A Hodge pessary is inserted and worn for 4-6 weeks following correction. Admission to hospital is advised and an indwelling catheter kept in situ for 48 hours until bladder tone is regained.

Danger. If no attempt at correction is made, sacculation of the anterior uterine wall will result, which means that it enlarges into a pouch to contain the fetus. Rupture of the bladder is possible. These are extremely rare situations and should not occur in today's obstetric and midwifery practice.

Anterior obliquity of the pregnant uterus

Definition
The fundus of the uterus leans forward and the abdomen is unduly prominent.

Pendulous abdomen occurs when the rectus muscles separate widely and the uterus leans so far forward that it hangs downwards (Fig. 24.2).

Causes
Laxity of the abdominal wall leads to failure of the support necessary for the pregnant uterus. This is most frequently seen in women of high parity whose abdominal wall has become lax due to repeated childbearing. In a primigravida, anterior obliquity can indicate a pelvic or spinal deformity which has reduced the space available for the pregnant uterus.

Management
Discomfort and pain experienced during pregnancy can be relieved to some extent by good

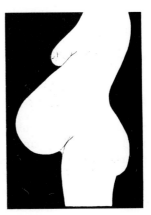

Fig. 24.2
Pendulous abdomen.

support. This will be achieved by wearing a well-fitting maternity corset. Malpresentations may occur and lead to associated problems during labour. In labour, the force of the uterine contractions will be misdirected and this leads to a prolonged labour with engagement of the head delayed. A firm binder worn during labour might help to some extent. Some authorities advise that the woman should draw her uterus upwards with each contraction in an attempt to direct the uterine force downwards in the correct direction. Careful monitoring must be carried out by the midwife to determine whether the fetal head enters the pelvis. The lack of a well-fitting presentation will predispose to early rupture of the membranes and associated cord prolapse.

Prolapse of the pregnant uterus

Definition
The uterus descends down the vaginal canal so that it lies below its normal position in the pelvis. Various degrees of uterine prolapse may occur. The minor degrees normally regress during pregnancy as the uterus rises in the pelvis drawing the cervix upwards.

It is very unusual for a woman with a marked degree of prolapse to become pregnant.

Management
In minor degrees no treatment is necessary; a ring pessary might be advised until the uterus rises. If the prolapse is such that the cervix protrudes

through the vagina, the woman should be confined to bed and strict asepsis maintained.

PELVIC TUMOURS

Fibroids (fibromyomata)

These are firm tumours of muscular and fibrous tissue, ranging from the very small to the very large. They are most frequently found in women at the older end of the childbearing age range. Both primigravid and multigravid women may have a pregnancy complicated to some extent by these.

Types

Fibroids are named according to their position. If situated immediately beneath the surface of the endometrium (or decidua) the fibroid is termed *submucous*, and if beneath the serous coat of the uterus, *subserous*. A fibroid confined to the myometrium is termed *intramural*. Occasionally subserous or submucous fibroids develop stalks and are called *pedunculated*. Fibroids can be found in both upper and lower uterine segments and may be singular or multiple (Fig. 24.3).

Effect on pregnancy, labour and puerperium

The effect of fibroids on pregnancy, labour and the puerperium depends greatly on whether they lie in the upper or lower segment and which layer of the uterus they occupy. Where numerous fibroids exist, subfertility may result. This depends on the area of the endometrium involved. Abortion may occur if multiple fibroids are present. As pregnancy advances, the fibroids will enlarge due to increased vascularity and the effects of oestrogen and progesterone.

Red degeneration. This occasionally occurs giving rise to pain and uterine tenderness. The cause of this is unclear but necrosis occurs. The mother is treated with analgesia and rest and normally the pain regresses after a few days. The diagnosis may be confused with appendicitis or even placental abruption.

Torsion of pedunculated fibroid. If a fibroid becomes twisted on its pedicle it will give rise to acute pain.

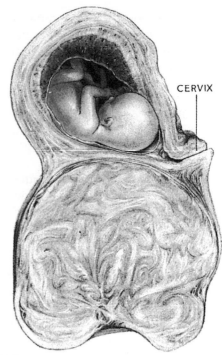

CERVIX

Fig. 24.3
Fibroid tumour in pregnant uterus. The fibroid, being in the lower segment of the uterus and measuring 11–12 cm, would have filled the pelvic cavity and obstructed labour.

Most fibroids cause little trouble except to make the uterus larger than would be expected for the stage of pregnancy. However a fibroid in the lower uterine pole may cause an abnormal lie or malpresentation of the fetus. In labour, obstruction may occur if the fibroid is in the lower pole and poor uterine activity may occur if the myometrium is the location of large or numerous fibroids. Postpartum haemorrhage may be caused by fibroids, especially if situated in the placental area. As involution occurs during the puerperium, fibroids reduce in size but may cause subinvolution and prolonged red lochia.

Ovarian cysts

Ovarian tumours are rarely found in pregnancy and malignant tumours account for only a small number of these. Most tumours are cystic with dermoid cysts found in about 25% of cases (Llewellyn-Jones 1990). During pregnancy the cyst does not alter in size but displacement may cause it to become more evident. Haemorrhage into the cyst and infection in the puerperium are possibilities.

Effect on pregnancy and labour

The cyst can occupy the pelvic cavity and cause obstruction.

If a fluctuating swelling is found alongside the uterus, the midwife should seek medical aid. If the cyst is large, pressure symptoms will exist and if torsion of a pedunculated cyst occurs, acute pain and vomiting result.

Management

Removal of the cyst is indicated because of the possibility of malignancy. Surgical removal of the cyst is performed between the 12th and 28th week. After 28 weeks, there is some technical difficulty in removal therefore surgery may be delayed until the fetus is delivered.

ABNORMALITIES OF THE BONY PELVIS

The normal gynaecoid pelvis is the one most suited to successful childbearing and variation in shape or size can lead to complications, particularly during labour. Where there is a deviation from the normal gynaecoid type, the possibility of a contracted pelvis exists.

Contracted pelvis

This is a pelvis in which one measurement or more is at least 1 cm less than the lower limit of normal. This causes delivery of a normal sized fetus to be difficult or impossible. A lesser degree of contraction, if combined with an unfavourable pelvic feature, may also give rise to difficulty in labour. If undiagnosed, the woman will undergo a prolonged labour, which may become obstructed. This can result in damage to both mother and child and it is imperative that the midwife recognises the possibility of contraction of the pelvis in any woman under her care.

Abnormally shaped pelves

The four basic pelvic types have already been described in Chapter 2. Every woman has a pelvis based on one of these four types and the vast majority are normal in shape and function. Where the features are exaggerated or combined with an abnormality of development or if deformity is caused by accident or disease, problems may ensue. The particular characteristics which may cause difficulty are discussed below.

Android pelvis

The heart-shaped brim favours a posterior position of the occiput. This is the result of insufficient space for the biparietal diameter in the narrow forepelvis, combined with the fact that the greater space lies in the hindpelvis. Funnelling in the cavity may hinder progress in labour. At the pelvic outlet, the prominent ischial spines sometimes prevent complete internal rotation of the head and the anteroposterior diameter becomes caught on them, causing a deep transverse arrest. The narrowed sub-pubic angle cannot easily accommodate the biparietal diameter, which displaces the head backwards (Fig. 24.4). (Posterior positions of the occiput are described in Chapter 26.)

Anthropoid pelvis

It is rare for the features of this oval-brimmed pelvis to cause any problems. Direct occipito-posterior or direct occipito-anterior positions are common. In either case, rotation of the head is

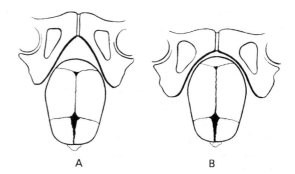

A   B

Fig. 24.4
(A) Outlet of android pelvis. The head does not fit into the acute pubic arch and is forced backwards onto the perineum. (B) Outlet of gynaecoid pelvis. The head fits snugly into the pubic arch.

unlikely and the position adopted for engagement will persist to delivery.

Platypelloid pelvis

The kidney-shaped brim with a reduced antero-posterior diameter often causes the fetus to negotiate the brim by a process known as asynclitism. This is described with the rachitic pelvis below. The divergent side walls and increased outlet diameters mean that problems rarely occur once the brim has been negotiated.

Justo minor pelvis

This is described as a gynaecoid pelvis in miniature. All diameters are reduced but are in proportion. It is normally found in women of small stature, less than 1.5 m in height with small hands and feet but is occasionally found in women of normal stature.

The outcome of labour in this situation depends on the fetus. If the fetal size is consistent with the size of the maternal pelvis, normal labour and delivery will take place. Often these women have small babies and the outcome is favourable. However, if the fetus is large, a degree of cephalo-pelvic disproportion will result. The same is true when a malpresentation or malposition of the fetus exists.

High assimilation pelvis

This occurs when the 5th lumbar vertebra is fused to the sacrum and the angle of inclination of the pelvic brim is increased. Engagement of the head is difficult but, once achieved, labour progresses normally.

Naegele's and Robert's pelves

Both these rarities are due to failure in development. In the Naegele pelvis one sacral ala is missing and the sacrum is fused to the ilium, causing a grossly asymmetric brim. The Robert pelvis is similar but bilateral. In both instances the abnormal brim prevents engagement of the fetal head.

Dietary deficiency

Deficiency of vitamins and minerals necessary for the formation of healthy bones is less frequently seen today than in the past but might still complicate pregnancy and labour to some extent. The midwife must be alert for them especially in immigrant populations.

Rachitic pelvis

Rickets in early childhood can lead to gross deformity of the pelvic brim. The weight of the upper body presses downwards on to the softened pelvic bones. The sacral promontory is pushed downwards and forwards and the ilium and ischium are drawn outwards. This results in a flat pelvic brim similar to that of the platypelloid pelvis. The sacrum tends to be straight with the coccyx bending acutely forward. Because the tuberosities are wide apart, the pubic arch is wide. With the improvements in child care seen throughout the world, this type of pelvis should be infrequently seen. The clinical signs of rickets, bow legs and spinal deformity, can occasionally be seen in immigrant mothers.

Outcome of labour. If severe contraction is present then caesarean section is required to deliver the baby. The fetal head will attempt to enter the pelvis by lateral tilting of the head referred to as *asynclitism.*

Anterior asynclitism. The anterior parietal bone moves down behind the symphysis pubis until the parietal eminence enters the brim. The movement is then reversed and the head tilts in the opposite direction until the posterior parietal bone negotiates the sacral promontory and the head is engaged.

Posterior asynclitism. The movements of anterior asynclitism are reversed. The posterior parietal bone negotiates the sacral promontory prior to the anterior parietal bone moving down behind the symphysis pubis.

Once the pelvic brim has been negotiated, descent progresses normally accompanied by flexion and internal rotation.

Complications of labour such as face or brow presentation and cord prolapse are risks associated with this type of pelvic brim (Fig. 24.5).

Osteomalacic pelvis

The disease osteomalacia is rarely encountered in Britain but may be found in immigrant popu-

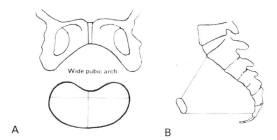

Fig. 24.5
Rachitic flat pelvis. (A) Note wide pubic arch and kidney-shaped brim. (B) The lateral view shows the diminished anteroposterior diameter of the brim and the increased anteroposterior diameter of the outlet.

lations. It is due to an acquired deficiency of calcium and occurs in adults. All bones of the skeleton soften due to the gross calcium deficiency. The pelvic canal is squashed together until the brim becomes a Y-shaped slit. Labour is impossible and caesarean section would be performed. In early pregnancy incarceration of the gravid uterus may occur because of the gross deformity.

Injury and disease

Trauma
A pelvis which has been fractured will develop callus formation or may fail to unite correctly. This may lead to reduced measurements and therefore to some degree of contraction. Conditions sustained in childhood such as fractures of the pelvis or lower limbs, congenital dislocation of the hip and poliomyelitis may lead to unequal weight-bearing which will also cause deformity. The child puts her weight on the stronger leg and that side of the pelvis is pressed inwards leading to flattening of the pelvic brim. With the expert orthopaedic care today, this should be less frequently seen.

Spinal deformity
If kyphosis (forward angulation) or scoliosis (lateral curvature) is evident, or suggested by a limp or deformity, the midwife must refer the woman to a doctor. Pelvic contraction is likely in these cases and the outcome of pregnancy is dependent on the degree.

Diagnosis of contracted pelvis

General observation of the woman will lead the midwife to suspect contracted pelvis. The woman who is of short stature or who walks with a limp or abnormal gait should be referred to an obstetrician. Medical history of injury or disease involving spine or pelvis is significant.

Obstetric history
Where a history of difficult labour, forceps delivery, caesarean section or stillbirth is given, the cause of the difficulty should be sought. A woman who has previously given birth to a baby of normal size with no difficulty is unlikely to have a contracted pelvis but it should be remembered that subsequent babies may be larger and cause new problems.

Examination
The problems outlined above will give an indication to the midwife as to when she should suspect a contracted pelvis. It is important that every pregnant woman is examined to assess pelvic capacity (see Ch. 10), but vital for the obstetrician to evaluate the probable outcome of labour when pelvic contraction is present. Digital examination of the pelvic canal will be carried out initially and X-ray pelvimetry may follow. This consists of a lateral view of the pelvis with the woman standing upright, which shows the anteroposterior dimensions of the pelvis and the relation of the fetal head to the brim. Towards term a final decision must be made as to the most suitable plan for delivery, for example trial of vaginal delivery or caesarean section. Admission at or before term is usual.

Management of labour
When contracted pelvis is suspected, labour must be managed with considerable care. If the degree of contraction is such that it is obvious that labour cannot progress satisfactorily, then a caesarean section will be the mode of delivery.

   Trial of vaginal delivery. If the degree of contraction is minor and the obstetrician is of the opinion that a normal outcome is possible, the woman is allowed to labour. (In the past this has been referred to as a Trial of Labour.)

The outcome is dependent on:

- the effectiveness of the uterine contractions
- the 'give' of the pelvic joints
- the degree of moulding of the fetal head
- flexion of the fetal head.

These factors are unpredictable until labour is established hence the reason for the 'trial'. If at any stage during this labour, the mother or fetus is under stress, a caesarean section will be performed. Labour should not be permitted to continue until signs of maternal and fetal distress are displayed. The aim is to ensure a live mother and child who have sustained minimal trauma.

Management. The woman, who is usually a primigravida, will continue her pregnancy to term and may enter labour spontaneously. However, labour may be induced if indicated for some other obstetrical reason. Constant supervision and expert care will be given in a unit which is fully equipped for operative procedures. Progress is recorded on a partograph and any failure of progress noted, reported and dealt with. If, despite good uterine contractions, cervical dilatation is slow and the head fails to descend, the outlook for vaginal delivery is poor and the obstetrician must make a decision whether or not to allow labour to continue.

The midwife's care. On admission to the Labour Suite, the woman should be welcomed by the midwife. The midwife will make the necessary baseline recordings, including the results of abdominal examination. The presentation will be vertex and the position should be found (LOA is most favourable). The level of the head in relation to the pelvic brim should be noted and this can be confirmed on vaginal examination. Usually the head will not be engaged at the onset of labour. The degree of flexion of the head is an important observation and any overlap at the brim should be reported to the obstetrician.

Maternal condition. It is especially important for the midwife to ensure that the woman's morale is kept high and to avoid the suggestion of failure if vaginal delivery is not achieved. Routine care is carried out with a particular view to preventing ketoacidosis and treating it promptly if it occurs.

Fetal condition. In most cases the fetal condition will be monitored with the use of a cardiotocograph and early signs of fetal distress will be apparent immediately. In the absence of monitoring equipment, the midwife must record the fetal heart rate every 15 minutes and report any deviation from normal.

Progress of labour. Effacement and dilatation of the cervix will be assessed on vaginal examination and related to the length of time in labour and the strength of uterine contractions. Rupture of the membranes will be confirmed on vaginal examination and excessive moulding or a large caput succedaneum noted. Uterine action is monitored closely, if possible using a cardiotocograph. Descent and flexion of the head are assessed on abdominal and vaginal examination and recorded. Engagement of the head is a favourable sign as it denotes successful negotiation of the pelvic brim. It does not, however, rule out difficulties at the outlet.

If progress is poor despite good uterine contractions, the midwife must report to the doctor. In the event of signs of maternal or fetal distress, or if the presentation alters from a vertex to a face or brow, she must also inform the doctor.

Obstructed labour (see Ch. 25). If contraction of the pelvis is such that the fetus cannot negotiate it, there is the possibility of labour becoming obstructed. Obstruction can occur at any level of the pelvis but in a trial of vaginal delivery the vigilance of attending staff should prevent this dire obstetric emergency. Obstruction might also be caused by some localised fetal abnormality such as hydrocephaly (see Ch. 28).

Midwives must be on the alert for signs of obstruction in every labour, but particularly in those women who are suspected of having a contracted pelvis.

Reader Activities

Devise midwifery care plans for the following clients:

1. Mrs Sandal, a 36-year-old para 3+0 at 20 weeks of pregnancy, admitted to an antenatal ward with lower abdominal pain and an abnormal swelling in the pelvic cavity.
Consider the possible reasons for Mrs Sandal's condition.

2. Mrs Walters, a primigravida at 38 weeks of pregnancy who is admitted in labour and is considered to have a contracted pelvis.
What might have led to this tentative diagnosis in the case of Mrs Walters?

FURTHER READING

Cunningham F G, MacDonald P C, Gant N F 1989, Williams obstetrics, 18th edn. Appleton-Century-Crofts, New York

Llewellyn-Jones D 1990 Fundamentals of obstetrics and gynaecology, 5th edn. Faber, London, vols 1 & 2

Moore K C 1989 Before we are born — basic embryology and birth defects, 3rd edn. W B Saunders, Philadelphia

25

Prolonged pregnancy and disorders of uterine action

JOSEPHINE WILLIAMS

This chapter opens with a section on the diagnosis and management of prolonged pregnancy, detailing the various investigations that may be used both to estimate fetal maturity and to monitor both fetal and maternal conditions. It includes discussion of the complications that may arise in such a pregnancy, and mentions the risk factors that may be relevant. It continues with the related subjects of induction and acceleration of labour, examining in some detail the indications for and against such procedures, before discussing the various methods used and their complications. The chapter examines the types of abnormal uterine action, their causes, management and complications, and concludes with the similar study of prolonged labour and obstructed labour. Throughout the chapter the emphasis is on the involvement of the woman and her partner in the care provided; although much of the content involves complications of pregnancy and labour, this very fact increases the importance of the role of the midwife in the care provided.

PROLONGED PREGNANCY

Prolonged or post-term pregnancy is considered to be a pregnancy which continues for over 294 days (42 weeks) from the first day of the last menstrual period or 280 days from conception; it occurs in approximately 10% of pregnancies.

Diagnosis of prolonged pregnancy

Expected date of delivery

A pregnancy cannot be termed 'prolonged' unless the expected date of delivery (EDD) has been predicted accurately. The methods used for calculation before 20 weeks' gestation are the most reliable.

Last menstrual period. The EDD is normally calculated by counting forward 280 days from the first day of the last menstrual period (see Ch. 10). For this to be accurate, the woman must be certain of this date, the period must have been of normal length, her cycle regular and she must not have conceived immediately after discontinuing the oral contraceptive pill. In addition if her normal cycle exceeds 28 days, the extra days must be added to the calculation; if it falls short of 28 days the deficit is subtracted. When the cycle is irregular, the EDD calculated in this way is unreliable.

Vaginal assessment of uterine size. Bimanual examination of the uterus within the first 12 weeks provides a more accurate estimation of uterine size than that obtained from abdominal palpation at a more advanced stage of pregnancy. It has the disadvantage of being uncomfortable for the woman and occasionally may provoke miscarriage.

Ultrasound examination (see also Ch. 41). Before 20 weeks' gestation the maturity of the fetus can be estimated with an accuracy of plus or minus 7 days. The crown–rump length can be measured from as early as 6 weeks' gestation and the biparietal diameter from 9 weeks' gestation. Ultrasound examination also gives the woman an opportunity to identify with the fetus at an early stage of her pregnancy.

Quickening. This observation involves the mother and is a useful method of estimating the duration of pregnancy. Fetal movements are first felt by primigravidae at 18–20 weeks' gestation and by multigravidae at 16–18 weeks. As it is subjective it is not completely reliable.

Estimation of fetal maturity

When the EDD is uncertain, fetal maturity must be determined by other methods. This is particularly necessary if the woman has booked late or received little antenatal care. It is essential to have this information before induction of labour is considered.

Abdominal examination. Estimation of the fundal height, the size of the fetus and the relationship of the presenting part to the pelvic brim permit fetal maturity to be assessed with a fair degree of reliability. Allowance must be made for variation in maternal size and the possibilities of a growth-retarded fetus or a multiple pregnancy.

The fundal height may be measured from the symphysis pubis. Between 20 and 36 weeks' gestation this distance should equal in centimetres the approximate gestation in weeks. Its apparent attractiveness as an objective measurement must be weighed against variation between observations on different occasions.

Ultrasound examination. A single examination will only provide an accurate estimation of the EDD after 20 weeks' gestation if fetal growth is progressing normally. Serial scans (at least three at fortnightly intervals) reveal the rate of growth and allow the EDD to be plotted with greater accuracy. It is also helpful to compare several measurements, such as head circumference, abdominal circumference, biparietal diameter, femur length and crown–rump length.

X-ray. Radiological examination can detect ossification centres of the femoral and tibial epiphyses. There is considerable variation in the time of appearance; the femoral epiphyses appear between the 35th and 40th week of pregnancy and the tibial epiphyses between the 37th and 42nd week. In most centres this test has been replaced by ultrasound which is more reliable and does not carry the hazards of X-rays.

Amniocentesis. The lecithin:sphingomyelin ratio (L:S ratio) in the amniotic fluid reflects the pulmonary maturity of the fetus and correlates well with gestational age. A ratio of 2:1 or more indicates that the lungs are mature. The L:S ratio does not show postmaturity.

Signs of placental deterioration

If the pregnancy is to be allowed to continue beyond term, it should be carefully monitored for signs of possible placental deterioration.

Static maternal weight or weight loss suggests cessation of fetal growth.

Diminishing amount of liquor. This may be detected either on abdominal palpation by the same observer on successive examinations or by ultrasound scan.

Diminished secretion of hormones. Serial estimations of urinary or plasma oestriols or of serum human placental lactogen (HPL) may be made. A fall is taken to indicate placental insufficiency. These tests have proved disappointing as an assessment of fetal risk.

Reduced fetal movements (see 'Kick charts' Ch. 10). A reduction in the number of fetal movement felt by the woman indicates deteriorating placental function. When less than ten movements are felt during a 12-hour period, the fetus is considered to be at risk.

Abnormal fetal heart patterns. If the fetal heart rate fails to accelerate in response to fetal movement or Braxton-Hicks contractions this may be an early indication of placental insufficiency. Loss of baseline variability has more serious implications and in a prolonged pregnancy would be an indication for induction of labour. Decelerations between uterine contractions indicate that the fetus is at considerable risk and early delivery, often by caesarean section, is indicated.

Meconium-stained liquor can be detected while the membranes are still intact by using an amnioscope. Oligohydramnios can also be identified. Amnioscopy is uncomfortable for the woman and the investigations mentioned above are preferred.

Maternal complications

Psychological

Prolongation of pregnancy tends to increase the anxiety felt by the woman, who is tired of being pregnant, feels at her most ungainly and is apprehensive to a degree about labour. Her subconscious fears regarding the health of the baby may become more overt. The reality of having a baby may seem to be receding further from her as each day passes. Such feelings of anxiety can make it more difficult to cope with the pain of labour and in extreme cases could precipitate a depressive illness.

Labour

There is a slight increase in the incidence of inefficient uterine action which may lead to prolonged labour. A large fetus may cause cephalo-pelvic disproportion.

Delivery

The fetal skull continues to ossify as time passes. As the membrane between the skull bones diminishes, overriding is restricted. The combination of increased head size and reduced moulding may lead to operative delivery with a consequent risk of trauma to the woman and child. Shoulder dystocia may also occur.

Fetal complications

Placental insufficiency

This is the main complication affecting the fetus. All placentae start to decline at a variable rate after term. Some continue to function satisfactorily up to 43 or 44 weeks' gestation. Insufficiency only occurs when the placental reserve has been used up. After this, placental dysfunction leads to a decreased supply of oxygen and nutrients. The effects are determined by the extent of insufficiency.

Intra-uterine death can result from acute fetal hypoxia but if hypoxia is chronic and continues over a long period, it can cause mental retardation.

Fetal distress. The effect of uterine contractions on an already compromised placenta may cause fetal hypoxia severe enough to warrant caesarean section.

Meconium aspiration. Where there is meconium-stained liquor as a result of fetal distress the fetus may aspirate it into the lungs either in utero or at delivery. This can result in pneumonitis, respiratory distress and pneumonia.

Delivery trauma

Operative deliveries are more common following prolonged pregnancy and may result in birth injuries (see Ch. 37). There is also a greater risk of shoulder dystocia.

Factors increasing risk

If the pregnancy continues beyond term the following factors increase the risk to the fetus, usually because of placental insufficiency.

The older primigravida. There is an increased incidence of placental insufficiency in primigravid women over 35 years of age, especially in those who also have a history of infertility.

Poor obstetric history. A history of stillbirth or intra-uterine growth retardation increases the likelihood of placental insufficiency. Maternal cigarette smoking increases the hazard.

Pre-eclampsia. This often causes placental insufficiency but it is unlikely that the pregnancy will be allowed to continue beyond term because of the risks to the mother (see Ch. 20).

Diabetes mellitus can result in the paradox of a large fetus, which may cause difficulties at delivery, combined with placental insufficiency, which may result in stillbirth.

Previous large baby. Fetal size tends to increase with successive pregnancies and a history of a previous baby weighing over 4 kg increases the risk of difficulty at delivery if the pregnancy is allowed to continue beyond term.

Management

Conservative management of prolonged pregnancy is becoming more common in the absence of other complications. The midwife must remain alert for signs of deterioration in the maternal and fetal conditions.

Referral to an obstetrician is usually made after 40 weeks' gestation if labour is not imminent. He or she will assess maternal and fetal well-being and discuss management of the remainder of the pregnancy. If any additional risk factors are present, labour is induced at term.

The women should visit the antenatal clinic weekly in order that both maternal and fetal conditions can be carefully monitored.

Maternal condition. Sudden weight gain, rising blood pressure and proteinuria would indicate pre-eclampsia. The midwife must also assess the woman's psychological condition and keep her fully informed of her progress.

Fetal condition. Fetal growth is monitored by abdominal examination and ultrasound scan. Fetal well-being may be assessed by means of a fetal activity chart which is kept by the mother and shows frequency of fetal movement. After 42 weeks' gestation, and earlier if thought advisable, antenatal cardiotocography is carried out twice a week, and more often if necessary, to exclude any fetal heart irregularities.

If either fetal or maternal condition gives cause for concern, induction of labour will be considered.

INDUCTION OF LABOUR

Induction is the initiation of labour by artificial means. Labour should only be induced for medical or obstetric reasons. The overall induction rate is between 10% and 30%, depending on the population involved.

Indications

Labour is induced when it is considered that the health or well-being of mother or fetus would be adversely affected if the pregnancy continued. In some cases both of them benefit from the pregnancy being terminated.

Prolonged pregnancy

After 42 weeks' gestation the rate of placental deterioration accelerates and the pregnancy is considered to be prolonged. Pregnancy is usually allowed to continue unless there are signs that fetal or maternal well-being is compromised.

Pre-eclampsia

In this condition maternal health is at risk from the effects of pre-eclampsia (see Ch. 20) and the fetus from placental insufficiency which usually accompanies it. The timing of induction depends on the severity of the symptoms. It is often necessary to weigh the risks of allowing pregnancy to continue against those of delivering a very immature fetus. When it is necessary to effect delivery before 30 weeks' gestation or if the cervix is unfavourable for induction (see below), caesarean section is sometimes preferred.

Evidence of diminished fetal well-being

Placental insufficiency severe enough to affect fetal well-being is characterised by intra-uterine growth retardation. This may be detected by the same observer measuring the fundal height at successive antenatal visits or, more reliably, by serial ultrasound scans. Additional factors which indicate the need for induction are falling hormonal assays, reduced fetal movements and abnormalities of the fetal heart found on cardiotocography.

The older primigravida

Placental insufficiency is more common in primigravidae aged over 35 years. For this reason it is usual to recommend induction of labour at term to avoid additional risk to the fetus.

Poor obstetric history

Stillbirth or intra-uterine growth retardation in a previous pregnancy is an indication for induction of labour at term, as placental insufficiency tends to recur in subsequent pregnancies.

Spontaneous rupture of membranes

If the membranes rupture spontaneously after 36 weeks' gestation and labour does not commence within 24 hours, it should be induced. A prolonged period of ruptured membranes can lead to intra-uterine infection.

Previous large baby

A previous baby whose birthweight was over 4 kg may indicate the need for induction between 38 and 40 weeks' gestation. Fetal size tends to increase with successive pregnancies and induction before term may prevent a difficult delivery caused by an abnormally large baby.

Diabetes mellitus

It is no longer considered necessary to induce labour between 36 and 38 weeks' gestation for fear of intra-uterine death occurring after this time in a diabetic pregnancy. Improved control of the diabetes is now possible. The fetal macrosomia which is often found in diabetic pregnancies if good control is not achieved can cause difficulties at delivery. Some obstetricians prefer planned induction in order to be assured of good control of blood glucose levels throughout labour. Caesarean section should only be performed on obstetric grounds.

Rhesus iso-immunisation

The use of Anti-D gamma globulin to prevent the formation of antibodies has made Rhesus iso-immunisation uncommon. When Rhesus antibodies are present in the maternal serum and the titre is sufficiently high to suggest a severe haemolytic process in the fetus, it may be necessary to induce labour. It is then possible to arrest the haemolysis and rectify its effects before irreversible damage occurs.

Unstable lie

If placenta praevia and pelvic abnormalities have been excluded as causes of unstable lie, labour may be induced after the lie has been corrected and made longitudinal. Cephalic presentation is preferred to breech as there is less risk of cord prolapse following rupture of the membranes.

Genital herpes (see Ch. 19)

In a woman with a history of genital herpes, labour is frequently induced, if the disease is in remission, after 38 weeks' gestation. This avoids caesarean section for active herpes at the onset of spontaneous labour.

Previous precipitate labour

As precipitate labour tends to recur in succeeding pregnancies, induction is sometimes performed at 38 weeks to ensure that labour takes place in safe surroundings.

Placental abruption

Once maternal shock has been treated by intravenous fluid replacement it is usual to induce labour by artificial rupture of the membranes. This relieves increased intra-uterine pressure caused by retroplacental haemorrhage and controls bleeding by allowing the uterus to contract and empty. Minor degrees of abruption occurring before 37 weeks' gestation may be treated conservatively if fetal and maternal conditions are stable.

Social reasons

Sometimes a woman may wish the baby to be born for family reasons or simply because she is fed up. In these cases labour should only be induced when the pregnancy is at term and assessment indicates a favourable outcome. It is never justifiable to plan the timing of deliveries simply for the convenience of maternity unit staff.

Intra-uterine death

Labour may be induced once intra-uterine death has been confirmed if the woman, in her distress, requests delivery. There is a risk of coagulation defects occurring if the pregnancy continues for a long period.

Fetal maturity and viability

Before inducing labour it is necessary to be certain of the length of gestation and the maturity of the fetus in order to avoid inadvertently delivering a baby which is more immature than was estimated.

When a deterioration in maternal health or placental function indicates a need for delivery before term, an amniocentesis may be performed. The lecithin:sphingomyelin ratio in the liquor is calculated in order to estimate fetal pulmonary maturity. When the ratio is less than 2:1, this indicates that the lungs are not mature and induction may be delayed. In some units a course of steroids is given to the mother to stimulate the fetal lungs to produce surfactant which reduces the risk of idiopathic respiratory distress syndrome developing after birth.

Contra-indications

Unreliable EDD

When the fetal and maternal conditions are satisfactory, induction for prolonged pregnancy should not be performed unless the estimated date of delivery is considered reliable.

Malpresentation

Oblique or transverse lie is an absolute contra-indication to induction of labour because of the risk of cord prolapse and of obstruction. Opinion varies as to whether labour should be induced when the breech is presenting; a spontaneous on-set of labour or an elective caesarean section is sometimes preferred. If induction is decided upon, care must be taken to avoid cord prolapse by delaying artificial rupture of the membranes until labour is established and the breech well down in the pelvis.

Cephalopelvic disproportion

Although induction of labour may be performed in cases of a minor degree of cephalopelvic disproportion, if a major degree of disproportion between fetal head and maternal pelvis is demonstrated, vaginal delivery will be impossible. An elective caesarean section should be carried out at about 38 weeks' gestation in order to pre-empt labour.

A previous caesarean section for disproportion is an indication for a repeat operation. If the caesarean section was performed for other reasons, induction may be considered but the scar may be vulnerable to rupture if contractions are excessive.

Fetal compromise

Caesarean section is preferable to induction of labour if the fetus would not tolerate the stress of uterine contractions due to extreme immaturity or placental insufficiency.

Psychological

In all instances the woman's consent and co-operation must be secured before labour is induced. If she and her partner feel strongly against induction their wishes must be respected. If either mother or fetus would be put at risk by continuation of the pregnancy the position should be carefully explained to the woman in the hope that she will change her mind.

A few women become tired with pregnancy and demand induction several weeks before term. In the absence of any real indication these wishes should be resisted because of the risk to the baby if he is delivered prematurely. This should be explained to the woman. A prematurely induced labour is likely to be longer and more painful than one which commences spontaneously at full term and therefore should be avoided unless absolutely necessary.

The midwife will need to call upon her greatest skills to discuss such decisions with the parents objectively and sympathetically and without applying undue pressure. In either situation the couple will need considerable emotional support.

Favourable factors

Gestation
When gestation is more than 38 weeks, induction of labour is more likely to be successful as the nearer to term a pregnancy is, the more sensitive is the uterus to induction.

Bishop score
The Bishop score is an objective method of assessing whether the cervix is favourable for induction of labour. Five different features are considered and each is awarded a score of between 0 and 3. When the total score is six or over, the prognosis for induction of labour is good.

Table 25.1
Modified Bishop's pre-induction pelvic scoring system

Inducibility features	0	1	2	3
Dilatation of cervix in cm	0	1–2	3–4	5–6
Consistency of cervix	firm	medium	soft	—
Cervical canal length in cm	>2	1–2	0.5–1	<0.5
Position of cervix	posterior	mid	anterior	—
Station of presenting part in cm above or below ischial spines	–3	–2	–1, 0	+1, +2

Level of presenting part
When three-fifths of the head or less is palpable above the pelvic brim or when, in a breech presentation, the breech is engaged, success is more likely.

Preparation

Psychological
The decision to induce labour should only be made with the informed consent of the woman and great care should be taken to ensure that she fully understands the reasons for it and the procedures to be followed. Women today prefer labour to commence naturally and this climate of opinion has resulted in a fall in the number of inductions. Most women will accept the necessity for induction when the health of mother or fetus is thought to be at risk.

Liaison with other departments
When complications are anticipated during labour or delivery which may involve specialists such as the paediatrician, the haematologist or the diabetic team, the date of induction should be arranged with them beforehand.

Bowel preparation
A loaded rectum leaves less room in the pelvis for the fetal head and may also result in defaecation at delivery. Routine evacuation of the lower bowel on admission to hospital is now considered unnecessary: if a woman is constipated, or if she expresses concern over possible incontinence of faeces during labour, the bowel may be emptied with the aid of suppositories or an enema.

Methods

Induction is frequently divided into medical, or more aptly medicinal, induction in which drugs alone are used and the amniotic sac remains intact, and surgical induction in which the membranes are artificially ruptured. It is usual for a combination of the two methods to be employed.

Prostaglandin E$_2$
This may be used to ripen an unfavourable cervix (Bishop score 5 or less) prior to amniotomy or to induce labour by stimulating uterine contractions.

Vaginal prostaglandin. Prostaglandin may be used in the form of pessaries (2.5–5 mg), vaginal tablets (3–6 mg) or in a gel (2.5–5 mg). The latter is administered through a Kwill or nelaton catheter attached to a syringe. The dosage varies according to parity, the Bishop score of the cervix and differences in maternity unit policies. It should only be administered when the membranes are intact because of the risk of infection and the increased sensitivity of the cervix after the membranes have ruptured. A few units do use vaginal prostaglandins to induce labour after spontaneous rupture of membranes.

Prostaglandin is inserted into the posterior vaginal fornix and the woman is requested to remain in bed for 1 hour afterwards to permit maximum absorption of the prostaglandin. During this time continuous cardiotocography is performed in order to monitor the reaction of the fetal heart to the contractions which are stimulated by the prostaglandin. After this period, provided that there are no abnormalities of the fetal heart trace, the mother is encouraged to get up and walk about. Observations are carried out as in normal labour.

If labour is not established 4 hours after insertion of the prostaglandin, a vaginal examination is performed. The state of the cervix is assessed and progress evaluated in order to decide further management. If there is no change in the Bishop score, more prostaglandin may be administered. If there has been progress, the membranes may be ruptured artificially and an intravenous infusion of Syntocinon commenced.

Endocervical prostaglandin. This involves insertion of 0.5 mg prostaglandin in a viscous gel into the cervical canal. It may be preferred when cervical ripening, rather than induction of labour, is the objective.

Extra-amniotic prostaglandin. Prostaglandin gel may be introduced into the extra-amniotic space through a fine nelaton catheter and the dose varies between 2.5 and 5 mg as mentioned above. A continuous infusion of prostaglandin solution may be administered through a Foley catheter at a pre-set rate using a syringe pump. The woman remains in bed and continuous cardiotocography is performed in order to detect variations in the fetal heart pattern or hyperstimulation of the uterus.

Oral prostaglandin. Prostaglandin tablets, each containing 0.5 mg of prostaglandin E_2 may be given to induce labour following rupture of the membranes. One tablet is swallowed at hourly intervals up to a maximum of ten tablets or until labour is established. Occasionally these tablets cause diarrhoea, in which case their administration should be stopped.

Oral prostaglandin is the least invasive method used and it allows the woman to remain mobile. Observations of the fetal heart rate and maternal condition should be made at least half-hourly as in normal labour.

Complications of prostaglandin induction. The woman may suffer discomfort and may find that the contractions are painful. The attempt at induction may be ineffective which is disheartening for her. The most serious complication is overstimulation of the uterus causing fetal distress, precipitate labour or a ruptured uterus. The midwife should be especially alert in monitoring uterine action in order to avoid administering an excessive dose of prostaglandin.

Prostaglandin increases the sensitivity of the uterus to Syntocinon. It is necessary to allow at least 2 hours to elapse between the last dose of prostaglandin and the commencement of an intravenous infusion of Syntocinon.

Intravenous oxytocin infusion (Syntocinon)

An intravenous infusion of Syntocinon in an isotonic solution is used to stimulate uterine contractions following rupture of the membranes. It may be used to ripen the cervix prior to amniotomy but prostaglandin is more commonly employed for this purpose. The dilution used varies between maternity units. The dose is measured in milliunits per minute (Table 25.2). Using a standard administration set, 15 drops per minute equals a rate of 1 ml per minute.

The drip rate is increased arithmetically at intervals until contractions are occurring every 3 minutes and lasting between 45 and 50 seconds. Each individual will respond slightly differently because the sensitivity of the uterus to oxytocin varies.

Table 25.2
Dose of Syntocinon in milliunits per minute at different infusion rates (1 unit Syntocinon = 1000 milliunits)

Syntocinon in 500 ml	1 ml/min	2 ml/min	4 ml/min
		(= milliunits/min)	
1 unit Syntocinon	2	4	8
2 units Syntocinon	4	8	16
4 units Syntocinon	8	16	32
8 units Syntocinon	16	32	64
10 units Syntocinon	20	40	80

It is vital that the infusion rate is carefully controlled and accurately administered. This may be achieved either by using a drip rate counter or infusion pump, or by an observer counting and adjusting the drip rate manually. Care must be taken not to infuse too much fluid in case water intoxication occurs. A Y-connection should be added to the intravenous cannula so that a second, additive-free infusion is in situ and may be commenced if it is necessary to stop the intravenous Syntocinon.

Syntocinon may also be administered in concentrated form using automatic infusion equipment such as a syringe pump which uses smaller volumes of fluid. With certain types the woman may be able to move about freely and this may add to her comfort.

Once labour is established the rate should not be further increased and may be decreased because the uterus becomes more sensitive to Syntocinon as labour progresses. Increased stimulation is counter-productive and results in more frequent but weaker contractions which do not dilate the cervix but may cause a degree of fetal hypoxia. If the uterine contractions become too frequent or too long the infusion should be slowed down but it may take 30 minutes for this reduction to affect uterine activity.

The principle which the midwife should follow is that she should administer the lowest dose of Syntocinon which will maintain effective, well-spaced uterine contractions.

Observation of mother and fetus.

The fetal heart rate is continuously monitored in order to detect signs of fetal distress caused by the uterine stimulation. A fetal scalp electrode gives the most satisfactory recording. If a cardiotocograph is not available, the fetal heart rate should be recorded on the partograph every 15 minutes.

Uterine contractions may be felt on palpation and their frequency, duration and strength should be recorded on the partograph every 15 to 30 minutes. Continuous tocography is employed if possible and the most accurate results are obtained if an intra-uterine catheter is used. The midwife should be in constant attendance while the Syntocinon dosage is being increased and should use 'fingertip' palpation (Fig. 25.1) to test the uterine tone both during and between the contractions. The urine is tested for ketones which may signify the development of keto-acidosis which requires treatment. A fluid balance chart should be kept to ensure that the woman is neither becoming dehydrated nor overloaded with intravenous fluid. Equally important is the woman's reaction to the pain caused by the contractions as many women find the rapid build-up in the frequency of Syntocinon-stimulated contractions difficult to cope with. The midwife must be aware of the woman's need for pain relief and be generous in her encouragement.

Progress in labour. Before commencing the infusion the abdomen will have been examined to ascertain the position of the fetus and its relationship to the pelvic brim. A vaginal examination will have been performed to assess the state and dilatation of the cervix. During labour, progress is monitored by noting the descent of the head on abdominal palpation and assessing cervical dilatation on vaginal examination. All findings are plotted on the partograph. The use of Studd's curve to evaluate the cervicograph demonstrates if progress is within normal limits. Vaginal examinations are usually performed 4-hourly but if progress is slow, or high doses of Syntocinon are used, more frequent examinations may be made, for example 2-hourly.

After delivery the infusion is continued for 1 hour as prophylaxis against postpartum haemorrhage.

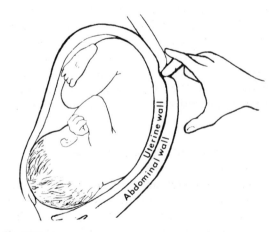

Fig. 25.1
Testing uterine tone.

Complications of Syntocinon infusion. *When these arise the infusion must be stopped.*

Overstimulation of the uterus is the main complication; this may cause the uterus to contract for several minutes together (tonic contraction) or may result in strong contractions which last more than 60 seconds and occur more frequently than every 2 minutes. Relaxation between contractions is inadequate. In either case the infusion is stopped and the doctor is summoned. In the case of a tonic contraction two puffs of a Ventolin inhaler may be administered to the mother while awaiting medical aid. (Women who regularly use a Ventolin inhaler as treatment for asthma should be given appropriate advice when receiving a Syntocinon infusion as it may counteract the effect.)

A ruptured uterus may result from overstimulation if any cephalopelvic disproportion is present. Syntocinon is contra-indicated in cases of absolute disproportion and must be used with great caution in the presence of a uterine scar. In the latter case the midwife must observe the mother carefully for any signs of impending rupture of the uterine scar.

Amniotic fluid embolism is a rare complication which may be caused by strong, tumultuous contractions.

Fetal distress may be caused by overstimulation of the uterus and this may resolve spontaneously if contractions lessen. In cases of placental insufficiency or preterm labour fetal distress may arise without uterine action being excessive. If this occurs the Syntocinon infusion should be turned off and medical aid summoned. The woman should be turned onto her left side, and in severe fetal distress where there are prolonged decelerations or bradycardia of 100 beats a minute or less, oxygen may be administered to the woman by face mask at 4 litres a minute.

Artificial rupture of the membranes (amniotomy)

Rupture of the membranes is performed to stimulate uterine contractions and is often used in conjunction with prostaglandin or Syntocinon infusion or both. At amniotomy, the forewaters are usually ruptured using an Amnihook or amniotomy forceps. In cases of polyhydramnios the hindwaters may be ruptured first, using a Drew-Smythe cannula. This carries a risk of puncture of the placenta should it be low-lying and for this reason is rarely used today.

Amniotomy has the additional attraction of enabling the colour of the liquor to be seen so that any meconium staining is revealed at an early stage of labour. It also allows a fetal scalp electrode to be applied to monitor the fetal heart rate accurately in cases where continuous monitoring is considered necessary. These are not in themselves sufficient indications to rupture the membranes without other supporting reasons.

Procedure. An explanation is given to the woman about what is to be done. She is asked to empty her bladder. The lie, the presentation, level of the presenting part and the fetal heart rate are determined by abdominal examination. The woman may be placed in the lithotomy position for the procedure but she will find this both uncomfortable and undignified and it should be maintained for the shortest time possible. If the cervix is easily reached and favourable the amniotomy may be performed with the woman in the dorsal position.

The colour of the liquor is observed for the presence of meconium.

The fetal heart rate is auscultated on completion of the procedure and at 15-minute intervals for the next hour. The frequency of subsequent recordings will depend on whether labour has commenced or an oxytocin infusion is in progress.

Complications are largely preventable as the circumstances causing them should be recognised before amniotomy is performed. If any of the causative factors is present, induction should be carried out with extreme caution, if at all.

Cord prolapse may occur when the presenting part is ill-fitting or not well down in the pelvis.

Placental separation may be caused by the sudden reduction in intra-uterine size following amniotomy. This is most likely to occur when polyhydramnios is present. In this instance a controlled rupture of the membranes is performed in which the liquor is drained slowly.

Infection is not usually a problem unless the membranes are ruptured for more than 24 hours before delivery. In order to avoid this, prostaglandin may be used to ripen an unfavourable cervix prior to amniotomy. A Syntocinon infusion is often commenced immediately following artificial rupture of the membranes with the object of reducing the induction–delivery interval. If this is not done straight away it will be considered if contractions have not begun within 4–6 hours.

Strict aseptic precautions are observed in order to minimise the risk of infection.

An intra-uterine death predisposes to infection once the membranes are ruptured and an alternative method of induction should be used.

Pre-existing vaginal infections such as genital herpes or gonorrhoea are liable to infect the fetus during delivery and caesarean section may be preferred to induction.

ACCELERATION OF LABOUR

Acceleration or augmentation of labour differs from induction in that labour starts spontaneously. The process aims to increase the efficiency of uterine contractions when progress in labour is slow. Any method which is used to induce labour, with the exception of vaginal or extra-amniotic prostaglandin, may also be used to accelerate it. The policy of active management of labour employs acceleration techniques if the rate of progress, as plotted on the partograph, falls more than 2 hours behind Studd's curve.

ABNORMAL UTERINE ACTION

Inefficient uterine action

Uterine action is said to be inefficient when the contractions do not effectively dilate the cervix. Progress in labour is slow and the length of labour prolonged. It may arise either because the contractions are too weak or because the parts of the uterus do not act in harmony with one another.

Hypotonic uterine action

The contractions are weak, short and infrequent. The result is slow dilatation of the cervix or none. The woman is not distressed by the contractions nor is the fetus adversely affected by them. Hypotonic action may be *primary*, occurring from the onset of labour, or *secondary*, developing during the course of a previously normal labour. The cause of primary hypotonic uterine action is unknown but it is most commonly found in primigravidae. Secondary hypotonic uterine action may be due to cephalopelvic disproportion, malpresentation or malposition of the fetal occiput. Uterine action may also diminish in the presence of maternal dehydration or keto-acidosis and sometimes following the commencement of epidural analgesia.

Management. The woman often becomes tired and dispirited through the lack of progress in labour and she requires considerable support and encouragement from the midwife. A vaginal examination is performed to exclude disproportion or malpresentation, both of which require delivery by caesarean section. The membranes are ruptured artificially if still intact, an intravenous infusion of Syntocinon is commenced and continuous cardiotocography is instituted. The woman's fluid and electrolyte balance is maintained and analgesia is given as required. Cervical dilatation is assessed on vaginal examination at 2–4-hourly intervals and the findings are recorded on the partograph.

Inco-ordinate uterine action

In each type of inco-ordinate uterine action there is alteration in the polarity of the uterus and often an increase in the resting tone. The cervix dilates slowly despite frequent, painful contractions and on vaginal examination it feels tight and unyielding. Characteristic contraction patterns are seen on cardiotocography (see Fig. 25.2).

Causation is poorly understood but there appears to be an association with malposition of the fetal occiput and minor degrees of disproportion.

Hypertonic lower uterine segment (reversed polarity). Fundal dominance is lost and the contractions start and last longest in the lower segment. The cervix fails to dilate but the woman is very distressed and complains of pain, particularly backache, which she feels before and after the contraction is palpable abdominally.

Colicky uterus. The different parts of the uterus contract independently and consequently are ineffective in dilating the cervix. The resting tone of the uterus is high and may reduce the placental blood flow, which leads to fetal distress. Pain continues between contractions.

Management of inco-ordinate uterine action is the same for both types. Cephalopelvic disproportion and malpresentation are excluded by abdominal and vaginal examination. The woman may well have been in labour for some time and consequently be tired and dehydrated as well as disheartened and in pain. She needs encouragement from the midwife, who must use all her skills to make her as comfortable as possible. Dehydration and keto-acidosis are corrected by an intravenous infusion of Hartmann's solution. A strict fluid balance chart is kept and all specimens of urine are tested for the presence of ketones. Frequent mouthwashes are given so that the woman's mouth remains moist and fresh.

Adequate pain relief is essential and may enable the woman to sleep; this in turn will help the contractions to become more co-ordinated. Epidural analgesia is the method of choice and is very effective in promoting more normal uterine action. When this is not available, or if the woman does not wish it, pethidine may be used either in an intravenous infusion or as an intramuscular injection in a dose of 150 mg which may be combined with a sedative such as promazine 50 mg.

The fetal heart and uterine contractions are monitored continuously as this condition often results in fetal distress which may necessitate early delivery. Once adequate analgesia has been achieved, the membranes, if still intact, are ruptured artificially and a low-dose Syntocinon infusion may be commenced to stimulate normal uterine contractions. Vaginal examinations are performed at 2–4 hourly intervals to assess progress,

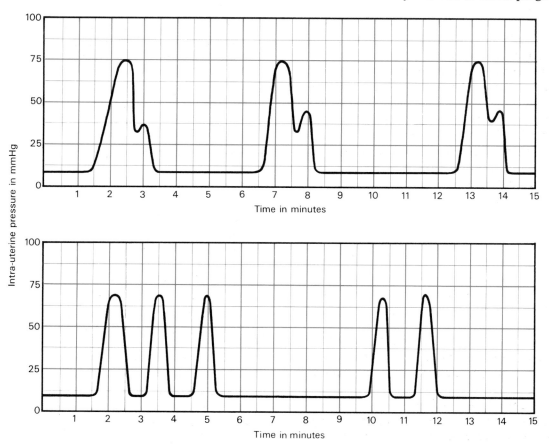

Fig. 25.2
Characteristic tocographic pattern of inco-ordinate uterine action.

which is plotted on the partograph. If after 4–6 hours of Syntocinon, labour is not progressing, a caesarean section is performed.

Constriction ring dystocia. This is localised spasm of a ring of muscle fibres which usually occurs at the junction of the upper and lower segments of the uterus. It is rare, affecting less than 1 in 1000 labours, and may arise during any stage of labour, although it is most common in the third stage. When it occurs in the first or second stage of labour the constriction ring often embraces a narrow part of the fetus such as the neck.

The immediate cause is hypertonic, colicky uterine action. This may arise spontaneously following early rupture of the membranes which leads to the uterus being moulded round the fetus. Alternatively it can be caused by mishandling of the uterus, intra-uterine manipulations or overdosage of Syntocinon.

First and second stages of labour. Constriction ring is rarely diagnosed during the first stage but may be suspected in the second stage when there is no advance of the presenting part and the upper segment is tender on palpation. The constriction ring may be felt on examination per vaginam. The only treatment prior to delivery is to achieve relaxation of the constriction ring by the administration of a deep general anaesthetic, after which forceps delivery is usually possible. Failing this a caesarean section is necessary, possibly with a classical incision.

In the third stage of labour constriction ring is known as an hour-glass contraction and prevents delivery of the placenta. Immediate relaxation of the constriction ring may be effected by inhalation of 1 ampoule of amyl nitrite but if this is unsuccessful a general anaesthetic will be needed.

Cervical dystocia

Rigid cervix. In this rare condition the cervix fails to dilate despite normal uterine contractions. The first stage is characterised by severe, persistent backache. On vaginal examination the cervix initially feels thin, tight and unyielding but may become thick and oedematous. The woman is often a primigravida and the problem is not repeated in a subsequent labour.

Annular detachment of the cervix. Prolonged pressure of the head on a rigid cervix, in rare instances, produces an ischaemic area which inhibits dilatation. Bearing down during the first stage may be a contributory factor. The necrosed ring of cervix becomes detached and expelled. It constitutes a uterine rupture.

Oedematous anterior lip of cervix. When the anterior part of the cervix is nipped between the fetal head and the pelvic brim it may become swollen. This prolongs the first stage of labour as an oedematous cervix does not dilate easily. It may be felt on vaginal examination as a firm ridge, sometimes as thick as a finger, and on occasions the glistening blue cervix may be seen at the vulva between the fetal head and the symphysis pubis.

Disproportion may be the cause but it is more likely to be due to the woman bearing down before the cervix is fully dilated, a problem particularly associated with a posterior position of the fetal occiput.

Management. The woman is encouraged to lie on her side and to use inhalational analgesia during contractions which will help her to refrain from pushing. The foot of the bed may be elevated to relieve some of the pressure on the cervix. When the midwife is unable to prevent the woman pushing, epidural analgesia may be effective. It is sometimes possible to ease the cervix up over the head but care must be taken not to cause lacerations.

Excessive uterine action

Precipitate labour

The contractions are strong and frequent from the onset of labour, which results in abnormally rapid progress and delivery within an hour of its commencement.

Maternal complications. Cervical and perineal lacerations may be caused by the rapid delivery, which is also very frightening for the woman. The uterus may fail to retract during the third stage which may lead to a retained placenta or a postpartum haemorrhage.

Fetal complications. The frequency and strength of the contractions may cause fetal hypoxia. Rapid moulding and alteration in intracranial pressure during delivery may cause intra-cranial haemorrhage. The baby may be injured by rapid delivery onto a hard surface or infected following delivery into the toilet. The cord may snap with a consequent risk of cord haemorrhage.

Future pregnancies. Precipitate labour tends to recur and the woman should be offered admission to hospital at 38 weeks' gestation so that she is in a suitable place for delivery. Induction may be considered in order to pre-empt labour but this must be undertaken with great caution.

Overstimulation of the uterus

Excessive use of Syntocinon or prostaglandin may result in tetanic contractions with inadequate periods of relaxation between them.

Complications. Uterine spasm may cause fetal hypoxia due to reduction in placento-fetal oxygen transfer which, if untreated, will lead to fetal death. Overstimulation of the uterus may provoke a precipitate labour: more often it results in frequent but ineffective contractions which fail to dilate the cervix. Retraction may also be lost and progress is slow because the contractions lack strength. If there is a degree of disproportion, the uterus may rupture.

Management. The administration of Syntocinon or prostaglandin must be stopped at once. The woman should be nursed on her left side and the fetal heart monitored continuously. If tonic contractions are present, she may be given 2 puffs of a Ventolin inhaler. If fetal bradycardia is present, oxygen should be administered to the mother. The doctor should be summoned and may obtain a fetal blood sample in order to determine the pH. If this is low, delivery may be expedited.

Tonic contractions

The contractions become progressively longer, stronger and more frequent until they merge into a state of almost continuous uterine contraction with only brief spells of partial relaxation every few minutes.

In a spontaneous labour the usual cause is disproportion. In a multigravida the uterine response to obstruction is to increase the strength and frequency of contractions in an effort to overcome that obstruction. In a primigravida, the uterus

initially ceases to contract but after a period of inertia tonic contractions may ensue.

Management. Any oxytocic drugs are discontinued and a doctor is summoned. The fetal heart and maternal pulse and blood pressure are carefully monitored and the woman may be given 2 puffs of a Ventolin inhaler. A vaginal examination is performed to assess the stage of labour and to diagnose any disproportion.

Maternal complications. Ruptured uterus due to disproportion is the main complication and is more commonly found in multigravidae.

Fetal complications. Hypoxia is caused by prolonged contractions and may result in fetal death.

PROLONGED LABOUR

Traditionally labour is prolonged if it exceeds 24 hours. When labour is actively managed, it is termed prolonged if delivery is not imminent after 12 hours of established labour.

The first stage

The partograph will illustrate slow progress or delay in the first stage of labour (Fig. 25.3). Action should be taken before complications arise.

Prolonged latent phase

The latent phase lasts from the onset of labour until the rate of cervical dilatation increases, which usually begins when the cervix is 3 cm dilated. The latent phase is considered prolonged if over 20 hours in primigravidae or 14 hours in multigravidae.

Primary dysfunctional labour

This describes a situation in which progress in the active phase of labour is slow and the cervix dilates at less than 1 cm an hour.

Secondary arrest

After normal progress in early labour, cervical dilatation is arrested in the active phase.

Causes

Uterine contractions ('powers'). Inefficient uterine contractions are the most common cause

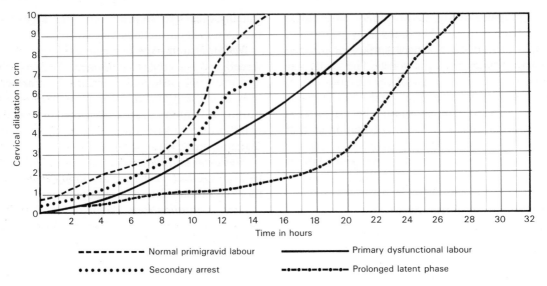

Fig. 25.3
Partographic illustration of delay in the first stage of labour.

of prolonged labour. The cervix dilates slowly or not at all.

Pelvic abnormalities ('passages'). A contracted pelvis and pelvic tumours prevent normal progress in labour.

The fetus ('passenger'). A large fetus, malposition of the occiput or malpresentation inhibit the progress of labour.

Psychological causes. Abnormally tense or apprehensive women tend to have prolonged labours. This phenomenon affects primigravidae more often than multigravidae.

Management

When progress in labour is slow, the cause must be identified before deciding on management. Weak uterine action may be rectified with a Syntocinon infusion. If, however, there has been no progress despite good uterine contractions, it is pointless to further stimulate the uterus and labour must be terminated by caesarean section. Obvious disproportion or malpresentation of the fetus likewise indicate the need for operative delivery.

Maternal condition. The woman is likely to be demoralised by lack of progress. She may also be exhausted, dehydrated and ketotic and may be suffering severe pain.

The midwife should help her to adopt a comfortable position and should assist the partner to provide continual support and encouragement. Adequate analgesia should be offered. An epidural block is beneficial because it will enable her to rest.

An intravenous infusion is commenced to correct fluid and electrolyte balance and to supply energy. The woman should be encouraged to empty her bladder regularly and the urine is tested for ketones. A fluid balance chart is kept. Sips of water only are allowed in case a general anaesthetic is required for delivery. Oral ranitidine 150 mg 6-hourly is prescribed to reduce gastric secretions.

If labour is prolonged due to abnormal uterine action the appropriate mangement is initiated. The midwife maintains careful observation and records.

If the membranes have been ruptured for more than 24 hours a high vaginal swab may be taken for culture and sensitivity if signs of infection are present. Broad-spectrum antibiotics may be prescribed prophylactically in the hope of preventing maternal uterine infection and congenital pneumonia in the baby.

Fetal condition. The fetal heart is monitored continuously and the amniotic fluid is observed for the presence of meconium. If meconium is present measures must be taken to prevent aspiration at delivery.

The second stage

Provided that fetal and maternal conditions are satisfactory there is little cause for concern if the latent phase of the second stage of labour takes some time. Once the woman has entered the active or perineal phase the midwife should expect to see continuous descent and advance of the fetal head. Less attention is paid to the actual passage of time than formerly.

Causes of a prolonged second stage of labour

Hypotonic contractions. Secondary hypotonic contractions may cause delay. An intravenous infusion of Syntocinon is commenced in order to stimulate adequate contractions.

Ineffective maternal effort. Fear, exhaustion or lack of sensation may inhibit a woman's ability to push and cause delay, especially in a primigravida. The midwife should ensure that the presenting part is visible before pushing is encouraged. If an epidural block is in progress the midwife may need to teach the woman when to push as she will lack the normal urge.

In the absence of fetal distress the woman may be turned on her side and encouraged to rest for up to 30 minutes. The change of position may be beneficial; kneeling or an upright position may also assist progress.

A rigid perineum may prevent the advance of the fetus during the perineal phase. If this is evident an episiotomy is performed under local anaesthesia.

Reduced pelvic outlet. An android pelvis is the most likely cause of obstruction at the outlet due to its prominent ischial spines and narrow sub-pubic arch. A forceps delivery is performed if possible or, in severe cases, caesarean section.

A large fetus or one with large presenting diameters as in a malposition or malpresentation may account for delay. An operative delivery will be necessary. If the occiput is in any position other than anterior, rotation will be required prior to delivery. Kielland's forceps or a vacuum extractor may be used. In cases of a very large fetus or malpresentation, a caesarean section may be necessary.

Complications

Maternal. Prolonged pressure of the fetal head on the vaginal walls and pelvic floor may cause oedema, increasing the likelihood of lacerations. Overstretching of the pelvic floor and uterine ligaments may lead to subsequent uterine prolapse, cystocele or rectocele. A urethra which is persistently compressed by the fetal head becomes bruised and this may cause retention of urine and possibly urinary tract infection during the puerperium.

Fetal. Prolonged head compression, a difficult instrumental delivery or hypoxia may lead to intracranial haemorrhage.

OBSTRUCTED LABOUR

Labour is said to be obstructed when there is no advance of the presenting part despite strong uterine contractions. The obstruction usually occurs at the pelvic brim but may occur at the outlet, for example deep transverse arrest in an android pelvis.

Causes

Cephalopelvic disproportion. The fetus may be large in relation to maternal size, such as the fetus of a diabetic mother, or the pelvis may be contracted. A previously fractured pelvis may also result in problems during labour.

Deep transverse arrest. This outcome of an occipitoposterior position causes obstructed labour.

Fetal abnormalities. A hydrocephalic fetus may result in cephalopelvic disproportion. Conjoined twins are a rare cause of obstruction.

Locked twins are a rare cause of obstruction.

Malpresentations. Vaginal delivery is impossible in cases of shoulder or brow presentation or persistent mentoposterior position.

Pelvic tumours. In rare instances cervical fibroids, an ovarian tumour or a tumour of the bony pelvis prevent the head from entering the pelvis.

Signs of obstructed labour

Early signs. The presenting part does not enter the pelvic brim despite good contractions.

The midwife must exclude the possibilities of a full bladder, a loaded rectum and a large amount of amniotic fluid as causes of non-engagement.

The cervix dilates slowly and hangs loosely like 'an empty sleeve' because the presenting part cannot descend and become applied to it. The forewaters tend to form a large elongated bag or to rupture early.

Late signs arise only in a badly managed or neglected labour and obstruction should be diagnosed before they are seen.

On general examination the woman is dehydrated, ketotic and in pain. Her pulse is rapid and she is pyrexial. Urinary output is poor and, as well as containing ketones, the urine is concentrated and often blood-stained. There are usually signs of fetal distress.

The uterus becomes moulded round the fetus and does not relax properly between contractions. These become stronger and more frequent until the uterus is in a state of virtually continuous tonic contraction. This results in the lower segment becoming progressively thinner and longer and the upper segment becoming shorter and thicker. The retraction ring may be seen abdominally as an oblique ridge above the symphysis pubis and marks the junction between the upper and the ballooned-out lower segment. A visible retraction ring is called Bandl's ring. It is of similar appearance to a full bladder, except that the ridge is at an oblique angle across the abdomen and on catheterisation the bladder is found to contain little urine. Uterine exhaustion, in which contractions cease for a while before recommencing with renewed vigour, may occur in a primigravida.

The vagina is hot and dry, the presenting part is high and feels wedged and immovable. There is excessive moulding of the fetal skull and a large caput succedaneum is present.

Management

If the obstruction cannot be overcome by manipulation or instrumental delivery, caesarean section should be performed as soon as possible.

The mother and her partner should be reassured as they will understandably be very anxious. An intravenous infusion is commenced to correct dehydration and blood is cross-matched in case it is required at delivery. Antibiotic therapy is instituted to combat infection.

If the fetus is alive, he is likely to be delivered in an asphyxiated and shocked condition. Neonatal resuscitation facilities should be available at delivery and a paediatrician should be present.

Complications

Maternal. Intra-uterine infection may follow prolonged rupture of the membranes. Trauma to the bladder may occur as a result of pressure from the fetal head during labour or as a result of injury at delivery.

Neglected obstruction will result in a ruptured uterus due to excessive thinning of the lower segment. This leads to haemorrhage and shock and may end in maternal death.

Fetal. Intra-uterine asphyxia may lead to stillbirth or permanent brain damage. Intracranial haemorrhage may be caused by asphyxia or trauma sustained during a difficult instrumental delivery. Ascending infection may cause neonatal pneumonia which may also result from meconium aspiration.

Prevention

Note should be made of any history of previous prolonged labours or difficult deliveries or of babies weighing over 4.5 kg at birth. Malpresentations should be detected antenatally and external cephalic version may be attempted. An unengaged head in a primigravida at term should be investigated. Some obstetricians routinely perform pelvic assessment at 36 weeks' gestation to determine whether the pelvis is adequate.

In cases of suspected disproportion of a minor degree, labour may be induced at 38 weeks so that the fetus does not grow too large or his skull bones become too hard.

Careful monitoring of progress in labour should detect lack of descent of the presenting part before labour becomes obstructed. This is aided by observation of both fetal and maternal conditions and of the length, strength and frequency of contractions.

If disproportion is suspected, a planned trial of labour may be undertaken with well defined limits.

Caesarean section must be performed as soon as any signs of obstruction become apparent.

If the presenting part fails to advance during the second stage of labour despite good contractions, labour may be obstructed and medical aid should be summoned.

Reader Activities

- Ascertain what methods are commonly used, or are available, in your antenatal clinic to estimate fetal maturity reliably.
- Determine how the fetal condition has been monitored after 40 weeks' gestation in a woman you have cared for who delivered at 42 weeks' gestation or later.
- Find out the induction rate in your maternity unit; what methods of induction are commonly used there?
- Compare and contrast the experiences of labour of women who have had:
  — spontaneous onset of labour
  — labour induced with vaginal prostaglandin
  — labour induced with intravenous oxytocin infusion.
- Examine the contraction pattern on the cardiotocographic trace of a woman with prolonged labour to see if it demonstrates any abnormal uterine action.
- Examine the partographs of several women whose labour has been accelerated to see what effect this had on the rate of cervical dilatation.

FURTHER READING

Altman D E, Hytten F 1989 Assessment of fetal size and fetal growth. In: Chalmers I, Enkin M, Keirse M J N C (eds) Effective care in pregnancy and childbirth. Oxford University Press, Oxford, vol 1, ch 26, p 411–418

Bakketeig L, Bergsjo P 1989 Post-term pregnancy: magnitude of the problem. In: Chalmers I, Enkin M, Keirse M J N C (eds) Effective care in pregnancy and childbirth. Oxford University Press, Oxford, vol 1, ch 46, p 765–775

Bishop E H 1964 Pelvic scoring for elective induction. Obstetrics and Gynaecology 24(2): 266–268

Cardozo L, Studd J 1985 Abnormal labour patterns. In: Studd J (ed) The management of labour. Blackwell Scientific Publications, Oxford, ch 12, p 171–187

Crowley P 1989 Post-term pregnancy: induction or surveillance? In: Chalmers I, Enkin M, Keirse M J N C (eds) Effective care in pregnancy and childbirth. Oxford University Press, Oxford, vol 1, ch 47, p 776–791

Grant J, Keirse M J N C 1989 Prelabour rupture of the membranes at term. In: Chalmers I, Enkin M, Keirse M J N C (eds) Effective care in pregnancy and childbirth. Oxford University Press, Oxford, vol 2, ch 64, p 1112–1117

Keirse M J N C, Chalmers I 1989 Methods for inducing labour. In: Chalmers I, Enkin M, Keirse M J N C (eds) Effective care in pregnancy and childbirth. Oxford University Press, Oxford, vol 2, ch 62, p 1057–1079

Keirse M J N C, van Oppen A C C 1989 Preparing the cervix for induction of labour. In: Chalmers I, Enkin M, Keirse M J N C (eds) Effective care in pregnancy and childbirth. Oxford University Press, Oxford, vol 2, ch 61, p 988–1056

Lewis T L T, Chamberlain G N P (eds) 1990 Obstetrics by ten teachers, 15th edn. Edward Arnold, London, p 132–133, 179–182, 209–211, 275–277

Llewellyn-Jones D 1990 Variations in duration of pregnancy: fetal maturity. In: Fundamentals of obstetrics and gynaecology. Vol 1 Obstetrics, 5th edn. Faber & Faber, London, ch 35, p 269–276

Llewellyn-Jones D 1990 Dystocia: faults in the powers. In: Fundamentals of obstetrics and gynaecology. Vol 1 Obstetrics, 5th edn. Faber & Faber, London, ch 44, p 339–346

Miller A W F, Callender R 1989 Abnormal labour. In: Miller A W F, Callender R (eds) Obstetrics illustrated, 4th edn. Churchill Livingstone, Edinburgh, ch 12

26

Malposition of the occiput and malpresentations

JOSEPHINE WILLIAMS

Occipitoposterior positions

Face presentation

Brow presentation

Breech presentation

Shoulder presentation

Unstable lie

Compound presentation

Occipitoposterior positions are the commonest type of malposition of the occiput. This chapter outlines their causes, diagnosis, the effects on and management of labour and the possible outcomes of these positions. The midwife's skills are fully utilised in such labours, which tend to be prolonged (see also Ch. 25). The chapter goes on to discuss face and brow presentations, both of which may develop during labour from an occipitoposterior position. Breech presentation is discussed very comprehensively in the next section, which includes detailed, well-illustrated guidelines for the management of a breech delivery. The final malpresentation examined is shoulder presentation, and the chapter concludes with the related subjects of unstable lie and compound presentation.

OCCIPITOPOSTERIOR POSITIONS

Although a vertex presentation is normal, labour can be adversely affected when the occiput lies in the posterior rather than the anterior part of the pelvis. In consequence, the head is deflexed and larger diameters of the fetal skull present. These positions occur in approximately 10% of labours.

Causes
The direct cause is sometimes unknown, but it may be associated with an abnormally shaped pelvis.

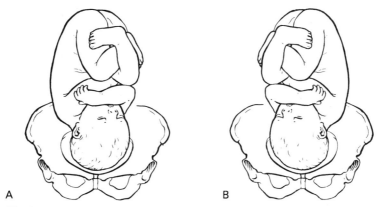

Fig. 26.1
(A) Right occipitoposterior position. (B) Left occipitoposterior position.

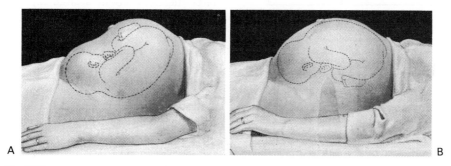

Fig. 26.2
Comparison of abdominal contour in (A) posterior and (B) anterior positions of the occiput.

Abnormal pelvis. In an android pelvis the fore-pelvis is narrow, and the occiput tends to occupy the roomier hind-pelvis. The oval shape of the anthropoid pelvis, with its narrow transverse diameter, favours a direct occipitoposterior position.

pitofrontal (11.5 cm), will not enter the pelvic brim until labour begins and flexion occurs allowing engagement of the suboccipitofrontal diameter (10 cm). The occiput and sinciput are on the same level.

The cause of deflexion is the straightening of the fetal spine against the lumbar curve of the

Antenatal diagnosis

Abdominal examination

On inspection. There is a saucer-shaped depression at or immediately below the umbilicus, because, when the back is not anterior, there is a 'dip' between the head and lower limbs of the fetus. The high unengaged head with the depression above it looks rather like a full bladder.

On palpation, the *head is high*, a posterior position being the most common cause of non-engagement in a primigravida at term. This is because the large presenting diameter, the occi-

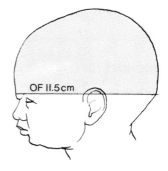

Fig. 26.3
Engaging diameter of a deflexed head: occipitofrontal 11.5 cm.

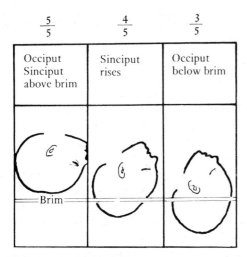

$$\frac{5}{5} \qquad \frac{4}{5} \qquad \frac{3}{5}$$

Occiput Sinciput above brim	Sinciput rises	Occiput below brim

Brim

Fig. 26.4
Flexion with descent of the head.

maternal spine. This makes the fetus straighten his neck and adopt a more erect attitude.

The back is difficult to palpate, as it is well out to the side and sometimes almost adjacent to the maternal spine.

Limbs are felt on both sides of the midline.

On auscultation the fetal heart will be heard most easily in the flank on the same side as the back but may also be found in the midline because when the back is not well flexed the fetal chest is thrust forward and the heart can be heard through the front of it.

Diagnosis during labour

Clinical features

The woman complains of continuous backache, worsening with contractions, which are felt mainly in the back. The contractions may be inco-ordinate (see Ch. 25) due to the irregularly-shaped presenting circumference not fitting well onto the cervix, and progress in labour is slow. The membranes tend to rupture spontaneously at an early stage. Descent of the head is slow, even when there are good contractions. There is a strong urge to push at the end of the first stage because the occiput is pressing on the rectum.

Vaginal examination (Fig. 26.5)

The findings will depend on the degree of flexion of the head; locating the anterior fontanelle in the anterior part of the pelvis is diagnostic but in the later stages of labour a large caput succedaneum may be present, making it difficult to define the position.

Management of labour

Labour may be prolonged because the deflexed head does not fit well onto the cervix and stimulate effective uterine contractions; instead they are painful and inco-ordinate. The head has to flex and rotate, which also increases the length of labour.

First stage of labour

The woman complains of continuous backache which, as well as being painful, is tiring and demoralising, especially if progress in labour is slow. The midwife will need to utilise all her skills in helping the woman to cope with this. A warm bath can be very soothing and massage of the woman's back in the lumbar region by her partner or midwife can be helpful during a contraction.

ANTERIOR

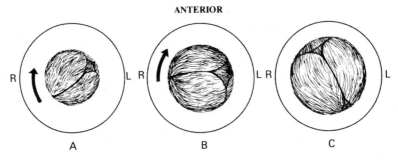

Fig. 26.5
Vaginal touch pictures in a right occipitoposterior position (A) Anterior fontanelle felt to left and anteriorly. Sagittal suture in the right oblique diameter of the pelvis. (B) Anterior fontanelle felt to left and laterally. Sagittal suture in the transverse diameter of the pelvis. (C) Following increased flexion the posterior fontanelle is felt to the right and anteriorly. Sagittal suture in the left oblique diameter of the pelvis. The position is now right occipito-anterior.

The mother should be encouraged to remain mobile for as long as possible and to adopt whatever position she finds most comfortable. Many women find that the all-fours position relieves much discomfort. It may also aid rotation of the fetal head. Routine observations of the maternal and fetal conditions are made as in normal labour (see Ch. 12).

When labour is prolonged, an intravenous infusion may be necessary to correct dehydration and, if the contractions are ineffectual and cervical dilatation slow, labour may be accelerated with an intravenous infusion of Syntocinon (see Ch. 25). Adequate analgesia should be given, an epidural anaesthetic often being the most effective kind. There is an increased likelihood of the woman needing an anaesthetic, and a prophylactic dose of oral ranitidine 150 mg every 6 hours may be prescribed. There is often a strong urge to push before the cervix is fully dilated due to the occiput pressing on the rectum. The woman should be helped to resist this urge in order to prevent the development of an oedematous anterior lip of cervix (see Ch. 25) which delays the onset of the second stage.

Second stage of labour

Full dilatation of the cervix may need to be confirmed by vaginal examination because excessive moulding and a large caput succedaneum may bring the vertex into view while an anterior lip of cervix remains. Maternal and fetal conditions are closely observed throughout the second stage.

If the head is not visible at the onset of the second stage, the woman may be encouraged to use Entonox during contractions to help her to refrain from pushing until the head rotates and descends. The all-fours position may help to bring this about.

If the contractions are weak, the woman should lie on her side or adopt the erect position. If this is ineffective, Syntocinon should be commenced to stimulate adequate contractions and achieve advance.

If, 30 minutes after confirmation of full dilatation of the cervix, and in the presence of good contractions, the vertex has not become visible or is not advancing, the doctor should be informed, as an operative delivery may be needed.

Mechanism of right occipitoposterior position (long rotation)

The lie is longitudinal
The attitude of the head is deflexed
The presentation is vertex
The position is right occipitoposterior
The denominator is the occiput
The presenting part is the middle or anterior area of the left parietal bone
The occipitofrontal diameter, 11.5 cm, lies in the right oblique diameter of the pelvic brim. The occiput points to the right sacro-iliac joint and the sinciput to the left iliopectineal eminence.

Flexion. Descent takes place with increasing flexion. The occiput becomes the leading part.

Internal rotation of the head. The occiput reaches the pelvic floor first and rotates forwards 3/8 of a circle along the right side of the pelvis to lie under the symphysis pubis. The shoulders follow, turning 2/8 of a circle from the left to the right oblique diameter.

Crowning. The occiput escapes under the symphysis pubis and the head is crowned.

Extension. The sinciput, face and chin sweep the perineum and the head is born by a movement of extension.

Restitution takes place and the occiput turns 1/8 of a circle to the right and the head rights itself with the shoulders.

Internal rotation of the shoulders. The shoulders enter the pelvis in the right oblique diameter, the anterior shoulder reaches the pelvic floor first and rotates forwards 1/8 of a circle to lie under the symphysis pubis.

External rotation of the head. At the same time the occiput turns a further 1/8 of a circle to the right.

Lateral flexion. The anterior shoulder escapes under the symphysis pubis, the posterior shoulder sweeps the perineum and the body is born by a movement of lateral flexion.

Possible course and outcomes of labour

Long internal rotation

This is the commonest outcome, with good uterine contractions producing flexion and descent of the

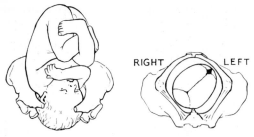

Fig. 26.6 Head descending with increased flexion. Sagittal suture in right oblique diameter of the pelvis.

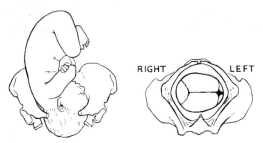

Fig. 26.7 Occiput and shoulders have rotated 1/8 of a circle forwards. Sagittal suture in transverse diameter of the pelvis.

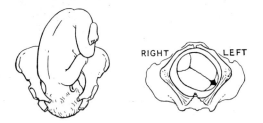

Fig. 26.8 Occiput and shoulders have rotated 2/8 of a circle forwards. Sagittal suture in the left oblique diameter of the pelvis. The position is right occipito-anterior.

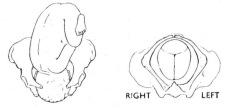

Fig. 26.9 Occiput has rotated 3/8 of a circle forwards. Note twist in neck. Sagittal suture in the anteroposterior diameter of the pelvis.

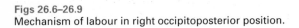

Figs 26.6–26.9
Mechanism of labour in right occipitoposterior position.

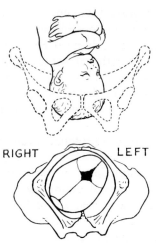

Fig. 26.10
Persistent occipitoposterior position before rotation of the occiput: position right occipitoposterior.

head so that the occiput rotates forward 3/8 of a circle as describe above.

Short internal rotation — persistent occipitoposterior position

The term 'persistent occipitoposterior position' indicates that the occiput fails to rotate forwards. Instead the sinciput reaches the pelvic floor first and rotates forwards. The occiput goes into the hollow of the sacrum. The baby is born facing the pubic bone (face to pubis).

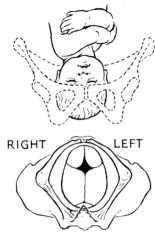

Fig. 26.11
Persistent occipitoposterior position after short rotation: position direct occipitoposterior.

Cause. *Failure of flexion.* The head descends without increased flexion and the sinciput becomes the leading part. It reaches the pelvic floor first and rotates forwards to lie under the symphysis pubis.

Diagnosis. *In the first stage of labour* signs are those of any posterior position of the occiput, namely a deflexed head and a fetal heart heard in the flank or in the midline. Descent is slow.

In the second stage of labour delay is common. On vaginal examination the anterior fontanelle is felt behind the symphysis pubis, but a large caput succedaneum may mask this. If the pinna of the ear is felt pointing towards the mother's sacrum, this indicates a posterior position.

The long occipitofrontal diameter causes considerable dilatation of the anus and gaping of the vagina while the fetal head is barely visible and the broad biparietal diameter distends the perineum and may cause excessive bulging. As the head advances, the anterior fontanelle can be felt just behind the symphysis pubis; the baby is born facing the pubis. Characteristic upward moulding is present with the caput succedaneum on the anterior part of the parietal bone.

Management of delivery. The sinciput will first emerge from under the symphysis pubis as far as the root of the nose and the midwife maintains flexion by restraining it from escaping

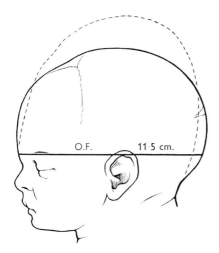

Fig. 26.12
Upward moulding (dotted line) following persistent occipitoposterior position.

O.F.   11·5 cm.

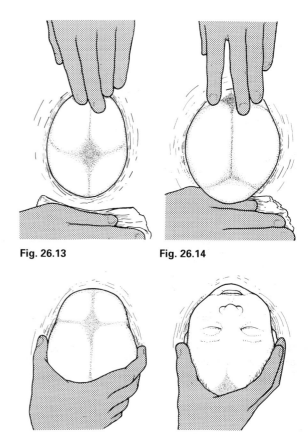

Fig. 26.13   Fig. 26.14

Fig. 26.15   Fig. 26.16

Fig. 26.13 Allowing the sinciput to escape as far as the glabella.
Fig. 26.14 The occiput sweeps the perineum, sinciput held back to maintain flexion
Fig. 26.15 Grasping the head to bring the face down from under the symphysis pubis.
Fig. 26.16 Extension of the head.

Figs 26.13–26.16
Delivery of head in a persistent occipitoposterior position.

further than the glabella, allowing the occiput to sweep the perineum and be born. She then extends the head by grasping it and bringing the face down from under the symphysis pubis. Due to the larger presenting diameters, perineal trauma is common and the midwife should watch for signs of rupture in the centre of the perineum ('button-hole' tear). An episiotomy may be required.

Undiagnosed face to pubis. If the signs are not recognised at an earlier stage, the midwife may first be aware that the occiput is posterior

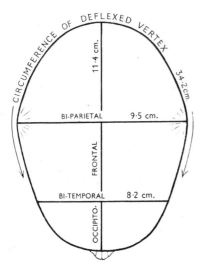

Fig. 26.17
Presenting dimensions of a deflexed head.

when she sees the hairless forehead escaping beneath the pubic arch. She may have been misguidedly extending the head and should therefore now flex it towards the symphysis pubis.

Deep transverse arrest

The head descends with some increase in flexion. The occiput reaches the pelvic floor and begins to rotate forwards. Flexion is not maintained and the occipitofrontal diameter becomes caught at the narrow bispinous diameter of the outlet. Arrest may be due to weak contractions, a straight sacrum or a narrowed outlet.

Diagnosis. The sagittal suture is found in the transverse diameter of the pelvis and both fontanelles are palpable. Neither sinciput nor occiput leads. The head is deep in the pelvic cavity at the level of the ischial spines although the caput may be lower still. There is no advance.

Management. The doctor should be informed. Meanwhile the midwife should encourage the woman to inhale Entonox during contractions. Pushing will not resolve the problem but the woman may find it difficult to overcome the urge to bear down. The midwife should help her to refrain with a change of position and 'SOS' breathing (see Ch. 40). The fetal heart should be continuously monitored. The doctor

will need to rotate the head, either manually or using Kielland's forceps, to an occipito-anterior position prior to a forceps delivery. This procedure may be undertaken under pudendal nerve block, or preferably under an existing lumbar epidural block or, more rarely, caudal anaesthesia. Sometimes a general anaesthetic is given. The condition of the fetus must be taken into account in making the choice.

Conversion to face or brow presentation

When the head is deflexed at the onset of labour, extension occasionally occurs instead of flexion. If extension is complete, a face presentation results, but if incomplete, the head is arrested at the brim, the brow presenting. This is a rare complication of posterior positions, and is more commonly found in multiparous women (see also below).

Complications associated with occipitoposterior positions

Apart from prolonged labour with its attendant risks to mother and fetus (see Ch. 25) and the increased likelihood of instrumental delivery, the following complications may occur.

Obstructed labour (see Ch. 25)

This may occur when the head is deflexed or partially extended and becomes impacted in the pelvis.

Maternal trauma

Forceps delivery may result in perineal bruising and trauma. Delivery of a fetus in the persistent occipitoposterior position, particularly if previously undiagnosed, may cause a third degree tear.

Cord prolapse (see Ch. 27)

A high head predisposes to early spontaneous rupture of the membranes which, together with an ill-fitting presenting part, may result in cord prolapse.

Cerebral haemorrhage (see Ch. 37)

The unfavourable upward moulding of the fetal skull, found in an occipitoposterior position, can cause intracranial haemorrhage, due to the falx cerebri being pulled away from the tentorium cerebelli. The larger presenting diameters also predispose to a greater degree of compression. Cerebral haemorrhage may also result from chronic hypoxia which may accompany prolonged labour.

FACE PRESENTATION

When the attitude of the head is one of complete extension, the occiput of the fetus will be in contact with its spine and the face will present.

The incidence is about 1:500 and the majority develop during labour from vertex presentations with the occiput posterior; this is termed *secondary face presentation*. Less commonly the face presents before labour; this is termed *primary face presentation*. The are six positions in a face presentation (Figs 26.18–26.23); the denominator is the mentum and the presenting diameters are the submentobregmatic (9.5 cm) and the bitemporal (8.2 cm).

Causes

Anterior obliquity of the uterus. The uterus of a multiparous woman with slack abdominal muscles and a pendulous abdomen will lean forward and alter the direction of the uterine axis. This causes the fetal buttocks to lean forwards and the force of the contractions to be directed in a line towards the chin rather than the occiput, resulting in extension of the head.

Contracted pelvis. In the flat pelvis, the head enters in the transverse diameter of the brim and the parietal eminences may be held up in the obstetrical conjugate; the head becomes extended and a face presentation develops. Alternatively, if the head is in the posterior position, vertex presenting, and remains deflexed, the parietal eminences may be caught in the sacrocotyloid dimension, the occiput does not descend, the head becomes extended and face presentation results. This is more likely in the presence of an android pelvis in which the sacrocotyloid dimension is reduced.

Polyhydramnios. If the vertex is presenting

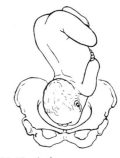

Fig. 26.18 Right mentoposterior.

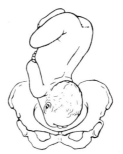

Fig. 26.19 Left mentoposterior.

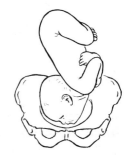

Fig. 26.20 Right mentolateral.

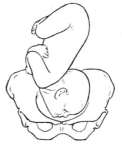

Fig. 26.21 Left mentolateral.

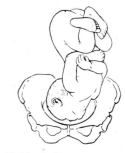

Fig. 26.22 Right mento-anterior.

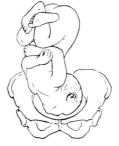

Fig. 26.23 Left mento-anterior.

Figs 26.18–26.23
Six positions of face presentation.

and the membranes rupture spontaneously, the resulting rush of fluid may cause the head to extend as it sinks into the lower uterine segment.

Congenital abnormality. Anencephaly is the commonest fetal cause of a face presentation. In a cephalic presentation, because the vertex is absent, the face is thrust forward and presents. More rarely a tumour of the fetal neck may cause extension of the head.

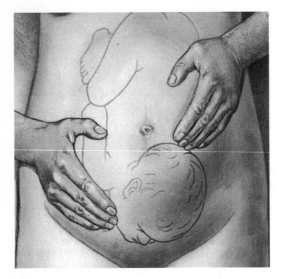

Fig. 26.24
Abdominal palpation of the head in a face presentation.
Position right mentoposterior.

Antenatal diagnosis

Antenatal diagnosis is rare since face presentation develops during labour in the majority of cases. A cephalic presentation in a known anencephalic fetus may be presumed to be a face presentation.

Intrapartum diagnosis

On abdominal palpation

Face presentation may not be detected especially if the mentum is anterior. The occiput feels prominent, with a groove between head and back, but it may be mistaken for the sinciput. The limbs may be palpated on the side opposite to the occiput and the fetal heart is best heard through the fetal chest on the same side as the limbs. In a mentoposterior position the fetal heart is difficult to hear because the fetal chest is in contact with the maternal spine.

On vaginal examination

The presenting part is high, soft and irregular. When the cervix is sufficiently dilated, orbital ridges, eyes, nose and mouth may be felt. Confusion between mouth and anus could arise, but the mouth will be open, and the hard gums diagnostic. The fetus may suck the examining finger. As labour progresses the face becomes oedematous, making it more difficult to distinguish from a breech presentation. To determine position the mentum must be located and if it is posterior, the midwife should decide whether it is lower then the sinciput; if so, it will rotate forwards if it can advance. In a left mentoanterior position, the orbital ridges will be in the left oblique diameter of the pelvis (see Fig. 26.25). Care must be taken not to injure or infect the eyes with the examining finger.

Mechanism of a left mento-anterior position

The lie is longitudinal
The attitude is one of extension of head and back
The presentation is face
The position is left mento-anterior
The denominator is the mentum
The presenting part is the left malar bone.

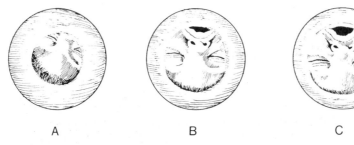

A   B   C

Fig. 26.25
Vaginal touch pictures of left mento-anterior position. (A) Mentum felt to left and anteriorly.
Orbital ridges in left oblique diameter of the pelvis. (B) Following increased extension of the head,
the mouth can be felt. (C) Face has rotated 1/8 of a circle forwards. Orbital ridges in transverse
diameter of the pelvis. Position direct mento-anterior.

Extension. Descent takes place with increasing extension. The mentum becomes the leading part.

Internal rotation of the head occurs when the chin reaches the pelvic floor and rotates forwards 1/8 of a circle. The chin escapes under the symphysis pubis.

Flexion takes place and the sinciput, vertex and occiput sweep the perineum; the head is born.

Restitution occurs when the chin turns 1/8 of a circle to the woman's left.

Internal rotation of the shoulders. The shoulders enter the pelvis in the left oblique diameter and the anterior shoulder reaches the pelvic floor first and rotates forwards 1/8 of a circle along the right side of the pelvis.

External rotation of the head occurs simultaneously. The chin moves further 1/8 of a circle to the left.

Lateral flexion. The anterior shoulder escapes under the symphysis pubis, the posterior shoulder sweeps the perineum and the body is born by a movement of lateral flexion.

Possible course and outcomes of labour

Prolonged labour

Labour is often prolonged because the face is an ill-fitting presenting part and does not therefore stimulate effective uterine contractions. In addition the facial bones do not mould and in order to enable the mentum to reach the pelvic

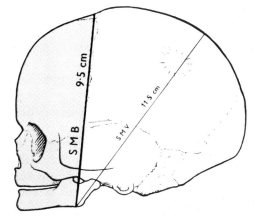

Fig. 26.26
Diameters involved in delivery of face presentation. Engaging diameter, submentobregmatic 9.5 cm. The submentovertical diameter, 11.5 cm, sweeps the perineum.

floor and rotate forwards, the shoulders must enter the pelvic cavity at the same time as the head. The fetal axis pressure is directed to the chin and the head is extended almost at right angles to the spine, increasing the diameters to be accommodated in the pelvis.

Mento-anterior positions

With good uterine contractions descent and rotation of the head occurs (see above) and labour progresses to a spontaneous delivery.

Mentoposterior positions

If the head is completely extended, so that the mentum reaches the pelvic floor first, and the contractions are effective, the mentum will rotate forwards and the position becomes anterior.

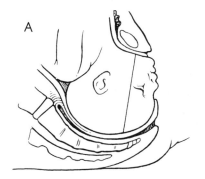
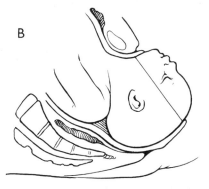

Fig. 26.27
Birth of head in mento-anterior position. (A) Chin escapes under symphysis pubis. Submentobregmatic diameter at outlet. (B) Head is born by a movement of flexion.

Persistent mentoposterior position

In this case the head is incompletely extended and the sinciput reaches the pelvic floor first and rotates forwards 1/8 of a circle which brings the chin into the hollow of the sacrum. There is no further mechanism. The face becomes impacted because in order to descend further, both head and chest would have to be accommodated in the pelvis. Whatever emerges anteriorly from the vagina must pivot around the subpubic arch; if the chin is posterior this is impossible because the head can extend no further.

Management of labour

First stage

When she diagnoses a face presentation, the midwife should inform the doctor of this deviation from the normal. Routine observations of maternal and fetal conditions are made as in normal labour (see Ch. 12), with continuous monitoring of the fetal heart. A fetal scalp electrode should not be applied, and care should be taken not to infect or injure the eyes during vaginal examinations.

Immediately following rupture of the membranes a vaginal examination should be performed to exclude cord prolapse as such an occurrence is more likely because the face is an ill-fitting presenting part. Descent of the head should be observed abdominally, and a vaginal

examination performed every 2–4 hours to assess cervical dilatation and descent of the head.

In mentoposterior positions the midwife should note whether the mentum is lower than the sinciput since rotation and descent depend on this. If the head remains high in spite of good contractions caesarean section is likely. The woman should be prescribed oral ranitidine 150 mg 6-hourly throughout labour as a preparation for anaesthetic.

Delivery

When the face appears at the vulva extension must be maintained by holding back the sinciput and permitting the mentum to escape under the symphysis pubis before the occiput is allowed to sweep the perineum. In this way the submentovertical diameter (11.5 cm) distends the vaginal orifice instead of the mentovertical diameter (13.5 cm). Because the perineum is also distended by the biparietal diameter (9.5 cm),

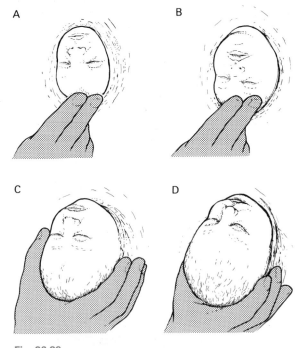

Fig. 26.29
Delivery of face presentation. (A) Sinciput held back to increase extension until the chin is born.
(B) Chin is born. (C) Flexing the head to bring the occiput over the perineum. (D) Flexion completed. The head is born.

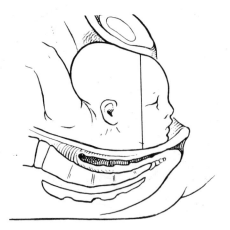

Fig. 26.28
Persistent mentoposterior position.

an elective episiotomy may be performed to avoid extensive perineal lacerations.

If the head does not descend in the second stage, the doctor should be informed. In a mento-anterior position it may be possible for him to deliver the baby with forceps; when rotation is incomplete, or the position remains mento-posterior, a rotational forceps delivery may be feasible. If the head has become impacted, or there is any suspicion of disproportion, a caesarean section will be necessary.

Complications

Obstructed labour (see Ch. 25)
Because the face, unlike the vertex, does not mould, a minor degree of pelvic contraction may result in obstructed labour. In a persistent mento-posterior position the face becomes impacted and caesarean section is necessary.

Cord prolapse (see Ch. 27)
A prolapsed cord is more common when the membranes rupture because the face is an ill-fitting presenting part. The midwife should always perform a vaginal examination when the membranes rupture in order to detect such an occurrence.

Facial bruising
The baby's face is always bruised and swollen at birth with oedematous eyelids and lips. The head is elongated (Fig. 26.30) and the baby will initially lie with his head extended. The midwife should warn the parents in advance of the baby's 'battered' appearance, reassuring them that this is only temporary, and that the bruising and oedema will disappear within 2 or 3 days.

Cerebral haemorrhage
The lack of moulding of the facial bones can lead to intracranial haemorrhage caused by excessive compression of the fetal skull or by rearward compression in the typical moulding of the fetal skull found in this presentation (see Fig. 26.30).

Maternal trauma
Extensive perineal lacerations may occur at delivery due to the large submentovertical and biparietal diameters distending the vagina and perineum. There is an increased incidence of operative delivery, either forceps delivery or caesarean section, both of which increase maternal morbidity.

BROW PRESENTATION

In the brow presentation the fetal head is partially extended with the frontal bone, which is bounded by the anterior fontanelle and the orbital ridges, lying at the pelvic brim. The presenting

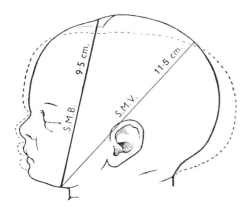

Fig. 26.30
Moulding in a face presentation (dotted line).

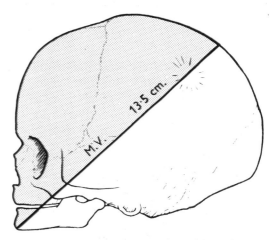

Fig. 26.31
Brow presentation. Mentovertical diameter, 13.5 cm, lies at the pelvic brim.

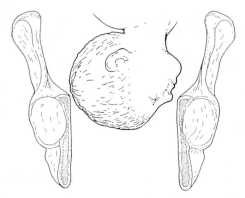

Fig. 26.32
Brow presentation.

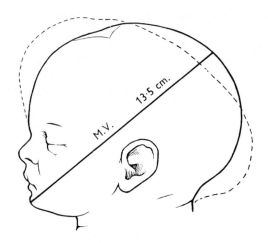

Fig. 26.33
Moulding in a brow presentation (dotted line).

diameter is the mentovertical (13.5 cm), which exceeds all diameters in an average-size pelvis. This presentation is rare, with an incidence of approximately 1 in 1000 deliveries.

Causes

These are the same as for a secondary face presentation (see above); during the process of extension from a vertex presentation to a face presentation, the brow will present temporarily and in a few cases this will persist.

Diagnosis

Brow presentation is not usually detected before the onset of labour.

On abdominal palpation. The head is high, appears unduly large and does not descend into the pelvis despite good uterine contractions.

On vaginal examination. The presenting part is high and may be difficult to reach. The anterior fontanelle may be felt on one side of the pelvis and the orbital ridges, and possibly the root of the nose, at the other. A large caput succedaneum may mask these landmarks if the woman has been in labour for some hours.

Management

The doctor must be informed immediately this presentation is suspected. Vaginal delivery is extremely rare and obstructed labour usually results. It is possible that a woman with a large pelvis and a small baby may deliver vaginally. When the brow reaches the pelvic floor the maxilla rotates forwards and the head is born

by a mechanism somewhat similar to that of a persistent occipitoposterior position. The midwife should never expect such a favourable outcome.

If there is no fetal distress the doctor may allow labour to continue for a short while in case further extension of the head converts the brow presentation to a face presentation. Occasionally spontaneous flexion may occur, resulting in a vertex presentation. If the head fails to descend and the brow presentation persists, a caesarean section is performed.

Complications

These are the same as in a face presentation, except that obstructed labour requiring caesarean section is the probable rather than a possible outcome.

BREECH PRESENTATION

The fetus lies longitudinally with the buttocks in the lower pole of the uterus. The presenting diameter is the bitrochanteric (10 cm) and the denominator the sacrum. This presentation occurs in approximately 3% of pregnancies at term. In mid-trimester the frequency is much higher because the greater proportion of amniotic fluid facilitates free movement of the fetus.

Types of breech presentation

Breech with extended legs (frank breech)

The breech presents with the hips flexed and legs extended on the abdomen. 70% of breech presentations are of this type and it is particularly common in primigravidae whose good uterine muscle tone inhibits flexion of the legs and free turning of the fetus.

Complete breech

The fetal attitude is one of complete flexion, hips and knees both flexed and the feet tucked in beside the buttocks.

Footling breech

This is rare. One or both feet present because neither hips nor knees are fully flexed. The feet are lower than the buttocks, which distinguishes it from the complete breech.

Knee presentation

This is very rare. One or both hips are extended, with the knees flexed.

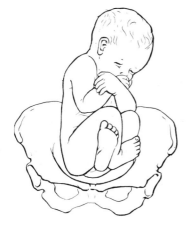

Fig. 26.34   Complete breech.

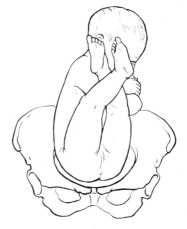

Fig. 26.35   Frank breech.

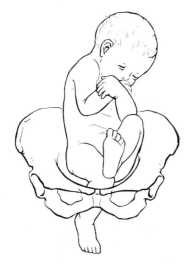

Fig. 26.36   Footling presentation.

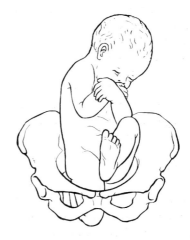

Fig. 26.37   Knee presentation.

Figs 26.34–26.37
Types of breech presentation.

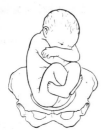

Fig. 26.38 Right
sacroposterior.

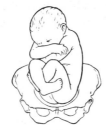

Fig. 26.39 Left
sacroposterior.

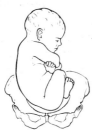

Fig. 26.40 Right
sacrolateral.

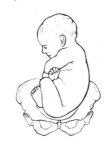

Fig. 26.41 Left
sacrolateral.

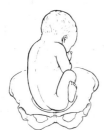

Figs 26.42 Right
sacro-anterior.

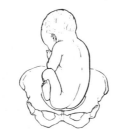

Fig. 26.43 Left sacro-
anterior.

Figs 26.38–26.43
Six positions in breech presentation.

Causes

Often no cause is identified but the following circumstances favour breech presentation.

Extended legs

Spontaneous cephalic version may be inhibited if the fetus lies with the legs extended, 'splinting' the back.

Preterm labour

As breech presentation is relatively common before 34 weeks' gestation, it follows that breech presentation is more common in preterm labours.

Multiple pregnancy

Multiple pregnancy limits the space available for each fetus to turn, which may result in one or more fetuses presenting by the breech.

Polyhydramnios

Distension of the uterine cavity by excessive amounts of amniotic fluid may cause the fetus to present by the breech.

Hydrocephaly

The increased size of the fetal head is more readily accommodated in the fundus.

Uterine abnormalities

Distortion of the uterine cavity by a septum or a fibroid may result in a breech presentation.

Placenta praevia

Some authorities believe this may be a cause of breech presentation but there is some disagreement on this.

Antenatal diagnosis

Abdominal examination

Palpation. In primigravidae, diagnosis is more difficult because of their firm abdominal muscles. On palpation the lie is longitudinal with a soft presentation which is more easily felt using Pawlik's grip. The head can usually be felt in the fundus as a round hard mass which may be made to move independently of the back by ballotting it with one or both hands. If the legs are extended, the feet may prevent such nodding. When the breech is anterior and the fetus well flexed, it may be difficult to locate the head but use of the combined grip in which the upper and lower poles are grasped simultaneously may aid diagnosis. The woman may complain of discomfort under her ribs, especially at night, due to pressure of the head on the diaphragm.

Auscultation. When the breech has not passed through the pelvic brim the fetal heart is heard most clearly above the umbilicus. When the legs are extended the breech descends into the pelvis easily. The fetal heart is then heard at a lower level.

Ultrasound examination

This may be used to demonstrate a breech presentation.

X-ray examination

Although largely superseded by ultrasound, X-ray has the added advantage of allowing a pelvimetry to be performed at the same time.

Diagnosis during labour

A previously unsuspected breech presentation may not be diagnosed until the woman is in established labour. If the legs are extended, the breech may feel like a head abdominally and also on vaginal examination if the cervix is less than 3 cm dilated and the breech is high.

Abdominal examination

Breech presentation may be diagnosed on admission in labour.

Vaginal examination

The breech feels soft and irregular with no sutures palpable, although occasionally the sacrum may be mistaken for a hard head and the buttocks mistaken for caput succedaneum. The anus may be felt and fresh meconium on the examining finger is diagnostic. If the legs are extended the external genitalia are very evident but it must be remembered that these become oedematous. An oedematous vulva may be mistaken for a scrotum.

If a foot is felt, the midwife should differentiate it from the hand. Toes are all the same length, they are shorter than fingers and the big toe cannot be opposed to the toes. The foot is at right angles to the leg, and the heel has no equivalent in the hand.

Presentation may be confirmed by ultrasound scan or X-ray.

Antenatal management

If the midwife suspects or detects a breech presentation at 32 weeks' gestation or later, she should refer the woman to a doctor. The presentation may be confirmed by ultrasound scan or occasionally by abdominal X-ray. There are differing opinions amongst obstetricians as to the management of breech presentation during pregnancy and a decision on management is usually deferred until near term.

External cephalic version

Turning the fetus from a breech to a cephalic presentation before 37 weeks' gestation does not reduce the incidence of breech birth or rate of caesarean section as it is likely to turn itself back spontaneously. External cephalic version at term, using tocolytic drugs to relax the uterus, has been more successful in attaining both of these objectives (Hofmeyr 1989).

Method. The procedure and the reasons for it should be explained to the woman. The bladder should be empty. The woman lies in a supine position and is asked to relax. The foot of the bed may be elevated to free the breech from the pelvic brim. The abdomen is palpated to ascertain the fetal position and the fetal heart is auscultated. The abdomen may be dusted with talcum powder prior to version being attempted (Figs 26.46–26.48).

If the woman is Rhesus negative an injection of anti-D immunoglobulin is given as prophylaxis against iso-immunisation caused by any placental separation. If the version is performed immediately prior to the onset of labour, this can be delayed until after delivery when the blood group of the baby is known. In this case anti-D must be given within 72 hours of the *version.*

If the fetus does not turn easily, the procedure should be abandoned. When the version is completed, the fetal heart is again

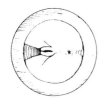

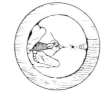

Fig. 26.44   No feet felt. Legs extended.

Fig. 26.45   Feet felt. Complete breech presentation

Figs 26.44 & 26.45
Vaginal touch pictures of left sacrolateral position.

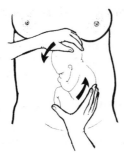

Fig. 26.46 Right hand lifts breech out of pelvis. Left hand makes head follow nose. Flexion of head and back maintained throughout.

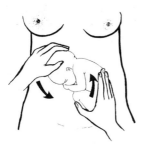

Fig. 26.47 Flexion is continued. Left hand brings head downwards. Right hand pushes breech upwards.

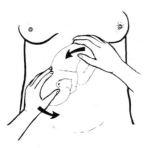

Fig. 26.48 Pressure is exerted on head and breech simultaneously until head is lying at the pelvic brim.

Figs 26.46–26.48
External cephalic version.

auscultated and ideally a 30-minute cardiotocograph recording should be made. It is usually for the heart rate to slow transiently but it should quickly return to normal.

Complications.
Knotting of the umbilical cord should be suspected if bradycardia persists. The fetus is immediately turned back to a breech presen-

tation. The woman is admitted for observation and, if necessary, caesarean section.

Separation of the placenta. The midwife should watch for vaginal bleeding during and after the procedure.

Rupture of the membranes. If this occurs the cord may also prolapse because the head is not engaged.

Preterm labour. This may be precipitated by performing a version.

Contra-indications to external version.
Pre-eclampsia or hypertension because of the increased risk of placental abruption.

Uterine scar, for example from previous caesarean section, in case it ruptures during the procedure.

History of premature labour as the procedure may initiate this.

Multiple pregnancy.

Oligohydramnios because too much force has to be applied directly to the fetus and the version is likely to be unsuccessful.

A hydrocephalic fetus. If a vaginal delivery is contemplated in preference to a caesarean section, the second stage is managed more easily when the fetus presents by the breech.

Persistent breech presentation
When external version has been unsuccessful or has not been attempted, a decision should be made before the onset of labour as to whether to perform an elective caesarean section or to attempt a vaginal delivery.

Planned caesarean section. Some obstetricians believe that the risks to the fetus of a breech delivery are such that all cases of breech presentation should be delivered by caesarean section and some would not attempt an external version. Others will resort to caesarean section for primigravidae but allow multigravidae to deliver vaginally, while yet others assess each case on its individual merits, resorting to elective caesarean section only in cases of known disproportion.

Assessment for vaginal delivery. Any doubt as to the capacity of the pelvis to accommodate the fetal head must be resolved before the buttocks are delivered and the head attempts to enter the pelvic brim. At this point the fetus begins to be deprived of oxygen and a last-minute decision to perform caesarean section may be too late.

Fetal size, especially in relation to maternal size, can be assessed on abdominal palpation but is most accurately judged on ultrasound examination.

Pelvic capacity can be judged on vaginal assessment (see Ch. 10), but it is usual to perform a lateral pelvimetry. This will show the shape of the sacrum and give accurate measurements of the anteroposterior diameters of the pelvic brim, cavity and outlet. In a multigravida information about the type of delivery and the size of previous babies when compared with the size of the present fetus can be helpful.

Mechanism of left sacro-anterior position

The lie is longitudinal
The attitude is one of complete flexion
The presentation is breech
The position is left sacro-anterior
The denominator is the sacrum
The presenting part is the anterior (left) buttock
The bitrochanteric diameter, 10 cm, enters the pelvis in the left oblique diameter of the brim. The sacrum points to the left iliopectineal eminence.

Compaction. Descent takes place with increasing compaction, due to increased flexion of the limbs.

Internal rotation of the buttocks. The anterior buttock reaches the pelvic floor first and rotates forwards 1/8 of a circle along the right side of the pelvis to lie underneath the symphysis pubis. The bitrochanteric diameter is now in the anteroposterior diameter of the outlet.

Lateral flexion of the body. The anterior buttock escapes under the symphysis pubis, the posterior buttock sweeps the perineum and the buttocks are born by a movement of lateral flexion.

Restitution of the buttocks. The anterior buttock turns slightly to the mother's right side.

Internal rotation of the shoulders. The shoulders enter the pelvis in the same oblique diameter as the buttocks, the left oblique. The exterior shoulder rotates forwards 1/8 of a circle along the right side of the pelvis and escapes under the symphysis pubis, the posterior shoulder sweeps the perineum and the shoulders are born.

Internal rotation of the head. The head enters the pelvis with the sagittal suture in the transverse diameter of the brim. The occiput rotates forwards along the left side and the sub-occipital region (the nape of the neck) impinges on the undersurface of the symphysis pubis.

External rotation of the body. At the same time the body turns so that the back is uppermost.

Birth of the head. The chin, face and sinciput sweep the perineum and the head is born in a flexed attitude.

Management of labour

When the breech is presenting, there is a possibility of a need for caesarean section. For this reason and because of the risks to the fetus, labour should take place in a consultant obstetric unit. Labour is sometimes induced after 38 weeks' gestation in order to deliver the fetus before it becomes too large or the skull too ossified but some obstetricians believe that spontaneous onset of labour is safer.

First stage

Basic care during this stage is the same as in normal labour (see Ch. 12). It is usual to monitor the fetal heart and uterine contractions by continuous cardiotocography once labour is established. Although the breech with extended legs fits the cervix quite well, the complete breech is a less well-fitting presenting part and the membranes tend to rupture early. For this reason there is an increased risk of cord prolapse and a vaginal examination is performed to exclude this as soon as the membranes rupture. If they do not rupture spontaneously at an early stage, it is considered safer to leave them intact until labour is well established and the breech at the level of the ischial spines. Meconium-stained liquor is sometimes found due to compression of the fetal abdomen and is not always a sign of fetal distress.

An epidural block is usually offered to a woman with a breech presentation because, as well as providing excellent analgesia, it inhibits the urge to push prematurely and allows better control of the delivery. It may also enable a manipulative delivery to be performed without a general anaesthetic. In view of the possibility of general anaesthesia, oral ranitidine 150 mg should be prescribed 6-hourly throughout labour.

Second stage

Full dilatation of the cervix should always be confirmed by vaginal examination before allowing the woman to push. This is because in a footling presentation a foot may appear at the vulva when the cervix is only partially dilated; or when the legs are extended, particularly if the fetus is small, the breech may slip through an incompletely dilated cervix. In either case, the head may be trapped by the cervix when the fetus is partially delivered.

The obstetrician should be informed of the onset of the second stage, a paediatrician should be present for delivery and it is usual to inform the anaesthetist in case a general anaesthetic is required. Active pushing is not commenced until the buttocks are distending the vulva. Failure of the breech to descend onto the perineum in the second stage despite good contractions may indicate a need for caesarean section.

Types of delivery

Spontaneous breech delivery. The delivery occurs with little assistance from the attendant.

Assisted breech delivery. The buttocks are born spontaneously, but some assistance is necessary for delivery of extended legs or arms and the head.

Breech extraction. This is a manipulative delivery carried out by an obstetrician and is performed to hasten delivery in an emergency situation such as fetal distress.

Management of delivery. The midwife should discuss this with the woman beforehand so that she understands the need of the attendance of the doctors. The delivery is explained in order to help her to appreciate the importance of not pushing until full dilatation of the cervix has been confirmed.

When the buttocks are distending the perineum the woman is placed in the lithotomy position (unless an upright position is chosen — see below) and the vulva is swabbed and draped with sterile towels. The bladder must be empty and it is usually catheterised at this stage. If epidural analgesia is not being used, the perineum is infiltrated with up to 10 ml of 0.5% plain lignocaine prior to an episiotomy being performed. (Pudendal block is sometimes used by a doctor.)

The woman is encouraged to push with the contractions and the buttocks are delivered spontaneously. If the legs are flexed, the feet disengage at the vulva and the baby is born as far as the umbilicus. A loop of cord is gently pulled down to avoid traction on the umbilicus. Spasm of the cord vessels can be caused by manipulating the cord or by stretching it. If the cord is being nipped behind the pubic bone it should be moved to one side. The midwife should feel for the elbows which are usually on the chest. If so, the arms will escape with the next contraction. If the arms are not felt, they are extended (see below).

Delivery of the shoulders. The uterine contractions and the weight of the buttocks will bring the shoulders down onto the pelvic floor where they will rotate into the antero-posterior diameter of the outlet.

The midwife now grasps the baby by the iliac crests with her thumbs held parallel over his sacrum and tilts the baby towards the maternal sacrum in order to free the anterior shoulder. It is helpful to wrap a small towel around the baby's hips which preserves warmth and improves the grip on the slippery skin.

When the anterior shoulder has escaped, the buttocks are lifted towards the mother's abdomen to enable the posterior shoulder and arm to pass over the perineum. As the shoulders are born the head enters the pelvic brim and descends through the pelvis with the sagittal suture in the transverse diameter. The back must

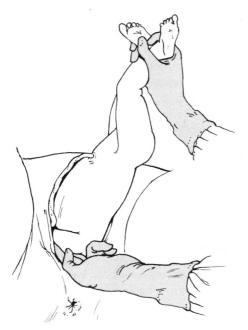

Fig. 26.49
Delivery of the posterior shoulder in a breech
presentation.

remain lateral until this has happened but will
afterwards be turned uppermost. If the back is
turned upwards too soon, the anteroposterior
diameter of the head will enter the anteroposterior diameter of the brim and may become
extended. The shoulders may then become
impacted at the outlet and the extended head
may cause difficulty.

Delivery of the head. When the back has
been turned the infant is allowed to hang from
the vulva without support. His weight brings
the head onto the pelvic floor on which the
occiput rotates forwards. The sagittal suture is
now in the anteroposterior diameter of the outlet. If rotation of the head fails to take place, two
fingers should be placed on the malar bones
and the head rotated. The baby can be allowed
to hang for 1 or 2 minutes. Gradually the neck
elongates, the hair-line appears and the suboccipital region can be felt. Controlled delivery
of the head is vital to avoid any sudden change
in intracranial pressure and subsequent cerebral
haemorrhage. There are three methods used.

Forceps delivery. Most breech deliveries are
performed by an obstetrician, who will apply

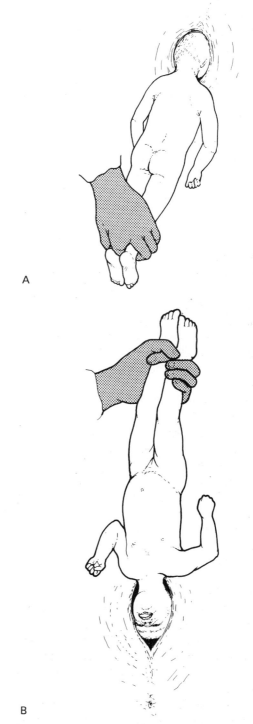

A

B

Fig. 26.50
Burns Marshall method of delivering the after-coming
head of a breech presentation. (A) Baby grasped by the
feet and held on the stretch. (B) Mouth and nose are free.
Vault of the head is delivered slowly.

forceps to the after-coming head to achieve a controlled delivery.

Burns Marshall method. The midwife or doctor stands facing away from the mother and, with the left hand, grasps the baby's ankles from behind with forefinger between the two (Fig. 26.50). The baby is kept on the stretch with sufficient traction to prevent his neck from bending backwards and being fractured. The suboccipital region, and not the neck, should pivot under the apex of the pubic arch or the spinal cord may be crushed. The feet are taken up through an arc of 180° until the mouth and nose are free at the vulva. The right hand may guard the perineum in order to prevent sudden escape of the head. An assistant may now clear the airway and the baby will breathe. The mother should be asked to take deliberate, regular breaths which allow the vault of the skull to escape gradually taking 2 or 3 minutes.

Mauriceau-Smellie-Veit manoeuvre (jaw flexion and shoulder traction — Fig. 26.51). This is mainly used when there is delay in descent of the head due to extension. Excessive shoulder traction may cause Erb's palsy.

The baby is laid astride the right arm with the palm supporting the chest. Two fingers are inserted well back into the mouth to pull the jaw downwards and flex the head. (If they can be accommodated, two fingers may be placed on the malar bones with the middle finger in the mouth.) Two fingers of the left hand are hooked over the shoulders with the middle finger pushing up the occiput to aid flexion. Traction is applied to draw the head out of the vagina and, when the suboccipital region appears, the body is lifted to assist the head to pivot around the symphysis pubis. The speed of delivery of the head must be controlled so that it does not emerge suddenly like a cork popping out of a bottle. Once the face is free the airways may be cleared and the vault is delivered slowly.

Alternative positions. When the woman has chosen to deliver in an alternative position, it is the upright or supported squat which is the most suitable. The delivery techniques described above will be adapted accordingly and the mid-wife will observe and encourage the spontaneous mechanism of delivery.

Use of oxytocics for third stage. These are withheld until the head is delivered.

Delivery of extended legs. The frank breech descends more rapidly during the first stage of labour. The cervix dilates more quickly and there is a risk of the cord becoming compressed between the legs and the body. Cord prolapse is less likely than in other breech presentations because the frank breech is a better-fitting presenting part. Delay may occur at the outlet because the legs splint the body and impede lateral flexion of the spine.

The baby can be born with his legs extended but assistance is usually required. When the popliteal fossae appear at the vulva, two fingers are placed along the length of one thigh with the finger tips in the fossa. The leg is swept to the side of the abdomen (abducting the hip) and the knee is flexed by the pressure on its under surface. As this movement is continued the lower part of the leg will emerge from the vagina (Fig. 26.52). This process should be repeated in order to deliver the second leg. The knee is a hinge joint which bends in one direction only. If the knee is pulled forwards from the abdomen, severe injury to the joint can result.

Delivery of extended arms. Extended arms are diagnosed when the elbows are not felt on the chest after the umbilicus is born. Prompt action must be taken to avoid delay and consequent hypoxia. This may be dealt with by using the Løvset manoeuvre (Fig. 26.54). This is a combination of rotation and downward traction which may be employed to deliver the arms whatever position they are in. The direction of rotation must always bring the back uppermost and the arms are delivered from under the pubic arch.

When the umbilicus is born and the shoulders are in the anteroposterior diameter, the baby is grasped by the iliac crests with the thumbs over the sacrum. Downward traction is applied until the axilla is visible.

Maintaining downward traction throughout, the body is rotated through half a circle, 180°,

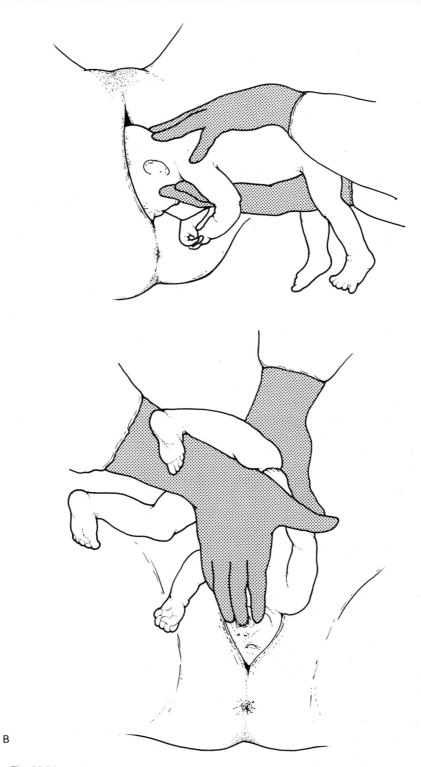

Fig. 26.51
Mauriceau-Smellie-Veit manoeuvre for delivering the after-coming head of breech presentation (see text). (A) Hands in position before the body is lifted. (B) Extraction of the head.

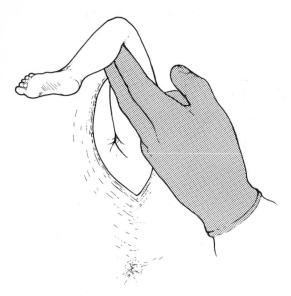

Fig. 26.52
Assisting delivery of extended leg by pressure on popliteal fossa.

starting by turning the back uppermost. The friction of the posterior arm against the pubic bone as the shoulder becomes anterior sweeps the arm in front of the face. The movement allows the shoulders to enter the pelvis in the transverse diameter.

The arm which is now anterior is delivered. The first two fingers of the hand which is on the same side as the baby's back are used to splint the humerus and draw it down over the chest as the elbow is flexed.

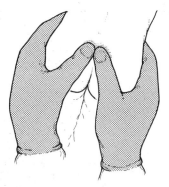

Fig. 26.53
Correct grasp for Løvset manoeuvre.

The body is now rotated back in the opposite direction and the second arm delivered in a similar fashion.

Delay in delivery of the head.
Extended head. If, when the body has been allowed to hang, the neck and hair-line are not visible, it is probable that the head is extended. This may be dealt with by the use of forceps or the Mauriceau-Smellie-Veit manoeuvre. If the head is trapped in an incompletely dilated cervix, an air channel can be created to enable the baby to breathe pending intervention. This is done by inserting two fingers or a Sim's speculum in front of the baby's face and holding the vaginal wall away from the nose. Moisture is mopped away.

Posterior rotation of the occiput. This malrotation of the head is rare and is usually the result of mismanagement, for the back should be turned upwards after the shoulders are born.

To deliver the head with the occiput posterior, the chin and face are permitted to escape under the symphysis pubis as far as the root of the nose and the baby is then lifted up towards the mother's abdomen to allow the occiput to sweep the perineum.

Complications of breech presentation

Apart from those difficulties already mentioned, other complications can arise, most of which affect the fetus. Many of these can be avoided by allowing only an experienced operator, or a closely supervised learner, to deliver the baby.

Impacted breech
Labour becomes obstructed when the fetus is disproportionately large for the size of the maternal pelvis.

Cord prolapse (see Ch. 27)
This is more common in a flexed or footling breech, as these have ill-fitting presenting parts.

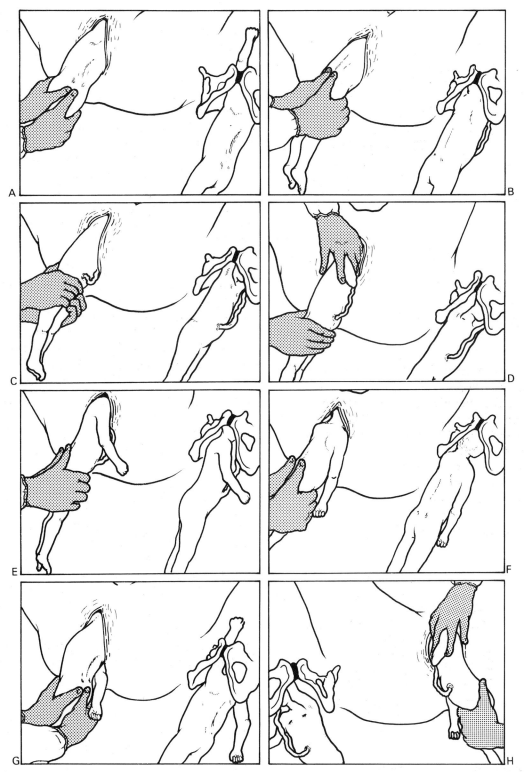

Fig. 26.54
Løvset manoeuvre for delivery of extended arms (see text).

Birth injury

If the delivery is performed correctly the following should not occur.

Fractures of humerus, clavicle or femur or dislocation of shoulder or hip caused during delivery of extended arms or legs.

Erb's palsy caused by the brachial plexus being damaged by twisting the neck.

Trauma to internal organs especially a ruptured liver or spleen produced by grasping the abdomen.

Damage to the adrenals by grasping the baby's abdomen, leading to shock caused by adrenaline release.

Spinal cord damage or fracture of the spine caused by bending the body backwards over the symphysis pubis while delivering the head.

Intracranial haemorrhage caused by rapid delivery of the head which has had no opportunity to mould. *Hypoxia* may also cause intracranial haemorrhage.

Soft tissue damage. Oedema and bruising of the baby's genitalia may be caused by pressure on the cervix. In a footling breech a prolapsed foot which lies in the vagina or at the vulva for a long time may become very oedematous and discoloured.

Fetal hypoxia

This may be due to cord prolapse or cord compression or to premature separation of the placenta.

Premature separation of the placenta

Considerable retraction of the uterus takes place while the head is still in the vagina and the placenta begins to separate. Excessive delay in delivery of the head may cause severe hypoxia in the fetus.

Maternal trauma

The maternal complications of a breech delivery are the same as found in other operative vaginal deliveries (see Ch. 28).

SHOULDER PRESENTATION

When the fetus lies with its long axis across the long axis of the uterus (transverse lie) the shoulder is most likely to present. Occasionally the lie is oblique but this does not persist as the uterine contractions during labour make it longitudinal or transverse.

Shoulder presentation occurs in 1:250 pregnancies near term and the majority are in multigravidae. The head lies on one side of the abdomen, with the breech at a slightly higher level on the other. The fetal back may be anterior or posterior (see Figs 26.55 & 26.56).

Causes

Maternal

Lax abdominal and uterine muscles. This is the most common cause and is found in multigravidae, particularly those of high parity.

Uterine abnormality. A bicornuate or subseptate uterus may result in a transverse lie as,

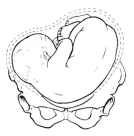

Fig. 26.55
Shoulder presentation, dorso-anterior.

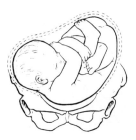

Fig. 26.56
Shoulder presentation, dorsoposterior.

more rarely, may a cervical or low uterine fibroid (see Ch. 24).

Contracted pelvis. Rarely this may prevent the head from entering the pelvic brim.

Fetal

Preterm pregnancy. The amount of amniotic fluid in relation to the fetus is greater, allowing the fetus more mobility than at term.

Multiple pregnancy. There is a possibility of polyhydramnios but the presence of more than one fetus reduces the room for manoeuvre when amounts of liquor are normal. It is the second twin which more commonly adopts this lie after delivery of the first fetus.

Polyhydramnios. The distended uterus is globular and the fetus can move freely in the excessive liquor.

Macerated fetus. Lack of muscle tone causes the fetus to slump down into the lower pole of the uterus.

Placenta praevia. This may prevent the head from entering the pelvic brim.

Diagnosis

Antenatal

On abdominal palpation. The uterus appears broad and the fundal height is less than expected for the period of gestation. On pelvic and fundal palpation neither head nor breech is felt. The mobile head is found on one side of the abdomen and the breech at a slightly higher level on the other.

Ultrasound may be used to confirm the lie and presentation.

Intrapartum

On abdominal palpation the findings are as above but when the membranes have ruptured the irregular outline of the uterus is more marked. If the uterus is contracting strongly and becomes moulded around the fetus, palpation is very difficult. The pelvis is no longer empty, the shoulder being wedged into it.

On vaginal examination. *This should not be performed without first excluding placenta praevia.* In early labour the presenting part may not be felt. The membranes usually rupture early because of the ill-fitting presenting part with a high risk of cord prolapse.

If the labour has been in progress for some time the shoulder may be felt as a soft irregular mass. It is sometimes possible to palpate the ribs, their characteristic grid-iron pattern being diagnostic. When the shoulder enters the pelvic brim an arm may prolapse; this should be differentiated from a leg. The hand is not at right angles to the arm, the fingers are longer than toes and of unequal length and the thumb can be opposed. No os calcis can be felt and the palm is shorter than the sole. If the arm is flexed, an elbow feels sharper than a knee.

Possible outcome

There is no mechanism for delivery of a shoulder presentation. If this persists in labour, delivery must be by caesarean section to avoid obstructed labour and subsequent uterine rupture (see Ch. 27).

Whenever the midwife detects a transverse lie she must obtain medical assistance.

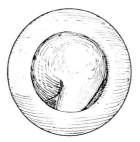
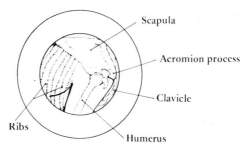

Fig. 26.57
Vaginal touch picture of shoulder presentation.

Management

Antenatal

A cause must be sought before deciding on a course of management. Ultrasound examination can detect placenta praevia or uterine abnormalities, whilst X-ray pelvimetry will demonstrate a contracted pelvis (see Ch. 24). Any of these causes requires elective caesarean section. Once they have been excluded, external version (see above) may be attempted. If this fails, or if the lie is again transverse at the next antenatal visit, the woman is admitted to hospital while further investigations into the cause are made. She frequently remains there until delivery because of the risk of cord prolapse if the membranes rupture.

Intrapartum

If a transverse lie is detected in early labour while the membranes are still intact, the doctor may attempt an external version followed, if this is successful, by a controlled rupture of the membranes. If the membranes have already ruptured spontaneously, a vaginal examination must be performed immediately to detect possible cord prolapse.

Immediate caesarean section must be performed:

- if the cord prolapses
- when the membranes are already ruptured
- when external version is unsuccessful
- when labour has already been in progress for some hours.

Complications

Prolapsed cord (see Ch. 27)

This may occur when the membranes rupture.

Prolapsed arm

This may occur when the membranes have ruptured and the shoulder has become impacted. Delivery should be by immediate caesarean section.

Neglected shoulder presentation

The shoulder becomes impacted having been forced down and wedged into the pelvic brim. The membranes have ruptured spontaneously and if the arm has prolapsed it becomes blue and oedematous. The uterus goes into a state of tonic contraction, the overstretched lower segment is tender to touch and the fetal heart may be absent. All the maternal signs of obstructed labour are present (see Ch. 25) and the outcome, if not treated in time, is a ruptured uterus and a stillbirth.

With adequate supervision both antenatally and during labour this should never occur.

Treatment. An immediate caesarean section is performed under general anaesthetic regardless of whether the fetus is alive or dead, as attempts at manipulative procedures or destructive operations can be dangerous for the mother, resulting in uterine rupture.

UNSTABLE LIE

The lie is defined as unstable when after 36 weeks' gestation, instead of remaining longitudinal, it varies from one examination to another between longitudinal and oblique or transverse.

Causes

Any condition in late pregnancy that increases the mobility of the fetus or prevents the head from entering the pelvic brim may cause this.

Maternal causes
Lax uterine muscles in multigravidae
Contracted pelvis.
Fetal causes
Polyhydramnios
Placenta praevia.

Management

Antenatal

The woman is admitted to the hospital at 37–38 weeks of pregnancy and remains there until she is delivered in order to avoid the unsupervised onset of labour with a transverse lie and to receive the essential expert supervision necessary prior to and throughout the labour. Ultrasonography is used to rule out placenta praevia.

Further attempts are made to correct the abnormal presentation by external version. If unsuccessful, caesarean section is considered.

Intrapartum

Many obstetricians induce labour after 38 weeks' gestation, having first ensured that the lie is longitudinal. This is usually performed by firstly commencing an intravenous infusion of Syntocinon to stimulate contractions. When these are established, a controlled rupture of the membranes is performed so that the head enters the pelvis. The midwife should ensure that the woman has an empty rectum and bladder before the procedure, as a loaded rectum or full bladder can prevent the presenting part from entering the pelvis.

She should palpate the abdomen at frequent intervals to ensure that the lie remains longitudinal and to assess the descent of the head. Labour is regarded as a trial (see Ch. 24) and the fetal heart is continuously monitored because of the risk of cord prolapse.

Complications

If labour commences with the lie other than longitudinal, the complications are the same as for a transverse lie.

COMPOUND PRESENTATION

When a hand, or occasionally a foot, lies alongside the head, the presentation is said to be compound. This tends to occur with a small fetus or roomy pelvis and seldom is difficulty encountered except in cases where it is associated with a flat pelvis. On rare occasions, head, hand and foot are felt in the vagina, a serious situation which usually occurs with a dead fetus.

If diagnosed during the first stage of labour, medical aid must be sought. If, during the second stage, the midwife sees a hand presenting alongside the vertex, she could try to hold the hand back, directing it over the face.

Reader Activities

- Evaluate the effectiveness of the different types of pain relief used by a woman in your care who feels her contractions mainly as backache.
- Compare the length of labour of a primigravida where the head is not engaged at the onset of labour with one where it is engaged.
- Ascertain the elective caesarean section rate for breech presentation in your maternity unit; does this demonstrate the existence of a definite policy on breech deliveries and, if so, is this policy the same for primigravidae and multigravidae?
- Examine, with your eyes closed, the heads of several newborn babies who have been delivered with a large caput succedaneum and/or marked moulding present. Practise defining the sutures and fontanelles you are feeling.
- Learn to differentiate by feeling, with your eyes shut, a baby's hand from his foot.
- Explain the management of a woman you have cared for with an unstable lie, with particular emphasis on the role of the midwife.

REFERENCE

Hofmeyr G J 1989 Breech presentation and abnormal lie in late pregnancy. In: Chalmers I, Enkin M, Keirse M J N C (eds) Effective care in pregnancy and childbirth, Oxford University Press, Oxford.

FURTHER READING

Lewis T L T, Chamberlain G V P (eds) 1990 Fetal malposition and malpresentation. In: Obstetrics by ten teachers, 15th edn. Edward Arnold, London, ch 5, p 182–201

Miller W F, Callander R 1989 Unstable lie. In: Miller W F, Callander R (eds) Obstetrics illustrated, 4th ed. Churchill Livingstone, Edinburgh, ch 10, p 239

Miller W F, Callander R 1989 Malposition and malpresentation In: Miller W F, Callander R (eds) Obstetrics illustrated, 4th edn. Churchill Livingstone, Edinburgh, ch 12, p 296–325

27

Obstetric emergencies

JOSEPHINE WILLIAMS

The immediate management of all the emergencies discussed in this chapter is reliant upon prompt action by the midwife; the speed of this action will often help determine the outcome for the mother and/or fetus. The chapter begins with discussion of presentation and prolapse of the cord, the predisposing factors to these emergencies and the immediate action and subsequent management required. It continues with the subject of vasa praevia and then covers the rare, but potentially catastrophic, condition of amniotic fluid embolism. Rupture of the uterus is the next emergency examined, a condition that, with good intrapartum care, should not occur. The chapter concludes with, what is for the midwife perhaps the most acute emergency covered in this chapter, shoulder dystocia.

PRESENTATION AND PROLAPSE OF THE CORD

Cord presentation
This occurs when the umbilical cord lies in front of the presenting part with the membranes still intact.

Cord prolapse (Fig. 27.1)
In this case the cord lies in front of the presenting part and the membranes are ruptured.

Occult cord prolapse. The cord lies alongside but not in front of the presenting part.

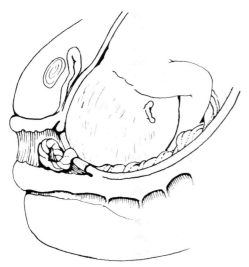

Fig. 27.1
Prolapsed cord.

Predisposing factors

These are the same for both cord presentation and cord prolapse. They include any condition in which the presenting part is not well applied to the lower uterine segment or well down in the pelvis. The space allows a loop of cord to slip down in front of the presenting part.

Multiparity
This is a contributory factor because the head may not be engaged when the membranes rupture and lax uterine and abdominal muscles make malpresentation more common.

High head
If the membranes rupture spontaneously when the fetal head is still high, the cord may prolapse. This is more common in multigravidae (see above). Artificial rupture of the membranes should not be performed when the head is high in order to avoid causing cord prolapse.

Prematurity
Cord prolapse is more common in preterm labours because there is more room between the small fetal head and the maternal pelvis and a loop of cord may prolapse.

Malpresentations
Breech presentation. Cord prolapse is more likely to occur with a complete or a footling breech than with a frank breech or a vertex presentation. Both of the former are ill-fitting presenting parts and in addition the umbilicus is nearer to the buttocks than to the head. The prognosis is fairly good, because the presenting part is soft and does not compress the cord as the head would.

Shoulder presentation or transverse lie. This, of all malpresentations, is the most likely to cause cord prolapse. It usually occurs when the membranes rupture spontaneously.

Face and brow presentations are less common causes of cord prolapse.

Polyhydramnios
The cord is liable to be swept down in a gush of liquor if the membranes rupture spontaneously; a controlled artificial rupture of the membranes is sometimes performed in order to prevent this happening.

Multiple pregnancy
Malpresentation is more common, particularly of the second twin (see Ch. 26), which makes cord prolapse more likely to occur when the membranes rupture.

Cord presentation

This is diagnosed on vaginal examination when the cord is felt behind the intact membranes. It is, however, rarely detected.

Management
Under no circumstances should the membranes be ruptured artificially, although spontaneous rupture may occur at any time. This is an acute emergency because of the risk to the fetus of hypoxia due to cord compression. Management is the same as for cord prolapse.

Cord prolapse

Diagnosis
Whenever there are factors present which predispose to cord prolapse, a vaginal examination should

be performed immediately following spontaneous rupture of the membranes in order to feel for the cord. An abnormal fetal heart rate, particularly bradycardia, may also indicate that the cord has prolapsed. Occasionally a loop of cord is visible at the vulva. It is more common to feel it during vaginal examination, either lying in the vagina or, if the presenting part is very high, lying in the os.

Immediate action

When a prolapsed cord is diagnosed the midwife should call for urgent assistance. At the same time she should reassure the woman and her partner by explaining what has happened and the emergency measures that will be needed. She will have assessed the amount of cervical dilatation, and identified the presenting part. She will feel whether the cord is pulsating but it should be handled as little as possible so as not to cause spasm of the cord vessels. An assistant should be asked to auscultate the fetal heart with a Sonicaid. If the cord is lying outside the vagina it should be gently replaced in it to keep it warm in order to prevent spasm of the vessels which results if the cord becomes cold or is subject to friction.

Pressure on the cord must be relieved. In order to do this, the midwife keeps her fingers in the vagina and holds the presenting part off the cord, especially during a contraction. The woman is positioned with her buttocks higher than her shoulders, causing the fetus to gravitate towards the diaphragm. This position may be achieved by elevating the foot of the bed or placing the woman in the knee-chest position (Fig. 27.2) or an exaggerated Sims position (Fig. 27.3). These measures must be continued until the fetus is delivered.

Management

The risks to the fetus are hypoxia and death as a result of cord compression. The risks are greatest in a cephalic presentation and least in a complete or footling breech. 10 minutes is the maximum time a fetus can be expected to survive cord occlusion but if pressure can be relieved the likelihood of survival is greatly increased. The speed with which treatment is initiated is vital. Once pressure on the cord is relieved, oxygen adminis-

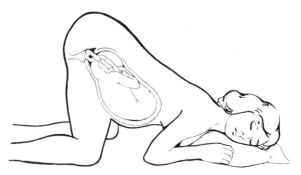

Fig. 27.2
Woman in the knee–chest position. Thighs must be straight. The fetus gravitates towards the fundus and pressure on the cord is relieved. This position is not useful during transportation.

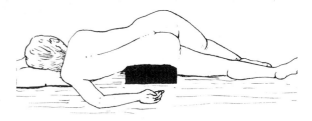

Fig. 27.3
Woman in the exaggerated Sims' position. Two large foam-rubber wedges or pillows elevate the buttocks further.

tered to the woman by face mask at 4 ℓ/min can reduce fetal hypoxia.

In the first stage of labour an immediate caesarean section is performed if the fetus is still alive.

In the second stage of labour, the lie is a deciding factor. If the lie is longitudinal, a forceps delivery or a breech extraction may be performed. If there is any possibility that a vaginal delivery may be difficult, a caesarean section should be performed. In the case of a multiparous woman, the midwife may encourage the mother to push and may expedite delivery by performing an episiotomy.

In the community. If the fetus is alive the woman should be transferred to hospital by ambulance immediately, while the midwife relieves pressure on the cord as described above. The knee–chest position is uncomfortable for the woman to maintain for any length of time; an exaggerated Sims' position is preferable. The consultant unit staff should be informed of the situation so that a caesarean section can be performed immediately on arrival at the hospital.

VASA PRAEVIA

This term is used when a fetal blood vessel lies over the os in front of the presenting part. This can only occur when a fetal vessel runs through the membranes between a velamentous insertion of the cord and the placenta and is positioned over the os. Vasa praevia may sometimes be palpated on vaginal examination when the membranes are still intact. If it is suspected, a speculum examination should be made.

Ruptured vasa praevia

When the membranes rupture in a case of vasa praevia, a fetal vessel may also rupture. This disaster leads to exsanguination of the fetus unless delivery follows within minutes.

Diagnosis
Slight fresh bleeding vaginally, particularly if it commences at the same time as rupture of the membranes, may be due to a ruptured vasa praevia. If, on monitoring the fetal heart rate, there are signs of fetal distress disproportionate to the amount of blood loss, this diagnosis should be considered. To determine whether the blood loss is fetal or maternal in origin, Singer's alkali-denaturation test may be performed but in practice there is rarely time.

Management
The midwife should summon a doctor urgently and continue to monitor the fetal heart. If the woman is in the second stage of labour, she is encouraged to push. In the first stage of labour, emergency caesarean section is performed if the fetus is alive. A paediatrician should be present for delivery. Cord blood is taken for haemoglobin estimation at birth. The baby will require a blood transfusion if he is fortunate enough to survive.

AMNIOTIC FLUID EMBOLISM

This rare, but potentially catastrophic, condition occurs when amniotic fluid is forced into the maternal circulation via the uterus or placental site forming an embolus which obstructs one of the pulmonary arterioles or alveolar capillaries.

Predisposing factors

Rapid or precipitate labour
This is considered to be the most common cause. The tumultuous contractions which occur in this type of labour force amniotic fluid into the maternal circulation through a break in the membranes or placenta. The forewaters may be intact but it may also occur when they have ruptured. Amniotic fluid embolism may also occur at caesarean section.

Multiparity
Amniotic fluid embolism rarely occurs in primigravidae, as tumultuous contractions are unlikely to occur except in multigravidae.

Overstimulation of the uterus
Excessive use of oxytocic drugs or prostaglandins may cause hypertonic uterine action (see Ch. 25).

Uterine trauma
Before the amniotic fluid can enter the maternal circulation there must be a laceration in the membranes. This can occur at caesarean section, in a ruptured uterus, during intra-uterine manipulation, such as internal podalic version, or during insertion of an intra-uterine catheter. It can also occur during manual removal of a retained placenta.

Diagnosis

This condition can only be diagnosed with certainty if amniotic fluid is detected in the maternal circulation. This is most commonly found in the lungs at postmortem examination, but occasionally may be discovered in blood aspirated from a central venous pressure catheter. Fetal squames have also been found in maternal sputum when stained with Nile blue.

Presenting signs and symptoms

Sudden onset of maternal respiratory distress. This often follows a rapid, tumultuous labour. The woman becomes severely dyspnoeic and cyanosed, and pulmonary oedema may be present. A chest X-ray may show widespread opacities.

Cardiovascular collapse. The woman will exhibit tachycardia and profound hypotension which bear no relation to the amount of blood lost. An electrocardiograph may show right-sided heart failure which may be followed by cardiac arrest.

Convulsions. These occur in a few women and may precede the onset of respiratory symptoms.

Haemorrhage. This is usually the result of disseminated intravascular coagulation which is a complication of amniotic fluid embolism. It may sometimes be the presenting symptom.

Emergency action

Any one of the above symptoms is indicative of an acute emergency. The mother is likely to be in a state of collapse and the doctor should immediately be summoned. This is also a frightening situation for the woman's partner. While she is dealing with the emergency, the midwife should try to explain what is happening and the procedures being undertaken. It may be expedient for him to leave the room but he should not be left unsupported. If the fetus is undelivered, steps will be taken to expedite delivery as soon as the mother's condition allows.

Treatment of respiratory distress or cardiovascular collapse

Oxygen is administered by face mask at 4 ℓ/min. Suction apparatus and resuscitation equipment should be to hand for use in case of cardiac arrest. If the woman is undelivered, the fetal heart rate should be monitored continuously.

Treatment of haemorrhage (see Ch. 29)

In the case of amniotic fluid embolism this occurs after placental separation and is often severe. The midwife should be prepared for the onset of postpartum haemorrhage which may ensue within an hour if the woman survives the initial collapse. Emergency treatment is as for any postpartum haemorrhage but infusion of clotting factors will be needed in an attempt to counteract disseminated intravascular coagulation (see below).

Complications

The mortality rate of this condition is very high and has been stated to be as great as 86%, with 25% of deaths occurring in the first hour.

Cardiopulmonary collapse

Severe hypoxia, frequently followed by cardiac arrest, is usually the first complication to occur.

Treatment. Oxygen is administered by face mask and if necessary the cardiac arrest team summoned. Once initial resuscitation has been successful, the woman may need to be transferred to an intensive care unit for artificial ventilation until her condition improves. Intravenous aminophylline may be administered to relieve bronchial spasm and hydrocortisone to counteract the effects of the amniotic fluid on the lung tissue.

Disseminated intravascular coagulation (see Ch. 21)

This invariably accompanies amniotic fluid embolism and is caused by the presence of amniotic fluid, which is rich in thromboplastin, in the maternal circulation. In women who survive the initial collapse, consumptive coagulopathy usually develops, which aggravates the situation. The treatment is dealt with fully in Chapter 21.

Acute renal failure

This is a complication of the excessive blood loss and prolonged hypovolaemic hypotension. The possibility of it occurring should be remembered and the midwife must keep accurate records of fluid intake, urinary output and urinalysis. Continuous urinary drainage and accurate measurements are maintained until the acute stage of this condition is past. A urinary output of less than 30 ml an hour should be reported, as should the presence of proteinuria.

Treatment. Renal dialysis may be required if the kidneys fail to respond to the stimulation of diuretic drugs such as mannitol.

RUPTURE OF THE UTERUS

This is one of the most serious complications met in obstetrics; it is often fatal for the fetus and may be so for the mother. With good antenatal and intrapartum care it should be avoided but is still not uncommon in developing countries.

Causes

Weak uterine scar

This is usually a caesarean section scar (Fig. 27.4) but may, less commonly, be due to a previous hysterotomy or other uterine surgery. Classical caesarean section scars are much more likely to rupture than those in the lower uterine segment. Factors which predispose to rupture of the scar are:

- impaired healing of the scar
- interpregnancy interval of less than 6 months
- overdistension of the uterus as with subsequent multiple pregnancy or polyhydramnios
- obstructed labour
- incorrect use of oxytocin
- trauma during manipulations.

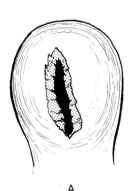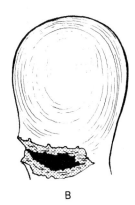

A   B

Fig. 27.4
(A) Rupture through a classical caesarean section scar.
(B) Transverse rupture of lower segment.

Obstructed labour (see Ch. 25)

The uterus ruptures because of excessive thinning of the lower uterine segment. The factors predisposing to rupture from this cause are:

Multiparity. The reaction of the multigravid uterus to obstruction is to contract more strongly in an effort to overcome the obstruction (see Ch. 25). This causes the lower segment to become progressively thinner until rupture occurs, usually at the junction of the upper and lower uterine segments. Women of high parity are particularly at risk.

Overstimulation of the uterus with oxytocics in the presence of undiagnosed cephalopelvic disproportion or malpresentation.

Cervical dystocia (see Ch. 25).

Incorrect use of oxytocic drugs
(see also Ch. 25)

Excessive or injudicious use of oxytocic drugs can cause hypertonic uterine action resulting in uterine rupture. Factors which predispose to rupture in these circumstances are:

Disproportion. In the presence of cephalopelvic disproportion, the use of drugs which stimulate uterine contractions may cause the uterus to rupture.

Obstructed labour (see above).

Multiparity. The multigravid uterus is more sensitive to oxytocin and hypertonic contractions are more easily stimulated.

Rupture during manipulation

If internal podalic version is carried out in an attempt to correct a shoulder presentation, or to correct the lie of a second twin, it may result in rupture of an already scarred uterus or one with an excessively thin lower segment, especially if the membranes were not intact immediately prior to the procedure. The chances of this happening are greater in the presence of the following factors:

Uterine scar which may rupture during the manipulation.

Obstructed labour which leads to the lower segment becoming very thin and overdistended; it is likely to rupture during any intra-uterine manipulation.

Extension of a cervical laceration

A severe cervical laceration may extend upwards

into the lower uterine segment. Although this more commonly occurs as a result of forceps being applied before full dilatation of the cervix, it may also be caused by the mother pushing the baby out through an incompletely dilated cervix.

Uterine rupture during the antenatal period

Rupture of the uterus prior to labour is a rare event. It invariably involves rupture of a caesarean section scar (usually a classical scar) and occurs in the last 4 weeks of pregnancy.

Signs and symptoms

This type of rupture is insidious in onset and is sometimes referred to as a *silent rupture*. The woman complains of intermittent right-sided abdominal pain for several days; it is not always severe and is due to the peritoneal irritation caused by bleeding from the uterine scar. As this progresses the abdominal tenderness increases and the woman may eventually become shocked. Intrauterine death is common.

Diagnosis

This is difficult but should be suspected when a woman known to have a uterine scar presents with the above symptoms. The diagnosis may only be confirmed at laparotomy.

Treatment

A hysterectomy is sometimes necessary although it may be possible to repair the scar. If the woman wishes to have another baby, she should be advised not to become pregnant for at least a year in order to allow the scar to heal completely. Any future pregnancies should be carefully monitored and the woman admitted to hospital for rest from 36 weeks' gestation. Delivery should be by caesarean section.

Intrapartum rupture of a caesarean section scar

Signs and symptoms

Abdominal pain. The woman may complain of severe, constant lower abdominal pain, which worsens during contractions. This may be accompanied by vomiting and she may also complain of tenderness suprapubically.

Pulse rate. This begins to rise but shock associated with this condition tends to increase slowly.

Blood loss. There may be some fresh blood loss but this is only slight and may be mistaken for a 'show'.

Progress in labour. Contractions may continue but the cervix fails to dilate during the first stage and the fetus fails to advance significantly in the second stage.

Fetal heart rate abnormalities. Signs of fetal distress, such as fetal tachycardia or fetal heart rate decelerations, are frequently present.

Cessation of contractions. Occasionally the scar ruptures at the height of a strong contraction, whereupon the contractions cease and the woman rapidly becomes shocked.

If labour is being conducted under epidural analgesia the earlier warning signs of abdominal pain and tenderness may be missed and for this reason some authorities believe that the presence of a uterine scar is a contra-indication to epidural analgesia.

Diagnosis

As the signs of impending rupture are sometimes masked by labour itself or by epidural analgesia, extreme vigilance is required by the midwife caring for a woman with a uterine scar. Such a woman should be cared for in a consultant obstetric unit and her labour managed as a trial of labour (see Ch. 24). A history of classical caesarean section, although now uncommon, is often considered to be an indication for an elective caesarean section because of the high risk of the uterine scar rupturing in labour.

Treatment

An immediate caesarean section is performed in the hope of delivering a live baby. Following delivery of the fetus and placenta the extent of the rupture can be assessed and either the scar is resutured or, if the tear is too extensive and difficult to repair, a hysterectomy is performed. The woman is likely to be shocked and a blood transfusion is usually necessary.

Uterine rupture following obstructed labour

The midwife should be able to detect the signs of obstructed labour (see Ch. 25) and seek medical assistance before uterine rupture occurs.

Warning signs and symptoms

All the signs of obstructed labour are present such as a rising pulse rate and tonic contractions and Bandl's retraction ring may be seen abdominally.

Signs of actual rupture

Severe, constant abdominal pain.

Vaginal blood loss. This is not always present.

Severe fetal distress. This may rapidly lead to fetal death if delivery by caesarean section is not effected quickly.

Irregular uterine outline and palpation of fetal parts. If the rupture is extensive the fetus may be expelled into the peritoneal cavity, and fetal parts may be easily felt through the abdominal wall.

Maternal shock. The rate of onset of shock depends on the extent of the rupture and the attendant blood loss. Onset may be slow and develop progressively or the woman may rapidly become profoundly shocked.

Treatment

Medical aid is summoned. Intravenous fluid replacement therapy is given urgently. A blood transfusion is usually necessary.

The fetal heartbeat, if still present, is continuously monitored, and the woman is prepared for immediate caesarean section. This situation is an acute emergency but the midwife must endeavour to keep the woman, if conscious, and her partner fully informed of what is happening. Following delivery of the fetus and placenta the uterine rupture is repaired if not too extensive; otherwise a hysterectomy is performed.

Incomplete rupture

In this condition the endometrium and myometrium are ruptured, and the perimetrium remains intact. This type of rupture may be discovered at caesarean section (when it is usually of a previous uterine scar) or it may occur at the end of the second stage and the baby may be delivered vaginally.

Signs and symptoms following vaginal delivery

Whenever shock during the third stage is more severe than the type of delivery or the blood loss warrants or if the woman does not respond to the treatment given, the possibility of incomplete uterine rupture should be considered.

Treatment

This is the same as for complete rupture.

SHOULDER DYSTOCIA

Pre-disposing factors

- Large baby
- Failure of the shoulders to rotate into the anteroposterior diameter of the outlet following delivery of the head.

Prevention

When delivering a fetus presenting by the vertex, the midwife must wait for the shoulders to rotate into the anteroposterior diameter of the pelvic outlet before attempting to deliver them. This rotation accompanies the external rotation of the head which occurs after restitution (see Ch. 14).

Recognition

Failure of the head to advance with crowning, a head which is large in size and difficulty in delivering the face and chin are warning signs of possible shoulder dystocia.

Management

When attempting to deliver the fetus in cases of shoulder dystocia, care must be taken not to twist the neck and as far as is possible excessive traction on the head should be avoided because of the risk to the fetus of damage to the brachial plexus.

If the shoulders are in the anteroposterior diameter of the outlet, attempt first to deliver them in the normal way. If this fails, ensure that a hand is not alongside the head posteriorly, as this can prevent delivery of the anterior shoulder.

If this is found, the posterior shoulder and hand are eased out first by using traction towards the mother's abdomen. The anterior shoulder can then be delivered easily.

Position of the mother. A position should be chosen which allows space for manoeuvring the baby towards the mother's sacrum. If she is on a bed turn the mother into the left lateral position with her buttocks at the edge of the bed. If the lithotomy position is used, the buttocks should be slightly beyond the end of the bed. In many cases a change in position is the only treatment required.

Medical aid. As soon as difficulty is experienced, the obstetric registrar and a paediatrician should be called.

Episiotomy. Unless an episiotomy has already been made, one should be performed in order to enlarge the outlet and reduce pressure from the pelvic floor. An existing episiotomy may need to be enlarged.

If the shoulders fail to rotate into the antero-posterior diameter of the outlet, the midwife should attempt to correct the position by hooking two fingers into the anterior axilla and rotating the shoulder forwards under the pubic arch. Traction should not be applied. If the anterior shoulder is caught above the pelvic brim, an assistant should try to push the shoulder behind the pubic bone by applying suprapubic pressure.

Delivery of the posterior shoulder first. If suprapubic pressure fails to enable delivery of the anterior shoulder, the posterior shoulder may be delivered first by drawing the head in an upward curving direction, while the assistant continues to apply suprapubic pressure on the anterior shoulder. Four fingers are inserted behind the posterior shoulder and an attempt made to rotate it into the hollow of the sacrum. Further traction can be applied by placing the fingers in the axilla of the posterior arm. If the posterior shoulder is successfully delivered, the anterior shoulder should follow.

Rotation of the shoulders. If the attempted delivery of the posterior shoulder fails, it may be possible to pass a hand along the back of the fetus and to try and rotate the shoulders 180°, thus making the posterior shoulder anterior. As the posterior shoulder is lower than the anterior, this manoeuvre brings it out from under the pubic arch.

Delivery of the posterior arm. This is the last resort, other than cleidotomy, and is a very difficult manoeuvre. The whole hand is inserted into the hollow of the sacrum, two fingers splint the humerus of the posterior arm, flex the elbow, sweep the forearm over the chest and bring the hand out. If, after delivering the arms, difficulty is still experienced, the midwife should suspected abdominal ascites or a tumour.

Reader Activities

- Working with a colleague, practise placing her in the knee–chest and exaggerated Sims' positions.
- Working on the supposition that you have diagnosed a cord prolapse on vaginal examination, work out a plan of action to cover the period from when you first feel the cord until the baby is delivered.
- Devise an intrapartum care plan for a woman who has had a previous caesarean section for placenta praevia.
- Ascertain the policy in your maternity unit, and the reasons for it, on the use of epidural anaesthesia in labour for women who have had a previous caesarean section.
- Ensure that you are aware of the arrangements in your maternity unit for obtaining assistance rapidly for a case of shoulder dystocia.

FURTHER READING

Hibbard B M 1988 Amniotic fluid embolism. In: Principles of obstetrics, Butterworth, London, ch 39, p 698–699

Hickman M A 1985 Presentation and prolapse of the umbilical cord. In: Midwifery, 2nd edn. Blackwell Scientific, Oxford, p 281–284

Kadar N 1985 Shoulder dystocia. In: Studd J (ed) The management of labour. Blackwell Scientific, Oxford p 281–282

Letsky E 1989 Amniotic fluid embolism. In: de Swiet M (ed) Medical disorders in obstetric practice, 2nd edition. Blackwell Scientific, Oxford, ch 3, p 127–128

Llewellyn-Jones D 1990 Rupture of the uterus. In: Fundamentals of obstetrics and gynaecology. Vol 1 Obstetrics, 5th edn. Faber & Faber, London, p 364–366

Morgan M 1979 Amniotic fluid embolism. Anaesthesia 34: 20–32

28

Obstetric anaesthesia and operations

RUTH BEVIS

Complications may arise in any labour. The aim of this chapter is to give a concise, factual overview of obstetric and anaesthetic interventions, to help the midwife become a knowledgeable, competent member of the team in an emergency.

OBSTETRIC ANAESTHESIA

Some definitions

It is important to distinguish between anaesthesia and analgesia. These terms are defined as follows:

>*Anaesthesia* means absence of sensation and therefore implies freedom from pain.
>*Analgesia* means freedom from pain.

Anaesthesia may be described under the headings of:

>*General anaesthesia* when a state of unconsciousness is induced, but which may also involve giving some analgesia.
>*Regional anaesthesia* when a group of nerves is anaesthetised, so giving an area of anaesthesia.
>*Local anaesthesia* when a small specific area is anaesthetised.

Anaesthesia will now be discussed under these general headings.

GENERAL ANAESTHESIA IN OBSTETRICS

General anaesthesia for the woman in the second and third trimesters of pregnancy, or who is newly delivered, is fraught with risks and is dangerous in unskilled hands. Factors connected with general anaesthesia have been a significant cause of maternal deaths in otherwise healthy women until very recently. In the triennium 1985–87, one in twelve maternal deaths in the United Kingdom was due to a direct anaesthetic factor or had some anaesthetic contribution (DH 1991).

It is essential for the midwife to be aware of these risks and why they occur, so that she may give intelligent help to the anaesthetist if required.

Problems in obstetric anaesthesia

The problems which arise in obstetric anaesthesia are due to:

- the effects of progesterone on the mother
- the pressure from the gravid uterus
- the presence of two patients rather than one.

Mendelson's syndrome

The effects of progesterone on the gastro-intestinal tract lead to delayed emptying of the stomach at term, particularly in the woman in labour. Narcotic analgesics such as pethidine given in labour will further delay gastric emptying. Because the stomach contents do not move on quickly they tend to be strongly acid in reaction. Pressure from the gravid uterus at term readily causes reflux of these acid stomach contents, especially when the woman lies recumbent. When general anaesthesia is induced, *silent regurgitation* may easily occur unnoticed and if acid stomach contents are then aspirated into the lungs, a condition known as Mendelson's syndrome results. Acid aspiration causes a chemical pneumonitis, damaging the alveoli so that gaseous exchange is impaired; if this is severe it is impossible to oxygenate the woman adequately and death may result.

Prevention

Antacid therapy. In order to try to prevent this condition occurring, women in labour are usually given antacid therapy. Certainly any woman who is about to undergo general anaesthesia will be given an oral antacid preparation such as sodium citrate. In order to inhibit the production of further hydrochloric acid most anaesthetists now give ranitidine or cimetidine prior to general anaesthesia.

'Crash induction'. This is a rather colloquial term used to describe the sequence of events occurring when giving general anaesthesia to an unprepared patient, for example the victim of a road traffic accident whose surgery cannot be delayed. Because even the prepared obstetric patient is liable to have acid stomach contents present, the

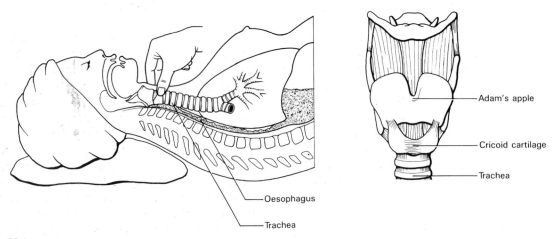

Fig. 28.1
Cricoid pressure, showing occlusion of the oesophagus by pressure applied to the cricoid cartilage.

same technique is employed. 'Crash induction' always includes endotracheal intubation with the use of cricoid pressure. A cuffed tracheal tube protects the lungs; even if silent regurgitation occurs, the acid contents cannot be aspirated past the cuff into the lungs.

Cricoid pressure is a technique which utilises the one complete ring of tracheal cartilage, the cricoid cartilage, to occlude the oesophagus, so preventing acid reflux. The anaesthetist will require his assistant to maintain cricoid pressure until the tracheal tube is in position and he has been able to check that the seal provided by the cuff is effective. The correct application of cricoid pressure is essential, and may prevent a mother's death.

Failed intubation

Almost every pregnant woman at term is likely to have some degree of oedema, including laryngeal oedema. The anaesthetist may have difficulty in visualising the vocal cords and introducing the tracheal tube. Incorrect application of cricoid pressure may compound the problem. Because the woman has been given a muscle relaxant in order to intubate the trachea, she cannot be oxygenated while attempts to intubate continue. Her oxygen needs are increased by the presence of the fetus, so that prolonged attempts to intubate may prove fatal to both.

Prevention

It is now common practice to 'pre-oxygenate' every pregnant woman prior to induction of anaesthesia. This procedure prolongs significantly the period of time which the anaesthetist may spend attempting to intubate her without cyanosis ensuing. Pre-oxygenation involves giving oxygen by face mask for an uninterrupted period, usually about 4 minutes. Some women, already stressed by the thought of an emergency caesarean section, find this procedure difficult to tolerate, as they may feel stifled by the mask, but calm careful explanation will help to allay their fears and many anaesthetists will allow the woman to hold the mask herself.

Pre-oxygenation also causes stress in the obstetrician, particularly if there is severe fetal distress,

and delivery is an urgent procedure. It may feel like an unnecessary waste of time.

Correct application of cricoid pressure is essential and the midwife should not be afraid to ask the anaesthetist for help if she is asked to assist him in this way but feels uncertain of her ability to perform the technique.

It is usual to have a *failed intubation drill*. Various factors will influence the anaesthetist's decision. If he is able to maintain a clear airway he may proceed using a face mask and Guedel airway with his assistant maintaining cricoid pressure throughout the anaesthetic. Spinal anaesthesia is another possibility. Epidural anaesthesia is not considered to be an option in this situation since if the stressed anaesthetist were unfortunate enough to perform an inadvertent *total spinal* he would need to intubate the trachea in order to prevent maternal death (see below). The midwife working in the operating theatre must understand clearly the failed intubation drill and the rationale behind it. Failed intubation is an emergency situation demanding prompt, appropriate action; most maternal deaths due directly to anaesthesia are caused by a misplaced tracheal tube (DH 1991).

Aortocaval occlusion

This is sometimes referred to as *supine hypotensive syndrome* but this can be misleading, since a fall in blood pressure may be a later sign of the problem and is often preceded by compromise of placental perfusion.

The problem is caused by the weight of the gravid uterus partially occluding the vena cava. Venous return is then reduced, followed by a fall in cardiac output. This sequence of events is not only associated with general anaesthesia but may occur at any time in late pregnancy or during labour. It will always occur if the woman lies supine in late pregnancy. Fortunately most women at term do not find it comfortable to lie flat but the midwife must take steps to ensure that the woman in labour does not do so. If emergency caesarean section is being performed because of fetal distress, aortocaval occlusion will increase the fetal distress and cause further fetal hypoxia.

Prevention

Whenever the woman in labour needs to lie flat the midwife should ensure that she is tilted laterally, either by means of a small rubber wedge under the mattress or by placing a folded blanket under the buttocks. It is usual to tilt the woman to the left and an angle of 15° is sufficient. Modern delivery beds and chairs have this facility, as does every operating table. The ideal means of prevention is to encourage the woman in labour to be upright as much as possible.

Maternal awareness

Most of the drugs given to the mother during general anaesthesia (except the muscle relaxants) will cross the placental barrier and affect the fetus, if only for a short time. In order to prevent a sleepy baby being delivered the anaesthetist will give the mother as light an anaesthetic as possible. The woman's level of consciousness may sometimes become sufficiently light for her to recall events which occurred during the operation but because she is paralysed, in order to allow the light level of anaesthesia, she is unable to give any indication of this. (With this light level of anaesthesia the obstetrician would experience difficulty with access to the abdominal cavity without muscle relaxation, and tracheal intubation is better tolerated.) Many women who have suffered awareness have not recalled pain but have recounted accurate details of conversations held in the operating theatre. This is a terrifying experience for the woman, who may well have opted for general rather than epidural anaesthesia because she wanted to know nothing of what was happening. The anaesthetist will make every effort to prevent awareness in the mother, but it does still occur occasionally.

Prevention

The likelihood of maternal awareness has been reduced significantly by giving the woman an opiate by intravenous injection as soon as the baby is delivered. The anaesthetist can also increase the amount of nitrous oxide given at this stage, as the woman's oxygen requirements are reduced when the baby is born. This will not prevent awareness prior to delivery.

The well-being of the fetus is of vital importance during caesarean section and the anaesthetist has to remember this as he treats the mother. In summary, the most important points are prevention of maternal and therefore fetal hypoxia, prevention of Mendelson's syndrome and aortocaval occlusion and avoidance of too deep a level of anaesthesia in the mother.

REGIONAL ANAESTHESIA

Epidural block

Epidural analgesia may be described as lumbar or caudal, depending on the site used when approaching the epidural space.

The epidural space is situated around the dura mater and contains blood vessels and fatty tissue, as well as the spinal nerves which pass through it. Because of the generalised venous engorgement which occurs in pregnancy, the space tends to be rather smaller in the pregnant woman than it is in other adults and during a uterine contraction, when the veins become more engorged, the space is even further reduced. The aim of the anaesthetist performing epidural anaesthesia is to introduce local anaesthetic solution into the epidural space so that it will surround the fibres of specific spinal nerves and anaesthetise them so achieving a selective block.

Lumbar epidural block

This is the commonest type of approach and there are different techniques which may be used. The anaesthetic is introduced between lumbar vertebrae 3 and 4 or 2 and 3.

A *single shot epidural* is one where the local anaesthetic is introduced using a Tuohy needle, but no catheter is inserted for 'top up' purposes.

A *continuous technique* is one where a fine polyethylene or nylon catheter is inserted into the epidural space so that further doses of local anaesthetic may be given when required. It may be more appropriate to call this an intermittent technique, since some anaesthetists favour a truly continuous technique, where a very dilute solution of local anaesthetic is infused via the epidural catheter using an intravenous infusion line attached to an electronic drip counter. The advantage of this is that inadvertent introduction of the local anaesthetic solution into the subarachnoid space is likely to have less sudden or dramatic results. (Complications of epidural block are discussed in more detail below.)

Caudal epidural block

This technique is not popular in obstetric practice in the UK. It is less easy to secure an epidural catheter safely and comfortably. A large amount of local anaesthetic solution is required in order to give effective analgesia and it is not easy to obtain a predictable, selective block. The woman may be required to lie in the knee–chest position during the procedure itself, which is uncomfortable and impractical for a woman in labour. The epidural needle is introduced between the sacral vertebrae and the coccyx, through the sacral hiatus. The complications which may be seen are similar to those in lumbar epidural block but because higher doses of local anaesthetic solution are required, toxicity is more likely.

Indications for epidural analgesia

Maternal request is probably the commonest indication for epidural analgesia. Many consultant obstetric units in the UK are now able to offer an epidural service to all or most mothers who wish to have this form of pain relief. Safety must always be the first consideration and if there are not sufficient anaesthetists for an experienced person to be readily available to the obstetric unit the epidural service will be restricted.

Although epidural analgesia is never performed without the mother's consent and it is unwise to persuade a reluctant subject, there are certain medical and obstetric conditions where an epidural block may be advised.

Malposition. For the woman with an occipitoposterior position where a long, exhausting labour is anticipated, an epidural block may be the ideal form of analgesia, although it may not be possible to relieve the severe backache completely.

Malpresentation. Epidural analgesia is helpful for the woman with any form of malpresentation. It is particularly valuable in a breech presentation when the obstetrician requires a well-relaxed mother if he has to perform an assisted breech delivery. Because she will usually be completely free of pain, this is also ideal from the mother's point of view. When an assisted breech delivery is anticipated, the epidural is 'topped up' so that anaesthesia is more profound than for a normal vaginal delivery. An effective epidural block may also be augmented sufficiently to perform caesarean section, if required, without undue delay.

Multiple pregnancy. An epidural block is advantageous for the woman with a twin pregnancy because of the possibility of manipulative delivery.

Pregnancy-induced hypertension. Epidural analgesia is *not* advised in this instance for the hypotensive side-effect. However, pain and tension will tend to exacerbate the hypertension and effective analgesia is an important part of the woman's treatment.

Effective analgesia. The woman who is not obtaining adequate pain relief from other analgesic methods, and who is tense and distressed, may need gentle guidance and the suggestion of an epidural block.

Contra-indications

The main contra-indications to epidural analgesia are usually cited as maternal reluctance, bleeding disorders, any infection near the site of the epidural, or any systemic infection. Existing central nervous system disease such as multiple sclerosis is usually regarded as a relative contra-indication. This is not because it has any known adverse effect on the disease, but because any exacerbation suffered by the woman may cause her to regret her decision. Abnormalities of the spine may make it very difficult for the anaesthetist to perform the epidural block, and it may not be fully effective.

Complications

Hypotension. Local anaesthetic solution blocks transmission of nervous impulses along motor and sensory nerves and also has an effect on the sympathetic nervous system. The vasodilation resulting from this will lead to a fall in blood pressure unless this is prevented by giving a rapid infusion of intravenous fluid prior to establishing the block. This rapid infusion is commonly known as a *pre-load*; it is common to give between 500 and 1000 ml of Hartmann's solution. A functioning intravenous infusion is essential before epidural analgesia can be commenced in order to prevent hypotension.

Dural tap. If the anaesthetist inadvertently punctures the dura mater this is known as a *dural tap*. It is usually recognised when a few drops of cerebrospinal fluid (CSF) leak through the Tuohy needle. It is essential that this problem is recognised promptly.

The anaesthetist will normally resite the epidural catheter in an adjacent space. The obstetrician is informed and a forceps delivery will be planned in order to prevent the woman from pushing and possibly forcing more CSF through the dural puncture. A reduction in volume of CSF usually results in a headache which is often severe and distressing. Another measure designed to minimise leakage of CSF is to leave the epidural catheter in position and infuse normal saline through it with the help of an infusion pump. This is normally continued for 24 hours and it is usual to keep the woman lying flat.

A headache resulting from a dural tap will resolve spontaneously within a week but will be incapacitating. Lying flat will give considerable relief, but this does not help the woman to enjoy her baby and the headache may be a lasting memory in place of what should have been a normal experience. The anaesthetist may therefore decide to perform a 'blood patch'. This involves taking between 10 and 20 ml of venous blood from the woman's antecubital vein, under strict asepsis, and introducing it into the epidural space via the intervertebral space nearest the dural puncture. Two anaesthetists will normally perform this procedure together. This treatment often has dramatic results, and the headache is cured almost immediately. The woman is asked to rest quietly for an hour or two, to avoid disturbing the blood clot which has sealed the dural puncture. Some anaesthetists will not carry out this procedure immediately, as there is some risk of infection. The success rate is reported to be approximately 90%

on the first occasion and 98% if the procedure has to be repeated.

Total spinal block. This is a rare complication but is seen if a dural puncture is not recognised and the anaesthetist proceeds to inject the local anaesthetic solution. The result will be a profound and rapid motor and sensory block with a dramatic fall in blood pressure. The mother collapses and cardiac arrest often follows. Immediate resuscitation is essential and ventilatory support is required. If maternal hypoxia can be prevented and normal blood pressure restored quickly, the baby may later be delivered unscathed.

Very occasionally this effect may be seen following a later *top-up* and not during the initial stages of the epidural analgesia. The reasons for this are largely unclear but in some cases the epidural catheter is thought to have 'migrated'. The midwife who tops up an epidural must therefore be vigilant and must be aware of the possible complications, their detection and immediate treatment.

Bloody tap. If the anaesthetist punctures one of the epidural veins, blood is seen in the epidural cannula or in the catheter and this is known as a *bloody tap*. The epidural catheter is resited in order to prevent intravenous injection of local anaesthetic solution. If local anaesthetic solution does enter the circulation, toxicity may result. The woman may complain of tingling or numbness of the mouth and tongue and of dizziness; her speech may become slurred and finally she may have a convulsion.

Patchy block. An epidural block may sometimes be more effective on one side of the body or it may be completely unilateral, for no obvious reason. Sometimes it may be impossible to provide analgesia for one particular area. The anaesthetist should always be informed if this occurs since adjustment of the epidural catheter may be effective.

Disadvantages

During labour the woman may find the loss of sensation and motor function in her legs unpleasant.

She will not be aware if her bladder becomes full and may find it difficult or impossible to pass urine, although this is common in any labour.

Even if the epidural is managed well, there is an increased likelihood of a forceps delivery being necessary due to lack of an urge to push.

The aim is to achieve a spontaneous delivery whenever possible, in the interests of reducing complications for both mother and baby and to give the mother the satisfaction she will enjoy following a normal delivery. Since time constraints on the duration of the second stage have been removed, the woman is not encouraged to bear down until she feels the urge to do so or until the presenting part distends the perineum. This makes normal delivery more likely. It is probable that maintaining an adequate level of analgesia (without profound motor block) rather than withholding top-ups during the second stage is more likely to allow the woman a normal delivery.

Certain symptoms which occur in the postnatal period may be attributed to the epidural block. These include:

- impaired bladder function
- marked perineal pain
- backache which may be due in part to local bruising where the Tuohy needle was introduced, especially if the anaesthetist had difficulty locating the epidural space.

Drugs used in epidural analgesia

Local anaesthetics

Bupivacaine (Marcain). The local anaesthetic drug most commonly used in the UK is bupivacaine (Marcain). It is marketed in strengths of 0.25% and 0.5% and these concentrations are modified in practice as required by dilution with normal saline. (0.75% bupivacaine is also available but is banned from use in obstetrics in the UK.)

Bupivacaine is effective within 10–20 minutes of administration and the effect lasts for about 2 hours during labour. The total dose given is therefore not excessive, unless labour is unduly prolonged, and toxicity is not common. The drug does cross the placenta but there are no gross effects on the fetus.

Bupivacaine is available with added adrenaline and this preparation is sometimes used in obstetrics.

Lignocaine. This is also available for epidural administration. It gives effective anaesthesia in a short time but has a short duration of action. This makes it unsuitable for use throughout labour since a large total dose would be required and toxicity is therefore a risk. However, if a woman is very distressed it may be used for the initial dose, with bupivacaine being used thereafter.

Toxicity. If the woman has received a large total dose of local anaesthetic solution or if some of the solution has passed directly into the circulation, she may complain of tingling or numbness of the mouth and tongue, dizziness and tinnitus. This may be followed by drowsiness, muscle twitching and slurring of the speech. Finally convulsions may occur, with cardiac arrest ensuing.

Opiates

Several of the opiate drugs have been used in the epidural space including diamorphine, morphine, pethidine, and more recently fentanyl. They give good postoperative analgesia without motor or sympathetic block and do not produce hypotension to any extent. They are not as effective as might be expected in relieving the pain of labour but are used by some anaesthetists following caesarean section. There is some risk of respiratory depression but this is not as great a risk in the young, fit woman as in the elderly patient following surgery. Drugs such as diamorphine produce a pleasant feeling of well-being.

Combined local anaesthetic agents and opiates

Epidural opiates used alone give disappointing results in labour, but a combination has been found to be very effective.

The greatest advantage is a marked reduction in motor blockade, as only a dilute solution of local anaesthetic, usually bupivacaine, is needed to give good analgesia.

The opiate most commonly used is fentanyl, and this has not been shown to have any adverse effects on the fetus or newborn baby. There is interest in other similar drugs, but their effect on the baby has not yet been investigated fully.

Preparation of the mother

The woman and her partner should receive information about epidural analgesia during the

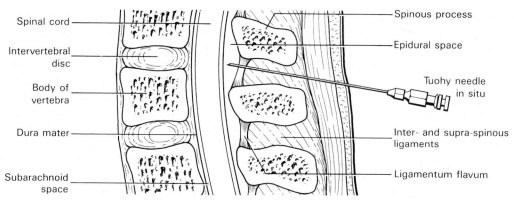

Fig. 28.2
Sagittal section of the lumbar spine with Tuohy needle in position.

antenatal period so that they have time to consider this option and to ask any questions.

The woman in labour who opts for epidural analgesia in desperation rather than as a planned measure, should be given as much information as she can absorb but she must be informed of the risks involved. She must then give her consent to the procedure.

An intravenous infusion is established, using a wide bore cannula so that fluid may be infused quickly if necessary. The midwife measures and records the woman's blood pressure.

The procedure

The woman is positioned either on her left side or sitting upright with her buttocks on the edge of the bed nearest the anaesthetist.

The skin of the lumbar area is cleaned by spraying with a preparation such as chlorhexidine in spirit.

The anaesthetist 'scrubs up' and puts on sterile gown and gloves. He places a sterile towel over the lumbar area, exposing the intervertebral space which he intends to use and infiltrates the skin and deeper tissues with local anaesthetic solution.

When this is effective he 'nicks' the skin with a sterile scalpel and introduces the Tuohy needle. He advances the needle cautiously. It passes through the tough ligamentum flavum before reaching the epidural space. Pressure within the epidural space is atmospheric or slightly negative and so he tests for 'loss of resistance' to check if the needle has passed through the ligamentum

flavum. Even slight movement by the woman at this stage may result in dural puncture and she must lie still.

Once the tip of the Tuohy needle lies in the epidural space the anaesthetist threads the epidural catheter through the needle which is then withdrawn.

He introduces a test dose of 3–4 ml of local anaesthetic solution; its purpose is to ensure that the solution is not in the subarachnoid space (see below).

The epidural catheter is secured firmly with adhesive tape and an anti-bacterial filter attached to the distal end. The woman is positioned as requested by the anaesthetist. The blood pressure is recorded 5 minutes after the test dose was given.

If this reading is satisfactory and no motor block has developed the remainder of the first full dose is given. The blood pressure is usually recorded every 5 minutes for 20 minutes, then 15 minutes later. Between top-up doses of local anaesthetic solution half-hourly recordings are usually sufficient.

After about 20 minutes, when the local anaesthetic solution is likely to have settled, the woman may be helped to find a comfortable position.

Subsequent care

The anaesthetist takes overall responsibility for the establishment of the epidural block but he will then delegate certain aspects of its maintenance to the midwife.

She is responsible for ensuring that adequate analgesia is maintained, whether or not she tops up the epidural block herself. She should report any hypotension, any areas of unsatisfactory analgesia and any symptoms of excessive block or of toxicity. She has a responsibility to ensure that she is adequately trained to care for a woman with an epidural block and she must follow hospital procedures and policies.

She must give particular attention to bladder care during labour. Immobile legs must be positioned with care, in order to avoid nerve damage and pressure.

The epidural top-up

The midwife may be trained to top up the epidural block by giving a further dose as prescribed by the anaesthetist. She is personally responsible for ensuring that she is competent to carry out the procedure. The same observations are made as with the initial dose. She should be aware of the possible dangers and complications and their immediate and subsequent treatment. It is important to prevent aortocaval occlusion since this would compound the effect of any hypotension occurring as a result of the epidural block.

Continuous epidural infusion (see also p. 444)

Good analgesia is afforded by continuous infusion of dilute local anaesthetic solution, with or without opiates. This is given by infusion pump into the epidural catheter. Occasional top-ups may still be needed but generally this technique avoids the peaks and troughs of analgesia afforded by the intermittent top-up technique. The midwife must still observe the woman carefully.

There has been some research in the USA into giving women some control over their epidural infusion (patient-controlled epidural analgesia). Certain restraints are built in, just as with patient-controlled intravenous analgesia, such as the Cardiff Palliator.

Epidural anaesthesia for caesarean section

Epidural anaesthesia for caesarean section must be more profound and more extensive than for labour. Sensation should be blocked to the level of the nipples (T4), and a good block is required in the pelvic area. If the motor block rises above the level of T6 the woman may have difficulty breathing.

Attaining this extensive block necessitates the use of a larger volume of the stronger local anaesthetic solution (commonly 0.5% bupivacaine). The risk of hypotension is therefore greater and a preload of at least a litre of intravenous fluid (usually Hartmann's solution) is required. Hypotension may still occur and ampoules of ephedrine should be ready for immediate use. Some women experience uncontrollable shivering during induction of epidural anaesthesia and this may be due in part to the rapid infusion of intravenous fluid. Some women dislike the complete motor block of the legs.

The greatest advantage for the woman is being able to see and cuddle the baby immediately. In many centres her partner can also be present. The mother does not have to recover from the effects of general anaesthesia and she is up and about very quickly in the postoperative period, especially if epidural opiates are used for postoperative analgesia.

The woman is not exposed to the risks of general anaesthesia although there is always the possibility that general anaesthesia may have to be induced at some stage, if the epidural block is not satisfactory. The anaesthetist is always prepared for this, and women should be warned that it is occasionally necessary. If a woman is slightly apprehensive about having an epidural for caesarean section she may be relieved to know this.

Spinal anaesthesia

Spinal anaesthesia must be distinguished from epidural anaesthesia.

Spinal anaesthesia is a technique by which local anaesthetic solution is injected into the subarachnoid space, that is, into the cerebrospinal fluid. It is quick and relatively easy to perform and is almost always completely effective. The onset of anaesthesia is almost immediate. The approach is similar to that for performing lumbar puncture.

A continuous or intermittent technique is not considered practicable by many anaesthetists and its greatest use is for shorter procedures such as manual removal of the placenta, suturing of a third degree perineal tear or forceps delivery.

It is possible to perform caesarean section using spinal anaesthesia, but there is a risk that the anaesthetic will have worn off before the end of the procedure, especially if some unexpected complication occurs. In developing countries the obstetrician may have to rely solely on spinal anaesthesia, which he performs himself prior to delivering the baby by caesarean section. In this situation the obstetrician may also use local anaesthetic solution for infiltration over the incision site.

The needle used for spinal anaesthesia is very fine so that leakage of CSF is minimal.

A very small amount of local anaesthetic solution is required. Between 1.5 and 2 ml is usually sufficient to give anaesthesia. Due to the fact that the drug is being injected into another fluid its location of action can be influenced by two factors:

- use of a hyperbaric or 'heavy' solution: if the drug being injected has a specific gravity greater than that of the CSF it will settle at the lowest possible point within the subarachnoid space. Examples of local anaesthetic solutions used in this way are heavy cinchocaine and amethocaine.
- positioning the woman: if a hyperbaric solution is used and the woman is positioned carefully, a specific block may usually be obtained without difficulty. Position is also important when an isobaric solution is used (that is, one with a specific gravity similar to that of the CSF).

The woman will have total motor and sensory block over and below the anaesthetised area. It is difficult to control the level of the block.

There is a greater risk of hypotension with spinal than with epidural block. The blood pressure is monitored carefully. Care of the bladder is also important in this instance.

Combined spinal and epidural anaesthesia

This technique is gaining in popularity. It is used because there is a risk that spinal block will not be sustained throughout caesarean section if the procedure is prolonged for any reason. Immediate anaesthesia is obtained by spinal blockade. A Tuohy needle and epidural catheter are then inserted in an adjacent intervertebral space and local anaesthetic solution is injected as necessary in order to maintain anaesthesia and provide postoperative pain relief.

Long-term sequelae

Research undertaken into long-term health problems following childbirth (MacArthur et al 1991) has revealed that the number of women who suffer from backache after epidural or spinal anaesthesia is almost double the number who do so after a normal delivery. This backache may be accompanied by shoulder ache, limb weakness or tingling in the limbs. It is postulated that the cause may be positional and care should therefore be taken to vary the position of the mother from time to time.

Pudendal block

This is a technique used to anaesthetise the specific area served by the pudendal nerve.

Local anaesthetic solution is injected adjacent to the pudendal nerves as they pass close to the ischial spines. The pudendal nerves are sensory nerves serving the lower vagina, the perineum and vulva. Pudendal block is notoriously unreliable and often does not give adequate analgesia. It may be more effective on one side than the other.

A guarded needle such as the Oxford needle is used. The more common approach is transvaginal. The ischial spines are palpated and the injection made on each side. The transperineal approach may be used if the presenting part is very low.

Paracervical block

In this technique the paracervical plexuses are blocked. This gives pain relief for the first stage of labour but each injection is only effective for about 3 hours. The local anaesthetic solution is injected using a guarded needle to prevent deep penetration of the tissues. The uterine artery passes close to the nerve plexus and inadvertent intra-arterial injection of even a small amount of local

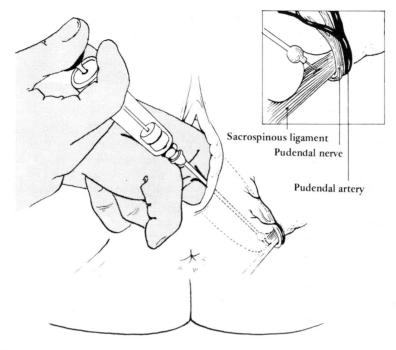

Sacrospinous ligament
Pudendal nerve

Pudendal artery

Fig. 28.3
Locating the pudendal nerve per vaginam.

anaesthetic solution may lead to fetal bradycardia or possibly intra-uterine death. The technique is not popular in the UK although it may be more widely used elsewhere.

LOCAL ANAESTHESIA

Perineal infiltration

This is the most common instance of local anaesthesia for the midwife, who may undertake it herself prior to performing or repairing an episiotomy.

The midwife should be aware of safe dosages and possible side-effects of the drug she is using.

The drug in most common use is lignocaine. There is a real risk of toxic reaction if more than 200 mg is given to the woman (the equivalent of 20 ml of 1% solution). For this reason the amount that the midwife may use on her own responsibility is considerably less than this.

The technique used will depend on the type of episiotomy favoured and on local policy and practice. The principles involved include:

- giving effective analgesia
- minimising the risk of intravenous injection.

It is therefore common practice to insert the needle, aspirate to ensure that the tip of the needle is not in a blood vessel, and inject the local anaesthetic solution as the needle is withdrawn. This may be repeated to give either a fan-shaped or a star-shaped pattern of infiltration (see also Ch. 14).

OBSTETRIC OPERATIONS

Forceps delivery

Forceps delivery is a means of extracting the fetus with the aid of obstetric forceps when it is inadvisable or impossible for the mother to complete the delivery by her own effort. Forceps can also be used to assist the delivery of the after-coming head of the breech and on occasion to withdraw the head up and out of the pelvis at caesarean section.

Formerly forceps deliveries were classified by the level of the head at the time the forceps were applied, i.e. high-cavity, mid-cavity or low-cavity. The last one of these is now the only one frequently performed as caesarean section is usually preferred to the more traumatic high- and mid-cavity operations.

Low-cavity forceps deliveries can be divided into rotational and non-rotational. The former refers to a manoeuvre of the fetal head from a malposition into a more favourable position with the aid of specially designed forceps, usually Kielland's. In unskilled hands this is a dangerous procedure and some obstetricians prefer to rotate the head manually prior to applying conventional forceps for the delivery.

Types of obstetric forceps

Obstetric forceps consist of two separate blades, each with a handle. Each blade is marked 'L' (left) or 'R' (right). They are inserted separately either side of the fetal head and locked together by means of the English or Smellie lock. (Rotational forceps have a sliding lock.) The blades are spoon-shaped to accommodate the baby's head, but fenestrated, to minimise trauma and for lightness. The spoon shape of the blades is called the 'cephalic curve'. In most modern obstetric forceps the blade is attached to the handle at an angle which corresponds to the pelvic curve. When the blades are correctly placed on the fetal head the handles will be neatly aligned.

There is a wide variety of forceps designs.

Non-rotational. Some examples are:

- Wrigley's forceps: short, stubby-handled forceps used for very low forceps deliveries, for the after-coming head of a breech delivery or at caesarean section.
- Simpson's forceps: standard, low-cavity forceps.
- Neville-Barnes', Haig-Ferguson's, Milne-Murray and Anderson's forceps: these were all originally designed for high- and mid-cavity forceps deliveries and have axis traction handle attachments to allow downward traction of a high head into the pelvis. These attachments are rarely, if ever, used and the forceps are used for low-cavity deliveries.

Rotational. One design is in common use:

- Kielland's forceps: for use when the head is in an occipitolateral or occipitoposterior position. Since the blades are applied to the head which is then rotated to an occipito-anterior position they have no pelvic curve, because this could cause trauma to the birth canal. In malposition there may also be asynclitism and their sliding lock allows this to be corrected. When the Kielland's forceps are applied there is a gap between the handles. There is a danger that if they are squeezed together pressure can be applied to the fetal head. Some operators like to rotate the head with the Kielland's forceps and deliver with non-rotational forceps.

Prerequisites for forceps delivery

There are certain conditions which must exist before forceps delivery can be performed:

- full dilatation of the cervix
- ruptured membranes
- positive identification of presentation and position
- no appreciable cephalopelvic disproportion
- definite engagement of the head.

Preparation of the woman

A woman about to be delivered with forceps will often be relieved to know that her baby is about to be born. The woman and her partner should have been fully informed throughout labour of progress and developments and her care should have been discussed with them. Ideally she should be prepared in advance for the possibility of a forceps delivery if this looks likely. Full explanation of the procedure itself and the need for it is likely to result in greater retrospective satisfaction.

Once the joint decision has been made, adequate and appropriate analgesia must be offered.

When such analgesia has been instituted and the obstetrician is ready to proceed the woman's legs are placed in the lithotomy position. Both legs must be positioned simultaneously to avoid strain on the woman's lower back and hips. This is an undignified and uncomfortable position, especially for a tired woman with a weighty gravid uterus who is in advanced labour. Both medical staff and midwives should try to minimise the woman's loss of dignity when they perform what is, for them, a routine procedure. The woman's legs should not be placed in the stirrups for longer than is necessary, and the vulval area should remain covered whenever possible. The minimum number of staff should be present, and interruptions should be discouraged. The woman will find it helpful to realise that the staff are aware of her probable discomfort and embarrassment.

She should be tilted towards the left at an angle of 15° to prevent aortocaval occlusion. (This is usually achieved by the use of a rubber wedge under the mattress; an operating table has the facility for lateral tilt.)

Preparations must also have been made for the baby and resuscitation equipment checked and in working order. In many centres the paediatrician will be present.

Procedure

The woman's vulval area is thoroughly cleaned and draped with sterile towels using aseptic technique; the bladder is emptied with a Jaques catheter. The obstetrician will perform a vaginal examination in order to confirm the station and

exact position of the fetal head. It is usual to positively identify the forceps blades (as left and right) by assembling them briefly before proceeding.

Positioning the forceps. The aim in positioning the forceps is to place them alongside the head over the ears. Myerscough (1982) describes this as being along an imaginary line running from the point of the chin to a point on the sagittal suture near the posterior fontanelle. The left blade is passed gently between the perineum and the fetal head with the first two fingers of the operator's right hand lying alongside the fetal head protecting the maternal tissue. The tip of the forceps blade slides lightly over the head, into the hollow of the sacrum and is then 'wandered' to the left side of the pelvis where it should sit alongside the head. The procedure is repeated with the right blade until it sits on the right of the pelvis. It should then be easy to lock the two blades and there should be little or no gap between the handles. A significant gap suggests that the forceps are wrongly positioned and they should be re-applied after carefully checking the position of the head.

During this time the woman needs the full attention and support of the midwife whom she

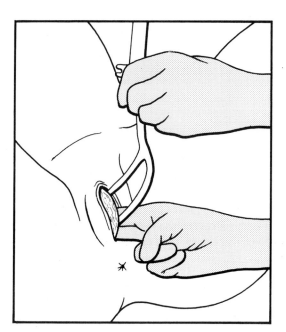

Fig. 28.4
Left blade being inserted. The fingers of the right hand guard the vaginal tissue.

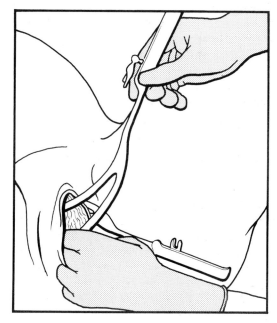

Fig. 28.5
Right blade being inserted.

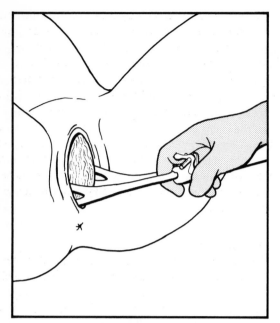

Fig. 28.6
Traction of the head is downwards until this point; when the head is low, the direction of pull is outward, towards the operator.

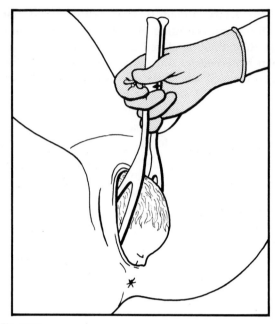

Fig. 28.7
As the head crowns it is lifted upwards.

has already come to know during her labour. The fetal heart rate is monitored throughout. As soon as the operator is ready and the uterus contracts the woman is encouraged to push; to supplement her expulsive effort the obstetrician places steady, downward traction on the forceps. Traction is released between contractions. The fetal heart is monitored carefully throughout. Intermittent traction is continued in a downward and backwards direction until the occiput can be felt below the symphysis pubis. When the head distends the perineum, an episiotomy is performed. Most obstetricians deliver the head using the forceps, as they feel this gives greater control, while others prefer to remove them and control delivery of the head as in a normal delivery. Once the body is delivered, unless the baby requires active resuscitation, he is handed straight to his mother and is dried thoroughly to prevent chilling.

After completion of the second and third stages the episiotomy is sutured as quickly as possible and the woman made comfortable.

Manual rotation of the fetal head. Some obstetricians prefer to rotate the fetal head manually in cases of occipitoposterior position as this is likely to be less traumatic than instrumental rotation. The exact position of the fetal head must be determined. The obstetrician grasps the head, usually by the sinciput, and rotates it encouraging flexion. It may be possible to lodge a finger on the edge of the anterior fontanelle or the overriding bone on the frontal suture and apply gentle, steady pressure to rotate the head. One disadvantage is that upward displacement of the head may be necessary in many instances in order to grasp it, but there is then no facility for downward traction. A large hand will take up more space within the birth canal than a pair of obstetric forceps.

Indications for forceps delivery
- Fetal distress in the second stage of labour.
- Delay in the second stage of labour.
- Malposition: occipitolateral, occipitoposterior positions.
- Maternal exhaustion or distress.
- Breech presentation: forceps are usually used to deliver the after-coming head in a controlled fashion.
- Preterm delivery: this is still a matter of debate, but some obstetricians and paediatricians like

to protect the fetal head, with its soft skull bones, if delivery occurs before about the 36th week of gestation.

- Conditions in which pushing is undesirable, such as dural tap, some cardiac conditions or moderate to severe hypertension.

Complications

Failure. Undue force should never be used. If the head does not advance with steady traction the attempt is abandoned and the baby is delivered by caesarean section.

In the infant:

Bruising. Severe bruising will cause marked jaundice which may be prolonged. (Forceps marks are almost always present on the face: parents may be reassured that although these will become more florid in the first few hours of life they will then fade uneventfully over some months.)

Cephalhaematoma. See Chapter 37.

Cerebral irritability. A traumatic forceps delivery may cause cerebral oedema or haemorrhage (see Ch. 37).

Tentorial tear. This may result from compression of the fetal head by the forceps. The compression causes elongation of the head and consequent tearing of the tentorial membrane.

Facial palsy. Occasionally the facial nerve may be damaged since it is situated near the mastoid process where it has little protection.

In the mother:

Bruising and trauma to the urethra. This may cause dysuria and occasionally haematuria or a period of urinary retention or incontinence.

Vaginal and perineal trauma. The vaginal wall may be torn during forceps delivery and the vagina must be inspected carefully, using a good light, prior to perineal repair. The episiotomy may extend or be accompanied by a further perineal tear and these must be repaired with care. As with any damaged perineum there may be bruising, oedema or occasionally haematoma formation.

Vacuum extraction (ventouse delivery)

The ventouse or vacuum extractor consists of a cup which is attached to the fetal scalp by suc-

tion. Traction is applied by means of a chain and the fetal head is drawn out of the vagina. It takes 10–15 minutes to apply. Its advantages are that it can be applied before the cervix is fully dilated, it does not add to the presenting diameters and, if correctly positioned, it brings about flexion of the head and natural rotation. Its main drawback is that the operator may be too hasty in applying traction before the suction has been built up, so that the cup comes off. It is useful in remote areas and midwives working in developing countries without medical support successfully perform vacuum extractions.

The equipment

The original vacuum extractors were of a very simple design, with a device similar to a bicycle pump being used to obtain the vacuum. Modern vacuum extractors use an electrical pump, which has much more sensitive controls.

A metal or hard rubber cup is applied to the fetal head; a vacuum is created inside this cup, which is connected to the pump by rubber tubing, and traction is then applied. Inside the rubber tubing is a metal chain designed to take the strain of traction, with a metal handle to give the operator a good grip. There are various sizes of cup.

It is possible to apply it to the breech but this is rarely done.

Indications

- Mild fetal distress.
- Delay in the second stage of labour or late first stage.
- Malposition: occipitolateral and occipitoposterior positions.
- Maternal exhaustion.

The procedure

The prerequisites are as for forceps delivery, with the possible exception of full dilatation of the cervix (see above). It is possible to apply the ventouse before full dilatation of the cervix and traction of the head against the cervix will stimulate uterine contractions. The head must be engaged.

The woman is positioned and prepared as for forceps delivery (see above).

The position of the fetal head is determined and an appropriately sized cup selected. The cup is placed against the fetal head as near to the occiput as possible, ensuring that no cervix is trapped beneath it.

The vacuum is then built up gradually, usually starting at 0.2 kg/cm^2 and increasing the pressure slowly until a vacuum of 0.8 kg/cm^2 is reached after 5–10 minutes. Once this pressure has been obtained the operator exerts steady, gentle traction on the fetal head, in conjunction with uterine contractions and the mother's expulsive efforts.

With descent of the head rotation to an occipito-anterior position may be effected if necessary. Because there is no part of the instrument between the head and the vaginal wall an episiotomy may not always be judged necessary and vaginal trauma should not occur. As with a forceps delivery, traction is exerted in the direction of the curve of Carus and the head is controlled carefully at crowning. Traction should not be maintained for too long a period but clearly a ventouse delivery will take longer than a forceps delivery, because of the time required to build up the vacuum.

Complications

Failure. An attempted vacuum extraction may be unsuccessful. Exerting too much traction will result in the cup coming off. In unskilled or impatient hands, the cup is also likely to come off.

Maternal. Trauma to the mother is rare, if the cup is applied carefully.

Fetal. The most common complication of ventouse delivery is trauma to the fetal scalp and some obstetricians prefer not to use it for this reason.

'Chignon'. Because the vacuum cup is applied to the slightly mobile scalp, all babies delivered with the ventouse will have a 'chignon'. This is an area of oedema and bruising where the cup was applied. These normally subside uneventfully but they may occasionally become infected.

Cephalhaematoma. Some babies will develop a cephalhaematoma.

Cerebral trauma. A few babies will suffer some degree of cerebral trauma, such as tentorial tear.

Caesarean section

There are two types of caesarean section: lower segment and classical.

The lower segment of the uterus forms after about 32 weeks' gestation and is less muscular than the upper segment of the uterus. In a lower segment caesarean section a transverse incision is made in the lower segment; this heals more rapidly and successfully than an incision in the upper segment of the uterus. There is less muscle and more fibrous tissue there which reduces the risk of rupture in a subsequent pregnancy.

Classical caesarean section is rarely performed. Indications for this approach are gestation of less than about 32 weeks before the lower segment has formed, placenta praevia which is anteriorly situated, in order to avoid incision of the placenta, and hour-glass contraction (constriction ring).

A longitudinal midline abdominal incision does not necessarily imply a longitudinal uterine incision. A lower segment caesarean section is most

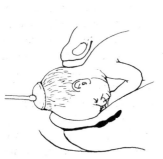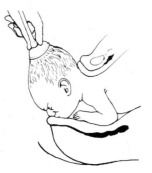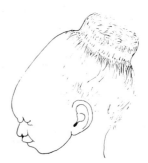

Fig. 28.8
Diagrams showing the application of the ventouse cup and the chignon which usually results.

commonly performed through a transverse incision, the Pfannenstiel or 'bikini-line' incision, but on occasions a midline incision may be preferred. A classical caesarean section is always performed through a midline incision.

Indications for caesarean section

Elective caesarean section. The term *elective* indicates that the decision to deliver the baby by caesarean section has been made during the pregnancy and before the onset of labour. While some indications are absolute, others will depend on a combination of factors and on the views of the obstetrician concerned.
Definite indications include:

- cephalopelvic disproportion
- major degrees of placenta praevia
- multiple pregnancy with three or more fetuses.

Possible indications include:

- the primigravida and often the multigravida with a breech presentation
- moderate to severe pregnancy-induced hypertension
- diabetes
- intra-uterine growth retardation
- antepartum haemorrhage.

If the indication for caesarean section pertains specifically to one pregnancy, such as placenta praevia, vaginal delivery may be expected on subsequent occasions. Certain conditions, however, warrant repeated caesarean section. Cephalopelvic disproportion due to contracted pelvis will recur and a uterus which has been scarred twice or more carries a greater risk of uterine rupture.

Emergency caesarean section is performed when adverse conditions develop during labour. Definite indications include:

- cord prolapse
- uterine rupture (dramatic) or scar dehiscence (may be less acute)
- cephalopelvic disproportion diagnosed in labour
- fulminating pregnancy-induced hypertension
- eclampsia
- failure to progress in the first or second stage of labour
- fetal distress, if delivery is not imminent.

Psychological preparation of the mother

Some women welcome caesarean section as a means of escaping the rigours of labour; others feel disappointed that they have not had the experience of a normal delivery and have not enjoyed the accompanying sense of achievement.

Different women require differing levels of information. While some feel reassured by a detailed description of what is to happen, others find it distressing and prefer to leave everything in the hands of the professionals.

The midwife must be sensitive in her dealings with women, whether in a group situation or in speaking to individuals. If a woman is to have an elective caesarean section it may be helpful to give information in stages. She should certainly be given the opportunity to ask whatever questions she wishes and should not be made to feel ridiculous in any way. Women are likely to have friends or relatives who have had caesarean sections, and this usually helps to reduce anxiety. It may be helpful for a woman to meet another person who has had the same experience recently.

If the possibility of caesarean section arises during labour, the midwife should begin to prepare the woman for this eventuality. The couple should be kept fully informed of events and progress during labour and should be given every opportunity to ask questions.

Physical preparation

Antacid therapy. It is now common practice in the UK for women to receive regular antacid therapy throughout labour. If this has not been given it should certainly be prescribed and administered once the decision to proceed with caesarean section has been made. Antacid preparations such as sodium citrate are effective in neutralising the stomach acid but do not prevent its secretion. In order to minimise production of gastric acid the anaesthetist may also prescribe a preparation such as ranitidine or cimetidine. The woman who is likely to need a caesarean section should only be permitted fluids in labour.

Intravenous infusion. If an intravenous infusion has not already been established or is not running freely, it is sited or resited.

Pubic shave. This is still usually considered necessary, though research suggests that tiny skin cuts predispose to infection. The use of a depilatory cream is likely to become more common.

Bowel care. If caesarean section is elective it is usual to give two glycerine suppositories the evening before operation in order to empty the rectum.

Bladder care. The bladder must be empty prior to caesarean section. This may be achieved by passing a catheter which is then removed, or by inserting an indwelling catheter into the bladder. This may be done before or after induction of anaesthesia; if epidural block is used the woman will be less distressed if the catheter is passed after the block has become effective.

Clothing and valuables. The woman is dressed in a clean operation gown and any valuables are placed in safe keeping according to hospital policy. Any rings or bracelets which cannot be removed are covered with adhesive strapping.

Anatomy

If the midwife is to assist at caesarean section as scrub nurse, it is important that she should understand the anatomy involved.

The most confusing aspect of the layers involved is the presence of two layers of peritoneum. The non-pregnant uterus is a pelvic organ and is closely covered by a layer of pelvic peritoneum. When the pregnant uterus grows up into the abdomen this peritoneum rises up with the uterus and comes into contact with the abdominal peritoneum. Each of these must be incised and repaired separately. The abdominal peritoneum is situated below the abdominal muscle layer.

The anatomical layers are:

- skin
- fat
- rectus sheath
- muscle (rectus abdominis)
- abdominal peritoneum
- pelvic peritoneum (perimetrium)
- uterine muscle.

The surgeon usually incises the rectus sheath, but divides the rectus muscle digitally. Care is taken to avoid trauma to the bladder and the ureters. The scrub nurse must avoid contamination of the sterile field and keep close account of all swabs, instruments and needles.

When the uterine cavity is opened, the amniotic fluid escapes and is aspirated. The baby is delivered in much the same way as in a vaginal delivery but through the uterine incision; obstetric forceps are often used to extract the head from the pelvis. When the baby is born, an oxytocic drug is administered before the placenta and membranes are delivered. The mother may now be given a slightly deeper anaesthetic and the operation proceeds at a more leisurely pace. The uterus bleeds freely at this stage and the surgeon will quickly apply the special haemostatic Green-Armytage forceps. The uterine muscle is sutured in two layers. The pelvic peritoneum is then sutured, followed by the abdominal peritoneum. Repair of the rectus sheath also brings the rectus abdominis into alignment. Sometimes the subcutaneous fat is sutured and finally the skin is closed with sutures or clips. A vacuum drain, such as a 'Redivac' drain, may be inserted beneath the rectus sheath to prevent the formation of a haematoma.

Immediate postoperative care

The care of the woman who has had a caesarean section is the same as that following any major abdominal surgery with one or two added considerations.

Observations. The blood pressure and pulse are recorded every quarter-hour in the immediate recovery period. The temperature is recorded every 2 hours. The wound must be inspected every half-hour to detect any blood loss. The lochia are also inspected and drainage should be small initially. Following general anaesthesia the woman is nursed in the left lateral or 'recovery' position until she is fully conscious, since the risk of regurgitation and silent aspiration of stomach contents is still present.

Analgesia is prescribed and is given as required. If the mother intends to breast feed, the baby should be put to the breast as soon as possible. This can be achieved with minimal disturbance to the mother.

Care following regional block. Following epidural or spinal anaesthesia the woman may sit up as soon as she wishes. All observations are recorded as described in the previous paragraph. Fluids are introduced gradually followed by a light diet. Although the woman may feel very hungry, there is a risk of paralytic ileus due to handling of the bowel and food is not permitted until bowel sounds are heard. The intravenous infusion remains in progress for the same reason. Care must be taken to avoid any damage to the legs which will gradually regain sensation and movement. Postoperative analgesia may be given in a variety of ways:

- an epidural top-up of local anaesthetic solution
- an epidural opiate
- intramuscular analgesia.

As it is possible that an opiate administered via the epidural route may cause some respiratory depression, the woman's respiratory rate must be recorded. This means of pain relief offers the advantage of excellent analgesia without motor block and also seems to give a feeling of well-being. Women are usually able to become mobile very quickly which reduces the risk of deep vein thrombosis.

Ideally the baby should remain with his mother and they should be transferred to the postnatal ward together as soon as possible.

Care in the postnatal ward. When mother and baby are transferred to the postnatal ward, the blood pressure, temperature and pulse are usually checked every 4 hours. The baby should remain with his mother, and the midwife should offer extra help to ensure that the mother has adequate rest. The mother is encouraged to move her legs and to perform leg and breathing exercises. The physiotherapist will usually teach these and will give chest physiotherapy. The woman is helped to get out of bed as soon as possible following caesarean section, and is encouraged to become fully mobile.

Urinary output must be monitored carefully; women may have some difficulty with micturition initially and the bladder may be incompletely emptied. Any haematuria must be reported to the doctor.

Women who have had a general anaesthetic for caesarean section may feel very tired and drowsy for hours or even days. A woman may complain of a feeling of detachment and unreality and may feel that she does not relate well to the baby. The woman who is concerned should be reassured and be given the opportunity to talk freely.

Appropriate analgesia must be given as frequently as necessary. It is usual to give intramuscular opiates for up to 48 hours and then to give oral analgesics.

The mother must be encouraged to rest as much as possible and tactful advice may need to be given to her visitors. If the mother becomes too tired, help is needed with care for the baby. This should preferably take place at the mother's bedside and should include support with breast feeding.

Some women may have a lingering feeling of failure or disappointment at having had a caesarean section and may value the opportunity to talk this over with a sympathetic listener.

Destructive operations (Embryotomy)

It may occasionally be necessary, in the interests of saving the mother's life, to destroy the fetus.

In the UK these drastic measures will only be undertaken if there is gross fetal abnormality causing fetopelvic disproportion. The alternative is caesarean section but although this is a relatively safe procedure in the 1990s, it still carries attendant risks and vaginal delivery may be preferred. The fetus may be equally difficult to deliver abdominally and may still need to be destroyed first. Whatever the situation it is traumatic for all concerned and calls for sensitive support of both the family and the staff.

In developing countries, these distressing procedures may have to be performed because of the non-availability or refusal of a caesarean section. A uterine scar carries a risk of uterine rupture in a subsequent pregnancy which may be fatal in an area remote from obstetric help. The woman may present with exhaustion from prolonged or obstructed labour or may have a uterine infection; the fetus may have been dead for some time.

The instruments used for destructive operations are of necessity brutal and must be used with great care to avoid injuring the mother.

Craniotomy is probably performed most commonly for hydrocephalus. Release of cerebrospinal fluid and brain tissue causes collapse of the skull bones and allows vaginal delivery. If fetal death has already occurred craniotomy may be used to overcome disproportion due to a brow presentation. In the case of hydrocephalus it is often sufficient to perforate the head and allow escape of CSF; forceps may be applied if the fetus does not deliver spontaneously. If more drastic measures are required instruments such as the cranioclast and cephalotribe may be used to crush and then deliver the head. A blunt hook, known as a crotchet, may be used to extract the aftercoming head of the breech.

Decapitation may be necessary when a shoulder presentation has become impacted. The Blond Heidler wire saw and thimble is usually used. There are also various types of decapitating hooks and knives which may be encountered.

Cleidotomy. In this procedure the clavicles are cut to reduce the width of the shoulder girdle. Heavy, long, straight scissors are used.

Evisceration. It may be necessary to remove the abdominal or thoracic contents in some cases of gross fetal abnormality. If the presentation is cephalic this is difficult but it is more feasible in a breech presentation. The abdomen or chest is opened using a perforator and the contents removed manually.

Supporting the family. It is impossible to summarise this briefly since cultural factors and expectations play an important part in the reactions to the loss of a child. In a developing country atti-

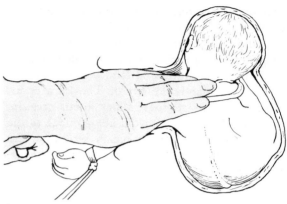

Fig. 28.10
Jardine's decapitation hook round the neck of the fetus. Traction on an arm by an assistant brings the neck within reach and fixes the head and trunk.

tudes are very different from those in the West and it may be accepted as a normal life event with very little grief apparent. In countries where infant survival is taken for granted, parents are likely to be devastated and the process of grieving should be encouraged. Many questions will be asked and opportunities for free discussion should be given. Parents will question their own actions and may feel intensely guilty at producing an abnormal fetus or perhaps refusing antenatal care. A feeling of anger is a normal part of the grieving process and parents should be allowed to express it. Midwives should not feel threatened by this unless of course there is some justification. Referral to an organisation such as the 'Compassionate Friends' may be helpful in the long term; such a traumatic

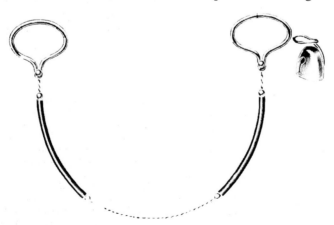

Fig. 28.9
Blond Heidler wire saw decapitator. (Reproduced by courtesy of Down Bros. and Mayer and Phelps Ltd, Mitcham, Surrey.)

experience may cause great stress in the couple's relationship (see also Ch. 49).

Symphysiotomy

This procedure enables a vaginal delivery in cases of minor cephalopelvic disproportion in areas of the world where caesarean section is not an option or a woman is not likely to seek obstetric care in a future pregnancy. The woman is usually primigravid and the operation is performed late in labour.

Both the pubic area and the perineum must be infiltrated with local anaesthetic as a generous episiotomy will be needed to avoid excessive pressure by the fetal head on the urethra and bladder. A firm catheter is inserted into the bladder to allow it to empty. It is held to one side during the incision which protects the urethra.

The fibro-cartilage is incised over the centre of the symphysis pubis while two assistants hold and abduct the legs. A vacuum extractor is often used to facilitate delivery.

Following the operation broad strips of Elastoplast are applied around the pelvis to give support and the legs are usually bandaged together. A self-retaining catheter remains in position for 4 to 5 days because the area is usually oedematous.

The woman may have backache and experience difficulty in walking but in most cases the pelvic girdle regains its stability.

Reader Activities

Epidural analgesia was once seen by women as heralding a new era of painless labour for all mothers (Morgan 1990).

Prepare a discussion considering the following points:

- what were the flaws in this supposition?
- to what extent do women expect or want a painless labour today?
- do we give appropriate preparation for labour pain in the antenatal period; if not how could we improve on this?

Prepare a leaflet for women who are likely to have a caesarean section, which they could read in the antenatal period. Include:

- what will happen in the ward and the anaesthetic room beforehand
- a description (at an appropriate level!) of induction of general and regional anaesthesia — find out and discuss how these procedures feel
- a discussion of how women feel about caesarean section afterwards — consult women who have had the experience, and find some appropriate research papers.

It is sometimes said that giving a woman epidural analgesia results in a 'cascade of intervention'.

- Discuss this statement with colleagues on the labour ward.
- Are there ways of minimising this effect?
- How can midwives influence the outcome of such a labour to the woman's benefit?

FURTHER READING

Anaesthetic services for obstetrics: a plan for the future 1988 The Association of Anaesthetists of Great Britain and Ireland 9 Bedford Square, London WC1B 3RA and The Obstetric Anaesthetists Association

Bevis R 1984 Anaesthesia in midwifery. Baillière Tindall, London

British National Formulary 1986 British Medical Association and Pharmaceutical Press, London

Department of Health et al 1991 Report on confidential enquiries into maternal deaths in the United Kingdom 1985–87. HMSO, London

Donald I 1979 Practical obstetric problems, 5th edn. Lloyd-Luke, London

Llewellyn-Jones D 1986 Fundamentals of obstetrics and gynaecology, 4th edn. Faber & Faber, London

MacArthur C, Lewis M, Knox E G 1991 Health after childbirth. HMSO, London

Moir D D 1980 Obstetric anaesthesia and analgesia, 2nd edn. Baillière Tindall, London

Morgan B 1990 Controversies in obstetric anaesthesia. Edward Arnold, London

Myerscough P R 1982 Munro Kerr's operative obstetrics, 10th edn. Baillière Tindall, London

Ostheimer G W (ed) 1984 Manual of obstetric anaesthesia. Churchill Livingstone, New York

Reynolds F (ed) 1990 Epidural and spinal blockade in obstetrics. Baillière Tindall, London

UKCC handbook of midwives rules 1991 HMSO, London

29

Complications of the third stage of labour

JENNIFER SLEEP

Postpartum haemorrhage

Acute inversion of the uterus

Shock

Emergency obstetric unit

POSTPARTUM HAEMORRHAGE

Postpartum haemorrhage is one of the most alarming and serious emergencies which a midwife may face and is especially terrifying if it occurs immediately following a straightforward delivery. It may also prove a frightening experience for the mother and can undermine her confidence, influence her attitude to future childbearing and delay her recovery. Although the number of maternal deaths from postpartum haemorrhage in the United Kingdom has fallen to a very low level (Department of Health et al 1991), this emergency still poses a major threat to the lives of women living in developing countries and may account for as many as a quarter to one-third of mortalities (Maine et al 1987).

The midwife is often the first and possibly the only professional person present so that her prompt, intelligent action will be crucial in controlling blood loss and safeguarding the mother's life.

Postpartum haemorrhage is defined as excessive bleeding from the genital tract at any time following the baby's birth up to 6 weeks after delivery. If it occurs during the third stage of labour or within 24 hours of delivery it is termed primary postpartum haemorrhage. This is usually a consequence of hypotonic uterine action or trauma. If bleeding occurs subsequently it is termed secondary postpartum haemorrhage.

Primary postpartum haemorrhage

Attempts have been made by several authors to define the actual quantity of blood loss to be regarded as excessive, during the first hour or two after birth. Fluid loss is extremely difficult to measure with any degree of accuracy especially when it has soaked into dressings and linen. Several studies have highlighted the resultant gross under-estimation which may represent only 50% of the true blood loss (Levy & Moore 1985, Newton et al 1961, Prendiville et al 1988). It should also be remembered that measurable solidified clots only represent about half the total fluid loss.

With these factors in mind, the best yardstick is that any blood loss, *however small*, which adversely affects the mother's condition constitutes a postpartum haemorrhage. Much will therefore depend upon the woman's general well-being. In addition, if measured loss reaches 500 ml, it must be treated as a postpartum haemorrhage, irrespective of maternal condition.

Atonic uterus

This is a failure of the myometrium at the placental site to contract and retract and to compress torn blood vessels and control blood loss by a living ligature action (see Ch. 15). When the placenta is attached, the volume of blood flow at the placental site is approximately 500–800 ml per minute. Upon separation, the efficient contraction and retraction of uterine muscle staunches the flow and prevents the dangerous haemorrhage which would otherwise ensue with horrifying speed.

There are several reasons why atonic uterine action may occur (Table 29.1).

Table 29.1
Causes of atonic uterine action

Incomplete separation of the placenta
Retained cotyledon, placental fragment or membranes
Precipitate labour
Prolonged labour resulting in uterine inertia
Polyhydramnios or multiple pregnancy causing overdistension of uterine muscle
Placenta praevia
Placental abruption
General anaesthesia especially halothane or cyclopropane
Mismanagement of the third stage of labour
A full bladder
Aetiology unknown

● **Incomplete placental separation.** If the placenta remains fully adherent it is unlikely to cause bleeding. However, once separation has begun, maternal vessels are torn. If placental tissue remains partially embedded in the spongy decidua, efficient contraction and retraction is interrupted.

● **Retained cotyledon, placental fragment or membranes** will similarly impede efficient uterine action.

● **Precipitate labour.** When the uterus has contracted vigorously during the first and second stages of labour (hypertonic action) then the muscle has insufficient opportunity to retract.

● **Prolonged labour** may result in uterine inertia due to muscle exhaustion.

● **Polyhydramnios or multiple pregnancy.** The myometrium becomes excessively stretched and therefore less efficient.

● **Placenta praevia.** The placental site is partly or wholly in the lower segment where the thinner muscle layer contains few oblique fibres: this results in poor control of bleeding.

● **Placental abruption.** Blood may have seeped between the muscle fibres, interfering with effective action. At its most severe this results in a Couvelaire uterus (Ch. 21).

● **General anaesthesia.** Anaesthetic agents may cause uterine relaxation, in particular the volatile inhalational agents, for example halothane.

● **Mismanagement of the third stage of labour.** It is salutory that this factor remains a frequent cause of postpartum haemorrhage. 'Fundus fiddling' or manipulation of the uterus may precipitate arrhythmic contractions so that the placenta only partially separates and retraction is lost.

● **A full bladder.** If the bladder is full, its proximity to the uterus in the abdomen on completion of the second stage may interfere with uterine action. This also constitutes mismanagement.

● **Aetiology unknown.** A precipitating cause may never be discovered.

There are in addition a number of factors which do not directly *cause* a postpartum haemorrhage but they increase the likelihood of excessive bleeding (Table 29.2).

● **Previous history of postpartum haemorrhage or retained placenta.** There is a risk of

Table 29.2
Predisposing factors which may increase the risks of postpartum haemorrhage

---

Previous history of postpartum haemorrhage or retained placenta
High parity resulting in uterine scar tissue
Presence of fibroids
Maternal anaemia
Keto-acidosis

---

recurrence in subsequent pregnancies. A detailed obstetric history taken at the first antenatal visit will ensure that arrangements are made for such a mother to give birth in a Consultant Unit.

- **High parity.** With each successive pregnancy fibrous tissue replaces muscle fibres in the uterus reducing its contractibility and the blood vessels become more difficult to compress. Women who have had three or more deliveries are at increased risk.
- **Fibroids.** These impede efficient uterine action.
- **Anaemia.** Women who enter labour with re-duced haemoglobin concentration (below 10 g/dl) will succumb more quickly to any subsequent blood loss, however small. Anaemia is associated with debility which is a more direct cause of uterine atony.
- **Ketosis.** The influence of ketosis upon uterine action is still unclear. Foulkes & Dumoulin (1983) demonstrated that in a series of 3500 women, 40% had ketonuria at some time during labour. They reported that if labour progressed well this did not appear to jeopardise either fetal or maternal condition. However, there was a signi-ficant relationship between ketosis and the need for Syntocinon augmentation, instrumental delivery and postpartum haemorrhage when labour lasted more than 12 hours. Correction of ketosis is therefore advisable.

Prophylaxis

In view of the serious consequences of post-partum haemorrhage, the midwife must identify women at risk and recognise causative factors. In some instances preventive measures are possible.

During the antenatal period a thorough and accurate history of previous obstetric experiences will identify risk factors, e.g. previous postpartum haemorrhage, precipitate labour. Arrangements can then be made for delivery to take place in a unit where facilities for dealing with emergencies are available. The reasons should be carefully explained. It would be most unwise to book such a woman for confinement at home or in a General Practitioner Unit.

The early detection and treatment of anaemia will help ensure that women enter labour with a haemoglobin in excess of 10 g/dl. The midwife should check that blood tests are taken regularly and the results recorded. If necessary, action is taken to restore the haemoglobin level before delivery. Mothers more prone to anaemia should be closely monitored, e.g. those with multiple pregnancies. During labour, good management of the first and second stages is important to prevent prolonged labour and keto-acidosis. A mother should not enter the second or third stage with a full bladder. An oxytocic agent may be used prophylactically for the third stage, either by intramuscular injection or intravenous infusion. Two units of cross-matched blood should be kept available for any woman known to have a placenta praevia.

Signs of postpartum haemorrhage

These may be obvious such as:

— visible bleeding
— maternal collapse.

However, more subtle signs may present:

— pallor
— rising pulse rate
— falling blood pressure
— altered level of consciousness: may become restless or drowsy
— enlarged uterus as it fills with blood or blood clot. It feels 'boggy' on palpation, i.e. soft and distended and lacking tone. There may be little or no visible loss.

Treatment

Three basic principles apply:

1. Call a doctor
2. Stop the bleeding
3. Resuscitate the mother.

Call a doctor. This is an important initial step so that help is on the way whatever transpires. If the bleeding is brought under control before the doctor arrives, his presence may appear unnecessary, but a mother's condition can deteriorate very rapidly, in which case his assistance will be required urgently. If the mother is at home or in a General Practitioner Unit, the emergency obstetric unit should be summoned.

On no account must a woman in a collapsed condition be moved prior to resuscitation.

Stop the bleeding. The initial action is always the same, regardless of whether bleeding occurs with the placenta in situ or later.

- Rub up a contraction
- Give an oxytocic
- Empty the uterus.

The skilled midwife will treat the uterus with the greatest respect. The fundus is first felt gently with the fingertips to assess its consistency. If it is soft and relaxed, the fundus is massaged with a smooth, circular motion, applying no undue pressure. When a contraction occurs, the hand is held still.

Meanwhile an oxytocic agent may be given to sustain the contraction. In many instances, Syntometrine 1 ml has already been administered and this may be repeated. Alternatively, ergometrine 0.25–0.5 mg may be injected intravenously, which will be effective in 45 seconds. No more than two doses of ergometrine should be given (including any dose of Syntometrine) as it may cause pulmonary hypertension. Several reports have described the dramatic haemostatic effects of prostaglandins used in cases of uterine atony but there is no evidence generated from controlled trials (Thiery 1986). Nevertheless its obvious benefits make it worthy of note for use in this dire emergency. The baby may be put to the breast to enhance the physiological secretion of oxytocin from the posterior lobe of the pituitary gland.

Once the midwife is satisfied that it is well contracted, she should ensure that the uterus is emptied. If the placenta is still in the uterus, it should be delivered; if it has been born, any clots should be expelled by firm but gentle pressure on the fundus.

If bleeding continues, urgent steps must be taken to prevent further deterioration of the mother's condition.

Resuscitate the mother. An intravenous infusion should be commenced while peripheral veins are easily negotiated. This will provide a route for Syntocinon infusion or fluid replacement. Both may be necessary to safeguard a mother's life. As an emergency measure the mother's legs may be lifted up in order to allow blood to drain from them into the central circulation. The foot of the bed should *not* be raised as this encourages pooling of blood in the uterus which prevents the uterus contracting.

It is usually expedient to catheterise the bladder in order to minimise trauma should an operative procedure be necessary and to exclude a full bladder as a precipitating cause of further bleeding.

The flow chart (Fig. 29.1) briefly sets out the possible courses of action which may be taken dependent upon whether or not bleeding persists. If the above measures are successful in controlling any further loss, Syntocinon, 40 units in a litre of dextrose/saline infused slowly over 8–12 hours, will ensure continued uterine contraction. This will help to minimise the risk of recurrence. Before the infusion is connected 10 ml of blood should be withdrawn for haemoglobin estimation and for cross-matching compatible blood. If bleeding continues uncontrolled, the choice of further action will depend largely upon whether the placenta remains undelivered.

Placenta delivered. If the uterus is atonic following delivery of the placenta, light fundal pressure may be used to expel residual clots whilst a contraction is stimulated. If an effective contraction is not maintained 40 units of Syntocinon in 1 litre of intravenous fluid should be commenced. The placenta and membranes must be re-examined for completeness since retained fragments are often responsible for uterine atony.

Bimanual compression. If bleeding continues bimanual compression of the uterus may be necessary in order to apply pressure to the placental site. It is desirable for an intravenous infusion to be in progress. The fingers of the right hand are inserted into the vagina like a cone; the

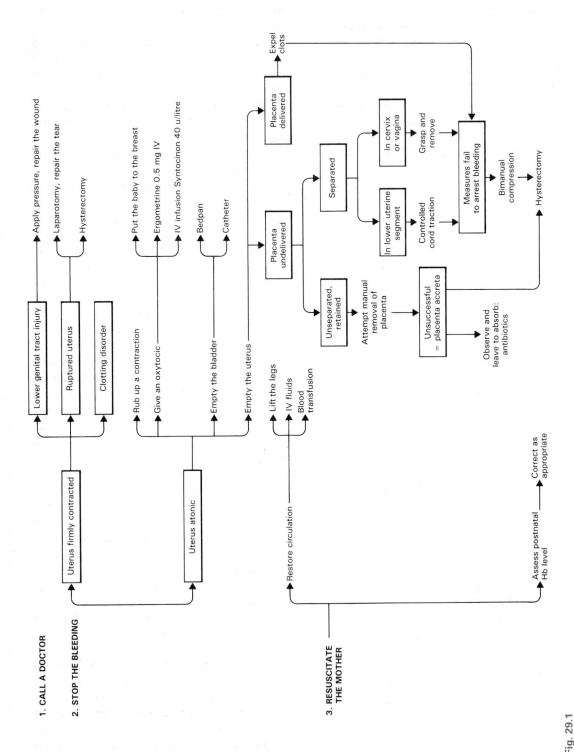

1. CALL A DOCTOR

2. STOP THE BLEEDING

Uterus firmly contracted

Lower genital tract injury → Apply pressure, repair the wound

Ruptured uterus → Laparotomy, repair the tear → Hysterectomy

Clotting disorder

Uterus atonic

Rub up a contraction

Give an oxytocic → Put the baby to the breast → Ergometrine 0.5 mg IV → IV infusion Syntocinon 40 u/litre

Empty the bladder → Bedpan → Catheter

Empty the uterus

Placenta undelivered → Placenta delivered → Expel clots

Separated → In cervix or vagina → Grasp and remove → Measures fail to arrest bleeding → Bimanual compression → Hysterectomy

In lower uterine segment → Controlled cord traction

Unseparated, retained → Attempt manual removal of placenta → Unsuccessful = placenta accreta → Observe and leave to absorb: antibiotics

3. RESUSCITATE THE MOTHER

Restore circulation → Lift the legs → IV fluids → Blood transfusion

Assess postnatal Hb level → Correct as appropriate

Fig. 29.1
Management of primary postpartum haemorrhage.

hand is formed into a fist and placed into the anterior vaginal fornix, the elbow resting on the bed. The left hand is placed behind the uterus abdominally, the fingers pointing towards the cervix. The uterus is brought forwards and compressed between the palm of the left hand and the fist in the vagina (Fig. 29.2). If bleeding persists, a clotting disorder must be excluded before exploration of the vagina and uterus is performed under a general anaesthetic.

Placenta undelivered. The placenta may be partially or wholly adherent.

Partially adherent. When the uterus is well contracted an attempt should be made to deliver the placenta by applying controlled cord traction. If this is unsuccessful a doctor will be required to remove it manually.

Completely adherent. Bleeding does not usually occur if the placenta is completely adherent. However, the longer the placenta remains in situ the greater the risk of partial separation which may give rise to profuse haemorrhage.

Retained placenta

This diagnosis is reached when the placenta remains undelivered after a specified period of time (usually half to 1 hour following the baby's

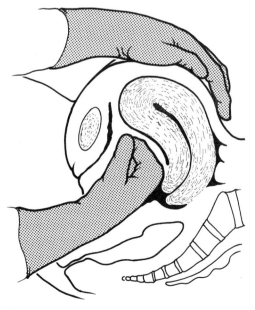

Fig. 29.2
Bimanual compression of the uterus.

birth). The conventional treatment is to digitally separate the placenta from the uterine wall, effecting a manual removal. Selinger et al (1986) noted that waiting for 1 hour before resorting to this intervention will almost halve the number of women who will require manual removal with its accompanying risks.

Manual removal of the placenta should be carried out by a doctor. An intravenous infusion must first be sited and an effective anaesthetic be in progress. The choice of anaesthesia will depend upon the mother's general condition.

If an effective epidural anaesthetic is already in progress, a top-up may be given in order to avoid the hazards of general anaesthesia. A spinal anaesthetic offers an alternative but otherwise a general anaesthetic will be induced. Details of obstetric anaesthesia are given in Chapter 28.

Management. Manual removed is performed with full aseptic precautions. With the left hand, the umbilical cord is held taut while the right hand is coned and inserted into the vagina and uterus following the direction of the cord. Once the placenta is located the cord is released so the left hand may be used to support the fundus abdominally so preventing rupture of the lower uterine segment (Fig. 29.3). The operator will feel for a separated edge of the placenta. The fingers of the right hand are extended and the border of the hand is gently eased between the placenta and the uterine wall, with the palm facing the placenta. With a sideways slicing movement the placenta is carefully detached. When the placenta is completely separated, the left hand rubs up a contraction and expels the right hand with the placenta in its grasp. The placenta should be checked immediately for completeness so that any further exploration of the uterus may be carried out without delay. An oxytocic drug is given upon completion, usually intravenous ergometrine maleate 0.25 mg.

In very exceptional circumstances when no doctor is available to be called, a midwife would be expected to carry out a manual removal of placenta. In the rare instances when this is necessary the midwife must act swiftly once she has diagnosed a retained placenta as the cause of postpartum haemorrhage in order to empty the uterus before the onset of shock and exsanguination. It

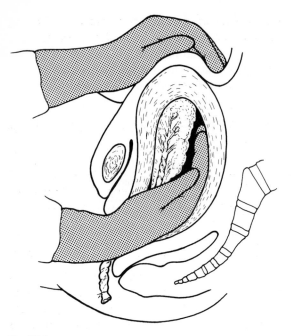

Fig. 29.3
Manual removal of placenta.

must be remembered that the risk of inducing shock by performing a manual removal of placenta is greater when no anaesthetic is given. *A Midwife's Code of Practice* (UKCC 1989) states that the midwife is unlikely to find herself dealing with this situation within the United Kingdom.

At home. If the placenta is retained following a home confinement, the emergency obstetric unit must be summoned. *Under no circumstances should a mother be transferred to hospital* until an intravenous infusion is in progress and her condition stabilised. Insufficient resuscitative measures prior to transfer have been cited as 'avoidable factors' in maternal deaths from postpartum haemorrhage (DHSS 1982).

It is advisable for the placenta to be removed in the place of delivery.

Upon completion of the third stage the mother should be transferred to a Consultant Unit for continued observation. The baby should accompany her.

Morbid adherence of placenta. Very rarely, the placenta remains morbidly adherent: this is known as *placenta accreta*. If it is totally adherent then bleeding is unlikely to occur and it may be left in situ to absorb during the puerperium. If, however, only part of the placenta remains embedded, the risks of fatal haemorrhage are high and an emergency hysterectomy may be unavoidable.

Trauma as a cause of haemorrhage

If bleeding occurs despite a well-contracted uterus it is almost certainly the consequence of trauma to the uterus, vagina, perineum or labia, or a combination of these.

In order to identify the source of bleeding the mother is placed in the lithotomy position, under a good directional light. An episiotomy wound or tears to the anterior labia, clitoris and perineum often bleed freely. These external injuries are easily identified and torn vessels may be clamped with artery forceps prior to ligation.

Internal trauma to the vagina, cervix or uterus more commonly occurs following instrumental or manipulative delivery. A speculum is inserted to enable the cervix and vagina to be clearly visualised and examined. Tissue or artery forceps may be used to apply pressure prior to suturing under general anaesthesia. If bleeding persists when the uterus is well contracted and no evidence of trauma can be found, uterine rupture must be suspected. Following a laparotomy, this is repaired but if bleeding remains uncontrolled a hysterectomy may become inevitable.

Blood coagulation disorders

As well as the causes already listed above, postpartum haemorrhage may be the result of coagulation failure which is fully discussed in Chapter 21. The failure of the blood to clot is such an obvious sign that it can be overlooked in the midst of the feverish activity which accompanies torrential bleeding. It can occur following severe pre-eclampsia, antepartum haemorrhage, amniotic fluid embolus, intra-uterine death or sepsis. Fresh blood is usually the best treatment as this will contain platelets and the coagulation factors V and VIII. The expert advice of a haematologist will be needed in assessing specific replacement products such as fresh frozen plasma and fibrinogen.

Observation of the mother following postpartum haemorrhage

Once bleeding is controlled the total volume lost must be estimated as accurately as possible. Large amounts appear less than they are in reality.

Maternal pulse and blood pressure are recorded quarter-hourly and temperature taken 4-hourly. The uterus should be palpated frequently to ensure that it remains well contracted and lochia lost must be observed. Intravenous fluid replacement should be carefully calculated to avoid circulatory overload. Monitoring the central venous pressure will provide an accurate assessment of the volume required especially if blood loss has been severe. Fluid intake and urinary output are recorded as indicators of renal function. The output should be accurately measured on an hourly basis by the use of a self-retaining urinary catheter.

The mother will usually remain in the labour ward until her condition is stable. This allows her progress to be closely monitored and, if further medical help is needed, facilities are at hand.

All records should be meticulously completed and signed as soon as possible.

Continued vigilance will be important for 24–48 hours. As this mother will need a quiet period for recuperation, a single room may be offered and visiting may be restricted to close family members. She will not be suitable for early transfer home.

Secondary postpartum haemorrhage

Secondary postpartum haemorrhage is bleeding from the genital tract more than 24 hours after delivery of the placenta and may occur up to 6 weeks later. It is most likely to occur between 10 and 14 days after delivery. Bleeding is usually due to retention of a fragment of the placenta or membranes, or the presence of a large uterine blood clot. The lochia are heavier than normal and will consist of a red loss which typically has recurred during the second week. They may also be offensive if infection is a contributory factor. Subinvolution, pyrexia and tachycardia are usually present.

The mother will be extremely alarmed by fresh bleeding if it occurs at a time when she is beginning to recover and gain in confidence following childbirth and when she is usually at home.

Management

The following steps should be taken:

- call a doctor
- rub up a contraction by massaging the uterus if it is still palpable
- express any clots
- encourage mother to empty her bladder
- give an oxytocic drug such as ergometrine maleate by intravenous or intramuscular route
- keep all pads and linen to assess the volume of blood lost
- if bleeding persists, prepare mother for theatre.

If the bleeding occurs at home and the woman has telephoned the midwife, she should be told to lie down flat until the midwife arrives (the front door should be left unlocked if the woman is alone). On arrival the midwife will assess the amount of blood loss and the mother's condition and attempt to arrest the haemorrhage. If the loss is severe or uncontrolled she will call the emergency obstetric unit and prepare mother and baby for transfer to hospital. The doctor who attends will commence an intravenous infusion and ensure that the mother's condition is stable first.

Careful assessment is usually expedient before the uterus is explored under general anaesthetic. The use of ultrasound as a diagnostic tool is invaluable in minimising the number of mothers who have operative intervention. If retained products of conception cannot be seen on scan the mother may be treated conservatively with antibiotic therapy and oral ergometrine. The haemoglobin should be estimated prior to discharge. If it is below 9 g/dl a replacement blood transfusion may be indicated. The need for a transfusion should always be thoroughly discussed with the mother and her consent obtained before proceeding.

Haematoma formation

Postpartum haemorrhage may also be concealed as the result of progressive haematoma formation. This may be obvious at such sites as the perineum or lower vagina but more difficult to diagnose if it occurs into the broad ligament or vault of the vagina. A large volume of blood may collect insidiously (up to $1\frac{1}{2}$ l). Involution and lochia are usually normal, the main symptom being increasingly severe maternal pain. This is often so acute that the haematoma has to be drained in theatre under a general anaesthetic. Secondary infection is a high possibility.

Care after a postpartum haemorrhage

Whatever the cause of the haemorrhage a mother will need the continued support of her midwife until she regains her confidence. Her partner may also be fearful of a recurrence and need much reassurance. If the mother is breast feeding, lactation may be impaired but this will only be temporary and she should be encouraged to persevere.

ACUTE INVERSION OF THE UTERUS

Inversion means that the uterus has turned inside out and it is a serious complication of the third stage (Fig. 29.4). In serious cases the inner surface of the fundus appears at the vaginal outlet. In less severe instances the fundus is dimpled.

This condition occurs in approximately 1 in 100 000 deliveries and remains a potential cause of death. A midwife's awareness of the precipitating factors enables her to take preventive measures to avoid this emergency.

Causes

Causes are all connected to applying force to the uterine fundus when it is relaxed:

- exerting controlled cord traction when the uterus is relaxed especially if the placenta is centrally sited in the fundus
- forcibly attempting to expel the placenta by using fundal pressure when the uterus is atonic
- combining fundal pressure and cord traction to deliver the placenta
- spontaneous occurrence, the cause being unknown although it is more likely to follow a delivery where a multiparous mother has pushed vigorously, or possibly has coughed or sneezed.

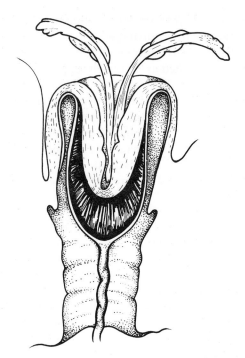

Fig. 29.4
Uterine inversion.

The first three of these causes are the *result of mismanagement* and are therefore avoidable.

Recognition

Sudden onset of shock is the outstanding sign accompanied by severe pain which is caused by the ovaries being dragged into the inverted fundus. Bleeding may or may not be present depending upon the degree of placental adherence to the uterine wall. The cause may not always be readily apparent as only in extreme cases is the fundus visible outside the vagina. Partial inversion may be present where the fundus does not pass through the cervix; it may however have extruded into the vagina. Upon palpation a concave shape will be felt at the fundus; if the inversion is complete, none of the uterus will be palpable. A vaginal examination will reveal the inversion.

Midwifery care

The best chance of replacing the uterus occurs immediately following the inversion and the midwife may need to seize this opportunity. Pressure is applied first to the part nearest the cervix, working upwards to the fundus on the principle of 'last out, first in'. No attempt is made to remove the placenta until the uterus is the right way out, otherwise haemorrhage cannot be controlled. An inverted uterus cannot contract and retract. Urgent assistance must be summoned meanwhile. If replacement of a totally inverted uterus is not possible it should be gently placed inside the vagina to relieve traction on the ovaries and fallopian tubes. Raising the foot of the bed will also help to relieve the tension and alleviate shock.

Severe shock is an immediate consequence so resuscitative meaures must be initiated prior to operative intervention. Blood is taken for cross-matching. An intravenous line must be established before the veins collapse and an infusion is commenced. Intramuscular morphine 15 mg is given for pain relief. Once the mother's condition is stable the uterus may be replaced manually under general anaesthetic or by using hydrostatic pressure. In the latter method several litres of warm saline or intravenous solution are run into the vagina via a douche nozzle held in the posterior fornix. The operator's forearm effectively seals the vaginal outlet. As the fluid pressure within the vagina rises, the uterus returns to its normal position. Intravenous ergometrine 0.25 mg should be given to secure a good contraction before the hand is withdrawn.

This manoeuvre may be complicated by the development of a retraction ring between the upper and lower segments.

The inhalation of amyl nitrite vapour may successfully relax uterine tone or a deep general anaesthetic may be necessary. In extreme cases, a hysterectomy may be considered.

SHOCK

Shock is collapse caused by failure of the mother's circulatory system to meet the body's need for oxygen, nutrients and the removal of waste substances. Shock can be acute and if quickly rectified, adverse effects may be reversed with little detriment to the mother. However, if unrecognised or inadequately treated, a chronic condition develops which leads to the residual problems of cortical or pituitary necrosis and even death. The midwife's alert observation and intelligent action are paramount in preventing or minimising the consequences.

Physiological response to shock

Sympathetic nervous system
As the pressure in the large arteries and veins falls, the sympathetic nervous system is stimulated to produce adrenalin which causes peripheral vasoconstriction. This enables blood to be shunted away from the superficial tissues (such as skin) in order to maintain the supply to the vital organs (such as the brain, heart and kidneys).

Signs. A greyish-blue skin pallor. The mother may feel cold and shivery and a sweat may be noticed on her face. Her mouth may become dry.

Respiration
The reduced blood flow through the chemoreceptors in the aortic and carotid bodies stimulates breathing.

Signs. Rapid, shallow respirations. As the mother's condition deteriorates her breathing becomes deeper and slower. She may lose consciousness.

Blood pressure
As circulating blood volume, venous return and cardiac output fall, a compensatory mechanism of arteriolar constriction initially maintains the blood pressure at normal levels; later it falls.

Signs. Blood pressure is not a reliable index of maternal condition especially if a hypertensive state already exists. Blood pressure readings may be normal, masking the severity of the collapse. Blood volume has to be reduced by 20% before blood pressure begins to fall; it only becomes unrecordable after 40% volume loss.

Pulse
The pulse rate rises in an attempt to maintain oxygenation of the tissues.

Signs. Rapid, weak pulse because stroke volume is low.

Renal system

Hypotension results in poor renal perfusion. Increased production of aldosterone and anti-diuretic hormone leads to water and salt conservation.

Signs. Reduced urinary output. In severe haemorrhage the blood supply to the kidneys may be drastically reduced. However, once blood pressure is restored to a normal level, urinary output can rapidly rise. If hypotension persists, irreversible damage and renal failure may occur.

Management

Determining the *cause* of the collapse is not of prime importance. Urgent resuscitative measures are needed before the condition becomes irreversible. In hospital, the emergency team may be summoned. If at home, the emergency obstetric service should be called.

Full assessment is urgently needed in order to take appropriate action, which is based on the need to restore maternal condition.

Maintain airway. If the mother is severely collapsed she should be turned on to her side and oxygen administered. An airway should be inserted if she is unconscious.

Replace fluids by the intravenous route having first obtained blood for cross-matching. Fresh frozen plasma or a plasma-expanding product such as Haemaccel is given until whole blood of the correct group and Rhesus factor is available.

Avoid warmth. Constriction of the peripheral blood supply is part of the physiological response to shock. Keeping the mother warm may interfere with this compensatory mechanism and cause her condition to deteriorate still further.

These life-saving measures should be taken prior to an investigation of the cause of the catastrophe.

Causes of shock

Haemorrhage

The main causes and initial treatment have been dealt with earlier in the chapter. Prompt and vigorous resuscitation and careful monitoring of the mother's condition are critical factors in helping to avert a potential disaster. The midwife's role is crucial.

In the presence of acute peripheral circulatory failure which accompanies severe shock, the monitoring of central venous pressure (CVP) aids assessment of blood loss and indicates the fluid replacement required. In such a situation it is extremely dangerous to base an intravenous regimen on guesswork. Hyper- or hypovolaemia, cardiac and renal failure may result. CVP is the pressure in the right atrium. For practical purposes it is taken as the pressure recorded in one of the great veins, usually the inferior or superior vena cava. It is an indicator of the volume of blood returning to the heart. Normal pressure varies between 5 and 10 cm H_2O. In shock, the pressure will be persistently low, i.e. below 5 cm and may even register a negative reading, indicating hypovolaemia. The correct volume of replacement fluids may then be assessed with greater accuracy.

Method of measuring central venous pressure (CVP). The mother should lie supine and remain in this position. A long-line, wide-bore catheter, for example a silastic catheter, size 14G, 36 cm length is used. This is passed into an accessible large vein such as the subclavian or external jugular vein and advanced into the right atrium. It is then connected to a manometer and an infusion apparatus with a three-way tap. The calibrating tape is adjusted to the drip stand so that 0 cm of water is at the level of the right atrium. The saline in the manometer will fall and rise in response to respiratory effort. The height of the fluid in the manometer above the mid-axillary line equals the CVP and thus indicates how much replacement fluid is required (Fig. 29.5).

The manometer requires close and constant supervision. Potential complications include air embolus, pneumothorax, hydrothorax, thrombosis, infection and trauma to lung or veins. Cardiac arrhythmia during insertion is not uncommon. The expert care required may necessitate this mother's transfer to an intensive therapy unit.

Endotoxic shock

Endotoxic shock is caused by septicaemia. Gram-negative organisms such as *Escherichia coli*,

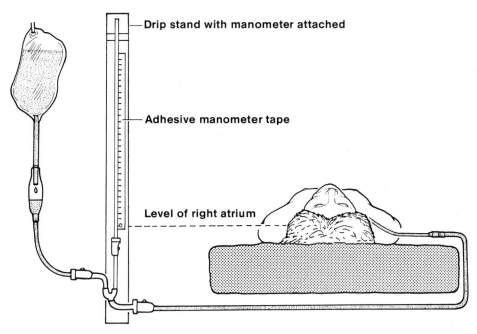

Drip stand with manometer attached

Adhesive manometer tape

Level of right atrium

Fig. 29.5
Monitoring central venous pressure.

Bacillus proteus and *Pseudomonas pyocyaneus* are common pathogens present in the genital tract. When their cell walls are destroyed they release endotoxins. The precise action of these substances is unclear but they are cytotoxic to the leucocytes and cause severe vasoconstriction. Disseminated intravascular coagulation may ensue.

The place of entry is usually the placental site especially following septic abortion, prolonged rupture of the membranes, obstetric trauma or retained placental tissue.

Signs. All the signs of shock are present although initially the skin may be flushed and the mother pyrexial and alert. Haemorrhage may be superimposed.

Management. This is based on preventing further deterioration by restoring circulatory volume and eradicating infection. A full infection screen should be carried out including a high vaginal swab, midstream specimen of urine and blood cultures. Carefully calculated bolus doses of intravenous antibiotics are usually given with due regard to the nephrotoxic effects of such drugs as gentamicin. An ultrasound scan will reveal whether products of conception are retained

in the uterus prior to attempted evacuation. Urinary output must be accurately measured and recorded.

Amniotic fluid embolism

This is a very rare occurrence, 1:60 000 maternities, but the fatality rate is as high as 86% (Mulder 1985). Amniotic fluid may enter the maternal circulation during separation of the placenta. It usually occurs as a consequence of hypertonic uterine contractions in multiparous labours. Other factors are the injudicious use of oxytocics, polyhydramnios and placental abruption. Amniotic fluid contains high levels of thromboplastins which precipitate intravascular coagulation. The signs are of dramatic onset followed by a profound degree of shock. Tragically the diagnosis is most often confirmed on postmortem examination by the presence of amniotic squamous cells, lanugo and possibly even meconium in the occlusive thrombi most clearly evident in the lungs.

The *Report on Confidential Enquiries into Maternal Deaths in the United Kingdom* 1985–87 (DH et al 1991) cites nine direct deaths due to amniotic fluid embolism confirmed on histological examination. In realistic terms, this may be an underestimation as amniotic fluid embolus may have been the underlying cause of some of the reported cases of fatal blood coagulation defect.

Signs. These may present during labour or may be delayed, notably following caesarean section. The condition is characterised by shivering, sweating and coughing with ensuing pink, frothy sputum. Severe chest pain and dyspnoea may occur as the result of the occlusion of pulmonary vessels. If the mother survives the cardiopulmonary collapse, intravascular coagulation and haemorrhage usually develop (Ch. 27).

Treatment. Oxygen therapy and the restoration of circulatory volume are urgent. Fresh frozen plasma or fresh whole blood is used to supply much-needed clotting factors. Intravenous heparin may also be given to prevent further abnormal clotting although its use is debatable and controversial. Morphia should be given to relieve pain. Intravenous oxytocic agents are used if there is uterine atony, to secure good uterine contraction.

Coincidental shock

This may be due to factors not directly associated with pregnancy including coronary thrombosis, pneumothorax, cerebrovascular accident and abdominal emergencies such as ruptured ovarian cyst. Adverse reaction to a blood transfusion and anaphylactic shock during Imferon infusion should not be overlooked.

Water intoxication

This occurs as a consequence of interventionalist obstetrics and is a relatively recent complication of labour. The main causes are interrelated:

Prolonged infusion of Syntocinon. This oxytocic drug has an anti-diuretic action which leads to hyponatraemia. Feeney (1982) suggests that the quantity of infused fluid is more important than the oxytocin concentration. However, the two factors appear to be linked and can increase the risks of water intoxication.

Prolonged administration of intravenous dextrose. Dahlenburg et al (1980) found significantly lower sodium levels in both mother and

fetus in those women receiving more than 3500 ml of dextrose solution during labour. Water intoxication may be a consequence. Particular caution is needed in expanding intravascular volume in women with pre-eclampsia, especially if urinary output is poor.

Signs. The signs include generalised oedema, tachycardia, increasing drowsiness, fits and coma as a result of cerebral oedema. These latter signs are similar to those of eclampsia. Differential diagnosis is confirmed by blood electrolyte estimations. Great accuracy in the calculation and monitoring of intravenous fluids and recognition of the avoidable risks of overtransfusion are therefore important responsibilities for the midwife.

Complications of shock

If the signs of maternal collapse are not swiftly recognised, reversed and the underlying cause corrected, irreversible damage may occur. Even if death is averted, increased morbidity can drastically reduce the quality of life of the individual with tragic consequences for the entire family.

Anaemia. This is easily remedied. A haemoglobin estimation must be made 3–4 days following delivery. If below 9 g/dl, then blood transfusion may be indicated. If above this level, oral iron or i.m. Jectofer will probably be adequate.

Acute renal failure. This may occur as the result of the hypovolaemia which leads to tubular necrosis. Very small volumes of bloodstained urine are passed followed by anuria. Spontaneous and complete recovery may occur due to regeneration of the damaged tubules. In severe cases there is renal cortical necrosis which is irreversible and usually fatal due to uraemia unless regular dialysis is available.

Sheehan's syndrome due to anterior pituitary necrosis. This is a rare complication associated with prolonged shock. Death may occur soon after delivery or the onset of symptoms may be delayed for several years. All the endocrine functions of the anterior pituitary gland are disturbed giving a clinical picture of Simmond's disease. Prolactin deficiency causes lactation to fail, lack of thyrotrophic hormone results in lethargy, sensitivity to cold and weight gain, and deficiency of gonadotrophic hormones leads to amenorrhoea and atrophy of the breasts. The woman ages prematurely. Once necrosis has occurred, supplementary endocrine substitutes may be given to maintain the mother in health. The disaster of anterior pituitary necrosis can be prevented by the prompt and vigorous treatment of maternal shock.

Infection. This is a very real danger following invasive procedures especially intra-uterine manipulation and urinary catheterisation. The effect is to delay the mother's recovery and reduce her chances of successful breast feeding. Bacteriological culture and sensitivities should be requested prior to the use of antibiotics to reduce the risk of resistant strains of bacteria developing.

Psychological effects. Any complication which occurs during labour is a frightening experience. When it arises following an apparently safe delivery the effects can be devastating. Fear of a recurrence may reduce the mother's confidence to move around and care for herself and her baby. Great support and understanding are required to build up physical strength and emotional security. Adequate sleep and a good nutritious diet are positive aids to recovery. A careful explanation of events must be offered to both partners and should include discussion of future pregnancies. This mother may benefit from postnatal midwifery care for the full 28 days.

EMERGENCY OBSTETRIC UNIT

This rapidly vanishing service is a feature of obstetric practice in Britain where women may deliver their babies at home or in small units where emergency obstetric cover is not available round the clock. The service is usually manned by staff from a nearby Consultant Unit who are alerted by telephone. The team comprises a senior obstetrician, an anaesthetist, an experienced midwife and a paediatrician. The emergency equipment usually includes anaesthetic facilities, intravenous infusion pack, blood of group O Rh negative, Hartmann's solution, oxytocic agents and equipment for instrumental delivery and manual removal of placenta. A full range of maternal and pae-

diatric resuscitative drugs is also available: expiry dates must be monitored and fresh supplies obtained as needed. A portable incubator may be taken if a paediatric emergency arises. All equipment must be checked frequently. Transport is usually supplied by the ambulance service or in some instances a specially equipped car is available.

The most common emergencies for which this service is alerted are antepartum and postpartum haemorrhages. A midwife may summon the obstetric flying squad at her own discretion. Clear travelling directions must be given to avoid unnecessary delay in reaching the home.

Meticulous record keeping of all events and exact times is essential.

In areas where the emergency obstetric unit has been withdrawn, the ambulance service usually provides specially trained paramedic teams.

Reader Activities

- What special advice could be given to reassure a woman who presents with a history of an acute emergency during a previous delivery? What steps can be taken to minimise the risks of recurrence?
- Wherever you work, is information related to the local incidence of both primary and secondary postpartum haemorrhage made available to the midwives? Can you think of a way in which these data could be used as the basis for discussion on issues of management by you and your colleagues? This may require obtaining statistics about gynaecology as well as maternity admissions.
- In your unit, what advice is given to women in relation to their general health following a postpartum haemorrhage?

REFERENCES

Dahlenburg G W, Burnell R H, Braybrook R 1980 The relation between cord serum sodium levels in newborn infants and maternal intravenous therapy during labour. British Journal of Obstetrics and Gynaecology 87: 519–522

Department of Health and Social Security 1982 Report on confidential enquiries into maternal deaths in England and Wales 1976–78. HMSO, London

Department of Health, Welsh Office, Scottish Home and Health Department, Department of Health and Social Services, Northern Ireland 1991 Report on confidential enquiries into maternal deaths in the United Kingdom 1985–87. HMSO, London

Feeney J G 1982 Water intoxication and oxytocin. British Medical Journal 285: 243

Foulkes J, Dumoulin J G 1983 Ketosis in labour. British Journal of Hospital Medicine 29(6) June: 562–564

Levy V, Moore J 1985 The midwife's management of the third stage of labour. Nursing Times 81(39): 47–50

Maine D, Rosenfield A, Wallace M, Kimball A M, Kwast B, Papiernik E, White S 1987 Prevention of maternal deaths in developing countries: program options and practical considerations. Centre for Population and Family Health, University of Colombia, New York

Mulder J I 1985 Amniotic fluid embolism: an overview and case report. American Journal of Obstetrics and Gynecology 152(4): 430–435

Newton M, Mosey L M, Egli G E, Gifford W B, Hull C T 1961 Blood loss during and immediately after delivery. Obstetrics and Gynaecology 17(1): 9–18

Prendiville W J, Elbourne D R, Chalmers I 1988 The Bristol third stage trial: active versus physiological management of the third stage of labour. British Medical Journal 297: 1295–1300

Selinger M, MacKenzie K, Dunlop P, James D 1986 Intra-umbilical vein oxytocin in the management of retained placenta. A double blind controlled study. Journal of Obstetrics and Gynaecology 7: 115–117

Thiery M 1986 Prostaglandins for the treatment of hypotonic postpartum haemorrhage. Prostaglandin Perspectives 2: 10

United Kingdom Central Council for Nursing, Midwifery and Health Visiting 1989 A midwife's code of practice. UKCC, London (Reprinted 1991)

FURTHER READING

Clayton S G, Lewis J L T, Pinker G (eds) 1980 Postpartum haemorrhage and abnormalities of the third stage. In: Obstetrics by ten teachers, 13th edn. Edward Arnold, London

Hibbard B 1981 Shock in obstetrics. Nursing Mirror 153 (11) Sept 9: ix–xiv

Hibbard B 1981 Complications associated with shock in obstetrics. Nursing Mirror 153 (11) Sept 9: xv–xvii

Prendiville W, Elbourne D 1989 Care during the third stage of labour. In: Chalmers I, Enkin M, Keirse M J N C (eds) Effective care in pregnancy and childbirth. Oxford University Press, Oxford

30

Complications of the puerperium

JEAN A. BALL

Maternal complications may arise during the puerperium as a result of trauma sustained during labour, disorders of the circulatory system or psychological disorders. The secret of effective care lies in the prevention of complications wherever possible and in the identification of problems so that prompt treatment can be given.

EFFECTS OF TRAUMA SUSTAINED DURING LABOUR

The soft tissues of the reproductive and urinary tracts may sustain trauma as a result of pressure from the presentation during labour and delivery. The soft tissues include muscle layers and blood vessels which may suffer bruising and oedema. Trauma may be particularly marked when manipulation of the fetus has been necessary. Recent research suggests that vacuum extraction involves less trauma than the use of forceps for delivery (Vacca & Keirse 1989).

All soft tissue trauma produces devitalised tissue which provides an ideal environment for pathogenic organisms and this may lead to puerperal infection. Trauma also increases the likelihood of clot formation and thrombo-embolic disorders.

Trauma to the perineum, vulva, vagina and anus

Tears of the perineum are graded according to their severity:

First degree tears involve the vaginal mucosa and the skin of the perineum.

Second degree tears involve the deeper layers of perineal muscle.

Third degree tear or an extended episiotomy is one in which the anal margin has been involved.

Fourth degree tears involve the anal sphincter and mucosa.

Other areas of trauma may be the cervix and extended tears of the vagina, neither of which may be readily visible when inspecting the perineum following delivery. Minor trauma to the cervix does not usually cause complications but larger tears give rise to persistent bleeding. A cervical tear may be diagnosed when the woman continues to bleed per vaginam even when the uterus is well contracted. Such bleeding can lead to hypovolaemic shock, so the condition requires prompt attention. Vaginal tears cause considerable pain although the amount of subsequent blood loss is variable.

Occasionally, rupture of a blood vessel may lead to the formation of a vulval haematoma. This takes the form of a tender purple swelling in the vulva or occasionally in the vagina itself. Large haematomas cause severe pain and may lead to shock.

The repair of any perineal tear requires skilled technique if permanent damage is not to be sustained. Scar tissue may cause pain during coitus and predispose to further tears in subsequent labours. A third degree tear may lead to the formation of a rectovaginal fistula.

Repair of trauma

It is very important that the various layers are sutured carefully in order to prevent scarring.

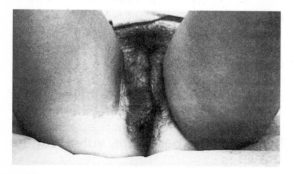

Fig. 30.1
Extensive bruising of the vulva, vagina and perineum following evacuation of a vulvovaginal haematoma.

Effective anaesthesia is essential before undertaking any repair. Second degree tears are generally sutured following perineal infiltration (see Ch. 14): the repair of third or fourth degree tears is usually carried out under general anaesthetic.

Recent research (Grant 1989, Sleep 1990) has shown that polyglycolic acid sutures (Dexon or Vicril) inserted as continuous, sub-cuticular stitches produce less discomfort than chromic catgut and interrupted stitches. The former technique, however, requires considerable skill.

Vulval or vaginal haematomas are treated by evacuation of the clot under general anaesthetic. If the bleeding blood vessel can be found it is ligatured. Firm pressure is put on the area. When severe bleeding has occurred a blood transfusion may be necessary.

Continuing care

Care should be directed to the relief of pain and discomfort, the prevention of infection and promotion of healing. Sleep (1990) has identified effective and ineffective methods of pain relief.

Oral analgesia. Paracetamol is the analgesic of choice in most cases. Ibuprofen is also effective and may be prescribed. Preparations containing codeine should be avoided because they cause constipation.

Topical methods. Sleep (1990) found that mothers said that soaking in a warm bath produced the most effective relief of pain and was preferred to the use of a bidet. The use of crushed ice may impair the healing process and should be used with caution. Local anaesthetic such as 5% lignocaine spray or gel is also effective and gives relief over a longer period of time. Steroid preparations should be avoided.

Physiotherapy. In recent years the application of Megapulse (pulsed electromagnetic energy), infra-red heat and ultrasound have been used by physiotherapists to relieve pain and promote healing. At present there are scanty research data to support these techniques. An intensive programme of pelvic floor exercises appears to result in reduced pain.

However, as Sleep (1990) points out, any or all of these measures provide a vehicle for sympathetic, individualised concern and this attention and care brings benefit to the mother.

Promoting healing. Careful hygiene is important; the mother should be encouraged to bathe as frequently as she wishes in order to ensure a clean wound and relief of discomfort. Care should be taken to dry the perineum after bathing. Mothers should be encouraged to walk about as they feel able. Sitting is often uncomfortable and discomfort may be relieved by the use of air rings or cushions. Mothers may find that lying on one side in bed is the most comfortable position for feeding the baby.

Care of third and fourth degree tears

Women who have sustained third degree tears are usually given a low residue diet for the first few days in order to prevent any further damage due to straining to pass a stool. After 3 days a glycerine suppository may be given to aid defaecation. It is usual thereafter to encourage a high residue diet in order to produce a bulky stool which is easier to expel. The main danger of a third degree tear is the formation of a rectovaginal fistula, leading to the expulsion of faeces per vaginam. This is not a common occurrence in the Western nations, but may be seen more frequently in the Third World where traumatic interference in labour may occur. The formation of a fistula is more likely in debilitated or malnourished women. Such a fistula is extremely difficult to heal and causes considerable distress to any woman. In certain cultures it may lead to her rejection and isolation.

Lack of healing

If the perineal wound becomes infected or if sloughing appears, some of the sutures may be removed to allow any pus or fluid to drain away from the wound. When the perineum does not heal by first intention the mother will need careful attention for some time. The perineum may heal but take a number of weeks to do so. Alternatively it may need to be re-sutured under general anaesthetic. If this occurs it is usual to wait for the resolution of any infection before the scar is incised and the tissues re-aligned and re-sutured.

Trauma in the urinary tract

During prolonged labour the presentation may cause considerable pressure upon the urethra and the base of the bladder, leading to bruising and oedema and this may lead to spasm of the internal sphincter. Severe pressure may lead to necrosis of the internal tissues and cause the formation of a vesicovaginal fistula.

Retention of urine. Any trauma may lead to retention of urine and chronic loss of muscle and sphincter tone. Retention of urine is most marked immediately after delivery. It causes considerable discomfort and if not relieved may go on to the stage of retention with overflow. When this occurs there is leaking of urine from the overdistended bladder. Such distension will put further strain upon the internal sphincter muscles predisposing to chronic urinary incontinence.

Catheterisation. Where retention with overflow or severe retention occurs it is usual to treat it by inserting a self-retaining catheter. If the bladder contains in excess of 1 litre of urine, it is not emptied immediately. The catheter is spigotted and released at intervals to drain a further half litre at a time. When the bladder is empty the catheter may be left open to drain freely into a collection bag for 24 hours. Prior to removal, the catheter is closed off and released intermittently to follow the normal pattern of the bladder being filled and emptied which aids the recovery of muscle tone. The catheter is usually removed after 48 hours.

Re-establishing micturition. Micturition may be painful after the removal of the catheter but the mother must be urged to pass urine frequently in order to maintain the regained tone and prevent further distension. A woman requires a great deal of encouragement because she may fear that she has lost control over her bladder, and it must be remembered that the psychological and reflex control of micturition is as important as the physical control.

The woman's intake and output of fluids should be measured and recorded in order to make certain that an appropriate volume of urine is being expelled. Ambulation should be encouraged.

PUERPERAL PYREXIA AND INFECTION

Puerperal pyrexia

A raised temperature accompanied by a rising pulse rate is a cardinal sign of puerperal infection.

In some cases the tachycardia may be the primary indicator.

Puerperal pyrexia arises from infection of the genital or urinary tract or the breasts, or inflammation of the veins. Mild pyrexia may be associated with breast engorgement or with intercurrent infections such as the common cold.

Although it is no longer notifiable, the midwife should inform the doctor if pyrexia occurs.

The use of antibiotics has greatly reduced the number of deaths due to puerperal pyrexia but the midwife and doctor must not become complacent about this condition and overlook its potential danger. Infection can still be a fatal condition in spite of widespread use of antibiotics. Four women died of genital tract sepsis in the puerperium during the triennium 1985–87 in the UK, two of them following caesarean section. Onset can be insidious and fever is not always present (DH 1991).

Investigations by the midwife

Upon discovery of a puerperal pyrexia, the midwife must examine the mother carefully to elicit any signs which will help to locate the site of infection. She will interview the woman to ask her how she feels and to identify any symptoms which are significant such as headache, sneezing, coughing, burning on micturition, painful breasts and so on. She makes a physical examination which includes inspection and palpation of the breasts, palpation of the uterus to see whether it is tender or bulky, inspection of the lochia and perineum and examination of the legs. It is often an established policy that the midwife will proceed to collect laboratory specimens such as throat swab, high vaginal swab and midstream specimen of urine. The midwife reports any abnormalities to the doctor.

Puerperal infection

Puerperal infection arises as a result of the invasion, incubation and multiplication of an organism and does not therefore normally occur until 24 hours or more after delivery. The effects which an infection has will depend upon the virulence of the causative organism and the mother's degree of resistance.

Causative organisms

These are classified in two groups: endogenous organisms and exogenous organisms.

Endogenous organisms are normally present in the body, where they do no harm and have a role to play in the ecology of the body. *Escherichia coli* inhabits the bowel and the healthy vagina, *Streptococcus faecalis* lives in the anus and on the perineum, anaerobic streptococci and *Clostridium welchii* are found in the vagina. Some organisms are called anaerobic because they flourish in the absence of oxygen. The presence of bruised, lacerated and oedematous tissue therefore provides an ideal environment for them to multiply. For this reason puerperal infection caused by these organisms is most likely to occur in women who have had a difficult forceps delivery or an emergency caesarean section and in those who are debilitated and anaemic.

Exogenous organisms, as their name implies, come from sources outside the body and are usually transmitted by another person. The source of puerperal infection arising from their activity may be the midwife, doctor, other attendants, other patients or visitors. These organisms are spread by touch or by droplet infection and are also found in the dust of hospitals.

Haemolytic streptococcus A is still a potential source of grave infection in vulnerable, debilitated patients. A member of staff or a visitor to the ward may be harbouring a virulent strain of this organism in a sore throat and such a source may easily infect a whole ward.

Staphylococcus aureus is often the cause of septic spots and minor skin infections. Most breast infections are staphylococcal. The organism is commonly found in dust and has developed considerable resistance to antibiotics in recent years.

Signs and symptoms of genital tract infection

Pyrexia is usually the first sign, occurring 24 hours or more after delivery and accompanied by a rising pulse rate. The onset may be sudden and accompanied by rigor or may be more gradual with the temperature and pulse rate rising each day. The pulse rate is significant and in the case of infection by *haemolytic streptococci* a rising pulse rate may be the first sign occurring before pyrexia is manifested. In some cases of infection by *haemolytic streptococci*, no marked rise in the temperature is seen.

The uterus is tender on palpation. The lochia *may be offensive* and suppuration of lacerations and of the suture line may be visible.

In the case of infection by *haemolytic streptococci*, the lochia will be scanty only 24 hours after delivery and may not be at all offensive initially. There may be little sign of external infection and indeed the woman may develop serious pelvic infection or septicaemia whilst the perineum continues to heal.

In the case of infection due to *Clostridium welchii*, the onset may be heralded by collapse, blood in the urine and a developing jaundice.

Effects of genital tract infection

Localised infection is seen in infected wounds and occasionally abscesses form.

Pelvic infection occurs as a result of ascending spread of infection from the perineum, vagina or cervix to the uterine cavity. From there it may spread to the fallopian tubes causing salpingitis and possible blockage of the tubes. It may also spread into the peritoneum. A patient who develops salpingitis or peritonitis becomes severely ill, with a thready pulse, pain on abdominal palpation, vomiting and diarrhoea leading to rapid dehydration. Lateral spread invades the parametrium and leads to pelvic cellulitis.

A virulent strain of *haemolytic streptococcus A* may rapidly infect the entire peritoneal cavity and gain access to the systemic circulation via the placental site causing septicaemia and haemolytic anaemia. The patient becomes acutely ill from the toxins produced by the organism and the pericardium, pleura and even the synovial membranes of the joints may be involved. Septicaemia causes rigor and persistent high fever, and the patient is gravely ill.

Investigations, treatment and prevention of spread

Any pyrexia following birth or miscarriage which persists for 24 hours should be regarded as an infection of the genital tract until proved otherwise.

Investigation

A full general examination is made by the doctor.

A high vaginal swab and midstream specimen of urine are sent to the laboratory. In taking a high vaginal swab the midwife or doctor should use a speculum to distend the vagina and enable the sample to be taken as high in the vagina and as near to the cervix as possible. No antiseptic lotion or cream should be applied and the midwife must use sterile gloves.

The purpose of these samples is to establish the source and cause of the infection and the sensitivity of the causative organisms to various antibiotics.

The culture of the organisms which is necessary to obtain this information will take 48 hours and the doctor may prescribe a broad spectrum antibiotic such as ampicillin or co-trimoxazole (Septrin) in the meantime.

Treatment

Antibiotic therapy should be commenced as soon as possible. Careful records should be kept of fluid intake and output. If the woman is severely ill and has been dehydrated an intravenous infusion may be necessary.

Analgesics may be given to relieve pain.

The woman's haemoglobin estimation should be checked to exclude anaemia as a predisposing or complicating factor. Where anaemia is present, appropriate treatment should be commenced and in cases of serious infection a blood transfusion may be given.

If there are signs of suppuration of lacerations or incisions of the vagina and perineum the sutures should be clipped in order to allow drainage. Localised infections and sloughing may be treated by applications of hydrogen peroxide.

The mother needs good nursing care and regular bathing or sponging to reduce pyrexia and increase comfort. If the mother is able to use the bidet or bath she should have one reserved for her use only. The vulval pads must be changed frequently. A light nourishing diet should be given and the mother protected from any unnecessary stress and overtiredness. The baby should not be removed from the mother's bedside unless she is severely ill but the midwife or other nursing staff should undertake most of the care of the baby.

Women diagnosed as suffering from puerperal infection are normally isolated from other mothers until such time as the cause has been identified, treatment has commenced and the temperature has returned to normal. The length of isolation will depend upon the severity of the infection and the causative organism. Every effort must be made to prevent cross-infection and in some cases it will be necessary to institute barrier nursing techniques.

Breast infection

Acute puerperal mastitis is inflammation of the breast. It is extremely painful and may lead to abscess formation.

The most common infecting organism is *Staphylococcus aureus*. The most likely source of the infection is the baby and outbreaks of skin and eye infections among babies are frequently due to *Staphylococcus aureus*. Organisms are transmitted by cross-infection and can easily affect a whole ward.

Mastitis arises in two ways: infection may enter via a cracked nipple and spread through the inter-lobular tissue or it may arise from a multiplication of organisms already present in the breast itself. This may happen when the breast has been bruised by careless handling or when there has been engorgement and stasis of milk.

Signs and symptoms

Mastitis may arise at any time in the puerperium but it is unusual to find it occurring before the 8th postnatal day. The onset is rapid with a sharp rise in the temperature which can reach as high as 40°C. The pulse is rapid and the woman complains of throbbing pain and tenderness in the affected breast. On examination a wedge-shaped, indurated and reddened area of the breast is seen.

Investigations and treatment

A sample of breast milk is sent for bacteriological examination and a broad spectrum antibiotic is given until the causative organism is known.

Breast feeding should be suspended if pus is found in the milk and the breast is emptied by the gentle use of a breast pump or hand expression. The breast must be gently but firmly supported and large pads of cotton wool used to protect the painful infected area. If the infection is mild, breast feeding may be continued as the anti-infective properties of the milk protect the baby.

Breast abscess

Acute puerperal mastitis may lead to abscess formation. If this occurs the affected breast is extremely painful, oedema is usually present and the breast becomes tense and red. The axillary glands become tender and enlarged. The abscess must be incised and drained to prevent spread into other areas of the breast which would cause damage.

Prevention

Breast infections are a serious and painful complication of the puerperium. The best method of treatment lies in prevention. The organisms causing breast infections are usually passed from baby to mother. It follows that scrupulous attention to hand washing and hygiene will both lower the incidence of infection among babies and reduce the risk of breast infection in mothers. Rooming-in has the effect of partially isolating the mother and baby together. Midwives and doctors must be aware that they are a potential means of cross-infection and they must maintain cleanliness and wash their hands before attending to a mother or a baby.

Urinary tract infection

Urinary tract infection is a common problem during pregnancy (see Ch. 22). Its cause lies in the stasis of urine which occurs during pregnancy and encourages the formation of a reservoir of organisms. Trauma during labour or inadequate vulval hygiene leading to an ascending infection predisposes to its recurrence during the puerperium. Such recurrent infections may lead to chronic pyelonephritis. The causative organism is usually *Escherichia coli.*

Signs and symptoms

Mild infection gives rise to malaise, aches and pains in the back and loins, and in some cases pain on micturition. The temperature may not be raised.

More severe infection may consist of either acute cystitis, characterised by scalding on micturition, or pyelonephritis which causes a raised temperature, pain over the kidney and haematuria.

Investigation and treatment

A midstream specimen of urine is obtained for bacteriological investigation. The infection is treated by the use of the appropriate antibiotic: ampicillin, nitrofurantoin (Furadantin) or nalidixic acid (Negram).

A well tried and useful method of additional treatment is the oral administration of potassium citrate mixture. *E. coli* thrives in acid urine; the mixture makes the urine alkaline which inhibits its growth.

Prevention

Chronic pyelonephritis leads to damage in the kidney. It may be prevented by the prompt treatment at the first indication of a urinary tract infection and by ensuring that the woman completes the course of prescribed antibiotic. It has been found that many women have a reservoir of organisms present in their urine but these do not cause any signs or symptoms of disease (Wang & Smaill 1989). These organisms may multiply and cause infection when the woman is less fit than normal or in the presence of stale urine or ascending infection. This condition is known as asymptomatic bacteriuria and should be screened for in early pregnancy. A bacterial count of 100 000 per ml of urine is considered significant and treatment by a course of antibiotics should be given. The bacterial count should then be re-assessed and the treatment repeated until the bacterial count is satisfactory.

THROMBO-EMBOLIC DISORDERS

Thrombosis

Thrombosis in the parturient woman is significant because of the risk of pulmonary embolism, still one of the major causes of maternal death, chiefly in the puerperium.

Pulmonary embolism is caused by the detachment of the whole or part of a large clot from the thrombosed vein which enters the cardiovascular system and causes obstruction of the pulmonary circulation. If the clot or thrombus is large, death may occur without any warning. In other cases pulmonary embolism causes severe chest pain, dyspnoea and shock. The patient is in great danger and requires urgent assistance and treatment.

Causes of thrombosis in pregnancy and the puerperium

Research indicates that thrombosis is five times more likely to occur in pregnant and parturient women than in non-pregnant women of the same age group (Letsky 1985).

This is due to the increased clotting tendency of the blood which is found during pregnancy in addition to the venous stasis which occurs because of progesterone activity. A fast-flowing bloodstream inhibits clotting; stasis favours it. (Refer to Ch. 21 for a full explanation of clotting.)

Predisposing factors

The evidence arising from the investigation of maternal deaths indicates that certain conditions increase the likelihood of venous thrombosis and the danger of pulmonary embolism. These are:

— caesarean section
— age over 35 years
— high parity
— obesity
— the use of oestrogens to suppress lactation.

In addition, general predisposing factors should be borne in mind, such as:

— smoking
— immobility
— trauma to the legs.

Prevention of thrombosis

Activity and exercise. All women should be encouraged to be as active as possible during pregnancy and in the later stages, when walking becomes uncomfortable, to sit with feet raised and to do leg and ankle exercises.

After delivery, mothers should be encouraged to walk about as soon as possible and to do post-natal exercises. It is important that mothers move about rather than sit at the bedside. The use of loose flat slippers in which the mother has a shuffling rather than a walking gait should be discouraged.

Women who have had caesarean sections or who are unable to move about freely because of peri-neal trauma should be encouraged to do leg and ankle exercises whilst lying in bed.

Prevention of trauma to lower limbs and pelvic veins. During labour exhaustion and de-hydration should be avoided. If necessary, intra-venous fluids should be given. Care must be taken to avoid trauma to the veins of the legs by careless handling or by pressure from the stirrups used to hold the legs in lithotomy position. No woman should be placed in the lithotomy posi-tion unnecessarily nor left there longer than is absolutely essential.

It is particularly important that care is taken to avoid bruising the legs of an unconscious or heavily sedated woman when moving her from the trolley to the theatre table or delivery bed and that the legs or feet of an unconscious woman are not allowed to lie heavily upon one another.

Prophylactic treatment. In women whose his-tory suggests that they may be particularly at risk of thrombosis, prophylactic treatment with low doses of anticoagulants may be given. The pre-ferred anticoagulant is heparin because its effects can be more readily reversed than those of oral preparations such as warfarin.

During early and late pregnancy warfarin is also contra-indicated because it passes the placental barrier. If antepartum or intranatal haemorrhage occurs due to the heparin its effect can be reversed by giving protamine sulphate solution 10 mg/ml. The dosage depends on the amount of heparin given and the time lapse since administration.

Anticoagulant therapy is then continued during the puerperium. The effects of anticoagulant therapy are carefully monitored by assessment of the clotting time of the blood and the dosage is regulated according to the results.

Identification of early signs of thrombosis

Successful treatment of thrombosis and prevention of embolism depends upon early diagnosis and prompt action.

An examination of the legs and enquiry about any pain or discomfort in the calves should form part of the midwife's daily postnatal examination of the mother. Unfortunately, however, some thromboses give rise to neither signs nor symptoms.

The risk of thrombosis and the action to be taken to prevent it should be part of the mother's postnatal care plan.

There are two main types of thrombosis during the puerperium:

- superficial thrombophlebitis
- deep vein thrombosis.

Superficial thrombophlebitis

This affects the superficial veins of the legs and can be plainly seen. The vein is tender; it becomes red and hard. The temperature and pulse may be raised. This form of thrombophlebitis mainly affects varicose veins. It does not normally lead to pulmonary embolism. However, it is more likely to occur in older, more overweight women who may also be of high parity. It is important therefore that the diagnosis of superficial thrombophlebitis does not obscure the possibility that such women may also develop deep vein thrombosis.

Superficial thrombophlebitis should be treated by applying a supportive bandage. The application of a preparation of glycerine and ichthyol to the affected vein reduces pain and redness. There is no need for exercise to be restricted but it is helpful if the legs are elevated when the mother is sitting. Anticoagulant therapy is not necessary.

Deep vein thrombosis

It is thrombosis of the deep veins of the calf, thigh or pelvis which gives rise to the danger of pulmonary embolism. The clinical signs of a deep vein thrombosis depend upon the extent of the thrombosis and whether or not phlebitis is also present. If the clot or thrombus is not obstructing the blood vessel there may be no clinical signs at all. Unfortunately, it is this type of thrombus which is most likely to become detached.

Deep vein thrombosis is usually manifest during the first 2 weeks after delivery. There may be pain or discomfort in the calf or thigh and this is increased when dorsiflexion of the foot is undertaken (Homan's sign). There may also be some swelling of the area and this can be identified by taking the measurements around the leg. The affected leg may be 2 or 3 centimetres larger than the non-affected leg. The temperature may be slightly raised.

The diagnosis of deep vein thrombosis based upon clinical signs alone can be very difficult. More conclusive methods of diagnosis include:

— ultrasound examination using the Doppler effect to study flow sounds in the femoral vein
— venography, in which radio-opaque medium is injected into the veins prior to X-ray.

Treatment

Treatment is by anticoagulant therapy and by restriction of movement until the clotting time has shown signs of improvement.

The anticoagulant drugs heparin and warfarin do not dissolve the clot but act by preventing its continued formation. Heparin is given intravenously and may be administered continuously using a pump or intermittently by bolus injection. The dosage will depend upon the estimation of the clotting time which should be done daily. This regime can be continued for a number of days. In some cases intravenous heparin is followed by oral warfarin, or warfarin alone may be the preferred method of treatment. The dosage of warfarin is monitored by estimation of the prothrombin time of the blood.

Side-effects of anticoagulants. The use of anticoagulants must be carefully controlled. There is a danger of haemorrhage occurring from the placental site and of the formation of haematomas.

If this occurs the anticoagulant therapy must be stopped and its effects counteracted. The effect of heparin is reversed by an intravenous injection of protamine sulphate. The effect of warfarin is counteracted by the use of vitamin K (Konakion) which is given in a slow intravenous infusion.

Restriction of exercise

Whenever deep vein thrombosis is suspected, the woman should not be allowed to walk about. Once the diagnosis has been made and treatment commenced the doctor's instructions as to the degree of movement allowed must be sought.

It is usual to confine the woman to bed until swelling has subsided and the anticoagulant therapy has had some time to take effect. It is important that detachment of the extensive thrombus is not caused by unnecessary movement.

Pulmonary embolism

Signs and symptoms of small pulmonary emboli are:

— pain in the chest
— dyspnoea
— slight haemoptysis.

Any such symptoms, however slight, must be reported at once to the doctor.

The signs and symptoms of major pulmonary embolism are:

— sudden collapse
— dyspnoea
— cyanosis
— hypotension
— marked distress.

Respiratory failure and cardiac arrest may follow within seconds.

Medical aid must be summoned at once. Oxygen is given meanwhile and intravenous heparin is administered as soon as possible and continued via intravenous infusion. Pain is relieved by morphine or diamorphine given intravenously.

The woman's condition will usually improve within a few hours, and the anticoagulant therapy and monitoring of the blood clotting time will then continue until treatment is complete. If the woman does not respond to this therapy, an intravenous infusion of streptokinase may be given in order to help break up the clot. In this situation the advice of a specialist in vascular disorders will be sought.

Occasionally the operation of pulmonary embolectomy may be necessary.

POSTPARTUM HAEMORRHAGE

There are two types of postpartum haemorrhage:

Primary postpartum haemorrhage occurs within the first 24 hours after delivery of the baby.

Secondary postpartum haemorrhage occurs at any time after 24 hours and up to 6 weeks following delivery of the baby.

The midwife responsible for postnatal care may encounter either of these, the first shortly after transfer from the delivery room and the second commonly during the second postnatal week. Postpartum haemorrhage is dealt with fully in Chapter 29; points relevant to the puerperium follow below:

Causes

Postpartum haemorrhage is caused by factors which interfere with normal uterine muscle contraction or as a result of laceration of the birth canal, especially cervical tears or extended vaginal tears.

Signs and symptoms

The most obvious sign is that of the bleeding itself. However not all uterine bleeding is overt; it is possible for blood to be retained in the uterus causing further disturbance of uterine contraction. When this occurs it can be detected by an increase in the height of the fundus and by distension of the uterus.

The blood pressure falls and the pulse rate is raised. The woman complains of feeling faint and ill and she may complain of low backache, especially if the blood is retained in the uterus.

Treatment

Treatment is directed to arresting the bleeding, initially by rubbing up a contraction if the uterus is still palpable. The midwife must send urgently for medical aid, and give an injection of ergometrine 0.5 mg intramuscularly or intravenously. The woman's bladder should be emptied. In cases of severe haemorrhage, bimanual compression of the uterus may be undertaken as an emergency measure.

Medical treatment continues by inducing contraction of the uterus and replacing blood loss. Intravenous Syntocinon is given in a dextrose or sodium chloride infusion and a blood transfusion is commenced as soon as possible. The cause of the bleeding must be established and treated.

The record of placental separation and the condition of the placenta must be checked. If the cause is thought to be the retention of placental tissue, a gentle exploration under general anaesthetic will enable the doctor to remove the retained products. Lacerations of the birth canal are sutured under anaesthetic. Occasionally, severe haemorrhage, which cannot easily be controlled, may necessitate a hysterectomy being performed.

Secondary postpartum haemorrhage is most commonly associated with retained placental tissue and an associated puerperal infection. Occasionally it may be due to lack of healing of a cervical laceration and haemorrhage ensues when the debris sloughs off. The most common time for secondary postpartum haemorrhage is between the 7th and 14th postpartum days. It may therefore occur after the woman has returned home. The midwife must send urgently for medical aid and if necessary call the obstetric flying squad in order that remedial measures can be taken before the woman is transferred to hospital for further treatment.

PSYCHIATRIC DISORDERS OF THE PUERPERIUM

There are two distinct types of psychiatric disorder associated with the puerperium and these are:

— postnatal depression
— puerperal psychosis

Postnatal depression

Research indicates that approximately 10% of all mothers develop clinical depression following childbirth and that a further 10% exhibit considerable emotional distress (Cox 1986).

The onset is gradual and the condition may

last for 3–6 months. In some cases it will persist throughout the first year of the baby's life.

Such depression is disabling for the mother and causes considerable disruption of family life and maternal–child relationships. There is some evidence that depression in the mother has an adverse effect upon her baby's performance in developmental tests at 9 months old (Murray 1988).

Causes

Postnatal depression is a reactive illness and its causes are complex. Research has shown that it is associated with a number of stress-inducing factors including marital tension, moving house, moving away from the family network and giving up a career. Low self-esteem and the lack of close support networks are contributory factors as is conflicting advice from midwives (Ball 1989, Holden 1990).

Symptoms

The symptoms of postnatal depression differ from those of 'normal' depression. The woman is usually able to sleep but continues to feel tired and exhausted in spite of adequate periods of rest. Most depressed patients feel worst in the morning and improve as the day goes on: women suffering postnatal depression feel well in the morning and become worse as the day goes on.

Management

Early detection. Early treatment brings the best prognosis, and therefore the midwife must be alert for signs of early depression. The onset is gradual and possible depression should be suspected when a mother continues to feel despondent about her ability to care for the baby adequately, when she constantly complains of tiredness or expresses the need for more help than she is receiving from family and friends. The normal anxiety which all mothers feel about their ability to cope normally passes as the baby settles down and the mother becomes more confident. Depressed women, however, continue to express anxiety in spite of evidence that the baby is well and thriving.

Reduce stress. Wherever possible, stress should be alleviated by providing continued help, which may need to extend well beyond the normal period of postnatal care. The midwife should ensure that members of the family are aware of the mother's needs and do not make excessive demands upon her.

Treatment. It must be emphasised that the danger of this condition lies in its non-recognition or in delay of treatment until the depression has become severe.

In mild cases, treatment with mild tranquillisers such as nitrazepam 10 mg at night or diazepam 5 mg three times daily may be prescribed and further support given by the community psychiatric nurse. In more severe cases, admission to a mother and baby unit in the local psychiatric hospital results in good recovery.

Holden (1990) found marked improvement in depressed women who were allocated to an experimental group who received directive counselling from specially trained health visitors.

When depression has occurred, the information must be recorded in order to give an opportunity for planning increased support and early alleviation of symptoms in any subsequent pregnancy.

Puerperal psychosis

This severe form of mental illness affects approximately one or two mothers in every 1000.

The onset is rapid and usually occurs within the first few days after delivery. The symptoms are those of a depressive psychosis, manic illness or in some cases schizophrenia. This illness most often affects primiparae.

Signs and symptoms

The affected woman shows bizarre behaviour, loses touch with reality and may suffer from hallucinations. The onset of these symptoms may be heralded by a time of acute restlessness and inability to sleep. Frequently, the mother may deny that her baby belongs to her and in rare cases she may harm the baby.

Treatment

The illness must be treated promptly by admission to a psychiatric unit under the care of a consultant.

In most cases the baby will be able to accompany his mother into hospital and this should be encouraged if at all possible. Within the postnatal period the midwife will continue to visit. Because of the extreme nature of the symptoms, medical help is usually summoned as a matter of urgency but there may be some reluctance to involve the psychiatrist. However, prompt psychiatric care is vital and skilled psychiatric nursing care is required. With prompt treatment the prognosis is good but, unfortunately, it is likely that further episodes of the illness will occur throughout the woman's life and there is a high risk of recurrence in subsequent pregnancies.

Reader Activities

- Read further texts about postnatal perineal care. Make a list of care techniques which have:
  — been demonstrated by research to be beneficial
  — been shown to be of little value or detrimental, or for which no research data are available.
- Enquire which methods for care of perineal wounds are most frequently used in your hospital and community service. Discuss with your colleagues which methods they favour and why. Explore with them Sleep's (1990) findings and her suggestion that the most important aspect of care is individualised attention and sympathy for the mother concerned.
- Draw a care plan for encouraging ambulation in a mother who has had an emergency caesarean section following a failed forceps delivery. Consider how you can balance the need to reduce the risk of thrombo-embolic complications against the fact that moving about will be painful.

REFERENCES

Ball J A 1989 Postnatal care and adjustment to motherhood. In: Robinson S, Thomson A M (eds) Midwives, research and childbirth. Chapman & Hall, London.

Cox J L 1986 Postnatal depression: A guide for health professionals. Churchill Livingstone, Edinburgh

Department of Health et al 1991 Report on confidential enquiries into maternal deaths in the United Kingdom 1985–1987. HMSO, London

Grant A 1989 Repair of perineal trauma after childbirth. In: Chalmers I, Enkin M, Keirse M J N C (eds) Effective care in pregnancy and childbirth. Oxford University Press, Oxford, ch 68

Holden J M 1990 Emotional problems associated with childbirth. In: Alexander J, Levy V, Roch S 1990 Midwifery practice: postnatal care. Macmillan, Basingstoke

Letsky E A 1985 Coagulation problems during pregnancy. Churchill Livingstone, Edinburgh

Murray L 1988 Effects of postnatal depression on infant development: the contribution of direct studies of early mother–infant interaction. In: Kumar R, Brockington I (eds) Motherhood and mental illness. John Wright, London, vol 2

Sleep J M 1990 Postnatal perineal care. In: Alexander J, Levy V, Roch S 1990 Midwifery practice: postnatal care. Macmillan, Basingstoke

Vacca A, Keirse M J N C 1989 Instrumental vaginal delivery. In: Chalmers I, Enkin M, Keirse M J N C (eds) Effective care in pregnancy and childbirth. Oxford University Press, Oxford, ch 71

Wang E, Smaill F 1989 Infection in pregnancy. In: Chalmers I, Enkin M, Keirse M J N C (eds) Effective care in pregnancy and childbirth. Oxford University Press, Oxford, ch 34

7

The Newborn Baby

31

The baby at birth

MAUREEN M. MICHIE

Immediate care of baby at birth

Adaptation to extra-uterine life

Early parent–infant relationships

Asphyxia and resuscitation

The transition from intra-uterine to extra-uterine existence is a dramatic one and demands considerable and effective physiological alterations by the baby in order to ensure survival. The fetus leaves an environment which has been completely life-sustaining, where his needs for oxygenation, nutrition, excretion and thermoregulation have been met with minimal effort on his part. The aquatic amniotic sac has permitted movement but freedom to extend his limbs has been limited towards the end of pregnancy as his size has increased in relation to the capacity of the uterus. Though the fetus is sensitive to sound, the uterine environment has dulled the impact of the noise of the outside world where daylight also contrasts sharply with the dim interior of the uterus.

Subjected to intermittent diminution of his oxygen supply during uterine contractions, compression followed by decompression of his head and chest, and extension of his limbs, hips and spine during delivery, the baby emerges from his mother to encounter light, noises, cool air, gravity and tactile stimulus for the first time. Simultaneously he has to make major adjustments in his respiratory and circulatory systems as well as control his body temperature. These initial adaptations are crucial to his subsequent well-being and should be facilitated by the midwife at the time of birth.

IMMEDIATE CARE OF BABY AT BIRTH

As the baby's head is born, excess mucus may be wiped gently from his mouth. Care must be taken to avoid touching the nares as such action may stimulate reflex inhalation of debris into the trachea.

Gentle handling during the delivery is essential, the baby being drawn up towards and, if wished by the parents, onto the mother's abdomen. (Maternal posture during delivery may necessitate modification of this manoeuvre.) The time of birth, and sex of the baby are noted and recorded once the baby has been completely expelled from his mother.

Clearing the airway

Although fetal pulmonary fluid is present in the mouth most babies will achieve a clear airway unaided. Mechanical clearing of the baby's airway can interfere with normal physiology and can be considered to constitute an assault on the baby. If necessary, the airway can be cleared with the aid of a mucus extractor or soft rubber catheter with a single end hole attached to low pressure (10 cm water) mechanical suction. It is important to aspirate the oropharynx prior to the nasopharynx so that, when the baby gasps as his nasal passages are aspirated, mucus or other material is not drawn down into the respiratory tract. Deep suction is neither necessary nor desirable as trauma or laryngospasm and bradycardia may result.

Cutting the cord

Separation of the infant from the placenta is achieved by dividing the umbilical cord between two clamps which should be applied approximately 8–10 cm from the umbilicus. Application of a gauze swab over the cord while cutting it with scissors will prevent blood spraying the delivery field. *The cord should not be cut until it has been clamped securely. Failure to comply with this procedure will result in exsanguination of the baby.*

The timing of clamping of the cord is not crucial unless asphyxia, prematurity or Rhesus incompatibility is present (see Ch. 34 and Ch. 35). Some centres advocate delay until respirations are established and cord pulsation has ceased thus ensuring

that the infant receives a placental transfusion of some 70 ml of blood. This view is countered by those who maintain that the placental transfusion so acquired may predispose to neonatal jaundice (see Ch. 32). Prior to clamping the cord, if the infant is held above the level of the uterus blood will gravitate to the placenta and if the infant is held below the level of the uterus an increased placental transfusion will result. The ensuing anaemia in the former instance and polycythaemia with increased viscosity of the blood in the latter can compromise the cardiopulmonary status of the infant.

Identification

When babies are born in hospital it is necessary that they are readily identifiable one from another. Various methods of indicating identity can be employed, e.g. name bands, china bead necklets. In the UK name bands are applied, usually one on the infant's wrist and one on the ankle, each of which should indicate *legibly* in indelible pen the family name, sex of the infant and date and time of birth. In some centres, the name bands are number-coded with the infant's case records, in others the number coding corresponds with that of the mother. The amount of information written on the name bands may vary slightly according to local policy. It is the practice in many units to apply the name bands to the infant *before* the cord is cut. The mother and/or father should verify that the information on the bands is correct prior to their being applied to the baby. The midwife should ensure that the name bands are fastened securely and are neither too tight, impeding circulation or likely to excoriate the skin, nor too loose risking loss of the means to identification which should remain on the baby until his discharge from hospital.

Assessment of the baby's condition

Provided the baby is seen to be making some respiratory effort, the midwife can proceed to dry the infant gently while attending also to the foregoing procedures. At 1 minute after the baby's birth, she will make an assessment of his general condition and will repeat this assessment at 5 minutes. This involves consideration of five signs and the degree to which they are present or absent. The factors assessed are heart rate, respiratory effort, muscle tone, reflex response to stimulus and colour. A score of 0, 1 or 2 is awarded to each of the signs in accordance with the guidelines in Table 31.1. This scoring system, the Apgar score (Apgar 1953) is recognised and used universally. Of the five signs the heart rate and respiratory effort are the most important. Colour is least important and some centres have discontinued the recording of this part of the score making the maximum score 8 rather than 10. Documentation of this modified system requires to be indicated, e.g. 'Apgar minus colour' score = 7. The colour of babies with pigmented skin is best assessed by inspecting the colour of the mucous membranes.

Table 31.1
The Apgar score. Score is assessed at 1 minute and 5 minutes after birth. Medical aid should be sought if the score is less than 7. 'Apgar minus colour' score omits the fifth sign. Medical aid should be sought if the score is less than 6.

Sign	Score		
	0	1	2
Heart rate	absent	less than 100 beats/minute	more than 100 beats/minute
Respiratory effort	absent	slow, irregular	good or crying
Muscle tone	limp	some flexion of limbs	active
Reflex response to stimulus	none	minimal grimace	cough or sneeze
Colour	blue, pale	body pink, extremities blue	completely pink

A normal infant in good condition at birth will achieve an Apgar score of 7–10. A score below 7 indicates that the baby requires some form of resuscitation.

ADAPTATION TO EXTRA-UTERINE LIFE

Onset of respiration

The initiation and establishment of respiration is of paramount importance to the survival of the neonate. Most infants achieve sustained regular respiration within 60 seconds of complete expulsion from the mother, many taking their first breath as soon as the head is delivered.

Effective establishment of respirations necessitates that the respiratory, cardiovascular and central nervous systems of the neonate are both structurally and functionally normal. A patent airway is necessary to enable ventilation of the lungs. The episodic shallow fetal breathing movements must be replaced by regular rhythmic respirations following lung expansion, and an increased pulmonary blood flow is required to facilitate gaseous exchange in the alveoli and the removal of lung fluid.

At term, approximately 100 ml of lung fluid is present within the respiratory tract. During delivery compression of the chest wall assists in the expulsion of some of this fluid, the remainder of which is absorbed by the pulmonary circulation and lymphatic system after birth. (Infants delivered by caesarean section are denied the benefits of chest compression and therefore expression of lung fluid. Residual lung fluid may contribute to transient tachypnoea of the newborn.)

The presence of surfactant in the lungs reduces surface tension, assisting expansion and preventing adherence of the alveoli following expiration (see Ch. 5).

The first breath which the infant takes is stimulated by the effect of cool air on his face. Initial

Transient tachypnoea of the newborn
This condition is characterised by rapid respirations of up to 120 per minute. The baby may be cyanosed but maintains normal blood gases apart from pO_2. Little or no recession of the rib cage is evident and the baby does not grunt on expiration. The respiratory rate may remain elevated for up to 5 days. Treatment consists of oxygen therapy to maintain adequate oxygenation and tube feeding to prevent aspiration of feeds. It is essential that other causes of respiratory distress are excluded especially infective causes (which mimic this condition) and respiratory distress syndrome (see also Ch. 35).

heat loss by evaporation from the skin at birth is thought to provide some continuing stimulus to respiratory efforts.

Compression of the chest wall during delivery followed by elastic recoil of the thorax as the body is delivered stimulates stretch receptors in the lungs. Considerable negative intrathoracic pressure of up to 9.8 kPa (100 cm water) is exerted as the first breath is taken. The effectiveness of the first breath is enhanced by a pulmonary reflex which stimulates additional inspiratory effort prior to exhalation. Pressures exerted to effect inhalation diminish with each breath taken until only 5 cm water pressure is required to inflate the lungs. This is as a result of surfactant lowering surface tension thus permitting residual air to remain in the alveoli between breaths.

Compression and decompression of the baby's head during delivery is thought to stimulate the respiratory centre in the brain which in turn maintains the stimulus to respiratory effort. The role of chemoreceptors in stimulating the onset of respiration is not clear though it is suggested that the alteration in the blood gas state of the fetus during labour is influential. Carotid baroreceptors, sensitive to changes in pressure, may also contribute to respiratory stimulus by their response to the circulatory changes which take place when the placental circulation ceases.

Tactile stimulus is considered to be of minimal importance. However, pain caused by extension of the hitherto flexed limbs, joints and spine is thought to contribute to the initial responses of the infant to extra-uterine life. The sensations of cold, gravity, noise, light and odours have also been suggested as significant sensory stimuli.

Sustained regular respirations are established normally within 60 seconds of delivery.

Circulatory changes

Separated from his life support system, the placenta, the baby must make major adjustments within his circulatory system in order to divert de-oxygenated blood to the lungs for re-oxygenation. This involves several mechanisms which are influenced by the clamping of the umbilical cord and also by the lowered resistance in the pulmonary vascular bed.

During fetal life (see Ch. 5) only approximately 10% of the cardiac output is circulated to the lungs through the pulmonary artery. With the expansion of the lungs and lowered pulmonary vascular resistance, virtually all of the cardiac output is sent to the lungs. Oxygenated blood returning to the heart from the lungs increases the pressure within the left atrium. At almost the same time, pressure in the right atrium is lowered because blood ceases to flow through the cord. As a result, a functional closure of the foramen ovale is achieved. During the first days of life this closure is reversible and re-opening may occur if pulmonary vascular resistance is high, resulting in transient cyanotic episodes in the baby. The septa usually fuse within the first year of life forming the inter-atrial septum though in some individuals perfect anatomical closure may never be achieved.

The ductus arteriosus, which is nearly as wide in lumen as the aorta, provides a diversionary route to bypass the lungs of the fetus. Contraction of its muscular walls occurs almost immediately after birth. This is thought to occur because of sensitivity of the muscle of the ductus arteriosus to increased oxygen tension and reduction in circulating prostaglandin (Heyman 1989). As a result of altered pressure gradients between the aorta and pulmonary artery, a temporary reverse left-to-right shunt through the ductus may persist for a few hours though there is usually functional closure of the ductus within 8–10 hours of birth. Anatomical closure with the formation of the ligamentum arteriosum takes several months. Persistence or re-opening of the ductus may occur if pulmonary vascular resistance is high. Cyanosis or cyanotic attacks will be evident as a result. This is a common problem in preterm infants with respiratory distress syndrome (see Ch. 35).

Persistence of the foramen ovale and/or ductus arteriosus may be life-saving in some forms of congenital heart abnormality (see Ch. 38).

The remaining temporary structures of the fetal circulation — the umbilical vein, ductus venosus and hypogastric arteries — close functionally within a few minutes after birth and clamping of the cord. Anatomical closure by fibrous tissue occurs within 2–3 months resulting in the formation of the ligamentum teres, ligamentum venosum and the obliterated hypogastric arteries. (The proximal portions of the hypogastric arteries persist as the superior vesical arteries.)

The cardiopulmonary adaptations which take place at birth are interdependent. Failure to establish respirations and satisfactory tissue oxygenation presents a life-threatening situation and is exacerbated by hypothermia.

Thermal adaptation

Vacating a thermoconstant environment of 37.7°C the baby enters a much cooler atmosphere at delivery. A delivery room temperature of 21°C contrasts sharply with intra-uterine temperature and causes rapid cooling of the infant as amniotic fluid evaporates from his skin. The infant's large *surface area : body mass* ratio potentiates heat loss, especially from his head which comprises 25% of his size. His subcutaneous fat layer is thin and provides poor insulation allowing transfer of core heat to the environment and also cooling of his blood.

In addition to heat loss by *evaporation* further heat will be lost by *conduction* when the baby is in contract with cold surfaces, by *radiation* to cold objects in the environment and by *convection* caused by currents of cool air passing over the surface of his body (this is increased by the air conditioning systems in some modern delivery rooms).

The heat-regulating centre in the baby's brain has the capacity to promote heat production in response to stimuli received from thermoreceptors. However, this is dependent on increased metabolic activity compromising the baby's ability to control his body temperature, especially in adverse environmental conditions. Unlike adults or even older children, the baby cannot shiver nor is he able voluntarily to increase his muscle activity in order to generate heat. This means that he must depend on his ability to produce heat by metabolism which in turn requires an increase in oxygen consumption.

The normal neonate, in common with some other young mammals, is endowed with brown adipose tissue which assists in the rapid mobilisation of heat resources, i.e. free fatty acids and

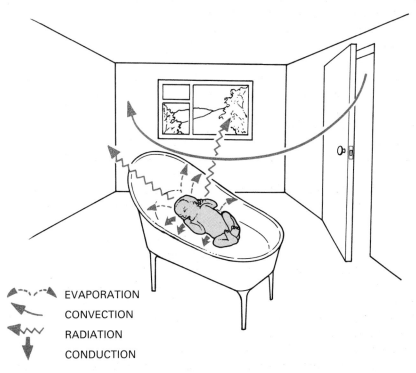

EVAPORATION
CONVECTION
RADIATION
CONDUCTION

Fig. 31.1
Modes of heat loss in the neonate.

glycerol, in times of cold stress. This mechanism is called non-shivering thermogenesis (Dawkins & Hull 1964). Brown adipose tissue is found in the mediastinum, around the nape of the neck, between the scapulae, along the spinal column and suprarenally. These deposits of brown fat have rich vascular and nerve supplies and are capable of increasing heat by up to 100%. Reserves of brown fat, however, are depleted rapidly with cold stress. Continued cold stress results in increased oxygen consumption as the infant strives to maintain sufficient heat for survival. This has the undesired effect of diverting oxygen and glucose from vital centres, e.g. the brain and cardiac muscle. Vasoconstriction occurs also, thus reducing pulmonary perfusion, and respiratory acidosis develops as the pH and pO_2 of the blood decrease and the pCO_2 increases. This plus the reduction in pulmonary perfusion may result in the re-opening or maintenance of the right-to-left shunt across the ductus arteriosus. Anaerobic glycolysis (i.e. the metabolism of glucose in the absence of oxygen) resulting in the production of acids compounds the situation by adding a metabolic acidosis. Protraction of cold stress therefore should be avoided.

The peripheral vasoconstrictor mechanisms of the baby are unable to prevent the fall in core body temperature which occurs during the first few hours after birth. It is important, therefore,

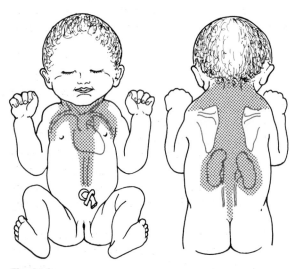

Fig. 31.2
Sites of brown fat.

for midwives to ensure that they employ measures to minimise heat loss at delivery (Dahn & James 1972, Rutter 1986). This is achieved by ensuring that the delivery room temperature is 21–24°C and that any fans are switched off prior to delivery thus minimising heat loss by convection; drying the baby as soon as possible to prevent heat loss by evaporation; providing a pre-warmed cot and blankets and encouraging skin-to-skin contact with the mother to promote heat gain; and avoiding heat loss by conduction following contact between the warm baby and cold surfaces. Delivery rooms which do not have outside windows help to reduce heat loss by radiation which, unlike the other methods, is unaffected by the ambient temperature. Loose clothing, swaddling and cuddling of the baby all help to maintain body heat. Covering of the baby's head is of particular importance.

The air conditioning systems in some modern delivery suites can compromise the infant's ability to maintain his body temperature without effort. Early transfer of the baby to a postnatal ward or nursery has been advocated as a means of minimising this problem. Transfer to the nursery or ward should be in a warmed cot or cuddled in the mother's arms to prevent heat loss while passing through corridors. In some hospitals, the provision of overhead radiant heaters within labour rooms has helped to avoid hypothermia, the heater being placed above the baby while he is in his cot or in his mother's arms covered with a blanket. Care must be taken to avoid overheating when using radiant heaters. Electric heating pads within babies' cots must be used with care to avoid burning. Hot water bottles used to pre-warm cots must be removed before the baby is placed in the cot.

It is preferable that the baby should remain with his mother during the first few hours of life whenever possible, that is, providing both mother and baby are in good condition, as this is the time when parent–infant interactions are initiated and the reality of parenthood begins.

Continued care of baby

Prior to transfer of the baby to the ward with his mother, the midwife replaces the initial cord clamp with another method of securing haemostasis by applying a disposable plastic clamp (or rubber band or 3 cord ligatures) approximately 2–3 cm from the umbilicus and cutting off the redundant cord. (Further care is discussed in Chapter 32.)

Instillation of eyedrops as prophylaxis against gonococcal infection is not practised in the UK though drops or antibiotic ointment may be instilled in other parts of the world. Localised reactions to silver nitrate drops have been shown to impair eye-to-eye contact with the mother (de Château 1987).

EARLY PARENT–INFANT RELATIONSHIPS

The safe delivery of a healthy baby engenders considerable emotion in most parents and indeed in attendants at the birth. The efforts of the preceding hours are temporarily forgotten as the mother sees her baby for the first time. Characteristically her first query relates to the sex of the infant speedily followed by an anxious enquiry about the infant's state of health — 'Is he all right?'. Reassured on these points, a mother progresses to an examination of her baby, which follows a fairly predictable pattern unless the condition of either the mother or the baby has been affected adversely by the process of labour or by narcotic drugs. Fathers too are involved in this early exploration of the newborn infant. The response of both parents is coloured not only by their prenatal understanding and previous experiences with babies but also by the appearance, behaviour and responses of their baby who takes an active part in the proceedings (White & Woollet 1987, Salariya 1990).

The mother. The first hour after birth is a time of particular sensitivity for the mother. Close contact with her baby during this time facilitates the attachment process.

Regardless of age, parity or marital status, mothers are likely to display a similar behavioural pattern when touching their babies for the first time. This sequence of touching behaviour is enhanced if the baby is naked. The mother begins her examination of her baby by exploring his extremities and head with her fingertips. Thereafter, she caresses her baby's body with her entire hand before gathering her baby in her arms often in the *en face* position where eye-to-eye contact can be established. She talks to her baby in a high pitched voice commenting on his appearance and behaviour to him, her partner and other birth attendants (Klaus et al 1975).

Her emotions at this time may be mixed. She may display great excitement and happiness — laughing, talking or even crying with joy. She may feel too tired to react positively towards her baby or may display disappointment or even anger towards her baby showing disinclination to touch him. Factors which may predispose to this latter reaction include prolonged labour, instrumental delivery, baby of the 'wrong' sex or congenital abnormality. Lack of support from partner or parents may influence the behaviour of an unmarried mother and for some mothers high parity may dampen their response. Childhood deprivation can inhibit some women from reacting in the anticipated manner.

For some mothers, the sight of an unwashed, wet and sometimes bloody infant is profoundly distasteful and they are not appreciative of skin-to-skin contact with a baby in this condition. A good midwife will ascertain the mother's attitude during pregnancy or early labour. This will allow her to modify her delivery technique and immediate care of the baby to meet the mother's wishes and so assist the mother to feel comfortable at her first meeting with her baby.

Some, though not all, mothers are keen to encourage their babies to suckle at birth. This practice should be facilitated and encouraged by the midwife as it helps not only to promote good mother–baby relationships, but also good lactation (Salariya et al 1979). (See also Chapter 33.)

The father. Many fathers are surprised at their profound emotional response to the birth of their babies. Sometimes a man's reactions are stronger than those of his wife or partner who may be rather tired initially.

The father feels a sense of deep satisfaction and self-esteem and is elated and keen to touch and hold his baby and his wife (Bedford & Johnson 1988).

Intimacy shared between the father and mother at this time is extended to include their new baby within an exclusive family group, often oblivious to their surroundings.

The baby. The baby at birth is alert and wakeful, reactive to his surroundings. His rounded, soft features provide an appealing image to which other human beings react protectively. The reaction of his parents is increased by their emotional ties with their baby.

Having accomplished his immediate physiological adaptations of respiration and circulation, the baby displays interest in sound, light and nutrition, responding to his mother's voice by moving his limbs in synchrony. His response to touch is illustrated in his grasp reflex and in his suckling of the breast if offered — or his own fist. He appears to focus on his mother's face at a distance of 20 cm and responds to movement of bright shiny objects such as his mother's eyes, by tracking them visually. These responsive behaviours evoke reinforcing responses from his parents thus promoting the interactions essential to his survival which is dependent on good parenting. A slightly darkened delivery room encourages the baby to open his eyes widely and look around him whereas bright lights cause him to frown. The midwife's understanding of these responses allows her to create optimum conditions for interaction to occur.

Bonding and promotion of parent–baby interaction

The term 'bonding' has been used to describe the establishment of parent–baby relationships in the early neonatal period. The implication of the desirability to feel instant love for one's child can lead to feelings of guilt in some parents who do not identify a strong emotional tie with their baby at birth. It is important to recognise that, as individuals, parents develop a loving relationship with their child at their own pace, some taking longer than others — days, weeks or months. Parents should feel able to express their disappointments as well as their joys without fear of being thought a 'bad' parent (Sluckin et al 1984, Herbert & Sluckin 1985, Parkinson & Harvey 1987).

A good rapport between the parents and the midwife should enable the development of their love for their baby to progress happily and at its own speed. However, the midwife must be alert to report and document marked negative reactions from either or both parents as this may be an early sign of future parenting difficulties. Adverse behaviours of note include hostile verbal or non-verbal attitude, lack of supportive interaction between the parents, failure to touch or hold the baby, disparaging remarks about the baby or marked disappointment about the sex of the baby.

Involvement of the father in the delivery of the baby's body, clamping of the cord and early bathing have been introduced in some centres to help to promote father–baby relationships. The midwife can do much to promote the beginnings of loving relationships by encouraging both parents to handle and examine their baby, by her positive comments about the baby, and by examining the baby beside the parents.

Privacy to talk, touch and be alone together with their baby is a privilege which most parents should be able to enjoy whether their baby is born at home or in hospital. The midwife should be sensitive to this often unexpressed need and leave the family alone together for some time before progressing with further care of the baby.

ASPHYXIA AND RESUSCITATION

Although the majority of infants gasp and establish respirations within 60 seconds of birth, some do not. This failure to initiate and sustain respiration at birth is known as asphyxia neonatorum. Mild asphyxia at birth is thought to be one of the factors involved in initiating respiration, as previously described. However, continued failure to breathe necessitates prompt and effective intervention if death or handicap is to be avoided. Midwives must therefore be aware of the predisposing factors and causes of asphyxia and be proficient in the resuscitative measures which can be employed in the absence of medical aid.

Intra-uterine hypoxia

Oxygenation of the fetus is dependent on oxygenation of the mother, adequate perfusion of the placental site, placental function, fetoplacental circulation and adequate fetal haemoglobin. Absence or impairment of any of these factors will result in a reduction of oxygen supply to the fetus (Fig. 31.3).

Oxygenation of the mother may be impaired as a result of cardiac or respiratory disease, an eclamptic fit, or during induction of general anaesthesia if difficulties arise during intubation. Perfusion of the placental site is dependent on satisfactory blood supply. This may be reduced in the presence of maternal hypertension or if hypotension occurs in response to haemorrhage, shock or aortocaval occlusion. Hypertonic uterine action, when uterine resting tonus is elevated, will impede the blood supply to the placental site. This is sometimes due to hyperstimulation of the uterus by Syntocinon and necessitates discontinuation of the oxytocic agent to allow the uterus to relax thus restoring circulation to the placental bed. The umbilical cord transports oxygenated blood to the fetus. If

prolapsed outside the uterus (causing vasoconstriction) or if compressed, fetal oxygenation will be reduced. The transport of oxygen within the fetus necessitates the availability of adequate haemoglobin which may be reduced if Rhesus incompatibility is present. Abnormal fetal cardiac function may also diminish the supply of oxygen to the fetal brain.

The fetus responds to hypoxia by accelerating his heart rate in an effort to maintain supplies of oxygen to the brain. If hypoxia persists, glucose depletion will stimulate anaerobic glycolysis resulting in a metabolic acidosis. Cerebral vessels will dilate and some brain swelling may occur. Peripheral circulation will be reduced. As the fetus becomes acidotic and cardiac glycogen reserves depleted, bradycardia develops, the anal sphincter relaxes and the fetus may pass meconium into the liquor. Gasping breathing movements triggered by hypoxia result in the aspiration of meconium-stained liquor into the lungs which presents an additional problem after delivery.

Auscultation of the fetal heart, use of cardiotocography and observation of meconium staining of the liquor draining per vaginam alert the midwife to fetal distress (see Ch. 12). Subsequent fetal blood sampling by the doctor may confirm a compromised fetus by revealing acidosis. However, Apgar scores do not always correlate with these findings (Silverman et al 1985, Jacobs & Phibbs 1989).

Birth asphyxia

Respiratory depression by fetal hypoxia is an important cause of birth asphyxia. However, it is only one factor to be considered when the baby does not breathe at birth (Roberton 1986).

Obstruction of the baby's airway by mucus, blood, liquor or meconium is one of the most common reasons for a baby failing to establish respirations. Rarely, a congenital abnormality, such as choanal or tracheal atresia, may be present. Immaturity of the infant causes mechanical dysfunction because of underdeveloped lungs, lack of surfactant and a soft pliable thoracic cage. Depression of the respiratory centre may be due to the effects of drugs administered to the mother,

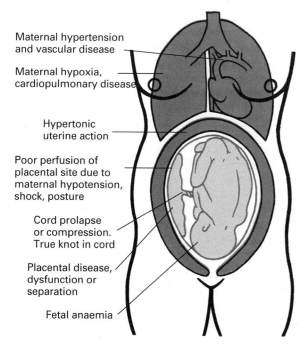

Maternal hypertension and vascular disease

Maternal hypoxia, cardiopulmonary disease

Hypertonic uterine action

Poor perfusion of placental site due to maternal hypotension, shock, posture

Cord prolapse or compression. True knot in cord

Placental disease, dysfunction or separation

Fetal anaemia

Fig. 31.3
Causes of intra-uterine hypoxia.

e.g. narcotic drugs, diazepam or chlormethiazole (Heminevrin), or to cerebral damage during labour or traumatic delivery. Respiratory function may be compromised by major congenital abnormalities such as congenital heart defects, abnormalities of the central nervous system or abnormalities within the respiratory tract, e.g. hypoplastic lungs co-existing with diaphragmatic hernia or renal agenesis. Intranatal pneumonia can inhibit successful establishment of respirations and should be considered especially if the membranes have been ruptured for some time.

Degrees of asphyxia

The length of time to which the fetus or neonate is subjected to hypoxia determines the outcome. It is considered that the human neonate responds to hypoxia in a similar manner to other young mammals (Cockburn 1971). This involves an initial response of gasping respirations followed by a period of apnoea lasting $1-1\frac{1}{2}$ minutes — *primary apnoea* — which, if not resolved by intervention techniques, is followed by a further episode of gasping respirations which accelerate while diminishing in depth until, approximately 8 minutes after birth, respirations cease completely — *terminal apnoea*. This suggests that it should be possible to determine the degree of asphyxia by assessment of the infant's condition at birth. The Apgar score provides a guide to the severity of birth asphyxia (Table 31.2) though does not necessarily reflect the metabolic status of the infant. This presents a dilemma for the birth attendant who may be uncertain as to whether primary or secondary (terminal) apnoea is present at birth. It is advisable therefore to be prepared to undertake specific resuscitative measures for any infant who is asphyxiated at birth.

Preparation for the reception of an asphyxiated baby

Though birth asphyxia may be anticipated in circumstances previously described, there are occasions when a baby is born in an asphyxiated condition without forewarning. It is essential that resuscitation equipment is always available and in working order and that personnel in attendance at the delivery of a baby are familiar with the equip-

Table 31.2
Degrees of birth asphyxia

Mild asphyxia	*Severe asphyxia*
Heart rate not severely depressed (60–80 bpm)	Slow feeble heart rate (less than 40 bpm)
Short delay in onset of respiration	No attempt to breathe
Good muscle tone	Poor muscle tone
Responsive to stimuli	Limp, unresponsive to stimuli
Deeply cyanosed	Pale, grey
Apgar score 5–7	*Apgar score less than 5*
No significant deprivation of oxygen during labour	Oxygen lack has been prolonged before or after delivery, circulatory failure is present, baby is shocked

ment, resuscitation techniques and local policies regarding the provision of medical aid.

In some units resuscitation of babies is undertaken in a specific area, whereas in others each delivery room is equipped to deal with this emergency. Whenever birth asphyxia is anticipated, e.g. preterm delivery, instrumental or breech delivery, or fetal distress, it is desirable that a paediatrician, paediatric nurse or midwife experienced in resuscitation techniques is present at the delivery. (In some centres an anaesthetist may be the person responsible for neonatal resuscitation.)

Management of birth asphyxia

The aims of resuscitation are:
— to establish and maintain a clear airway, ventilation and oxygenation
— to ensure effective circulation
— to correct acidosis
— to prevent hypothermia, hypoglycaemia and haemorrhage.

As soon as the baby is born, the clock timer should be started. The Apgar score is assessed in the normal manner at 1 minute. In the absence of any respiratory effort, resuscitative measures are not delayed however. The baby's upper airways should be cleared by gentle suction of the oro- and nasopharynx and the presence of an apex beat verified. The baby is dried quickly and transferred

Resuscitation equipment

Resuscitaire with overhead radiant heater and light, piped oxygen, manometer, suction and clock timer. The shelf should provide a firm surface and enable a 15° head tilt to be achieved

Two straight-bladed infant laryngoscopes, spare batteries and bulbs

Neonatal endotracheal tubes (with shoulders) 2.5 mm and 3.0 mm and connectors

Neonatal airways sizes 0, 00, 000

Mucus extractors

End hole suction catheter sizes 6, 8, 10 FG

Neonatal bag and mask and face masks of assorted sizes

Syringes 5 ml and 2 ml and assorted needles

Drugs
— naloxone hydrochloride (Narcan Neonatal) 200 μg/ml in 2 ml ampoules
— sodium bicarbonate 8.4% and 4.2%
— dextrose 10% and 5%
— vitamin K_1 1 mg ampoules
— normal saline
— THAM 7%

Stethoscope

Cord clamps

to a well-lit resuscitation area where he should be placed on a flat, firm surface at a comfortable working height and under a radiant heat source to prevent hypothermia. The baby's shoulders may be elevated on a small towel to straighten the trachea by slight extension of the head. Hyperextension is unnecessary. It is not desirable to hold the baby upside down as this causes a sharp rise in cerebral venous pressure, hyperextends and stretches the spine and hips which is painful, and risks the infant being dropped.

Clearing the airway

If meconium is present in the airway, suction under direct vision should be performed by passing a laryngoscope and visualising the larynx (Roberton 1986). Care should be taken to avoid touching the vocal cords as this may induce laryngospasm, apnoea and bradycardia. Mechanical suction, if used, should not exceed 10 cm water pressure and should be applied in short 10-second periods

as the catheter is withdrawn. End hole catheters minimise the risk of trauma. No force should be exerted while passing the catheter as this could cause trauma to the mucosa predisposing to oedema, bleeding and increased secretions. Thick meconium may require to be lavaged out of the trachea with normal saline through an endotracheal tube.

Stimulation

Rough handling of the infant merely serves to increase shock and is unnecessary. Gentle stimulation by drying the baby and clearing the airway should suffice. Directing a low flow (2–4 litres/min) of oxygen over the baby's face may stimulate a gasp reflex.

Warmth

Hypothermia exacerbates hypoxia as essential oxygen and glucose are diverted from the vital centres in order to create heat for survival. Wet towels should be removed and the baby's body and head should be covered with a prewarmed blanket leaving only the chest exposed. N.B. It is hazardous to use a silver swaddler under a radiant heater because it could cause burning.

Ventilation and oxygenation

If the baby fails to respond to clearing of his airway, assisted ventilation is necessary. This can be achieved in a variety of ways.

Neonatal bag and mask. A close-fitting mask is applied over the baby's nose and mouth taking care not to encroach on his eyes. Oxygen or air is blown through the mask by means of a bag which has a self-limiting pressure valve of 2.9 kPa (30 cm water), e.g. Ambu or Cardiff bag. The baby's jaw must be held forward and supported to maintain the airway. Insertion of a neonatal airway helps to prevent obstruction by the baby's tongue. Note that overextension of the baby's head causes airway obstruction. Ventilation at a rate of 40 respirations per minute is applied by squeezing the bag. A longer inspiration phase improves oxygenation. Higher inflation pressures may be required to produce chest movement (Milner 1991). If the infant is attempting to breathe out, his efforts at expiration may be foiled as the operator inflates the chest with positive pressure. This technique therefore requires a skilled operator to achieve success.

Endotracheal intubation. If the baby fails to respond to intermittent positive pressure ventilation (IPPV) by bag and mask, or if bradycardia is present, an endotracheal tube should be passed without delay. Intubating a baby is different from intubating an adult and requires special skill. The skill once acquired must be practised to be retained. Midwives can learn this skill by practice on models. (Practising resuscitation techniques on stillborn infants, while realistic, poses ethical questions, especially with regard to parental consent (Carlisle 1992).)

Technique of intubation. The blade of the laryngoscope is introduced over the baby's tongue into the pharynx until the epiglottis is seen. Elevation of the epiglottis by the tip of the laryngoscope reveals the vocal cords. Any mucus, blood or meconium which is obstructing the trachea should be cleared by careful suction prior to passing the endotracheal tube a distance of 1.5–2 cm into the trachea. (Pressure on the cricoid cartilage may facilitate visualisation of the larynx. Intubation may be easier if a cold tube which has been in the refrigerator is used.) After the laryngoscope is removed, oxygen is administered by IPPV to the endotracheal tube via the Ambu bag or Y-piece connector attached to the manometer. A maximum of 30 cm water pressure should be applied — there is risk of rupture of alveoli or tension pneumothorax if higher pressure is applied. The rise and fall of the chest wall should indicate whether the tube is in the trachea. This can be confirmed by auscultation of the chest. Distension of the stomach indicates oesophageal intubation necessitating resiting of the tube.

Mouth-to-face resuscitation. In the absence of specialised equipment, assisted ventilation can be achieved by mouth-to-face resuscitation. The operator places her mouth over the infant's mouth and nose and, using only the air in her buccal cavity, blows gently into the baby's airway at a rate of 20 breaths per minute allowing the infant to exhale between breaths.

External cardiac massage

If bradycardia persists or the heart rate is less than 40 beats per minute, external cardiac massage may be applied. This is achieved either by placing the tips of the index and middle fingers of one hand over the middle of the sternum or by encircling the baby's chest with the fingers on the spine and thumbs on the lower mid-sternum (Roberton 1986, Graves 1988, Milner 1991) and depressing the chest at a rate of 100–120 times per minute. (Excessive pressure over the lower end of the sternum may cause rib, lung or liver damage.)

Use of drugs

Naloxone hydrochloride — up to 400 µg (or approximately 100 µg per kg body weight) may be administered intravenously (through the umbilical vein) or intramuscularly to reverse the effects of maternal narcotic drugs. *It must not be given until respiration is effected.* Naloxone has the advantage of not having a respiratory depressant effect itself therefore no harm arises if it is given in the absence of narcotic analgesia. The dose can be repeated safely.

Sodium bicarbonate — 5ml of 4.2% or 8.4% solution given intravenously assists in the correction of metabolic acidosis. It should be administered slowly — 1 ml per minute — in order to avoid rapid elevation of serum osmolality with the attendant risk of intracranial haemorrhage (Howell 1987). *It should not be given prior to ventilation being established.* THAM may be used in preference to sodium bicarbonate (Roberton 1986).

Dextrose — 5 ml of 5% or 10% solution may be given intravenously to correct or prevent hypoglycaemia.

Konakion (vitamin K_1) — up to 1 mg may be given intramuscularly to reduce the risks associated with haemorrhage. Some centres give vitamin K orally.

Dexamethasone — 1–2 mg may be given intravenously or intramuscularly to minimise the risk of cerebral oedema if severe asphyxia is present.

Observations and after-care

Throughout the resuscitation procedure the baby's response should be monitored and recorded, making special note of the time when spontaneous respirations are established. The endotracheal tube may be left in place for a few minutes after the baby starts to breathe spontaneously. Suction may be applied through the endotracheal tube as it is removed. Careful documentation of all drugs given and of serial Apgar scores is essential.

A baby whose Apgar score was less then 6 at 5 minutes or who was slow to respond to resuscitation should be transferred to the neonatal unit for a period of observation in order to monitor behaviour (see Ch. 37).

Explanation about the resuscitation and the need for transfer to the special nursery must be given to the parents and, providing the baby's condition permits, the mother should have the opportunity to see and hold her baby prior to being separated from him. This assists the attachment process.

Babies who respond quickly to resuscitation can be reunited with their parents, remaining in the delivery room until the usual transfer time to the postnatal ward where their care continues as normal (see Ch. 32).

Reader Activities

In each of the following activities, repeating it more than once will add to the information and experience gained.

- Observe and record the time of the first gasp and onset of spontaneous breathing in babies delivered: (a) by spontaneous vertex delivery; (b) by forceps delivery; (c) by caesarean section. Compare the responses of these babies to one another.
- When you are present at a birth but are not delivering the baby, record the Apgar score of the newborn. Which of the five factors appear the most informative?
- What does a baby normally do during the first hour of life? Make observations to decide what may influence behaviour, such as handling, maternal sedation during labour or other factors.
- Take an opportunity to watch the interactions between a mother and father and their baby at and just after birth.

Compare the reactions and behaviour of the mother with those of the father. Compare reactions of first-time parents with those of experienced parents.

- Compare the temperature of the baby after birth with the temperature recorded 1 hour, then 2 hours, later.
- Attend the resuscitation of a baby by a paediatrician or a specialist midwife. Record the baby's response to treatment. Review the labour record to find out what signs of hypoxia were observed before birth.
- Using a model, practise mouth-to-face resuscitation; bag and mask resuscitation; intubation and intermittent positive pressure ventilation. This experience will hopefully stand you in good stead when, under supervision, you undertake the resuscitation of an infant with respiratory depression.
- Monitor the subsequent behaviour of a baby who required resuscitation. Compare this with the observations of normal behaviour that you made earlier.

REFERENCES

Apgar V 1953 A proposal for a new method of evaluation of the newborn infant. Current Research in Anaesthesiology and Analgesics 40: 340

Bedford V, Johnson N 1988 The role of the father. Midwifery 4: 190–195

Carlisle D 1992 A secret procedure? Nursing Times 88(35): 16–17

Cockburn F 1971 Resuscitation of the newborn. British Journal of Anaesthesia 43: 886–902

Dahn L S, James L S 1972 Newborn temperature and calculated heat loss in the delivery room. Pediatrics 49: 504–506

Dawkins M, Hull D 1964 Brown adipose tissue in the response of newborn rabbits to cold. Journal of Physiology 172: 215–238

de Château P 1987 Promotion of mother–infant relationship during delivery. In: Harvey D (ed) Parent–infant relationships. Wiley series on perinatal practice Vol 4, John Wiley, Chichester

Graves B 1988 Challenges of neonatal resuscitation for nurse-midwives. Journal of Nurse-Midwifery 33(5): 217–224

Herbert M, Sluckin A 1985 A realistic look at mother–infant bonding. In: Chiswick M (ed) Recent advances in perinatal medicine 2. Churchill Livingstone, Edinburgh

Heyman M 1989 Arachidonic acid derivatives in the perinatal period. In: Barness L, De Vivo D, Morrow G, Oski F, Rudolph A (eds) Advances in pediatrics 36. Year Book Medical, Chicago, p 151–176

Howell J 1987 Sodium bicarbonate in the perinatal setting — revisited. Clinics in Perinatology 14(4): 807–816

Jacobs M, Phibbs R 1989 Prevention, recognition and treatment of perinatal asphyxia. Clinics in Perinatology 16(4): 785–807

Klaus M H, Trause M A, Kennell J H 1975 Does human maternal behaviour after delivery show a characteristic pattern? In: CIBA Foundation Symposium 33, Parent–infant interaction. Associated Scientific, Amsterdam

Milner A D 1991 Resuscitation of the newborn. Archives of Disease in Childhood 66: 66–69

Parkinson C E, Harvey D 1987 Child development and the maternal–infant relationship. In: Harvey D (ed) Parent–infant relationships. Wiley series on perinatal practice Vol 4, John Wiley, Chichester

Roberton N R C 1986 Resuscitation of the newborn. In: Roberton N R C (ed) Textbook of neonatology. Churchill Livingstone, Edinburgh

Rutter N 1986 Temperature control and its disorders. In: Roberton N R C (ed) Textbook of neonatology. Churchill Livingstone, Edinburgh

Salariya E, Easton P, Cater J 1979 Early and often for best results. Nursing Mirror 148(22) 15–17

Salariya E 1990 Parental–infant attachment. In: Alexander J, Levy V, Roch S (eds) Postnatal care — a research based approach. Macmillan, Basingstoke

Silverman, F, Suidan J, Wasserman J, Antoine C, Young B 1985 The Apgar score: Is it enough? Obstetrics and Gynaecology 66: 331–336

Sluckin W, Sluckin A, Herbert M 1984 On mother-to-infant bonding. Midwife, Health Visitor and Community Nurse 20(11): 404–407

White D G, Woollet E A 1987 The father's role in the neonatal period. In: Harvey D (ed) Parent–infant relationships. Wiley series on perinatal practice Vol 4, John Wiley, Chichester

Bloom R S, Cropley C (eds) 1987 Textbook of neonatal resuscitation. American Heart Association/American Academy of Pediatrics, Dallas

Brant H 1985 Childbirth for men. Oxford Medical, Oxford

D'Souza S W 1983 Neurodevelopmental outcome after birth asphyxia. In: Chiswick M (ed) Recent advances in perinatal medicine 2. Churchill Livingstone, Edinburgh

Harvey D (ed) 1987 Parent–infant relationships. Wiley series on perinatal practice Vol 4, John Wiley, Chichester

Hull D 1976 Temperature regulation and disturbance in the newborn infant. Clinics in Endocrinology and Metabolism 5: 39–53

Low J, Muir D, Pater E, Kachmar E 1990 The association of intrapartum asphyxia in the mature fetus with newborn behavior. American Journal of Obstetrics and Gynecology 163: 1131–1135

Moir D 1986 Pain relief in labour, 5th edn. Churchill Livingstone, Edinburgh

Olds S, Loudon M, Ladewig P, Davidson S 1988 Maternal/newborn nursing, 3rd edn. Addison Wesley, Menlo Park, California

Portman R, Carter B, Gaylord M, Murphy M, Thieme R, Merenstein G 1990 Predicting neonatal morbidity after perinatal asphyxia: a scoring system. American Journal of Obstetrics and Gynecology 162: 174–182

Roberton N R C (ed) 1986 Textbook of neonatology. Churchill Livingstone, Edinburgh

Shah P M 1990 Birth asphyxia: a crucial issue in the prevention of developmental disabilities. Midwifery 6: 99–107

Winkler C, Hauth J, Tucker J, Owen J, Brumfield C 1991 Neonatal complications at term as related to the degree of umbilical artery acidemia. American Journal of Obstetrics and Gynecology 164(2): 637–641

FURTHER READING

American Academy of Pediatrics Committee on Fetus and Newborn 1986 Use and abuse of the Apgar score. Pediatrics 78(6): 1148–1149

32

The normal baby

MAUREEN M. MICHIE

Extra-uterine life presents a challenge to the newborn infant. The most important changes, those in the heart and lungs, take place at birth (see Ch. 31). However, continued adaptations are necessary in the first weeks of life as the infant assumes independence from the maternal and placental nurturing which he enjoyed before birth. He remains dependent on his mother or other caregiver for nutrition and protection but is responsible for his own metabolism and homeostasis among other functions essential to survival.

GENERAL CHARACTERISTICS

Appearance

A normal full-term infant weighs approximately 3.5 kg, when fully extended measures 50 cm from the crown of his head to his heels, and has an occipitofrontal circumference of 34–35 cm. His head comprises one-quarter of his size. He is plump and has a prominent abdomen. He lies in an attitude of flexion — in the supine position with his head turned to one side and one shoulder elevated off the mattress, in the prone position with his buttocks elevated, his knees drawn up under his abdomen, and his head turned to one side. With his arms extended his fingers reach to mid-thigh level. He has a lusty cry which he uses to evoke a response from his attendants with a view to controlling his environment.

Skin

Vernix caseosa, a white sticky substance present on the baby's skin at birth, is absorbed within a few hours. It is thought to have a protective function.

The skin of a newborn baby is thin, delicate, and easily traumatised by friction, pressure or substances with a different pH. This renders the skin prone to blistering, excoriation and infection. The skin is colonised by flora within 24 hours of birth. Downy hair, lanugo, covers the skin and is plentiful over the shoulders, upper arms and thighs. The general colour of the skin depends on the baby's ethnic origin ranging from pink and white to olive or dark brown. Peripheral cyanosis is common. Pigmentation of nipples and genitalia is deeper in babies with darker skins and a linea nigra may be present. Another feature of racial origin is the Mongolian blue spot which presents as a diffuse bluish-black area usually over the sacral region. Dark-skinned babies become more pigmented in the first weeks of life though the palms of the hands and soles of the feet remain paler than the rest of the body.

Sebaceous glands, though present in the skin, are relatively inactive. Distended glands may be present over the nose and cheeks. These are called milia. Sweat glands are present but inactive in the first days of life.

A mature baby has plentiful skin creases on the palms of his hands and soles of his feet. His nails are fully formed and adherent to the tips of the fingers, sometimes extending beyond the finger tips. His hair is soft and silky: some babies have virtually no hair and appear somewhat bald, whereas others have plentiful straight or curly hair. Eyebrows and eyelashes present a similar variation. The cartilage of the ears is well formed.

The umbilical cord stump necroses and separates by a process of dry gangrene usually within the first 10 days of life.

Genitalia and breasts

Both boys and girls have a nodule of breast tissue around the nipple. In boys the testicles are descended into the scrotum which has plentiful rugae. The prepuce is adherent to the glans penis. In girls the labia majora cover the labia minora and the hymen may appear disproportionately large.

Eyes

Most babies have dark blue-grey eyes. Permanent colouring of the iris is not manifest for weeks, months or even several years. Dark-skinned babies may have brown eyes though this varies according to the racial origins of the parents. The shape of the baby's eyes also reflects racial origin, for instance the epicanthic folds of Oriental babies alter the appearance of the orbital region. No tears are present in the eyes of a newborn baby and they become infected easily.

PHYSIOLOGY

Respiratory system

At birth the respiratory system is developmentally incomplete, growth of new alveoli continuing for several years. The lumen of the peripheral airways is narrow which predisposes to airway obstruction. Respiratory secretions are more plentiful than in an adult and the mucous membranes are delicate and sensitive to trauma, the area below the vocal cords being particularly prone to oedema.

Babies are obligatory nose-breathers and do not convert automatically to mouth breathing when nasal obstruction occurs.

The normal baby has a respiratory rate of 30–60 breaths per minute. His breathing is diaphragmatic, chest and abdomen rising and falling synchronously. The breathing pattern is erratic. Respirations are shallow and irregular being interspersed with brief 10–15 second periods of apnoea. This is known as periodic breathing. Apart from the initial profound respiratory efforts at birth, no nasal flaring, sternal or subcostal recession or grunting is present. The pattern of respiration alters during sleeping and waking states. Respiratory difficulties can occur due to neurological, metabolic, circulatory or thermoregulatory dysfunction as well as infection, airway obstruction or abnormalities of the respiratory tract itself (see relevant chapters).

The baby's cry is normally loud and of medium pitch unless neurological damage, infection or hypothermia is present, when the cry may be high pitched or weak. Transient cyanosis may arise in the first few days when the baby is crying and altered pressure gradients recreate right-to-left shunts within the heart and great vessels.

Cardiovascular system and blood

The changes in the infant's heart at birth have been described in Chapter 31. The heart rate is rapid, 120–160 beats per minute, and fluctuates in accordance with the baby's respiratory function and activity or sleep state. Peripheral circulation is sluggish. This results in mild cyanosis of hands, feet and circumoral areas and in generalised mottling when the skin is exposed. Blood pressure fluctuates according to activity and rises from 50/25 mmHg to 70/40 mmHg in the first 10 days of life.

The total circulating blood volume at birth is 80 ml/kg body weight. However, this may be raised if there is delay in clamping of the umbilical cord at birth. The haemoglobin level is high (15–20 g/dl). 70% is fetal haemoglobin. Conversion from fetal to adult haemoglobin which commenced in utero is completed in the first 1–2 years of life. Haemoglobin, red cell count ($5–7 \times 10^{12}/\ell$) and haematocrit (55%) levels decrease gradually during the first 2–3 months of life during which time erythropoiesis is suppressed.

Breakdown of excess red blood cells in the liver and spleen predisposes to jaundice in the first week. Prothrombin levels are low owing to lack of vitamin K. This inhibits blood clotting during the first week (colonisation of the intestine by bacteria which synthesise vitamin K is delayed until feeding is established). Platelet levels equal those of the adult.

The white cell count is high initially ($18.0 \times 10^9/\ell$) but decreases rapidly.

Renal system

Though the kidneys are functional in fetal life, their workload is minimal until after birth. The urine is dilute, straw coloured and odourless. Cloudiness caused by mucus and urates may be present initially until fluid intake increases. Urates may cause pink staining which is insignificant. The glomerular filtration rate is low and tubular resorption capabilities are limited. The infant is not able to concentrate or dilute the urine very well in response to variations in fluid intake, nor can he compensate well for high or low levels of solutes in the blood. The ability to excrete drugs is also limited.

Urine is voided by reflex emptying of the bladder. The first urine is passed at birth or within the first 24 hours and thereafter with increasing frequency as fluid intake rises. As the neonatal pelvis is small, the bladder becomes palpable abdominally when full.

Gastro-intestinal system

The gastro-intestinal tract of the neonate is structurally complete though functionally immature in comparison with that of the adult. The mucous membrane of the mouth is pink and moist. The teeth are buried in the gums and ptyalin secretion is low. Small epithelial pearls are sometimes present at the junction of the hard and soft palates. Sucking pads in the cheeks give them a full appearance. Sucking and swallowing reflexes are co-ordinated.

The stomach has a small capacity (15–30 ml) which increases rapidly in the first weeks of life. The cardiac sphincter is weak, predisposing to regurgitation or posseting. Gastric acidity, equal to that of the adult within a few hours after delivery, diminishes rapidly within the first few days and by the 10th day the infant is virtually achlorhydric which increases the risk of infection. Gastric emptying time is 2.5–3 hours.

In relation to the size of the infant the intestine is long, containing large numbers of secretory glands and a large surface area for the absorption of nutrients.

Enzymes are present though there is a deficiency of amylase and lipase which diminishes the infant's ability to digest compound carbohydrates and fat.

When food enters the stomach a gastrocolic reflex results in the opening of the ileocaecal valve. The contents of the ileum pass into the large intestine and rapid peristalsis means that feeding is often accompanied by reflex emptying of the bowel.

The gut is sterile at birth but is colonised within a few hours. Bowel sounds are present within 1 hour of birth. Meconium, present in the large intestine from 16 weeks gestation, is passed within the first 24 hours of life and is totally excreted within 48–72 hours. This first stool is blackish-green in colour, is tenacious and contains bile, fatty acids, mucus and epithelial cells. From the 3rd–5th day the stools undergo a transitional stage and are brownish-yellow in colour. Once feeding is established, yellow faeces are passed. The consistency and frequency of stools depend on the type of feeding. Breast milk results in loose, bright yellow and inoffensive stools. The baby may pass eight to ten stools a day or alternatively pass stools as infrequently as every 2 or 3 days. The stools of the bottle-fed infant are paler in colour, semi-formed and have a slightly sharp smell. The baby passes four to six stools a day but there is an increased tendency to constipation.

Physiological immaturity of the liver results in low production of glucuronyl transferase for the conjugation of bilirubin. This, together with a high level of red cell breakdown, may result in a transient jaundice which is manifest on the 3rd–5th days. Glycogen stores are rapidly depleted, so early feeding is required to maintain normal blood glucose levels (2.2–4.4 mmol/l). Feeding stimulates liver function and colonisation of the gut which assists in the formation of vitamin K. Infant feeding practices are designed to meet the physiological needs and capabilities of the baby and are discussed in Chapter 33.

Temperature regulation

Thermal control in the neonate remains poor for some time. Initial thermal adaptation and modes of heat loss and gain have been described in Chapter 31. Due to the immaturity of the hypothalamus, temperature regulation is inefficient and the infant remains vulnerable to hypothermia particularly when exposed to cold or draughts, when wet, when unable to move about freely, or when deprived of nutrition. As a baby who is cold is unable to shiver, he will attempt to maintain his body heat by adopting a flexed fetal posture, increasing his respiratory rate and activity, and he may cry. These activities increase calorie consumption and may result in hypoglycaemia which in turn will compound the effects of hypothermia as do hypoxia, acidosis and hyperbilirubinaemia (see Ch. 38).

The infant's normal rectal temperature is 36–37°C. A healthy, clothed, term infant will maintain this body temperature satisfactorily provided his environmental temperature is sustained between 18° and 21°C, his nutrition is adequate and his movements are not restricted by tight swaddling. However, like adults, babies are individuals with differing metabolic rates. This makes finite statements of thermoneutral range difficult. Hyperthermia can occur when the infant is exposed to a radiant heat source. Sweating may occur especially over the forehead, although the neonate's ability to sweat is limited. An unstable temperature may indicate infection.

Immunological adaptations

Neonates demonstrate a marked susceptibility to infections particularly those gaining entry through the mucosa of the respiratory and gastro-intestinal systems. Localisation of infection is poor, 'minor' infections having the potential to become generalised very easily.

The baby has some immunoglobulins at birth, but the sheltered intra-uterine existence limits the need for learned immune responses to specific antigens. There are three main immunoglobulins, IgG, IgA and IgM, and of these only IgG is small enough to cross the placental barrier. It affords immunity to specific viral infections. At birth the baby's levels of IgG are equal to or slightly higher than those of the mother. This provides passive immunity during the first few months of life.

IgM and IgA do not cross the placental barrier but can be manufactured by the fetus. Levels of IgM at term are 20% those of the adult, taking 2 years to attain adult levels (elevation of IgM levels at birth are suggestive of intra-uterine infection). This relatively low level of IgM is thought to render the infant more susceptible to enteric infections. IgA levels are very low and produced slowly although secretory salivary levels attain adult values within 2 months. IgA protects against infection of the respiratory tract, gastro-intestinal tract and eyes.

Breast milk, and especially colostrum, provides the infant with passive immunity in the form of *Lactobacillus bifidus*, lactoferrin, lysozymes and secretory IgA among others (see Ch. 33).

The thymus gland, where lymphocytes are produced, is relatively large at birth and continues to grow until 8 years of age.

Reproductive system

Spermatogenesis in boys does not occur until puberty, but the total complement of primordial follicles containing primitive ova is present in the ovaries of girls at birth. In both sexes withdrawal of maternal oestrogens results in breast engorgement sometimes accompanied by secretion of 'milk' by the 4th or 5th day. Baby girls may develop pseudomenstruation for the same reason. This is short-lived.

Skeletomuscular system

The muscles are complete, growth occurring by hypertrophy rather than by hyperplasia. The long bones are incompletely ossified to facilitate growth at the epiphyses. The bones of the vault of the skull also reveal lack of ossification essential for growth of the brain and facilitating moulding during labour. Moulding is resolved within a few days of birth. The posterior fontanelle closes at 6–8 weeks. The anterior fontanelle remains open until 18

months of age making assessment of hydration and intracranial pressure possible by palpation of fontanelle tension.

Neurological system

In comparison with the other body systems the nervous system is remarkably immature both anatomically and physiologically at birth. This results in predominantly brain stem and spinal reflex activity with minimal control by the cerebral cortex in the early months though social interaction occurs early. After birth brain growth is rapid requiring constant and adequate supplies of oxygen and glucose. The immaturity of the brain renders it particularly vulnerable to hypoxia, biochemical imbalance, infection and haemorrhage. Temperature instability and unco-ordinated muscle movement reflect the incomplete state of brain development and incomplete myelination of nerves.

The neonate is equipped with a wide range of reflex activities the presence of which at varying ages provides indication of the normality and integrity of the neurological and skeletomuscular systems.

Moro reflex. This reflex occurs in response to a sudden stimulus. It can be elicited by holding the baby at an angle of 45° and then permitting the head to drop 1 or 2 cm. The infant responds by abducting and extending his arms with his

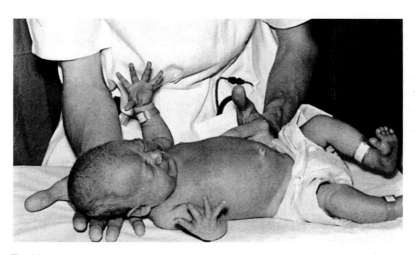

Fig. 32.1
Moro reflex.

fingers fanned sometimes accompanied by a tremor. The arms then flex and embrace the chest. A similar response may be seen in the legs which, following extension, flex onto the abdomen (Fig 32.1). The reflex is symmetrical and is present for the first 8 weeks of life. Absence of the Moro reflex may indicate brain damage or immaturity. Persistence of the reflex beyond the age of 6 months is suggestive of mental retardation.

Rooting reflex. In response to stroking of the cheek or side of the mouth the baby will turn towards the source of stimulus and open his mouth ready to suckle.

Sucking and swallowing reflexes are well developed in the normal baby and are co-ordinated with breathing. This is essential for safe feeding and adequate nutrition.

Gag, cough and sneeze reflexes protect the infant from airway obstruction.

Blinking and corneal reflexes protect the eyes from trauma.

Grasp reflexes. A palmar grasp is elicited by placing a finger or pencil in the palm of the baby's hand which is grasped firmly. A similar response can be demonstrated by stroking the base of the toes (plantar grasp).

Walking and stepping reflexes. When supported upright with his feet touching a flat surface the baby simulates walking. If held with the tibia in contact with the edge of a table the infant will step up onto the table (limb placement reflex).

Asymmetrical tonic neck reflex. In the supine position the limbs on the side of the body to which the head is turned extend while those on the opposite side flex.

Traction response. When pulled upright by the wrists to a sitting position the head will lag initially then right itself momentarily before falling forward on to the chest.

These reflexes are only a few of the many present at birth and assist in the attachment process to the mother who views these responses as indications of communication by her baby.

PSYCHOLOGY AND PERCEPTION

The newborn baby is alert and aware of his sur-roundings when he is awake. Far from being impassive he reacts to stimuli and begins at a very early age to amass information about his environment (Brazelton 1984).

Special senses

Vision
Though immature, the structures necessary for vision are present and functional at birth. The baby is sensitive to bright lights, which cause him to frown or blink. He demonstrates a preference for bold black and white patterns and the shape of the human face. His focusing distance is 15–20 cm which allows him to see his mother's face when being nursed. He can track a moving object briefly within the first 5 days. His ability to establish eye contact with his mother helps to enhance bonding. By 2 weeks of age he can differentiate his mother's face from that of a stranger. Interest in colour, variety and complexity of patterns develops within the first 2 months of life.

Hearing
The baby turns his eyes towards sound. On hearing a high pitched sound he first stills and then becomes agitated. He is comforted by low pitched sounds. A sudden sound elicits a startle or blink reflex. He prefers the sound of the human voice to other sounds and within a few weeks the patterns of adult speech are mimicked in his movements. He can discriminate between voices and prefers his mother's (DeCasper & Fifer 1987). This, too, promotes mother–baby interaction.

Smell and taste
Babies prefer the smell of milk to that of other substances and show a preference for human milk. Within a few days the baby can differentiate the smell of his mother's milk from that of another woman (MacFarlane 1975). He turns away from unpleasant smells. His preference for sweet taste is demonstrated by vigorous and sustained sucking and a speedy grimacing response to bitter, salty or sour substances.

Touch
Infants are acutely sensitive to touch, enjoying

skin-to-skin contact, immersion in water, stroking, cuddling and rocking movements. The baby withdraws from painful stimuli and cries vigorously. A puff of air on his face induces an inspiration or gasp reflex. His curving response to touch and his grasp reflexes enhance his relationship with his mother.

Habituation

If a stimulus is repeated several times in succession it will eventually fail to elicit a response from the infant unless his responding behaviours are reinforced in some way. It has been suggested that some habituation may be initiated in utero (Damstra-Wijmenga 1991). Babies learn quickly and soon demonstrate individuality in the way they become irritable or can be soothed. This influences the responses of their parents.

Sleeping and waking

Following the initiation of respiration at birth, the baby remains alert and reactive for a period of approximately 1 hour after which he relaxes and sleeps. The length of this first sleep varies from a few minutes to several hours and is followed by a second period of reactivity during which mucus accumulation in the oropharynx may occur causing choking or gagging. Subsequent sleeping and waking rhythms show marked variations and the baby takes some time to settle into his individual pattern. Initially waking periods are related to hunger, but within a few weeks the waking periods last longer and meet the need for social interaction.

Sleep states

Two sleep states are identifiable.

In *deep sleep*, the baby's eyes are closed, respirations are regular, no eye movements are present, response to stimuli is delayed and is quickly suppressed. Jerky movements may occur at intervals.

In *light sleep*, rapid eye movements are observable through the closed eyelids. Respirations are irregular and sucking movements occur intermittently. Response to stimuli occurs more readily and may result in an alteration of sleep state. Random movements are noted.

Awake states

A wider range of awake states are observed ranging from drowsiness to crying.

In the *drowsy state*, the baby's eyes may be open or closed with some fluttering of the eyelids. Smiling may occur. Limb movements are variable, generally smooth, but are interspersed by startle responses. Alteration in state occurs more readily following stimulation.

In the *quiet alert state*, though motor activity is minimal, the baby is alert to visual and auditory stimuli.

In the *active alert state*, the baby is generally active and reactive to his environment.

In the *active crying state*, the baby cries vigorously and may be difficult to console. Muscular activity is considerable.

The amount of time that the baby spends in each state varies tremendously and influences the way in which he responds to stimuli, whether visual, auditory or tactile (Brazelton 1984).

Crying

The crying repertoire of the baby distinguishes different needs, and is the way in which he communicates discomfort and summons assistance. With experience it is possible to differentiate the cry and identify the need which may be hunger, thirst, pain, general discomfort (e.g. wanting a change of position or feeling too cold or too hot), boredom, loneliness or a desire for physical and social contact. Maternal anxiety and difficulties related to infant crying can be allayed by information and advice from the midwife. The mother needs to learn how to comfort her baby. Rapid rocking induces sleep, swaddling and an upright position appear to be soothing (Downey & Bidder 1990).

Growth and development

Because of his physiological limitations, the baby is dependent on his mother for his continued survival, growth and development. These will progress satisfactorily only if he is physiologically and neurologically normal, he is in a safe environment, his nutritional needs are met, and his psychological development is promoted by appropriate stimulation and loving care. Abnormality of the infant's body systems, inadequate nutrition or emotional deprivation will compromise the baby's ability to grow and develop to his full potential. His relatively immature organ functions and his vulnerability to infection and hypothermia demand that his care must be designed to meet his needs and capabilities.

OBSERVATION AND CARE

Screening

Normality of the baby is assessed by a variety of means. This assessment begins at birth.

Examination at birth

Following a period of socialisation with his parents, the baby is examined carefully by the midwife to ascertain that externally at least, the baby is normal. If any defects are identified, medical assistance can be sought early.

Examination of the baby, whenever possible, should be performed beside the parents. The midwife should talk to them as she proceeds, explaining her findings. Prior to examining the baby the midwife should wash her hands to prevent infection. Her hands should be warm to prevent chilling of the infant. During the examination the baby should be naked in a warm, draught-free environment. There should be sufficient light to allow the midwife to see the baby clearly. The examination is performed in an orderly manner from the head of the infant to his feet. Overall symmetry should be verified and skin blemishes or abrasions noted.

Face, head and neck. After a general impression of the facies is gained, the eyes and mouth of the infant are examined first. Each eye should be visualised to confirm that it is present and that the lens is clear. The baby may open his eyes spontaneously if held in an upright position. Any slight oedema or bruising is noted but may be insignificant. The normal space between the eyes is up to 3 cm.

The mouth can be opened easily by pressing against the angle of the jaw. This allows inspection of the tongue, gums and palate. The palate should be high arched, intact and the uvula central. Epithelial pearls may be observed. The midwife uses her little finger to feel the palate for any submucous cleft. A normal baby will respond by sucking the finger. Precocious teeth may protrude through the central part of the lower gum. (Though usually covered by epithelial tissue, such teeth may have erupted and be loose, requiring extraction in the early neonatal period to prevent their inhalation.) A tight frenulum will give the appearance of tongue tie: no treatment is necessary for this. The frenum of the upper lip should be central.

During quiet breathing the baby breathes through his nose. If one nostril is blocked, occlusion of the other results in cyanosis and unsuccessful attempts to breathe through the mouth, culminating in crying. Bilateral obstruction has the same effect.

The ears are inspected, noting their position. The upper notch of the pinna should be level with the canthus of the eye. Patency of the external auditory meatus is verified. Accessory auricles, small tags of tissue, are sometimes noted lying in front of the ear.

By palpating the vault of the skull the midwife can determine the degree of moulding by the amount of overriding of the bones at the sutures and fontanelles. The bones should feel hard in a full-term infant. A wide anterior fontanelle and splayed sutures may indicate hydrocephalus or immaturity. The shape of the baby's head as a result of moulding gives indication of the presentation in utero (Fig. 32.2). An oedematous swelling, caput

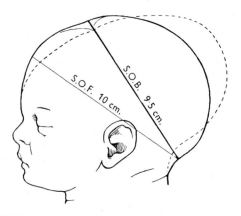

Fig. 32.2
Type of moulding in a vertex presentation.

succedaneum, may be noted overlying the part that was presenting. This is a result of pressure from the cervical os and will disappear spontaneously within 24 hours (see Ch. 37).

The short thick neck of the baby must be examined to exclude the presence of swellings and to ensure that rotation and flexion of the head is possible.

Chest and abdomen. Observation of respiratory movement should reveal that chest and abdominal movements are synchronous. The respirations may still be irregular at this stage. Spacing of the nipples should be noted, widely spaced nipples being associated with chromosomal abnormality.

The shape of the abdomen should be rounded. The midwife notes any variation, including a scaphoid (boat-shaped) abdomen or any protrusions particularly at the base of the umbilical cord.

The artery forceps securing the umbilical cord should be replaced by a plastic disposable clamp applied approximately 2 cm from the umbilicus. Excess cord is discarded. Normally three cord vessels are present. Absence of one of the arteries is associated with renal or cardiac anomalies and must be brought to the attention of the paediatrician.

Genitalia and anus. The genitalia should be examined carefully. If the sex is uncertain, the paediatrician will initiate investigations. The baby's temperature is taken rectally to detect any excessive cooling and to confirm patency of the anus.

Limbs and digits. In addition to noting length and movement of the limbs it is essential that the digits are counted and separated to ensure that webbing is not present. The hands should be opened fully as any accessory digits may be concealed in the clenched fist. The axillae, elbows, groins and popliteal spaces should also be examined. Normal flexion and rotation of the wrist and ankle joints should be confirmed.

Spine. With the baby lying prone the midwife should inspect and palpate the baby's back. Any swellings, dimples or hairy patches may signify an occult spinal defect.

Hips. It is essential that all babies undergo a specific examination (Ortolani's test) to detect congenital dislocation of the hips (Watson 1990).

In some centres this is performed by the midwife, in others the paediatrician is the person responsible for this.

To examine the hips the examiner must place the baby on a firm flat surface at waist height. The baby's legs are grasped with the flexed knees in the palms of the examiner's hands and the femur splinted between the index and middle fingers and the thumb. The baby's thighs are flexed onto the abdomen and rotated and abducted through an angle of 90° towards the examining surface. *No force should be exerted.* If the hip is dislocated a 'clunk' will be felt as the head of the femur slips into the acetabulum.

Barlow's test is a similar examination used in many centres.

Early referral to a paediatrician is essential if effective treatment is to be achieved (see Ch. 38).

Measurements. The baby's head circumference, length and weight are measured to provide parameters against which future growth can be monitored.

The head circumference is measured encircling it at the occipital protuberance and the supraorbital ridges with a measuring tape. Moulding may reduce this measurement and for this reason this estimate is sometimes delayed until the 3rd day when the head shape has resumed its normal contours.

The length of the baby is calculated in two stages, firstly by measuring from the crown of the head to the base of the spine, then from the base of the spine to the heels when the legs are extended. The practice of suspending the baby upside down for measuring purposes is outmoded and hazardous for the reasons stated in Chapter 31.

The baby is weighed and the identity bands are rechecked prior to his being dressed and wrapped in warm blankets.

Documentation. The midwife records her findings in the case notes and any abnormalities are brought to the attention of the paediatrician and of the receiving midwife in the postnatal ward.

Examination by the paediatrician

All newborn babies should be examined by a paediatrician (or other medical practitioner if a paediatrician is not available) within the first 24 hours of life and again prior to transfer home. Moss et al (1991) assert that a second examination is of little value, apart from a repeat examination of the hips. The mother should be present. Some aspects of the examination duplicate that of the midwife and so only the medical aspects are considered here. A general appraisal of the baby's colour, overall appearance and muscular activity is made throughout the examination.

Neurological assessment. The baby's reflex responses are elicited in order to establish normality of the neurological system. These are tested while the baby is in a quiet alert state. Absent or weak responses may indicate immaturity, cerebral damage or abnormality.

Auscultation. The paediatrican listens to the heart and lung sounds. A heart murmur may be present for some days after birth.

Palpation. The abdominal organs, particularly the liver, spleen and kidneys, are palpated noting any enlargement. Femoral pulses are assessed ensuring that they are full and of equal strength. The hips are re-examined.

Blood tests

Certain inborn errors of metabolism and endocrine disorders are detected by means of a blood test (Danks 1981). Blood, obtained from a heel prick with a stilette, is dripped onto circles on an absorbent card onto which full details of the baby's identity are entered. For detection of phenylketonuria, the baby must have had at least 48 hours of milk feeding and if for any reason the infant is receiving antibiotics himself or via breast milk, this information should be included. The blood collection may be delayed until the 6th or 7th day in order to test for hypothyroidism. Some centres test routinely for galactosaemia as well. (See Chapter 38 for details of these conditions and tests.)

Child health surveillance

Following discharge from the care of the midwife into that of the health visitor the screening of the baby is continued on a regular basis at the child health clinic (see Ch. 45).

Protection and safety

Prevention of infection is one essential aspect of the infant's protection and safety. Additional considerations are prevention of asphyxia, hypothermia, haemorrhage, injury and accident.

The midwife receiving the baby from the delivery suite staff should verify the baby's identification, sex and the date and time of birth. These details are entered on a cot card. The baby should be warmly dressed and placed in a prewarmed cot beside his mother to allow him to rest until he awakes to feed. During these first few hours after birth especially, the midwife should observe frequently that the baby's colour remains pink, his airway unobstructed, and that the umbilical cord clamp is secure. His temperature should be monitored to ensure that it is maintained within the normal range.

The mother's wishes regarding feeding should be determined so that the midwives are aware of her plans for the baby's nutrition (see Ch. 33).

Prevention of infection

Each baby should be provided with equipment for his sole use. Adequate linen supplies are essential. Members of staff who are liable to be a source of infection should not handle babies, and friends and relatives, especially children, who have colds should not visit.

Staphylococcal infection can be a particular problem in hospitals. For this reason hexachlorophane preparations are used for handwashing by personnel handling babies. In some centres hexachlorophane-based soap or liquid preparations (maximum concentration 3%) are used for cleansing the baby's skin (excluding the face).

Daily bathing is not essential but the mother should be given sufficient opportunities to bath the baby in order to increase her confidence. 'Topping and tailing', i.e. washing the baby's face, skin flexures and napkin area, should be carried out once or twice a day.

Cleanliness of the umbilical cord is essential. Minimal handling with washed hands, cleansing with tap water and keeping the cord dry have been shown to promote separation. This may include application of 0.33% hexachlorophane powder

(Mugford et al 1986, Salariya & Kowbus 1988, Rush 1990). It is advisable to ensure that the cord is not enclosed within the baby's napkin where contamination by urine or faeces may occur. The cord clamp is removed on the 3rd day provided the cord is dry and necrosed.

The baby's buttocks must be washed and dried carefully at every napkin change. Petroleum jelly applied to the buttocks will prevent meconium adhering to the skin and causing excoriation. Regular use of a barrier cream is recommended by some people. Sore buttocks may occur if the stools are loose or the skin is traumatised by over-enthusiastic rubbing.

The baby's eyes do not need to be cleansed unless a discharge is present. Hair is washed and dried carefully at the first bath but need not be washed daily.

Prevention of asphyxia

Choking can occur during feeding if co-ordination is poor and also following vomiting or regurgitation. When in his cot the baby should be laid on his back or side. A mucus extractor should be readily available so that aspiration of the baby's airway can be instituted quickly.

Prevention of hypothermia

Overexposure of the baby should be avoided. The room temperature should be maintained at 18°–21°C. The infant should be dressed in a cotton gown and covered by two cellular blankets. An additional blanket underneath the bottom sheet will provide extra warmth for babies who are having difficulty in maintaining their temperature. At home, additional clothing may be required. Overheating should be avoided (Hull & Chepallah 1983, Rutter 1986, Bacon 1991). Bath water should be warm, 37°C, and wet clothing should be changed as soon as possible. Swaddling should be loose enough to permit movement of arms and legs.

Prevention of haemorrhage

Haemostasis of the umbilical cord is vital. A blood loss of 30 ml from a baby is equivalent to almost half a litre of blood from an adult. In some hospitals prophylactic vitamin K 1 mg is given orally or intramuscularly to promote prothrombin formation (Jørgensen et al 1991).

Prevention of injury and accident

Sensible precautions should be observed by all staff in their own practice and taught to the mother. A baby should not be left unattended unless in his cot as vigorous activity may result in his falling off a bed or table. The temperature of bath water should be tested prior to immersing the baby and the temperature of a bottle feed tested before it is offered to the baby.

A baby should be moved from place to place in his cot rather than in arms and the bassinet of the cot should be flat, not elevated, to prevent dropping him if uneven floors are encountered.

If safety pins are used to secure the napkin they should be inserted into the cloth with one hand protecting the baby's abdomen to avoid penetration of the skin or genitalia.

If the baby's nails are long or ragged he may scratch his face. Mittens should be worn to prevent this. Such mittens should be made from cotton material with French seams to prevent loose threads entwining the fingers and occluding the circulation.

Babies do not require a pillow until the age of 2 years. Mothers should be advised that placing a pillow behind the baby's head is unsafe and an unnecessary decoration in pram or cot.

Polythene bags or sheeting should not be used near a baby. Waterproof mattress covers should enclose the mattress completely to prevent suffocation.

Advice should also be given to mothers about safety in the home, e.g. use of cat-nets, fireguards, cooker guards and stair gates.

Observation of behaviour

Observation of the baby's behaviour provides information about his general well-being.

Feeding

During feeds the midwife should observe the baby's eagerness or reluctance to feed and the co-ordination of his sucking and swallowing reflex. She should note the frequency with which he demands feeds. While feeding the baby clenches his fists, tucks them under his chin and wriggles his toes. He may grasp his mother's fingers during feeding. Eye contact also occurs, which enhances communication between mother and baby. Sucking is interspersed with rest periods. Abnormal feeding behaviours may signify cerebral damage, congenital abnormality or illness. See also Chapter 33.

Excretion

Observation of the phases of the stools and of any vomiting helps to identify abnormalities of the gastro-intestinal tract, inborn errors of metabolism and infection.

Sleeping and waking

A newborn baby usually sleeps for most of the time between feeds but should be alert and responsive when awake. Erratic sleep patterns may prove disconcerting to new parents (Booth 1985). Undue lethargy or irritability may indicate cerebral damage or sepsis.

Daily examination

Each day, the baby should be examined by a midwife to evaluate his progress and identify problems as they arise. The examination is similar to that undertaken at birth but is now concerned with monitoring daily changes in the baby and detecting any signs of infection.

The examination begins by noting the baby's posture and his colour and respirations. Any cyanosis should be reported to the paediatrician immediately. Jaundice may be noted from the 3rd day, and is abnormal if it arises earlier, deepens, or persists beyond the 7th day.

Palpation of the head permits assessment of the anterior fontanelle, which should be level, resolution of caput succedaneum and moulding, and identification of any new swellings, e.g. cephalhaematoma (see Ch. 38).

The baby's eyes and mouth are inspected for signs of infection. Sticky eyes are cleaned with normal saline after obtaining a swab for culture and sensitivity. The mouth should be clean and moist. Adherent white plaques indicate oral thrush infection.

Sucking blisters on the baby's lips may be observed, especially if he has been fed recently. These do not require any treatment.

As the baby is undressed his response to handling can be observed, his identity bands inspected and his responses to the midwife's voice noted as she talks to him and explains her actions to his mother.

The skin, especially in flexures and between the digits, is inspected for septic spots or abrasions. The fingertips and toes are examined for rag nails and paronychia. Skin rashes such as erythema toxicum, a red blotchy rash, are of little significance. Sometimes a harlequin colour change may be noted when the infant is lying on his side, the dependent part of the body appearing pinker than the rest with a clear line of demarcation down the centre of the body. This is caused by vasomotor instability and is of little importance. However, its appearance is startling and can alarm the mother.

Septic spots must be differentiated from milia which do not require treatment. Even a few septic spots must be taken seriously. The paediatrician may prescribe topical applications or systemic antibiotics and consider possible isolation of the baby.

Areas that rub on cot sheets may become excoriated. If this occurs the affected part should be protected from further friction.

The umbilical cord base is inspected for redness and the mother is reminded about care.

In some areas the baby's temperature is recorded with a low-recording thermometer. This may be taken under the axilla, in the groin or rectally, inserting the bulb 2.5 cm into the rectum. If the rectal route is used it is essential that the baby's legs and the thermometer are held to prevent sudden movement of the baby which could cause the thermometer to break and perforate the rectum.

Sore buttocks may be treated by exposure to the air but care must be taken to avoid chilling and the infant should be nursed on his side to prevent excoriation of his knees.

The stools are observed and compared with expectations in relation to the baby's age and feeding method. Constipation may be alleviated by offering the baby water between feeds. Loose watery stools may signify sugar intolerance or infection. The frequency of passing urine and stools in the preceding 24 hours should be noted.

Breast engorgement and pseudomenstruation require no treatment but explanation to the mother is essential.

If the baby is to be weighed, this is done before he is dressed and the result compared with his birthweight. A common regime is weighing every 3rd day. Weight loss is normal in the first few days but more than 10% bodyweight loss is abnormal and requires investigation. Most babies regain their birthweight in 7–10 days, thereafter gaining weight at a rate of 150–200 g per week.

All findings at the daily examination are entered in the baby's records and abnormalities reported.

Promotion of maternal confidence

Parent–infant attachment

Positive responses from the baby to the attention or care given by the parents reinforce parental attachment and stimulate further interaction. Knowledge of the reflexes, general abilities and sleep and awake states of babies enables the midwife to teach the parents how to take advantage of the occasions when their baby is likely to be most responsive. The resulting interactions continue the process of attachment initiated at delivery (see Ch. 31). Admiration of the baby's best features, use of his given name and requesting the mother's permission to handle the baby help the woman to perceive herself as a mother.

It is important, however, not to overemphasise 'bonding' as this can create non-productive guilt feelings in parents who do not experience instant love for their child. This may result in negative attitudes towards the baby (Sluckin et al 1984, Parkinson & Harvey 1987).

The foregoing discussions in this chapter have endeavoured to illustrate how the midwife can enhance the mother–baby relationship. Her teaching, support and encouragement of the mother as she learns to provide for her baby's needs is of paramount importance and should culminate in a happy, confident and competent mother being discharged from the midwife's care. The midwife can also do a great deal to encourage a father's interaction with his baby and should take every opportunity to do so. These aspects of midwifery practice are described more fully in Chapter 16 (see also Richards 1986).

Reader Activities

The mother's agreement should be obtained before undertaking these activities. Repeating the activity will help you notice differences between babies.
- Compare the examination of the baby's head on day 1 and day 4 with regard to (a) fontanelle size; (b) overriding of the sutures; (c) measurement of occipito-frontal circumference.
- Keep a detailed record of the umbilical cords of up to ten babies with regard to (a) treatment–type, frequency, number of persons involved; (b) day of cord separation; (c) mother's reaction to the cord; (d) the sex of the baby.
- Observe a baby who is awake. Is the baby in a drowsy, quiet alert, active alert or active crying state? Relate the awake state to the timing of the last feed or period of handling.
- Examine a baby in a quiet alert state and endeavour to elicit (a) Moro reflex; (b) grasp, stepping and walking reflexes; (c) rooting reflex. Involve the mother in your observations.
- Observe a sleeping baby. Determine whether the sleep is light or deep. Shine a light on the baby's face and observe the response. Repeat the action and note habituation. Repeat the exercise using sound, e.g. clapping your hands. Explain the baby's behaviour to the mother.
- Observe crying babies and note (a) crying pattern; (b) colour; (c) mother's reaction. Does it make a difference if the mother has had a baby before? What strategies appear to soothe babies most? What is your own reaction to persistent crying?
- Ascertain the addresses of local support groups for mothers of crying babies, e.g. CRY-SIS. Do the mothers in your care know about this help-line?

- Compare five breast-fed and five bottle-fed babies with regard to (a) stool pattern — colour, consistency, odour and frequency; (b) sleep/awake pattern; (c) feeding behaviour — sucking pattern, co-ordination between sucking, swallowing and breathing — does the baby behave the same at each feed? Is the baby held in the same way at each feed? How much eye contact is made with the mother?
- Observe and record the interaction of ten babies with their parents — five first babies, and five later babies. Note the response of each baby to the mother's voice in comparison with others; observe the baby's visual tracking; compare the patterns of stroking and touching by both parents.

REFERENCES

Bacon C J 1991 The thermal environment of sleeping babies and possible dangers of overheating. In: David T J (ed) Recent advances in paediatrics. Churchill Livingstone, Edinburgh, p 123–136

Booth K 1985 Babies' sleeping patterns, parental opinions and low sleeping infants. Health Visitor 58: 17–18

Brazelton T B 1984 Neonatal behavioural assessment scale, 2nd edn. Spastics International Medical Publications, Blackwell Scientific, London

Damstra-Wijmenga S M I 1991 The memory of the new-born baby. Midwives Chronicle and Nursing Notes March 1991: 66–69

Danks D 1981 Diagnosis of metabolic diseases after birth: neonatal screening and the investigation of symptomatic patients or babies at genetic risk. In: Hull D (ed) Recent advances in paediatrics — 6. Churchill Livingstone, Edinburgh

DeCasper A, Fifer W 1987 Of human bonding: newborns prefer their mother's voices. In: Oates J, Sheldon S (eds) Cognitive development in infancy. Lawrence Erlbaum Associates in association with the Open University, Hove

Downey J, Bidder R T 1990 Perinatal information on infant crying. Child: Care, Health and Development 16(2): 113–121

Hull D, Chepallah G 1983 On keeping babies warm. In: Chiswick M (ed) Recent advances in perinatal medicine — 1. Churchill Livingstone, Edinburgh

Jørgensen F S, Felding P, Vinther S, Andersen G 1991 Vitamin K to neonates. Peroral versus intramuscular administration. Acta Paediatrica Scandinavica 80: 304–307

MacFarlane A 1975 Olfaction in the development of social preferences in the human neonate. In: Parent–infant interaction. CIBA Foundation Symposium 33, Elsevier, Amsterdam

Moss G D, Cartlidge P H T, Speides B D, Chambers T L 1991 Routine examination in the neonatal period. British Medical Journal 302: 878–9

Mugford M, Somchiwong M, Waterhouse I 1986 Treatment of umbilical cords: a randomised trial to assess the effect of treatment methods on the work of midwives. Midwifery 2: 177–186

Parkinson C E, Harvey D 1987 Child development and the maternal–infant relationship. In: Harvey D (ed) Parent–infant relationships. Wiley series on perinatal practice Vol 4, John Wiley, Chichester

Richards M 1986 Psychological aspects of neonatal care. In: Roberton N C R (ed) Textbook of neonatology. Churchill Livingstone, Edinburgh

Rush J 1990 Care of the umbilical cord. In: Alexander J, Levy V, Roch S (eds) Midwifery practice: postnatal care: a research-based approach. Macmillan, Basingstoke

Rutter N 1986 Temperature control and its disorders. In: Roberton N C R (ed) Textbook of neonatology. Churchill Livingstone, Edinburgh

Salariya E, Kowbus N 1988 Variable umbilical cord care. Midwifery 4: 70–76

Sluckin W, Sluckin A, Herbert M 1984 On mother-to-infant bonding. Midwife, Health Visitor and Community Nurse 20(2): 404–407

Watson J 1990 Screening for congenital dislocation of the hip. Maternal and Child Health 15(10): 310, 312–314

FURTHER READING

Behrman R E, Vaughan V C 1983 Nelson textbook of paediatrics, 12th edn. W B Saunders, Philadelphia, p 13–16 and ch 7

Clarke A M, Clarke A D B 1976 Early experience: myth and evidence. Open Books, London

Harvey D (ed) 1987 Parent–infant relationships. Wiley series on perinatal practice Vol 4, John Wiley, Chichester

Illingworth R S 1987 The development of the infant and young child, 9th edn. Churchill Livingstone, Edinburgh

Jensen M, Bobak I 1985 Maternal and gynaecologic care (the nurse and the family), 3rd edn. Mosby, Boston

Klaus M H, Kennell J H 1982 Parent–infant bonding, C V Mosby, St Louis

Reeder S, Mastroianni Jr L, Martin L 1987 Maternity nursing, 16th edn. Lippincott, Philadelphia

Roberton N C R (ed) 1986 Textbook of neonatology, Churchill Livingstone, Edinburgh

Rutter M 1981 Maternal deprivation reassessed, 2nd edn. Penguin, London, ch 10

Salariya E 1990 Parent–infant attachment. In: Alexander J, Levy V, Roch S (eds) Postnatal care — a research based approach. Macmillan, Basingstoke

Sluckin W, Herbert M, Sluckin A 1983 Maternal Bonding. Basil Blackwell, Oxford

Stratton P (ed) 1982 Psychobiology of the human newborn. (Developmental psychology series) John Wiley, Chichester

Whaley L, Wong D 1991 Nursing care of infants and children, 4th edn. Mosby, St Louis

33

Feeding

CHLOE FISHER

The World Health Organization's definition of a midwife includes the skilled supervision, care and advice to be given to the mother during the post-partum period and the care to be given to the newborn baby and the young infant. Responsibility for the initiation of infant feeding and lactation therefore lies with the midwifery profession. The International Confederation of Midwives adopted a policy about breast feeding in 1984 which clearly defines the midwife's responsibility in this field and describes the 'unique and vital role of the midwife in the promotion of breast feeding' (ICM 1985).

Many hours of the mother's time, day and night for many months, will be spent feeding the baby. She should be supported in the feeding method of her choice and enabled to accomplish it with skill, knowledge, confidence and pleasure. A firm mother–baby attachment can be forged during these frequent encounters, provided that they proceed without anxiety. When breast feeding goes well, there is the added advantage of the mother's sense of achievement and satisfaction. For these reasons alone, breast feeding must be the ideal way to feed a baby.

THE BREAST AND BREAST MILK

In developing countries, where the knowledge and skills of breast feeding have been retained within society, women consider it the normal thing to do. In these countries midwives will encourage mothers to breast feed because of the protection against infection conferred on the baby and breast feeding will have an excellent chance of being successful. On the other hand, in the so-called developed world, the midwife should recognise that the majority of women who choose to breast feed do so because they regard it as the fulfilment of motherhood and are less conscious of the benefits of human milk for their babies. Unfortunately there is currently a high failure rate which must in part be attributed to lack of knowledge and loss of skills. It is most important for midwives to understand the benefits of human milk for human babies because this will help to inspire them in their supportive role (Howie et al 1990, Lucas & Cole 1990). This knowledge should be shared with mothers where it is appropriate but should not be used to put undue pressure on them.

Anatomy and physiology of the breast

The breasts are compound secreting glands, composed mainly of glandular tissue which is arranged in *lobes*, approximately 20 in number. Each lobe is divided into *lobules* that consist of *alveoli* and *ducts*. The alveoli contain *acini cells* which produce milk and are surrounded by *myo-epithelial cells* which contract and propel the milk out. The breasts are richly supplied with blood. Small *lactiferous ducts*, carrying milk from the alveoli, unite to form larger ducts: one large duct leaves each lobe and widens to form a *lactiferous sinus* or *ampulla* which acts as a temporary reservoir for milk. A *lactiferous tubule* from each sinus emerges on the surface of the nipple. Each breast functions independently of the other.

The *nipple*, composed of erectile tissue, is covered with epithelium and contains plain muscle fibres which have a sphincter-like action in controlling the flow of milk. Surrounding the nipple is an area of pigmented skin called the *areola* which contains *Montgomery's glands*. These produce a sebum-like substance which acts as a lubricant during pregnancy and throughout breast feeding. Breasts, nipples and areolae vary considerably in size from one woman to another.

The breast is supplied with blood from the internal and external mammary arteries and branches

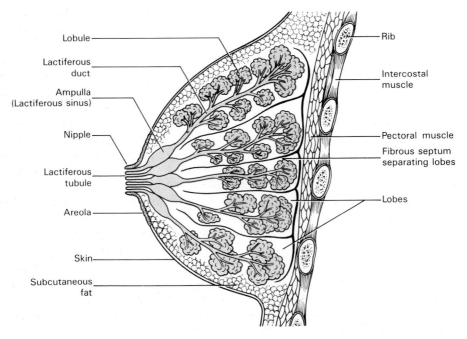

Fig. 33.1
Lactating breast.

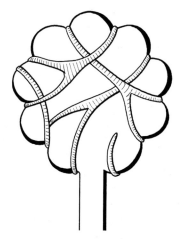

Fig. 33.2
Alveoli surrounded by myo-epithelial cells which propel the milk out of the lobule.

from the intercostal arteries. The veins are arranged in a circular fashion around the nipple.

Lymph drains freely between the two breasts and into lymph nodes in the axillae and the mediastinum.

During pregnancy, oestrogens and progesterone induce alveolar and ductal growth as well as stimulating the secretion of *colostrum*. Other hormones are also involved and they govern a complex sequence of events which prepare the breast for lactation. The production of milk is held in abeyance until after delivery, when the levels of oestrogens fall. This allows the level of prolactin to rise and milk production to commence. Continued production of prolactin is caused by the baby feeding at the breast, with concentrations highest during night feeds. (Prolactin suppresses ovulation and causes some women to remain anovulatory until lactation ceases, although for others this effect is not so prolonged.) If breast feeding (or expressing) has to be delayed for a few days, lactation can still be initiated.

Milk release is under *neuro-endocrine control*. Tactile stimulation of the breast stimulates the production of oxytocin causing contraction of the myoepithelial cells. This process is known as the *'let-down'* or *'milk ejection' reflex* and makes the milk available to the baby. In the early days of lactation this reflex is unconditioned and is therefore unlikely to be inhibited by anxiety. Later it becomes a conditioned reflex responding to the baby's cry (or other circumstances associated with the baby or feeding). At this stage it could be inhibited to some extent by anxiety. Milk is transferred to the baby by a combination of the milk ejection reflex and active removal of milk by the action of the baby's tongue and jaw. Removal of milk is the most important factor in the maintenance of milk production, because without it prolactin will not be released and the supply will diminish.

Properties and components of breast milk

Human milk varies in its composition with the time of day, with the stage of lactation, in response to maternal nutrition and because of individual variations. Fore-milk, at the beginning of the feed, differs from hind-milk, towards the end of the feed. Samples obtained for research may not represent the milk obtained by the baby because of the methods used for collection. Comparison with the milks of other animals shows human milk to be unique. It meets all the nutritional requirements of the new baby and has many other important properties as well.

Fat provides the baby with more than 50% of his calorific requirements (Helsing & Savage King 1982). The fat content in human milk has diurnal variations, being lowest in the morning and highest in the afternoon. The proportion of fat in the milk increases during the course of the feed, sometimes increasing to five times the initial value. It is utilised very rapidly because of the action of the enzyme *lipase* which is present in the milk in a form which only becomes active in the infant's intestine. Pancreatic lipase is not plentiful in the newborn baby.

Lactose. There is more lactose in human milk than in any other mammalian milk. It is converted into galactose and glucose by the action of the enzyme *lactase* and these sugars provide energy to the rapidly growing brain. Lactose enhances the absorption of calcium and also promotes the growth of lactobacilli which increase intestinal acidity, thus stemming the growth of pathogenic organisms.

Protein. Human milk contains less than half the amount of protein contained in cow's milk but because of its easy digestibility it provides the baby with the ideal quantity. Human milk forms soft, flocculent curds when acidified in the stomach. The predominant protein is *lactalbumin (whey protein)* and *caseinogen* is present in lower quantities. This provides a continuous flow of nutrients to the baby. Two amino acids, cystine and taurine, are found in human milk but not in cow's milk. The first is important for growth and the second for the development of the brain. Colostrum contains nearly three times the amount of protein that is present in mature milk and contains all the ten essential amino acids. It also contains secretory IgA and *lactoferrin* (see below).

Vitamins, minerals and trace elements

There are four fat-soluble vitamins, A, D, E and K:

Vitamin A. Mature human milk contains 280 international units (IU) of vitamin A and colostrum contains twice that amount. Cow's milk contains only 180 IU.

Vitamin D. It is now believed that both water-soluble and fat-soluble vitamin D are present in human milk. Provided that the mother's diet is adequate and that the baby can be exposed to the sun, supplementation with vitamin D is not necessary. Dark-skinned babies living in temperate zones and preterm babies are the exceptions.

Vitamin E. Human colostrum is rich in vitamin E and the levels in mature human milk are higher than in cow's milk. Its main function is to prevent haemolytic anaemia but it also helps to protect the lungs and retina from oxidant-induced injury.

Vitamin K. This vitamin is essential for the synthesis of blood-clotting factors. It is present in human milk and absorbed efficiently. Recent research suggests that the breast-fed baby may receive more vitamin K than has previously been demonstrated because it has been discovered that levels are higher in colostrum and, in the early days, in the high fat hind-milk (Kries et al 1987). Later, levels depend on maternal dietary intake. Babies who are at risk of haemorrhage, such as the preterm and those delivered precipitately or instrumentally, usually receive a prophylactic dose, usually by intramuscular injection. Many paediatricians consider that all other babies should receive an oral dose soon after birth. After a few days the baby's gut flora will synthesise vitamin K. Colonisation of the gut may be aided by encouraging the mother not to wash her breasts, or otherwise clean them before a feed.

Vitamin B complex. All of the B vitamins are present at levels which are believed to provide the baby with his necessary daily requirements.

Vitamin C. Human milk contains 43 mg/100 ml of vitamin C compared with 21 mg/100 ml in fresh cow's milk. The amount in the mother's milk reflects the dietary intake and it is advisable for her to increase her intake during lactation. Vitamin C is essential for collagen synthesis.

Iron. Normal full-term babies are usually born with a high haemoglobin level (16–22 g/dl) which decreases rapidly after birth. The iron recovered from haemoglobin breakdown is utilised again. They also have ample iron stores which last from 4–6 months. Human milk and cow's milk contain small quantities of iron (0.5–1 mg/1). 49% of the amount available in human milk is utilised, whereas only 4% is absorbed from cow's milk (Saarinen & Siimes 1977). The difference is due to the high levels of vitamin C and lactose in human milk which facilitate absorption. Babies who are fed cow's milk may become anaemic because of microhaemorrhages of the bowel. Preterm babies do not have good iron stores and may need supplementation with oral iron.

Zinc. This trace mineral is essential to humans. A deficiency may result in failure to thrive and typical skin lesions. Although there is more zinc present in cow's milk than in human milk, the bio-availability is greater in human milk.

Other minerals. Human milk has significantly lower levels of calcium, phosphorus, sodium and potassium than cow's milk. Breast milk therefore imposes a lower solute load on the neonatal kidney than does unmodified cow's milk. If a baby is fed on 'doorstep' milk, he will become dehydrated due to hypernatraemia (excess sodium). The breast-fed baby does not ingest an overload of salts and is therefore unlikely to need additional water under most conditions (Almroth 1978, Goldberg & Adams 1983, Sachdev et al 1991).

Other important properties

Anti-infective factors. During the first 10 days there are more white cells per ml than there are in blood.

Macrophages and neutrophils are amongst the most common leucocytes in human milk and they surround and destroy harmful bacteria by their phagocytic activity.

Secretory IgA and interferon are important anti-infective agents produced in abundance by lymphocytes in human milk.

Immunoglobulins IgA, IgG, IgM and IgD are all found in human milk. Of these the most important is IgA, which appears to be both synthesised and stored in the breast. It 'paints' the intestinal epithelium and protects the mucosal surfaces against entry of pathogenic bacteria and enteroviruses. It affords protection against *Escherichia coli*, salmonellae, shigellae, streptococci, staphylococci, pneumococci, poliovirus and the rotaviruses.

Lysozyme is present in breast milk in concentrations 5000 times greater than in cow's milk. It is a well known general anti-infective agent and its activity appears to increase during lactation.

Lactoferrin is abundant in human milk but is not present in cow's milk. It effects the absorption of enteric iron, thus preventing pathogenic *E. coli* from obtaining the iron they need for survival.

The bifidus factor in human milk promotes the growth of Gram-positive bacilli in the gut flora, particularly *Lactobacillus bifidus*, which discourages the multiplication of pathogens. Babies who are fed on cow's milk formula have Gram-negative (potentially pathogenic) bacilli in their gut flora.

Anti-allergic factors. Allergic problems occur less frequently in breast-fed babies than in bottle-fed babies. This may be because the infant's intestinal mucosa is permeable to proteins before the age of 6–9 months and proteins in cow's milk can act as allergens.

Occasionally a baby may become allergic to substances in his mother's milk which come from her diet. This is rare and can be circumvented by the mother avoiding the foods which cause the trouble so that she may continue to breast feed.

MANAGEMENT OF BREAST FEEDING

Medical involvement in infant feeding is known to have occurred throughout the history of the human race. Modern medicine entered the 'scientific' era early this century and, as a result, many practitioners came to believe that they had knowledge which would enable them to improve upon nature and they applied this belief to the management of breast feeding. Unfortunately, they were unaware of the fact that each mother–baby pair is unique and that the 'rules' that they evolved would be inappropriate for the majority. Another unfortunate fact is that when information is published in a medical textbook, it is repeated in further editions as well as in textbooks by other authors. In this manner, an idea that may have been speculative and never tested soon becomes an accepted 'truth'.

There are many examples of ideas about breast feeding which originated in the first 20 years of this century and were never properly tested. Some are to be found in textbooks in use in the 1990s. A few *fallacies* will serve to illustrate this point:

- During the first few days of breast feeding, the length of the feed should be limited to prevent sore nipples. (This must have been based on a mistaken belief that the baby fed from the nipple, not the breast.)
- That both breasts must be used at each feed.
- That the baby should feed for 10 minutes at each breast or that feeds should last only 20 minutes.
- That the breast must be held away from the baby's nose during a feed.
- That the baby should feed at regular intervals (King 1913).

These are the most common *errors* that have been perpetuated over a period of more than 60 years. They have been repeated in both medical and midwifery textbooks because the authors relied on the writings of other 'experts' rather than common sense or research evidence. Such evidence is now available.

Antenatal preparation

The majority of women who choose to breast feed know before they conceive that they want to breast feed their babies. A few may not make this choice until after giving birth, so it is important that the midwife should have a sensitive approach and not require a definite decision. Time should be taken during antenatal classes to talk about the day-to-day progress and management of early breast feeding, so that after the baby is born these concepts will be familiar to the mother. This does not mean that she will not require to be taught about the major details of management *after* the baby is born because pregnant women find it difficult to project their thoughts forward to the time beyond the birth.

Breasts and nipples are altered by pregnancy (see Ch. 8). Increased sebum secretion obviates the need for cream to lubricate the nipple. A comfortable brassière that does not compress the breast may be worn to support the increasing weight: this will not affect the changes in the shape of the breast which occur as a result of pregnancy. Anatomically small nipples cannot be altered by preparation but they are no bar to satisfactory breast feeding. Women who have inverted and non-protractile (flat) nipples often find that they improve spontaneously during pregnancy (Hytten & Baird 1958). If not, help given with positioning the baby at the breast after birth often results in successful breast feeding (Hytten 1954). Wearing breast shells inside a brassière and gentle stretching of the breast tissue at the base of the nipple (Hoffmann's exercises (Hoffmann 1953)) have both been recommended for many years. These practices are being evaluated (Alexander et al 1991); at present there is no evidence to support their routine use.

Education of the mother is better preparation than any physical exercises. If she understands how milk is produced and has an opportunity to observe babies feeding, she will be well on the way to success with feeding her own.

Technique

The commencement of breast feeding

The first feed is a profoundly important experience for the mother and her baby. If it proceeds without pain and if the baby is allowed to terminate the feed naturally, both will have been helped to begin the learning process necessary for good breast feeding in a happy and positive way. This feed should be supervised by the midwife.

Early feeding contributes to the success of breast feeding but the time of the first feed should, to a large extent, depend on the needs of the baby. Some may demonstrate a desire to feed almost as soon as they are born. Many midwives use this as a means to facilitate uterine contractions during the third stage of labour and thereby reduce blood loss. Other babies may show no interest until they are an hour or so old (Widström et al 1987, Righard & Alade 1990). Babies of mothers who have received narcotics during labour may sleep for some time before wanting to feed.

Whenever the first feed takes place, the quality of that experience is of the utmost importance. Mothers who receive the right help and education at the start will require less support and remedial intervention later.

They should be told about the cause, and therefore prevention, of sore nipples (see below). They should be urged to seek help if problems do arise. They should be told about the changes that will take place in their breasts during the next few days. An explanation about the changes in the

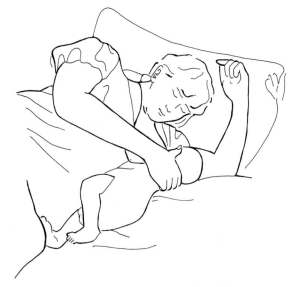

Fig. 33.3
Mother lying comfortably on her side.

pattern of feeds and the reasons for the variation in the length of feeds will enable them to greet these changes with confidence. Helping them to understand that breast feeding is a learned, not an instinctive, skill will enable them to be patient with themselves and their babies during this time.

Positioning the mother

There are two main positions for the mother to adopt while she is breast feeding. The first is lying on her side and this may be appropriate at different times during her lactation (Fig. 33.3). If she has had a caesarean section, or if her perineum is very painful, this may be the only position she can tolerate in the first few days after birth. She will need assistance in placing the baby at the breast because it will be difficult for her to manipulate him skilfully. When feeding from the lower breast it may be helpful to raise her body slightly by tucking the end of a pillow under her ribs. Later she may choose to feed lying down after she and her baby have learned how to breast feed, either during the day because she finds it

more comfortable and restful or at night because it is more convenient.

The second position is sitting up. In the early days it is particularly important that the mother's back is upright and at a right angle to her lap (Fig. 33.4). This is not possible if she is sitting in bed with her legs stretched out in front of her (though she might be able to achieve it sitting cross-legged) or if she is sitting in a chair with a deep backward-sloping seat and a sloping back.

Both lying on her side and sitting correctly in a chair (with her back and feet supported) enhance the shape of the breast and also allow ample room in which to manoeuvre the baby.

Positioning the baby's body

The baby's body should be turned towards the mother's body (Fig. 33.5). The baby's mouth should be opposite the nipple and the neck should be slightly extended (Fig. 33.6).

Positioning (or attaching or latching) the baby's mouth onto the breast

The baby should be supported across his shoulders, so that the slight extension of the neck can be

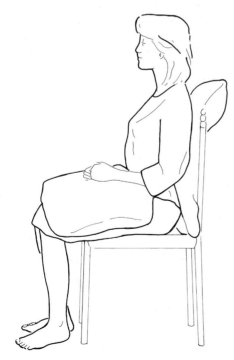

Fig. 33.4
Mother sitting with upright back and flat lap.

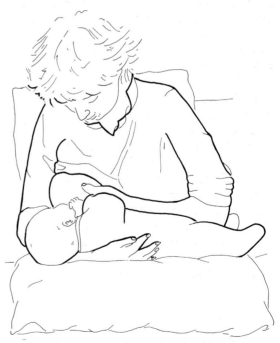

Fig. 33.5
The baby's body turned towards the mother's body.

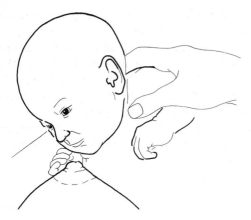

Fig. 33.6
The baby's mouth opposite the nipple, the neck slightly extended.

maintained. The head may be supported by the extended fingers of the supporting hand (Fig. 33.7) or on the mother's forearm (Fig. 33.8). It may be helpful to wrap the baby firmly in a small sheet so that his hands are by his sides (Fig. 33.9). If the baby's mouth is moved gently but persistently against his mother's nipple he will open his mouth wide (Fig. 33.10). This is termed the *rooting reflex*. Mothers may find the suggestion that they should try to stroke the top lip against the nipple helpful (Prechtl 1958). As his

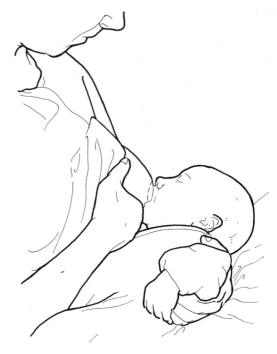

Fig. 33.8
The baby's head supported on the mother's forearm.

mouth gapes, he is moved quickly to the breast. The aim is to position the bottom lip at least $\frac{1}{2}$ inch (1.5 cm) away from the base of the nipple. This allows the baby to draw some of the breast tissue into his mouth with his tongue and lower jaw. If correctly positioned, the baby will have formed a teat from the breast and the nipple. The lactiferous sinuses will now be within the baby's

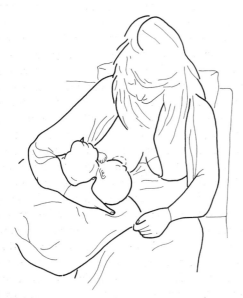

Fig. 33.7
The baby's head supported by the mother's extended fingers.

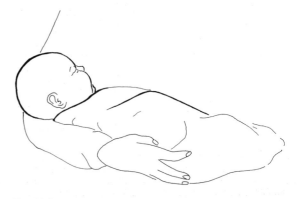

Fig. 33.9
The baby wrapped firmly with hands by sides.

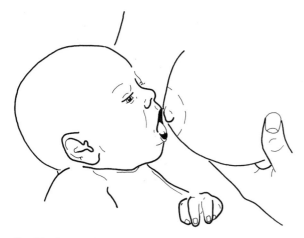

Fig. 33.10
Wide gape, with tongue down and forward.

mouth (Fig. 33.11) (Woolridge 1986). The nipple will extend back as far as the soft palate and make contact with it. It is this contact which triggers

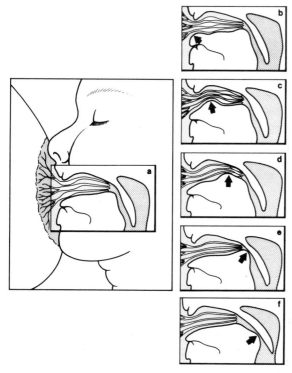

Fig. 33.11
The baby has formed a 'teat' from the breast and the nipple, which causes the nipple to extend back as far as the junction of the hard and soft palates. The lactiferous sinuses are within the baby's mouth. A generous portion of areola is covered by the bottom lip. (Reproduced from Woolridge 1986.)

the *sucking reflex*. The baby's lower jaw closes on the breast tissue, suction is exerted so that the nipple is held well within the mouth and the tongue applies rhythmical cycles of compression so that milk is stripped from the ducts. Although the mother may be startled by the physical sensation, she should not experience pain. Some women experience feelings of sexual arousal or even orgasm due to the stimulation of the nipple, though this is probably rare.

The role of the midwife

The midwife's role during the first few feeds is two-fold. First, she must ensure that the baby is adequately fed at the breast. Second, she must help the mother to develop the necessary skills so that she is able to feed her baby by herself. Some mothers will need more teaching and support than others; even women who have breast fed previously may require help with their new babies. Correct attachment of the baby to the breast prevents many breast-feeding problems.

In practical terms it may be necessary for the midwife to help attach the baby to the breast for several feeds. She should think of her own comfort, as well as that of the mother and her baby, because she will be much less capable of providing skilled help if she is strained and uncomfortable. She should also consider which hand guides the baby most skilfully and use it for preference. For example, she may be helping a mother who is lying on her left side and have successfully attached the baby to the left breast with her right hand (Fig. 33.12). Instead of asking the mother to turn on her right side she could raise up the baby on a pillow and attach him to the right breast, again using her right hand (Fig. 33.13). If the mother is sitting up, she could consider placing the baby under the mother's arm on the side she finds less easy (Fig. 33.14). Some midwives feel more comfortable if they stand behind the mother so that they get the same view as she does. Once the baby has fed efficiently he is likely to do so again with little difficulty and it is from this point that the mother can begin to learn how to feed her baby by herself.

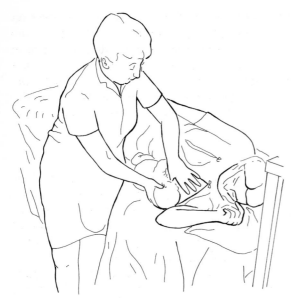

Fig. 33.12
The mother lying on her left side with the midwife helping her baby to feed at the left breast.

The midwife must give the mother positive, correct advice. *The baby feeds from the breast* rather than from the nipple and the mother should guide her baby towards her breast without distorting its shape. *The baby's neck should be slightly extended* and *the chin should be in contact with the breast.* A generous portion of areola should be taken in by the lower jaw but the baby is often unable to draw in the whole of the areola.

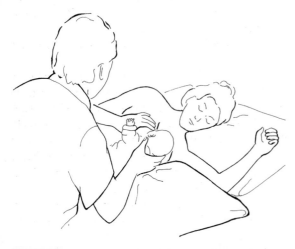

Fig. 33.13
The mother still on her left side with the midwife helping the baby to feed from the right breast.

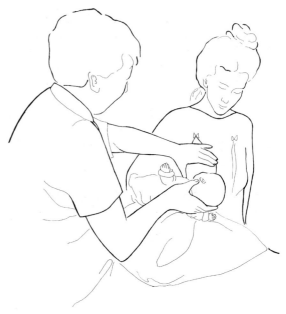

Fig. 33.14
The baby placed under the mother's arm with midwife helping.

Feeding behaviour

When the baby first goes to the breast he feeds vigorously, with few pauses. As the feed progresses, pausing occurs more frequently and lasts longer. Pausing is an integral part of the baby's feeding rhythm and should not be interrupted. The midwife should simply encourage the mother to allow herself to be paced by the baby. The change in the pattern probably relates to milk flow. The *fore-milk* which he obtains first is more generous in quantity but more dilute than the *hind-milk* delivered at the end which is high in calories (Woolridge & Fisher 1988).

Finishing the first breast and finishing a feed

The baby will release the breast when he has had sufficient milk from it. His ability to know this may be controlled either by the calories he has received or by the change in the volume available. The baby should be offered the second breast after he has had the opportunity to bring up wind. Sometimes in the early days the baby will not need to feed from the second breast. Taking the baby off the first breast before he has finished may cause two problems. Firstly, the baby is deprived of the high-calorie hind-milk and second-ly, if adequate milk removal has not taken place, milk stasis may occur leading to mastitis or dimi-nution of secretion. Provided that the baby starts each feed on alternate sides, both breasts will func-tion equally. If the baby does not release the breast or will not settle after a feed, the most likely reason is that he had not been correctly attached to the breast and was therefore unable to strip the milk efficiently.

Other reasons for coming off the breast
- The baby may not have been correctly attached.
- The baby may need to let go and pause if the milk flow is very fast.
- The baby may have swallowed air with the generous flow of milk that occurs at the begin-ning of a feed and need an opportunity to bring it up.

Timing and frequency of feeds
If the length of the feed is determined by the baby from the beginning, the feed lengths will be fairly long, as will the intervals between. This is described as *baby-led feeding* which is a term pre-ferable to 'demand feeding'. It is not unusual in the first day or two for the baby to have 6–8 hour gaps between good feeds (Waldenström & Swensen 1991). This is normal and provides an excellent opportunity for the mother to rest. As the milk volume increases, the feeds become more fre-quent and a little shorter. It is unusual for a baby to feed less often than 6 times in 24 hours from the third day. If he demands fewer feeds he may also be taking less than he needs at each feed. Reasons for this include drowsiness, immaturity and illness. Each possibility should be investigated. The feeding technique and the weight should be monitored. Individual mother–baby pairs develop their own unique pattern of feeding and, provided the baby is thriving, there can be no valid reason for attempting to change it.

Volume of the feed
No precise information is available on the actual volume of breast milk which an individual baby requires in order to grow satisfactorily. Previous recommendations (150 ml per kg) were based on the requirements of artificially fed babies, and these can therefore be used only as a guideline. If the baby's initial weight loss exceeds 10%, this indicates an inadequate intake. If the baby has regained his birth weight by the 10th day, this indicates that his intake has been adequate.

Expressing breast milk

Expressing the breast should not be part of the normal management of lactation. The balance between the volume of milk produced and the requirement of the baby, which results from correct feeding, prevents the occurrence of problems that would require artificial removal of milk.

The situations where expressing is necessary result from the absence of a baby feeding at the breast. Examples are as follows:

- Where there are major problems in attaching the baby to the breast.
- Where the baby is separated from the mother, due to prematurity or illness.
- Later in lactation, when the mother may be separated temporarily because of work.

Manual expression of milk. This method is not commonly practised where electric breast pumps are available but it has several advantages over mechanical pumping. It costs nothing and can be practised anywhere. It causes a higher level of prolactin release which will help to main-tain lactation over a longer period.

Expressing with a breast pump. There are several types:

Electrical. There are several designs available. Some pumps provide a regular vacuum and release cycle, with variability in the strength of the suc-tion. Some vary the frequency of the cycle as well. Some simpler models provide only continuous suction, so that the mother has to take her finger off a hole to release it. Women can be very adapt-able and make all of these work. The size of the breast cup may be the determinant of success and it is important to encourage the mother to experiment.

Manually controlled breast pumps. There are many designs. Most manually operated pumps are not efficient enough to allow initiation of full lactation but they can be useful when expressing is necessary in well established lactation. It is helpful to mothers to explain that the pumps function most efficiently if the vacuum phase is considerably longer than the release phase.

Care of the breasts

Daily washing is all that is necessary for breast hygiene. The normal skin flora are beneficial to the baby. Brassières may be worn in order to provide comfortable support and are useful if the breasts leak and breast pads are used. They should be large enough not to compress the breasts.

Breasts should be examined daily by the midwife. If the mother does not complain of any problems the examination will probably show that the breasts are soft and are free from lumps, redness and soreness.

Breast problems

Sore and damaged nipples

These two conditions occur so commonly in developed countries that many health professionals believe them to be inevitable. The cause is almost always trauma from the baby's mouth and tongue which results from incorrect positioning of the baby's mouth at the breast. Correcting this will provide immediate relief from pain and will also allow rapid healing to take place. It is thought that there may be healing properties contained in fresh human milk and saliva which aid this process. 'Resting' the nipple also enables healing to take place but makes the continuation of lactation much more complicated because it would be necessary to express the milk and to use some other means of feeding it to the baby. The use of nipple shields does not solve the problem either, because they do not allow the mother to learn how to feed her baby correctly and the feeds may both continue to be painful and to cause trauma to the nipple.

Better understanding of the cause of these problems enables midwives to be proficient at helping women with these distressing conditions.

Other causes of soreness

Infection with **Candida albicans** (thrush) can occur, although it is not common during the first week. It frequently follows a period of trouble-free feeding. The nipple and areola are inflamed and shiny and pain persists throughout the feed. The baby may show signs of oral or anal thrush. Both mother and baby should receive fungicidal treatment (nystatin: see Ch. 34) and it may take several days for the pain in the nipple to disappear.

Sensitivity may develop to topical applications such as creams, ointments or sprays. The mother with sore nipples should be questioned about the use of such products.

Feeding difficulties due to the mother

Abnormal nipples

Long nipples. These can lead to poor feeding because the baby is able to latch onto the nipple without drawing breast tissue into his mouth. The mother may need to be shown how to help the baby to grasp a sufficient portion of the breast.

Short nipples. As the baby has to form a teat from both the breast and nipple, short nipples should not cause problems and the mother should be reassured of this.

Abnormally large nipples may cause difficulties. If the baby is small, his mouth may not be able to get beyond the nipple and on to the breast. Lactation could be initiated by expressing, although pumps may not be of any use because the nipple may not fit into the breast cup. As the baby grows and the breast and nipple become more protractile, breast feeding may become possible.

Inverted and flat nipples. As stated earlier, there is no clear evidence that physical preparation during pregnancy can effect a change in the nipples. Many babies are able to attach to the breast, even if the nipple is considered to be unfavourable, and are able to feed adequately. In more difficult cases it may be necessary to initiate lactation by expressing and to delay attempting to attach the baby to the breast until lactation is established and the breasts have become soft and the nipples more protractile.

Complications of breast feeding

Engorgement

This condition occurs around the third or fourth day postpartum. The breasts are hard, painful and sometimes flushed. The mother may develop a pyrexia. Engorgement results from an increase in the blood volume in the breast with accompanying oedema and indicates that the baby is not in step with the stage of lactation. Research published in the early 1950s demonstrated that the incidence was greatly reduced when restrictions on the duration of the early feeds were removed; early unrestricted feeding helps to prevent engorgement (Illingworth & Stone 1952). The condition may also occur when the baby is unable to feed efficiently because he is not correctly attached to the breast.

Management should be aimed at enabling the baby to feed well. Pushing away the oedema by gently manipulating the tissue that lies under the areola may be all that is required. Sometimes a breast pump can be used for the same purpose. Quicker resolution will occur if the baby is allowed to feed completely from the first breast before being offered the other one. In severe cases the only solution will be the gentle use of a pump. The mother's fluid intake should not be restricted, as this has no direct effect on breast function.

Mastitis

Mastitis means inflammation of the breast. It may occur as the result of an infective process but in over 50% of cases there is no infective component initially (Thomsen et al 1984). Typically, one or more adjacent segments are inflamed and appear as a wedge-shaped area of redness and swelling.

Non-infective (acute intramammary) mastitis. This condition results from milk stasis. It may occur during the early days as the result of unresolved engorgement or at any time when poor feeding technique results in one or more segments of the breast not being efficiently stripped by the baby. Pressure from fingers or clothing have been blamed for causing the condition without any supporting evidence. The mother may have a pyrexia and general malaise.

It is extremely important that breast feeding from the affected breast continues, otherwise milk stasis will increase further and provide ideal conditions for pathogenic bacteria to replicate. An infective condition may then arise which could, if untreated, lead to abscess formation, causing much pain and distress to the mother.

Where close supervision is available, 6–8 hours could be allowed to elapse to ascertain whether the process can be reversed by instructing the mother on good feeding technique and encouraging her to allow the baby to finish the first breast first. If supervision is not available, or if no improvement occurs during that period, antibiotics should be given prophylactically (RCM 1991).

Infective (superficial) mastitis. The main cause of infection is damage to the epithelium which allows bacteria to enter the underlying tissues. The damage results from incorrect attachment of the baby to the breast which has caused trauma to the nipple. The mother therefore urgently needs help to improve her technique. Multiplication of bacteria may be enhanced by the use of breast pads or shells. In spite of antibiotic therapy, abscess formation may occur.

Breast abscess. A fluctuant swelling develops in a previously inflamed area. Pus may be discharged from the nipple. Simple needle aspiration may be effective or incision and drainage may be necessary (Dixon 1988). It may not be possible to feed from the affected breast for a few days but breast feeding should be commenced as soon as practicable because this has been shown to reduce the chances of further abscess formation (Benson & Goodman 1970). A sinus which drains milk may form but it is likely to heal in time. Bilateral or multiple abscesses may sometimes occur.

Feeding difficulties due to the baby

Cleft lip

Provided that the palate is intact, the presence of a cleft in the lip should not interfere with breast feeding because the vacuum that is necessary to keep the baby attached to the breast is created within the oral cavity.

Cleft palate

Though there are cases documented which suggest that it is possible to breast feed if the baby has a cleft of the palate, a closer look indicates that the babies were able to obtain milk only as the result of the mother's milk ejection reflex. This would suggest that it is rarely likely to be completely successful. Because of the cleft, the baby is unable to form a teat out of the breast and nipple. The use of an orthodontic plate is unlikely to help because the baby is unable to feel the breast against the soft palate and this is necessary to elicit the sucking response.

Many mothers have expressed their milk and used various techniques to feed it to their babies. Some have maintained their lactation until the baby has had a surgical repair and have then succeeded in breast feeding.

Blocked nose

Babies normally breathe through their noses. If there is an obstruction, they have great difficulty with feeding because they have to interrupt the process in order to breathe. A blockage caused by mucus may be relieved by instilling drops of normal saline before a feed. Choanal atresia is a rare abnormality causing obstruction to the nasal passage and the baby is unable to feed successfully before corrective surgery.

Down's syndrome

Babies with this condition can be successfully breast fed, although extra help and encouragement may be necessary initially.

Prematurity

Preterm infants who are sufficiently mature to have developed sucking and swallowing reflexes may successfully breast feed. Breast feeding has been shown to suit the preterm baby because it is less tiring than bottle feeding and because the milk is adapted to the individual baby in composition (Meier & Cranston-Anderson 1987). If the reflexes are not strongly developed the baby may tire

before the feed is complete and complementary tube feeding may be necessary.

Less mature babies who are unable to suck or swallow at all will be dependent on artificial methods such as tube feeding and intravenous alimentation.

Illness or surgery

Babies recover quickly following illness or surgery. If they have never been to the breast, or if feeding has been interrupted for a long period, the mother may require skilled help to initiate or re-establish feeding.

Contra-indications to breast feeding

Drugs

Breast feeding may have to be suspended temporarily following the administration of certain drugs or following diagnostic techniques which use radioactive isotopes. Some drugs, such as those used to treat cancer and certain hormones, are an absolute contra-indication to breast feeding. Most regions have drug centres where advice may be sought about the safety of drugs for lactating women.

Cancer

If the mother has cancer, the treatment she receives will make it impossible to breast feed without harming the baby. If she has had a mastectomy, she may feed successfully from one breast. Following a lumpectomy for cancer she may also be able to breast feed. She should seek advice from her surgeon.

Breast surgery

Neither breast reduction nor augmentation is an inevitable contra-indication to breast feeding, but much depends on the techniques used. Where possible, advice should be sought from the surgeon. If, for instance, the nipple has been displaced the duct system is not likely to be patent. No harm can result from testing the breast by allowing the baby to suck.

Breast injury

Injuries caused by scalding in childhood may cause such severe scarring that breast feeding is impossible. Burns or other accidents may also cause serious damage.

AIDS

The human immunodeficiency virus (HIV) may be transmitted in breast milk and breast feeding may not be advisable if the mother is HIV positive (see Ch. 19).

Cessation of lactation

Suppression of lactation

If a mother chooses not to breast feed or if she has a late miscarriage or stillbirth, lactation may need to be suppressed. The most common management is to do nothing. Most women complain of discomfort for a day or two but if unstimulated the breasts will naturally cease to produce milk. Very rarely severe discomfort with engorgement occurs. Expressing small volumes of milk once or twice can afford great relief and leads to rapid regression of the condition. The mother will be more comfortable if her breasts are supported but it is doubtful if binding the breasts contributes anything towards suppression.

Midwives should resist the temptation to advise restricting fluid intake and should not seek a prescription for a diuretic. These measures merely add to the woman's discomfort by making her thirsty.

Suppression with hormones is effective. Bromo-criptine acts as a suppressant for prolactin. It is very expensive and may lead to rebound lactation when it is stopped. Stilboestrol and related preparations also suppress lactation but are no longer used because of the risk of thrombosis.

Discontinuation of breast feeding

Stopping lactation abruptly once breast feeding has become established may cause serious problems for the mother. She could develop engorgement or mastitis or even a breast abscess. She should be encouraged to mimic normal weaning by expressing her breasts but reducing the frequency over a few days. The reduction in the stimulation of the breasts will lead to a diminution in the production of milk. After a few days she should be encouraged to express only if she feels uncomfortable. The most tragic circumstance under which this advice might be required follows the death of a baby.

Weaning from the breast

When the mother or the baby decides to stop breast feeding, feeds should be tailed off gradually. Breast feeds may be omitted, one at a time, and spaced further apart. Adding supplementary foods should not begin until 4–6 months of age.

Complementary and supplementary feeds

Complementary feeds are given after a breast feed. A widely held belief that these feeds were frequently necessary became firmly established over a period of many years. This practice probably had its origin at the turn of the century, when it was recommended that the duration of the early feeds should be severely restricted and that the baby should be given complementary feeds of cow's milk 'until its mother is able to nurse it' (Vincent 1904). It has become possible only in recent times in the developed world to see how unnecessary this practice is when feeding is unrestricted from the beginning.

There may be rare occasions when problems, such as small-for-dates babies, lethargic, jaundiced babies or even difficulties in attaching babies to breasts, make the giving of a complementary feed necessary. Ideally this should be the baby's own mother's milk. Alternatively donor milk from a human milk bank could be used. Donors must have been screened for HIV antibodies and a negative result received before their milk can be accepted. There is no evidence that water or glucose solutions are of any value in these circumstances.

The use of formula feeds based on either cow's milk or soya 'milk' should be avoided whenever possible. Their use may cause sensitivity to either product to occur later in the child's life and may cause changes in the flora of the baby's gut which may take some time to revert to the pre-complementary feed status.

The routine use of complementary feeds interferes with the establishment of lactation and causes confusion in the baby because he has to try to adapt to two different methods of feeding. It also has a damaging effect on the mother's confidence in her ability to feed her baby herself.

Supplementary feeds are given in place of a breast feed. There can be no justification for their use except in extreme circumstances, because each breast feed missed by the baby will interfere with the establishment of lactation and damage the mother's confidence.

Return to work

If the breast feeding mother returns to work her baby will have to be fed in her absence (unless she is fortunate enough to have a crèche at work or a child minder close at hand). She may wish her baby to have her own milk at all times and she may express for this purpose. Her baby may refuse a bottle but he can be fed with a cup or spoon. On the other hand, she may find it difficult to provide her own milk and her baby may receive a formula feed while she is away but she may continue to breast feed at all other times. Midwives should help mothers to understand that returning to work does not mean that breast feeding has to be terminated.

ARTIFICIAL FEEDING

The amazing adaptability of the human infant has been demonstrated by the fact that adequate growth and development can take place in spite of being fed on a formula based on the milk of another species, even one which is deficient in many of the properties and components found in human milk.

Most women who artificially feed their babies belong to one of two distinct groups and it is important for midwives to understand the difference. The first group comprises mothers who have chosen to feed their babies this way; those in the second group have been forced into doing so because they have not been able to establish successful breast feeding. A much smaller group wishes to breast feed but cannot do so because of contra-indications (see above).

Reasons for the primary choice

Research has show that women who choose to feed their babies by this method have not chosen it because they believe it is best for their babies, but because they do not want to breast feed (Hally et al 1984). Many will have experienced the disappointment felt by relatives or friends who failed to breast feed because of unresolved problems. Some state that they find the idea of using their breasts for this function repulsive or 'animal-like', others that they would be embarrassed to breast feed in front of relatives or in public. A few may state that their partners do not wish them to breast feed.

Midwives should support this choice and help the mother to make bottle feeding as satisfying for herself and her baby as possible. It must be accepted that, under the right conditions, formula milk provides a safe alternative to breast feeding.

Cow's milk

The chart in Figure 33.15 shows that, when compared with human milk, unmodified cow's milk contains more protein. It also contains more

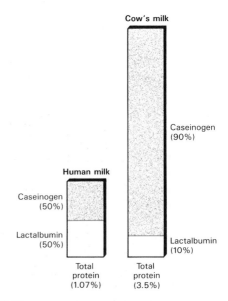

Fig. 33.15
Diagrammatic representation of ratio of caseinogen to lactalbumin in human and cow's milk.

minerals, less lactose (sugar) and about the same amount of fat.

Cow's milk *protein* contains 90% caseinogen and 10% lactalbumin, whereas human milk contains equal proportions of each. The proportion of amino acids is completely different from that in human milk (Fig. 33.16).

The proportion of *minerals*, compared with human milk, is almost twice the quantity. There is three times as much sodium.

The *fat* in human milk is easily digested because it is accompanied by lipase. *Cow's milk fat* is poorly digested and absorbed. Human milk contains much more cholesterol and it has been speculated that this suppresses the body's own synthesis of cholesterol, an effect which may last throughout life.

Until the early 1970s most infant formulae consisted of crudely modified dried cow's milk with added vitamins. It became evident that their high solute loads contributed to infantile hypocalcaemia and to hypernatraemic dehydration. This led to the development of a new generation of infant formulae. The older types were phased out, including National Dried Milk which was withdrawn in 1977.

Modified cow's milk formulae

The two main components used are skimmed milk (a by-product of butter manufacture) and whey (a by-product of cheese manufacture). Other substances used are not products of the dairy industry. They include maltodextrin, vegetable oils, animal fats, mineral salts and vitamins. Midwives must be aware that some animal fats may be unacceptable to mothers of certain faiths. In particular Hindus eschew beef fat.

There are now two main types of formula: whey-dominant and casein-dominant.

Whey-dominant formulae. These are recommended for use from birth for the first few weeks. A small amount of skimmed milk is combined with demineralised whey. Added fats are vegetable oils and animal fats. The ratio of proteins in the formulae resembles the ratio of whey protein (lactalbumin) to casein found in human milk. The use of demineralised whey reduces the mineral content which then closely

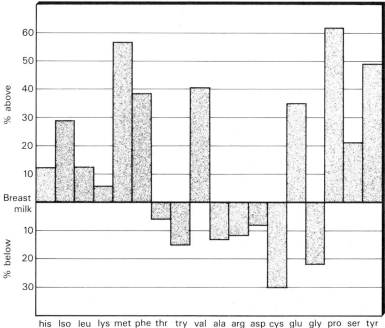

Fig. 33.16
The amino-acid profile of cow's milk compared with breast milk (from Food and Agriculture Organization (1970). Nutritional studies: amino-acid content of foods. FAO/WHO and Jelliffe & Jelliffe, 1978.)

resembles the concentration found in mature human milk. These feeds are more readily digested than the casein-dominant formulae. This leads to feeding patterns that closely resemble those of breast-fed babies.

Casein-dominant formulae. These are recommended for use after the first few weeks and the baby should continue to be fed on this type of milk formula until he is about 1 year old, after which household milk can be used. The casein-dominant formulae contain skimmed milk with added carbohydrates and fats and a mixture of vegetable and animal fats.

Non-cow's milk formulae

There are soya-based milk substitutes which approximate to the compositional guidelines for infant formulae and which are suitable as the sole source of nourishment for young infants. They should not be used unless there is a clear indication that a cow's milk formula would be unsuitable for the baby, because babies can become sensitive to soya as well as to cow's milk. They contain only vegetable fats.

Babies intolerant of standard formulae

For the small number of babies who are unable to tolerate either cow's milk or soya-based formulae there are expensive feeds based on protein hydrolysate or comminuted chicken and these are available on prescription.

Preparation of the mother for artificial feeding

There is debate concerning the most appropriate time to demonstrate the preparation of a feed and the sterilisation of feeding utensils. Ideally, only those women who have chosen this method of feeding from the beginning should be shown routinely. Demonstrations may be given when appropriate for those who decide to change their method of feeding at a later stage.

Clear instructions about the volumes of powder and water are provided on the container but the midwife should ensure that the mother understands them, as inaccurate measurements occur frequently (Lucas 1991).

The effective cleaning of all utensils used must be demonstrated and the method of sterilisation discussed. If boiling is to be used, full immersion is essential and the contents of the pan must be boiled for at least 5 minutes. If cold sterilisation using a hypochlorite solution is the method of choice, the utensils must be fully immersed in the solution for the recommended time. Where the risk of cross-infection is high, namely in hospitals or in unhygienic home conditions, no rinsing should take place before the equipment is used. Otherwise it is recommended that rinsing with recently boiled water should be carried out. Equipment that sterilises by steam is now available. Microwave sterilisation is not efficient and is not recommended.

Ready-to-feed bottles, as supplied to mothers in many hospitals, should not be used a second time. They are not intended to be resterilised and the measurement marks are not accurate.

Mothers should be warned about the dangers of 'bottle propping', and told that the baby must never be left unattended while feeding from a bottle. They should be told about the need of the baby to relate to a small number of caregivers, and that he should not be passed from person to person for feeding.

Concern has been voiced about the nitrosamine content of rubber teats: in some countries mothers have been urged to boil the teat several times with fresh water before using. Silicone teats are now available but, as these have been known to split, the mother should be urged to check for signs of damage in order to ensure that the baby does not swallow any fragments.

A mother should try to simulate breast-feeding conditions for the baby by holding him close, maintaining eye-to-eye contact and allowing him to determine his intake.

In some developed countries formulae come ready made in cans or cartons but most are available in powdered form. The milk must be reconstituted accurately, using the precise amounts of powder and water specified by the manufacturers. It is essential that the water used is free from bacterial contamination and any harmful chemicals. In some areas of the UK mothers who are artificially feeding their babies have to be provided with a separate supply of water because the tap water is not suitable for babies' consumption. If bottled water is used, a still, non-mineralised variety suitable for babies must be chosen and it should be boiled as usual. Softened water is usually unsuitable.

Modern formulae do not, when correctly prepared, cause hypernatraemia as the older types did. There is therefore no need to give the babies extra water.

The stools and vomit of a formula-fed baby have an unpleasant sour smell. The stools tend to be more formed than those of a breast-fed baby and, unlike a breast-fed baby, there is a real risk that the artificially fed baby may become constipated.

The size of the hole in the teat causes much anxiety to mothers. It is probably a good idea to have several teats with different sized holes so that they can be changed throughout the feed as necessary. A useful test for the correct hole size is to turn the bottle upside down: the feed should drip at a rate of about one drop per second.

There is now some evidence that old fashioned modified liquid cow's milk formula contained some anti-infective properties that are not present in modern whey-based formulae. The mechanism for this effect is not at present understood.

If an emergency artificial feed has to be prepared from liquid pasteurised milk, it should be made as follows: 2/3 full cream milk, 1/3 water, 1 level teaspoonful of sugar. The milk should be boiled for 2 minutes so as not to overconcentrate it before adding the previously boiled water and the sugar.

Midwives and the WHO Code

In 1981, the combined forces of the World Health Organization (WHO) and the United Nations Children's Fund (UNICEF) produced the WHO International Code of Marketing of Breast Milk Substitutes. This Code was adopted by the Health Assembly of the WHO at its 34th World Health Assembly. The Code has major implications for the work of midwives. Although it is at present a voluntary code in most countries, some countries have implemented their own legal version. The existence of international recommendations for the practice of infant feeding must affect the work of midwives.

Recommendations in the Code include:

- No advertising or promotion directly to the public (this includes posters in hospitals and advertisements in mother-and-baby books).
- No free samples of breast milk substitutes to be given to mothers.
- No free gifts to mothers, including discount coupons or special offers.
- Information provided by manufacturers to health workers should include only scientific and factual material and should not create or imply a belief that bottle feeding is equivalent or superior to breast feeding.
- No financial or material gifts should be given to health workers for the purpose of promoting products.
- Health workers should encourage and protect breast feeding.

The code does not prevent mothers from bottle feeding, but rather seeks to contribute to safe, adequate nutrition for infants and to promote and protect breast feeding.

Reader Activities

- A mother has no access to clocks. How does she know:
  — When to feed her baby
  — When her baby has had sufficient.
  Provide at least two factors for each.
- The baby is not correctly attached to the breast. List at least four problems which might arise in:
  — the mother
  — the baby.
- Interview a recently delivered mother who is breast feeding. Identify what advice she has received and ascertain, from your own reading, whether it is based on research and knowledge of physiology. If it is not, identify its source if possible. What action could you take?

REFERENCES

Alexander J M, Grant A M, Campbell M J 1991 The antenatal management of inverted and non-protractile nipples in women who intend to breastfeed: a randomized trial. Abstract from the Proceedings of the Conference 'Research in Midwifery — the state of the art?', June 1991, Birmingham

Almroth S G 1978 Water requirements of breastfed babies in a hot climate. American Journal of Clinical Nutrition 31: 1154–1157

Benson E A, Goodman M A 1970 An evaluation of the use of stilboestrol and antibiotics in the early management of acute puerperal breast abscess. British Journal of Surgery 57: 258

Dixon J M 1988 Repeated aspiration of breast abscess in lactating women. British Medical Journal 297: 1517–1518

Goldberg N M, Adams E 1983 Supplementary water for breastfed babies in a hot dry climate — not really a necessity. Archives of Disease in Childhood 58 (January): 73–74

Hally M R, Bond J, Crawley J et al 1984 Factors influencing the feeding of first-born infants. Acta Paediatrica Scandinavica 73: 33–39

Helsing E, Savage King F 1982 Breast-feeding in practice. Oxford University Press, Oxford, p 175

Hoffmann J B 1953 Suggested treatment for inverted nipples. American Journal of Obstetrics and Gynecology 66: 346

Howie P W, Forsyth J S, Ogston S A et al 1990 Protective effect of breast feeding against infection. British Medical Journal 300: 11–16

Hytten F E 1954 Clinical and chemical studies in human lactation, IX Breast feeding in hospital. British Medical Journal 4902: 1447–1452

Hytten F E, Baird D 1958 The development of the nipple in pregnancy. The Lancet 7023: 1201–1204

Illingworth R S, Stone D G H 1952 Self-demand feeding in a maternity unit. The Lancet i: 683–687

International Confederation of Midwives 1985 I C M speaks out on breast feeding. Midwifery 1, 47

Jelliffe D B, Jelliffe E F P 1978 Human milk in the modern world. Oxford University Press, Oxford

King F T, 1913 Feeding and care of the baby. Society for the Health of Women and Children, London

Kries R V, Shearer M, McCarthy P T et al 1987 Vitamin K_1 content of maternal milk: influence of the stage of lactation, lipid composition, and Vitamin K_1 supplements given to the mother. Pediatric Research 22(5): 513–517

Lucas A 1991 Milk for babies and children. Correspondence. British Medical Journal 301: 350–351

Lucas A, Cole T J 1990 Breast milk and neonatal necrotising enterocolitis. The Lancet 336: 1519–1523

Meier P, Cranston-Anderson J 1987 Responses of small preterm infants to bottle and breast-feeding. Maternal–Child Nursing Journal 12: 97–105

Prechtl H F R 1958 The directed head turning response and allied movements of the human baby. Behaviour 13: 212–242

Righard L, Alade M O, 1990 Effect of delivery room routines on success of first breast-feed. The Lancet 336: 1105–1107

Royal College of Midwives 1991 Successful breast feeding, 2nd edn. Churchill Livingstone, Edinburgh

Saarinen U M, Siimes M A, 1977 Iron absorption from infant formula and the optimal level of iron supplementation. Acta Paediatrica Scandinavica 66: 719

Sachdev H P S, Krishna J, Puri R K 1991 Water supplementation in exclusively breastfed infants during the summer in the tropics. The Lancet 337: 929–933

Thomsen A C, Espersen M D, Maigaard S 1984 Course and treatment of milk stasis, noninfectious inflammation of the breast, and infectious mastitis in nursing women. American Journal of Obstetrics and Gynecology 149: 492–495

Vincent R 1904 The nutrition of the infant. Baillière Tindall and Cox, London, p 40

Waldenström U, Swensen Å 1991 Rooming-in at night in the postpartum ward. Midwifery 7: 82–89

Widström A M, Ransjo-Arvidson A B, Christensson K et al 1987 Gastric suction in healthy newborn infants. Acta Paediatrica Scandinavica 76: 566–578

Woolridge M W 1986 The 'anatomy' of sucking. Midwifery 2: 164–171

Woolridge M W, Fisher C 1988 'Overfeeding' and symptoms of malabsorption in the breast-fed baby: a possible artefact of feed management? The Lancet ii: 382–384

World Health Organization 1981 International code of marketing of breast-milk substitutes, WHO, Geneva

FURTHER READING

Akre J 1990 (ed) Infant feeding: The physiological basis. Supplement to vol 67, 1989, Bulletin of the World Health Organization. WHO, Geneva

DHSS 1988 Present-day practice in infant feeding: third report. HMSO, London

Chalmers I, Enkin M, Keirse M J N C (eds) 1989 Effective care in pregnancy and childbirth. Oxford University Press, Oxford

Fisher C 1981 Breast feeding: a midwife's view. Maternal and Child Health 6: 52–57

Fisher C 1984 The initiation of breastfeeding. Midwives Chronicle 97: 39–41

Greaseley V 1986 Breastfeeding. Nursing 3(2): 63–70

Helsing E, Savage King F 1982 Breast-feeding in practice: a manual for health workers. Oxford University Press, Oxford

Howie P W 1985 Breast feeding: a new understanding. Midwives Chronicle 98: 184–192

Inch S 1990 Postnatal care relating to breastfeeding In: Alexander J, Levy V, Roch S (eds) Midwifery practice. Postnatal care. A research-based approach. Macmillan Education, Basingstoke

Palmer G 1988 The politics of breastfeeding. Pandora Press, London

Renfrew M, Fisher C, Arms S 1990 Bestfeeding. Celestial Arts, Berkeley

Woolridge M W 1986 Aetiology of sore nipples. Midwifery 2: 172–176

World Health Organization 1989 Protecting, promoting and supporting breast-feeding: the special role of maternity services. A joint WHO/UNICEF Statement. WHO, Geneva

If passage through the gut is slow, some of the bilirubin will be acted on by β glucuronidase which unconjugates it, making it fat-soluble again, as it is reabsorbed from the gut. It enters the portal circulation and is returned to the liver for re-conjugation.

In the healthy baby the level of bilirubin in the blood will not exceed 250 μmol/ℓ during the first week of life. This depends on a normal amount of bilirubin production, normal conjugation and efficient excretion.

JAUNDICE

Jaundice is a yellow discolouration of the skin, sclera and mucous membranes due to an increase in the serum bilirubin level. This will not become clinically apparent until the serum bilirubin reaches a level of about 80 μmol/ℓ.

Associated signs are connected with the effect of bilirubin on the brain and include lethargy and disinclination for feeds.

'Physiological' jaundice

Most babies, during their first few days of life, become jaundiced to some extent. It is usually a normal happening, but as it may indicate a serious condition, the midwife must be aware of the parameters of normality. These are as follows for a full-term baby:

- It never appears before 24 hours of age.
- The serum bilirubin level never exceeds 250 μmol/ℓ.
- The highest serum bilirubin level occurs on the 3rd or 4th day of life.
- The jaundice fades by the 7th day of life.
- The baby is otherwise well.

Aetiology of physiological jaundice

Red cell breakdown. In utero the fetus requires a high level of haemoglobin (18–22 g/dl) in order to attract sufficient oxygen across the placenta. After birth the baby no longer needs this high level and the excess must be broken down and removed. Neonatal red blood cells also have a shorter life span (60–70 days) than those of the adult. These two factors increase the need for haemolysis and consequently result in a higher production of bilirubin.

Liver immaturity. The neonatal liver may not produce sufficient glucuronyl transferase to cope with the large amount of bilirubin which must be conjugated. This shortage gives rise to the term *enzyme deficiency jaundice* which is favoured as an alternative term for physiological jaundice.

Reabsorption of bilirubin from the gut. Peristalsis is slow until feeding is established and the newborn gut is not yet colonised with the normal bacteria which will be responsible for converting bilirubin diglucuronide to stercobilinogen. These allow the opportunity for reabsorption of unconjugated bilirubin.

Management

Early feeding of the baby encourages gut motility and supplies glucose for the manufacture of liver enzymes. It also helps the gut to become colonised. The midwife should therefore encourage early feeding as a preventive measure but if jaundice occurs, the frequency of feeding should be increased in order to supply glucose to the liver and to ensure that peristalsis is adequate. Giving the baby extra water may achieve the latter objective but may also prevent him from taking adequate nourishment.

The degree of jaundice must be observed. If it appears to exceed normal, the serum bilirubin level should be measured. If the parameters of physiological jaundice are surpassed, investigations should be instituted to identify the cause. In this case the jaundice can no longer be regarded as physiological.

Jaundice of the preterm baby

The preterm baby is more prone to jaundice than the full-term baby but this may be regarded as an extension of physiological jaundice. The parameters are slightly different. Jaundice tends to occur earlier, peak later and last longer than in the full-term baby.

Haemolysis occurs in the same way but the life of the red cells is shorter (30–40 days).

There is likely to be a delay in feeding of the preterm baby, especially if he is sick. The immaturity of the gut in very preterm infants is an additional factor which will further reduce peristalsis.

Albumin-binding capacity is affected by an increased tendency to hypoxia, acidosis, hypothermia, hypoglycaemia and hypoalbuminaemia.

The immature liver is even less able to deal with the large amount of bilirubin which requires conjugation.

The preterm infant is more prone to the complications of jaundice and requires treatment at lower serum bilirubin levels than the full-term baby.

Pathological jaundice

Causes

The causes of pathological jaundice can be linked to the stages in the metabolism of bilirubin.

Bilirubin production. Jaundice can be caused by an excess of bilirubin production due to haemolysis. This may occur as a result of an excess in the number of red cells or due to the red cells meeting a hostile antibody or as a result of an abnormality of the red cells themselves which

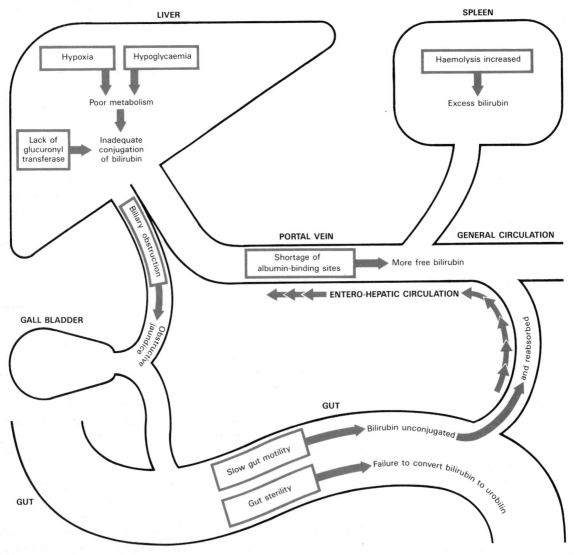

Fig. 34.2
Sites of events leading to jaundice.

makes them fragile. Excessive haemolysis eventually leads to anaemia.

Haemolysis also occurs where there is an extravasation of blood such as a haematoma or internal haemorrhage.

Albumin-binding capacity. If plasma albumin is insufficient to carry the circulating unconjugated bilirubin, jaundice is more likely. The actual amount of albumin may be deficient or the binding sites may be occupied by competing substances, usually drugs.

Conjugation. There are a number of factors which interfere with the normal conjugation of bilirubin including metabolic disorders and deficiency of glucuronyl transferase.

Hypoglycaemia and hypoxia both inhibit the normal conjugation of bilirubin as glucose and oxygen are essential to the process.

Biliary excretion. Rarely, conjugated bilirubin is unable to escape via the biliary system and is returned to the bloodstream. It remains conjugated and water-soluble and it can be passed out of the body in the urine albeit slowly.

Intestinal reabsorption. Any condition which slows down peristalsis allows more time for reabsorption and unconjugation of bilirubin. This does not add to the overall amount of bilirubin but leads to some being conjugated twice and increases the load on the liver.

HAEMOLYTIC JAUNDICE

Rhesus incompatibility

The Rhesus (Rh) factor is an antigen carried on the red blood cells of 83% of the Caucasian population; these people are said to be *Rhesus positive*. The 17% of the population who do not have this antigen are said to be *Rhesus negative*. The Rhesus factor is made up of several antigens, Cc Dd Ee. C, D and E are dominant; c, d and e are recessive. Those who are Rh positive carry the D antigen.

When there is Rhesus incompatibility between a mother and her fetus, *haemolytic disease of the newborn* may occur. This incompatibility occurs when the mother is Rh negative and her fetus is Rh positive, having inherited the gene for the Rhesus factor from his father.

Inheritance of the Rhesus factor

The fetus inherits a gene for the Rhesus factor from each parent. If either or both of these is the dominant D, he is Rh positive, Dd or DD; if he inherits two recessive genes, dd, he is Rh negative. The Rhesus genotypes DD and dd are homozygous, while Dd is heterozygous.

Figure 34.3 shows the possible inheritance patterns for the Rhesus factor in unions between: Rh negative (dd) female and homozygous positive male (DD); Rh negative (dd) female and heterozygous positive male (Dd); female and male who are both heterozygous Rh positive (Dd).

Rhesus iso-immunisation

An individual who is Rh negative does not naturally carry antibodies to the Rhesus factor. If by some means Rh positive red blood cells enter her circulation they alert the immune system and antibodies may be produced in order to destroy the foreign protein. This is most likely to occur if blood from a Rh positive fetus leaks across the placental barrier and enters a woman's bloodstream. It may also occur as a result of a mismatched blood transfusion. The process is termed iso-immunisation.

There is normally no mixing of fetal and maternal blood during pregnancy and labour but when the placenta begins to separate and the chorionic villi tear, the risk of a fetomaternal transfusion increases. In many cases between 0.5 and 5 ml of fetal blood enters the maternal circulation and Rhesus antigens on the fetal red cells stimulate the production of maternal Rh antibodies. The first encounter may not result in actual antibody formation but the woman will be sensitised; on a second encounter, antibodies are produced in abundance. Once formed, these antibodies are permanent.

Other occasions on which a fetomaternal transfusion may occur are at abortion, amniocentesis, external cephalic version or antepartum haemorrhage.

In any pregnancy subsequent to Rhesus iso-immunisation these small antibodies, which are of the type immunoglobulin G (IgG), will cross the placenta. If the fetus is Rh positive they will attach themselves to some of his Rhesus antigens, resulting in haemolysis.

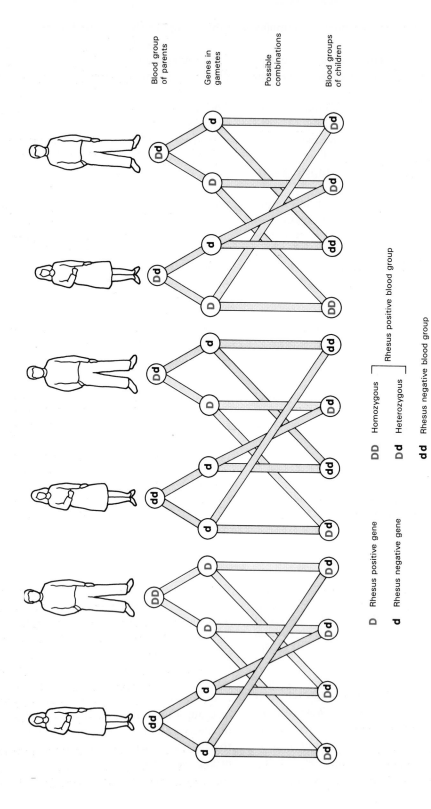

Fig. 34.3
Patterns of Rhesus factor inheritance.

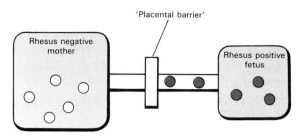

Fig. 34.4 Normal placenta with no communication between maternal and fetal blood.

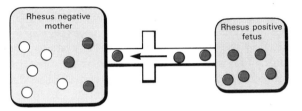

Fig. 34.5 Fetal cells enter maternal circulation through 'break' in 'placenta barrier', e.g. at placental separation.

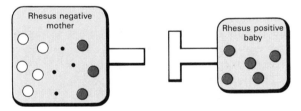

Fig. 34.6 Maternal production of Rhesus antibodies following introduction of Rhesus positive blood.

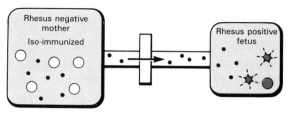

Fig. 34.7 In a subsequent pregnancy maternal Rhesus antibodies cross the placenta resulting in haemolytic disease of the newborn.

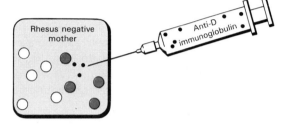

Fig. 34.8 Anti-D immunoglobulin administered within 72 hours of birth or miscarriage.

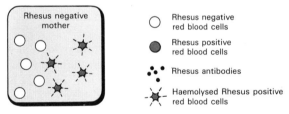

Fig. 34.9 Anti-D immunoglobulin has destroyed fetal Rhesus red cells and prevented iso-immunisation.

Figs 34.4–34.9
Rhesus iso-immunisation and its prevention.

If ABO incompatibility exists between mother and fetus, the naturally-occurring maternal antibodies (anti-A or anti-B) may destroy the escaped fetal red cells before the maternal immune system is alerted.

Prevention of maternal iso-immunisation

There are three ways of preventing a woman from producing Rhesus antibodies:

- avoiding transfusion of Rh positive blood
- prevention of avoidable fetomaternal transfusion
- administration of anti-D immunoglobulin.

Avoiding transfusion of Rh positive blood. Even a small amount of Rh positive blood introduced into the circulation of a Rh negative person will result in sensitisation. Children should be discouraged from playing games which involve so-called 'blood pacts'. Rh positive blood should never be administered if the individual's blood group is unknown and whenever possible cross-matching should be undertaken prior to blood transfusion.

Prevention of avoidable fetomaternal transfusion. Whereas it is not possible to avoid every instance of fetal blood leaking into the maternal circulation, care should be taken to ensure that it is not unnecessarily provoked. Placental localisation by ultrasound should be undertaken before amniocentesis in order to avoid penetrating the placenta. Procedures such as external cephalic version or manual removal of the placenta should be performed with gentleness in order to reduce the risk of damaging placental tissue and allowing fetal blood to escape into the maternal sinuses. In cases of placental abruption, abdominal palpation should be reduced to a minimum.

Administration of anti-D immunoglobulin. If Rh positive fetal cells do escape into the maternal circulation, the immune reaction can be forestalled by giving the woman a dose of Rhesus antibodies (anti-D immunoglobulin). This will coat the fetal red cells and destroy them before the woman's immune system has time to recognise the foreign protein and react to it. The immunoglobulin must be given within 72 hours of the leak if it is to be effective. In effect this bestows on the woman a passive immunity to the Rhesus factor and as such it will last for about 3 months. Passive immunity is temporary and it will not affect a future pregnancy.

The normal dose of anti-D immunoglobulin is 500 IU after delivery or following an abortion which takes place after 20 weeks' gestation. In cases of earlier abortion, 250 IU is given. If there is thought to be a risk of sensitisation during pregnancy, for example following amniocentesis or external cephalic version, anti-D immunoglobulin may be ordered.

In some cases, when the fetomaternal transfusion has been particularly large, one dose of anti-D immunoglobulin is insufficient. The number of fetal cells in the maternal circulation is estimated by means of the Kleihauer test which is performed on a sample of maternal blood obtained after delivery. The laboratory will inform the doctor if a second dose is recommended.

Antenatal management

Every pregnant woman has her blood grouped for ABO and Rhesus types. Women with Rh negative blood group are screened for Rhesus antibodies with an indirect Coombs' test. If there are no antibodies, the blood will be retested at 28 and 34 weeks of pregnancy. If antibodies are found at any stage, a further test is made to estimate the quantity by titration and the titre is monitored at regular intervals thereafter. Antibody estimation does not give an accurate indication of fetal well-being but a rise to a critical level suggests a need for amniocentesis.

Spectrophotometric scanning of the amniotic fluid measures its optical density and shows the amount of bilirubin being excreted into the liquor amnii by the fetus. The value of gaining this information must be weighed against the risk of causing a further fetomaternal transfusion by performing amniocentesis. The investigation is usually delayed if possible until 26 weeks' gestation or later. The specimen of amniotic fluid must be protected from light while being conveyed to the laboratory, as light will alter the result. Discovery of bilirubin in the liquor amnii is significant because unless the amount of bilirubin produced by the fetus is excessive, the mother is able to excrete it all.

The level of bilirubin shown by analysis of the amniotic fluid must be assessed with regard to the period to gestation. Management is determined by plotting the result on a Liley chart which gives an estimate of possible outcome.

The possible courses of action are:

- to allow pregnancy to continue but to repeat the amniocentesis at intervals in order to assess bilirubin levels. If the bilirubin level rises, intervention may be necessary.
- to deliver the fetus if it is dangerous to continue pregnancy. Delivery should be in a consultant unit with facilities for neonatal intensive care.
- to administer an intra-uterine transfusion to the fetus in order to prolong life until he is mature enough to survive.

Intra-uterine transfusion. The transfusion may be into the peritoneum or into the umbilical vein via fetoscopy. The fetus is given a transfusion of Rh negative packed cells which are usually blood group O. The amount given will depend on the gestational age, the antibody titre and the bilirubin level and is between 40 and 120 ml. Further transfusions are given at 2-weekly intervals until delivery.

This type of treatment can only be given in specialist centres.

Care at delivery

Immediately the baby is born, the cord must be clamped in order to prevent any further Rhesus antibodies from entering the circulation. A sample of cord blood is needed in order to estimate the condition of the child. The cord blood must be free of contamination by maternal blood or Wharton's jelly and is best collected by syringe and needle from a surface vein on the placenta. The needle is removed before transferring blood into the appropriate bottles in order to avoid haemolysis.

Tests performed on cord blood:
- ABO blood group and Rhesus type
- direct Coombs' test to detect the presence or absence of maternal antibodies on fetal red cells
- haemoglobin estimation which will indicate the degree of haemolysis
- serum bilirubin level.

Cord blood is taken for testing from the babies of all Rh negative mothers but the serum bilirubin is only estimated if the mother has Rh antibodies.

Rhesus haemolytic disease

Transference of maternal Rh antibodies to the fetus during pregnancy will result in destruction of some of his red cells (haemolysis) and consequently in anaemia and jaundice. The degree of haemolysis and the number of maternal antibodies remaining in his circulation determine the condition of the baby.

Degrees of haemolytic disease:

Congenital haemolytic anaemia. This arises when haemolysis is minimal. It causes anaemia of slow onset but little jaundice. The liver and spleen are enlarged. The baby's haemoglobin level must be monitored and if necessary a small transfusion of 30 ml packed cells is given.

Icterus gravis neonatorum (severe jaundice of the newborn). Haemolysis has been taking place in the fetus and the baby is born with a low haemoglobin level. During intra-uterine life, however, the mother is able to excrete most of the bilirubin so that the baby is not jaundiced at birth. There may be staining of the umbilical cord due to bilirubin in the liquor amnii.

After delivery the baby cannot cope with the large amount of bilirubin from red cell breakdown and he rapidly becomes jaundiced.

Treatment must restore the haemoglobin level, reduce the bilirubin level and remove maternal Rh antibodies.

Hydrops fetalis. This condition is one of congestive heart failure due to gross haemolytic anaemia. At birth the baby is extremely pale, has severe oedema and ascites and may be stillborn. His most immediate need is for blood to transport oxygen and he must be given a replacement transfusion of packed cells. Later an exchange transfusion will also be needed to remove bilirubin and maternal antibodies. The placenta is also large and pale and has fluid oozing from it.

Postnatal management. All babies whose mothers have Rh antibodies should be transferred to a neonatal intensive care unit until the results of cord blood tests are known and further management has been planned.

If the baby is of blood group Rh negative he will suffer no ill-effects from the iso-immunisation of his mother.

If the baby is Rh positive, management will depend on his clinical appearance, his haemoglobin and bilirubin levels at birth and the rate of rise in the serum bilirubin level.

ABO incompatibility

In this condition the mother is classically group O and the baby is group A or less often B. The mother has naturally occurring antibodies anti-A and anti-B. These are of the type IgM and are too large to cross the placenta. If the immune system produces small antibodies (IgG) similar to anti-A and anti-B, these will be able to cross the placenta and become attached to fetal red cells and destroy them. The condition may affect the first-born as much as a subsequent child.

The jaundice is usually mild but may appear within the first 24 hours of life. If this happens, blood must be taken for grouping and Coombs' test, although the latter is usually negative. Bilirubin levels are estimated. Treatment depends on the serum bilirubin level and its rate of rise.

Other causes of haemolytic jaundice

Other antibodies

Rarely, haemolytic disease of the newborn is caused by the other Rhesus antibodies (C,c,E,e) or by Kell, Lewis or Duffy antibodies.

Polycythaemia

This is a condition in which the blood contains too many red cells and the haematocrit (packed cell volume) exceeds 65%. Babies affected are:

- recipients of a twin-to-twin transfusion
- recipients of a large maternofetal transfusion
- infants of diabetic mothers
- light-for-dates babies (see also Ch. 35).

Polycythaemia is a cause of neonatal jaundice as the baby must destroy the excess red cells. In extreme cases it may be necessary to perform a partial exchange transfusion using plasma in order to reduce the haematocrit.

Extravasation of blood

If blood escapes from its vessels in bruising or haematomas, the collected blood will be destroyed and the resulting bilirubin must be excreted. The main example of this is cephalhaematoma but it also occurs from such injuries as bruising at breech delivery. The level of bilirubin may be sufficient to cause jaundice and the haemoglobin level should also be monitored.

Septicaemia

Some types of sepsis will cause haemolysis and therefore predispose to jaundice.

Glucose 6-phosphate dehydrogenase (G6PD) deficiency

This is a rare hereditary condition caused by a deficiency of a red cell enzyme (G6PD). The enzyme maintains the stability of the red cell membrane. When it is absent the cell is fragile and will be destroyed when certain conditions prevail. It is a possible cause of neonatal jaundice in Mediterranean, oriental or African peoples.

Spherocytosis

The red cells are of an abnormal spherical shape in this autosomal-dominant inherited condition. It may cause jaundice during the first 48–72 hours of life. This is usually mild but may require exchange transfusion.

OTHER TYPES OF PATHOLOGICAL JAUNDICE

Reduced albumin-binding capacity

Bilirubin which is unable to find albumin-binding sites is free to escape to nervous and fatty tissue. The danger of this situation is that the basal ganglia of the brain may become stained and damaged irreparably. This is termed *kernicterus*.

Binding sites may be occupied by drugs such as diazepam, Synkavit, sulphonamides, steroids and salicylates.

Hypoxia, hypoglycaemia, hypothermia, acidosis and hypoalbuminaemia also reduce the available albumin.

Defective conjugation

Several conditions interfere with the ability of the liver to conjugate bilirubin. The liver requires adequate fluid and carbohydrate in order to function normally, therefore dehydration and starvation may cause jaundice.

Hereditary glucuronyl transferase deficiency is a rare condition which prevents adequate conjugation. So-called breast-milk jaundice appears to be caused by the excretion of a steroid in the breast milk which competes with bilirubin for conjugation. In this case the jaundice persists while the baby is taking breast milk but it fades when he is not. It causes no harm and once the diagnosis is made, breast feeding may be resumed.

Infection also may interfere with conjugation. The TORCH (Toxoplasmosis, Others, Rubella, Cytomegalovirus, Herpes) infections cause jaundice, usually accompanied by hepatosplenomegaly and thrombocytopenia.

Inborn errors of metabolism such as galactosaemia, cystic fibrosis and congenital hypothyroidism must also be borne in mind when seeking the cause of jaundice.

Obstructive jaundice

This term refers to obstruction of the biliary channels which allow the bile to drain from the liver into the gut. The bilirubin in bile is conjugated and water-soluble. If its level in the blood is raised, it does not carry the same danger as high levels of unconjugated bilirubin.

The cause is either hepatitis or atresia of the bile ducts. Both are rare. Jaundice is accompanied by pale stools and dark urine.

Hepatitis is either acquired from the mother or results from an ascending infection from the umbilical cord. Prognosis is poor but two-thirds of these infants recover completely.

If the biliary ducts are not patent, the prognosis depends on the site of the atresia. Within the liver there is little that can be done; atresia of the larger bile ducts outside the liver may be amenable to surgery in some cases especially if carried out before 8 weeks of age (Kay 1990).

Early identification is crucial and midwives should alert mothers to the danger of late jaundice. If jaundice persists until 14 days of age, especially if the urine is yellow rather than clear and the stools are *not* yellow or green, the urine should be tested for bilirubin and serum conjugated bilirubin should be measured. Hussein and colleagues (1991) plead for the date of the well-baby check to be brought forward to 4 weeks after birth in order to detect biliary atresia.

MANAGEMENT OF PATHOLOGICAL JAUNDICE

Phototherapy

Phototherapy is a treatment which provides an alternative way of dealing with bilirubin in the blood when the liver is unable to conjugate the quantities produced. Bilirubin in the skin and superficial capillaries is converted to a water-soluble form during exposure to light in the blue part of the spectrum. It was first noticed as an effect of sunlight but in cold climates it is applied by high-density fluorescent lights, using blue or white tubes.

Indications for phototherapy
- Serum bilirubin exceeding 250 μmol/l in a full-term baby or a level determined by the baby's gestation if he is preterm.
- Jaundice appearing before 24 hours of age.

Phototherapy is ineffective before the baby is clinically jaundiced (about 80–100 μmol/l). It is therefore not a prophylactic method although early use in babies with known haemolytic disease will help to control serum bilirubin levels. In babies without Rhesus disease early use of phototherapy at low levels of bilirubinaemia has no advantage (Lancet 1991).

Management of the baby receiving phototherapy

The naked baby is exposed to the light and should be turned at regular intervals. It is usual to cover his eyes to prevent retinal damage. The eyes are an important means of communication with the mother and the light should be switched off and the eye pads removed during feeding so that she can converse with her baby. Temperature control is important because the baby may become too cold from being uncovered or too hot as a result of radiant heat coming from the light. Fluid may be lost by perspiration from the skin and by intestinal hurry due to the effects of the phototherapy. Extra fluid must therefore be given to the baby.

Phototherapy may be given at the mother's bedside if the baby is otherwise well. This helps to overcome the fears and distress which the treatment arouses for the parents. The mother should be encouraged to touch and speak to her baby even during treatment periods and to lift him and feed him as often as necessary. If the baby is unable to control his own temperature, it may be possible to nurse him in an incubator at the bedside.

The treatment may be given continuously, interrupted only for care and feeding, or intermittently for periods of 6 hours on and 6 hours off.

Exchange transfusion

This is a transfusion where the baby's blood is gradually removed and replaced with fresh, Rhesus negative, ABO-compatible blood. This has the effect of washing out excess bilirubin and the unwanted antibodies and also increases the haemoglobin level. An amount equivalent to twice the baby's blood volume needs to be used. Rhesus negative blood is used so that there is no Rhesus antigen to attract the antibodies. It does not alter the baby's blood group; he will continue to produce Rhesus positive blood cells.

Indications for exchange transfusion

Babies who are anaemic, who have a high or rising serum bilirubin level or in whom there is evidence of a reduced albumin-binding capacity may need an exchange transfusion. The indications are summarised in Table 34.1.

Preparation for exchange transfusion

Before this procedure is carried out it must be carefully explained to the parents and their permission must be obtained. They need to be informed of the baby's condition at frequent intervals.

A trolley is prepared with the equipment required for an exchange transfusion. In addition a cardiorator, a blood warmer and an overhead radiant heater will be needed.

Management of an exchange transfusion

The transfusion is given by umbilical vein. A catheter is passed through the vein and the ductus venosus into the inferior vena cava (Fig. 34.10). 10 ml of blood is withdrawn and used for determining levels of serum bilirubin, haemoglobin and glucose before the transfusion. This deficit is

Table 34.1
Indications for exchange transfusion

Anaemia: haemoglobin < 10 g/dl in cord blood
Hyperbilirubinaemia:
    serum bilirubin exceeding 100 to 135 µmol/l at birth
    serum bilirubin rising at 17 µmol/l per hour or faster
    serum bilirubin 340 µmol/l at any time (in preterm infants exchange transfusion should be carried out at lower levels — see Table 34.2)
Evidence of reduced albumin-binding capacity, e.g. use of a drug which competes for binding sites or hypoproteinaemia

Table 34.2
Approximate indication levels for exchange transfusion in preterm infants

Gestation in weeks	Serum bilirubin level
27 weeks or less	250 µmol/l
28–30 weeks	280 µmol/l
31–34 weeks	310 µmol/l
35 weeks or more	340 µmol/l

not immediately replaced, in order to avoid overloading of the circulation. The transfusion itself is accomplished by removing and discarding 5 or 10 ml of blood and immediately replacing it with a similar amount of fresh blood. This procedure is repeated until the calculated volume has been exchanged. A double-volume exchange results in a replacement of about 90% of the baby's blood. A continuous slow infusion of calcium may be given concurrently in order to counteract any hypocalcaemia due to the citrate in the stored blood. The procedure takes up to about 2 hours. At the conclusion the last syringeful of blood removed is preserved for post-transfusion tests.

The process is very repetitive and tedious and the personnel must be especially careful about the accuracy of their recordings.

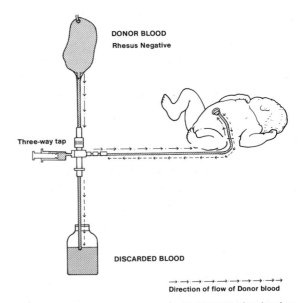

Fig. 34.10
Diagram showing apparatus for performing an exchange transfusion.

- An accurate record must be made of each aliquot of blood withdrawn or replaced. A special chart is used.
- The heart rate must be monitored with a cardiorator or electrocardiograph. Any changes are reported as well as being recorded.
- The baby's temperature is monitored in order to avoid the development of hypo- or hyperthermia.
- Any cyanosis, greyness or pallor is noted as these could indicate heart failure or collapse.
- Respirations are recorded and any signs of tachypnoea, rib recession or grunting on expiration are reported.
- Abnormal movements such as jitteriness or twitching may indicate hypoglycaemia or hypocalcaemia.

Post-transfusion care

The baby is returned to his warm cot or incubator and observed closely for 6–8 hours. Besides his general condition, his umbilicus is inspected for bleeding every half hour for the first few hours and then 4-hourly. Serum bilirubin levels are estimated 4-hourly. Capillary blood glucose is estimated at similar intervals, using test strips. Calcium levels may be estimated and the slow calcium infusion continued for a while after the exchange transfusion.

Phototherapy may be given because the serum bilirubin level will rebound as antibodies in the tissues return to the circulation and haemolyse further red blood cells. The parents are encouraged to visit.

Follow-up

Babies who have suffered hyperbilirubinaemia in the neonatal period should be followed up and examined regularly in case they develop anaemia, deafness, cerebral palsy or mental retardation.

BILIRUBIN TOXICITY

Kernicterus

If unconjugated bilirubin escapes into the basal ganglia of the brain it can cause irreversible damage. Only free, unconjugated bilirubin is harmful because bilirubin which is bound to albumin cannot leave the blood spaces. Conjugated bilirubin does not damage the brain.

Kernicterus is difficult to diagnose in the neonate but he may show signs of hypotonia, lethargy, poor sucking and an abnormal Moro reflex. Later he develops other signs of cerebral irritation and athetoid cerebral palsy.

It is important to treat jaundice at an early stage in order to prevent this condition. If early toxic effects appear, treatment should be continued as it will minimise the damage.

NEONATAL INFECTION

Vulnerability of the newborn to infection

The defence mechanisms of the newborn infant are imperfectly developed. This is more pronounced in the preterm baby. Babies who are small for gestational age or born after a prolonged labour or prolonged rupture of the membranes are also more vulnerable to infection.

- Skin and mucous membranes are thin and easily damaged.
- The baby is virtually free from organisms and lacking a protective resident flora.
- There is decreased cellular immunity due to a reduced number of T-cell lymphocytes.
- Phagocytosis is less efficient.
- Immunoglobulins (Ig) are deficient. Only IgG is transported across the placenta from the mother in the second half of pregnancy. This protects the baby against those infections to which his mother is immune. IgM is only produced by the fetus if he is exposed to intrauterine infection and IgA is not manufactured until after birth.

Modes of acquiring infection

The baby may acquire infection as a fetus by pathogens transmitted across the placenta or ascending via the mother's genital tract. He may also become infected during labour and delivery or after birth.

Prevention of infection

Prior to conception, rubella vaccination is offered to mothers who are not already immune. Care should be taken of the mother's general health during pregnancy and any infections should, if possible, be treated before delivery. Occasionally it is advisable to perform a caesarean section in order to avoid passage through an infected vagina. In labour it is important to keep intervention to a minimum in order to reduce the risk of introducing organisms into the genital tract.

Once the baby is born the principles of preventing infection are to protect and reinforce his ability to defend himself and to limit the opportunities of infection gaining access to the baby. In practical terms this is achieved by:

- encouraging breast feeding in order to take advantage of the many anti-infective properties of breast milk (see Ch. 33)
- avoidance of trauma to skin and mucous membranes
- administration of immunoglobulin in specific instances
- maintaining a safe environment by provision of adequate ventilation and sufficient space, the use of cleaning techniques which reduce dust, attention to sinks and pipes, regular changing of equipment and clothing for baby and cot
- hand washing, which is outstandingly important in that hands easily convey organisms from one site to another
- individual equipment for each baby and the use of disposables
- exclusion of infected persons from the vicinity of the baby
- isolation of infected babies
- avoidance of over-use of antibiotics which may reduce their effectiveness.

Recognition of infection

Signs of infection in the newly born baby are often non-specific, and in the early stages the midwife may simply notice that the baby does not seem well, without identifying any clear pointers to distinguish the diagnosis from other neonatal problems (Cerase 1989).

Any history of maternal infection, pyrexia, offensive amniotic fluid or prolonged rupture of the membranes will alert the midwife to a risk of perinatal infection. Infection of early onset is usually derived from the mother. Signs are a low Apgar score, respiratory distress, labile temperature and possibly apnoeic spells, a rash, shock or sclerema.

Infection of late onset (after 48 hours) is usually characterised first by lethargy and loss of appetite. In addition the baby may fail to thrive and gain weight and be unable to tolerate milk and may vomit. He may be pale or jaundiced and look anxious. The temperature may be low, high or unstable but may be normal. Convulsions may occur.

Infection screening

A neonate often does not display localised signs of infection and the clinical features are general. In order to identify the exact site of the infection it is necessary to carry out a full infection screen on the baby. This involves taking swabs from the nose, throat and umbilicus and obtaining specimens of urine, meconium and blood for culture. In addition, some paediatricians will carry out a lumbar puncture on all babies showing signs of infection while others restrict this examination to babies with specific signs of meningitis. If there are local lesions such as pustules, swabs will be taken from these. In cases of early onset of infection, a specimen of amniotic fluid may give valuable information. This is obtained from a specimen of gastric aspirate prior to feeding or from a deep ear swab. A full blood count is usual and a chest X-ray may be useful.

Transplacental infection

Most bacteria are too large to cross the placenta. Viruses, being very small, may cross the placental barrier and the spirochaete of syphilis has the ability to penetrate membranes. Protozoa, such as *Toxoplasma gondii*, may also infect the fetus.

Rubella virus causes an insignificant infection in the adult but is potentially teratogenic to the embryo and fetus. If the infection is acquired during the early weeks of pregnancy, cell division is inhibited in the embryonic organs, particularly the eyes, ears, heart and brain. The earlier the infection, the more disastrous are the consequences. The baby may be born with one or more of the following defects: cataract, deafness, heart anomalies, mental subnormality. If the mother contracts the infection after the 3rd month her baby should be screened for deafness which may occur as a single defect.

The diagnosis of maternal rubella is confirmed by virological tests. A rising antibody titre is proof of infection and may be considered sufficient grounds for termination of pregnancy.

An infant may be born with *congenital rubella* in which case he is highly infectious and must be isolated. Birth weight may be low and a purpuric rash may be evident in addition to possible congenital defects. The child may harbour the virus for up to 1 year. The mortality rate is high in babies who show signs of acute disease at birth.

Prophylaxis consists of rubella vaccination which is given at 12–18 months as part of the MMR (see Ch. 45) and also to non-immunised girls aged 13 years. In addition pregnant women are often screened at booking and, if non-immune, offered vaccination during the postnatal period. After vaccination a reliable contraceptive must be used for 3 months to avoid any risk of damage to a developing embryo. Those working with mothers and babies should also have their antibody titres estimated and be offered vaccination if necessary. They may be a hazard to women in early pregnancy if they are incubating rubella and their own embryos may be at risk if they are in contact with cases of congenital rubella.

Cytomegalovirus (CMV) is one of the herpes virus group. Infection is more common in the lower socio-economic groups and is usually asymptomatic. In pregnancy CMV may cause abortion, preterm labour, intra-uterine growth retardation or fetal death. The greatest risk to the fetus occurs if the mother is infected during the first 20 weeks of pregnancy. Hepatic and neurological damage, microcephaly and respiratory difficulty may be evident. Nerve deafness and mental retardation may be diagnosed later. Diagnosis is confirmed by culturing the virus from a specimen of urine or a throat swab, isolating inclusion bodies in renal tubular cells in the urine and the presence of a raised CMV antibody titre. If the infection is acquired perinatally the prognosis is very good.

There is no specific treatment available but, as these infants are highly infectious, they should be isolated.

Toxoplasmosis. This infection is caused by the protozoon *Toxoplasma gondii* which may be found in dog and cat faeces and uncooked meat. Maternal infection is difficult to recognise although it may cause lymphadenopathy. About 0.2% of all pregnant women will have toxoplasmosis and about 36% of these will produce affected babies. Some women may request screening, treatment with spiramycin if infected and cordocentesis to test if the fetus is infected. Termination of pregnancy may be considered.

Clinical features in the baby are microcephaly, hydrocephaly, cerebral calcification and hepatosplenomegaly with or without jaundice. Diagnosis is made if high concentrations of toxoplasma antibody are detected in the baby's blood.

Syphilis has become a rarity in the neonate. It is caused by the spirochaete *Treponema pallidum* which may cross the placenta during pregnancy. Screening in pregnancy leads to an opportunity to treat the infected mother and fetus simultaneously. Syphilis may cause late abortion, preterm labour, stillbirth or the child may be born with syphilis.

Acquired immune deficiency syndrome (AIDS) is caused by the *human immunodeficiency virus (HIV)*. It can be transmitted via the placenta during pregnancy (see Ch. 19 for details).

Listeria monocytogenes is a bacillus which may be transmitted across the placenta or intrapartum. Pets and farm animals may be the source of the infection which causes a mild 'flu'-like illness or urinary tract infection in the mother. When babies are found to be affected, investigation of the history often reveals a maternal pyrexia a few days before delivery. The neonate may develop a serious respiratory disease or meningitis from which the mortality is high. Treatment is with ampicillin and gentamicin.

Intrapartum transmission of infection

Once the membranes have ruptured there is a risk of ascending infection which is greater if they have been ruptured for more than 24 hours. Infection may also be acquired by direct contact with the maternal passages during birth.

Herpes simplex is caused by Type II (genital) *Herpesvirus hominis*. If the mother has active lesions at the time of delivery the baby is at high risk of acquiring the infection and should be delivered by caesarean section. The signs may be non-specific at first. Herpes simplex should be suspected if the baby develops blisters, a papular vesicular rash or the more serious signs of neonatal sepsis. These usually occur within a week of birth but may appear as late as 3 weeks of age. The virus may be cultured from vesicles, urine, eye lesions or cerebrospinal fluid. Treatment is with acyclovir.

Hepatitis B. If the mother has symptoms of hepatitis her baby is also at risk. He should receive hepatitis B hyperimmune globulin and be vaccinated at birth, 1 month and 6 months old.

Candida albicans (monilia) is the organism which causes thrush. Oral thrush should be suspected if a baby who has been feeding well for the first 3 or 4 days becomes reluctant to feed. Examination of the mouth will reveal greyish-white patches on the inside of the cheeks, on the gums, palate and tongue. They may be distinguished from milk curds by signs of inflammation, spots of blood or lesions on the edge of the tongue where milk curds would have been removed by sucking. A drink of cooled, boiled water would also remove milk curds and this could aid diagnosis. The midwife should not attempt to remove the lesions as this would leave a raw area. Peri-anal thrush presents as a red rash over the napkin area. The organism may descend from the mouth into the lungs or intestinal tract particularly in a baby receiving antibiotic therapy or parenteral nutrition or in the preterm baby, for whom it may be fatal.

Diagnosis should be confirmed by taking swabs from affected areas. Blood and urine samples may also be taken for culture.

Treatment of topical lesions is by oral nystatin and local application of nystatin cream. Exposure of sore buttocks may aid healing. Amphotericin may be given intravenously for systemic candidiasis.

Ophthalmia neonatorum is defined in England as any purulent discharge from the eyes of an infant within 21 days of its birth and in Scotland as any inflammation that occurs in the eyes of an infant within 21 days of birth which is accompanied by a discharge. There are several possible causative organisms including *Staphylococcus albus* or *aureus*, *Escherichia coli*, *Bacillus proteus*, *Pseudomonas aeruginosa*, *Chlamydia trachomatis* and *Neisseria gonorrhoeae*. Gonococcal ophthalmia is the most dreaded because of its destructive action; chlamydia is widespread and difficult to identify and treat. Treatment of vaginal discharges in pregnancy will help to prevent some cases of ophthalmia. Postnatally educating the mother in correct hygiene will help to reduce the incidence of eye infection.

A swab must be taken from any purulent discharge for culture and sensitivity, and a doctor notified immediately. The swab may be placed in Stuart's medium for transport to the laboratory. Depending on the result, the doctor will prescribe antibiotic eye drops or ointment. Chloramphenicol is commonly used but erythromycin or gentamicin should be used for chlamydial infection and polymixin for *Pseudomonas aeruginosa*. The baby should be isolated in a single room with his mother.

Eye care. The infected eye or eyes are cleaned with sterile swabs moistened with normal saline. Each swab will be used once only, wiping from the inner canthus outwards. If the nurse's hands become contaminated with the discharge, she must wash them again before continuing. The appropriate antibiotic drops or ointment are instilled. If only one eye is affected the baby should be laid on the side of the infected eye so that the discharge cannot run into the second eye and infect it. This should be repeated at least 4-hourly but in severe cases the treatment must be intensive and may be needed every few minutes as pus accumulates very rapidly.

Gonococcal ophthalmia. If ophthalmia is severe, gonococcal infection should be suspected. Onset may be as early as the 1st day but is likely to be later in the 1st week. The discharge may be watery at first but becomes copious and purulent later. The conjunctiva will initially be reddened; later it becomes congested and often oedematous. The eyes become swollen and are tightly shut. The baby may be transferred to an isolation unit. Penicillin is the antibiotic of choice and is administered both as eye drops and systemically. Blindness is a serious complication of gonococcal ophthalmia and is due to damage to and ulceration of the cornea.

Pneumonia occurs as an ascending or intrapartum infection. Causative organisms include beta-haemolytic streptococcus group B, *Escherichia coli* and *Pseudomonas aeruginosa*. The symptoms may be similar to those of respiratory distress syndrome (RDS) occurring about 4 hours after delivery. The baby will become cyanosed in air with nasal flaring. He will also be restless due to hypoxia. A chest X-ray will be performed but the picture may be identical to that seen in RDS. Culture of nose and throat swabs may help to identify the organism. If the baby develops signs soon after birth and before the first feed, a specimen of gastric aspirate should be cultured as it may contain infected amniotic fluid.

The infant will require intensive neonatal nursing care (see Ch. 36) and antibiotics should be commenced as soon as swabs have been taken. Penicillin and gentamicin are often chosen because group B streptococcus is the most likely organism.

Septicaemia may be caused by group B haemolytic streptococcus from the mother's vagina. Onset is rapid with mild respiratory distress and cyanosis occurring within 1–2 hours of birth. The condition quickly deteriorates and the mortality rate is high despite treatment with appropriate antibiotics.

Infections acquired after birth

These are acquired from the environment, from contaminated equipment and from the people handling the baby. Cross-infection from other babies is also significant.

Surface infections

Eyes. Mild infections of the eyes are common and will usually respond to cleansing with normal saline. If there is a discharge which persists, swabs are taken and appropriate antibiotic therapy is prescribed by the doctor. Ophthalmia neonatorum (see above) may occasionally be the result of postnatal infection for instance with the staphylococcus.

Mouth. Thrush is usually contracted from the mother's vagina but may be transmitted by the hands of attendants, from improperly washed and sterilised teats or from the infant himself. Antibiotic therapy predisposes to candida.

Buttocks. Peri-anal thrush may cause soreness of the buttocks and is secondary to oral infection. The skin is extremely red and the affected area may involve the flexures and extend as far as the umbilicus. Topical application of nystatin or amphotericin cream is indicated in addition to oral administration.

Skin. Most skin infections in the newborn baby are staphylococcal in origin and many of the hygiene measures which are routine in neonatal care were devised to combat the spread of this organism. Antibiotic therapy is usually appropriate and flucloxacillin is effective against the *Staphylococcus aureus*.

Septic spots. Isolated pustules may resolve if swabbed with a cotton wool swab soaked in chlorhexidine 0.5% in spirit. If the pustules persist or appear in clusters, a swab should be taken for culture and sensitivity and an appropriate antibiotic commenced.

Paronychia. Injury to the folds of skin surrounding the finger- or toenails may result in infection. In the early stages, dabbing with chlorhexidine 0.5% in spirit may be sufficient to dry up the whitlow. The baby's hand should be enclosed in a mitten in order to prevent him from touching his eyes with it. In severe cases, pus may need to be released by surgical incision but this is rare.

Pemphigus neonatorum. This is a rare, highly contagious skin disease characterised by watery blisters. If it is suspected, a doctor should be summoned, the baby isolated and swabs taken from the lesions. Antibiotics may be given intravenously. A very severe form of pemphigus, termed *toxic epidermal necrolysis* (Ritter's disease), results in exfoliation of the skin over a wide area.

Omphalitis is infection of the umbilicus. It is suspected if there is any inflammation, discharge or offensive odour. There is a possibility of cellulitis developing around the base of the cord and also of spread via the umbilical vein to the liver causing hepatitis and septicaemia. Bacteriological investigation will establish the correct antibiotic to use. Neomycin-bacitracin (Cicatrin) powder is applied locally.

Neonatal mastitis. This condition should not occur. It is due to squeezing breasts which are enlarged due to the effect of maternal hormones. If an abscess forms, incision and drainage are necessary and antibiotic therapy is given.

Respiratory infection

Infection of the respiratory tract is usually caused by airborne organisms transmitted by parents, visitors or staff. Upper respiratory tract infection must be treated promptly because it may be the cause of more severe, life-threatening respiratory infection.

Nasopharyngitis causes snuffles in the baby. If it spreads downwards the cry becomes hoarse. Mother and baby should be nursed in a single room and the baby given extra fluids.

Rhinitis is an inflammation of the mucous membrane of the nose, caused by staphylococci. Nose and throat swabs should be taken for culture and sensitivity prior to commencing the appropriate antibiotic. The nasal passages should be kept clear, if necessary by administering ephedrine nasal drops 0.25%, as babies are compulsive nose-breathers.

Pneumonia. While congenital pneumonia (see above) presents in the first 24 hours, if a baby presents with pneumonia after the first 48 hours of life, it is probable that the infection has been acquired postnatally and is due to staphylococci. It may be a complication of endotracheal intubation, mechanical ventilation, inhalation of vomit or meconium aspiration. Treatment is with gentamicin and flucloxacillin and chest physiotherapy is given.

Gastro-intestinal tract infections

Infection in the gastro-intestinal tract is dangerous because diarrhoea and vomiting rapidly dehydrate the baby. Wholly breast-fed infants are virtually never affected because of the protective anti-infective factors in breast milk. All diarrhoea in the newborn must be regarded as transmissible

until several negative stool cultures have been obtained.

Gastro-enteritis. Many cases are due to rotavirus and a bacterial pathogen will not be found. In those cases which are bacterial in origin possible organisms include shigellae, salmonellae and pathogenic *Escherichia coli*. The condition is not common in the newborn.

The clinical features of gastro-enteritis are profuse vomiting, loose, watery, offensive stools, weight loss, dehydration and electrolyte imbalance. The treatment is to stop oral feeding and administer fluid intravenously. Blood should be taken for estimation of electrolytes and the appropriate supplements such as sodium and potassium added to the infusion. Culture of a stool specimen may reveal the pathogen. Antibiotics are not given unless the baby has septicaemia.

After 48 hours, if diarrhoea has ceased, oral feeding may be gradually resumed, possibly commencing with half-normal saline or dextrose. If, when milk is re-introduced, the condition recurs, milk intolerance should be suspected.

Necrotising enterocolitis (NEC) is a condition in which the gut mucosa is damaged due to reduced perfusion; necrosis results and the bowel is invaded by gas-forming organisms. It has only been recognised in recent times since tiny babies have benefited from intensive supportive care. The precise cause of NEC is uncertain but it is clear that some babies are particularly vulnerable to it especially those of very low birth weight and those who have undergone procedures which affect blood flow, such as umbilical catheterisation. It is best understood by recognising that factors which damage the mucosa are responsible, such as hypotension and hypoperfusion or injury from umbilical catheters or hypertonic feeds.

The baby may show some early signs of infection such as unstable temperature, lethargy, reluctance to feed and abdominal distension due to paralytic ileus. In addition he will pass small amounts of blood in the stool. As the disease progresses, the baby becomes pale and mottled with increased distension. Gastric emptying is delayed and there is bile-stained vomit. Bowel sounds are absent. An X-ray will reveal gas in the bowel wall or portal venous system and fluid levels in the abdomen. Further deterioration may be the result of perforation of the bowel wall.

This very ill baby will need intensive nursing care with special attention to maintaining a stable temperature. Oral feeds are stopped immediately and a nasogastric tube passed to relieve distension. Intravenous fluids must be commenced. Antibiotics are given intravenously, a typical combination being penicillin, gentamicin and metronidazole. If the condition is recognised promptly and treatment instituted without delay, the baby may recover with medical treatment alone. Perforation of the bowel necessitates surgery and the prognosis for these babies is poor.

Urinary tract infection

The baby shows general signs of infection. Diagnosis is confirmed by culture of a urine sample which is best obtained by a clean catch or suprapubic bladder aspiration rather than a bag specimen. Antibiotics are prescribed.

Meningitis

Meningitis is an extremely serious and potentially fatal infection. It is often accompanied by septicaemia. The organism responsible may be *Escherichia coli*, group B beta-haemolytic streptococcus, *Listeria monocytogenes*, *Pseudomonas aeruginosa* or *Bacillus proteus*. As with all other neonatal infections, signs may not be specific at first and the diagnosis may be made on routine lumbar puncture in a sick baby. Later, signs such as bulging fontanelles, head retraction and convulsions may develop. Treatment should be started without delay. Antibiotics are chosen which will cross the blood–brain barrier, such as intravenous penicillin, gentamicin or cephalosporin. Antibiotic therapy will be continued for at least 2 or 3 weeks.

The baby will require careful nursing. Fluid balance is particularly important. The blood pressure may be monitored and daily head circumference measurements should be recorded to observe for any increase. Ultrasound scanning can detect ventriculitis or hydrocephalus. CSF may be re-examined after 48 hours if there is no improvement (Han & Halliday 1992).

If the baby recovers he may be left with brain damage and remain handicapped.

Reader Activities

- Link up with the person who is responsible for monitoring neonatal infections. Ask her or him for recent records of micro-organisms identified as having caused various infections in babies:
  — in the maternity unit as a whole
  — in the neonatal intensive care unit.
  Find out to which antibiotics the organisms have been sensitive.
- Compare Table 34.2 with the policies of the neonatologists in your own unit.
- Talk to one or more mothers whose babies are receiving (or have received) phototherapy. How did the mothers feel about this treatment? Were there particular features of the regime that gave them cause for anxiety? How can the midwife help the mother overcome such anxieties?

USEFUL ADDRESS

The Toxoplasmosis Trust
61–71 Collier Street, London N1 9BE
Helpline 071 713 0599
Office 071 713 0663

REFERENCES

Cerase P A 1989 Neonatal sepsis. Journal of Perinatal and Neonatal Nursing 3(2): 48–57

Editorial 1991 Moderate neonatal hyperbilirubinaemia: hold tight. Lancet 338 (Nov 16): 1242–1243

Han K, Halliday H 1992 Treating meningitis in the neonate. Professional Care of Mother and Child 2(1): 18–22

Hussein M et al 1991 Jaundice at 14 days of age: exclude biliary atresia. Archives of Disease in Childhood 66(10): 1177–1179

Kay J 1990 The management of a baby with biliary atresia. Paediatric Nursing 2(10): 20–22

FURTHER READING

Ennever J F 1990 Treatment of neonatal jaundice. In: Maisels M J (ed) Clinics in perinatology: neonatal jaundice. June. Saunders, Philadelphia

Halliday H L 1989 Handbook of neonatal intensive care, 3rd edn. Baillière Tindall, London

Hodson W A, Truog W E 1989 Critical care of the newborn. Saunders, Philadelphia

Kelnar C J H, Harvey D 1986 The sick newborn baby, 2nd edn. Baillière Tindall, London

Newman T B, Maisels M J 1990 Does hyperbilirubinaemia damage the brain of infants? In: Maisels M J (ed) Clinics in perinatology: neonatal jaundice. June. Saunders, Philadelphia

Roberton N R C 1986 A manual of neonatal intensive care. Edward Arnold, London

Roberton N R C 1992 Textbook of neonatology. Churchill Livingstone, Edinburgh

Whittle M J 1992 Rhesus haemolytic disease. Archives of Disease in Childhood 67: 65–68

35

Small and large babies

ELIZABETH THOMSON

PRETERM BABIES

The last decade or so has produced, notably in Western nations, a significant increase in preterm infants, particularly those born weighing less than 1500 g and after less than 30 weeks' gestation. Concurrently, there has been an upsurge in technology which has enabled the survival of these babies, some of whom are born on the lower borders of viability, i.e. 22–26 weeks' gestation.

Greatly improved antenatal monitoring skills have permitted better control of many high risk women in order to retain and sustain their pregnancies towards a gestation when intervention can be planned for an optimal neonatal outcome. Such changes have inevitably resulted in a different stratum of babies in neonatal units producing an often overwhelming increment in the workload and demanding greater, more in-depth knowledge, skills and attitudes from the carers of the newborn.

Definitions

Preterm infant. A baby born before 37 completed weeks of pregnancy. Some preterm babies may also be growth-retarded and therefore small for gestational age. Others may be excessively large and therefore large for gestational age.

Low birthweight (LBW) baby. A baby whose birthweight is 2500 g or less.

Very low birthweight (VLBW) baby. A baby whose birthweight is 1500 g or less.

Causes

In many instances, the cause of preterm birth remains unknown although there are several factors which are considered to predispose to a shortened pregnancy.

Previous obstetric history

A history of previous mid-trimester miscarriage is not uncommon in women who have a preterm birth. Controversy continues regarding the effect of therapeutic abortion on subsequent pregnancy but in practice a proportion of women having had previous terminations do experience a preterm birth. It is possible that any cervical interference may give rise to cervical incompetence.

Maternal age

This is not considered to be a major factor in the duration of pregnancy although there does appear to be an increase in preterm birth outside the optimum childbearing age range of 20–35 years.

Social class

There seems to be an increased likelihood of women in social classes IV and V having a shorter gestation period though there may be other compounding factors present such as maternal illness.

Multiple pregnancy

Overdistension of the uterus not uncommonly results in spontaneous preterm labour but multiple births, especially when there are more than two babies, are now frequently elective preterm events.

Maternal disease in pregnancy

Pre-eclampsia, infection, antepartum haemorrhage, placenta praevia or placental abruption may prompt the decision to conclude the pregnancy early. Likewise, chronic maternal disease such as hypertension and renal disease may also be indications for obstetric intervention.

Fetal causes

Instances where the well-being of the fetus may be seriously compromised if the pregnancy were continued include placental insufficiency and Rhesus disease. The presence of congenital abnormalities possibly complicated by growth retardation may also be associated with preterm birth.

Appearance and neurological development, gestational age assessment

The appearance of the preterm infant can vary enormously according to the degree of intra-uterine growth. To assess growth, separate centile charts have been devised for boys and girls so that birthweight can be plotted against gestational age. Babies who have grown normally in utero

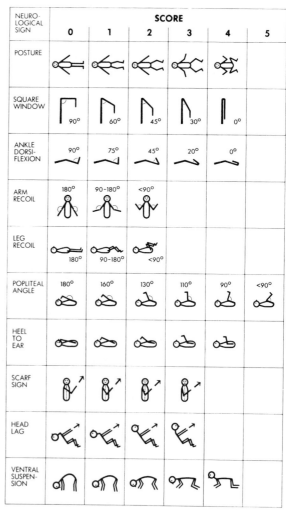

Fig. 35.1
Neurological criteria (Dubowitz et al 1970).

with a birthweight between the 10th and 90th centile are appropriate for gestational age (AGA). Babies whose intra-uterine growth has been retarded with a birthweight below the 10th centile are small for gestational age (SGA). Babies whose intra-uterine growth has been excessive with a birthweight above the 90th centile are large for gestational age (LGA). It is important therefore to differentiate between a preterm baby who is AGA and one who is SGA or LGA.

The preterm baby has soft skull bones surrounding a fragile brain and is therefore at greater risk of neurological damage from a traumatic delivery.

POSTURE: Observed with infant quiet and in supine position. Score 0: Arms and legs extended; 1: beginning of flexion of hips and knees, arms extended; 2: stronger flexion of legs, arms extended; 3: arms slightly flexed, legs flexed and abducted; 4: full flexion of arms and legs.

SQUARE WINDOW: The hand is flexed on the forearm between the thumb and index finger of the examiner. Enough pressure is applied to get as full a flexion as possible, and the angle between the hypothenar eminence and the ventral aspect of the forearm is measured and graded according to diagram. (Care is taken not to rotate the infant's wrist while doing this manœuvre.)

ANKLE DORSIFLEXION: The foot is dorsiflexed onto the anterior aspect of the leg, with the examiner's thumb on the sole of the foot and other fingers behind the leg. Enough pressure is applied to get as full flexion as possible, and the angle between the dorsum of the foot and the anterior aspect of the leg is measured.

ARM RECOIL: With the infant in the supine position the forearms are first flexed for 5 seconds, then fully extended by pulling on the hands, and then released. The sign is fully positive if the arms return briskly to full flexion (Score 2). If the arms return to incomplete flexion or the response is sluggish it is graded as Score 1. If they remain extended or are only followed by random movements the score is 0.

LEG RECOIL: With the infant supine, the hips and knees are fully flexed for 5 seconds, then extended by traction on the feet, and released. A maximal response is one of full flexion of the hips and knees (Score 2). A partial flexion scores 1, and minimal or no movement scores 0.

POPLITEAL ANGLE: With the infant supine and his pelvis flat on the examining couch, the thigh is held in the knee-chest position by the examiner's left index finger and thumb supporting the knee. The leg is then extended by gentle pressure from the examiner's right index finger behind the ankle and the popliteal angle is measured.

HEEL TO EAR MANŒUVRE: With the baby supine, draw the baby's foot as near to the head as it will go without forcing it. Observe the distance between the foot and the head as well as the degree of extension at the knee. Grade according to diagram. Note that the knee is left free and may draw down alongside the abdomen.

SCARF SIGN: With the baby supine, take the infant's hand and try to put it around the neck and as far posteriorly as possible around the opposite shoulder. Assist this manœuvre by lifting the elbow across the body. See how far the elbow will go across and grade according to illustrations. Score 0: Elbow reaches opposite axillary line; 1: Elbow between midline and opposite axillary line; 2: Elbow reaches midline; 3: Elbow will not reach midline.

HEAD LAG: With the baby lying supine, grasp the hands (or the arms if a very small infant) and pull him slowly towards the sitting position. Observe the position of the head in relation to the trunk and grade accordingly. In a small infant the head may initially be supported by one hand. Score 0: Complete lag; 1: Partial head control; 2: Able to maintain head in line with body; 3: Brings head anterior to body.

VENTRAL SUSPENSION: The infant is suspended in the prone position, with examiner's hand under the infant's chest (one hand in a small infant, two in a large infant). Observe the degree of extension of the back and the amount of flexion of the arms and legs. Also note the relation of the head to the trunk. Grade according to diagrams.

If the score for an individual criterion differs on the two sides of the baby, take the mean.

Fig. 35.2
Some notes on techniques of assessment of neurological criteria (Dubowitz et al 1970).

Gestational age assessment

The Dubowitz score has been found to be an accurate method of assessing gestational age providing it is undertaken within 48 hours of delivery (see Figs 35.1, 35.2, 35.3 and 35.4).

Potential problems

Asphyxia

Asphyxia is a major problem in the preterm infant because, being generally immature, he is less well equipped to cope with such a physiological insult. In utero the fetus is subjected to hypoxia and

EXTERNAL SIGN	SCORE				
	0	**1**	**2**	**3**	**4**
OEDEMA	Obvious oedema hands and feet; pitting over tibia	No obvious oedema hands and feet; pitting over tibia	No oedema		
SKIN TEXTURE	Very thin, gelatinous	Thin and smooth	Smooth; medium thickness. Rash or superficial peeling	Slight thickening. Superficial cracking and peeling esp hands and feet	Thick and parchment-like; superficial or deep cracking
SKIN COLOUR (Infant not crying)	Dark red	Uniformly pink	Pale pink: variable over body	Pale. Only pink over ears, lips, palms or soles	
SKIN OPACITY (trunk)	Numerous veins and venules clearly seen, especially over abdomen	Veins and tributaries seen	A few large vessels clearly seen over abdomen	A few large vessels seen indistinctly over abdomen	No blood vessels seen
LANUGO (over back)	No lanugo	Abundant; long and thick over whole back	Hair thinning especially over lower back	Small amount of lanugo and bald areas	At least half of back devoid of lanugo
PLANTAR CREASES	No skin creases	Faint red marks over anterior half of sole	Definite red marks over more than anterior half; indentations over less than anterior third	Indentations over more than anterior third	Definite deep indentations over more than anterior third
NIPPLE FORMATION	Nipple barely visible; no areola	Nipple well defined; areola smooth and flat diameter <0.75 cm.	Areola stippled, edge not raised; diameter <0.75 cm.	Areola stippled, edge raised diameter >0.75 cm.	
BREAST SIZE	No breast tissue palpable	Breast tissue on one or both sides < 0.5 cm. diameter	Breast tissue both sides; one or both 0.5–1.0 cm.	Breast tissue both sides; one or both > 1 cm.	
EAR FORM	Pinna flat and shapeless, little or no incurving of edge	Incurving of part of edge of pinna	Partial incurving whole of upper pinna	Well-defined incurving whole of upper pinna	
EAR FIRMNESS	Pinna soft, easily folded, no recoil	Pinna soft, easily folded, slow recoil	Cartilage to edge of pinna, but soft in places, ready recoil	Pinna firm, cartilage to edge, instant recoil	
GENITALIA MALE	Neither testis in scrotum	At least one testis high in scrotum	At least one testis right down		
FEMALES (With hips half abducted)	Labia majora widely separated, labia minora protruding	Labia majora almost cover labia minora	Labia majora completely cover labia minora		

Fig. 35.3
External (superficial) criteria (Dubowitz et al 1970).

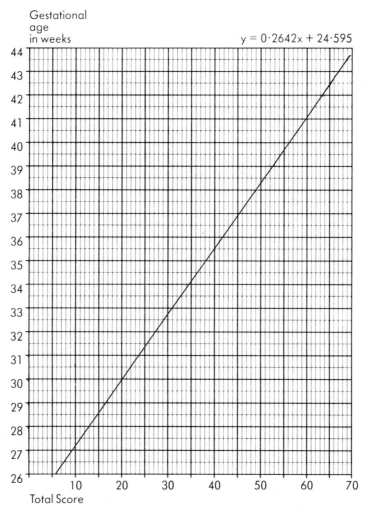

Fig. 35.4
Graph for reading gestational age from total score (Dubowitz et al 1970).

hypercapnia, both of which act as respiratory stimulants. However, during the latter part of the second stage of labour, fetal blood supply is diminished or terminated by cord compression, resulting in moderate asphyxia. The fetus responds by gasping for a short period before becoming apnoeic. This stage is referred to as primary apnoea, during which the heart rate and blood pressure may remain constant or become slightly elevated. Following an interval of a few minutes a second period of gasping commences and the heart rate and blood pressure fall quickly. After the last gasp, the fetus enters a stage of terminal apnoea. Most asphyxiated infants are born in primary apnoea and will commence spontaneous respiration if given air to breathe. Those born in terminal apnoea will require active intervention to avoid death (see also Ch. 31).

Apnoea

Apnoea is defined as the cessation of breathing for greater than 20 seconds. Commonly, preterm babies demonstrate irregular or periodic breathing with respiratory pauses lasting up to 15 seconds, a pattern which may continue for several weeks. Apnoea, which may or may not be accompanied by bradycardia, is frequently observed in preterm infants. The frequency and severity of apnoeic episodes decreases as gestational age progresses. Observations have shown that apnoea may be related to sleep state, with apnoeic attacks being seen more often during active, rapid eye movement (REM) sleep. It has also been noted that apnoea may occur, though less frequently, during quiet (non-REM) sleep. This is significant since preterm infants spend about 18 hours per day asleep.

Apnoea in an otherwise well preterm infant may be an indication of an impending disorder whilst apnoeic episodes in an already sick infant are often a signal of deterioration. Important respiratory causes of apnoea in the preterm include hyaline membrane disease (respiratory distress syndrome), exhaustion (often seen when weaning a baby off ventilation), pneumonia, vagal stimulation by suction and bolus orogastric tube feeds (possibly with milk aspiration).

Central causes of apnoea comprise cerebral birth trauma, cerebral haemorrhage, seizures, meningitis and oversedation. Metabolic disturbances such as hypoglycaemia, hypocalcaemia, metabolic or respiratory acidosis and hypothermia may also initiate apnoea. Additionally, the preterm infant is especially vulnerable to handling and apnoeic attacks may occur following physical examination, nappy changing or physiotherapy for example.

Transient tachypnoea of the newborn

Although this disorder is more commonly seen in near term babies, a brief outline is included to illustrate the differentiation from hyaline membrane disease. The cause of transient tachypnoea of the newborn is attributed to delayed clearance of lung fluid and is sometimes referred to as 'wet lung'. It is commonly associated with caesarean section where there has been no gradual chest compression. Clinically, the baby presents at about 2–4 hours of age with an increased respiratory rate greater than 60 per minute, possibly with chest recession, slight grunting and maybe mild cyanosis. Characteristically these signs subside after 24 hours (see also Ch. 31).

Hyaline membrane disease

Hyaline membrane disease (HMD) or respiratory distress syndrome (RDS) is the major cause of respiratory problems in babies of short gestation. Fundamentally, it is a disorder of lung immaturity caused by deficiency of surfactant. Although many affected infants appear satisfactory at birth with good Apgar scores, during the first few hours they develop signs of respiratory distress. Those infants who have been asphyxiated will usually exhibit signs of distress more rapidly. Classically, these respiratory problems include tachypnoea greater than 60 per minute, substernal and intercostal recession and an expiratory grunt and they increase in severity during the 24–48 hours after birth. Recovery usually occurs after 72 hours when the baby starts to synthesise surfactant.

Aetiology. To ensure normal lung function, adequate surfactant production is essential to reduce surface tension and keep the alveoli expanded following expiration. Surfactant is a complex phospholipid secreted by the type II alveolar cells from about 22 weeks' gestation though it is not usually seen in the lung fluid until after 30 weeks. Measurement of surfactant is expressed as the ratio between lecithin and sphingomyelin (L:S ratio) in tracheal fluid and results greater than 1.8:1 are indicative of lung maturity.

Physiological or clinical course. Tachypnoea is commonly the most pronounced feature of RDS accompanied by varying degrees of substernal and intercostal recession which is created by the inability to exert sufficient inspiratory pressure to expand the alveoli. The chest wall is very compliant and exhibits the tendency to collapse around the relatively stiff lungs. Expiratory grunting originates from an attempt to expire actively against a partially closed larynx, thus delaying alveolar collapse. As a consequence of these events, therefore, it can be seen that alveolar ventilation is progressively reduced with resultant hypoxaemia. Clinically, this presents as cyanosis and with increasing hypoxaemia there is retention of carbon dioxide producing a respiratory and metabolic acidosis which impedes surfactant synthesis.

A chest X-ray will demonstrate the characteristic diffuse granularity of the lung fields with a poorly defined cardiac border. In severe disease, the larger airways are visible against the opaque lung fields (air bronchogram) (Fig. 35.5).

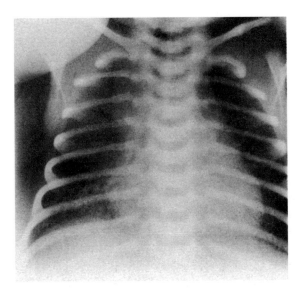

Fig. 35.5
Chest X-ray of hyaline membrane disease showing mild, diffuse granularity throughout both lung fields. (Reproduced by permission from D. Lindsell, Consultant Radiologist, John Radcliffe Hospital, Oxford.)

Jaundice

Jaundice is a problem of particular importance in the preterm baby because there is an increased risk of kernicterus developing. Along with other physiological processes, hepatic function in the preterm infant is reduced and enzyme systems are immature; in particular, the level of glucuronyl transferase production is low. Additionally, there is a deficiency in Y and Z carrier proteins and hypoalbuminaemia. These factors substantially reduce the ability of the preterm neonate to cope with bilirubin excretion (see also Ch. 34).

Infection

Infection poses a major problem to preterm babies because they are poorly equipped to combat the multitude of organisms in the environment. Significantly, the placental transfer of IgG is incomplete which makes them highly susceptible to many common bacteria and viruses. The preterm infant is also incapable of producing sufficient IgM making him especially vulnerable to Gram-negative bacterial infections.

The skin is a non-specific defence against infection but in preterm babies, particularly those of less than 28 weeks' gestation, the skin is very thin and easily damaged. Contributing towards this problem is the fact that often the treatment of a preterm infant requires invasive procedures such as endotracheal intubation or insertion of an intravenous cannula, many of which provide portals of entry for pathological organisms (see also Ch. 34).

Poor temperature control

Regulation of body temperature is difficult for the preterm baby chiefly because of the large surface area to body weight ratio. Stores of brown fat in the neck, around the aorta and between the scapulae are low which diminishes the baby's ability to produce heat. Additionally, there is a lack of subcutaneous fat and preterm babies tend to lie in a splayed out position which exposes more body surface and exaggerates heat loss.

Heat loss. Heat is lost in the following ways: conduction, convection, radiation and evaporation.

Conduction. Heat loss by conduction can occur if the baby lies on a solid surface which is cooler than himself. However, most babies lie on a mattress which provides insulation from a cool surface.

Convection. The transfer of heat from the baby to the surrounding cooler air constitutes convective heat loss. The rate at which heat is lost by this method will depend on the ambient temperature, the amount of the baby's skin exposed to the air and the speed of the air flow. Heat loss can be reduced by clothing the baby and increasing the air temperature.

Radiation. Heat loss by radiation involves the transfer of heat from the baby to cooler surrounding surfaces such as the walls of the incubator or the room. Radiant heat loss is independent of ambient air temperature.

Evaporation. Heat is lost in this manner when water evaporates from the skin or breath. Therefore, the amount of heat lost will be dependent on the water loss. At delivery when the baby is covered in amniotic fluid, heat loss occurs rapidly as the fluid evaporates. The skin of the preterm baby has greater permeability and is consequently more vulnerable to evaporative heat loss than that of a baby born at term.

Heat production. Babies produce heat by metabolic activity and are specially equipped for this purpose by the provision of brown fat. As a response to a fall in environmental temperature, cutaneous nerve endings are stimulated. Following a release of noradrenaline which initiates metabolic activity in the brown fat, heat is produced which subsequently warms the blood perfusing through the tissues.

Anaemia

Preterm babies are likely to develop iron deficiency anaemia because they have lost the opportunity to store iron by being born too soon. Supplements are not required until infants weigh about 2000 g and should be continued until weaning is established. Ankett et al (1986) indicate that there is cumulative evidence that iron deficiency anaemia in early life can retard psychomotor development.

Folic acid may need to be supplemented in order to avoid megaloblastic anaemia.

Vitamin E deficiency may cause a haemolytic anaemia and contribute to retinopathy of prematurity. An oral supplement should be given to infants of less than 2000 g.

Bone marrow function in the preterm baby may be slow to adjust to extra-uterine life with inadequate response to the postnatal fall in haemoglobin level. The preterm infant grows rapidly and there is a concurrent increase in circulating blood volume but the bone marrow is unable to match this demand with increased red cell production.

Problems of extreme immaturity

The extremely immature baby presents a range of difficult yet challenging problems to those involved in neonatal care. The degree of immaturity is currently the focus of controversy and extensive debate in relation to subsequent survival. The professionals face a dilemma regarding the initiation of intensive care in the case of babies of very short gestation and extremely low birthweight. Suffice it to say that such decisions should be made at consultant level taking into account the individual problems of the baby and parental feelings.

In essence, the problems of the extremely immature baby include those already mentioned in relation to the preterm baby but probably with exaggerated presentation. The very immature infant is even less robust. He will encounter serious difficulties if asphyxiated, with an increased likelihood of apnoeic episodes largely due to the curtailed intra-uterine existence. The majority of babies born at less than 28 weeks gestation will develop hyaline membrane disease on account of their lung immaturity. These babies will also be at greater risk of developing complications associated with ventilatory support (see also Ch. 36).

Jaundice practically always features as a complex problem of management in these babies and is attributable to the underdeveloped hepatic function and low level of plasma proteins. The problem of infection is almost overwhelming to these tiny babies whose immunological deficiency places them at considerable disadvantage in coping with extra-uterine life. Their wafer-thin and easily traumatised skin only contributes to the inadequacy of their defences.

Temperature control is yet another difficulty which at times borders on the insurmountable. Because of their multiple problems, immature infants require an active approach to their management which in itself, despite modern technology, may entail some compromise in the regulation of their thermal environment.

It is still not fully understood what are the optimal nutritional requirements for short gestation babies and there are obviously major difficulties in management for a protracted period. These difficulties are almost wholly due to the absence of sucking ability and poorly developed gastrointestinal function. Sometimes total parenteral nutrition is indicated which may entail a host of complications. Acid–base balance and fluid and electrolyte balance pose added stress to the extremely preterm infant whose respiratory, renal and cellular functions are already disordered.

Finally, in addition to these physiological considerations, there are the problems of separation and adjustment for the parents of an extremely immature baby. The lower the gestation, the greater the anxiety of the parents as their tiny baby moves unsteadily along the precipice between life and death (see also Ch. 36).

Management

Labour and delivery

Ideally, preterm labour and delivery should be managed in a consultant obstetric unit with full support facilities from pathological, radiological, pharmaceutical, blood transfusion and neonatal intensive care services. Therefore, it follows that all women likely to give birth prematurely should be transferred to such a centre so that perinatal events can be managed optimally. If preterm labour arises unexpectedly, the obstetric and neonatal flying squad services should be summoned without delay since delivery may be precipitous.

In pregnancies of less than 34 weeks' gestation, labour may be inhibited by an infusion of beta-mimetic drugs. This therapy is contra-indicated in the presence of maternal cardiovascular disease, pre-eclampsia, antepartum haemorrhage, amnionitis or diabetes mellitus.

Careful assessment of the strength and frequency of uterine contractions and of the degree of cervical dilatation and whether or not the membranes have ruptured are other factors to be considered. Of greater importance, however, is the status of the baby and clearly there is no point in prolonging the pregnancy if the fetus is abnormal. If fetal welfare is compromised the infant should be delivered in preference to inhibiting labour. Blood glucose levels should be monitored in babies whose mothers were given betamimetic drugs. Growth retardation and the possibility of intrauterine infection are other determinants requiring evaluation (Anderson & Turnbull 1982). Continuous fetal heart rate monitoring should be employed so that any variation from normal can be detected promptly and appropriate action taken. The use of epidural anaesthesia may be advisable as it avoids the need for narcotic drugs which may have a respiratory depressant effect on the fetus.

Early episiotomy and gentle application of forceps are usually chosen in order to prevent damage to the soft skull bones. It is obviously desirable for the baby to be received in the best possible condition and this may not be so if the infant has endured a vaginal delivery. There is a growing concern that, as far as is reasonable, preterm birth should not impose undue stress on the baby. On these grounds, elective caesarean section may well be considered and vaginal breech delivery, expect where unavoidable, should never be undertaken below 32 weeks' gestation.

Resuscitation at birth

Diligent thought and preparation should be applied to an imminent preterm birth to enable the baby to be born under the most favourable circumstances. The temperature in the delivery room or theatre should be at least 25°C. All resuscitation equipment is meticulously checked and prepared. The paediatrician is called in good time so that he or she may become fully acquainted with the pertinent details about mother and baby and may meet the parents.

Steps in resuscitation

1. After delivery of the face, gentle suction is applied to the oropharynx and nostrils.
2. The midwife receiving the baby will wrap him in warm towels and place him on the resuscitaire.
3. The clock is started.
4. The baby is dried thoroughly and placed in a fresh warm towel.
5. The oropharynx and nostrils are aspirated using a mucus extractor or mechanical suction.
6. The baby is observed carefully and the Apgar score is assessed at 1 minute.
7. If the score is 7 or above, no active intervention is required, though occasionally facial oxygen may be necessary for a short period.
8. An Apgar score of between 4 and 6 signifies moderate asphyxia and a laryngoscope is inserted and suction applied to the larynx under direct vision. An airway is inserted and 100% oxygen administered via a well-fitting mask with bag attachment, e.g. Penlon. It is important to compress the bag carefully with the thumb, index and middle fingers only (over-zealous ventilation may cause a pneumothorax) and inflate the lungs 30–40 times a minute to a pressure not exceeding 25 cm H_2O. The baby's response should be

observed by constantly listening to the heart rate and air entry. The apex beat should improve and spontaneous respirations become established after about 30 seconds. If after 1 minute there is no improvement, the colour deteriorates or the apex beat falls to below 100 beats per minute (bpm) immediate intubation is required.

9. Any baby with an Apgar score of less than 4 must be intubated immediately.

10. The Apgar score is re-assessed at 5 minutes and if the baby is slow to respond, again at 10 minutes.

Intubation. The baby is laid flat on the resuscitaire with slight extension of the neck. Taking a neonatal laryngoscope in the left hand, the blade is gently inserted along the right side of the mouth so that the tongue is displaced towards the left. The end of the blade should rest in the vallecula between the base of the tongue and the epiglottis. Carefully tilting the blade upwards, the glottis is visualised. Brief suction will clear secretions so that the vocal cords are seen. Gentle pressure on the cricoid cartilage may provide clearer vision. An endotracheal tube of the appropriate

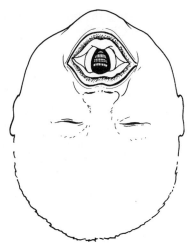

Fig. 35.7
View of the glottis.

size is inserted 1–2 cm beyond the glottis. The endotracheal tube is connected to the oxygen supply and resuscitation bag; ventilation is continued as previously described. The baby's chest should rise with each ventilation and air entry should be equal on both sides. If breath sounds are absent on the left side, the tube is withdrawn slightly as it may have been inserted into the right main bronchus.

If this procedure proves difficult at any stage, it is far better to insert an airway and use bag and mask ventilation until the arrival of more skilled assistance. Numerous attempts at intubation cause trauma and further deterioration in the baby's condition. Skilful intubation technique cannot be learnt from textbooks. It is helpful to practise on models or dead babies but there is no substitute for supervised experience in vivo.

Cardiac support. If at any stage during resuscitation the apex beat falls below 60 bpm, external cardiac massage must be instituted immediately. The index and middle fingers are placed on the middle of the sternum*. Applying downward pressure not exceeding 2 cm, the chest is compressed 100–120 times per minute in cycles of 3–6 chest compressions to one ventilation. Extreme caution must be exercised in synchronising these events because a pneumothorax could result if chest compression is accompanied by

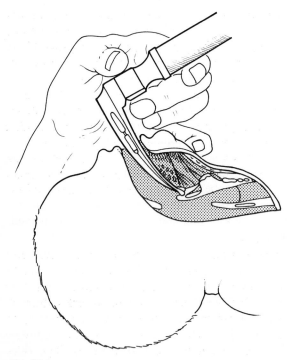

Fig. 35.6
Insertion of the laryngoscope blade.

*Some advise the lower sternum or slightly to its left.

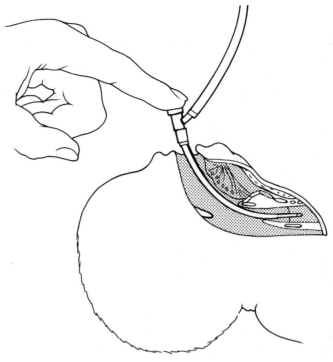

Fig. 35.8
Endotracheal tube in position.

ventilation. It is also important to remember that the newborn chest is very compliant and over-vigorous compression could cause fractures or laceration of abdominal organs.

Use of drugs. Drug administration constitutes a minor role in resuscitation since the over-whelming priority is to establish ventilation and circulation. The safest route of administration for any drugs required is via an umbilical venous catheter primed with normal saline and inserted in an aseptic manner. In the uncommon instances when sodium bicarbonate is required to correct acidosis, 2 ml/kg of 8.4% solution should be given diluted with 5% dextrose to double its volume. When severe asphyxia has occurred causing hypo-glycaemia, it is necessary to give 2 ml/kg of dextrose 10% with subsequent monitoring of capillary blood glucose at intervals. When the mother has been given pethidine shortly before delivery and the baby is slow to establish and sustain respirations, it may be necessary to give naloxone 0.01 mg/kg intramuscularly. A delayed response to resuscitation may be due to shock resulting from fetal haemorrhage. In such cir-cumstances, volume expansion can be achieved by giving 10–20 ml/kg of O Rhesus negative blood or fresh frozen plasma. The administration of vitamin K or cruel smacking of the soles of the feet or any other anatomical part are not con-stituents of resuscitation, since neither contributes to the paramount considerations of attaining optimal ventilatory and circulatory function.

Following resuscitation it is essential to talk with the parents and try if possible to let them cuddle the baby especially if he is to be transferred to the neonatal unit.

Transport
Transporting a preterm baby to the neonatal unit should be undertaken with the utmost care. In any circumstances the baby's condition must first be stabilised as far as possible as sick babies do not tolerate travel well. It is rarely necessary to travel at great speed; high velocity movement may be detrimental to the baby's status. The baby should be clearly identified with two name bands.

Transport within a hospital. Wherever possible, the parents should see, touch and hold their baby prior to transfer and be given an explanation regarding the baby's needs. Usually the delivery suite is situated fairly close to the neonatal unit but this is not always so and emergencies may arise anywhere in transit. The baby should therefore be accompanied by a paediatrician and at least one midwife. The baby is wrapped in a silver swaddler or insulating blanket and placed in a prewarmed portable incubator. If the baby requires ventilatory support he must be intubated and the endotracheal tube efficiently secured. Ventilation can be administered either via a Penlon bag or via an inbuilt portable ventilator. Air and oxygen supplies and resuscitation equipment will need to be readily available. The baby will require constant observation. Great care must be taken when manoeuvring the incubator around corners and in and out of lifts.

Hospital layout and local practice will dictate whether further resuscitative measures need to be undertaken prior to transfer.

Transport between hospitals. This is a potentially hazardous exercise and should only be undertaken by personnel experienced in neonatal intensive care, normally a paediatrician and a neonatal nurse or midwife. Even in the UK, neonatal transport may be over long distances by road, sea or air in an ambulance, hovercraft, helicopter or aircraft which may be military or commercial. Prevailing weather conditions and terrain will also influence the journey. Plainly, these factors will necessitate adjustments both for the baby and his caretakers. Where complex travelling arrangements are involved, it is imperative that good communications are established to avoid any untoward events.

Both parents should be seen by the paediatrician and neonatal nurse or midwife and a full explanation given to them regarding the need for transfer and how they can contact and reach the receiving hospital. Many neonatal units now have parents' booklets giving details concerning visiting, neonatal care, contacts and support available. If possible the parents should be given a photograph of the baby before they are separated.

Prior to transport, the baby's condition should be physiologically stable. If necessary he is intubated and ventilated; blood gas analysis is performed, and any ventilatory adjustments made. Clinical decisions regarding the need for insertion of umbilical arterial catheter, chest drain or intravenous cannula must be made and implemented before transportation as these procedures are extremely difficult to perform in transit. Throughout transportation the baby should be kept warm and disturbed minimally. Continuous cardiac, temperature and transcutaneous pO_2 monitoring will assist in achieving this goal: constant observation and recording of vital signs will be mandatory. Anticipation of problems will enable swift and skilful intervention to take place.

Admission to Neonatal Intensive Care Unit

Admission to a neonatal intensive care unit should be for sound medical reasons only, though this will include the majority of preterm infants. Where admission is indicated, discussion with the parents should occur at the earliest opportunity. Good communication between the delivery suite and the neonatal unit is essential so that the neonatal unit staff have time for adequate preparation. This is especially important in the case of a preterm multiple birth.

On arrival in the neonatal unit, the baby is moved smoothly from the transport incubator onto nearby scales and thence to a pre-warmed incubator or infant care centre. The delivery suite midwife should ensure that all relevant details are given verbally and in writing to the neonatal nurse or midwife assigned to the baby's care.

Baseline observations of vital signs are performed together with a capillary blood glucose estimation and calculation of fluid requirements. An apnoea monitor will be used and other monitoring and supportive therapy is initiated as indicated. The parents are encouraged to visit the baby as soon as possible and are given clear explanations from both the nursing and medical staff regarding their baby's problems and the future management.

Control of environment
See also Chapters 32 and 36.

Temperature. With the advent of more efficient

and sophisticated incubators, the problems relating to temperature control have been reduced. Nonetheless, vigilant scrutiny of environmental temperature remains important in the management of the preterm and it is the responsibility of the nurse or midwife assigned to the care of the individual baby. For each baby, there is a range of environmental temperature in which energy losses and oxygen consumption required to maintain body temperature within normal limits will be minimal. This is known as the neutral thermal environment and charts are available showing these ranges for both clothed and naked infants.

Since the head constitutes a proportionately large amount of the total body surface of the preterm baby, it should be covered with a wool bonnet. Clothing the baby will reduce heat loss though this is inadvisable with sick infants since it precludes optimal observation.

For babies who are intubated and nursed under radiant heaters, a polythene sheet laid over the baby may be useful in reducing evaporative water and heat loss. For non-intubated babies or babies in incubators, insulating bubble wrap sheets may be used to reduce heat loss.

Although useful in reducing heat loss, humidification of incubators is currently the subject of controversy and many units do not use humidity because of the problem of bacterial infection in the water tank.

Great care should be exercised in adjusting the environmental temperature of a cold baby; the aim is to increase body temperature by not more than 1°C per hour. If an infant is febrile, the environment is monitored to ensure that his temperature rises no further: the baby must not be over-swaddled, the temperature of his incubator must not be too high nor must he be subjected to sunlight. Modifications of the environmental temperature are obviously necessary according to day and night external temperature differences and seasonal variations.

Prevention of infection. The single most important factor in the prevention of infection is **scrupulous, obsessional hand washing.** Since the forearm, up to the elbow, enters the baby's incubator porthole, it must be included in washing. Liquid cleansing agents such as iodine- or chlorhexidine-based scrub solutions can be used and the hands and arms dried thoroughly with soft disposable handtowels. The frequent use of hand-cream will prevent the skin from becoming dry and cracked. Hand washing should take place before and after attending to each infant and after 'dirty' procedures such as nappy changing. Judicious use of elbow taps, porthole catches and pedal bins will also help to minimise the spread if infection. Gloves should be worn when handling body secretions.

Staff or visitors with herpes simplex, upper respiratory tract infections, gastro-enteritis or septic lesions should not enter the neonatal unit until they have been adequately treated. There should be sufficient space available between babies to avoid overcrowding and babies admitted from postnatal wards or other hospitals should be isolated if possible.

Each baby should have all his own equipment which can be stored in cupboards under the incubator or cot. Particular attention should be afforded to items such as transcutaneous pO_2 monitors and fibre-optic lights to ensure that they are thoroughly cleansed after use.

Disposable items are used wherever possible: extra storage space and safe disposal systems are needed.

A neonatal unit and staff displaying the highest standards of hygiene imaginable demonstrate that the needs of preterm infants are understood.

Noise and disturbance. A modern neonatal intensive care unit frequently operates with high noise levels and this is a problem of continuing concern. The latest incubators function fairly smoothly and quietly but should any malfunction develop it must be attended to promptly. All other equipment is fitted with audible alarms but babies and staff benefit if these are turned down to a low volume. Special care should be taken in such activities as closing portholes or cupboard doors and in moving incubators so as not to jolt the baby unnecessarily.

In order to meet the need of the preterm baby for rest and sleep, procedures can be grouped together and intervals allowed between interruptions.

LIGHT-FOR-DATES BABIES

The term 'light for dates' refers to those babies whose birthweight falls below the 10th centile for their gestational age. The term equates to 'small for gestational age'. If the gestational age of a light-for-dates baby is less than 37 weeks then he is both light for dates and preterm.

Causes

Certain causes may have been present for the entire duration of the pregnancy whilst others are largely influential in the third trimester.

Parity
First babies are normally lighter than those born subsequently.

Maternal age
There is a tendency for a mother below the age of 20 or over 35 years to have lighter babies.

Social class
Women in social classes IV and V are more likely to have light-for-dates babies than those in the higher social classes. However, other factors such as nutrition, smoking or ethnic origin may influence this pattern.

Multiple pregnancy
This is a well-recognised factor in connection with growth retardation and in general terms the greater the number of babies per pregnancy the lighter they are.

Maternal disease in pregnancy
Any disorder where there is interference in the maternal blood supply to the placenta is likely to result in the baby being light for dates. Such disorders include pre-eclampsia, antepartum haemorrhage, hypertension and renal disease.

Ethnic origin
Certain ethnic groups such as Asians have a tendency to have much smaller babies than Caucasians, although nutrition may be a complicating factor. Nevertheless, it is important to allow for possible ethnic variations when assessing such groups of babies because many centile charts are devised from Caucasian populations.

Smoking
Maternal smoking results in high levels of carbon monoxide in the circulation which approximate with levels found in cord blood samples. Elevated fetal carbon monoxide levels may result in hypoxia due to reduced availability of haemoglobin for oxygen transport. It is possible that this fetal hypoxia is the cause of growth retardation although it has been suggested that nicotine-induced placental vasoconstriction may impede the transfer of oxygen and nutrients. There is clear evidence that smoking is a causal factor in intra-uterine growth retardation and may precipitate a preterm delivery (Lumley & Astbury 1989). Passive and paternal smoking have also been identified as hazardous to the fetus. Evidence that these babies suffer from increased respiratory ailments postnatally is growing.

Drug addiction
Hypoplastic fetal growth has been attributed to maternal heroin and morphine addiction although poor maternal nutrition is considered to be an additional factor.

Fetal causes
Babies who have acquired an intra-uterine infection such as cytomegalovirus are often found to be growth-retarded. There also seems to be a link between the presence of congenital abnormalities, particularly chromosomal defects, and growth retardation.

Appearance and neurological development

Light-for-dates babies fall roughly into two categories regarding their appearance. Some are in proportion but appear generally small: these are babies whose growth has been retarded throughout pregnancy. In this group there is the possibility that brain growth, which is most rapid during the second and third trimesters, may have been affected. Other babies appear long, thin and scrawny, with a disproportionately large head. They have a lack of subcutaneous fat but are usually quite active and vigorous. (See symmetric and asymmetric growth retardation, Ch. 41.)

Problems

Asphyxia

(See also Asphyxia in preterm babies, above.)
Growth-retarded babies may have been subjected to hypoxia for some time prior to labour. Because of their diminished physical resources they find it difficult to cope with the additional stresses of the birth process. Consequently, recovery from this arduous journey is often difficult and may be impossible without intervention.

Meconium aspiration

Light-for-dates babies are specifically at risk of meconium aspiration because they are frequently subjected to intra-uterine hypoxia. In response to such hypoxia there is relaxation of the anal sphincter and release of meconium into the amniotic fluid. The distressed baby then displays reflex gasping and meconium enters the upper respiratory tract. Further aspiration into the bronchioles may occur during and after birth. As a consequence, fragments of meconium inevitably block the airways in a haphazard fashion. During inspiration when the bronchioles dilate, air may pass around these fragments but on expiration, air is unable to escape because of the reduced diameter of the bronchioles and the tenacity of the meconium. This is referred to as the ball-valve mechanism and results in overdistension of the terminal airways. Meconium may also completely block the airway, resulting in atelectasis. Together with this problem of obstruction, the meconium initiates an inflammatory response in the airways known as chemical pneumonitis. Such inflammation causes thickening of the alveolar walls which reduces oxygen diffusion. These events inhibit dilation of the pulmonary vascular bed and produce a right-to-left shunt via the ductus arteriosus. Clinically, the baby will display respiratory distress with tachypnoea greater than 60 per minute, sternal and intercostal recession

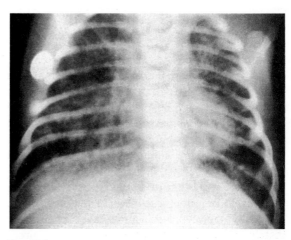

Fig. 35.9
Chest X-ray of meconium aspiration showing coarse nodular shadowing with linear shadowing radiating from the hilum. (Reproduced by permission of D. Lindsell, Consultant Radiologist, John Radcliffe Hospital, Oxford.)

with cyanosis is severe cases. Pneumothorax and pneumonia are common complications.

Hypoglycaemia

Light-for-dates babies are at significant risk of developing hypoglycaemia, principally because they have decreased hepatic glycogen stores and reduced subcutaneous fat stores which are quickly utilised. Hypoglycaemia in light-for-dates babies is often symptomatic. Jitteriness, apnoeic episodes, lethargy and poor feeding are the most common features. Untreated hypoglycaemia may cause brain damage, therefore prompt management is indicated (see also Ch. 38).

Infection

If meconium staining of the skin occurs, this poses a particular risk as it is an ideal medium for bacterial multiplication. Additionally, dry, cracked skin may assist the entry of pathological organisms thereby elevating the risk of systemic infection.

Temperature control

Because they have scant subcutaneous fat coupled with a large body surface area, light-for-dates babies find it difficult to conserve their body temperatures. (See also Ch. 31.)

Less common problems of light-for-dates babies

Polycythaemia

Polycythaemia is an increase in the haematocrit (packed cell volume) above 65% determined on a venous blood sample. Capillary samples may demonstrate an appreciably higher reading and are therefore inaccurate. When the haematocrit exceeds 65%, there is an increase in viscosity and blood flow becomes sluggish. In the light-for-dates baby intra-uterine hypoxia may initiate an increase in erythropoiesis causing polycythaemia. Clinically, polycythaemia may cause respiratory distress as cardiopulmonary function is impaired. Hyperbilirubinaemia may also result due to the increase in bilirubin from excessive breakdown of red blood cells.

Congenital abnormality

The incidence of congenital abnormality in the light-for-dates baby is significantly greater than in its appropriately grown counterpart. This is mainly due to cellular hypoplasia in early pregnancy. Such defects are usually manifest as chromosomal abnormalities, anencephaly and congenital heart disease.

Fetal alcohol syndrome

Although there is not a widely reported incidence of this problem in the UK it may become more extensive in the future. Fetal growth may be retarded due to maternal alcohol consumption. The baby of a chronic alcoholic mother may suffer acute withdrawal symptoms after birth. This is hardly surprising since alcohol reaches the baby in the same concentrations as those in maternal plasma. The baby quickly becomes agitated with hyperactivity and trembling. These features may continue for 2–3 days before gradually subsiding. Babies suffering from fetal alcohol syndrome commonly display dysmorphic features consisting of characteristic facial defects, hypoplastic development of the limbs and cardiac abnormalities. It is not clear to what extent these abnormalities relate to the amount of alcohol consumed or to the pattern of drinking. (See also Ch. 38.)

Twin-to-twin transfusion

In rare instances, there is an arteriovenous connection between the placental circulations of identical twins which results in blood passing from one baby into the other. The baby who has received the extra blood will be large and polycythaemic and will develop hyperbilirubinaemia. Cardiac overload may lead to congestive heart failure. In contrast, the other baby has suffered the blood loss and will be small, pale, anaemic and, if blood loss is severe, may be shocked.

Management

Labour and delivery

Resuscitation

Admission to Neonatal Intensive Care Unit

Control of environment

} See Preterm babies pages 567–571

Management of specific problems

Management of meconium aspiration

Meconium aspiration is life-threatening, therefore action is directed towards preventing meconium from entering the air passages. As soon as the head is born, meconium must be removed from the oropharynx and nostrils using a mucus extractor. Following separation from the mother, the baby's chest may be held to prevent gasping and a laryngoscope inserted which allows suction under direct vision. If it is apparent that meconium has been aspirated beyond the vocal cords, then an endotracheal tube is inserted. The resuscitator wears a double mask and applies mouth suction directly to the endotracheal tube. Whilst possibly indelicate, this is a highly efficient method of removing the thick, viscid plugs of meconium from the airways. In severe cases, the endotracheal tube will become blocked and require several replacements to ensure complete removal of all meconium.

Some centres use bronchial lavage. 1 ml normal saline is instilled down the endotracheal tube prior to suction and the procedure is repeated until the fluid is clear. When all meconium has been removed, oxygenation and ventilation are initiated and continued until respirations are established. Afterwards, the baby should be observed for signs of respiratory distress though this should not necessarily entail separation from the mother.

Hypoglycaemia

Hypoglycaemia is common in light-for-dates babies and therefore routine capillary blood glucose screening with test strips should commence at birth. Estimations should continue at 6-hourly intervals until the baby is 24 hours old then 12-hourly to 48 hours of age unless there is any reading below 2.5 mmol/ℓ in which case more frequent estimations will be required. Early and frequent feeding should be established within 1–2 hours of birth to avoid hypoglycaemia. If there is a capillary blood glucose estimation of 1.4 mmol/ℓ –2.5 mmol/ℓ, a feed should be given promptly and the estimation repeated 1 hour later. If the reading is again below 2.5 mmol/ℓ, medical advice should be sought without delay. In any instance where the recording is below 1.4 mmol/ℓ, medical aid must be summoned so that a laboratory estimation of blood sugar can be made. Where the blood sugar is below 1.4 mmol/ℓ or if symptoms are present, an intravenous infusion of dextrose 10% should be commenced preceded by a bolus dose of dextrose 20%. Very high concentrations of dextrose may overstimulate insulin production with a consequential rebound hypoglycaemia when the dextrose is discontinued. Capillary glucose monitoring is continued hourly until readings are 2.5 mmol/ℓ or above and subsequently 2-hourly, gradually decreasing the frequency as homeo-stasis is achieved. Oro- or nasogastric tube feeds or oral milk feeds should be gradually introduced. Once feeds are being absorbed adequately, intra-venous therapy can be reduced ensuring that the dextrose 10% is changed to dextrose 5% before discontinuation. Regular capillary glucose moni-toring should continue throughout this transition and after the intravenous therapy has been discontinued.

Twin-to-twin transfusion

If a large twin-to-twin transfusion has taken place, the polycythaemic twin may require a plasma exchange transfusion to reduce the haematocrit. Conversely, the small pale twin will need a blood transfusion to correct anaemia and restore blood volume to normal.

HEAVY-FOR-DATES BABIES

Definition

A heavy-for-dates baby is one whose intra-uterine growth has been excessive. His birthweight will be above the 90th centile and he is therefore termed 'large for gestational age'.

Causes

The principal cause of exaggerated intra-uterine growth is maternal diabetes mellitus or gestational diabetes. The macrosomia is considered to be due to maternal hyperglycaemia resulting in fetal hyperglycaemia which triggers off increased fetal insulin production. Hyperinsulinism in turn causes increased growth and fat deposition. The extent of the macrosomia will depend upon how well the maternal diabetes is controlled during pregnancy. Other causes of heavy-for-dates babies include the Beckwith-Wiedemann syndrome, an unusual disorder of uncertain aetiology and 'infant giants' who are infants of extremely high birth-weight in whom pancreatic hyperplasia has been described.

Appearance and relative maturity

Characteristically, the heavy-for-dates infant is large, fat and cherubic in appearance. However, many are also preterm and if so they adopt a splayed-out posture. Infants of diabetic mothers have a two- to threefold higher incidence of con-genital abnormality than their normal counter-parts. The features of the Beckwith-Wiedemann syndrome include the presence of an omphalocele, exomphalos or gastroschisis in conjunction with a large tongue (macroglossia) and enlarged kidneys and liver.

Problems

Hypoglycaemia

Where there has been prolonged fetal hyper-insulinism, islet cell activity will continue after birth. As a result, hypoglycaemia is very likely to occur because the maternal source of glucose has been lost.

Hyaline membrane disease

(See also Preterm babies, above.)
The infant of a diabetic mother suffers from delayed surfactant maturation and is at increased risk of developing hyaline membrane disease. In addition, some diabetic pregnancies are terminated at 36–37 weeks gestation or even earlier.

Polycythaemia

Babies of diabetic mothers are prone to polycythaemia and consequently jaundice. Occasionally plasma exchange transfusion may be needed.

Hypocalcaemia

Hypocalcaemia of late onset (5–10 days) is rare nowadays since the majority of artificial milk formulae have a calcium:phosphorus ratio closely matching that in human milk. (Excessive phosphorus in cow's milk prevents absorption of calcium.) Normal serum calcium levels are 1.75–2.25 mmol/ℓ. Early onset hypocalcaemia is seen in preterm infants, infants of diabetic mothers and asphyxiated babies. It is suggested that temporary hypoparathyroidism may be the cause. Generally, there are no specific symptoms and the calcium deficiency is only revealed on haematological investigation.

Infection

See Chapter 34 and also Preterm and Light-for-dates babies, above.

Management

Labour and delivery

If a large baby is expected it is important to verify that internal pelvic dimensions are adequate. If there is doubt a trial of labour may be planned or an elective caesarean section. If the former is chosen, careful fetal heart rate monitoring will be indicated and, if the mother has diabetes, blood sugar levels must be carefully controlled. A possible difficulty which may arise with a vaginal delivery is shoulder dystocia. This may be due to large fetal shoulders, small maternal pelvis or failure of the shoulders to rotate into the anteroposterior diameter of the pelvis. Immediate action is required in order to effect delivery before cord occlusion or placental separation or both result in irreversible asphyxia. Where such possibilities are foreseen it is judicious to call the paediatrician in time to prepare for resuscitation of the baby.

Prevention of hypoglycaemia

(See also Light-for-dates babies, above.)
Those infants of mothers whose diabetes has not been well controlled during pregnancy should be admitted to a neonatal unit for 24–48 hours to enable problems to be managed without delay. Hypoglycaemia is likely to arise very quickly after birth. Capillary blood glucose level should therefore be estimated on arrival and monitored at 2-hourly intervals. Early feeding should be initiated. Lin et al (1989) report that if the birthweight is more than 4000 g the baby is at high risk of developing asymptomatic hypoglycaemia within 4 hours.

Preconception counselling offers the best chance of preventing the congenital malformations which are problematic in infants of diabetic mothers. Good control achieved at this stage will be likely to be carried over through pregnancy and so reduce the risks to the infant. (See Chs 7 and 22.)

Hyaline membrane disease

See Chapter 36.

Hypocalcaemia

This is rectified by administering calcium supplements intravenously in the form of calcium gluconate 10% 1 mmol/kg in 24 hours which is added to the burette of the intravenous infusion. Continuous cardiac monitoring should be employed to detect any bradycardia. The site of the intravenous cannula needs careful observation as extravasation could cause tissue damage.

Once milk feeds are being absorbed supplements can be given orally. When the serum calcium levels have been restored to normal, the supplements can be discontinued.

Acknowledgement

Figures 35.1–35.4 are reproduced by permission of the author and publishers from Dubowitz L M S et al 1970 Clinical assessment of gestational age in the newborn infant. The Journal of Pediatrics 77(1): 1–10

Reader Activities

- Devise a teaching pack related to the cultural and religious groups encountered in your practice.
- Plan and implement a booklet for parents whose babies are in the neonatal unit.

REFERENCES

Anderson A, Turnbull A C 1982 Effect of oestrogens, progestogens and betamimetics in pregnancy. In: Enkin M, Chalmers I (eds) Effectiveness and satisfaction in antenatal care. Heinemann Medical, London, ch. 11, p 170–178

Ankett M A et al 1986 Treatment with iron increases weight and psychomotor development. Archives of Disease in Childhood 61: 849–857

Dubowitz L M S, Dubowitz V, Goldberg C 1970 Clinical assessment of gestational age in the newborn infant. Journal of Pediatrics 77(1): 1–10

Lin M S et al 1989 A five-year study of neonatal hypoglycaemia in Toa Payoh Hospital. Journal of the Singapore Paediatric Society 31(3–4): 116–121

Lumley J, Astbury J 1989 Advice for pregnancy In: Chalmers I, Enkin M, Keirse M J N C (eds) Effective care in pregnancy and childbirth. Oxford University Press, Oxford, ch 16, p 242–244

FURTHER READING

Avery G B (ed) 1987 Neonatology, pathophysiology and management of the newborn, 3rd edn. J B Lippincott, Philadelphia

Hill S 1990 Family. Viking Penguin, Harmondsworth

La Leche League 1983 Breast feeding your preterm baby. Information sheet No. 13 GB. LLL, London

Kelnar C J H, Harvey D 1987 The sick newborn baby. Baillière Tindall, London

Klaus M H, Fanaroff A A 1986 Care of the high risk neonate, 3rd edn. W B Saunders, Philadelphia

Korones S B 1986 High risk newborn infants, 4th edn. Mosby, St Louis

Midwives Information and Resource Service 1991 MIDIRS directory of maternity organisations. MIDIRS, Bristol

National Childbirth Trust 1983 Breast feeding if your baby needs special care. Leaflet No. 30. NCT, London.

Roberton N R C 1986 A manual of neonatal intensive care, 2nd edn. Edward Arnold, London

36

Intensive care of the newborn

ELIZABETH THOMSON
ELIZABETH TORLEY

PSYCHOLOGICAL EFFECTS OF ADMISSION TO THE NEONATAL INTENSIVE CARE UNIT

An era has now been entered in which the psychological needs of both baby and parents are increasingly the focus of attention. No longer is it acceptable merely to attend to physical needs. Proper emphasis must be afforded to mental and spiritual needs so that they become an integral part of total care.

Special and intensive care of the newborn

The admission of a baby to a neonatal intensive care or special care baby unit (NICU/SCBU) is a situation fraught with tension and anxiety for parents. As 2% of all live births at present need the specialist care offered by a NICU/SCBU this is obviously an area which merits close appraisal of the services offered.

Many factors impinge on the quality of care in a NICU/SCBU. Cultural factors can easily be misunderstood and lead to additional stress for a family, whilst the mental adjustment required may overwhelm the coping mechanisms of even the most robust family. The midwife requires not only to be competent in the physical aspects of care but also skilled in counselling, in order to cope with psychological, spiritual and cultural needs as they arise. It is also salutory to remember that the substantial emotional investment, which characterises the caring professions, is nowhere more manifest than in a NICU/SCBU. The vulnerability of staff in these situations has been demonstrated by research. Studies, particularly those relating to burnout and stress, should be perused and acted upon by all caregivers in NICU/SCBU settings.

The baby

The transfer from the well-protected, warm and passive sojourn in the uterus to the noisy, vulnerable exposure of extra-uterine existence is a difficult enough adaptation. The feeling of naked helplessness, dyspnoea and exhaustion, whilst tubes, catheters and cannulae are inserted into orifices and blood vessels with simultaneous prodding and poking of anatomical components is even more devastating. Nevertheless, neonates are extraordinarily versatile and resilient and this somewhat traumatic entrance into the world appears to have few long-term effects. Whilst in the uterus, the fetus has been accustomed to the maternal heart beat and rush of circulating blood, gastrointestinal activity and breathing, amniotic fluid movement and external noises. He has also been familiar with the maternal diurnal rhythm which possibly provides some guide for his own activity. The stimuli he receives in the neonatal unit are quite different. He is lying on a firm base, listening to the constant purr of the incubator punctuated by the intermittent alarms of the monitoring equipment. It is no longer dark for the environment is constantly illuminated.

Regularly, throughout the day, a succession of caretakers will attend to physical needs, touching, stroking and talking in high pitched tones. These interventions may be punctuated by painful stimuli such as heel pricks for blood sampling which are unpleasant. Even worse are the invasive procedures, necessary to sustain life, but nevertheless provoking considerable pain. Despite the increasing use of analgesia in neonatal care, it is difficult for the perceptions of the carer to match the actuality of the infant's pain. Therefore it is therapeutic for carers to gently stroke, comfort and, if possible, cuddle a baby to provide positivity following painful stimuli.

Sleep is intermittent and, although the preterm infant will attempt to spend a substantial part of the day in this state, it will be disordered by interventions. Full-term babies who are sick will have increased sleep needs and be resentful of disturbances. Maximising the time available for rest and sleep can be achieved by prudent grouping of interruptions.

Premature departure from the uterus signals the need for external warmth and protectiveness. The thermal and comfort properties of sheepskins and, more recently, heated water-filled mattresses have been demonstrated (Sarman et al 1989). Clothing can be worn in the recovery phase to minimise physical isolation.

The parents

The problems which face parents today are compounded by a heightened awareness of the achievements of neonatal intensive care together with an increase in public expectation. Perinatal mortality in the United Kingdom has improved so significantly that it is now much less than a third of the figure of 30 years ago and in some centres it is as low as 5.0 per thousand total births. The decline in perinatal mortality, however laudable, has cultivated a decreased recognition of the possibility of death. Furthermore, with improved techniques and management, the frontiers of viability have been pushed back to around 22 weeks' gestation and there is an ever-increasing population of babies emerging into society who were theoretically nonviable. Media coverage of these accomplishments raises expectations so substantially that many parents appear to believe, quite literally, that miracles can happen. In fact apparent miracles do occur occasionally but, more commonly, a great deal of realism has to be imparted.

Shock and numbness are amongst the first feelings to be experienced. Parents who have anticipated a sick or preterm baby as a pregnancy outcome may not endure the same intensity of feeling as those who have not shared that anticipation. Considerably more intense feelings may be experienced by parents whose baby was at the bedside initially but was precipitated into the neonatal unit by sudden deterioration. There is usually a period of mourning for the baby they perceived, pink, healthy and well grown, and until this is complete they cannot attach to the real baby who may be quite the opposite in appearance. Rejection of the real baby may also be felt because he is not the baby they had foreseen.

Feelings of guilt may also be borne (Was it their fault? Do they have some physical inadequacy? Are they being punished?). Fathers, particularly, may feel very angry and upset because they imagine the event to be an insult to their masculinity.

An additional burden is imposed by separation from the baby, a burden which may be the result of a reduced timespan in the uterus and which may be the harder because parents have a natural urge to be physically close to their child when he is ill. To add to their distress, they then find that their role as parents is usurped by a team of surrogate mothers and fathers who take care of their baby with almost alarming efficiency. The sight of their baby connected to numerous tubes and wires, surrounded by complex, sophisticated equipment with puzzling visual displays which emit alarm signals, can be extremely frightening to the uninitiated. During this most critical phase they are probably unable to hold their baby in their arms and this contributes to the remoteness and distance in the relationship. Some parents may find this crisis all but impossible to handle and they may not even attempt to attach to the baby for fear of further hurt if he dies.

Such difficulties may be manifest by infrequent visiting or overt lack of interest in the baby. Conversely, they may appear abnormally cheerful and casual, giving the impression that they are coping well.

Strategies for mitigating untoward effects

Until quite recently professional education was astonishingly devoid of emphasis on the importance of interpersonal skills in providing a supportive, sympathetic and empathetic response to family crises. Fortunately there is now a considerable amount of published literature, much written by parents themselves, describing the depth of their reactions and how they can best be supported. Disbelief, desperation, obsession with and fear of technology, unreality, guilt, self-blame, sadness and loss are some of the feelings described by parents who have had a baby being cared for in a NICU (Thompson 1990, Hill 1990).

One of the most important elements of this support occurs soon after birth. Whenever possible, and there are very few instances where it is *impossible*, the parents need to hold the baby in their arms. This is feasible even when the baby requires intubation and intermittent positive pressure ventilation. Subsequently the encouragement of physical contact (holding the baby's hand, touching and stroking the baby) will assist in the developing relationship. Parents also need to be persuaded to talk to their baby, although at first they may feel this is rather irrelevant.

A photograph of the baby serves as a positive and definite reminder at the mother's bedside. Parents can also be encouraged to take their own photographs of the baby, gradually building up an album of his progress. A booklet, briefly outlining the aims of care within the neonatal unit can be helpful in strengthening but not replacing the information given by staff on a regular daily basis. More detailed discussions and explanations from a consultant neonatal paediatrician will be necessary at intervals. The general tone of such interactions should be one of cautious optimism, giving frank and truthful information in small quantities. Parents experiencing such emotional turmoil have limited ability to assimilate factual material and there is often a need for repetition.

Unlimited visiting for parents, grandparents and siblings will help to reduce the anguish of separation. When parents phone the neonatal unit, whenever practicable, they should be able to talk personally to the midwife caring for their baby.

Involvement in the care of their baby is also beneficial in helping parents to channel their feelings. Most will be delighted to change the baby's nappy, perform mouth care or give a tube feed. Many parents also like to bring some small toys which can be kept inside the incubator. Some mothers like to make or buy special clothes for the baby which will contribute to reinforcing his identity.

Parents may wish to be resident in the hospital if their baby is seriously ill. Some units provide self-contained accommodation and it is more restful if such facilities are not in close proximity to a hot, stressful, noisy nursery.

Access to a social worker is also a priority as a multitude of unforeseen problems can be raised by an untimely birth or an unexpected serious illness. A health visitor who is familiar with the technology currently used in neonatal units and who understands the improved prognosis for these babies can also be very supportive (Stewart 1989). Likewise, where available, support groups can assist parents in coming to terms with their bewilderment. The organisation BLISS (Baby Life Support Systems) offers an information pack for those wishing to set up a parent support group.

Whatever the outcome, the impact of the experiences within a neonatal unit is likely to remain with the parents for the rest of their lives. It is for this reason that staff should diligently endeavour to make those experiences as positive and helpful as possible, even through the endurance of many critical periods. Overall, it is important to recognise that in many instances supporting the parents can be far more demanding of energy and emotionally harrowing than is caring for the baby.

INCUBATORS AND SPECIALISED EQUIPMENT

The use of incubators and other specalised equipment in neonatal units calls for a high degree of knowledge and skill. Such equipment is an adjunct to good nursing not a substitute for it. Midwives must be fully conversant with the functioning of all equipment before attempting to use it for the care of neonates. It is useful to keep a folder or file containing the manufacturer's operating manual for each piece of equipment in current use. This can be enhanced by specialist input from the unit technician or from representatives of equipment manufacturers. Anxiety and distress may be heightened if parents sense that staff are unsure of how equipment functions.

Incubators

Most babies who are preterm and those who are sick or cold will need to be nursed in an incubator at least initially. Modern incubators are highly developed technologically, incorporating accurate temperature controls with inbuilt alarm systems whilst providing good observation and accessibility.

The most common model in current use is the type shown in Figure 36.1. This incubator provides two different modes of operation. Firstly, there is the air mode whereby the air is warmed by a heating coil in the base and then circulated continuously within the perspex canopy by a fan. The heat is regulated by the digital controls set in 'A' mode at the desired environmental temperature on the operating panel. An audible alarm will operate if the air temperature exceeds 39°C, if the fan fails, if there is a fault in the probe or air temperature sensor, if there is electrical malfunction or if there is a power failure. Secondly, there is the baby mode in which warmed air is cir-

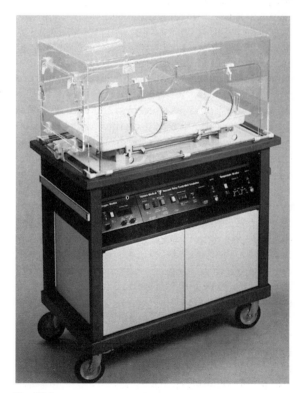

Fig. 36.1
Vickers Neocare incubator. (Reproduced by permission of Vickers Medical, Basingstoke.)

culated within the incubator in the manner just described but the controlling system is different. A temperature probe connected to the temperature monitor on the operating panel is taped to the baby's skin, usually on the lower abdomen. The digital controls are set to 'B' mode at the desired baby skin temperature. The heating system then warms the air until the set baby skin temperature is achieved. Should the baby skin temperature exceed the pre-set temperature, then the heating is reduced until the skin temperature adjusts to the pre-set level. Obviously, it is important to check that the skin probe does not become wet or detached or that the baby is not lying on the probe. An alarm will operate as in the 'A' mode setting.

The baby mode setting is sometimes preferred if the baby needs a high ambient temperature which the air mode cannot achieve. The major disadvantage is that it may mask a pyrexia. For detailed guidance the manufacturer's operating manual should be consulted.

For babies requiring intensive care, the extremely useful intensive care centre can be used (Fig. 36.2). This facilitates easy access to the baby during the most critical phase of illness whilst providing continuous, effective temperature regulation via an overhead radiant heater. The temperature probe inserted into the central panel is attached to the baby's abdomen with a special disc which protects the probe from external heat. The target baby skin temperature is set on the digital controls on the vertical operating panel. This must not be more than 0.5°C above or below the measured skin temperature at the time of setting. The overhead heater emits heat until the desired skin temperature is reached. When the baby skin temperature exceeds the pre-set level, the overhead heating is reduced, allowing the baby to cool. Again it is important to check that the skin probe does not become detached or wet or overlaid by the baby. An audible alarm system is incorporated which sounds when the baby skin temperature exceeds or falls below the pre-set level by 0.5°C. Alarms are also provided for probe and power failures.

A major advantage of the infant care centre is that it permits attention to very sick babies, for

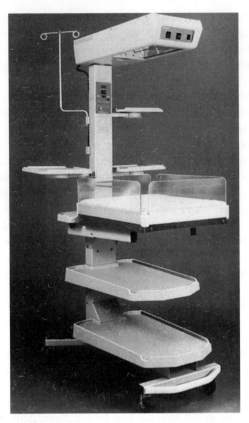

Fig. 36.2
Air Shields Infant Care Centre. (Reproduced by permission of V. A. Howe & Company Ltd, London.)

example during intubation, insertion of an umbilical arterial catheter and an intravenous cannula under maintained heating and without impairment of vision and access. Another asset of the infant care centre is that it allows unobstructed, close physical contact for the parents of the baby who is critically ill. Clearly this is vitally important at a time when their feelings towards the baby may be ambivalent and disordered.

The main disadvantage of the infant care centre is that the radiant heater causes significant insensible water loss. This may be overcome in part by placing a layer of clear plastic sheeting (intubated babies only) or bubble wrap (non-intubated babies) over the baby but fluid supplementation is also necessary (see nutritional needs). Another important factor to be borne in mind when infant care centres are used is that because of the intense heat generated, the carers themselves may become fluid-depleted. It is important that they recognise this possibility and ready access to fluid supplements will be essential.

Specialised equipment

Perspex heat shield. When working with incubators that do not have double walls, a perspex heat shield with one end closed can be used to reduce convective and radiative heat loss in babies. Care is needed to ensure that the baby's hands and feet do not become trapped under the edge of the perspex. Very small babies need additional observation as they have a tendency to wriggle down inside the shield. The head should always be outside the shield to avoid the possibility of hypoxia.

Perspex headbox. For babies requiring supplemental oxygen a perspex headbox can be used to maintain a stable concentration. These can be made in different sizes to accommodate large or small babies. Care should be taken to ensure that there is sufficient space around the neck in order to allow movement. Tubing from piped oxygen and air supplies is fitted onto the connection which is usually in a corner of the box. The oxygen and air mixture should be warmed and humidified to avoid unnecessary cooling of the head and evaporative heat loss from the airways. A thermometer or tempature probe is placed inside the headbox to enable hourly temperature recordings. A sufficient flow of gas is needed to provide adequate oxygenation and the individual volumes of oxygen and air have to be regulated accordingly.

Oxygen analyser. Any baby receiving oxygen therapy must have the oxygen concentration measured continuously and written recordings made every hour. Various models are available but all incorporate a sensor probe which is placed inside the headbox or incubator and connected to the monitor. Most operate on batteries which need to be checked regularly. The actual oxygen concentration inside the headbox or incubator is shown on the monitor either by a needle dial or digital display. Such monitors are delicate and sensitive in function and therefore require calibration at least once daily. Many analysers have inbuilt alarm limits which can be set: these are usually 5%

above and 5% below the desired concentration so that if these parameters are exceeded, an audible alarm will sound.

Apnoea monitor. This is an invaluable aid in the management of sick babies and should be used for all babies with respiratory problems, those requiring phototherapy, babies with infections or convulsions and in any other baby in whom there is a physiological disturbance. Basically there are two types, one which uses a pressure-sensitive pad and one with a sensor probe. The first kind consists of a sensor pad which is placed underneath the sheet and connected to a monitor which may function either from a battery or mains electricity. Each time the baby makes a respiratory movement, a light flashes on the monitor. There is also an alarm system which can be set for 10, 15 or 20 seconds. If there is no breathing within this time-span, the alarm will sound and a red light will be displayed on the monitor. After attending to the baby, the alarm is re-set. False alarms may be activated if the baby slips off the mattress or if the breathing is very shallow. The second type of apnoea alarm uses a probe which is taped to the baby's chest and is connected to a monitor which will sound an alarm if the baby is apnoeic beyond the pre-set time limits.

Tubing support. For babies receiving assisted ventilation, it is essential that the ventilator tubing is adequately supported and does not drag on the endotracheal tube. Various designs of tubing support are in use. Care must be taken to reposition the tubing each time the baby's position is changed.

Transcutaneous blood gas monitor. Transcutaneous monitors are now widely used in neonatal units for babies receiving supplemental oxygen therapy or in those whose blood gas status is dubious. Transcutaneous oxygen monitors have been used for many years and more recently transcutaneous carbon dioxide monitors have become available. The combined oxygen and carbon dioxide probes provide a non-invasive method of monitoring capillary pO_2 and pCO_2, and give a prompt indication of changes on a digital display and printed sheet. Following calibration, the probe is carefully applied to the baby's skin which is subsequently heated, normally to a temperature of 44°C. Heating of the skin dilates the capillaries and enables measurements of pO_2 and pCO_2 to be made transcutaneously via the probe mechanism. The audible and visual alarms can be adjusted to pre-set high and low limits so that deviations from normal are quickly noted and action taken. It is extremely important to change the probe site every 4 hours otherwise burns may result.

Transcutaneous monitoring is very dependent upon the quality of peripheral circulation and this factor needs to be constantly borne in mind in relation to the readings displayed. In babies who have poor peripheral circulation or a fluctuating status, precise results may not be achieved. Over-reliance on transcutaneous monitoring as an accurate reflection of blood gas status can be dangerous and arterial sampling should be employed for additional verification.

Pulse oximeters. Pulse oximeters provide continuous, non-invasive measurement of arterial oxygen saturation (SaO_2) and pulse rate by measuring the absorption of selected wavelengths of light. Oxygenated haemoglobin and reduced haemoglobin differ in their absorption of light. (Arterial blood high in O_2 saturation is red, venous blood low in O_2 saturation is blue.)

Pulse oximeters measure the absorption of red light. The light generated in the probe is converted into an electronic signal by a *photodetector*. The pulse oximeter consists of a probe, a central control processing unit and a display unit with high and low SaO_2 and pulse alarms.

Application procedure:

1. It is important to select a site that will allow the detector to be secured over a fleshy area. A foot, a finger or an ear lobe may be used in a neonate.

2. The probe must be carefully positioned so that the circulation is not restricted. It should be resited at least every 4 hours in order to avoid skin damage.

Special points to note:

1. Movement may cause large variations in photodetector signals. Careful and secure fixation of the probe is crucial to good recordings.

2. Intense light may also affect photodetector signals and the probe may have to be shielded from overhead heating and phototherapy lights.

Phototherapy (see also Ch. 34). Phototherapy units are commonly used in the management of jaundice in the newborn. Two types are currently used in neonatal units. The first is an independent unit which fits over the top of a conventional incubator. The second type consists of two separate units, one fitted to each side of the radiant heater of an infant care centre. Special precautions necessary when using phototherapy include placing the baby on an apnoea monitor and applying protection over the eyes. Constant observation of the baby's activities is also necessary to ensure that the eye protection does not occlude the nasal passages.

Cardiac monitor. Very many different models are in use, some of which also have facilities for monitoring respiration, blood pressure and blood gases. All sick babies and those whose condition is likely to fluctuate should have cardiac function monitored. When applying cardiac leads to babies, especially very tiny ones, it is vital to place the electrodes laterally on the chest wall so that they do not occlude important landmarks when X-rays are taken. The high and low alarm limits must be carefully set so that the audible and visual alarms will be activated when the heart rate is outside the normal range.

Blood pressure monitor. Comparatively few babies require regular or continuous blood pressure monitoring; nevertheless it is an important parameter to measure in specific neonates. These babies include those with arterial lines in situ and those who are exceedingly sick, for example following a pre- or postnatal haemorrhage. It is quite impossible to obtain accurate blood pressure recordings in babies using a sphygmomanometer. There are several automatic digital blood pressure monitors available which use infrasonic sound waves as a method of pulse detection. A special transducer is placed over the brachial artery and a neonatal cuff applied to secure it in position. The cuff is inflated and deflated automatically, following a specific press-button sequence, and the systolic and diastolic pressures are displayed visually.

More accurate measurements of blood pressure are achieved directly via an arterial line which is connected to a transducer and blood pressure monitor giving a continuous wave form pattern and a digital readout of systolic, diastolic and mean pressures.

Intravenous monitor and perfusor pump. If a baby requires intravenous fluids, this therapy must only be delivered via an electronic infusion monitor with a paediatric burette or a perfusor pump. This avoids the possibility of over-infusion which could be catastrophic. Perfusor pumps may also be used for intravenous blood administration, for perfusion of intra-arterial lines and for perfusion of milk feeds via orogastric or nasogastric feeding tubes. Meticulous care is necessary to ensure that there are no air bubbles in the system and that all connections are tight. Accurate calculation of fluid requirement is essential so that the correct amount is delivered hourly using the digital switches on the monitor or pump. An audible and visual alarm will be activated when the fluid volume is completed or if there is an equipment malfunction. This does not preclude the need for vigilant observation to ensure that there is no leakage, disconnection, blockage or extravasation of fluid.

Care of incubators and specialised equipment

All equipment should be used with great care especially when moving it around a neonatal unit. Jolting and collisions are not conducive to optimal functioning. Small but heavy items such as cardiac monitors should always be transported on trolleys in order to eliminate the possibility of back injuries. Since the majority of equipment functions from mains electricity, the plugs need to be placed logically, avoiding entanglement and in a manner unlikely to jeopardise others' safety at floor level.

Any piece of equipment found to be malfunctioning must be taken out of use immediately. It is highly beneficial to engage a unit technician who can repair faulty equipment quickly. An additional advantage is that he can keep detailed records of each piece of equipment, noting when repairs are completed, spare parts fitted and servicing due.

Following use, all equipment no longer required by an individual baby should be removed for thorough cleaning in accordance with local hospital policy, infection control guidelines and the manufacturer's instructions. Where possible, non-nursing staff specifically trained to clean, sterilise and maintain this equipment should be employed.

NURSING A BABY IN AN INCUBATOR OR INFANT CARE CENTRE

Nursing a baby in an incubator or infant care centre is often an exceedingly complex undertaking which requires careful thought and planning. Sick babies do not tolerate handling well and should only be disturbed minimally. Unfortunately, because they are sick, many interventions are often necessary to sustain their existence. Wherever possible these should be grouped together so that the baby is allowed intervals for recovery, rest and sleep. The midwife is in constant attendance throughout the 24-hour period and is in the unique position of always having first-hand knowledge of the individual baby's status. It is her responsibility as the baby's guardian to regulate interventions carefully so that the baby does not become unduly physiologically compromised.

Nursing should follow a problem-orientated approach to the management of the individual baby and his parents. The family should be considered in a holistic manner whereby their physical, mental and spiritual needs are perceived as inseparable, interrelated and interdependent. Following are guidelines for the needs of sick babies grouped under specific headings though it should be stressed that many of these needs and their management are interconnected and they should not be seen as separate entities divorced from one another.

Respiratory needs

In order to determine respiratory needs, an accurate hourly assessment of the neonate is made. The characteristics of the chest shape are noted, for instance overinflated, concave, or with symmetry of right and left sides. The colour of the baby and any colour change are observed. The rate and regularity of respiration are also noted together with breath sounds on auscultation, e.g.

unequal air entry, diminished sounds or wheezing. Depending on these findings, the need for suction can be determined. In all babies with breathing difficulties, gentle suction of the oropharynx and oral cavity will remove secretions. It is important to remember that suction removes air from the lungs and this may contribute to hypoxia.

Babies receiving oxygen-enriched air will need an assessment of the oxygen concentration, humidity, temperature and mode of administration. If a baby is ventilated a record must be made of the size of endotracheal tube, ventilator type, mode of ventilation and settings of positive end expiratory pressure, mean airways pressure, rate and inspiratory:expiratory ratio.

In addition to keeping records there is a need for constant vigilance in order to detect deviations from expected observations. Careful account is taken of all information when deciding upon appropriate intervention.

The most suitable position for nursing babies with respiratory problems is usually supine, alternating to the left and right sides. The tray of the incubator is slightly tilted upwards at the head end in order to prevent abdominal organs from pressing on the diaghragm. A small neck roll can be inserted to help maintain alignment of the airway.

Apnoea and bradycardia. Apnoea and bradycardia are very common problems in sick newborn babies and for the most part are managed by midwives or nurses. All sick babies should have continuous respiratory and cardiac monitoring which will promptly detect deviations from the normal. If an apnoeic or bradycardic episode occurs without spontaneous recovery, gentle stimulation may restore the respiratory and cardiac pattern. If there is little or no response, IPPV via a facemask with a hand resuscitator must be initiated (see Ch. 35). Most infants will recover within a short period. It is important that the stomach is emptied beforehand in order to avoid overdistension which may result in aspiration. Suction to the mouth and oropharynx may also be necessary. If there is no response to these measures, medical assistance must be sought and preparation made for intubation and continuous ventilation.

Special charts can be used to plot the incidence of apnoea and bradycardia so that a daily profile of episodes can be evaluated (Fig. 36.3).

Respiratory support

One of the factors that has contributed to increased survival in preterm infants has been the ability to offer ventilatory support. While general signs of respiratory distress such as expiratory grunting, increased work of breathing, decreased breath sounds, tachypnoea, bradycardia or apnoea suggest respiratory failure, the diagnosis is usually made by blood gas analysis which indicates an inability to achieve adequate oxygenation and/or carbon dioxide excretion. Respiratory failure in infants usually occurs as a result of one of the following:

- poor respiratory drive (due to birth asphyxia, extreme prematurity, surgery)
- abnormality of the lungs resulting in poor alveolar exchange (due to respiratory distress syndrome, pulmonary oedema)
- insufficient alveolar area for gas exchange (meconium aspiration, diaphragmatic hernia).

Modes of ventilation

Intermittent positive pressure ventilation (IPPV). This is administered as regularly timed breaths by a mechanical ventilator or inflation bag. The aim is to achieve synchronous respiration so that the baby is not fighting the ventilator, though spontaneous breaths may occur between cycles. Rates vary between 20 and 60 breaths per minute. The peak pressure used should be kept as low as possible but in exceptional instances may be as high as 40 cm H_2O. A base pressure is always used with babies, normally up to 5 cm H_2O, and is referred to as PEEP (positive end expiratory pressure). IPPV is used in any serious respiratory disease where spontaneous respiration does not provide adequate oxygenation.

Negative pressure ventilation. The infant is nursed in an airtight chamber, sealed around the neck, from which air is intermittently extracted, thus allowing chest expansion and air entry to the lungs. Although negative pressure ventilators provide the most physiologically sound method of

DATE OF BIRTH

DATE

DAY OF LIFE

NAME																							
HOUR	00/01	01/02	02/03	03/04	04/05	05/06	06/07	07/08	08/09	09/10	10/11	11/12	12/13	13/14	14/15	15/16	16/17	17/18	18/19	19/20	20/21	21/22	22/23	23/24
INDICATE ANY CHANGES IN THERAPY																								
TOTAL NUMBER OF BRADYCARDIAS																								
TOTAL NUMBER OF APNOEAS																								
0 - 5 mins																								
5 - 10 mins																								
10 - 15 mins																								
15 - 20 mins																								
20 - 25 mins																								
25 - 30 mins																								
30 - 35 mins																								
35 - 40 mins																								
40 - 45 mins																								
45 - 50 mins																								
50 - 55 mins																								
55 - 60 mins																								

Apnoea - not requiring stimulation - mark with blue dot.

Apnoea - requiring stimulation - mark with blue S (no dot)

Apnoea - requiring Penlon - mark with blue P (no dot)

Bradycardia - under 100 not requiring stimulation - mark with red dot.

Bradycardia - requiring stimulation - mark with red S (no dot)

Bradycardia - requiring Penlon - mark with red P (no dot)

Fig. 36.3
Apnoea and bradycardia chart. (Reproduced by permission of Andrew Wilkinson, Consultant Neonatal Paediatrician, John Radcliffe Hospital, Oxford.)

ventilation, since they require no artificial airway, they have not been popular. Since the mid-1980s, however, there has been increased interest in their use and multicentre randomised controlled trials have been initiated in order to compare their effectiveness with that of other current methods of respiratory support.

Intermittent mandatory ventilation (IMV). This is a mode whereby regularly timed breaths are delivered via a ventilator at a rate which allows for independent, spontaneous breathing by the baby between puffs. The rates used are usually between 5 and 18 per minute with a peak pressure below 25 cm H_2O. IMV is used in the process of weaning off the ventilator after a period of IPPV.

Continuous positive airways pressure (CPAP). In this mode, the baby breathes independently but a continuous distending pressure is exerted on the airways preventing alveolar collapse at the end of expiration. Normally, pressures up to 5 cm of water (H_2O) are used. CPAP is used mainly as the baby is weaned off the ventilator following a period of IPPV.

Ventilators in use

The ventilatory needs of sick babies are quite different from those of older children or adults. For this reason the only ventilators that should be used for neonates are those specially designed for the purpose. At present IPPV is used almost exclusively. A suitable model should be selected which meets safety standards. The ventilator needs a humidifier which will warm and moisten the gas and it should provide the facility for continuous gas flow to prevent the rebreathing of expired gases.

Ventilators may be *volume-controlled*, when a fixed volume of gas (oxygen and air) is delivered, or *pressure-controlled*, when a maximum pressure is delivered, in each inspiratory phase. Most neonatologists favour pressure-controlled ventilators. These may be either *pressure-cycled*, when inspiration ends as soon as a pre-set pressure is attained, or *time-cycled*, when once the pre-set pressure is reached it is maintained until a determined inspiratory duration is completed. Time-cycling allows maximum gaseous exchange in the infant with stiff lungs. A time-cycled, pressure-controlled

ventilator has been developed which is valveless and uses an air jet to provide the driving force. This air jet does not take part in the gaseous exchange. As yet it remains to be fully evaluated but would appear to represent an important advance in the management of infants with severe respiratory distress.

Complications of ventilation

Endotracheal tube obstruction or displacement. A blocked endotracheal tube can cause life-threatening airway obstruction. It is essential that the ventilation gases are adequately warmed and humidifed and that regular suctioning of the endotracheal tube is carried out. Endotracheal aspiration is a skilled procedure and should be carried out in accordance with local policy. Throughout the procedure the infant's heart rate and colour should be monitored closely. Both transcutaneous oxygen monitors and oxygen saturation monitors will give useful information about the effect of aspiration on the infant's oxygenation and can be valuable aids in teaching good technique.

Accidental extubation is another life-threatening complication. Regular inspection should be made of tube fixation and unstable tubes retaped at once. Equipment for re-intubation should be readily available and the size of each baby's endotracheal tube displayed prominently at the cotside.

Occasionally the tube may become displaced into the right main bronchus with consequent loss of air entry on the left side and an increase in ventilatory pressure. This may be rectified by withdrawing the tube about 1 cm and securing it firmly.

Air leaks. These are a fairly common and potentially serious complication of ventilation. They result from alveolar rupture with subsequent accumulation and retention of air. Frequently, air is released into the pleural space causing a pneumothorax. Rapid deterioration of the baby may follow with cyanosis and unequal chest movement being noticed. This can often be detected quickly by using a fibre-optic cold light to transilluminate the chest and by later confirmation with an X-ray (Fig. 36.4). When severe, an underwater seal chest

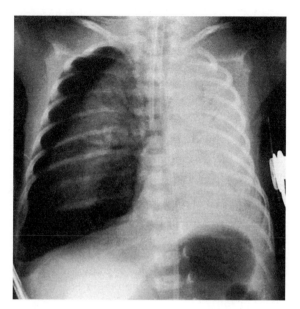

Fig. 36.4
Chest X-ray of baby with hyaline membrane disease showing air bronchogram and severe right-sided pneumothorax. (Reproduced by permission of D. Lindsell, Consultant Radiologist, John Radcliffe Hospital, Oxford.)

drain should be inserted without delay. If the drain is correctly placed, improvement is immediate.

Pneumonia. Although pneumonia can be acquired antenatally, it may develop during mechanical ventilation for several reasons. The sick preterm baby is already immunocompromised and the presence of an endotracheal tube bypasses the normal protective mechanisms in the respiratory tract. The risk of infection is increased by artificially warmed and moistened gases being delivered to the airways via a foreign body. Gram-negative organisms such as pseudomonas thrive in such a medium. If an infective process does ensue, antibiotic therapy will be required.

Cardiovascular needs

These are assessed by ascertaining the heart rate, rhythm and position of the greatest intensity of sound. Note is also taken of the baby's colour which may not always be uniform or constant. Babies requiring intensive or high-dependency care will have continuous cardiac monitoring with pre-set alarm limits of below 100 or above 180 beats per minute. Such monitoring requires regular observation so that deviation from the normal and reactions to interventions are noticed promptly. If the alarm signals, a correct assessment and clinical decision will be required. It is important to ensure that electrodes are placed securely, usually one placed laterally on each side of the chest, so as not to obscure the anteroposterior vision of the chest for X-rays, and one on a leg. Difficulties may arise in securing electrodes on extremely low birth-weight babies because of the shortage of smooth, flat surfaces for application. Certain neonatal cardiac monitors have the ability to monitor respirations simultaneously.

In sick babies, regular observation of blood pressure is essential either by using an infrasonic blood pressure monitor or directly via an arterial line. Specific norms of blood pressure in neonates are difficult to assess as they vary with gestation and age. Important to notice are differences, sometimes subtle, sometimes sudden, which are indicative of internal haemorrhage (e.g. periventricular haemorrhage) which may reduce circulating blood volume considerably.

Maintenance of correct blood volume is vital to the neonate; it is not always recognised that a blood loss which would be trivial to an adult may be major to a neonate. The circulating blood volume of a baby weighing 1000 g is only 85 ml. It follows therefore that such small amounts must be sustained and any significant subtraction replaced. Extreme care is required in obtaining blood samples by only extracting the absolute minimum and avoiding any leakage. Additionally, in babies who have intravenous or intra-arterial lines, a watchful eye is necessary to detect possible haemorrhage from loose connections. Top-up blood transfusions are a fairly regular requirement in babies who are critically ill and the utmost accuracy is essential in order that the exact amount of blood is transfused. Whilst reactions to blood transfusions are rare in babies, it is crucial that the circulation is not overloaded. Likewise, all fluid intake requires diligent calculation and administration to avoid compromising the cardiovascular system.

Thermoregulatory needs
(see also Ch. 35)

The midwife is potentially the most influential and instrumental member of the clinical team in meeting the thermoregulatory needs of the neonate. Sick newborn babies are at an even greater risk of heat loss, due in part to the many interventions which they have to withstand in relation to their physical nurture.

The ideal temperatures in which to nurse infants of differing birthweights have been identified and appropriate charts should be referred to when setting temperature controls on incubators. Some babies will have an abdominal temperature probe for servo-control of the incubator temperature. Where this is not required axillary temperature will be taken regularly according to the baby's individual needs. The thermometer must remain in the axilla for a full 5 minutes in order to obtain a true reading (Earnshaw 1978). Rectal temperature, although nearer to the core temperature, is not now taken because there is a risk of trauma and it is distressing for the baby (Earnshaw 1978). Peripheral temperature, for example of the big toe, is useful in situations where it is important to know if perfusion of the limbs is adequate, for instance after surgery or in other high-risk babies.

It is important to recognise the influence of humidification on body temperature. When oxygen is being administered it should first be humidified and warmed to a temperature at least equivalent to that inside the incubator. Furthermore babies, whether in incubators or cots, should not be placed near outside walls or draughts from doors, passages or air conditioning vents nor should they be in a position which is subjected to direct sunlight. Care also needs to be exercised when taking babies out of incubators or cots for feeding or cuddling. Such practices are emotionally beneficial to the baby but it is critical to check that the baby is well wrapped and wearing a bonnet and bootees if necessary.

Nutritional needs

The nutritional needs of the sick neonate are somewhat different from his healthy counterpart since he not only requires the nutrients necessary for growth and development but also some for tissue repair and sustenance throughout an often stormy course of physiological difficulties.

In 1977 the American Academy of Pediatrics stated that 'the optimal diet for the low birth-weight infant may be defined as one that supports a rate of growth approximately that of the third trimester of intra-uterine life without imposing stress on the developing metabolic and excretory systems.' Lucas (1986) argues that, as this statement is not supported by data on the outcomes of attempting to mimic fetal growth, it may be salutory to remember that a preterm baby is not a fetus and that he requires a diet which promotes adaptation to extra-uterine life. For a fuller discussion of the philosophies underpinning the feeding of at-risk infants the reader is referred to Lucas (1986).

Preterm infants have virtually no reserves of tissue and require urgent attention to their calorie needs if they are to avoid catabolism and hypoglycaemia.

Healthy, low birthweight infants should be fed naso- or orogastrically with expressed breast milk or a preterm formula milk.

Ziemer & George (1990) consider that human milk remains an important source of nutrition for the low birthweight infant, although supplementation of certain nutrients may be necessary. Enteral feeds should not be given to very sick infants because of the risk of paralytic ileus.

Feeding regimes and frequency of feeding
Feeding regimes vary from unit to unit but preterm babies require a higher volume of feed than full-term babies. A preterm baby nursed under a radiant heater requires an extra 40 ml per kg per day to compensate for insensible water loss. Normally, daily increases in fluid volume can be made until a total of 180 ml per kg per day is reached but the fluid requirements of very sick babies may need to be adjusted more slowly in accordance with their physiological status.

The route, frequency and method of feeding are largely a matter of clinical judgement and are amended according to the level of tolerance in the individual baby. Tolerance of feeds can be measured by aspirating the gastric contents every 3–4 hours. If these are excessive in relation to the amount and frequency of feeding, it may be necessary to commence or increase fluid intake by the intravenous route. A baby weighing below 1000 g has a very small gastric capacity and cannot tolerate feeds less frequently than hourly. An alternative in such babies is to try perfusor feeding which may be tolerated more readily than bolus feeding. Preterm infants have poor muscle tone in the cardiac sphincter and regurgitation with possible aspiration must be avoided.

Feeding methods

As the sucking and swallowing mechanisms are not usually developed until around 34 weeks' gestation, breast or bottle feeding is not normally possible for babies who are less mature. Even babies above this gestation are often too ill to attempt sucking. However, if a baby is able to suck and swallow without becoming exhausted, the mother should be encouraged to feed him by breast or bottle as she chooses.

Breast feeding (see also Ch. 33)

Successful breast feeding of a full-term baby is rarely established without at least a few problems and these are often exaggerated for the mother of a preterm or sick baby. The emotional trauma of a preterm birth may leave a mother feeling shocked and numb with associated denial, anger and depression. Additionally, anxiety and tiredness will not contribute to the successful establishment of lactation. Some mothers will have had no previous experience of breast feeding nor observed natural suckling at the breast. Many mothers suppose that having a preterm baby totally precludes successful breast feeding. It is hardly surprising therefore that a mother may be bewildered and somewhat ambivalent in her feelings concerning her ability to breast feed.

Such feelings are reinforced by the reality that her baby may be very small and sleepy, curling up into a ball easily and consequently difficult to position. There may also be mismatching in the size of the baby's mouth and the dimensions of the maternal breast. The baby will be unable to suck vigorously and feeding will take longer.

Inevitably many mothers are unable to feed their babies immediately and they need advice on milk expression at the earliest opportunity. Some find this process distinctly unappealing and feel that they become a 'milking machine'. It is preferable that a special room, tastefully decorated, is set aside for milk expression where the mother can relax in privacy. She may find it helpful to look at a picture of her baby, read or listen to some taped music whilst she is expressing her milk.

The establishment of a good rapport between the midwife and the mother and the inclusion of the partner will assist in building maternal confidence. Discussion in privacy with great sensitivity will enable the mother to appreciate that her efforts to breast feed are highly valued within the neonatal unit. The environment for breast feeding should be quiet and relaxing with comfortable chairs, stools and pillows available. Attractive decor, cushions, a coffee table and a selection of plants with all contribute towards a positive and supportive ambiance. Above all, the mother of a preterm or sick baby needs encouragement and praise in her efforts no matter how small. Advice must be consistent.

Bottle feeding (see also Ch. 33)

Bottle feeding for the preterm infant should not be introduced until there are adequate sucking and swallowing reflexes present, normally around the equivalent of 35–36 weeks' gestation though occasionally sooner. Attempting to bottle feed before this time may lead to inhalation of milk and cyanosis. The first bottle feed should always be given by an experienced midwife or at least be closely supervised by one. Special disposable preterm baby teats are now available which are suitable for the small infant and fit onto ready-to-feed bottles. As bottle feeds are introduced, the indwelling gastric tube is kept in situ since the whole feed is unlikely to be completed at the first attempt and topping-up will be necessary. Oral feeds should be introduced gradually. One per day is given for several days until the baby finishes a whole feed then 2 per day until these are completed and so on. It is inadvisable to rush this process as the baby's ability and enthusiasm for sucking may diminish rather than increase.

Tube feeding

The majority of sick preterm babies will require gastric feeding via an oral or nasal tube. For babies requiring oxygen supplementation, orogastric tubes are preferable since they permit easier breathing. In practice nasogastric tubes tend to be more stable and are certainly a satisfactory method for babies without respiratory problems. A size 5FG tube is used for either route and secured to the chin or cheek with hypo-allergenic tape, ensuring that the nostrils are not occluded, the mouth or ears covered or the lower eyelids displaced.

Jejunal feeding is practised in a few units though there can be difficulties with correct tube placement, which normally takes several hours. The rationale for choosing jejunal feeding may be that gastric feeds are poorly tolerated by the baby. However, if this is caused by reduced intestinal blood flow there is a risk of necrotising enterocolitis and jejunal feeding may be unwise. Also, the medium of the jejunum is alkaline and if the acid medium of the stomach is bypassed there is, theoretically, an increased likelihood of introducing pathogenic organisms into the small intestine.

Intravenous fluids

For the majority of sick babies initially, the intravenous route is the most appropriate method of supplying fluid, calories and electrolytes. Extracellular water content is approximately 90% in preterm infants as opposed to 70% in full-term infants and the possibility of dehydration is greater. Furthermore, the preterm infant's capacity for maintaining fluid and electrolyte balance is limited by the immaturity of the kidneys. Such babies will require their electrolyte levels to be estimated at least once daily.

Glucose (dextrose) 5% is the standard solution used although for babies with hypoglycaemia, glucose 10% may be necessary. It is preferable to use peripheral veins on the hand or foot. Scalp veins should only be used as a last resort because the head will need shaving and if extravasation occurs, if may produce scarring. Neither of these events is particularly pleasing to parents. Careful

siting of the cannula should be accompanied by meticulous splinting of the limb, ensuring that the cannula site is visible and that the strapping is not too tight. Frequent observation is essential to prevent the sequelae of extravasation (Fig. 36.5).

Once his condition is more stable, a sick baby may commence intragastric tube feeds, usually 1 ml hourly. The situation is reassessed after 4 hours following aspiration. Obviously extreme caution must be employed, especially if the baby is being ventilated, because overdistension of the stomach with subsequent inhalation of milk is to be avoided. Early feeding is advantageous in expediting the passage of meconium and reducing the degree of hyperbilirubinaemia in addition to initiating intestinal hormone release. Intravenous nutrition in tandem with intragastric feeding can continue until further stabilisation and improvement permit discontinuation of parenteral fluids.

Total parenteral nutrition (TPN)

Over the past 20 years parenteral nutrition has been acknowledged as having an important role in the management of some acutely ill neonates. Indications for its use include extreme prematurity, congenital abnormalities which require major resection of the small bowel, necrotising enterocolitis and intractable diarrhoea of infancy.

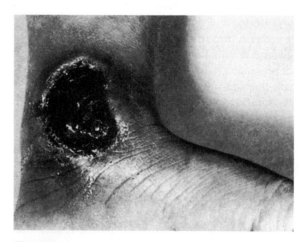

Fig. 36.5
Baby's foot showing tissue necrosis following extravasation of intravenous infusion. (Reproduced by permission of P. Jaffe, Consultant Paediatrician, Hillingdon Hospital, London.)

Parenteral fluids will include amino acids, glucose, minerals, vitamins and sometimes fat (lipids). These will be prescribed daily and prepared in the pharmacy in a laminar flow work situation using aseptic techniques. In neonatal practice, solutions are usually infused concurrently from two containers, one containing amino acids, dextrose, electrolytes and trace elements and the other, fat emulsion and vitamins. Although parenteral nutrition can be administered via a peripheral vein for short periods, because of the high osmolarity, the fluids are damaging to tissues and produce thrombophlebitis and tissue necrosis if extravasation occurs: it is therefore usual to use a central line. Potential complications of TPN include infection, hepatic dysfunction, hypoglycaemia, hyperglycaemia and central catheter complications.

A meticulous aseptic technique is required when handling infusion apparatus and protocols should be devised in relation to changing bags and care of the central line. Bacteriological and biochemical monitoring are essential. As parenteral feeding causes a reduction in the enzyme and hormone activity in the gut, early introduction of milk feeding is important. Oral feeds should be re-introduced slowly with parenteral back-up.

Spiritual needs

The UKCC Code of Professional Conduct states in clause 6 that the midwife will 'take account of

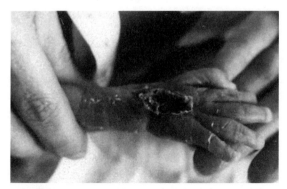

Fig. 36.6
Baby's hand following extravasation of total parenteral nutrition. Surrounding skin had contracted badly and venous return from fingers was obstructed. Baby lost full use of hand. (Reproduced by permission of P. Jaffe, Consultant Paediatrician, Hillingdon Hospital, London.)

the customs, values and spiritual beliefs of patients/ clients'. Despite being unable to communicate verbally, the sick neonate does have spiritual needs although in practice these may be reflected on the parents and perceived by caretakers to be parental needs. Nevertheless, they still constitute an integral part of the holistic approach and should not be neglected. It is obviously not possible for the midwife to be familiar with every religious persuasion, nevertheless the tenets of the major religions likely to be encountered should be known and every attempt made to meet individual needs. In times of great crisis even those who do not practise any religion may feel the desire for some spiritual comfort for their child. Parents of critically ill babies should always be consulted regarding their wishes concerning baptism or a naming ceremony. Individual needs may vary enormously even amongst those with similar religious beliefs. Some parents may hold unusual beliefs but they should be made to feel that their wishes are recognised, accepted and met as far as circumstances permit.

If time allows, baptism should be a pre-arranged event at which both parents are present along with other relatives if they desire. Despite practical difficulties, the ceremony should display the respect and reverence that one would experience inside a church because it is the equivalent of a church ceremony.

A tray or trolley should be prepared, covered with a white cloth, on which, neatly laid, there are a small font and teaspoon, a cross, a small vase of flowers and perhaps one of the baby's toys. At an often distressing time, it is vital to transmit to the family the caring recognition of the importance of this event. Clearly, a great deal of emotional support will be offered by the priest or minister but he is usually less well known to the family than the staff who should also provide appropriate support. Baptism is not an exclusively clerical responsibility: every midwife should be aware of this and conversant with the format of infant baptism in case clergy are not available.

Following the ceremony, the priest or minister will complete the baptismal register and give the parents a baptismal certificate. In more urgent circumstances such as sudden, unexpected deterioration, a midwife may have to baptise a baby and those working in neonatal units need to be familiar with the correct method of undertaking this ceremony.

Very great distress can be caused to families of certain Christian denominations should a baby die unbaptised. It is also important that this is carried out in accordance with the parents' wishes and that they are still given a baptismal certificate for it is no less valid than a pre-arranged ceremony.

Often, parents are reluctant to have their baby baptised in hospital because it is usually impossible for many of the family to attend. The parents may also perceive baptism as an indication of impending death which they have not yet accepted. Sensitive explanation is required to reduce their fears and anxieties, bearing in mind that no one is aware of the eventual outcome. When the baby has recovered, most clergy are willing to organise a ceremony of blessing in the church, at which all family members may be present. It is helpful if contact numbers of advisors from all religious persuasions are held at unit level for reference.

Skin care and prevention of infection

The prevention of iatrogenic skin problems in the low birthweight baby is an important nursing responsibility. The increasing use of technology which involves the application of monitoring devices to fragile skin and the survival of increasingly immature infants present a considerable challenge to the nurse's skill and ingenuity. Ramussen (1987) suggests that by the age of 21 days the skin characteristics of the preterm infant are comparable to those of the full-term baby regardless of the gestational age at birth. Particular vigilance is therefore called for in the early weeks of life when the use of monitoring and medical interventions tends to be at its peak. Problems include epidermal stripping caused by the application of tape, thermal injuries associated with transcutaneous monitoring, damage from the use of chemicals and warm ambient humidity, ischaemia and necrosis such as ulceration of the nares caused by improperly secured endotracheal tubes and extravasation injury. Research-based protocols related to the skin care of these vulnerable infants should be established more generally, as a means of improving and standardising care.

Whilst minimal handling remains a cardinal principle in the care of the preterm infant, daily care should include cord inspection and care, eye care, mouth care which includes the inspection of the mouth for monilial infection and a general inspection of the skin for trauma and infection. A swab should be taken of any localised septic foci and sent for culture and sensitivity.

When signs of infection are less specific, for instance behavioural changes, temperature instability or an increasing number of apnoeic episodes, a full infection screen is usually indicated. This will include nose, throat, umbilical and rectal swabs, a bladder tap, a lumbar puncture, a full blood count, differential white cell count, blood culture and a chest X-ray. It is mandatory that suspected infection be investigated promptly; initial signs may be insidious but progression very rapid.

Hand washing remains the single most important infection control measure. All staff and visitors, including children, must use appropriate hand-washing techniques.

Any staff member or visitor with an infection or infective lesion or who has been in contact with someone with an infection should seek specialist medical advice before entering the special care nursery.

COMPLICATIONS OF INTENSIVE CARE

While advances in neonatal intensive care have resulted in significant reductions in both neonatal morbidity and mortality, the technical interventions required to keep these babies alive are associated with complications arising from their application to immature body systems. Complications tend to occur quickly and there is little margin for error. Constant vigilance and attention to detail are necessary qualities in intensive care staff.

Bronchopulmonary dysplasia

This serious and increasingly prevalent chronic

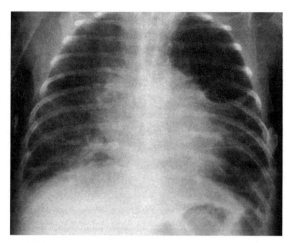

Fig. 36.7
Chest X-ray of baby with chronic lung disease
demonstrating overinflated lung fields and linear
shadowing with large, cystic spaces. (Reproduced by
permission of D. Lindsell, Consultant Radiologist, John
Radcliffe Hospital, Oxford.)

lung disorder is associated with prolonged mechanical ventilation in low birth weight infants.
While high ventilatory pressures (barotrauma) and
prolonged exposure to oxygen have been considered primary causes, other factors such as pulmonary immaturity, fluid overload, retention of
secretions and bronchospasm may all contribute
to the disease process. Clinically an affected baby
is difficult to wean off ventilation and quickly becomes hypoxic and apnoeic if this is attempted.
There is no specific treatment but the role of
drugs such as dexamethasone, diuretics and bron-
chodilators is currently being assessed. As alveolar
development continues in the child for the first 7
years of life bronchopulmonary dysplasia usually
improves spontaneously although respiratory support and oxygen supplementation may need to be
continued for many months. Home oxygen therapy
may be recommended in order to allow early discharge and to promote family integrity.

Retinopathy of prematurity (ROP)

Retinopathy of prematurity is characterised by
widespread vasoconstriction of the retinal capillaries. Later there is dilatation of the capillaries and
they become more numerous. Subsequently, retinal
oedema and haemorrhage occur resulting in retinal

detachment, scarring and eventual blindness. These
ocular changes occur in relation to high arterial
oxygen tension; other aetiological factors such as
shock, hypoxia and vitamin E deficiency have also
been suggested. There is no known maximum
oxygen concentration below which it is safe to
assume that ROP will not occur. Careful monitoring of the infant and of the arterial oxygen
tension is essential; special care is needed during
suctioning and feeding to ensure hypoxaemia does
not occur. All babies treated with oxygen should
have their eyes examined by an ophthalmologist
before discharge or transfer as should all babies
over the age of 6 weeks who are ventilator dependent. Recent advances include trials of large
prophylactic doses of vitamin E (100 mg); results
as yet are inconclusive. Cryotherapy may be used
to prevent progression of pathology.

Table 36.1
International classification of ROP

Stage no.	Characteristic	
1	Demarcation line	
2	Ridge	
3	Ridge with extraretinal fibrovascular proliferation	
4	Subtotal retinal detachment	
	a. extrafoveal	
	b. retinal detachment including fovea	
5	Total retinal detachment	
	Funnel:	*Anterior*	*Posterior*
		open	open
		narrow	narrow
		open	narrow
		narrow	open

Patent ductus arteriosus (PDA)

The mechanism by which the ductus arteriosus
closes in response to the increased arterial oxygen
tension which occurs at birth is complex and
involves autonomic activity, the ductal musculature
and the action of prostaglandins. Because the
ductal musculature develops from the 25th to the
37th week of intra-uterine life ductal closure may
be delayed or absent in preterm infants especially
those who suffer from hypoxia. The incidence of
patent ductus arteriosus is 32% in infants of less
than 36 weeks' gestation.

As pulmonary vascular resistance falls following birth left-to-right shunting develops with tachycardia, tachypnoea and dyspnoea. If the infant is ventilated it becomes difficult or impossible to wean the baby from the ventilator.

Restriction of fluids and diuretics may help to control heart failure but medical or surgical closure is usually necessary. Indomethacin (a prostaglandin synthetase inhibitor) given intravenously is usually the treatment of first choice. It has been reported as producing closure in 50% of cases. If medical management fails, small size is not a contra-indication to surgery. Ligation has been carried out on a 660 gram infant.

Necrotising enterocolitis

There is an increased likelihood of necrotising enterocolitis in any sick baby who receives intensive care. Whilst the aetiology is uncertain, two

factors, namely intestinal ischaemia and invasion of the bowel by gas-forming bacteria, seem instrumental in the pattern of the disorder. Episodes of hypoxia in which blood flow is directed away from the intestine to vital organs are clearly more probable in the high-risk infant. Following an ischaemic insult, it appears that the mucosal lining of the bowel is destroyed, thus reducing the secretion of protective mucus. Anaerobic organisms then invade the bowel wall causing inflammation and swelling. An abdominal X-ray will demonstrate *pneumotosis intestinales*, air in the bowel wall (Fig. 36.8). Further progression of the disease leads to severe necrosis of large segments of bowel with possible perforation and death (Figs 36.9 and 36.10).

The onset is often insidious with non-specific signs including apnoea, unstable temperature, vomiting, poor absorption of feeds and hypotension. Definitive signals of progressive deterioration

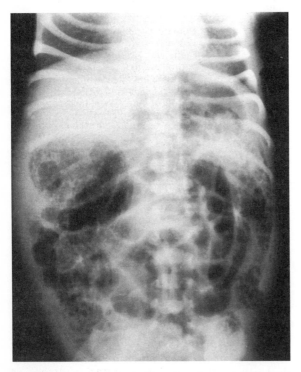

Fig. 36.8
Abdominal X-ray showing a diffuse bubbly pattern throughout the large bowel due to intramural blebs of gas. (Reproduced by permission of D. Lindsell, Consultant Radiologist, John Radcliffe Hospital, Oxford.)

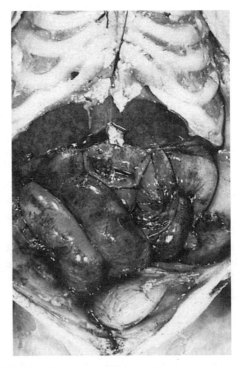

Fig. 36.9
View of abdomen at postmortem showing large, distended loops of inflamed bowel and perforation. (Reproduced by permission of J. W. Keeling, Consultant Paediatric Pathologist, John Radcliffe Hospital, Oxford.)

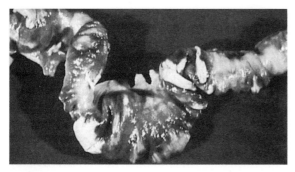

Fig. 36.10
Close-up view, necrotising enterocolitis, showing twisted loop of bowel with areas of inflammation, necrosis and obstruction. (Reproduced by permission of J. W. Keeling, Consultant Paediatric Pathologist, John Radcliffe Hospital, Oxford.)

are the presence of blood or mucus in the stools and abdominal distension. At this stage milk feeds should cease, enabling the bowel to rest, and total parenteral nutrition should be commenced. Broad-spectrum intravenous antibiotics are also indicated. Surgical intervention is not normally necessary unless there is perforation. However, reconstructive bowel resection may be required following recovery. Recognition of early signs with prompt commencement of therapeutic management may contribute to a better eventual outcome.

Complications of umbilical arterial catheter insertion

An umbilical arterial catheter can be a vital source of samples for the estimation of blood gas values in ventilated and sick babies. However, the insertion of a catheter is often extremely difficult even for an experienced operator and incorrect positioning can easily occur. The catheter should normally occupy the abdominal aorta: if it is misdirected down one of the internal iliac arteries, its diameter practically fills the lumen of the artery and blocks circulation. Additionally, micro-emboli may form around the catheter and enter the circulation undetected. As a consequence, varying degrees of necrosis ensue (Figs 36.11 and 36.12).

As a precautionary measure, the limbs and buttocks should be carefully inspected before any

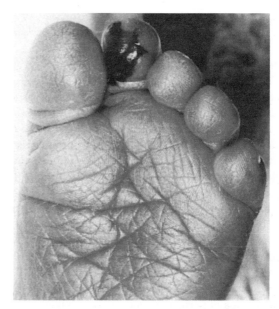

Fig. 36.11
Baby's foot showing necrotic portion of toe as a result of an embolus from an umbilical arterial catheter. (Reproduced by permission of P. Jaffe, Consultant Paediatrician, Hillingdon Hospital, London.)

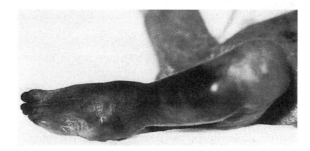

Fig. 36.12
Serious but rare necrosis of leg arising from emboli from umbilical arterial catheter. Leg had to be amputated below the knee. (Reproduced by permission of Karen Norton, Midwife, Neonatal Unit, Hillingdon Hospital, London.)

catheterisation is attempted in order to record the presence of any bruising which could be confused with cyanosis. Should any cyanosis develop distal to the catheter, the latter must be removed immediately. Regular inspection of the limbs for cyanosis, pallor and diminished pulses should be made as long as the catheter remains in situ. No heel stabs should be carried out.

Periventricular haemorrhage and leukomalacia

Periventricular haemorrhage (PVH)

This is a common early complication affecting low birthweight infants. 90% of these haemorrhages occur during the first week of life.

In the early months of intra-uterine brain development a structure called the germinal matrix is situated close to the ventricles. It contains developing brain cells and therefore receives a high blood flow rich in nutrients. Bleeding into and around this structure is much rarer in term babies, as by this time the developing cells have migrated to the cortex and the germinal matrix has regressed. PVH can be detected by cranial sonography in 35% of very low birthweight infants.

Levene et al (1982) have suggested the following grades of periventricular haemorrhage:

Grade 0 = Normal
Grade 1 = Mild haemorrhage encompassing the germinal matrix
Grade 2 = Haemorrhage into the ventricles
Grade 3 = Haemorrhage into the ventricles with extension into the cerebral parenchyma.

A clear picture of a Grade 2 haemorrhage is shown in Figure 36.13.

The aetiology is probably multifactorial. Prematurity and artificial ventilation for respiratory distress syndrome are strongly associated as are factors causing fluctuations in cerebral blood flow, such as acidosis, hypercapnia, hypoxia, hypotensive and hypertensive episodes. These are particularly significant as in preterm and asphyxiated infants cerebral auto-regulation does not occur.

Many prophylactic measures have been tried including surfactant therapy, ethamsylate (a platelet stabilising drug), phenobarbitone, vitamin E and pancuronium. The effectiveness of these treatments remains open to debate. The most important single factor in avoiding PVH appears to be careful attention to the finer details of neonatal intensive care, namely head positioning, the maintenance of synchronous ventilation, the avoidance of hypertensive peaks associated with tracheal suctioning and accurate maintenance of fluid balance.

Haemorrhages into the parenchyma are responsible for significant mortality. Obstructive hydrocephalus develops in 70% of patients with one-third of these requiring ventricular shunts.

Periventricular leukomalacia

Periventricular leukomalacia is characterised by cystic, ischaemic lesions appearing in the periventricular region (Fig. 36.14). Diagnosis can only be made by the use of real-time ultrasound scanning over a period of several weeks. Research so far suggests a high risk of cerebral palsy in babies with periventricular leukomalacia (Bozynski et al 1985, Weindling et al 1985).

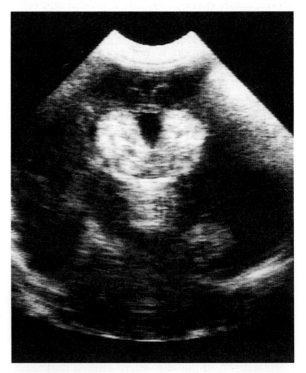

Fig. 36.13
Periventricular haemorrhage. Ultrasound scan of coronal section showing extensive intraventricular haemorrhage filling and dilating both lateral ventricles and extending into the third ventricle. (Reproduced by permission of M. J. Rochefort, Research Fellow, Neonatal Unit, John Radcliffe Hospital, Oxford.)

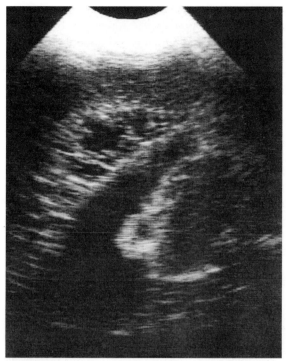

Fig. 36.14
Periventricular leukomalacia. Parasagittal scan showing cystic periventricular leukomalacia lying over the superior aspect of the lateral ventricle. (Reproduced by permission of M. J. Rochefort, Research Fellow, Neonatal Unit, John Radcliffe Hospital, Oxford.)

ADVICE TO PARENTS ON TAKING THEIR BABY HOME FROM NEONATAL INTENSIVE CARE

Probably one of the most valuable pieces of advice which can be given to parents in preparation for their baby's homecoming is that although he may have been extremely ill, it is now vitally important to treat him as a normal baby. Parents need reassurance that whatever the baby's previous problems were they are not going to recur.

It is also important that parental support throughout the time their baby has been in the neonatal unit has promoted maximal competence and confidence. Parents thus prepared are less likely to be anxious and apprehensive when they assume total responsibility for their baby.

Warmth

Parents should be advised to keep the baby's environment heated to 18–21°C. Even in a centrally heated house it will be necessary to have an additional, safe source of heating such as an electric fire. During very cold weather it is not necessary to bath a baby every day as this may cause rapid cooling. Parents often ask how they will know if the baby's temperature is satisfactory. They need to feel the baby carefully, centrally and peripherally and adjust the amount of clothing accordingly.

Clothing

The layette will need to include items of an appropriate size and there are now several companies producing preterm baby clothes which are available in shops or by mail order. These can be quite expensive, however, and have a limited period of usefulness. Several neonatal units have established clothes 'libraries' where parents can hire a set of preterm baby clothing on payment of a deposit and hiring fee, returning the clothes when their baby is large enough for the first newborn size. A support group may also help in supplying clothing at budget prices. Nimble-fingered parents and relatives may prefer to sew or knit their own clothes and special preterm baby sewing and knitting patterns are now available.

Disposable nappies may be desirable at least initially and their use will also reduce the amount of washing. Several baby goods manufacturers now offer bulk deliveries of nappies to the home which may be a convenience for parents.

Feeding

The neonatal unit staff will advise parents at discharge regarding the amount of milk to be offered at each feed time. This amount can be gradually increased according to the baby's needs, following a regime of 180 ml per kg per 24 hours. A mother who is breast feeding will be guided by the baby's perceived satisfaction, increasing the frequency of feeds as indicated. Those mothers who have had to supplement or complement breast feeds in hospital will probably find that their milk supply improves once they are more relaxed in their home environment. As the baby grows larger and the parents become confident and organised in his management, they can increase the volume of feeds and reduce their frequency which allows a longer period of sleep through the night. Caring for a preterm baby at home can be exhausting and emotionally draining and the need of the parents for sleep must be considered. The parents can easily become irritable and fractious and they need to be helped to attend to their own need for sleep and rest in order to retain the ability to cope with their tiny baby and to maintain family harmony and happiness.

Outings and integration into the family

Gradually the baby can be taken out unless it is foggy or extremely cold. Extra clothing will be essential in cooler weather but only light clothing on hot days. A canopy will prevent direct sunshine on the baby's skin which is very vulnerable to sunburn.

Pets may become jealous of the new arrival and react adversely. It is therefore advisable to keep the crib or cot raised off the floor and to observe the baby very closely whilst the cat or dog is in the same room. It is unwise for the baby to be in the same room as a caged bird as dust, excreta and feathers are regularly discharged into the atmosphere. Emphasis on hand washing between handling pets and the baby is important in order to prevent toxoplasmosis. When outside, a cat net fixed onto the pram will protect the baby from animals. Family and friends will undoubtedly want to cuddle the baby and this should be encouraged providing they do not have any signs of infection. Grandparents will want to participate in the care of the baby and this will further contribute to the establishment and continuation of a loving relationship. Siblings may find the adjustment to their new situation very difficult: careful handling is necessary if long term problems are not to ensue. The parents may be advised to incorporate them into caring for the new infant, to offer small gifts and to ensure that they get extra attention from grandparents or friends.

Reader Activities

- With reference to research findings reflect upon the psychological needs of infants and parents in a neonatal intensive care unit.
- Following a literature review formulate a protocol in relation to skin care for the low birthweight infant.
- Identify problems associated with intensive care of the neonate and discuss with a colleague nursing measures that might prevent or minimise their impact.
- Prepare a list of useful information and local addresses of organisations such as parent support groups to be offered to parents on discharge of an infant from the intensive care unit.

REFERENCES

American Academy of Paediatrics Committee on Nutrition 1977 Nutritional needs of low birthweight infants. Paediatrics 60(4): 519–530

Astbury J 1982 Determinants of stress for staff in a neonatal intensive care unit. Archives of Disease in Childhood 57: 108–111

Blisslink Information Pack of setting up a parent support group. Available from Bliss, 17–21 Emerald Street, London WC1 3QL

Bozynski M E A et al 1985 Cavitary periventricular leukomalacia, incidence and short term outcome in infants weighing less than 1200 grams at birth. Developmental Medicine and Child Neurology 27: 572–577

Catterson J 1988 Special care baby units study. Oxford Regional Health Authority, Old Road, Headington, Oxford OX3 7LF

Cook R W I 1981 Factors associated with intraventricular haemorrhage in very low birth weight infants. Archives of Disease in Childhood 50: 425

Earnshaw A 1978 Causes of respiratory distress in neonates. Journal of Royal Society of Medicine 71 (May): 388

Gladman G 1989 Advances in neonatal intensive care. The Practitioner 233 (May 8): 670–673

Gross S J, David R J, Bauman L, Tomarelli R M 1980 Nutritional composition of milk produced by mothers delivering preterm. Journal of Pediatrics 96: 641–644

Halliday H L, McClure G, Reid M 1989 Handbook of neonatal intensive care, 3rd edn. Baillière Tindall, London

Hill S 1990 Family. Viking Penguin, Harmondsworth

Jacobson S D 1978 Stressful situations for neonatal intensive care nurses. The American Journal of Maternal Child Nursing 3: 144–150

Kidd J F 1988 Pulse oximeters. Basic theory and operation. Care of the Critically Ill 4(1): 10–13

Levene M I, Fawer C-L, Lamont R F 1982 Risk factors in the development of intraventricular haemorrhage in the preterm neonate. Archives of Disease in Childhood 57: 410–417

Levene M I, Williams J L, Fawer C-L 1985 Ultrasound of the infant's brain. Blackwell, Oxford

Lucas A 1986 Infant feeding. In: Roberton N (ed) Textbook of neonatology. Churchill Livingstone, Edinburgh

Noyes J 1990 Respiratory failure in infants. Nursing Standard 4 (Aug 29): 49

Pope K E, Wigglesworth J S 1979 Haemorrhage, ischaemia and the perinatal brain. Spastics International Medical Publications, MacKeith Press, London

Ramussen J 1987 The skin structure, function and percutaneous absorption. In: Kelly V C (ed) Practice in paediatrics. Harper and Row, Philadelphia

Sarman I et al 1989 Rewarming preterm infants on a heated, water filled mattress. Archives of Disease in Childhood 64(5): 687–692

Stewart A 1989 Having a baby in the neonatal unit. Health Visitor 62(12): 374–377

Sleath K 1989 Breath of life. Nursing Times 85(44): 30

The Court Report 1976 Fit for the future. HMSO, London

Thompson J 1990 Early comfort. Nursing Times 86(30): 20

United Kingdom Central Council for Nursing, Midwifery and Health Visiting 1992 Code of Professional Conduct. UKCC, London

Walker C H M 1982 Neonatal intensive care and stress. Archives of Disease in Childhood 57: 85–88

Weindling A M, Rochefort M J, Calvert S A, Fok T–F, Wilkinson A 1985 Development of cerebral palsy after ultrasonographic detection of periventricular cysts in the newborn. Developmental Medicine and Child Neurology 27: 800–806

Ziemer M M, George C 1990 Breastfeeding the low birthweight infant. Neonatal Network 9(4): 33–38

FURTHER READING

Midwives Information and Resource Service 1991 MIDIRS directory of maternity organisations. MIDIRS, Bristol

National Childbirth Trust 1983 How to express and store breast milk. NCT Leaflet No. 22

37

Trauma and haemorrhage

MARGARET A. LANG

Birth injury

Haemorrhage in the newborn

Intracranial haemorrhage

Convulsions

The primary and only purpose of reproduction is to have a living healthy child (Walker 1985). At a time when there is worldwide emphasis on family planning, and population growth in some countries has reached close to zero (Rowley 1984), the quality of life for each survivor assumes increased importance, both within families and for society. While disabled or handicapped persons may in individual cases often be a source of joy, their birth or the diagnosis of their condition may be devastating to the parents and family. To society their care is both complicated and costly.

Birth trauma should be considered avoidable. It is the duty of midwives and obstetricians to do everything in their power to ensure that babies are born in as good a condition as possible while recognising that some will require the care of a paediatrician, for example if they are preterm.

Babies who are at particular risk of birth trauma include those who are:

- large in relation to the mother's pelvis
- growth-retarded
- preterm
- born by vaginal breech delivery
- twins or higher multiples.

The midwife must be as much concerned with prevention as with treatment, and the antenatal identification of the high risk pregnancy as well as the correct conduct of labour will continue to reduce the incidence of birth trauma.

BIRTH INJURY

Caput succedaneum and cephalhaematoma

Moulding of the baby's head varies according to the presentation, position and duration of labour. Damage may occur to the superficial tissues of the presenting part causing bruising or abrasion. When moulding is excessive cranial compression may take place and can lead to serious intracranial injury (see below). A large caput succedaneum, not to be confused with cephalhaematoma, is often present in such cases (Figs 37.1, 37.2, 37.4 and 37.5).

Mothers can be very distressed by the appearance of a caput or cephalhaematoma. They need reassurance as these injuries are rarely harmful on their own, should disappear completely, and will not compromise the baby's development.

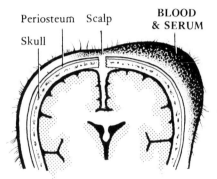

Fig. 37.1
Caput succedaneum.

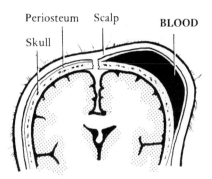

Fig. 37.2
Cephalhaematoma.

Caput succedaneum

A caput succedaneum is an oedematous swelling on the fetal skull, a serosanguinous (serum and blood) infiltration into the scalp tissue. Due to pressure by a *'girdle of contact'* which is usually the cervix; the venous blood return is retarded, and the area lying over the os becomes congested and oedematous.

A second caput may form:

1. In occipito-posterior positions when the occiput rotates forwards.
2. In cases where the head is held up on the perineum.

Is present at birth.
May cross a suture.
Tends to grow less.
Disappears within 36 hours.
Is diffuse, pits on pressure.
A double caput is always unilateral.

Cephalhaematoma

A cephalhaematoma is a swelling on the infant's skull, an effusion of blood under the periosteum covering it, due to friction between the skull and pelvis. It occurs in cases of cephalopelvic disproportion and precipitate labour, when tearing of the periosteum from the bone causes bleeding.

As the periosteum is adherent to the edges of the skull bones, the swelling is confined to one bone. Late-onset jaundice may occur.

No treatment is necessary, the blood is absorbed and the swelling subsides. A ridge of bone may later be felt round the periphery of the swelling, due to the accumulation of osteoblasts.

Appears after 12 hours.
Never crosses a suture.
Tends to grow larger.
Persists for weeks.
Is circumscribed, does not pit.
A double cephalhaematoma is usually bilateral (Fig. 37.5).

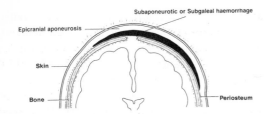

Fig. 37.3
Subaponeurotic haemorrhage.

Subaponeurotic haemorrhage

A subaponeurotic haemorrhage is occasionally seen following spontaneous delivery but more often is associated with vacuum extraction. Bleeding occurs below the epicranial aponeurosis (Fig. 37.3). It can be confused with a caput succedaneum as the swelling extends across the suture lines. The infant must be observed for signs of hyperbilirubinaemia and anaemia. If the haemorrhage is severe, a blood transfusion may be necessary. Death due to massive haemorrhage is a possibility.

Is present at birth.
Crosses suture lines.
Increases in size.
Resolves over 2–3 weeks.
Firm, fluctuent mass.
Can extend into subcutaneous tissue of neck and eyelids.
Bruising may be apparent for days and sometimes weeks.

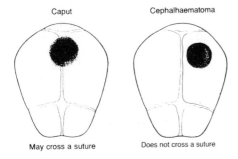

Fig. 37.4
Caput may cross a suture; Cephalhaematoma does not cross a suture.

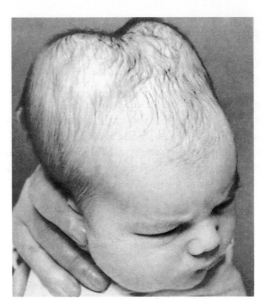

Fig. 37.5
Bilateral cephalhaematoma.

Subaponeurotic haemorrhage

Subaponeurotic haemorrhage is a potentially serious complication. This is rarely seen with good obstetric care.

Fractures

The most commonly affected bones are those of the skull, clavicle, humerus and femur.

Skull
Skull fractures are rare; the majority of fractures are linear and asymptomatic. An overlying cephalhaematoma or skull deformation may be the only feature. Occasionally they may be associated with intracranial haemorrhages, seizures and death as contusion of the underlying brain may have occurred. X-rays are usually required for the diagnosis of skull fractures. The majority of linear fractures in asymptomatic infants heal within 2 months and the prognosis is good. In cases of depressed fracture, infants may be asymptomatic and closed elevation of the fracture is still controversial. However, if depressed fractures are associated with neurological deficit, raised intracranial

pressure or the presence of bony fragments within the brain, open elevation of the fracture is indicated. Treatment of symptoms such as seizures and raised intracranial pressure is necessary. Leakage of cerebrospinal fluid from the auditory canal or nasal orifice necessitates antibiotic cover.

Clavicle

Fractures of the clavicle are often asymptomatic and initially may go undiagnosed unless a crack is heard during delivery or the injury is suspected in association with brachial plexus damage (see below). The clavicle which is fractured is usually the one which was nearest to the maternal symphysis. The fracture may be diagnosed by feeling the distortion at the break, by the presence of crepitus or, in the late phase, by callus formation. Treatment is seldom needed; very occasionally a figure-of-eight bandage may be applied if the infant shows signs of discomfort. A stable union of the break usually occurs within 7–10 days.

Humerus

Fractures of the humerus may occur in cases of shoulder dystocia or during the bringing down of an extended arm in a breech presentation. A crack may be heard at delivery or the infant may present with deformity or pseudoparesis of the upper arm secondary to pain. A proximal epiphyseal fracture should be differentiated from a dislocated shoulder. If a midshaft fracture occurs there may be damage to the radial nerve. Diagnosis of a fracture is confirmed by X-ray. Treatment is by splinting the upper arm, by applying a large crepe bandage or by bandaging the arm to the chest, first placing a pad in the axilla, and taking care not to embarrass respiration. A stable union usually occurs within 2 or 3 weeks.

Femur

Fractures of the femur can occur during delivery of extended legs in a breech presentation, often a crack being heard or felt at the time. The fractures are usually in the midshaft and present with deformity or pseudoparesis. Diagnosis is confirmed by X-ray. Treatment is by simple splinting, a crepe bandage being firmly applied to the upper leg for 2–3 weeks.

Spine

Spinal fractures are very rare: the vast majority occur in breech presentations with an extended head. Fetal cervical hyperextension also predisposes to injury even if delivery is by caesarean section. A loud pop may be heard at delivery. High cervical or brainstem injuries are usually incompatible with life. Lower lesions may allow long-term survival with handicap. Treatment consists of immediate immobilisation of head and trunk even before establishing an airway.

Nerve injuries

The most common are facial nerve and brachial plexus injuries.

Facial palsy

This is usually associated with forceps deliveries where the facial nerve has been compressed against the ramus of the mandible. There is unilateral facial weakness, the eyelid of the affected side remaining open while the mouth is drawn over to the normal side (Fig. 37.6). Minimal feeding difficulties occur. No treatment is required. Occasionally methyl cellulose eye drops may be required, usually if the eyelids remain open. Spontaneous improvement should be seen in 7–10 days. Non-traumatic causes of facial palsy include nuclear agenesis and primary muscle disorders. Recovery is poor in the latter cases.

Brachial plexus injuries

These are caused by stretching or disruption of

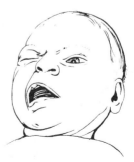

Fig. 37.6
Left-sided facial paralysis. Note that the eye is open on the paralysed side, the mouth drawn over to the non-paralysed side.

the nerves of the brachial plexus which is a group of nerves at the apex of the axilla, lying under the clavicle. Injuries can be caused by excessive lateral flexion of the head and neck in cases of shoulder dystocia or breech presentation. There are three main types of injury:

Erb's palsy (Fig. 37.7). This involves damage to upper roots of the brachial plexus. The baby's inwardly rotated arm lies limply by his side and he cannot flex his elbow or lift his arm, although there is movement of the arm and fingers. The half-closed hand is turned outwards (waiter's tip position).

Klumpke's palsy. Klumpke's palsy involves the lower arm, wrist and hand, with wrist drop and limp fingers caused by damage to spinal roots C8 and T1. The upper arm has normal movement.

Total brachial plexus palsy. In this injury there is loss of both proximal and distal muscle innervations.

These injuries require further investigation including X-rays of clavicle, arm, cervical spine and chest. Careful assessment of joints is particularly important. Treatment consists of resting the arm for 7–10 days followed by gentle physiotherapy to avoid contractures. Parents should be taught a full range of passive movements for shoulder, elbow and wrist. Complete spontaneous recovery is more common with Erb's than Klumpke's or total brachial plexus palsy but may take from several months up to 2 years. Follow-up is necessary as cases not recovering spontaneously have benefited from early surgical treatment. Advances in microsurgery have enabled surgeons to repair nerves and to use nerve grafts more precisely (Shenaq & Dinh 1990).

Incidence of birth injury

Table 37.1 gives the incidence of the foregoing birth injuries in Scotland.

Soft tissue injuries

These usually result from trauma during delivery particularly in cases of breech presentation. Serious injury is rare.

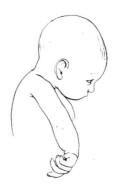

Fig. 37.7
Erb's paralysis.

Injury to the superficial tissues

Bruising can occur together with excoriation caused by damage to the superficial tissues when the presenting part is the face or the breech. With the former the face is congested and bruised and the eyelids and lips oedematous. Before seeing the baby mothers need reassurance that the bruising and oedema will subside over a few days. Mothers who are prevented from seeing the bruising for themselves will tend to imagine injury that is worse than the reality.

Following a breech delivery there is bruising and oedema of the vulval area in the female, and the scrotum in the male. Complications which can arise include:

— loss of blood into skin, subcutaneous tissue and muscle leading to hypovolaemia, anaemia and circulatory collapse; babies have been known to lose as much as 25% of their circulating blood volume
— trauma to the muscle leading to myoglobinuria and renal tubular infarction
— consumptive coagulopathy
— breakdown of blood cells leading to hyper-bilirubinaemia and hyperkalaemia.

Unless complications arise, no treatment is necessary. Again mothers need reassurance that the bruising and oedema will subside over a few days.

Liver and spleen

If injury presents as a subcapsular haematoma

Table 37.1
Selected diagnosis 1988/1989
(Information reproduced by courtesy of Dr S K Cole 1991, Information and Statistic Division, Common Services Agency, Scotland)

Diagnosis	ICD9 code	1988	1989
Subaponeurotic haemorrhage	767.14	0	0
Skull fracture (other injury to skeleton)	767.30	1	3
Clavicle fracture	767.2	20	11
Fractured femur	767.31	1	2
Fractured humerus (other long bones)	767.32	3	4
Spinal fractures	767.49	0	0
Facial injury (facial nerve injury)	767.5	37	31
Brachial plexus injuries (TOTAL)	767.6	47	53
— Erb's palsy	767.60	39	41
— Klumpke's palsy	767.61	0	2
— phrenic nerve injury	767.62	0	0
— other and unspecified	767.69	8	10
Horner's syndrome	337.9	0	0

Source: SMR11 Accumulated Totals Scotland 1988, 1989; SMR11 Diagnostic Index Scotland 1989.

there is often a delay in obvious signs but there may be a fall in haematocrit and haemoglobin levels. It can be diagnosed by ultrasound. If rupture occurs, massive haemorrhage can take place with resultant circulatory collapse. The abdomen may be distended, with bluish discolouration of the skin. Immediate resuscitative measures include restoration of the circulatory volume followed by laparotomy and repair.

Renal and adrenal glands

Slight injury to these organs may escape diagnosis. Massive haemorrhage presents with circulatory collapse and anaemia. Diagnosis is made by ultrasound. Treatment is usually supportive and includes blood transfusion. If adrenal insufficiency is suspected steroid replacement may be required.

Intestinal injury

This may present with a coagulopathy, bleeding per rectum, anaemia and feeding difficulties. Treatment includes correction of coagulopathy and perhaps a short period of intravenous fluids and nasogastric suction. The haematoma usually resolves. Surgery is rarely indicated.

Muscle injuries

Torticollis

Torticollis results from injury to the sternomastoid muscle during birth when either the muscle is torn or its blood supply is impaired. This may occur during delivery of the anterior shoulder in a vertex presentation or while rotating the shoulders during a breech delivery. It usually presents 1 or 2 weeks after birth as a small painless lump 2 cm or so in size, commonly on the left side of the neck. It is no longer thought to be a haematoma but is probably a mixture of blood and fibrous tissue. The swelling will resolve over several weeks. Muscle-stretching exercises should be taught to parents to prevent shortening. Infants should sleep on the opposite side to the injury to increase passive stretching.

Skin injuries

These are often iatrogenic caused by forceps blades, scalp electrodes, scalpels etc. Compression from forceps blades can cause an area of bruising or subcutaneous fat necrosis, usually on the face. There is no treatment as it is self-resolving, disappearing over a period of a few weeks or months. Abrasions can also be caused from forceps blades or the use of vacuum extractors. Death has occasionally occurred from massive scalp and intracranial haemorrhage following the use of the latter. In recent years with the increasing use of fetal monitoring equipment a new type of injury being seen is the puncture wound from a scalp electrode. Like any laceration or abrasion it is a potential source of infection which can lead on to abscess formation. The affected area should be kept clean. If an abscess develops, this may require incision and antibiotics. Occasionally when the uterus is incised during caesarean section, the scalpel may lacerate the baby's skin. This can occur anywhere on the body but is usually superficial. It usually only needs cleansing and closing with butterfly adhesive strips. Sutures may be required for deeper lacerations.

HAEMORRHAGE IN THE NEWBORN

Causes of bleeding in the neonate are haemorrhagic disease of the newborn, disseminated intravascular coagulation, thrombocytopenia and inherited coagulation factor deficiencies. Bleeding may also occur as a result of local trauma.

Haemorrhagic disease of the newborn

This is due to a deficiency of the vitamin-K-dependent coagulation factors II, VII, IX and X.

Predisposing factors include breast feeding (Chapter 33 discusses Vitamin K in human milk), asphyxia, hypoxia, liver damage, extreme prematurity and maternal anticonvulsant or anticoagulant therapy.

Bleeding usually presents in the first few days of life but may be delayed for a number of weeks. The baby may bleed from various sites including the umbilical stump, skin, nose, scalp and puncture sites. Gastro-intestinal bleeding is manifested as melaena and haematemesis. If the haemorrhage is severe, circulatory collapse occurs. Diagnosis is confirmed if blood tests reveal prolonged prothrombin and partial thromboplastin times. The platelet count is normal.

Currently research is looking into the aetiology

and management of this problem. Trials are being undertaken to establish whether effective prophylaxis can be achieved with oral vitamin K analogues. This would be preferable to the current practice of administering vitamin K_1 1 mg intramuscularly, to all babies.

Mild cases of haemorrhagic disease are treated with vitamin K systemically. In severe cases when coagulation is grossly abnormal and there is active bleeding into vital structures a transfusion of fresh frozen plasma is necessary to replace deficient clotting factors. If circulatory collapse and severe anaemia have occurred a transfusion of red cell concentrate will be required in addition to fresh frozen plasma. In all cases of severe haemorrhage the infant is nursed in an incubator to allow close observation, warmth and careful monitoring.

Disseminated intravascular coagulation (DIC)

DIC results from activation of the coagulation cascade resulting in widespread deposition of fibrin in the microcirculation. This has a number of consequences including a consumptive coagulopathy with abnormally low platelets and coagulation factors and also a haemolytic anaemia as red blood cells are fragmented by the fibrin deposits in blood vessels. Organ dysfunction may be caused by interference with blood supply to the organ.

It is now widely recognised as a disease secondary to other primary conditions and may be associated with:

— severe birth asphyxia
— severe respiratory distress syndrome
— severe infections, e.g. septicaemia
— hypothermia
— hypoxia
— hypotension.

Other consumptive coagulopathies are associated with:

— polycythaemia
— giant haemangiomas
— necrotising enterocolitis
— vascular thrombosis
— intraventricular haemorrhage.

The infant develops a generalised purpuric rash with bleeding from puncture sites and the umbilical stump leading to anaemia. DIC is often associated with intracerebral and pulmonary haemorrhage. Diagnosis is a combination of clinical signs and laboratory findings. Blood films show a low platelet count, distorted and fragmented red blood cells, and raised fibrin degradation products (FDPs) with a prolonged prothrombin time and partial thromboplastin time.

Treatment includes correction of the underlying cause if possible, transfusions of fresh frozen plasma, cryoprecipitate, concentrated clotting factors and platelets. In cases of anaemia transfusions of whole blood or red cell concentrate may also be required. Occasionally an exchange transfusion of fresh blood may be performed removing harmful substances at the same time as replacing the missing clotting factors and blood. Heparinisation treatment remains controversial but may be considered in persistent DIC. (See also Ch. 21.)

Thrombocytopenia

Thrombocytopenia is a low count of circulating platelets and results from a decreased rate of formation of platelets or an increased rate of consumption. Causes include:

- severe infection, congenital or acquired, e.g. syphilis, cytomegalovirus, rubella, toxoplasmosis, bacterial
- maternal causes, e.g. idiopathic thrombocytopenia, purpura, systemic lupus erythematosis, drug ingestion (thiazide diuretics), thyrotoxicosis
- isoimmune thrombocytopenia
- inherited thrombocytopenia.

A petechial rash appears soon after birth presenting in a mild case with a few localised petechiae and in a severe case with widespread and serious haemorrhage. Diagnosis is based on history, clinical examination and the presence of a reduced platelet count. It is differentiated from other haemorrhagic disorders because coagulation times, fibrin degradation products and red blood cell morphology are normal. In mild cases no treatment is required. In severe cases where there is haemorrhage and very low platelet counts, a transfusion of platelet concentrate may be required.

Inherited coagulation factor deficiencies

Conditions such as haemophilia (Factor VIII deficiency) and Christmas disease (Factor IX deficiency) rarely cause problems in the neonatal period but may present with excessive bleeding after birth trauma or surgical intervention, e.g. circumcision. If there is a known family history, close observation of the infant is necessary and follow-up is arranged after discharge home.

Local causes of haemorrhage

Umbilical haemorrhage
This usually occurs due to a poorly applied cord ligature. The use of plastic cord clamps has almost eliminated this type of haemorrhage, although care is required in case the clamp catches or pulls. Tampering with partially separated cords before they are ready to come off should be discouraged. Cord haemorrhage is a potential cause of death. A purse string suture should always be inserted if umbilical bleeding does not stop after 15 or 20 minutes. It is a simple, life-saving measure.

Vaginal bleeding
A discharge of blood-stained mucus is common and is due to withdrawal of maternal oestrogen. Parents need reassurance that it is harmless. Continued or excessive bleeding warrants further investigation to exclude a pathological cause.

Haematemesis and melaena
These usually result when the baby has swallowed maternal blood during delivery or from cracked nipples during breast feeding. The diagnosis must be differentiated from haemorrhagic disease of the newborn. Other causes of haematemesis include oesophageal, gastric or duodenal ulceration while intestinal duplications, haemangiomas within the gut, necrotising enterocolitis and anal fissures are causes of blood in the stool. Stools can be tested for blood by using the simple 'Haemoccult' card.

Haematuria

Haematuria can be associated with coagulopathies, urinary tract infections and structural abnormality of the urinary tract. Birth trauma may cause renal contusion and haematuria. Occasionally after suprapubic aspiration of urine, transient mild haematuria may be observed.

Catheters

Umbilical, arterial and venous catheterisation, central venous lines, radial and femoral artery lines, and peripheral venous infusion sites all carry the potential danger of severe haemorrhage resulting from dislodgement of the catheter from the vessel or from accidental disconnection of the catheter from the administration infusion set. Close observation and careful handling of these infants is imperative to prevent this potentially fatal haemorrhage.

INTRACRANIAL HAEMORRHAGE

There are three important and often interrelated causal factors, namely prematurity, anoxia and trauma. Other predisposing factors such as congenital anomalies of the brain or cerebral blood vessels must not be overlooked. The injuries that lead to permanent damage range from the immediately obvious, like massive subdural haemorrhage or spinal cord injury, through minor degrees of intraventricular bleeding or cerebral oedema to those still obscure adverse influences on the brain which result in cerebral palsies, mental retardation, minor brain dysfunction syndromes or even mental illness. It must be emphasised that trauma can be purely mechanical in origin. The associations between the main types of intracranial haemorrhage, gestational age and precipitating events are shown in Table 37.2.

All areas of the brain can be affected. Large fatal subdural haemorrhages are now less common and intraventricular haemorrhage is the main form of trauma seen at autopsy (Levene et al 1985).

Types of haemorrhage

Subdural haemorrhage

This almost exclusively traumatic lesion is seen both at term and preterm (Volpe 1981). The soft, compressible skull of the preterm infant, precipitate labour, cephalopelvic disproportion, excessive compression of the fetal head during labour and forceps manoeuvres are predisposing factors. In a flexed vertex presentation compression of the head occurs along the occipitofrontal diameter and in a face or brow presentation between vault and skull base (Menkes 1984). The tentorium, or more rarely the falx cerebri, is stretched and torn, usually where the two membranes join, causing rupture or thrombosis of engorged dural sinuses and cerebral veins. Excessive overriding of the parietal bones may lead to laceration of the sagittal sinus. Signs of subdural haemorrhage are those associated with severe asphyxia, cerebral irritation and a bulging anterior fontanelle due to cerebral oedema. Diagnosis is confirmed by ultra-

Table 37.2
The association between main types of intracranial haemorrhage, gestational age and precipitating events (Modified from Philip A G S and Allan W C 1985 Neonatal intracranial haemorrhage and cerebral oedema. In: Crawford J W (ed) Risks of labour. John Wiley & Sons Ltd.)

Type of haemorrhage	Gestational age			Precipitating events	
	Term	Preterm	Very preterm	Trauma	Hypoxia
Subarachnoid	s	s	s	s	s
Subdural	s	u	u	c	u
Intraparenchymal	u	u	s	s	s
Intracerebellar	s	u	s	c	u
Intra(peri)ventricular	u	s	c	u	c

Key: u = uncommon; s = sometimes; c = common

sound examination. Subdural taps may be required to drain large collections of blood. Supportive treatment is geared towards controlling the consequences of asphyxia and raised intracranial pressure. In survivors, residual symptoms may range from none (50–80%) to a hyperalert state and sometimes focal signs with paralysis.

Subarachnoid haemorrhage

This haemorrhage occurs when small amounts of a capillary or venous bleeding take place in the subarachnoid space following mild trauma or asphyxia at delivery. It often goes undiagnosed as many babies are asymptomatic; consequently this form of haemorrhage appears less common than it really is. The condition is suspected at lumbar puncture when the cerebrospinal fluid is uniformly blood-stained. A subarachnoid haemorrhage does not usually show up on ultrasound scan but a scan should still be performed to rule out other types of intracranial haemorrhage. Treatment involves the control of the consequences of asphyxia and the control of convulsions. Hydrocephalus is a complication of subarachnoid haemorrhage and regular measurements of the occipitofrontal circumference should be made and charted. Ultrasound examination of intracranial structures should be made if hydrocephalus is suspected.

Intraparenchymal haemorrhage

This is bleeding into the cerebral tissue and may be a complication of disseminated intravascular coagulopathy (see above), of a central nervous system malformation, of birth asphyxia or of the extension of a subependymal haemorrhage (see below). Signs include cerebral irritation and convulsions. Diagnosis is usually made by ultrasound examination and computerised tomography (CT) scan. Intraparenchymal haemorrhage may be complicated by destruction of cerebral tissue and the formation of porencephalic cysts, and optimism for the longer term must be guarded. Treatment is usually symptomatic and aimed at controlling convulsions and cerebral oedema.

Periventricular-intraventricular haemorrhage

This is the most common and serious of all intracranial haemorrhages. It is a common cause of death in preterm infants of less than 32 weeks' gestation. The infant particularly at risk is one for whom the delivery has been complicated by asphyxia or trauma and who then develops severe respiratory distress requiring ventilatory support.

The stage of brain development in the preterm infant is a crucial factor in the aetiology of the periventricular-intraventricular haemorrhage. The germinal matrix surrounding the ventricles of the premature infant's brain consists of actively dividing cells. The germinal matrix is sometimes called the *subependymal layer*. Between about 24 and 32 weeks' gestation the blood vessels supplying the matrix are very prominent as a large proportion of cerebral blood flows to this vital area. After 32 weeks' gestation the matrix becomes less and less prominent and by term has involuted almost completely.

Bleeding usually occurs from rupture of the very fine capillaries around the germinal matrix giving rise to a periventricular or subependymal haemorrhage. An intraventricular haemorrhage develops when the subependymal haemorrhage ruptures into the ventricular system. A subependymal haemorrhage can also extend into the cerebral tissue giving rise to a cerebral or intraparenchymal haemorrhage.

Predisposing factors include:

— birth asphyxia or trauma
— prematurity
— severe respiratory distress
— hypotension or hypertension
— hypoxia or hyperkapnia
— pneumothorax.

A small subependymal haemorrhage may have no clinical features. If the subependymal haemorrhage increases or extends, the clinical features may include the following:

— increasing frequency and severity of apnoeic episodes
— pallor
— poor peripheral circulation
— tonic convulsions
— decerebrate posturing
— the appearance of divergent squinting.

If the periventricular-intraventricular haemorrhage is large and sudden in onset, the infant may present with apnoea and circulatory collapse leading rapidly to death. If the baby's condition stabilises the fontanelle may be enlarged and tense and the baby will require active resuscitation and ventilatory support if he is to survive.

The clinical features of a severe haemorrhage are virtually diagnostic but suspicions may be confirmed by cranial ultrasound. The portable instruments in use today are so advanced that it is possible to grade the degree of haemorrhage:

Grade I	Germinal layer haemorrhage
Grade II	Intraventricular haemorrhage with normal ventricles
Grade III	Intraventricular haemorrhage with distended ventricles
Grade IV	Intraparenchymal extension.

This grading is important as the degree of haemorrhage correlates with the longer term outcome for the infant and in Grades III and IV the prognosis for the infant may be poor (see Figs 37.8–37.10). CT scanning, although another excellent means of diagnosis, is now less frequently used as it usually necessitates moving a critically ill infant to the X-ray department. Lumbar or ventricular puncture is seldom required.

Prevention plays as important a part as treatment. It begins with a high standard of midwifery

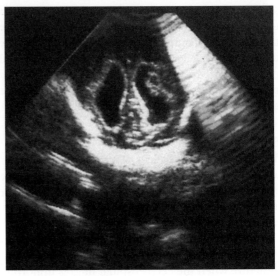

Fig. 37.9
Shows a subependymal haemorrhage extending into the lateral ventricle giving rise to an intraventricular haemorrhage. Both lateral ventricles are markedly dilated secondary to post-haemorrhagic hydrocephalus.

care aimed at avoiding asphyxia, followed by a high standard of neonatal intensive care aimed at preventing further extension of the haemorrhage. The latter includes minimal handling of the infant, secure stabilisation of the endotracheal tube, the use of appropriate ventilator settings and the use of pancuronium to reduce the risk of pneumothorax.

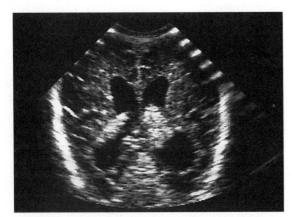

Fig. 37.8
Post-haemorrhagic hydrocephalus following intraventricular haemorrhage. Both lateral ventricles are markedly dilated.

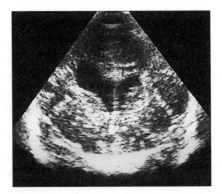

Fig. 37.10
Porencephalic cyst resulting from extension of liquified periventricular haemorrhage into the frontal horn of the left lateral ventricle.

Management includes nursing the infant in an intensive care area with full monitoring facilities. If possible, a quiet place is found where the infant is nursed naked in an incubator which will provide warmth and ease of observation. The use of apnoea mattresses, cardiorators, transcutaneous oxygen monitors and electronic blood pressure machines help to keep handling to a minimum. Resuscitation equipment and suction apparatus should always be at hand. Feeding may be given by tube and fluid requirements may be restricted initially. If oral feeds are not tolerated intravenous therapy may be necessary. Urinary output must be observed and if the baby is sedated his bladder may require manual expression. Care must be taken to prevent skin trauma from leads and probes and their position must be changed regularly. If the baby is anaemic a blood transfusion may be required. Acidosis may require correction. If convulsions occur, phenobarbitone and phenytoin may be given. In spite of good intensive care, babies with large haemorrhages usually die within 48 hours of the onset. Those who survive often develop hydrocephalus which, if severe, may require regular drainage of cerebrospinal fluid by ventricular puncture until surgery can be attempted and a shunt inserted.

Prognosis for babies with small haemorrhages is usually good even if there is ventricular dilatation. Babies with larger haemorrhages and no ventricular dilatation usually recover but if dilatation is present they do less well. Those infants with massive haemorrhages usually suffer from multiple seizures, cerebral atrophy or rapidly developing hydrocephalus. Long-term follow up is necessary and parents need much support.

Cerebral palsy

This is a neurological syndrome characterised by disordered movement, posture, tone and power and is often associated with intellectual deficit and epilepsy.

Perinatal asphyxia and prematurity are the two major presumptive causes. In a study carried out by the Scottish Council for the Care of Spastics which looked at the association between perinatal abnormality and cerebral palsy only 6% were caused by birth trauma.

The aim of modern management of the handicapped child is early recognition and full multidisciplinary assessment followed by appropriate therapy including counselling of the child's family. Obstetric practice is beset by worries about medical negligence; birth injury is a much less common cause of cerebral palsy than is often supposed and appears to have a minor role in its aetiology (Acheson 1991).

CONVULSIONS

Convulsions in the neonate can be more difficult to recognise than those of later infancy and childhood. They may be tonic when the body and limbs become stiff and rigid with arching of the back, or clonic in nature with repetitive movements and may be focal or generalised. They may be accompanied by apnoeic, cyanotic and bradycardic episodes which may be more obvious than the actual convulsion. In some cases abnormal eye movements and sucking movements will be the only indication.

The major conditions giving rise to neonatal convulsions are listed in Table 37.3.

As can be seen from Table 37.3 some of the predisposing factors can overlap making further investigation necessary.

Investigations include:

- blood glucose (test strip or in laboratory)
- plasma electrolytes
- plasma calcium and magnesium
- haemoglobin
- white blood count and differential
- blood culture
- lumbar puncture.

If the above investigations are inconclusive the following investigations may also be required:

- skull X-ray
- cranial ultrasound
- CT scan
- electro-encephalogram.

As the fits may differ in length, severity and type, it is important for the midwife to observe the

Table 37.3
Major causes of neonatal convulsions
(Reproduced with permission from Roberton N R C 1986 A manual of neonatal intensive care. Edward Arnold, London.)

Diagnosis	Age at presentation and type of fit	Differential diagnosis
Hypoxic-ischaemic encephalopathy	0–72 hours, usually clonic, may be tonic or subtle	History of intrapartum asphyxia
With cerebral oedema	As above	As above + bulging fontanelle, head retraction
With subarachnoid or subdural haemorrhage	As above	As above + blood on lumbar puncture
Periventricular-intraventricular haemorrhage	24–72 hours, usually subtle or short tonic	Rare >1.5 kg: often in infants with severe RDS or recurrent apnoea Decreased PCV. CSF blood-stained Blood in ventricles on ultrasound
Meningitis	Any time and any type of fit	Associated signs of sepsis: lumbar puncture
Metabolic Hypoglycaemic	Usually <72 hours; clonic	Small-for-dates infant, preterm baby. If later, suggests rare cause of hypoglycaemia
Hypocalcaemia	< 48 hours tonic or clonic 5–8 days, multifocal clonic	Usually seriously ill infant High phosphate intake
Hyponatraemia	Any age, usually clonic	Usually an oedematous, sick preterm baby
Hypernatraemia	Any age, usually clonic	Usually sick, dehydrated preterm baby
Rare inborn errors of metabolism	Usually <72 hours; any type of fit	Often apnoeic, hypotonic: positive family history
Kernicterus	Any time, any type of fit	Associated with severe jaundice
Congenital malformation	Any time, any type of fit	Other physical signs and stigmata
Drug withdrawal	Usually <1 week; usually clonic	Mother's drug history
Idiopathic	Any time, usually clonic	By exclusion

convulsions carefully and to note the infant's general behaviour. A typical chart for recording the findings is shown (Fig. 37.11). Jitteriness differs from convulsions, being characterised by fine tremor of the limbs as opposed to convulsive movements. It is often of no significance when seen in an agitated, hungry, alert baby. Unlike convulsions it is often stimulated or made worse by disturbance, and can be stopped by flexing the affected limb. However, it can be a sign of some pathological disorder and should not be entirely disregarded.

Date	Time	Type (clonic, tonic)	Region(s) involved	Apnoea	Cyanosis	Duration

Fig. 37.11
Convulsion chart.

Immediate treatment of the convulsion necessitates turning the infant to the semi-prone position, thereby keeping the tongue from falling back and obstructing the airway. Gentle oral suction removes any milk or mucus from the mouth and pharynx. If cyanosed, oxygen is given by face mask at a rate of 2–3 litres per minute. Medical aid will already have been summoned. Resuscitation equipment should be at hand in case apnoea and cyanosis persist. Capillary glucose should be estimated to exclude hypoglycaemia. Further management includes minimal handling and allowing the infant to rest. The baby should be nursed unclothed in an incubator for ease of observation and maintenance of a neutral thermal environment. Anticonvulsant therapy may be commenced. Drugs initially used may include phenobarbitone, phenytoin and paraldehyde. Other anticonvulsants such as diazepam should be held in reserve for cases in which control of seizures proves difficult. Restoring correct levels of blood sugar, electrolytes, calcium and magnesium may be the only treatment required. Parents require adequate explanation and support.

Reader Activities

- A mother is very anxious because her baby has a cephalhaematoma. Using a diagram, write down how you would explain to this mother what a cephalhaematoma is, any treatment required and the outcome.
- A mother you are looking after in the labour suite requests that her baby is not given an injection of vitamin K after he is born. Discuss with an experienced midwife the advice you would give this mother.
- Parents are visiting their baby in the Special Care Baby Unit. The baby suddenly has a generalised convulsion. Devise an immediate action plan. What reassurance can you give to the parents of this baby while they are waiting to speak to the paediatrician?

USEFUL ADDRESSES

Spastics Society
12 Park Crescent
London W1N 4EQ
Tel: 071 636 5020

Scottish Council for Spastics
22 Corstorphine Road
Edinburgh EH12 6HP
Tel: 031 337 9876

Haemophilia Society
123 Westminster Bridge Road
London SE1 7HR
Tel: 071 928 2020

REFERENCES

Acheson D 1991 Are obstetrics and midwifery doomed? Midwives Chronicle 104 (1241): 158–165
Levene M L et al 1985 Ultrasound of the infant brain. Spastics International Medical Publications, Oxford
Menkes J H 1984 Perinatal trauma and asphyxia. In: Avery M E, Taeusch H W (eds) Schaffer's Diseases of the newborn. W B Saunders, London, p 661–679

Philip A G S, Allan W C 1985 Neonatal intracranial haemorrhage and cerebral oedema. In: Crawford J W (ed) Risks of labour. John Wiley, Chichester, p 95–117
Roberton N R C 1986 A manual of neonatal intensive care, 2nd edn. Edward Arnold, London, p 236
Rowley J 1984 A watershed of ideas. People 11: 4–7
Shenaq S M, Dinh T A 1990 Paediatric microsurgery. Clinics in Plastic Surgery 17(1): 79–83
SMR11 Information, Courtesy of Dr S K Cole 1991
Volpe J J 1981 Neurology of the newborn. W B Saunders, Philadelphia
Walker C H M 1985 Birth trauma. In: Crawford J W (ed) Risks of labour. John Wiley, Chichester, p 71–93

FURTHER READING

Geirsson R T 1988 Birth trauma and brain damage. Clinical Obstetrics and Gynaecology 2(1): 195–212
Kelnar C J H, Harvey D 1988 The sick newborn baby, 2nd edn. Baillière Tindall, London
Roberton N R C 1986 A manual of neonatal intensive care, 2nd edn. Edward Arnold, London
Trip J H, Mc Ninch A W 1987 Haemorrhagic disease and vitamin K. Archives of Disease in Childhood 62: 436–437
Vulliamy D G 1987 The newborn child, 6th edn. Churchill Livingstone, Edinburgh

38

Metabolic disorders and congenital abnormalities

JOHNANNA MATTHEW

Metabolic disorders
Drug dependency
Congenital abnormalities

The birth of a child who has any sort of abnormality is devastating for the parents. The incidence of babies born with abnormalities is falling, due to prenatal screening (see Ch. 41) and terminations of pregnancy. Early postnatal screening can limit the damage associated with some metabolic disorders.

Preconception care (see Ch. 7) may offer ways of preventing abnormality. Parents are encouraged to avoid drugs, including nicotine and alcohol, which are harmful.

The midwife can educate parents to follow a healthy life-style before and during pregnancy. She may play a part in detecting abnormality and can be a tremendous support to parents who have to cope with an adverse diagnosis, by using listening and helping skills (see Ch. 49).

METABOLIC DISORDERS

Inborn errors of metabolism

An inborn error of metabolism is a permanent, inherited condition which is due to an enzyme abnormality. The result of this abnormality is an alteration in metabolic pathways causing increased or decreased levels of chemical compounds. Given the complex system of human metabolism it is not surprising that errors occur from time to time and many such errors have now been identified.

Some of these errors can lead to mental retardation and poor growth and development of the child unless treatment is initiated promptly. In this chapter the commonest of these inborn errors will be considered.

Screening

Procedures have been developed to detect the commoner conditions and this allows prompt initiation of the necessary treatment. The test most frequently used is the *Guthrie test* in which blood, dropped on to filter paper, is examined using microbiological techniques. The *Scriver test* involves chromatographic examination of blood.

Phenylketonuria

This is an autosomal recessive condition occurring in about 1 in 10 000 children but there is a geographical variation. Amino-acid metabolism is disordered because of the absence or deficiency of the enzyme *phenylalanine hydroxylase* which is normally responsible for the conversion of *phenylalanine* to *tyrosine* in the liver.

Because of the failure of conversion, phenylalanine levels rise and although some will be excreted in the urine, most is converted to *phenylpyruvic acid*, which is responsible for the mental retardation associated with this condition.

The rise of phenylalanine in the blood is found within a few days of birth after the baby is subjected to dietary protein. The build-up of the dangerous phenylpyruvic acid takes longer and without treatment mental retardation results.

Clinical features. At birth the baby looks and behaves normally. Often this infant has blue eyes and fair skin and hair. A 'musty' odour develops and often eczema is present.

Diagnosis is on routine blood collection for the *metabolic screening test*. This should be taken between the 6th and 14th days of life (normally Day 8) once the baby has been on milk feeds.

Management. A low phenylalanine diet is prescribed and milk substitutes have been developed for the newly born baby. *Minafen, Analog XP* and *Lofenalac* milks will be used with iron and vitamin supplements. During the school years the child can usually graduate to a normal diet but follow-up care is important.

Prognosis is good if parents adhere to the instructions given. In females, a return to the diet is essential prior to conception and during pregnancy. Fetal damage may be caused by exposure to high concentrations of phenylalanine and its metabolites in the mother.

Galactosaemia

This is also an autosomal recessive condition occurring in 1 in 66 000 children. There is an inability to convert *galactose* to *glucose* with resultant increased galactose and reduced glucose levels in the blood. Toxic by-products of galactose can damage the lens of the eye, the liver, the kidneys and the brain. In severe cases death will occur within a few weeks following liver failure. Mental retardation and behavioural problems can be the result of untreated galactosaemia.

Clinical features. At birth the baby appears normal although cataracts may be present. Once milk feeds (either breast or bottle) are given the infant's condition deteriorates. Reluctance to feed, vomiting and diarrhoea develop with resultant weight loss and dehydration. The liver is found to be enlarged and jaundice is persistent. Haemolysis and deficient clotting factors will lead to anaemia and purpura.

Diagnosis. Screening using the blood sample collected for the phenylketonuria screening test is normally carried out. Finding reducing substances in the urine of a sick baby will alert the paediatrician to a need for the blood test.

Management. *Galactomin 17* milk has been developed for these babies and all soya milk preparations may be used. As the baby grows, specially prepared low galactose foodstuffs are used. With the removal of galactose from the diet, the disease corrects itself, but damage to organs which has already been sustained, cannot be corrected.

Prognosis. It would appear that a life-long, galactose-free diet is indicated for those affected. Non-adherence to the diet has resulted in older children showing evidence of deterioration.

Hypothyroidism

Congenital hypothyroidism occurs in approximately 1 in 4000 children. Low circulating levels of thyroid hormone result in impaired intellectual and motor function because of abnormal brain development. This serious situation gives rise to the condition of cretinism.

When the low hormone levels are associated with abnormal thyroid function, the cause is metabolic in origin, and these have been found to have a strong familial tendency. Research indicates that this is an autosomal recessive condition. Failure of development of the thyroid gland may also occur and this is thought to be due to some genetic factor.

Clinical features. There are different degrees of hypothyroidism depending on the amount of thyroid hormone being produced. Severe cretinism shows a typical appearance of coarse facial expression with a low hairline. The forehead is wrinkled and the nasal bridge flat. The neck is short and thick and may disguise the goitre which is present. The extremities are broad. Untreated, cretinism is associated with severe mental defi-

ciency. Milder forms of cretinism may go unnoticed for some time.

Diagnosis. Screening can be conveniently carried out using blood collected for the phenylketonuria screening test and this type of screening procedure is well established in the UK. T4 (thyroid hormone) and TSH (thyroid stimulating hormone) assays will be carried out in all positive cases detected prior to treatment being commenced.

Treatment. Replacement treatment using thyroxine is started as soon as possible.

Prognosis. Normal or near-normal intellectual development can be expected if treatment is instituted quickly but those infants who have complete absence of thyroid tissue will have a less favourable outcome. Genetic counselling should be offered to parents before they embark on another pregnancy.

Neonatal thyrotoxicosis

This is a rare complication found in babies delivered of mothers suffering from hyperthyroidism. When the mother has been treated with antithyroid preparations during pregnancy the baby will take about 3 days to develop signs but in uncontrolled cases, hyperthyroidism is evident at birth.

Clinical features. The baby will be restless and may have exophthalmos. He will be flushed, warm and sweaty with tachycardia evident. A goitre will be seen. The baby's appetite is good but weight gain is poor. Diagnosis is made on checking serum levels of thyroid hormones.

Treatment and prognosis. Prognosis is good if treatment is started quickly. Potassium iodide is given but if serious signs are apparent, then carbimazole may be required.

Congenital adrenal hyperplasia

Adrenal hyperplasia is a rare autosomal recessive condition in which excessive growth of the adrenal cortex occurs. This can affect either sex but is more frequently seen in males. Abnormal genitalia are found due to excessive androgenic hormone production and an associated adrenal insufficiency can develop with resultant salt and water loss. The male child is more prone to this latter problem.

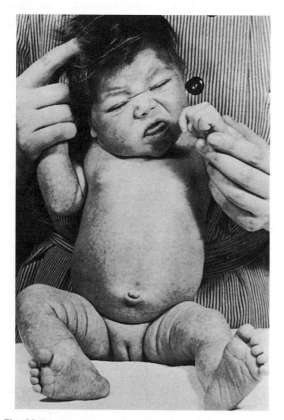

Fig. 38.1
Severe cretinism in 6-week-old infant. (Forfar & Arneil, vol 2, 1984).

Diagnosis. Abnormal genitalia may be found at birth in female children but in males, excessive growth of genitalia may not be noticed for some months. Poor weight gain might be the first indication of abnormality but if there is acute salt and water loss, dehydration will result and eventually peripheral vascular collapse. Confirmation of the diagnosis is made on biochemical investigation.

Management and prognosis. Correction of fluid and electrolyte balance is the first priority. Once the initial crisis is over, cortisone may be given to suppress the androgenic hormones. Prognosis is poor if untreated, but if corrected, these children will survive on a maintenance dose of cortisone and additional salt in their diet.

Acquired metabolic disorders

Hypoglycaemia

This is the commonest acquired metabolic disorder and is a consequence of insufficient stores of glycogen or of overuse of these stores. Neonatal hypoglycaemia occurs when blood sugar levels are less than 1.5 mmol/l in full-term infants (a level of 2.2 mmol/l after 72 hours).

In the first 72 hours of life there is normally a sharp drop in glycogen stores in the liver but the healthy newborn can compensate for this. Once oral feeding is established the baby can begin to store glycogen again.

Early detection of hypoglycaemia is necessary because it may cause brain damage.

Infants at risk.

- *Hypoxic infants*: carbohydrate metabolism is upset by oxygen lack and excessive metabolism of glycogen occurs.
- *Low birthweight babies*, especially light-for-dates infants, but also preterm babies whose glycogen levels are low.
- *Babies of diabetic mothers* who have been subjected in utero to high sugar concentrations from their mothers. Insulin production is high and takes some time after birth to return to normal.
- *Hypothermia*: metabolism is upset because glucose is consumed in order to produce energy for heat production.

Signs. The baby is lethargic and reluctant to feed. Jitteriness and irritability may be found in handling. Apnoeic attacks and convulsions may occur.

Management. The midwife must be aware of those infants who are at risk and use some form of screening test to detect this condition. The capillary blood glucose level can be estimated using a test strip such as Dextrostix or BM-Test-Glycemie. A true blood sugar estimation will be carried out if this test proves that blood glucose is low. The aim is to commence treatment before signs appear.

Treatment is by administration of glucose feeds by the oral or intravenous route, depending on the condition of the baby. This will be continued until the blood glucose levels are stable.

Prognosis is favourable unless the hypoglycaemia is particularly severe and symptomatic. Damage may not be found until the child is older, therefore there is a need for follow-up care. Later assessment sometimes shows poor scholastic performance.

Hyperglycaemia

Neonatal diabetes mellitus is very rarely seen. A blood sugar level of over 8.3 mmol/l would arouse suspicion. The cause is thought to be immaturity of the pancreatic islets with a resultant insulin deficiency. Treatment is with insulin, carefully monitored because of the danger of inducing hypoglycaemia. The treatment continues until the condition is resolved. This can take anything from a few days to several months. Iatrogenic hyperglycaemia may result from intravenous therapy.

Hypocalcaemia

This is a condition in which the serum calcium level falls below 1.8 mmol/l in babies fed on cow's milk and below 2.0 mmol/l in breast-fed babies.

It rarely occurs during the first 72 hours of life but may be found in low birthweight infants or infants who have been asphyxiated at birth. The prognosis for these infants is poor.

After 72 hours the cause is most likely to be an excess of phosphorus. Cow's milk has a high phosphorus content and any excess is normally excreted via the kidney. The neonatal kidney cannot cope with the high load presented to it and there is a build-up of phosphorus in the bloodstream. Normally phosphorus and calcium are kept in balance, but a high phosphorus level results in malabsorption of calcium.

The baby displays signs of irritability with fine, rapid, jerky movements and convulsions may occur.

Management is to give oral calcium gluconate as indicated.

Hypercalcaemia

Hypercalcaemia is a rare complication of the newborn infant in which there is an abnormal sensitivity to excessive vitamin D. The high calcium levels can lead to renal damage and pathological changes in the heart. Mild forms of this condition are not usually detected until the child is some months old but more severe states will be seen within the first month.

Management is with a low calcium diet (*Locasol* milk) and a reduction in vitamin D. Steroids may be used to impair absorption of calcium from the alimentary tract.

Hypomagnesaemia

This condition may occur along with hypocalcaemia and the signs are identical. When the serum calcium level is being checked it is usual to check the magnesium level as well. Newborn babies who vomit or have diarrhoea will deplete their magnesium stores.

Treatment is with intramuscular or intravenous magnesium sulphate after which a dramatic return to normal is seen. The prognosis is good.

Hyponatraemia

This occurs when the serum sodium concentration falls below 120 mmol/l. If the mother herself has had a low serum sodium level, the infant is likely to follow suit. Water retention or excessive salt loss during the neonatal period will also result in hyponatraemia.

Extremely low birthweight infants are particularly at risk because their immature kidneys allow high salt loss and have a limited ability to excrete water.

The infant may be lethargic, irritable and suffer tremors and convulsions.

Management. If the baby is oedematous, fluid intake will be limited and a saline solution can be given intravenously. If there is associated dehydration, both sodium and water are required. Very careful calibration of fluids is required.

Hypernatraemia

Hypernatraemia is the situation when the serum sodium level rises above 150 mmol/l. This may be due to excessive intake of sodium or to excessive water loss. The baby is usually dehydrated and may sustain a cerebral haemorrhage if the condition goes unchecked. This condition is unusual in the newborn infant but it can be found where there is increased insensible water loss which occurs in infants nursed under radiant heaters and in babies receiving phototherapy. The cause may be iatrogenic as a result of intravenous therapy or injudicious administration of sodium bicarbonate.

Management. Careful restoration of fluid and electrolyte balance must be attempted. Mortality rates are high and brain damage is common, despite treatment.

Prevention is of vital importance in this condition. Babies who are exposed to radiant heat or phototherapy need extra fluid. As the incorrect reconstitution of baby milks can result in a concentrated feed high in sodium, it is part of the midwife's role to educate parents to follow the manufacturer's instructions meticulously. Artificial milk products are safe if they are made up properly and it is the midwife's duty to ensure that all parents are able to cope with this task.

DRUG DEPENDENCY

There is an increasing incidence of babies being delivered of mothers who are addicted to narcotics. These infants are of low birthweight and exhibit withdrawal symptoms.

These symptoms are hyperirritability, restlessness, feeding difficulties, high pitched cry and convulsions. When complicated by prematurity they can be fatal. The onset of symptoms can occur any time from the 1st to the 3rd day of life and is possibly dependent on the time of the mother's last dose of narcotic, which may have been pethidine given during labour.

Management by weaning the child from the drug using methadone in decreasing amounts is less frequently used today. Anticonvulsant drugs are used when indicated. Once the child has been weaned from the narcotic influence, normal care is given. A social work report on suitability of the mother to care for her child is recommended. This baby may be at risk of maltreatment and malnourishment if the mother continues her habit.

Fetal alcohol syndrome

Over the past 25 years an increasing concern has been expressed about the effects of maternal alcohol use on the fetus. The term 'fetal alcohol syndrome' is used to describe the characteristic pattern of features displayed by infants delivered of women who consume alcohol to excess during pregnancy.

Clinical features

Marked intra-uterine growth retardation is found and subsequently all parameters of growth are reduced, especially length.

The eyes are small with exaggerated epicanthic folds. The philtrum is shallow or absent and the nasal bridge poorly formed. The ears appear large. The baby may show signs of alcohol withdrawal and can be fretful with resultant difficulty in feeding.

Between 29 and 50% have an associated heart defect and 40% a musculoskeletal abnormality. Other abnormalities have also been found such as cleft palate, atresias and skin lesions. The infants are found to be of low intelligence verging on moderate mental deficiency. They are clumsy children who may display tremors and have learning and behavioural problems.

Prevention

A 'safe' level of maternal alcohol consumption is still unknown. Alcohol crosses to the fetus once the placenta is formed and concentrations in the fetus have been found to be similar to those in the mother. It is as yet unclear how the damage to organs occurs. Unfortunately it is not always possible to identify those women at risk of producing an affected infant. Effective preconception care and careful antenatal screening would help to reduce the problems (see also Ch. 7).

Management of the baby

The baby suspected of having fetal alcohol syndrome should be closely monitored. It is likely that he or she will be raised in a poor environment, especially if parents continue to drink heavily. The infant's potential, both physically and mentally, is limited.

CONGENITAL ABNORMALITIES

All prospective parents look forward to the delivery of a healthy normal child and the delivery of an abnormal child brings with it acute feelings of disappointment, guilt and sometimes revulsion. The midwife must approach this situation with great care because the parents frequently suffer a reaction akin to the grief reaction (see Ch. 49) which requires careful handling. Attending staff also suffer because they too have had the expectation of a normal baby and recognition of this will help the midwife to cope with her own feelings in this stressful situation.

Any defect of form, structure or function occurring during conception or in fetal life is termed a congenital abnormality. Some of these are slight and cause little problem to the child or parents but some are profound and cause the daily care of the child to be fraught with difficulties. A few will require immediate surgery or other treatment which necessitates removal of the baby from its mother almost immediately after birth.

Recognition of abnormality often rests with the midwife who examines the baby at birth. Some defects are not detected until the baby is some days old and will be found on subsequent examination by the midwife. When the midwife finds any abnormal condition of the baby she must inform the doctor.

Causes of abnormality

The causes of abnormality are not fully understood but they can be divided into two important groups.

Genetic or inherited causes

When there is a defect in the genetic material contained in the ovum or sperm an abnormality will result. If the genetic mixture is particularly poor, the pregnancy will end in abortion. Less extensive defects will result in the birth of a child with an abnormality. Examples include Down's syndrome, achondroplasia and phenylketonuria.

Environmental factors

In intra-uterine life the developing embryo is dependent on its mother for all its sustenance, and deprivation of materials which are essential for normal development can lead to abnormality. The very small delicate organs have little resistance to infection or noxious substances which can reach them through the placenta. If an adverse factor reaches the embryo at a time when body organs are forming, these organs can be damaged.

Hypoxia. A constant supply of oxygen is essential for correct development and if some factor interferes with this supply the embryo is unable to develop normally. Maternal health is therefore vitally important to the health of her growing embryo.

Infection. Rubella, cytomegalovirus and Coxsackie B virus will all affect the unborn child. Immunisation of schoolgirls against rubella has prevented much of the abnormality from this condition but cardiac, eye and ear defects can still be found in the babies of non-immune mothers who contract rubella during pregnancy.

Radiation. Radio-active substances have a harmful effect on the fetus. Women whose work brings them into contact with radiation are advised to discontinue this employment prior to pregnancy. Diagnostic radiography is avoided in pregnancy as far as possible.

Drugs. Certain drugs taken by the mother in early pregnancy can cause abnormality. Great care is exercised when prescribing drugs for the pregnant woman and midwives should advise women not to take drugs or medicines unless prescribed by a doctor. Alcohol and nicotine use must be included in any discussion about drugs and midwives involved in preconception care (see Ch. 7) will advise parents about the possible harmful effects of these.

Detection of abnormality

Some abnormalities can be detected prenatally and screening procedures are now in use (see Ch. 41). Often, however, it is not until an infant is born that an abnormality is found. The urgency of diagnosis and treatment depends upon the degree of risk associated with the abnormality. The midwife must be able to recognise abnormalities and refer the baby promptly for appropriate care.

This chapter will concentrate on those conditions which the midwife must be able to recognise in order to give immediate, appropriate treatment.

Malformations of the central nervous system

Hydrocephaly. An excess of cerebrospinal fluid in the ventricles of the brain is caused by some obstruction in the cerebrospinal fluid pathway. This may be detected prenatally on ultrasound examination or in labour when, on vaginal examination, wide sutures and fontanelles are felt. However these fetuses frequently present by the breech and hydrocephaly may not be diagnosed until the head is unable to enter the pelvis during the second stage of labour.

Hydrocephaly may develop after birth and would be suspected when abnormal growth of the head is identified. Widening of the lambdoidal suture will be found. The increase in intracranial pressure causes the eyes to roll downwards giving them a 'setting sun' appearance (Fig. 38.2).

If this condition is diagnosed in labour a destructive operation may be necessary to effect delivery. If an infant born with hydrocephalus survives, he may be mentally subnormal. Draining of the excess fluid from the lateral ventricle of the brain into the right atrium can be achieved using a valve mechanism.

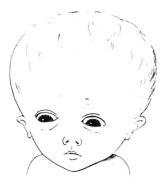

Fig. 38.2
'Setting-sun' eyes of hydrocephalic baby.

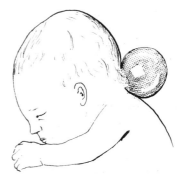

Fig. 38.4
Meningocele.

Anencephaly. This is a major malformation of the skull and brain which is incompatible with life. The cranial vault is missing and the cerebral hemispheres are missing or are reduced to small masses attached to the skull. This abnormality is easily identified by the midwife. Prenatal screening of maternal blood for raised alpha fetoprotein levels will suggest an open neural tube defect and if anencephaly is diagnosed on further investigation termination of pregnancy is offered (see Ch. 41). If pregnancy continues beyond 28 weeks' gestation, labour may be induced. The fetus often presents by the face or the breech and 75% are female. Parents should be gently encouraged

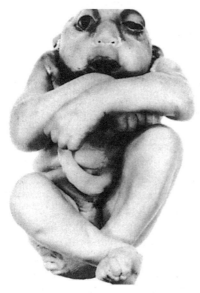

Fig. 38.3
Anencephalic baby.

to attend for genetic advice before embarking on another pregnancy (see Ch. 7).

Microcephaly. The vault of the skull is small and there is an associated reduction in the amount of brain tissue. This can be caused by rubella infection or it may be an autosomal recessive condition. The child will be mentally retarded.

Encephalocele. This tumour, covered with meninges, protrudes through the lambdoidal suture on the fetal skull. An encephalocele contains brain tissue. It pulsates, is opaque, does not fluctuate and usually has a pedicle. A similar swelling which contains no brain tissue but consists of meninges and contains cerebrospinal fluid is termed a *meningocele*. It is fluctuant, does not pulsate and becomes tense when the baby cries. Large meningoceles may rupture during delivery. The baby should be nursed prone with the sac covered with a sterile dressing until the doctor arrives. The meningocele may be aspirated.

Spina bifida. This is a defect in the vertebral column due to failure of the neural arches to unite. There are differing degrees of severity. In *occult spina bifida* the defect is small with no

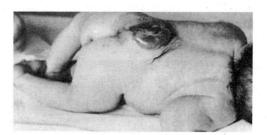

Fig. 38.5
Spina bifida.

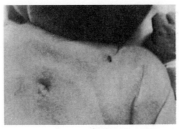

Fig. 38.6
Spina bifida occulta showing slight dimpling of skin.

herniation present; a slight dimpling of the skin may be evident. *Meningocele* is a herniation of the meninges and may be closed, i.e. covered with skin, or open.

A *myelomeningocele* is a protrusion of both meninges and spinal cord.

Open defects can be suspected prenatally when an increased alpha fetoprotein level is found in maternal serum (see Ch. 41).

Ultrasonography may also be useful in diagnosis. The commonest form is easily recognised at birth by the presence of a reddish mass in the sacrolumbar region. Movement of the lower limbs may be impaired and the presence of a patulous anus and continuously dribbling urine suggests damage to the nerves which supply the bowel and bladder.

The midwife must notify the doctor, apply a non-adherent dressing to any exposed tissue and observe the movements of the baby. Surgery may be possible if the degree of neurological involvement is not considered to be severe. Subsequent to the operation to repair a myelomeningocele half of the infants develop hydrocephaly. Parents should be directed towards preconception care before embarking on another pregnancy and may be interested in joining the local branch of the Association for Spina Bifida and Hydrocephalus (ASBAH).

Gastro-intestinal malformations

Cleft lip and palate

These are fairly common abnormalities of which the incidence is approximately 1 in 1000 births but there is geographical variation. Clefts occur due to failure of union in the development of the face and mouth. Defects may occur in the lip or palate alone or may be combined. Bilateral clefts are sometimes found.

The midwife will easily recognise cleft lip but cleft palate can be more difficult to identify.

Cleft lip is an unsightly abnormality and care should be taken when showing the baby to parents at birth. The immediate problem is one of feeding as it is difficult for the baby to suck and swallow. When the palate is affected, an orthodontic plate can provide a false palate. A flanged teat or a spoon may be used for feeding until a suitable plate is made.

Plastic surgery is required to correct the defects. An operation to close the cleft of the lip is usually carried out at 3–4 months of age while closure of the palate is deferred until 12–15 months. In order to allay some of their anxieties, parents can be shown 'after' and 'before' pictures of children who have had successful operations. Parents should also have adequate instruction and experience in feeding their baby prior to discharge.

Pierre Robin syndrome. The child with this syndrome has a central cleft palate and *micrognathia* (underdevelopment of the mandibular processes). The receding jaw leads to further difficulties in feeding and also respiratory problems.

The airway must be kept clear. It may be sufficient to nurse the infant in the prone position but it may be necessary to suspend the head in order to prevent the tongue from obstructing the airway until the lower jaw has grown to more normal proportions.

Atresias

Oesophageal atresia. This occurs when there is incomplete canalisation of the oesophagus in early intra-uterine development. It is commonly associated with a *tracheo-oesophageal fistula* which connects the trachea to the upper or lower oesophagus or occasionally both. The commonest type of abnormality is where the upper oesophagus terminates in a blind pouch and the lower oesophagus connects to the trachea.

This abnormality should be suspected in the presence of maternal polyhydramnios. At birth

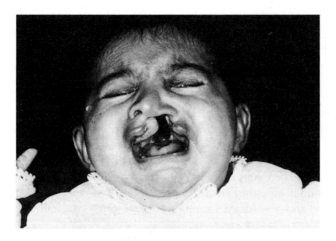

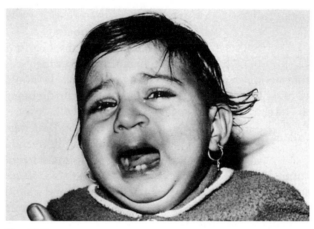

Fig. 38.7
Cleft lip and palate in an Asian child before and after operative correction. (Turner et al 1988.)

the baby has copious amounts of mucus coming from the mouth. Early detection is essential and an orogastric tube must be passed but it will travel less than 10–12 cm. Radiography will be used to confirm the diagnosis. *The baby must be given no oral fluid.* He should be transferred immediately to a paediatric surgical unit. It may be possible to anastomose the blind ends of the oesophagus. If the distance between them is too large, a transplant will be needed at a later date and the baby will be fed via a gastrostomy.

Duodenal atresia. Atresia may occur at any level of the bowel but the duodenum is the most common site. Persistent vomiting occurs within 24–36 hours of birth and is the first feature encountered. The vomit often contains bile. As

the obstruction is high up, abdominal distension may not be present and meconium may be passed.

Radiography is used to detect the obstruction and treatment is by surgical repair of the atresia. Prognosis is good if the baby is otherwise healthy but this abnormality is often associated with others (30% of cases occur in children with Down's syndrome).

Rectal atresia and imperforate anus. An imperforate anus should be obvious at birth on examination of the baby but a rectal atresia might not become apparent until difficulty is encountered when inserting a rectal thermometer. A recto-urethral fistula (in boys) or a recto-vaginal fistula (in girls) may complicate the situation. Surgery will be used to restore patency of the bowel and to close any fistulae.

Diaphragmatic hernia

Herniation of abdominal contents into the thoracic cavity occurs through a defect in the diaphragm. This is an acute emergency. Respiratory distress and cyanosis are present at birth and resuscitation is difficult. There will be reduced respiratory movement and heart sounds are displaced. X-ray will confirm the diagnosis. Continuous gastric suction should be commenced to prevent further distension and the infant immediately transferred for surgery. The mortality rate is high and death usually occurs because of underdevelopment of the lung.

Cardiac malformations

The signs of cardiac malformation may not be evident until some weeks after birth and heart murmurs found at birth might prove to be insignificant.

Cyanotic heart lesions

Fallot's tetralogy and transposition of the great vessels are the commonest causes of cyanotic lesions. The presence of cyanosis renders these abnormalities more easily recognisable than the acyanotic lesions although cyanotic heart defects account for only one-third of all cases.

Cyanosis occurs because blood bypasses the lungs and returns to the systemic circulation without being oxygenated. The severity is dependent on the pulmonary blood flow. Cyanosis in the newborn infant is a serious sign and the baby should be referred for cardiac assessment. Investigations include electrocardiogram, chest X-ray, ultrasound scan and cardiac catheterisation which will be carried out urgently. Corrective surgery will be carried out if and when the defect is amenable to it.

Acyanotic heart lesions

The most common acyanotic malformations are ventricular septal defect, patent ductus arteriosus, atrial septal defect, pulmonary stenosis, aortal stenosis and coarctation of the aorta.

These defects may be suspected on routine medical examination. Some babies present with a history of breathlessness and failure to thrive and some will display signs of congestive cardiac failure. Signs may appear in the first 24 hours of life but may not be found for some months. The earlier the onset of serious symptoms, the worse is the prognosis. If serious signs and symptoms develop, the baby will have a cardiac catheterisation and surgery is carried out to correct the defect. If the condition is not life threatening, surgery is deferred until the child is older.

Malformations of the genito-urinary system

Renal agenesis

Congenital absence of the kidneys is a serious malformation which is incompatible with prolonged survival. It should be suspected in cases of maternal oligohydramnios. The baby has a typical appearance with low set ears, wide set eyes, a beaked nose and micrognathia. The diagnosis can be made by intravenous pyelogram but ultrasonography is more frequently employed. No treatment is available. *Potter's syndrome* consists of renal agenesis and pulmonary hypoplasia.

Unilateral renal agenesis will not give rise to any signs if the single remaining kidney functions normally. It would be evident on ultrasonography. There may, however, be other associated abnormalities.

Bladder and urethra

Abnormalities of the bladder and urethra can lead to urinary obstruction which in turn leads to disordered renal function. Bladder distension should always be investigated and the midwife must call the paediatrician to see any baby who has not passed urine within 24 hours of birth.

Hypospadias and epispadias

Hypospadias is a malformation in which the urethral meatus opens onto the inferior aspect of the penis. Surgical correction should be carried out before the boy reaches school age. He must not be circumcised because the foreskin is needed for the repair. Epispadias, in which the urethral

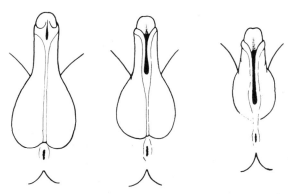

Fig. 38.8
Degrees of hypospadias. (Turner et al 1988.)

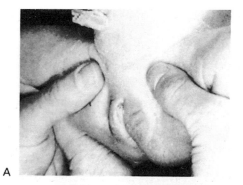

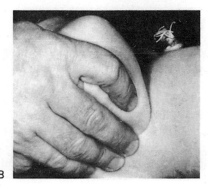

Fig. 38.9
Barlow's test for congenital dislocation of hip showing position of the hands.

meatus opens onto the superior aspect of the penis, is extremely rare and is often associated with complex pelvic abnormalities (see Fig. 38.8).

Doubtful sex

Ambiguous genitalia raise an immediate dilemma at birth because the parents seek to know the sex of the child. While the midwife will be supportive and explain gently to the parents, she should make no attempt to decide the matter but must refer the case to a paediatrician. The diagnosis of sex will be carried out using chromosomal studies and it will be some time before the parents have confirmation of the sex of their child. The infant may have one of a number of conditions.

Musculoskeletal malformations

Congenital dislocation of the hip

Unilateral or bilateral hip dislocation can be diagnosed soon after birth using Ortolani's or Barlow's test. If the diagnosis is missed the child will develop shortening and external rotation of the affected limb.

Barlow's test (a modification of Ortolani's test). The baby is placed on a firm surface with the legs pointing towards the examiner. The hips and knees are flexed. The examiner grasps the knees with the middle finger of each hand over the greater trochanter and the thumb of each hand applied to the inner side of the thigh approximately opposite the lower trochanter. The thighs are abducted and the middle finger of each hand pushes the greater trochanter forward. If the hip

is dislocated, the femoral head will be felt to enter the acetabulum with a 'clunk'. If no 'clunk' is felt the hip is stable.

If the hip is dislocatable, the femoral head can be displaced backwards out of the acetabulum by exerting minimal pressure when the hips are flexed and adducted (Barlow's sign).

This test is repeated at 3–6 months of age to detect missed cases. Each unit must have a policy which stipulates who may carry out the test in order to prevent the damage which may result from repeated testing. Diagnosis is confirmed by X-ray or ultrasound.

Treatment of congenital dislocation of the hip is by application of a splint which maintains flexion and full abduction of the hip. The splint should be adjusted weekly.

Club foot

Talipes equinovarus. In this condition the foot is bent downwards and inwards. It may affect one or both feet and is often a positional defect due to pressure from the uterus.

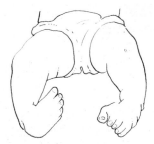

Fig. 38.10
Talipes equinovarus.

Treatment. Gentle manipulation every few hours commenced early and the physiotherapist instructs the mother how to carry this out. The feet can be held in the corrected position by adhesive strapping. Special splints may be applied. In most cases correction is achieved within the first year of life.

Talipes calcaneovalgus. The foot is turned upwards and bent outwards which is the opposite of talipes equinovarus. It is less severe and, unless the deformity is excessive, no treatment is required except to manipulate the foot gently into a normal position at frequent intervals.

Achondroplasia

This is a rare condition in which the limbs are short because of failure to form cartilage but the body is of normal length. The children are dwarfed permanently but will have normal mental development.

Polydactyly

This is the name given to a condition where there are extra digits on hand or foot. Fingers and toes should be counted by the midwife during routine examination at birth. The hand must be opened to find any digit folded into the fist. Polydactyly will be reported to the paediatrician and a decision will be made as to treatment.

Syndactyly

This term indicates fusion of digits which may be in the form of webbing between the fingers or toes or may be complete fusion. Separation will be carried out if the digits are otherwise normal.

Skin disorders

A variety of *birth marks* can be identified by the midwife when she examines the newborn baby. Small, flat, pinkish-red areas caused by an abnormal collection of small blood vessels are commonly seen on the eyelids and the nape of the neck. These will disappear in a few weeks and require no treatment.

Strawberry haemangioma

A haemangioma is bright red in colour, slightly elevated and sharply defined. It appears in the first week of life, increases in size until about 6 months and then regresses. By the 6th year it will have disappeared. No treatment is required but parents will be anxious during the first year and will require reassurance, especially if there is an unsightly swelling on the face.

Port wine stain (capillary haemangioma)

This deep purple discoloration is not raised and is frequently seen on the face. It can be extensive and disfiguring and is permanent. There is no satisfactory treatment, although the palest ones improve with age. Cosmetic preparations can be used to camouflage the haemangioma.

Pigmented naevi

Pigmented naevi or moles vary in size and may be covered with fine hair. No treatment is carried out in the neonatal period but excision and radiotherapy will be required later.

Epidermolysis bullosa

This rare, congenital skin disorder is often fatal. It resembles pemphigus neonatorum but is non-infective. The baby has large blisters all over the body and the skin is scaly. Treatment is aimed at protecting the skin and preventing infection.

Chromosomal abnormalities

Chromosomes are bodies which are carried in the nucleus of cells and which hold the elements of heredity in the form of genes. Abnormality can occur in various ways.

Non-disjunction: failure of chromosomes to separate during meiosis.

Trisomy: when there is an extra chromosome in addition to the normal complement, resulting in a particular chromosome being represented three times in the nucleus.

Deletion: breaking off or loss of part of a chromosome.

Translocation: transfer of material from one chromosome to another of a different kind.

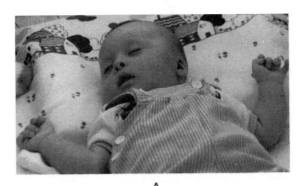

A

Trisomy 21 (Down's syndrome)

This condition is normally recognised at birth because of the characteristic appearance of the child. The head tends to be small with a flat occiput, the eyes slant upwards and the mouth is small with a short upper lip. The hands are short and a single tranverse palmar crease (simian crease) is present. The great toe is widely separated from the others. The baby tends to be hypotonic and may suffer other abnormalities such as cardiac defects.

These infants have three number 21 chromosomes. The condition is associated with ageing of the maternal ovaries. Investigative amniocentesis can be offered to mothers aged over 35–40 years (see Ch. 41). Study of the fetal cells will reveal the abnormality, and termination of pregnancy may be offered.

Although the diagnosis is normally apparent at birth, the midwife should first compare the baby's facial appearance with those of his parents. Confirmation of the diagnosis will be made on chromosomal analysis. Parents may suspect the diagnosis themselves, but definite information cannot be given until the results of the chromosomal studies are received. It will normally be the paediatrician who gives this information to the parents and the midwife should be available to offer support.

Parents may wish to be put in touch with the local branch of the Down's Syndrome Association.

Trisomy 18 (Edward's syndrome)

This condition is found in about 1 in 5000 births. An extra chromosome number 18 is responsible for the characteristic features. The life-span for

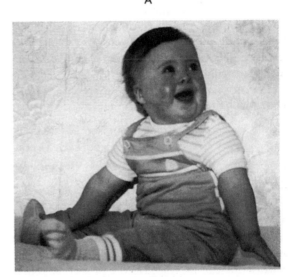

B

Fig. 38.11
(A) Baby with Down's syndrome — note slant of eyes and incurving of little fingers.
(B) With good parental involvement and stimulus these infants can reach maximum potential.

these children is short and the majority die during their first year.

The head is small with a flattened forehead, a receding chin and frequently a cleft palate. The ears are low set and maldeveloped. The sternum tends to be short. The fingers often overlap each other and the feet have a characteristic 'rocker bottom' appearance. Malformations of the gastrointestinal and cardiovascular systems are common.

Trisomy 13 (Patau's syndrome)

An extra chromosome on the 13 pair leads to multiple abnormalities. These children have a short life; only 5% live beyond 3 years. The infants affected are small and are microcephalic. Midline facial abnormalities are common and limb abnormalities are frequently seen. Brain, cardiac and renal abnormalities may co-exist with this trisomy.

Turner's syndrome (XO)

In this monosomal condition only one sex chromosome exists, an X. The absent chromosome is indicated by 'O'. The child is a girl with widely spaced nipples, oedematous feet and a short, webbed neck. The genitalia tend to be under-developed and the internal reproductive organs do not mature. The condition may not be diagnosed until puberty fails to occur. Congenital cardiac defects may also be found. Mental development is usually normal.

Genetic disorders

Genes are carried on the chromosomes, are composed of deoxyribonucleic acid and each is concerned with the transmission of one specific hereditary factor.

Dominant gene

A dominant gene will produce its effect even if present on only one chromosome of a pair. An autosomal dominant condition will result and usually this can be traced through several generrations. *Achondroplasia, Huntington's chorea, oesteogenesis imperfecta* and *polycystic kidneys* are examples of autosomal dominant conditions.

Genetic counselling should be offered (see Ch. 7).

Recessive gene

A recessive gene needs to be present on both chromosomes before producing its effect. Autosomal recessive conditions result, such as those already discussed in the section dealing with inborn errors of metabolism. Both parents are healthy but carry the affected gene and their children have a 1 in 4 chance of developing the condition.

The midwife's role in supporting parents

The immediate effect of the delivery of a child with physical or mental subnormality is distress both for the parents and in the attending staff. Midwives should give emotional support to the parents and help them to come to terms with the situation (see Ch. 49).

Practical advice about the day-to-day care of the child must be given and the parents are informed about the facilities provided by the Health and Social Services and other agencies. Self-help groups may also be available which provide parents with opportunities to meet others in a similar situation and share experiences.

Reader Activity

Arrange to visit a local self-help group for parents of children with a congenital abnormality. (These groups normally welcome professional observers.) When at the group, use your skills of communication to ascertain the particular concerns of the parents and whether they feel that they were given sufficient explanation at the time of diagnosis.

The results of this exercise might be useful for class presentation and subsequent discussion with your peers.

In discussion, try to determine how you would develop your approach to such parents subsequent to diagnosis.

REFERENCE

Turner T L, Douglas J, Cockburn F 1988 Craig's care of the newly born infant, 8th edn. Churchill Livingstone, Edinburgh

FURTHER READING

Forfar J O, Arneil G C 1984 Textbook of paediatrics, 3rd edn. Vols 1 & 2. Churchill Livingstone, Edinburgh
O'Doherty N 1985 Atlas of the newborn, 2nd edn. MTP Press, Lancaster
Roberton N R C (ed) 1988 Textbook of neonatology. Churchill Livingstone, Edinburgh
Schaffer A J 1984 Diseases of the newborn, 5th edn. Saunders, Philadelphia

8

39

Community midwifery

THELMA BAMFIELD

The community midwife has the privilege of building a relationship with women in their social and family context, and supporting them through a major life event. The care she offers is flexible and adapted to individual circumstances, though her work patterns are constantly modified by changes in maternity care provision.

THE COMMUNITY MIDWIFE

Role of the community midwife

Most commonly, the community midwife becomes involved after pregnancy is confirmed, but she may work in family planning or pre-pregnancy clinics and so follow a couple through the whole continuum of childbearing.

She provides antenatal care, often sharing this responsibility with general practitioners and/or consultant obstetricians; she may undertake monitoring of high-risk pregnancies at home.

She attends home births, though only about 1% of babies in the UK are now born at home. Schemes are being developed whereby community midwives accompany women in their care to hospital for delivery. These provide continuity for the women, and also help to maintain midwives' skills and increase their job satisfaction.

The length of postnatal stay in hospital is steadily reducing, due to pressure on beds as well as maternal choice. There is a corresponding increase in the workload of community midwives as they care for the new mother and baby at home.

Integral to the role of the community midwife is health education and preparation for birth and parenthood, both on a one-to-one basis and with groups. As well as in the home and at clinics, possible settings include schools, drop-in centres, and antenatal and postnatal classes. She is involved in the training of student nurses; she may become a teaching midwife and be allocated a student midwife undertaking community experience.

'Social and psychological support of pregnant women should be an integral part of all forms of care given during pregnancy and childbirth. Unfortunately it is not.' (Elbourne et al 1989)

Many women have little or no support from their immediate or extended family, due to moving house, marital discord or breakdown, or because they are single parents. Few mothers in developed countries have had any experience of looking after children before the birth of their own babies. Furthermore, many women feel that modern obstetric care ignores them as people and treats them as incubators. Surveys of women's views of maternity care (reviewed by Reid & Garcia 1989) highlight the need for realistic advice, respect from caregivers, for personal care, and for information.

It is also well known (Townsend & Davidson 1988; Garcia et al 1989) that social and ethnic background are associated with inequalities not only in health but also in the use of health care provision, notably antenatal care. Reasons for this include the attitudes of caregivers, a woman's own perception of needs and priorities, and difficulties in communication and obtaining information.

Elbourne et al (1989) discuss the results of 14 controlled trials of enhanced social and psychological support in pregnancy; the controls received 'normal' antenatal care. Women receiving enhanced support fared better on a whole range of outcomes, from feeling more in control and less worried during pregnancy and labour, and better able to communicate with staff, to being more likely to breast feed successfully. The baby's father was also more likely to be involved in his child's care.

While these results are undoubtedly a condemnation of standard antenatal care, the challenge for the community midwife is clear. Understanding the woman's social and family situation and with the opportunity to get to know her and develop a trusting relationship over time, she is in a unique position to offer social and psychological support according to individual need.

Work of the community midwife

The community midwife may be based in a hospital, a General Practitioner Unit or a health centre or she may work from home. She usually works in a team. The midwives relieve each other for days off, holidays, courses and on-call duties or while one of them is attending a woman in labour. Each midwife communicates with her colleagues in daily meetings or by telephone, backed up by answerphone, paging devices or two-way radio. Her work mainly consists of home visiting. A Crown car may be provided; a mileage allowance is payable if she uses her own vehicle.

Liaison with other professionals

The community midwife is part of the primary health care team. Effective communication between all members of the team is vital and the role of each must be clearly defined if mothers and babies are to receive the best possible care.

General practitioner (GP). The midwife may be allocated to a geographical area, to a group practice or to a number of individual GPs. She must get to know the doctors she is working with if communication between them is to be effective. The GP usually confirms the pregnancy but the midwife should be informed without delay if she is to have the opportunity to use her midwifery skills to the full. The GP is able to see a woman's pregnancy against the background of his knowledge of the family, while the midwife contributes her specific and specialised clinical expertise to the care of the woman. She may need to exercise her skills in diplomacy and negotiation in order that the woman may obtain maximum benefit from this shared care.

Health visitor. If a woman has other children the health visitor may be the first member of the team to know about her pregnancy. She may make a point of meeting all expectant mothers in order to lay the foundations for a relationship which will last until the child reaches school age. Mothers, and the professionals themselves, should be in no doubt about what the distinct roles and training of midwife and health visitor involve (see Ch. 45). Every effort must be made to avoid giving conflicting advice so that clients may have confidence in those responsible for their care.

Social worker. A pregnant woman should be referred to a social worker if she has problems with finance or accommodation or needs to arrange care for her existing children or for the one she is expecting. A girl under 16 must continue her education, either with a home tutor or at school. She may need to be placed in care if not supported by her parents. The social worker's help is also required if a baby is to be adopted.

A midwife may occasionally need to refer a woman for marriage guidance or psychosexual counselling or for other appropriate help.

Working in the home

Hospital and clinic are the territory of doctors and midwives where they are in control. In the woman's home the midwife is a guest and must behave accordingly. She has no authority to insist that things be done a particular way; she must rely on tact and persuasion. She may have to work hard at building up a trusting relationship in order to demonstrate to her clients that she has their interests at heart. Her privileged position gives her unequalled opportunities for getting to know and understand the families in her care and to assess their particular needs. She must tactfully and sensitively tailor her advice and health education to the situation she finds. A dogmatic or judgemental approach is inappropriate and will reduce her chances of helping the family.

The midwife working in the home must be accepting and adaptable. She must always seek to provide the highest standard of care even if facilities are inadequate. She must be prepared to improvise and offer practical suggestions about making plans for the baby and caring for him after his arrival.

The midwife's bags

Equipment carried by the community midwife will vary slightly according to individual circumstances and local policy. Minimum requirements are:

For antenatal visits
- Sphygmomanometer and stethoscope
- Fetal stethoscope
- Urine test strips.

For postnatal visits
- Clinical thermometers (one low-reading)
- Baby scales
- Equipment for neonatal screening tests
- Equipment for removing sutures.

Equipment for delivery is listed in the section on home birth.

The midwife will also carry an appropriate supply of stationery and maternity benefit forms.

The midwife has a duty to keep her bags and equipment in good order and her records up to date.

A practising midwife shall give to her supervisor of midwives, the relevant Board and the local supervising authority, every reasonable facility to inspect her methods of practice, her records, her equipment and such part of her residence as may be used for professional purposes. (Midwives' Rules 43(1): Inspection of premises and equipment. UKCC 1991)

ANTENATAL CARE

History-taking

Soon after pregnancy is confirmed, a full history is taken from the woman in order to assess her present state of health and to detect any factors which may affect the course or outcome of pregnancy. It will identify any physical, psychological or social needs and form the basis of her care plan.

This information may be sought separately by the GP, by the community midwife and at the hospital. One way to avoid this repetition is for a thorough history to be taken once only, preferably in the woman's own home, and for the woman to be responsible for her own notes throughout pregnancy, taking them with her whenever she attends for antenatal care.

History-taking may be stressful for the woman. It necessitates a number of personal and searching questions which should include an exploration of why the woman is pregnant, her attitudes to child-bearing and her own and her family's reactions to this pregnancy in particular. It must be done in private, with every effort made to ensure that the atmosphere is relaxed and unhurried. In a hospital clinic this can be difficult; however welcoming the staff, the hospital environment in itself may be unsettling.

In the woman's own home, the history-taking can become an integral part of the family's preparation for the baby. The woman will be at ease and communicate more readily. The midwife will develop a greater understanding of the woman if she talks with her in her own surroundings. The social history in particular will have far more relevance if the midwife can actually see the living conditions and meet other members of the family. With her knowledge of the local community she may be able to put the woman in touch with facilities such as playgroups, support groups and sources of reasonably priced baby equipment. Women who are still going out to work or who have just moved to the area may appreciate meeting mothers living nearby. Local parent education groups can help in this respect.

The initial home visit should form a sound basis for a satisfying and supportive relationship. Possible sources of stress can be identified and the plan of care can be tailored to individual circumstances.

Choosing the place of delivery

The decision about where to have her baby should be made by the woman herself in consultation with her community midwife, GP and, if necessary, the obstetrician. During labour she needs to feel at ease in her surroundings and have confidence in her attendants. The choice will be influenced by her past and current history and previous experiences, availability of beds and her home conditions.

Hospital booking under consultant care. The view favoured by most obstetricians that all births should take place in hospital means that a bed will probably be available for any woman who needs or wants one. There may be medical or obstetric reasons why hospital delivery is advisable and many women feel more secure knowing that emergency facilities are close at hand. Home conditions may be such that a few days away would benefit the mother and baby.

Indications for hospital delivery:

Medical
— cardiac disease
— renal disease
— diabetes mellitus
— essential hypertension
— tuberculosis
— habitual drug use
— sexually transmitted disease.

Past obstetric history
— uterine surgery
— difficult forceps delivery
— postpartum haemorrhage
— manual removal of placenta.

Current pregnancy
— cephalopelvic disproportion
— placenta praevia
— pregnancy-associated hypertension
— multiple pregnancy
— breech presentation
— preterm labour
— Rhesus iso-immunisation
— atypical antibodies.

Relative indications
— age under 18 or over 35
— parity 0 or more than 4
— height under 5' ($\leqslant$1.5 m)
— prolonged pregnancy.

The chief concerns that have been expressed about hospital delivery:

- multiplicity of carers
- the prevailing medical ideology with its implications of illness and abnormality which leads to use of technology and unnecessary interference
- the imposition of routine at the expense of the woman's individuality

- disruption of family life and disturbance to other children
- ambivalence of the father's role.

The use of birth plans should help to alleviate some of these problems if hospital staff are fully committed to them.

Some areas have schemes whereby community midwives conduct deliveries in hospital with consultant cover. This should ensure some continuity and reduce the routine use of intervention.

Dissatisfaction with the hospital service should ensure that other options for booking remain open, for example Domino schemes, General Practitioner Unit deliveries and home births.

Domino scheme. The Domino scheme (DOMiciliary IN and Out) combines some of the advantages of community care with the facilities of the obstetric unit. The consultant may wish to see the woman during pregnancy to agree her suitability for the scheme, but otherwise all her care is provided by the community midwife and GP.

The community midwife is called to the home at the onset of labour. When it is well established she accompanies the woman to the hospital where she conducts the delivery. Medical cover is provided by the GP who will indicate whether he wishes to be present at the birth. He is notified immediately if there is any deviation from the normal and arranges for the woman to be transferred to consultant care if necessary. If she is already in hospital this can be accomplished with little disturbance and the community midwife may remain with the mother rather than hand her over to strangers.

If the birth is uncomplicated, mother and baby go home between 2 and 6 hours afterwards or the following morning.

General Practitioner Units (GPUs) are either separate from or on the same premises as a consultant unit. They may have their own midwives or be staffed by community midwives on a rota system. Medical cover is provided by a woman's own GP or arrangements may be made with another local doctor.

The medical criteria for booking are the same as for home delivery. GPUs are most suitable for women with no foreseeable problems, for whom a stay away from home would be an advantage.

Advantages of the Domino scheme:
- continuity of care from community midwife and GP
- little contact with hospital routines
- minimal disruption of family life
- easy access to emergency facilities
- may provide an acceptable alternative for a woman who does not meet the criteria for home birth
- the community midwife maintains her delivery skills

The main disadvantages are the risk of deferring the transfer to the hospital too long and the upheaval of returning shortly afterwards.

The scheme is proving very popular with mothers and midwives in areas where it has been introduced.

Advantages of GPUs:
- friendly, relaxed atmosphere
- continuity of care from GP and possibly the community midwife
- GPUs separate from the main hospital may be more accessible for mothers and visitors
- some GPs are prepared to carry out minor obstetric interventions such as induction of labour or uncomplicated forceps deliveries
- GPUs on obstetric unit premises have easy access to emergency facilities
- mothers who are delivered in a consultant unit and need a long stay may benefit more from transferring to a GPU for a few days than remaining on a busy hospital postnatal ward

Disadvantages of isolated GPUs:
- they are not equipped to deal with complications — if problems arise, the woman is transferred to consultant care and the Emergency Obstetric Unit may have to be called
- they can be expensive to run.

For these reasons many isolated GPUs are being closed.

Home birth can be a uniquely satisfying experience for the mother, her family and the midwife. Every woman has the right to consider it amongst her options. The most commonly given reasons for choosing it are listed above under hospital booking. The central issue is one of control. Couples who seek a home delivery often do so because they wish to retain control of events surrounding the birth. They hope to enhance the quality of the birth experience not only for themselves but also, by minimising the use of drugs and intervention, for the baby. The effects on the future well-being of the family may be far-reaching.

The couple may feel that it is important for their child to be born into the same loving environment in which he was conceived, for the father to be free to demonstrate his affection and support and for other children to see birth as a normal, happy event.

There are certain medical and obstetric conditions which would make a home birth inadvisable (see indications for hospital booking). Few women intentionally put themselves or their babies at risk. The midwife must develop a good relationship with the family, based on mutual trust. She must spend some time with them exploring their feelings about childbirth and their hopes for the coming event. If the couple feel that the midwife is committed to helping them to achieve the kind of birth they want, conflict should be avoided if complications arise which make admission to hospital desirable.

Booking a GP for home birth. GPs vary considerably in their attitudes to home delivery. A woman has the right to engage the services of a different doctor for the duration of pregnancy and childbirth if her own GP does not wish to cover a home birth. She should therefore not sign the agreement between doctor and patient for provision of maternity services (form EC24) unless she is sure that the GP will provide the necessary medical cover. She is then free to approach any other doctor who is obstetrically ap-proved and ask if he will be prepared to supervise the pregnancy.

Failure to find a GP who is willing to accept a home delivery does not rule out a home birth.

The midwife notifies her Supervisor of Midwives and continues to give the necessary antenatal care. Arrangements will be made for a second midwife to be present for the delivery. Medical cover will be provided by a GP on the obstetric list or by the consultant obstetrician usually via the Emergency Obstetric Unit. Any GP who is called in an emergency is obliged to attend.

Plans for transfer home after the birth

If the woman is to be booked for a hospital or GPU delivery, the length of postnatal stay should be discussed with the community midwife, even though 'it appears to be determined more by fashion and the availability of beds than by any systematic assessment of the needs of recently delivered women and their new babies' (Rush et al 1989).

It has been assumed that primiparous mothers will benefit from a longer stay in a protected environment to gain confidence in caring for their babies, and that multiparous mothers will be anxious to return home quickly to their other children. However, a first-time mother may be very distressed at being away from her home and partner for longer than is absolutely necessary and the mother who already has a family may be in need of a complete rest away from her domestic responsibilities.

The most important consideration is whether adequate help is available in the home. A mother needs at least 10 days free from household duties and the care of other children in order to recover from the birth and lay the foundations of a good relationship with her baby. The community midwife may have to spend some time discussing the various options with the family and make sure that they understand that help must be effective, reliable, unobtrusive and non-threatening. The partner may be able to take paternity leave but many men who take time off work will either lose pay or use up limited holiday entitlement. The woman's mother or mother-in-law may be able to run the household but both may have work and domestic commitments of their own. Alternatively they may live at a distance which would necessitate coming to stay, an arrangement which is not always in the best interests of family harmony.

It may be possible to arrange a home help with the local Social Services department, but she will only be available for a short time daily. Other children may be taken into care if necessary, usually with foster parents.

Inevitably, help and support are sometimes limited but a woman cannot be expected to remain in hospital or to rest when there is no-one to look after her other children. The midwife can only advise and offer suggestions and support; there may ultimately have to be a compromise between the interests of the mother and those of her family.

The planned length of postnatal stay in hospital should be discussed early enough in pregnancy for satisfactory arrangements to be made. The partner may need time to improve his house-keeping skills and children may need a few practice visits in order to become used to staying with other adults.

The environment in which the new baby will be cared for must also be considered. If it is grossly inadequate the midwife should contact a social worker who may be able to obtain help with rehousing or repairs or with special payments for heating and equipment.

Whatever the conditions, the family must appreciate the need for heating day and night in cold weather, if neonatal hypothermia is to be avoided. The midwife may be able to make practical suggestions to save on heating bills. If there is no heating in the bedrooms, mother and baby could perhaps sleep in a downstairs room. Considerations of hygiene and safety can be tactfully mentioned of appropriate; parental backache can be prevented by planning for the baby to be bathed and changed at suitable heights. Other factors which affect the baby's welfare can also be discussed such as helping other children and family pets to adjust to the baby's arrival.

Follow-up antenatal care

Antenatal care may be organised in a number of different ways depending on where the woman is booked for delivery:

Hospital delivery + hospital antenatal care

Hospital delivery + shared antenatal care
Domino scheme ⎫
GPU delivery ⎬ + community antenatal care.
Home birth ⎭

Hospital antenatal care
Relatively few women nowadays attend hospital for all their antenatal care. Those who do are in particularly high-risk categories such as women with diabetes mellitus, or those who have conceived after treatment for subfertility.

Shared antenatal care
This combines the benefits of specialist supervision with the convenience and continuity of attendance at a local clinic. The woman attends the consultant unit for booking and again at around 32–36 weeks. The rest of her care is given by her community midwife and GP. She is referred back to the hospital in between if any complications arise.

Schemes are being developed by some health authorities to take consultant care into the community particularly in areas of social deprivation. This can provide an ideal solution to the inadequacy and expense of public transport and the reluctance of some women to attend hospital. An obstetrician visits peripheral clinics on a regular basis and any problems can be referred to him directly.

Community antenatal care
The woman may have an initial consultation with the obstetrician to assess her suitability for the Domino scheme, GPU or home birth and she will be referred to him if any complications develop. Otherwise she receives all her antenatal care from the community midwife and GP, either alternately or in joint clinics. Whatever the arrangement, the midwife should be using her skills to the full, not only to establish physical normality but also to discover how the woman is coping with the changes of pregnancy and the prospect of motherhood. She needs to encourage the woman to discuss her feelings and voice any anxieties in a supportive and confidential atmosphere.

During her pregnancy, if at all possible, the woman should meet all of the midwives who may subsequently be involved in her labour and post-natal care.

Antenatal care in the home

The community midwife may attend some pregnant women in their own homes. This may be because they find it difficult to attend the clinic due to illness, lack of transport, having no-one with whom to leave their children or simply through lack of motivation. Other women who have complications such as hypertension or a multiple pregnancy may be offered home antenatal care in order to avoid admission to hospital.

Follow-up of defaulters. The community midwife is informed if a woman fails to keep a clinic appointment. She makes a home visit at which an antenatal examination is made. The midwife tries to elicit the reasons for failure to attend. If there are practical problems she will try to find a solution. She explains the importance of antenatal care and encourages the woman to make every effort to keep future appointments and to contact her if there are problems in doing so.

INTRAPARTUM CARE

Home birth

Although the community midwife becomes adept at improvisation and has to work in all kinds of situations, when a home birth is being considered certain criteria should be specified. She must assure herself that there is safe and reliable heating, day and night during the winter, and even in the summer some form of heating should be available in the room where the birth is to take place. There must be running water, preferably hot as well as cold, and sanitation must be adequate. It is an advantage if the home is not too remote, particularly if the baby is due in the winter, and it should be reasonably clean. Access to a telephone is important.

Preparation of the family

It is essential that the family be committed to the idea of a home birth and willing and able to provide the necessary support. Most partners

nowadays want to be fully involved with the birth and to form a relationship with the baby from the beginning. This may be one of the reasons for choosing a home delivery. The midwife should make a point of meeting the partner during the antenatal period in order to discuss his part in the proceedings and allay any anxieties.

The question of running the household should be explored in some detail so that all the possible implications can be considered and a suitable support network organised. Although one of the advantages of home birth is that it minimises household disruption, a great deal of thought should still be given to arrangements for other children. Labour could start at any time of the day or night but a child's normal routine should be disturbed as little as possible. Small children have a very short attention span; if the woman's partner intends to be with her, someone else must take responsibility for the children during the hours of labour.

Children must be prepared for the event according to their age and understanding. Some children may be intrigued by the birth itself (and some parents may wish the whole family to be present) but they may become distressed if their mother appears to be in pain.

Preparation of the home

Practical details are mentioned during the initial home visit and discussed in more detail later in pregnancy. The midwife calls before the 37th week to check that satisfactory arrangements have been made.

If there is a choice, the room should be reasonably spacious and near the bathroom and lavatory. Any rugs should be lifted and a fitted carpet should be protected during the delivery by something waterproof and non-slip, such as PVC or heavy brown paper. A lamp with a strong bulb will be needed if lighting is dim or inconveniently placed.

The bed should preferably be accessible from both sides. A sagging mattress can be supported by placing a board underneath. A plastic sheet or mackintosh large enough to cover the mattress and tuck in on both sides is necessary and a polythene drawsheet is useful. Plenty of old, freshly-laundered bed linen should be available, also a number of pillows and possibly a bean bag.

Even if the woman intends to remain ambulant during the first stage of labour and wishes to give birth kneeling or squatting on the floor, the bed may be required for examinations and affords several options for change of position. The mattress protection should be left in place for the first one or two days postnatally.

A working area is needed, for example a small kitchen table. Any polished surfaces which are used must be well protected with towels or layers of newspaper covered with a clean piece of sheeting.

Other items provided by the mother
For delivery:
Washing-up bowl
2 towels — 1 for midwife, 1 for mother
Flannel
Soap
Dettol/Savlon
New nail brush and jam jar for antiseptic
    solution
Old nightdress/shirt/pyjama jacket for wear
    during labour
Sanitary belt or old pants
Sanitary towels
Plastic dustbin liner for soiled dressings
Emergency lighting (torch and spare
    batteries)
Bedpan or bucket.

For baby's immediate needs:
Soft towel to wrap baby in at birth
Cot and bedding
Set of baby clothes
Hot water bottle to warm the cot, towel and
    garments.

Some health authorities provide a maternity pack containing cotton wool, sanitary towels and absorbent pads.

Vaginal examination and delivery packs prepared by the Central Sterile Supply Department may be available. Otherwise equipment is boiled in a large saucepan, or in the steriliser incorporated in the delivery bag, on arrival at the home. It is left to cool in the covered receptacle and items are

---

Midwife's delivery bag
Plastic apron
Nail brush
Disposable gloves
Urine testing strips
Disposable enema
Disposable razor
Urinary catheters
Labour progress charts
Birth notification forms and envelopes
Fetal stethoscope
2 thermometers (one low-reading)
Scales
Tape measure
Disposable mucus extractors
Cord clamps
Lotions: Savlon; obstetric cream
Alcohol swabs
Drugs: pethidine obtained on midwives'
    supply order; naloxone (Narcan) neonatal;
    vitamin K; lignocaine 1% solution; oxytocic
    agents
Disposable syringes and needles
Entonox
Bag and mask for infant resuscitation
Baby oxygen cylinder
Bowl for lotion
Gallipot for obstetric cream
Kidney dish for placenta
Jug for measuring blood loss
2 pairs cord forceps; 1 pair cord scissors
1 pair episiotomy scissors
Sterile cotton wool balls
Perineal pads and dressing towels
Suturing equipment.

---

removed as needed. After the delivery the equipment is resterilised.

Management of the delivery

It is important that the family know exactly when and how to contact the midwife. Any midwife who may be called for the delivery should have met the family, and should know how to find the home.

The midwife visits to assess the situation as soon as she is called. If labour is not established and her continued presence is not required, she may leave but ensures that she can be contacted without delay. After the beginning of the second stage of labour she must stay with the woman until the expulsion of the placenta and membranes and as long afterwards as may be necessary.

The principles of care are the same wherever labour takes place. They are the provision of physical and emotional support, including pain relief, vigilant observation of the condition of mother and fetus and of the progress in labour and finally the safe conduct of the delivery. Full and accurate records are essential.

Plans for labour and birth will have been discussed in some detail beforehand. Many women choosing home birth are anxious to avoid the use of drugs and, as long as the attendants are calm and supportive, will usually succeed in remaining relaxed and in control. Midwife and partner can assist by massaging the woman's back or helping her to change position. The use of heat may be comforting, for example a hot water bottle, hot flannels above the symphysis pubis, in the small of the back or on the perineum, or sitting in a warm bath may help. If the mother can avoid the use of narcotics she escapes the drowsiness and detachment which they cause and the baby is also more alert at delivery.

The couple may have views regarding the routine use of oxytocics or the time of clamping of the cord. Circumstances where such interventions may be indicated in the interests of mother or baby should have been discussed beforehand to avoid conflict in an emergency.

At a convenient time after the birth the baby is examined, weighed and dressed and the mother is washed and made comfortable. The midwife tidies up the room and disposes of any sharps and soiled dressings safely. The midwife must make arrangements for the disposal of the placenta, either at the hospital or by burning. However, it belongs to the mother, who must be allowed to retain it if she wishes.

The midwife writes a detailed account of the delivery in her records. She remains at the home for an hour or two until she is satisfied that mother and baby can be safely left. She gives instructions about how she may be contacted if there is any cause for concern.

The first postnatal visit is made about 6 hours after the end of labour. Mother and baby are both given a full examination. The mother is helped to the lavatory if she has not already voided urine and at some time during the first day she is assisted to take a bath or shower.

The community midwife may occasionally be called to an unplanned home delivery. She should therefore be prepared for any eventuality and keep equipment for emergency situations ready in her car. Drug expiry dates should be checked regularly even if no home births have been booked.

Medical cover for home birth

When a GP is booked, the midwife will ascertain whether he wishes to be notified that the woman is in labour, in which case he may visit during labour or request to be called for the delivery. He may only wish to be called if there are any problems.

If no GP is booked, arrangements should have been made for cover to be provided by another GP or by the hospital.

If medical help is needed and the booked GP and his deputy are not available, the midwife calls in another GP, preferably one who is on the approved obstetric list, or, if necessary, the Emergency Obstetric Unit.

Transfer to hospital may occasionally be indicated, for example if there is fetal distress or failure to progress.

In emergencies such as postpartum haemorrhage or neonatal asphyxia it may be necessary to call the Emergency Obstetric or Paediatric Unit. The midwife should know how to arrange this herself in order to avoid any possible delay. She must state the nature of the problem accurately and concisely, giving directions to the home and any other relevant information. She ensures that the location can be easily identified by putting all the lights on or stationing someone outside to watch for the ambulance.

While awaiting their arrival, the midwife pays close attention to her patient's condition and administers appropriate emergency care. If possible she writes a concise history of the case. Supplies of hot and cold boiled water should be made available if appropriate. In the case of haemorrhage the pulse is checked and recorded at

5-minute intervals and the blood pressure every 15 minutes. The placenta, blood and bloodstained linen are kept for inspection.

Excerpt from *A Midwife's Code of Practice* (UKCC 1989)

4 Home Confinements

4.1 A midwife attending a mother having a home confinement should ascertain whether or not a registered medical practitioner is available for referral, to attend or be on call if required. The registered medical practitioner should preferably be from the obstetric list in those parts of the United Kingdom where such a list is held. In situations where the support of a registered medical practitioner is not available the midwife should discuss the situation with her supervisor of midwives and agree and record appropriate arrangements to provide advice and support when necessary.

4.2 In a situation where the midwife considers that home confinement is inappropriate and the mother refuses to take the advice of the midwife to receive care in a maternity unit the midwife must continue to give care and consult with her supervisor of midwives, making an appropriate record.

4.3 In some instances a midwife may require medical assistance for a mother booked for a home confinement but the mother or her partner may refuse to have the registered medical practitioner in attendance. If this situation arises the midwife must continue the care of the mother and consult as soon as possible with her supervisor of midwives, making an appropriate record.

4.4 It is the duty of the supervisor of midwives to ensure that agreed local policies are easily available to all practising midwives within their supervisory jurisdiction. The local policy should provide support for the midwife in the above or other difficult situations associated with home confinements, and enable the best possible arrangements to be made for the care of the mother and her baby.

POSTNATAL CARE

Transfer home

The decision about when to go home after a hospital birth should be made by the mother herself in consultation with both hospital and community midwives.

A substantial minority of women may have to or may decide to change the plans for postnatal hospital stay which they had made tentatively during pregnancy: women's physical, social and psychological circumstances after delivery vary greatly. It would seem sensible for professionals to be as flexible as possible in trying to respond to this variation. The exercise of choice may well be the crucial issue (Rush et al 1989).

The community midwife is given details of the delivery, its outcome, and any other relevant information. If requested, she will make an evening visit, otherwise she will visit the following morning.

Routine postnatal care

The Midwife's Code of Practice used to stipulate that a mother and baby should be examined morning and evening for the first few days after delivery and then at least daily. It is no longer so prescriptive and the midwife may use her discretion. The examination of the mother is described in Chapter 16 and that of the baby in Chapter 32.

The major differences between postnatal care in the home and in the hospital are the environment in which it takes place, and the fact that it is intermittent.

Room temperature should be maintained at 18–21°C to prevent neonatal hypothermia, and the baby's temperature is estimated, either by touch or using a low-reading thermometer. The midwife should also be aware of the dangers of hyperthermia.

The mother may have been shown how to bath her baby and change his nappy while in hospital, but the practicalities are rather different in the home. It may be necessary to demonstrate these procedures again, suitably adapted, and the mother, and indeed the father, may need to be supervised more than once, with encouragement and praise, until confidence is achieved.

Arrangements for sterilising bottles and making up feeds are discussed, if appropriate, and again the midwife may wish to demonstrate or supervise these procedures.

If the mother has a sore perineum, she may have appreciated frequent baths and using the bidet in hospital. These facilities may not be available at home. Improvising with a bath showerhead, or even a plant spray or soft plastic bottle, well rinsed and filled with warm water, after each use of the lavatory, can help ensure perineal cleanliness and comfort.

Many mothers have difficulty obtaining adequate rest on their return home. The midwife can do nothing about the domestic situation, but practical suggestions may help: a lot of housework can wait; this is not a time to be too proud to accept offers of assistance with chores or children and visitors can be tiring.

The community midwife comes across many challenging situations. She must always remain calm and non-judgemental. Any suggestions or advice offered must be realistic in the circumstances. She can teach by example, washing her hands before supervising a feed or after changing a nappy, and in her handling of the baby, talking to him and reacting patiently when he cries.

Because the midwife's visits are intermittent, she needs to give the family her full attention, alert to non-verbal and verbal clues about how they are adapting to the new situation. She observes the mother's mental state and her attitude to the baby, her partner and any other children. She notes the reactions of the other members of the family as they each come to terms with their altered roles. Signs of jealousy in siblings and even the partner are not unusual. There must be time at each visit for the parents to talk through how they feel, to express any anxieties about the baby, other children or their own relationship, and for the midwife to listen, giving unstinting support and encouragement.

The unsupported mother may be spared these particular concerns but will need extra help to boost her confidence in her ability to bring up her child alone.

At the end of each visit the midwife completes her notes, recording precisely any advice given so that if another midwife has to call, the possibility of conflicting advice is minimised. She also ensures that the family knows how to contact a midwife at any time before the next visit.

The neonatal screening test for metabolic disorders is carried out between the 6th and 14th day according to local policy. Parents may have to be reminded of the need to register the birth and the midwife should be aware of how, when and where this may be done.

Before the 10th day the midwife broaches the subject of family planning. She is in an ideal situation to encourage the mother to think positively about the timing of any subsequent pregnancies. If oral contraception is the method of choice, the mother is advised to visit the GP or Family Planning Clinic 2–3 weeks after the birth. If an intrauterine contraceptive device is to be fitted, arrangements can be made for this to be done at the 6-week postnatal examination. The midwife's relaxed attitude to sexuality will encourage the parents to discuss any concerns they may have about resumption of intercourse. The duration of the lochia and likely return of fertility and menstruation can be explained and physical and psychological ways of minimising perineal discomfort can be suggested.

The health visitor is informed of the birth by means of the birth notification and makes her first visit around the 11th day. The timing should be discussed with the midwife, so that they visit either together or separately by arrangement. The handover of care will take place either at this time or later on cessation of the midwife's visits, according to local practice or individual need. The midwife passes on all relevant information concerning the baby's welfare and how the mother is coping.

Medical cover in the postnatal period

The GP should call to see the mother and baby at least once and should thoroughly examine any baby born under his care as part of the maternity service he has agreed to provide. In most areas he carries out the postnatal examination at 6 weeks and some GPs are also involved in developmental screening programmes for babies.

He is notified immediately if any deviations from the normal occur in mother or baby. It may occasionally be necessary for one or other to be admitted to hospital. Conditions which warrant this include secondary postpartum haemorrhage or mental illness of the mother and convulsions or hypothermia of the baby. If at all possible, mother and baby should not be separated and arrangements should be made for both to be admitted if it is necessary for one of them.

Special situations

There are certain situations for which the community midwife needs to develop special skills.

'Failure' to produce a perfect healthy baby is traumatic for parents, a blow to their self-esteem and a cause of great distress. If the baby remains in hospital when the mother returns home there is a prolonged sense of unreality. Practical concerns about visiting the hospital, especially if there are other children needing attention, are added to their anxiety about the baby. The longer he remains in the Special Care Baby Unit the more difficulty the parents are likely to have in coping when he is finally discharged home, particularly if he is still very small or abnormal in some other way.

The birth of a handicapped baby is arguably the worst possible outcome of pregnancy, especially if the child survives. Not only do the parents need to work through their grief and dismay but they must also face an uncertain and difficult future. The midwife can prepare them for practical difficulties such as meeting neighbours and friends and may be able to help them to reconcile themselves to the situation. Parents who reject such a child may also need help in coming to terms with their decision.

Loss of a baby at any stage during pregnancy, or after birth, is increasingly recognised as calling for particular helping skills. A woman is usually sent home within a day or two of miscarriage or stillbirth. Her partner and parents will probably be unable to offer any support because of their own grief. Friends and neighbours may avoid her because they do not know what to say. GPs are busy, and the health visitor may not become in-

volved if this was the first baby. So it may fall to the community midwife to help the family to mourn. She should be notified of the woman's discharge from hospital in the usual way, whatever the stage of pregnancy. Visits should be made according to need, as for families with a baby.

The subject of counselling is dealt with in Chapter 49.

Reader Activities

Carry out a study of your local community. Identify, for example, the ethnic and social class mix, typical housing conditions, employment levels and types of employment, family structures, car ownership, public transport facilities.

- Taking into account the particular needs of pregnant women and mothers of young children, identify the quality and accessibility of local services. These could include shops, DSS office, Post Office, child care provision, and health care facilities, such as health centre or general practitioner surgery, maternity hospital, baby clinic, family-planning and well-woman services.
- How does the nature of the locality affect the work of the community midwife and other health professionals?
- What evidence is there that the needs of specific groups, such as teenage mothers, women from ethnic minorities and working mothers, are being identified and that attempts are being made by the health service to meet these needs?
- What patterns of maternity care are available to women in the locality?
- How are decisions made regarding types of antenatal care and place of birth? Do the women have a choice?

USEFUL ADDRESSES

Association for General Practice Maternity Care
Barncroft Surgery
Temple Sowerby
Penrith
Cumbria CA10 1RZ

Association for Improvements in the Maternity Services (AIMS)
21 Iver Lane
Iver
Buckinghamshire SL0 9LH
Tel: 0753 652781

Centre for Advice on Natural Alternatives (CANA)
Tydon Y Myndd
Llanelli Hill
Abergavenny
Gwent NP7 0PN

CRY-SIS
B. M. Cry-sis
London WC1N 3XX
Tel: 071 404 5011

Home Birth Centre
Flat 3
55 Elm Grove
Southsea
Hampshire PO5 1JF
Tel: 0705 864494

Independent Midwives Association (IMA)
94 Auckland Road
London SE19 2DB

International Home Birth Movement
22 Anson Road
London N7 0RD
Tel: 071 607 4137

Miscarriage Association
PO Box 24
Ossett
West Yorkshire WF4 4TP
Tel: 0924 830515

National Childbirth Trust
Alexandra House
Oldham Terrace
London W3 6NH
Tel: 081 992 8637

PARENTLINE (Organisations for Parents under Stress)
Rayfa House
57 Hart Road
Thundersley
Essex SS7 3PD
Tel: 0268 757077

Society to Support Home Confinements
Lydgate
Lydgate Lane
Wolsingham DL13 3HA
Tel: 0388 528044

Stillbirth and Neonatal Death Society (SANDS)
28 Portland Place
London W1N 4DE
Tel: 071 436 5881

Twins and Multiple Births Association (TAMBA)
59 Sunnyside
Worksop
Nottinghamshire S81 7LN
Tel: 0909 479250

REFERENCES

Elbourne D, Oakley A, Chalmers I 1989 Social and psychological support during pregnancy. In: Chalmers I, Enkin M, Keirse M J N C (eds) Effective care in pregnancy and childbirth. Oxford University Press, Oxford, vol 1, ch 15, p 233

Garcia J, Blondel B, Saurel-Cubizolles M J 1989 The needs of childbearing families: social policies and the organization of health care. In: Chalmers I, Enkin M, Keirse M J N C (eds) Effective care in pregnancy and childbirth. Oxford University Press, Oxford, vol 1, ch 14

Reid M, Garcia J 1989 Women's views of care during pregnancy. In: Chalmers I, Enkin M, Keirse M J N C (eds) Effective care in pregnancy and childbirth. Oxford University Press, Oxford, vol 1, ch 8

Rush J, Chalmers I, Enkin M 1989 Care of the new mother and baby. In: Chalmers I, Enkin M, Keirse M J N C (eds) Effective care in pregnancy and childbirth. Oxford University Press, Oxford, vol 2, ch 78, p 1341

Townsend P, Davidson N (eds) 1988 The Black report 1982. In: Inequalities in health. Pelican, Harmondsworth

United Kingdom Central Council for Nursing, Midwifery and Health Visiting 1989 A Midwife's Code of Practice. UKCC, London

FURTHER READING

Association of Radical Midwives 1986 The Vision: proposals for the future of the maternity services. ARM, Ormskirk

Campbell R, Macfarlane A 1987 Where to be born: the debate and the evidence. National Perinatal Epidemiology Unit, Radcliffe Infirmary, Oxford

Claxton R (ed) 1986 Birth matters: issues and alternatives in childbearing. Unwin Paperbacks, London

Cronk M, Flint C 1989 Community midwifery: a practical guide. Heinemann Nursing, Oxford

Davies J, Evans F 1991 The Newcastle community midwifery care project. In: Robinson S, Thomson A M (eds) Midwives, research and childbirth. Chapman and Hall, London, vol 2, ch 5

Flint C 1991 Continuity of care provided by a team of midwives — the Know Your Midwife Scheme. In: Robinson S, Thomson A M (eds) Midwives, research and childbirth. Chapman and Hall, London, vol 2, ch 4

Huntingford P Birth right: the parents' choice. BBC Publications, London

Inch S 1982 Birthrights: a parents' guide to modern childbirth. Hutchinson, London

Kitzinger S 1979 Birth at home. Oxford University Press, Oxford

Kitzinger S, Davis J A 1978 (eds) The place of birth. Oxford University Press, Oxford

Laryea M 1984 Postnatal care: the midwife's role. Churchill Livingstone, Edinburgh

Monaco M, Junor V 1980 Homebirth handbook. Junor, Monaco

Porter M, Macintyre S 1989 Psychosocial effectiveness of antenatal and postnatal care. In: Robinson S, Thomson A M (eds) Midwives, research and childbirth. Chapman and Hall, London, vol 1, ch 4

Rakusen J, Davidson N 1982 Out of our hands: what technology does to pregnancy. Crucible — Science in Society. Pan, London

Royal College of Midwives 1991 Towards a healthy nation: every day a birthday. RCM, London

Zander L, Chamberlain G (eds) 1984 Pregnancy care for the 1980s. Royal Society of Medicine and Macmillan, London

40

Special exercises for pregnancy, labour and the puerperium

EILEEN BRAYSHAW

Back care

Relief of aches and pains

Antenatal exercises

Teaching exercises

Stress, relaxation and respiration

Labour

Postnatal exercises

An obstetric physiotherapist is the ideal choice to teach physical skills required for parenthood. However, in areas where there is no physiotherapist available, midwives may find themselves responsible for physical preparation as well as parent education in antenatal classes. This chapter will give midwives an insight into the teaching of physical skills and information about exercise, relaxation and breathing for pregnancy, labour and the puerperium.

Preparation for parenthood classes provide the opportunity for talks, exercise and discussion sessions with a combined approach from midwives, physiotherapists, health visitors and other health care professionals. They should aim to create a learning environment with a relaxed atmosphere, where parents-to-be can enjoy developing a confidence to cope with pregnancy, labour, delivery and the early postnatal days. Specific therapeutic aims of physical preparation include the prevention or relief of minor discomforts such as backache, the teaching of coping strategies for labour, the promotion of a speedy postnatal recovery and the prevention of future gynaecological or orthopaedic problems. Exercise sessions should be designed to stimulate interest in the physical changes occurring, to promote body awareness and to facilitate physical and mental relaxation. Classes held early in pregnancy allow for advice and discussion relating to rest, anticipated postural changes and relief of minor discomforts. Sessions covering relaxation, positions for labour and postnatal exercises are more appropriate during the third trimester of pregnancy.

Gentle exercise during pregnancy stimulates circulation, helps to keep joints flexible, creates good muscle tone and promotes a general sense of well-being. It is advisable to avoid long periods of standing or sitting.

Walking in the fresh air remains the most natural and simplest form of exercise and should be encouraged. Exercise sessions should be interspersed with periods of rest and relaxation whenever possible.

Cycling is another popular form of exercise which allows for good mobility of the lower limbs with the body weight supported. It is an easy way to travel, although short distances are preferable. Steep hills should be avoided and it is advisable to stop before feeling tired.

Swimming is excellent exercise as water relieves the weight of gravity on the body and muscles can be strengthened and flexibility of joints retained without undue fatigue. It is important to avoid strenuous activities such as diving and crawl or butterfly strokes during pregnancy. Breast stroke is usually the most popular but has a tendency to aggravate backache. Leisurely back stroke with gentle supporting arm movements is often the most comfortable way to proceed.

In many areas local swimming pools hold *aquanatal classes*. If these are well designed and carefully supervised by a suitably qualified professional, they are an excellent and a very enjoyable way of keeping fit.

Energetic and competitive sports activities, such as squash, aerobics, horse riding, jogging and skiing are best avoided during pregnancy and it is not the time to take up new sports. Strenuous keep-fit exercises such as sit-ups and double leg lifts should *never* be performed as these may cause ligamentous strain and consequent back problems. For the same reason, pregnant women should avoid lifting heavy weights or objects.

Postural changes in pregnancy

Accompanying the gradual gain in weight in pregnancy and its centralising redistribution is

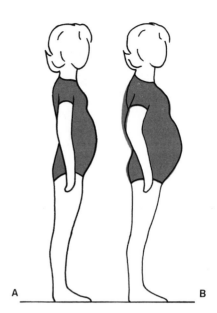

Fig. 40.1
(A) Posture in early pregnancy. (B) Posture in later pregnancy — note increased lordosis.

the hormonal influence on ligamentous structures. Both of these factors alter the posture of the pregnant woman (Fig. 40.1) and her self-image. The body's centre of gravity moves forwards and when this is combined with stretching of weak abdominal muscles it often leads to a subsequent hollowing of the lumbar spine with a rounding of the shoulders and the head poking forwards. There is a tendency for the back muscles to shorten as the abdominal muscles stretch, extra strain is placed on the ligaments and the end result is backache, usually of sacro-iliac or lumbar origin. Postural re-education, including correction of the 'pelvic tilt', should be taught preferably with the benefit of a full length mirror. The theme of back care must be developed with advice relating to comfortable positions in sitting, standing, lying, general mobility and how to lift correctly.

BACK CARE

Sitting. The pregnant woman should choose a comfortable chair which supports both back and thighs. She should sit well back and if necessary place a small cushion or folded towel behind the lumbar spine for additional comfort. The seat height should allow the feet to rest on the floor, or a small footstool or cushion may be placed under the feet to raise them slightly (Fig. 40.2). If relax-

ing in an easy chair, the head can be supported and the legs elevated on a stool.

Standing. The posture should be as tall as possible with both the abdomen and buttocks tucked in. Weight must be evenly distributed on both legs, to prevent undue strain on the pelvic ligaments, and spread between the heels and balls of the feet. High heels will throw the balance of the pregnant woman too far forward and are best discarded in favour of a medium- or low-heeled shoe which also gives support. Shoulders which are relaxed and down help to prevent thoracic aches.

Lying. Equal pressures on all parts of the body will lead to a good posture in lying with no undue strain on any one area. Lying flat on the back must be discouraged because of the danger of supine hypotension: three or four pillows or a wedge will raise the head and shoulders sufficiently to avoid that risk (Fig. 40.3). It may be more comfortable with a pillow placed under the thighs to reduce the tension behind the knees. Side-lying (coma position) with pillows under the top forearm and knee is a common posture adopted by pregnant women (Fig. 40.4).

Getting up from lying by bending the knees, rolling onto one side then using the arms to push up into a sitting or kneeling position will prevent strain on both the back and the abdominal muscles.

Household activities. Discussion needs to take place on the way in which the woman does her housework. Many tasks such as ironing or preparing food can be undertaken in a sitting position instead of standing. Working surfaces at the correct height or the use of a high stool will avoid the need to stoop and the subsequent backache which a stooping posture can bring about. Making beds or cleaning the bath in a kneeling position prevents lumbar strain.

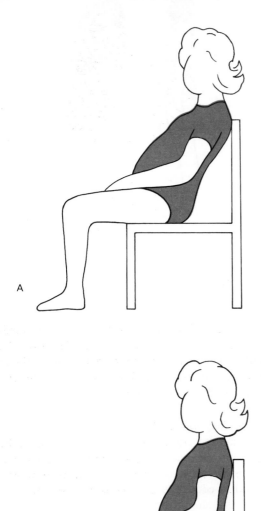

A

B

Fig. 40.2
(A) Poor sitting posture. (B) Good sitting posture.

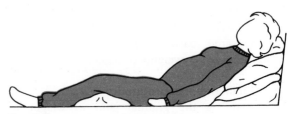

Fig. 40.3
Half back lying supported with pillows.

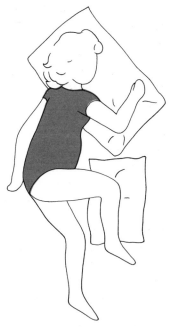

Fig. 40.4
Side lying supported with pillows.

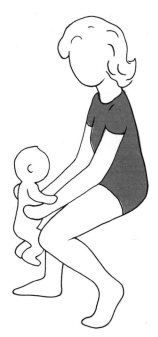

Fig. 40.5
Correct lifting.

Lifting heavy or awkward objects should be avoided during pregnancy if at all possible. If lifting is unavoidable then the object must be held close to the body with the knees bent and the back kept straight (Fig. 40.5). That way the strain is taken by the thigh muscles not those of the back. All twisting movements whilst lifting are dangerous and must not be executed.

RELIEF OF ACHES AND PAINS

Backache
This is a fairly common problem during pregnancy and can be helped by encouraging the mother to follow the advice on posture and encouraging practice of the pelvic tilting exercise in standing, sitting and lying positions.

Cramp
Prevention of cramp is helped by practising foot and leg exercises. To relieve sudden cramp in the calf muscles whilst in the sitting position the woman should hold the knee straight and stretch

the calf muscles by pulling the foot upwards (dorsiflexing) at the same time. Alternatively, standing firmly on the affected leg and striding forwards with the other leg, will stretch the calf muscles and solve the problem.

Rib stitch or discomfort
Discomfort around the rib cage can often be relieved by adopting a good posture, or by specifically stretching one or both arms upwards, depending on which side the pain is present.

Relief of sciatic discomfort
Suggest lying on the side away from the discomfort, so that the affected leg is uppermost. Pillows should be placed strategically to support the whole limb.

ANTENATAL EXERCISES

It is a fact that muscles of good tone are more elastic and will regain their former length more efficiently and more quickly after being stretched than muscles of poor tone. Exercising the *abdominal muscles* antenatally will ensure a speedy return to normal postnatally, effective pushing in labour and the lessening of backache in pregnancy. An important function of the abdominal muscles is the control of the pelvic tilt. As the ligaments around the pelvis stretch and no longer give such firm support to the joints, the muscles become the second line of defence, helping to prevent an exaggerated pelvic tilt and unnecessary strain on the pelvic ligaments. It must be remembered that overstretched ligaments during pregnancy can lead to chronic skeletal problems postnatally as well as backache antenatally. To prevent this and to maintain good abdominal tone the pelvic tilting exercise is taught.

Pelvic tilting or rocking

- Lie well supported with pillows, knees bent and feet flat. Place one hand under the small of the back and the other on top of the abdomen. Tighten the abdominals and buttocks, and press the small of the back down onto the underneath hand. Breathe normally, hold for 4 seconds then relax. Repeat five times.

Pelvic tilting can also be performed sitting or standing. It plays an important part in good posture.

A great strain is put on the muscles of the *pelvic floor* during pregnancy by both the weight of the developing fetus and the altered pelvic posture. It is important, therefore, to teach pregnant women pelvic floor exercises antenatally in order to maintain the tone so that these muscles

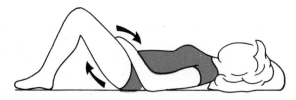

Fig. 40.6
Pelvic tilting exercise.

retain their functions, will relax during parturition and regain their former strength quickly during the puerperium. (For anatomy and functions see Ch. 2.)

All women should be able to perform this simple exercise which can be practised anywhere and at any time.

Pelvic floor exercise

- Sit, stand or lie with legs slightly apart. Close and draw up around the back passage as though preventing a bowel action then repeat around the front two passages as though preventing the flow of urine. Hold for as long as is comfortable, breathing normally, then relax. Repeat four times.

All women should practise this exercise very regularly antenatally, particularly after emptying the bladder. For those with diminished pelvic floor awareness, attempting to 'stop midstream' occasionally or 'gripping' on to an imaginary tampon which is slipping out may assist the ability to contract the correct muscles.

Foot and leg exercises

The circulation during pregnancy, particularly the venous return, is sluggish and this can lead to problems such as cramp, varicose veins and oedema. To help to prevent these the following simple exercises and advice will improve the circulation.

- Sit or lie with legs supported. Bend and stretch the ankles twelve times. Circle both feet at the ankle twelve times in each direction. Brace both knees, hold for 4 seconds, then relax. Repeat six times.

These exercises should be performed before getting up from resting, last thing at night and several times during the day. Women should be discouraged from standing unnecessarily and encouraged to put their feet up whenever possible. Crossing the legs at the knee or ankle will impede circulation further. If varicose veins or oedema are present, support tights may be prescribed with the appropriate advice to put them on before allowing the legs to drop over the edge of the bed.

Breathing awareness

It is important to be aware of one's own natural breathing rhythm.

- Sit comfortably with eyes closed. 'Listen in' to your breathing, concentrating especially on the outward breath, recognising the short pause before the inward breath naturally follows. Keep the movement fairly low down in the chest and be aware of your own breathing rate whilst resting.

A few deeper breaths now and again will help the venous return and aid the oxygen supply to both the pregnant woman and her baby but only three or four breaths at a time or hyperventilation may occur.

TEACHING EXERCISES

Anyone who is teaching exercises to others must first be proficient at performing those particular exercises herself. Next she must familiarise herself with instructions describing the execution of the exercise and practise teaching two or three colleagues or family members before introducing the teaching to a larger group. It is important to describe or demonstrate fully and to give relevant additional information which makes the topic more interesting and meaningful. When planning to teach specific exercises, such as foot and leg exercises, think in the following way:

Teaching foot and leg exercises

Why the exercise is relevant
- During pregnancy, circulatory changes occur which may lead to cramp, oedema or varicose veins.

What we hope to achieve
- Improvement in circulation and prevention or alleviation of cramp, oedema and varicose veins.

How
- Bend and stretch the ankles.
- Circle feet at the ankles.
- Brace knees and let go.
- Repeat ten times.

When
- Several times per day and always before getting up from resting and last thing at night.

Additional information
- Avoid long periods of standing, which may increase oedema, but encourage walking.
- Discourage sitting or lying with legs crossed, which can impede circulation.
- Describe how to relieve cramp.
- Advise on correct use of support tights.
- Stress the importance of supporting footwear of sensible height.
- Advise sitting with feet elevated wherever possible and heels higher than hips if oedema is present.

The positions pregnant women are asked to adopt for exercises should be carefully considered. The women should not be asked to lie flat because of the danger of supine hypotension, instead a half-lying position with the back raised to an angle of approximately 45° can be used. Foot and leg exercises and pelvic tilting can be performed in sitting or half-lying whereas pelvic floor exercises can be carried out in any position.

Remember before asking a group to exercise on the floor, the correct way of getting up and down must be demonstrated.

STRESS, RELAXATION AND RESPIRATION

The normal stresses of everyday life often lead to a build-up of tension within the body. If anxiety, fear or pain are present the body may unconsciously adopt a posture which is extreme. Relaxation is concerned with reducing body tension to a minimum and once learned can be used whenever increased tension is a problem. It can be particularly useful during pregnancy and labour and the early postnatal days. Tension manifests itself with muscle tightening and shows in the following ways:

Frowning face
Tense jaw
Hunched shoulders
Elbows bent and close to sides
Fingers gripping or tapping
Trunk bent forward
Legs crossed
Feet pulled up or tapping.

When tension increases, breathing often becomes shallow and rapid, or when severe, breath-holding may feature. The higher the stress level, the greater the degree of postural change that will be evident. Mental tension often leads to physical tension and a vicious circle is established.

Ideas about relaxation have been developed and exchanged over many years but today it is generally recognised that 'Relax' is a negative instruction and does not readily bring results for most individuals. Muscles can work singly but usually they work in groups and when any group of muscles is working, the opposite group relaxes. This is a physiological fact and is known as reciprocal inhibition or reciprocal relaxation. Try the following example:

● Concentrate on your right hand.
● Stretch your fingers really long. Hold for a moment.
   (This is tightening the muscles on the back of your hand and wrist.)
● Now stop stretching and feel the ease not only in the muscles you were stretching but in the palm of your hand and fingers.

Reciprocal relaxation ensures that when following a series of instructions for the whole body, one will be able to bring release of tension and relaxation to all areas.

There is continual interest in the practice of yoga and general body awareness and both these avenues are worth pursuing with alternative approaches to achieving relaxation.

Planning a scheme of relaxation

To be effective, relaxation must be practised regularly and it is important to develop a theme running through classes and to encourage daily practice at home. The environment should be relatively peaceful with no irritating distractions such as the telephone. An adequate supply of mats, blankets and pillows is essential. In order to convey an air of confidence in the subject it is advisable to have a clear outline plan of instructions or commands. This allows for fluency and a tension-free progression which also help to create a relaxed atmosphere. Participants should be encouraged to wear loose, comfortable clothing, to remove shoes and spectacles and then choose a comfortable position in which to relax. This could be side lying, half back lying or sitting with supporting pillows strategically placed.

Physiological relaxation

This technique consists of a series of instructions and movements which help the body to move away from the posture caused by tension and so achieve a position of comfort, ease and relaxation. Following each individual instruction and movement, any tension in that part of the body will disappear.

> For each part of the body where tension manifests itself there is a threefold instruction:
>
> * an order to the reciprocal muscle group to work strongly
> * a command to that muscle group to stop working
> * a direction to the brain to recognise the new position of ease and to remember it.
>
> As with exercises the teacher of relaxation techniques must first practise them herself.

● Lie down comfortably on a firm surface with pillows supporting your head and thighs or sit in a suitable chair, with head, shoulders, arms and thighs supported (Fig. 40.3).

● *Shoulders*. Pull your shoulders towards your feet, — stop pulling — concentrate on this new position of ease — your shoulders are relaxed and down.

- **Arms.** Push your elbows slightly out from your body as though straightening the elbows — stop pushing, think about this position — your arms are relaxed and comfortably supported.

- **Hands.** Let them rest on your tummy or thighs or the supporting surface — stretch the fingers really long and straight — stop stretching — feel the new position — comfortably supported and relaxed.

- **Hips.** Tighten your buttocks and press your knees out sideways — stop tightening, register this comfortable position — your hips are relaxed.

- **Knees.** Move your knees slightly — stop moving them — feel the comfort you have created in your knees and thighs.

- **Feet.** Press your feet down — away from your face — stop pressing — you now have comfortably relaxed feet.

- **Body.** Press your body into the support, i.e. floor, bed or chair — stop pressing — be aware of comfort and relaxation in your trunk.

- **Head.** Press your head into the support, i.e. pillow or chair — now stop pressing — notice how this movement has relaxed your neck and shoulders.

- **Face.** Close your eyes if you want to. Drop your lower jaw slightly so that your teeth are not touching. Make sure that your tongue is resting comfortably in the lower jaw and not stuck to the roof of your mouth. Imagine that someone is smoothing away the frown lines from your forehead.

- **Breathing.** Give a big sigh out and continue to breathe gently keeping the movement fairly low down in the chest; be aware of the outward breath. Your body is now in a position of ease and is as relaxed as is possible in that position and you are breathing at your normal resting rate.

- Never get up in a hurry after a spell of relaxation. Instead, gently exercise the hands and feet to stir the circulation and slowly roll over onto one side, getting up in the correct way.

- Relaxation can be adapted and used as labour progresses by combining the most comfortable positions with easy breathing.

When group participants are fluent in the practice of relaxation there is no need to go through the whole check list of instructions every time. Gradually shorten the list of instructions given and work towards the situation where relaxation can be achieved almost spontaneously. The shoulders, arms and hands are usually the first areas to respond to stress and the following can be practised to be used during contractions.

- Shoulders down
- Arms comfortably supported
- Easy breathing and **sigh out slowly**.

This can be practised for the approximate duration of a contraction with concentration on easy breathing which helps to achieve comfort and relaxation.

Respiration

Respiration is affected by stress and adapted breathing is one of the easiest ways of assisting relaxation. Breathing can be used to increase the depth of relaxation by varying its speed; slower breathing leads to deeper relaxation. Natural rhythmic breathing must not be confused with specific unnatural levels or rates of breathing which research has proved to be harmful to both mother and fetus. Women in labour frequently breathe very rapidly at the peak of a contraction but should be encouraged not to do so. Persistent rapid breathing or breath-holding is usually a sign of panic.

Very slow deep breathing can cause hyperventilation, which can produce tingling in the fingers and may proceed to carpopedal spasm and even tetany. Rapid shallow breathing or panting is only tracheal and can lead to hypoventilation with subsequent oxygen deprivation.

During pregnancy, labour and delivery, emphasis should be placed on easy, rhythmic breathing and on avoiding very deep breathing, shallow panting or long periods of breath-holding.

LABOUR

It is important to stress to the parents-to-be, the relevance of co-operation with the midwife and a policy of working together. During exercise sessions it is often necessary to give reminders about where contractions are felt, how often they occur and their progression. The need for relaxation and breathing techniques should be stressed together with how and when they can be used. Careful choice of words is essential when describing pain and pain relief. As individuals, we appear to experience discomfort and pain to varying degrees. With good training it is possible to raise the individual's threshold of tolerance. A positive and down-to-earth approach is desirable when explaining the benefits of using breathing and relaxation techniques. It must be remembered that continual support and reminding will be necessary as labour progresses, if the breathing and relaxation techniques are to achieve their maximum potential.

Early first stage of labour

A woman in labour should be encouraged to keep mobile and active if there are no complications. When discomfort increases, she should be encouraged to try alternative positions of ease and to concentrate on rhythmical easy breathing during contractions.

Coping with early first stage of labour

The following positions of ease may help during the early stages of labour and can be discussed and practised in the antenatal period:

- sitting against a table and relaxing forwards so that shoulders, arms and head are supported.
- standing, leaning backwards against the wall of the room.
- kneeling on all fours.
- kneeling on the floor and leaning forwards against a chair.
- leaning forward against a partner.
- sitting astride an armless chair with arms supported on the chair back and body relaxing forwards.

Pelvic rocking in any of these positions may be helpful. Deep massage of the lower back or gentle stroking of the abdomen soothes many women and can be taught to the partner at couples' classes.

Later first stage of labour

As labour progresses it becomes more difficult to find a comfortable position and frequent changes may be necessary. Many women, however, are content to sit back against pillows on the bed at this stage and concentrate on relaxation and breathing. As each contraction builds up, the speed and depth of breathing sometimes alter but mothers must be encouraged to keep it as natural and easy as possible. They may find that 'sighing out slowly' (SOS) helps to avoid panic breathing and also relaxes physical tension.

The emotional aspects of the end of the first stage of labour will be explained to couples antenatally and coping strategies need to be discussed. If there is a premature urge to push, an interrupted outward breath can be introduced (i.e. two shorter breaths out followed by a longer breath out). This is often known as pant, pant, blow or puff, puff, blow breathing and it prevents the diaphragm from fixing and a subsequent increase in intra-abdominal pressure. An alteration in position will take away some of the urge to push, for example side lying or prone kneeling with the forehead resting on the hands.

Second stage of labour

Positions for second stage will depend on individual choice, method of pain relief and obstetric factors but mothers should give some thought to alternatives available in their delivery suite. These may include:

- side lying
- kneeling and leaning forwards facing the backrest of the bed with pillows placed for comfort
- kneeling on all fours
- squatting on the bed or floor
- supported squatting — partner holding from behind

- sitting fairly upright against the backrest with knees bent and feet resting on the bed.

As the contraction starts, the mother is reminded to breathe in and out gently. When the urge to push becomes overwhelming she will tuck in her chin and bear down, keeping the pelvic floor relaxed. Breath-holding should not be encouraged because of the danger of fetal hypoxia (see Ch. 14). To prevent pushing whilst the head is delivered, SOS breathing can be practised.

POSTNATAL EXERCISES

These should be started as soon after delivery as possible in order to improve circulation, strengthen pelvic floor and abdominal muscles and prevent transient and long-term problems.

Circulatory exercises

Foot and leg exercises as described in the antenatal section must be performed very frequently in the immediate postnatal period to improve circulation, reduce oedema and prevent deep vein thrombosis (DVT). If oedema is present the foot of the bed may be raised slightly.

Pelvic floor exercises

The pelvic floor muscles have been under strain during pregnancy and stretched during delivery and it may be both difficult and painful to contract these muscles postnatally. Mothers should be encouraged to try the exercise as often as possible in order to regain full bladder control, prevent prolapse and ensure normal sexual satisfaction for both partners in the future. The exercise can be linked to, and performed during, everyday activities such as feeding, bathing, nappy changing and after each visit to the toilet.

The contraction, as described in the antenatal section, should be held for a few seconds if possible before relaxing, and repeated four times at any one time, breathing normally throughout.

Mothers should be encouraged to test their pelvic floor muscles after 2 to 3 months. With a full bladder they should be able to jump up and down with legs apart and cough deeply without leaking urine. If there is leakage then the exercise must be continued several times a day for a further 3 months and the test repeated. If leakage still occurs the mother should report back to her GP for a physiotherapy or gynaecological referral. Future pregnancies will exacerbate the problem. Even if there is no leakage on testing, every woman should exercise her pelvic floor muscles regularly to prevent gynaecological problems.

Abdominal exercises

The straight and oblique muscles need to regain tone as soon as possible after delivery in order to protect the spine, prevent back problems and help the mother regain her 'former figure'.

Pelvic tilting

Pelvic tilting as described in the antenatal exercise section will tone up the straight abdominal (rectus abdominis) muscles and will ease any postural backache which may occur in the first few days of the puerperium. As the abdominal muscles become stronger, the woman can progress to lifting the head and stretching the hands towards the knees whilst holding the pelvis tilted. This is known as a 'curl-up' but must always be performed with the knees bent (Fig. 40.7).

After 48 hours the rectus muscles (see Fig. 40.8A) should be checked for any undue diastasis. A gap of two knuckles at this stage is considered normal and the mother may progress to exercising the oblique abdominal muscles. However, if the gap is more than two knuckles' width and 'peaking' of the abdominals is visible on head-lifting, then the straight abdominals only should

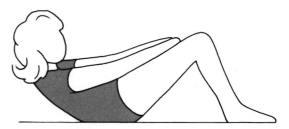

Fig. 40.7
Curl-up exercise.

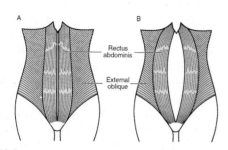

Fig. 40.8
(A) Rectus muscles before pregnancy. (B) Diastasis of rectus muscles after delivery.

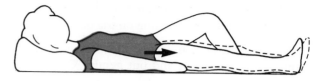

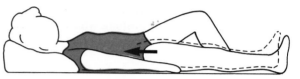

Fig. 40.9
Hip hitching (up-drawing) exercise.

be exercised until the gap reduces (Fig. 40.8B). An obstetric physiotherapist will advise on a regime of exercise and follow-up.

Knee rolling

This exercise will strengthen the oblique abdominal muscles.

- In back-lying with knees bent, pull in the abdomen and roll both knees to one side as far as is comfortable, keeping shoulders flat. Return knees to an upright position, then repeat to the other side. This exercise can be performed six to ten times.

Hip hitching

Also working the oblique abdominals, hip-hitching or leg-shortening is performed in back-lying with one knee bent and the other knee straight.

- Slide the heel of the straight leg downwards thus lengthening the leg. Shorten the same leg by drawing the hip up towards the ribs on the same side. Repeat six to ten times, keeping the abdomen pulled in. Change to the opposite side.

Exercises following caesarean section

Comfort is a high priority and can be achieved by the use of adequate pillows. These should preferably be three or four for the back, shoulders and head with an additional one under the thighs to take the strain from the sutures.

Foot and leg exercises as described earlier should be started as soon as possible especially after epidural anaesthesia as distal circulation will be especially sluggish. These may be followed by not more than four deep breaths to ensure full expansion of the lungs and pumping action on the inferior vena cava. If a general anaesthetic has been given, the mother may have extra secretions and needs to be taught how to clear them by coughing in a sitting position with the sutures supported by both hands or a pillow. Deep breathing and huffing will help to loosen the secretions.

To ease backache and flatulence the *pelvic tilting* and *knee rolling* exercises can be practised gently after 24 hours.

Mothers will progress to the *pelvic floor exercise*, *curl-ups* and *hip hitching* when they feel more comfortable, usually after 4–5 days.

Adequate rest is essential postnatally to allow the tissues to regain their normal function. After a caesarean section the woman has not only given birth but has also undergone major surgery yet she still has to cope with her baby. The midwife must take every opportunity to remind relatives of the need to help with chores and the organisation of rest periods for the mother.

Care of the back

It is several weeks before the ligaments resume their normal functions so it is vital that mothers receive advice on back care in relation to everyday activities at this time.

When feeding, the mother should sit back in a chair well supported with the baby raised up on pillows to prevent a slouched forward position. Nappy changing and bathing are best carried out at waist level or with the mother kneeling at a surface at coffee-table height.

Lifting should be avoided if at all possible but if unavoidable the object should be as light as possible and kept close to the body. The knees are bent and the back must be kept straight (Fig. 40.5).

Resuming sporting activities

The postnatal exercises illustrated are safe and effective and need to be practised regularly and increased gradually. Walking, cycling and swimming will increase general fitness but more strenuous keep-fit exercises, aerobics and competitive sports are best left until 10–12 weeks after delivery and then only resumed after ensuring the pelvic floor muscles are functioning effectively. **Double leg lifts and sit-ups should never be performed.**

Conclusion

During pregnancy, labour and the puerperium, midwives and other health care professionals have many opportunities to influence parents-to-be, incorporating a sensible approach to exercise within the broader sphere of healthy routines for all family members.

Relaxation, walking, cycling, swimming and other forms of exercise should be encouraged as part of a general lifestyle. Specific exercises for strengthening abdominal muscles or relieving aches and pains, e.g. cramp or backache, will have relevance far beyond the months of child bearing.

Parents-to-be are an extremely receptive audience. These opportunities to develop both specific and general health care measures should not be missed.

Reader Activities

- In any one day, write down all the stressful situations you have experienced.
- Observe others in stressful situations and note how the stress manifests itself.
- Practise physiological relaxation, repeating the instructions until you no longer need to read them. Teach your staffroom colleagues the method at lunch-time and explain the theory behind it.
- Perform each of the exercises in the ante- and postnatal sections. Memorise the instructions until you are ready to teach colleagues or family.
- Write down why, how, where and when each exercise should be performed.

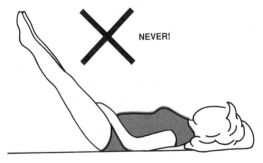

Fig. 40.10
Never attempt double leg lifts.

FURTHER READING

Mitchell L 1987 Simple relaxation. John Murray, London
Noble E 1990 Essential exercises for the childbearing year. Houghton Mifflin, Boston
Whitehead B, Polden M 1991 The postnatal exercise book. Frances, Lincoln

41

Specialised antenatal investigations

JEAN PROUD

Screening for congenital abnormalities

Ultrasound

Invasive procedures undertaken during pregnancy

Intra-uterine therapeutic procedures

Screening for intra-uterine growth retardation

Use of radiology in obstetrics

The provision of good antenatal care has always been a priority for the midwife. A healthy mother produces a healthy baby and midwives for generations have been involved in educating mothers on fitness both during pregnancy and prior to having a family. Early booking and the early detection of any abnormality during the pregnancy have always been thought to be important, as antenatal diagnosis of any maternal condition can lead to appropriate treatment of the mother, with obvious beneficial effect for the fetus.

In the past few years knowledge has vastly increased. It is now possible to diagnose conditions occurring in the fetus. This has largely been due to rapid advances in technology and new discoveries in genetics and biochemistry. In turn this has led to advances in such areas as treatment of the fetus in utero and also in neonatal surgery. A new branch of antenatal care has therefore evolved which offers prenatal diagnosis and treatment.

This rapid advance in knowledge, though obviously of great benefit to all involved, produces its own set of problems in the medical, ethical and social fields. The midwife will inevitably find herself involved in counselling parents faced with dilemmas which were not confronted a few years ago. It is therefore important that midwives keep up to date with advances in prenatal diagnosis so that they are in a position to advise and assist in counselling when problems arise.

Because of this increased knowledge, many mothers now have access to specialised screening programmes. From the first antenatal visit parents are therefore faced with decisions as to whether or not to avail themselves of the opportunity of screening. They also need to consider the implications involved if they do or if they decide to decline. Some of these investigations will be described in this chapter.

SCREENING FOR CONGENITAL ABNORMALITIES

Maternal serum screening

Alpha fetoprotein

This fetal protein is present in small amounts in the maternal serum during pregnancy. It is also present in the amniotic fluid. Normal values have been assessed in both the maternal serum and in the amniotic fluid in the mid-trimester of pregnancy. Levels of alpha fetoprotein in the maternal serum are highest in early pregnancy and decrease as the pregnancy advances. Levels higher than normal are found in cases of open defects of the fetus, since obviously there is a leakage of alpha fetoprotein into the amniotic fluid, some of which enters the maternal circulation. Measurement of the maternal serum alpha fetoprotein (MSAFP) can be undertaken to detect this type of abnormality. Recent studies have shown that in the absence of open defects high levels indicate such abnormalities as renal anomalies, Turner's syndrome and the so-called 'high risk' pregnancy.

This procedure has now been superseded by what has become known as the 'triple test', so called because the maternal serum is not only tested for alpha fetoprotein (AFP) concentration, but also for the concentration of unconjugated oestriol and human chorionic gonadotrophin (HCG).

A low level of MSAFP is associated with Down's syndrome in the fetus. A more accurate estimation of this risk can be obtained by combining the serum concentration of unconjugated oestriol, which has also been found to be low in such instances, together with the serum concentration of AFP and the maternal age. In this way 45% of affected pregnancies can be identified.

Further research has shown that by adding to this the concentration of HCG in the maternal serum, which is usually high in affected pregnancies, a risk factor can be obtained which leads to 60% of affected pregnancies being identified (Wald et al 1988a, 1988b).

The concentrations of these three substances in the maternal serum may be estimated from 15–20 weeks' gestation but they can be most accurately assessed between 16 and 18 weeks. A sample of maternal blood is obtained and the serum removed for examination.

Because of its value in picking up fetal anomalies many districts offer parents the triple test screening programme. Programmes vary greatly from one district to another depending on the facilities available. It is essential to have an ultrasound service alongside such a programme. Ultrasound scanning will give an accurate estimation of gestational age, identify multiple pregnancy or fetal death and examine the suspect fetus. The incidence of open neural tube defects varies from one geographical area to another. Wales, for example, is known to have a higher incidence of these abnormalities than East Anglia. This factor is taken into account when deciding whether routine screening should be offered.

Reasons for raised levels of AFP in the maternal serum are as follows:

- Over-assessment of gestational age.
- Multiple pregnancy, with the exception of monozygotic twins because there is more placental tissue than usual.
- Fetal death.
- An open defect of the fetus, e.g. anencephaly, open spina bifida, gastroschisis, exomphalos.
- More rarely, Turner's syndrome, associated with cystic hygroma.
- False positive result. (The rate is approximately 1:7.)

Reasons for low levels of AFP are:

- Under-assessment of gestational age.
- A possible association with Down's syndrome.

Taking this together with a low level of unconjugated oestriol and a high level of HCG, and taking into consideration the maternal age, an estimated risk factor can be given to the mother as to the possibility of her carrying a fetus suffering from Down's syndrome.

In the majority of programmes if the first result shows a raised level of MSAFP, a second sample of maternal serum is obtained and the two results are averaged. If the mean of the two results is above normal, there are two options:

- The fetus is examined by ultrasound.
- The patient undergoes amniocentesis, when a specimen of amniotic fluid is obtained and the level of alpha fetoprotein is measured.

In some centres both of these options are undertaken. An ultrasound scan does not only detect an abnormality of the fetus but can assess its type, extent and severity. The level of AFP in the amniotic fluid can be measured and this is a more accurate assessment than in the maternal serum. A further examination is performed which is more specific, namely estimation of the level of acetylcholinesterase in the amniotic fluid. This is determined by polyacrylamide gel electrophoresis which reveals distinguishing bands that confirm diagnosis of an open neural tube or an abdominal defect. False positive results are very rare.

If the triple test reveals that there is a high risk that the mother is expecting a baby suffering from Down's syndrome karyotyping of the fetal chromosomes is carried out. A risk factor of over 1:200 is usually considered positive. The risk of having a baby with Down's syndrome is considered to be 1:190 at the age of 36 years, if age alone is considered. The fetal chromosomes can be examined in the fetal cells present in the amniotic fluid or those in fetal blood. Amniocentesis or cordocentesis will therefore be necessary.

Further research is taking place which involves measuring an enzyme, urea-resistant neutrophil alkaline phosphatase (UR-NAP) (Wald et al 1988b). The activity levels of this enzyme are markedly raised in women expecting a baby with Down's syndrome. It is hoped that it will be possible to carry this out at an earlier gestational age, namely in the first 12–13 weeks of gestation (Wald et al 1988a, 1988b).

It will be seen that the period of waiting for these results will be one of great anxiety for the pregnant woman and her partner. The midwife should be very much aware of this and should be prepared for frequent enquiries. In centres which offer a particularly good ultrasound service, some of this anxiety may be reduced by scanning the fetus for any obvious abnormality.

Although in some centres the blood samples taken routinely at booking include sufficient for a specimen for the triple test, the implications of this test should first be discussed with the woman and, if possible, with her partner. It is very important that the couple is told exactly what abnormalities the test is able to detect, what the programme entails and the options available in the event of an abnormality being detected. This does not necessarily mean termination of pregnancy; parents for whom this would be unacceptable need not be excluded from the programme.

The explanation is likely to take place at the first visit to the GP's surgery or the first hospital antenatal clinic visit. It takes place in a strange environment and at a time when a lot of other equally important information is given to the mother. Much will be forgotten. It is helpful for her to have some written material to take away and refer to later. Many hospitals require written consent for the screening test.

If an abnormality is discovered and the type and severity assessed by ultrasound scan (USS), the parents can discuss the outcome of the pregnancy with the obstetrician.

- Termination of the pregnancy may be offered and accepted.
- Arrangements can be made for the birth of the affected infant to take place in a centre where specialised neonatal surgery can be performed.
- Genetic counselling may be appropriate.

Midwives may not be directly involved in these discussions but they need to be available to provide empathy and support and to answer any questions arising following the interview. It will be seen that a good counselling service is vital to back up a prenatal screening programme (see Ch. 49).

ULTRASOUND

During pregnancy most women are offered an ultrasound scan. In some districts this is a routine procedure, whilst others recommend its use only when there are clinical indications.

Indications for USS are a controversial issue, especially during pregnancy. Many obstetricians think that the advantages of routine scanning during pregnancy far outweigh the disadvantages. Others would argue that clinical skills are being lost because instant information is easily obtained from the 'scan'.

Advantages of USS

* It is a surgically non-invasive technique.
* The mother requires minimal preparation.
* It provides instant information.
* Movement can be observed, e.g.
  — heart valves
  — fetal behaviour.
* It promotes fetomaternal bonding and can allay some maternal anxiety.

Disadvantages of USS

* The possibility of exposing the fetus to some danger as yet unknown.
* Possible decline of clinical expertise.
* Overreliance on ultrasound findings.
* The impersonal approach of some operators, replacing the personal examinations by the midwife.

There is little doubt that ultrasound should be treated with a great deal of respect.

Since the introduction of ultrasound into medicine, numerous research programmes have been undertaken to detect possible dangers to the patient.

Observations during USS on fetal movement, fetal breathing and fetal heart rate have been done. A retrospective study of children who were exposed to ultrasound in the uterus is still being carried out.

Ultrasound operators need to keep abreast of all reports issued regarding research into possible hazards so that they can advise obstetricians and patients accordingly. In the meantime operators must adhere to the recommendations regarding the use of ultrasound. Mothers' exposure time should be kept to the minimum and USS should never be used for fun just to 'watch the baby'.

How does ultrasound work?

Sound emitted at a high pitch travels in a more or less straight line. At a low pitch it spreads out. Sound which is produced at a very high pitch (ultrasound) is therefore transmitted in a narrow beam. The sound is produced by a type of electric gong. This gong (known as the probe or transducer) is a thin disc to which a wire is attached.

The transducer transforms electrical energy to sound and back again. When the transducer is placed on the body a sound wave passes into the body and encounters a structure; a fraction of that sound is reflected back. The echo is detected electronically and transmitted onto the screen as a dot.

The amount of sound reflected from each organ varies according to the type of tissue encountered; strong echoes give bright, white dots, whereas weaker echoes give various shades of grey according to their strength. Fluid-filled areas cause no reflection and give rise to a black image.

Scanners and transducers

There are two main types of scanner:

* The static scanner, i.e., producing static pictures. There is a single transducer which is attached to a rigid mechanical frame. It is moved in a horizontal or vertical plane over the patient to produce a picture.
* The real-time scanner:
  — the linear array
  — the sector.

The principle of both is the same. Moving pictures are produced. Instead of a single crystal there are several. These are arranged in a row on the linear array and on a disc in the sector. Each transducer sends a sound pulse and collects the echoes one after the other very rapidly. In this way a moving picture is produced.

Uses of ultrasound in obstetrics

Ultrasound scanning has for some time been widely used for accurate assessment of gestational age. This has proved invaluable in an age when the oral contraceptive is popular and surprisingly few women know the date of their last menstrual period. Differentiation can therefore be made between the fetus suffering from intra-uterine growth retardation (IUGR) and the one who is immature. A variety of measurements is used in order to assess the growth and well-being of the fetus.

Women who definitely know the date of their last menstrual period, and especially those who know the date of conception, do not necessarily need an ultrasound scan to confirm gestational age. It must be remembered that there is a small percentage of women in whom it is unjustifiable to date the pregnancy by ultrasound despite the fact that the measurements of the fetus may not be average for menstrual age. Approximately 5% of normal fetuses lie above or below the two standard deviations of the normal charts.

Measurements in common use

It should be remembered that in every case a series of measurements is more informative than a single one.

Linear measurements

Crown–rump length (CRL). This is the length of the embryo from the top of the head to the rump or end of the sacrum. This is used in the first trimester for estimation of gestational age.

Biparietal diameter (BPD). This is the measurement between the two parietal eminences of the fetal skull. It is useful in assessing gestational age during the second trimester. It becomes less accurate later in pregnancy because the shape of the head can change. The head circumference is then thought to be a more accurate measurement.

Limb lengths. All limbs can be measured. Measurement of the femur helps in estimating gestational age. In addition fetal anomalies associated with abnormal limb lengths can be detected and any fractures will be apparent.

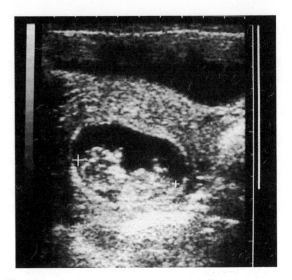

Fig. 41.1
USS showing crown–rump length.

Non-linear measurements

Head circumference (HC). Measurement of the circumference of the head is preferred in the third trimester when moulding may render the BPD less reliable. Because fetal growth is slower in the third trimester of pregnancy it is difficult to make a precise estimation of fetal age. However when gestation has been confirmed by USS in early pregnancy, HC is a useful measurement in help-

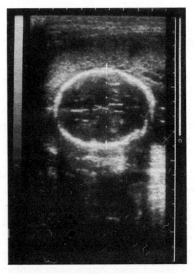

Fig. 41.2
USS showing biparietal diameter.

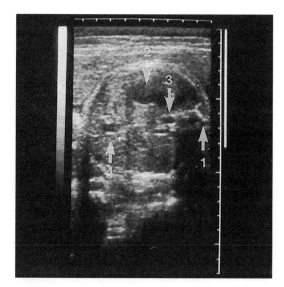

Fig. 41.3
USS showing abdominal circumference:
1 Spine; 2 Stomach; 3 Aorta; 4 Umbilical vein.

ing to detect intra-uterine growth retardation (IUGR).

Abdominal circumference (AC). This is measured at the level of the bifurcation of the main portal vein. The correct cross-section of the fetal trunk is obtained by bringing the bifurcation of the main portal vein, the fetal stomach and the fetal spine into view simultaneously. At this point the picture is frozen and the circumference measured. This is useful in screening for IUGR but not very accurate as a method of assessing gestational age.

The HC:AC ratio. The ratio between the two measurements described above helps in the diagnosis of growth retardation: if growth is retarded the abdomen will be affected before the head.

Area measurements can be calculated from the circumferences described above.

Volume measurements can be useful in some instances. These include sac volumes in very early pregnancy, which are used in the diagnosis of a blighted ovum. In later pregnancy pockets of amniotic fluid can be measured to give a guide to the total volume and may aid diagnosis of IUGR.

Nomograms are available for other measurements which are used in diagnosing fetal anomalies and are used by some centres. They include thigh measurements, intra-orbital distances and measurement of the cerebellum.

Scanning in early pregnancy

Ultrasound scanning in early pregnancy is usually a very rewarding experience both for the mother and the operator. It is especially delightful for a

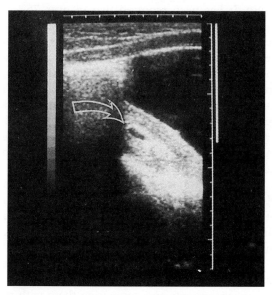

Fig. 41.4
USS showing early fetal sac.

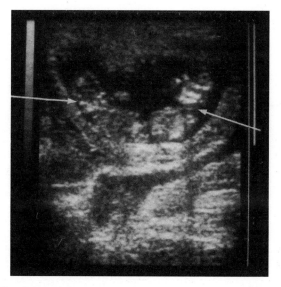

Fig. 41.5
USS showing twin pregnancy.

mother with a long history of infertility or one who has suffered the symptoms of a threatened abortion to see a live fetus moving on the screen.

A fetal sac can be seen from 5 weeks' gestation and a small embryo at 6 weeks' gestation including the movement of the fetal heart.

One can answer several useful questions by scanning in early pregnancy:

- Is the woman pregnant?
- Is the pregnancy intra-uterine?
- Is the pregnancy single or multiple?
- Is the fetus alive?
- What is the gestational age?
- Is there an associated pelvic mass? Fibroids or ovarian cysts can be diagnosed and measured. Luteal cysts are quite a common feature in early pregnancy.

Prenatal diagnosis of fetal abnormality

Ideally all mothers should have the opportunity of having an examination by ultrasound between 18 and 20 weeks' gestation, possibly in conjunction with a maternal serum screening programme. At this time an accurate assessment of gestational age can be made, multiple pregnancy can be diagnosed and the fetal anatomy can be checked for any abnormality. Some of these are quite obscure but a few of the more common ones are described here:

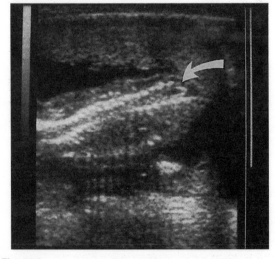

Fig. 41.6
USS showing fetal spine and spina bifida.

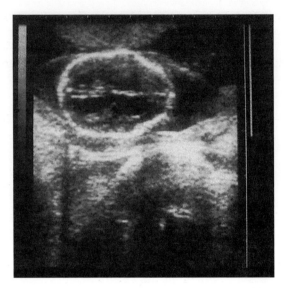

Fig. 41.7
USS showing hydrocephaly.

Craniospinal defects.

Anencephaly. Absence of the cranial vault can be detected as early as 12 weeks' gestation.

Spina bifida. The spine is examined to detect a neural arch that is not intact. A meningocele can be identified and the site, nature and extent of the lesion can be assessed.

Hydrocephaly and other disorders of the brain. It has been reported that in over 75% of cases of spina bifida there is associated hydrocephaly. Cases of isolated hydrocephaly can also be diagnosed. During a routine examination of the head, measurements of the ventricular hemispherical ratio (VHR) can be made. This is measured from the anterior horn of the lateral ventricle to the midline and expressed as a ratio over the width of the cerebral hemisphere. Similar measurements can be made from the posterior horn.

It is interesting to note that the BPD and the HC are not usually increased until the latter part of pregnancy in cases of hydrocephaly; indeed the BPD is usually small in comparison to other measurements such as CRL and AC.

Microcephaly. This is a difficult diagnosis to make by ultrasound. It is made by making serial HC measurements and comparing them with the fetal length and AC. The fetus with microcephaly can then be differentiated from the fetus suffering from IUGR.

Gastro-intestinal anomalies. Polyhydramnios is often the feature that alerts the ultrasound operator to consider atresia of the gastro-intestinal tract.

- In oesophageal atresia the stomach shadow is not seen except where there is an associated tracheo-oesophageal fistula.
- Atresias further down the tract are characterised by the appearance of cystic spaces: the lower the obstruction the more spaces seen.
- In cases of omphalocele and gastroschisis the MSAFP is raised and the anomaly can be seen outside the abdominal wall.
- Diaphragmatic hernia can be diagnosed by examination of the diaphragm and the chest.

If any of these conditions is detected the mother should be transferred to enable her to deliver in a unit where neonatal surgery is a specialty. Immediate care of the baby greatly increases the chances of a favourable outcome.

Renal tract anomalies. Oligohydramnios is the feature that indicates anomalies of the renal tract. As it is also present in severe cases of IUGR it is sometimes difficult to differentiate between the two. These cases are usually difficult to examine by USS because the black window provided by the amniotic fluid is absent.

Renal agenesis is characterised by the absence of kidney and bladder echoes. Polycystic kidneys can be diagnosed and also obstructive uropathies, where the enlarged bladder and sometimes hydronephrotic kidneys can be easily identified.

It should always be remembered that many structural defects are associated with chromosomal disorders. For example, many babies suffering from Down's syndrome have congenital heart defects. Detection of one fetal abnormality should always alert the ultrasonographer to look for another.

Chromosomal abnormalities. Many major structural abnormalities of the fetal heart can be detected by examination of the four chambers at the time of the 18–20 week scan. If more detailed examination of the vessels leading from and to the heart or exact diagnosis is required the woman should be referred to a specialist centre. Congenital heart defects, clefts of the lip and palate, cystic hygromas, choroid plexus cysts and many limb deformities can be detected by routine scanning. Many are 'markers' to certain chromosomal abnormalities. By careful examination of the fetus, therefore, a pattern of markers is produced so that a particular syndrome can be diagnosed and the parents counselled accordingly. Confirmation can be obtained by karyotyping of fetal cells.

Scanning the placenta

Localisation of the placenta

Since ultrasound became readily available it has been widely used to localise the placenta in cases of suspected placenta praevia, i.e. following antepartum haemorrhage or when the lie is abnormal or the presenting part is high at term.

It is common practice to comment in the scan report on the position of the placenta from 16 weeks' gestation. Women who are found to have a low-lying placenta at this time have a repeat scan in the last trimester to see whether its position relative to the cervical os has changed. Apparent movement or migration (as it has been called)

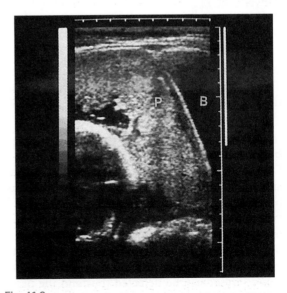

Fig. 41.8
USS showing low-lying placenta. P = Placenta, B = Bladder.

of the placenta occurs because of the growth of the uterus and formation of the lower segment which develops during the last trimester. Normally as the lower segment stretches and enlarges the lower edge of the placenta becomes more distant from the internal cervical os.

It has been found by ultrasonographers who have studied this phenomenon that approximately 20–30% of pregnant women are found to have a low-lying placenta in the second trimester but only about 0.5% have placenta praevia at term.

If a scan is being performed to localise the placenta, the woman's bladder must be reasonably full. It is necessary to note the relationship between the internal os and the lower edge of the placenta. The placenta is more difficult to locate if it is situated on the posterior uterine wall.

In instances where the placenta is found to be low-lying in the third trimester of pregnancy a diagnosis of placenta praevia is made. Repeat scans may be performed to obtain information about its exact position.

Placental abruption

A retroplacental clot can be visualised by ultrasound to give a diagnosis of placental abruption. It is also possible to see blood which has seeped between the membranes and uterine wall. Absence of these findings does not necessarily exclude placental abruption.

Trophoblastic disease or hydatidiform mole

The characteristic appearance of this rare condition is diagnostic.

Measurement of fetal and uteroplacental blood flow

During an ultrasound scan the fetal and uterine arteries can be observed and the movement of blood along them is visible.

In some units the blood flow in these vessels is measured by means of special equipment during the 18–20 week scan. There is much evidence to suggest that the fetus who is likely to become compromised can be detected thus and the pregnancy kept under close surveillance. This is useful in the diagnosis and management of IUGR.

Observation of fetal movement

One of the first questions asked at an antenatal clinic visit after 16 weeks' gestation is whether the mother is feeling the fetus move. Excessive fetal movements or reduced fetal movements signify fetal compromise.

Fetal movement can be observed on the screen of the real-time scanner as early as 7 or 8 weeks' gestation. This takes the form of total body movement, somersaulting, extension and flexion of the embryo. As the limbs become visible, their movements can be identified. Sucking, swallowing, and breathing movements can be observed; filling and emptying of the fetal stomach and bladder and rolling of the eyes can be seen at appropriate stages of gestation. Some of these observations have greater significance than others.

These observations are used, together with measurement of the liquor volume and examination of the texture of the placenta, to assess fetal well-being in the third trimester of pregnancy. The fetus is observed, usually for a period of half an hour, and a scoring system used to assess its condition. Low scores at this stage of pregnancy indicate the need for delivery.

The midwife's involvement in ultrasound scanning

The extent to which midwives are involved in ultrasound scanning varies widely. Some may never see an ultrasound scan at all whereas others are operators.

All midwives will be involved in the preparation of the mother and in counselling the parents when the findings are revealed. This can mean anything from giving a simple explanation of measurements and gestational age to offering support and advice when an abnormality is found.

Preparation of the woman
- It is desirable in most instances for the woman to have a reasonably full bladder.
- A gel is used as a couplant between the mother's skin and the transducer. It is inclined to stain and because of this some departments require the woman to wear a gown. Alternatively some

other protection must be provided to prevent the gel getting on her clothes.

- The mother should be given a full explanation of the procedure.

In most hospitals the mother can watch the screen during the ultrasound scan. Many units also welcome fathers and children, making the scan a delightful experience for the whole family and one that the mother looks forward to and remembers with joy.

Most ultrasound scanning takes place within an imaging department where the operator is usually a radiographer who is trained in all aspects of ultrasound. Besides scanning obstetric and gynaecological patients, he or she performs abdominal, ophthalmic and cardiac scans. In this case the mother will receive little information at the time and will be told the result of the scan later by her general practitioner or obstetrician.

In some units the obstetrician performs the ultrasound scan. Less commonly a midwife specially trained in the procedure will do so. This has the tremendous advantage that they can immediately apply their obstetric knowledge in interpreting the scan. The findings can be given to the mother immediately which eliminates any anxiety caused by delay.

Some imaging departments employ midwives to work alongside the radiographers. They are responsible for obstetric scanning only.

Depending on these arrangements, the responsible consultant may be a radiologist or an obstetrician.

The ultrasound scan operator has a great responsibility for promoting good relationships between the fetus and the family. In most instances this is a pleasant experience for all concerned. Difficulties arise when something abnormal is revealed on the screen. The mother very quickly becomes aware that something is wrong. Any one or a combination of the following events may occur:

- the operator's attitude changes and she or he may become quiet
- the atmosphere in the room becomes tense
- the mother may recognise the abnormality shown on the screen

- the operator hesitates to answer questions asked by the mother or her relatives.

The operator should always be completely honest with the woman in order to maintain her confidence, both in him- or herself and in the medical profession in general.

Definite guidelines must be laid down in advance of any such event in order to avoid difficulty. If the consultant obstetrician prefers disclosures of any abnormality to come directly from himself (or herself), he may give instructions to call him if a malformation is discovered. As this may be difficult to achieve, it has become the policy of many imaging departments to withhold the results and not to let the mother see the screen.

Midwife operators must be free to reveal the scan findings as they are bound to become involved in discussing the results. Midwives may be bombarded with questions after a couple have received news of an abnormality, even if they are not involved in the actual operation of the scan. They must therefore keep themselves up to date on the latest prenatal diagnoses, the treatments available and the possible outcomes of such pregnancies. In this way they are always in a position to give empathy and support.

INVASIVE PROCEDURES UNDERTAKEN DURING PREGNANCY

A mother who is to undergo an invasive investigative procedure will already be aware that there is some indication that the fetus may be abnormal. She and her partner are seeking assurance that this is not so.

Parents should be prepared carefully with a full explanation of the purpose of the investigation and a discussion of the hazards of the procedure itself (see below). They must weigh these against the risks of the suspected abnormality in order to arrive at their decision. Possible reasons for this type of procedure include:

- suspicion of Down's syndrome aroused by calculation of high risk following maternal serum screening
- a family history of fetal abnormality

- a family history of certain congenital abnormalities or medical conditions, e.g. Duchenne muscular dystrophy
- maternal illness which may affect the fetus
- Rhesus iso-immunisation in the mother
- raised maternal serum alpha fetoprotein
- suspicion of fetal abnormality on ultrasound scan.

Amniocentesis

Amniocentesis consists of withdrawing a sample of amniotic fluid through a transabdominal needle. Ultrasound has made this procedure a great deal safer because the placenta can be localised and avoided, a suitable pool of liquor can be identified and the depth of needle insertion can be measured. The scan should be performed immediately prior to insertion of the needle. With certain equipment the amniocentesis can be performed under direct visualisation, the needle being inserted through the ultrasound probe.

If fetal abnormality is suspected, amniocentesis is usually performed between 16 and 18 weeks' gestation. Earlier than this there is usually an inadequate pool of liquor and there are too few exfoliated fetal cells within it to be sure of getting a useful sample. Later than this there would be insufficient time to arrange a termination of pregnancy if this was desirable.

Indications for amniocentesis in early pregnancy

Chromosomal analysis. This may be done for chromosomal abnormalities, e.g. Down's syndrome or for fetal sexing in X-linked disorders, e.g. haemophilia. The incidence of chromosomal anomalies increases greatly with rising maternal age. The rate increases from 1.22% at a maternal age of 35 years to 9.7% at a maternal age of 47 years (Ferguson-Smith and Yates European Collaborative Study on Prenatal Diagnosis).

Neural tube defects. A raised level of alpha fetoprotein together with the presence of acetylcholinesterase in the amniotic fluid indicates a high probability of an open neural tube defect in the fetus (see above for details of the whole screening programme).

Inborn errors of metabolism. Examination of the liquor amnii for enzymes and metabolites can be helpful in the detection of certain inborn errors of metabolism but further work needs to be done in this area.

Deoxyribonucleic acid (DNA) analysis. Probes are now available which enable certain genes to be isolated from the DNA. This assists in the detection of such diseases as Duchenne muscular dystrophy, thalassaemia and sickle cell anaemia. As further probes are developed, it will become possible to identify more genetic disorders antenatally.

Indications for amniocentesis in later pregnancy

Rhesus iso-immunisation. Spectrophotometric scanning of the amniotic fluid is done in cases of fetal haemolytic disease to estimate the amount of bilirubin excreted by the fetus. This can be performed at frequent intervals to monitor the effect on the fetus of the rising antibody titre in the mother.

Assessment of fetal maturity. A sample of amniotic fluid is obtained in order to estimate the lecithin:sphingomyelin (L:S) ratio in the surfactant being produced by the fetal lungs. Surfactant is a surface-active phospholipid of which two components are lecithin and sphingomyelin. Its presence reduces surface tension within the alveoli and its lack is responsible for causing respiratory distress syndrome (RDS) (see Ch. 35).

The level of lecithin increases throughout pregnancy; the level of sphingomyelin remains constant. The ratio between these two phospholipids is a guide to fetal lung maturity. When the ratio reaches 2:1 the lungs are said to be mature and if the baby is delivered RDS should not develop. Since facilities for intensive care of the newborn have improved, this test has become infrequent.

Technique of amniocentesis

An ultrasound examination is performed, the placenta localised and a pool of liquor found. The woman's bladder should be empty and strict asepsis observed throughout the procedure. The skin is cleaned and dried and the doctor inserts a needle and stilette through the abdominal wall into the uterus. The needles most commonly used are 20 or 22 gauge spinal needles or a Medicut cannula. Local anaesthesia may be used but is not always considered necessary. 10–20 ml of amniotic fluid is withdrawn for analysis. If a stilette is not used, the first 2 ml may be contaminated with blood and should be discarded.

If the woman has a Rhesus negative blood group, a Kleihauer test for fetal red cells should be performed and anti-D immunoglobulin administered to the mother to prevent Rhesus iso-immunisation.

Following the procedure the fetal heart must be auscultated, if necessary with a Sonicaid. The woman must be given clear information about when to expect news of the result of the examination as there will be a delay of up to 5 weeks. The obstetrician may wish to advise her about her activities in the next few days.

Risks of amniocentesis

Maternal
Infection
Haematoma
Antepartum haemorrhage
Rhesus iso-immunisation
Fetal loss

Fetal
Death
Trauma
Haemorrhage
Abortion
Preterm labour
Amniotic fluid leakage
Respiratory problems
Orthopaedic abnormalities

Fetoscopy

This is a technique whereby direct visualisation of the fetus is undertaken via an endoscope. A cannula 2.4 × 3.0 mm in diameter with a selfoscope 1.7 mm in diameter, attached to a microscope and with a fine glass fibre light source is inserted transabdominally under local anaesthetic. An ultrasound scan is performed immediately

prior to the technique so that damage to placenta and fetus is kept to the minimum. The mother is usually sedated in order to reduce fetal and maternal movement. Fetoscopy is rarely performed: other procedures have proved less hazardous and equally effective.

The following samples can be obtained during fetoscopy:

* Fetal skin biopsy
* Fetal liver biopsy

Observations of maternal pulse, blood pressure and uterine activity and of the fetal heart rate are maintained for several hours following the examination. In addition, mothers with Rhesus negative blood must be given anti-D immunoglobin.

Risks of fetoscopy
Fetal loss 2–5%
Amniotic fluid leakage 4–5%
Preterm labour 8–10%.

Cordocentesis

This is a technique for sampling fetal blood during pregnancy in order to screen for chromosomal abnormalities, haemoglobinopathies and other disorders affecting the blood or cells.

A needle is guided to the base of the umbilical cord with the aid of ultrasound. It is also possible to sample the maternal placental blood from a sub-chorionic lake. This gives information about the oxygenation of the fetus. The procedure is simpler and less hazardous than fetoscopy and is becoming more widely used.

Blood can be taken during cordocentesis to screen for:

* haemophilia
* platelet disorders
* haemoglobinopathies
* severe combined immune deficiencies
* inborn errors of metabolism
* rapid karyotyping
* assessment of fetal anaemia in severe Rhesus iso-immunisation prior to intravascular transfusion

Reasons for performing a biopsy may include:
* DNA analysis
  — haemoglobinopathies
  — other genetic conditions
* Chromosomal analysis
  — fetal sexing
  — chromosomal abnormalities
* Enzymology
  — diagnosis of inborn errors of metabolism

Chorionic villus biopsy

This procedure is undertaken in the first trimester. Anaesthesia is not required. Under ultrasound guidance an endoscope is introduced vaginally or transabdominally. A sample of the chorionic villi is aspirated via a syringe or suction pump. Examination of the villi may yield information about congenital anomalies.

Advantages of chorionic villus biopsy over other invasive techniques are that it examines fetal tissue and quick diagnosis of many disorders can be obtained. The membranes are not punctured. It can be performed in the first trimester of pregnancy and if necessary an abortion can be offered before the pregnancy is known outside the family.

Disadvantages of chorionic villus biopsy include a spontaneous abortion rate which is higher than that following amniocentesis. There are risks of infection, intra-uterine death, haematoma, placental abruption and perforation of the uterus.

It is now known that the chromosomal constitution of the placental tissue may not reflect that of the fetus itself. False positive or false negative diagnoses may therefore be made. A recent study in Oxford has revealed a possible association between chorionic villus sampling in the first trimester and babies born with congenital defects.

INTRA-UTERINE THERAPEUTIC PROCEDURES

The introduction of ultrasound in the detection of fetal abnormality has led to the fetus being treated for a variety of conditions.

Rhesus haemolytic disease

Intraperitoneal transfusion is a much safer procedure now that it can be performed under ultrasound guidance.

Intravascular transfusion is now possible via the umbilical cord during fetoscopy. Blood sampling can be done at the same time.

Fetal obstructive uropathy

The presence of a urethral obstruction can be detected by ultrasound by visualising the distended bladder and ureters and by the presence of hydronephrosis. Under fetoscopy suprapubic catheterisation of the fetus can be performed and the urine drained into the amniotic fluid. As far as possible other abnormalities should be excluded before undertaking this procedure.

Fetal hydrocephalus

Methods of draining excessive cerebrospinal fluid (CSF) in cases of hydrocephalus are being developed at some centres. If a shunt can be inserted into the fetal ventricle to drain CSF into the amniotic fluid, severe brain damage will be prevented. Conventional shunts may be inserted at birth.

As techniques in fetoscopy and chorionic villus biopsy improve, many more disorders will be diagnosed antenatally. Intra-uterine therapies, including treatment for genetic conditions will be possible in the not too distant future.

SCREENING FOR INTRA-UTERINE GROWTH RETARDATION

Hormonal tests of placental function

Oestriol estimation

The ovary produces progesterones and oestrogens. The oestrogens are oestradiol, oestrone and oestriol. Oestriol is excreted in the urine in larger quantities than the other two hormones.

During pregnancy the fetus and the placenta are intimately associated in the production of oestrogens. In the fetal adrenals a steroid is metabolised and carried to the placenta where it acts as a precursor in the elaboration of oestriol. This hormone is excreted in the urine of pregnant women and the amount gives some indication of fetal well-being. During the third trimester, in screening for intra-uterine growth retardation (IUGR), assays are made of urinary oestriol.

Accuracy in collection of 24-hour specimens of urine is imperative. Prior to the commencement of the 24 hours the woman passes urine into the toilet. After this she must place all urine passed into a container. At the end of the 24-hour period she passes urine again and this is added to the specimen. A series of such assays gives a better indication than a single estimation.

Measurement of creatinine as well as oestrogen content in the urine obviates difficulties encountered with incomplete collection and gives a better assessment of a single assay. Creatinine is excreted at a constant rate and the ratio of oestrogen output:creatinine output is calculated.

In some centres, radio-immune assay of plasma oestriol is performed, the result being obtained more rapidly and therefore giving a more immediate picture of fetal condition. A series of assays gives a better indication of the functional ability of the fetoplacental unit. Very low values can indicate impending fetal death.

Human placental lactogen (HPL)

HPL is produced by the syncytiotrophoblast and is detectable in the plasma. The concentration rises steeply during pregnancy until 36 weeks, when it falls. Assays of serum HPL are utilised as a measure of placental function. Low levels can indicate:

- poor prognosis in cases of threatened abortion
- placental dysfunction with consequent risk to the fetus.

Serum HPL assays are used in assessment of IUGR. Obstetricians vary in their preference for oestriol or HPL estimations. Oestriol estimation is usually more popular. Prediction of fetal compromise has been disappointing and these tests are now less frequently used.

Ultrasound

The use of ultrasound in screening for congenital abnormalities and in assessing gestational age has already been described. These measurements can also be used in screening for IUGR.

Measurements used in the diagnosis of IUGR are usually the circumference and area measurements. Assessment of liquor volume and the textural appearance of the placenta are also useful.

The HC:AC ratio

The ratio between the head circumference (HC) and the abdominal circumference (AC) aids the diagnosis of growth retardation and the differentiation between the two types.

Symmetric growth retardation. Here both parameters (HC and AC) are reduced. It usually becomes apparent comparatively early in the pregnancy. The child takes some time to make up the growth deficiency after birth and may be developmentally slow and/or mentally retarded. It is often associated with chromosomal abnormalities.

Asymmetric growth retardation. This type of growth retardation usually becomes apparent later in the pregnancy. The abdominal circumference becomes reduced as liver stores are diminished. The head circumference continues to grow at the normal rate. This phenomenon is known as 'the brain-sparing syndrome'. Once the baby is delivered he feeds avidly and the liver stores are soon replenished.

Charting and use of measurements

It sometimes falls to the midwife to chart measurements and examine growth curves. The following points should be observed:

- the chart used must equate with the velocity of the machine used
- the method of 'plotting' growth curves must be consistent. The gestational age is either calculated from the mother's last menstrual period or from the measurements obtained from an early (first or second trimester) scan. Wrong plotting can be disastrous. A fetus suffering from IUGR can be missed or a perfectly normal fetus can be delivered prematurely because the curve appears to have fallen off.

The detection of IUGR by USS is said to be 95% accurate, whereas clinical assessment alone or in conjunction with hormonal tests of placental function is not so reliable.

THE USE OF RADIOLOGY IN OBSTETRICS

Radiology in obstetrics is used mainly to supplement and confirm findings which have been made on clinical examination during pregnancy. It is used less frequently now since ultrasound scanning has come into its own.

Radiation hazards

The risks involved in the use of radiology must be balanced against the advantages to mother and fetus.

An increased mutation rate in the germ cells of mother and child may affect future generations by causing congenital disease and abnormalities.

Attempts to prevent these dangers are being made by the use of modern radiological techniques, namely shielding of fetal and maternal gonads and shorter wavelengths. During childbearing years X-ray examinations of abdomen, pelvis and hips should only be made during the 10 days following a menstrual period to avoid the possibility of irradiation during early pregnancy.

Because of adverse publicity many mothers are worried about the hazards of radiography during pregnancy. They need a great deal of reassurance from the midwife and careful explanation as to why the investigation is thought to be necessary.

Lateral pelvimetry

Radiography to determine pelvic size and shape might be indicated in the following circumstances:

- history of injury or disease of pelvis and spine
- previous difficult delivery
- cases of maternal limp or deformity
- suspected cephalopelvic disproportion which may be indicated by any of the following:
  — history of caesarean section for contracted pelvis

  — high head or unstable lie in late pregnancy
  — unengaged head in labour
  — breech presentation.

Fetal abnormality

There are certain instances where a straight X-ray of the maternal abdomen may be used to confirm the diagnosis of fetal abnormality, e.g. achondroplasia or conjoined twins.

Infertility

In cases of infertility radio-opaque substances may be injected into the uterus and fallopian tubes (hysterosalpingogram) to demonstrate the patency or non-patency of the tubes (see Ch. 7).

FURTHER READING

Campbell S (ed) 1983 Ultrasound in obstetrics and gynaecology: recent advances. Royal College of Obstetricians and Gynaecologists, London

Campbell S et al 1983 New Doppler technique for assessing utero-placental blood flow. Lancet 1675

Enkin M, Chalmers I 1982 Effectiveness and satisfaction in antenatal care. Spastics International Medical Publications

Kalousey D K 1985 Mosaicism confined to chorionic tissue in human gestation. In: Fraccono M et al (eds) First trimester diagnosis. Springer Verlag, Berlin

Lilford R 1990 Prenatal diagnosis and prognosis. Butterworths, London

Manning F A et al 1980 Antepartum fetal evaluation: development of fetal biophysical profile. American Journal of Obstetrics and Gynecology 136: 787–795

Michael Y 1988 Intra-uterine growth retardation — a prospective study of the diagnostic value of real-time sonography combined with umbilical artery flow velocimetry. American Journal of Obstetrics and Gynecology 72(4): 611–615

Nicolaides K H et al 1986 Ultrasound-guided sampling of umbilical cord and placental blood to assess fetal wellbeing. Lancet (May 10): 1085–1087

Rodeck C H, Nicolaides K H (eds) 1983 Proceedings of the eleventh study group of the Royal College of Obstetricians and Gynaecologists. Royal College of Obstetricians and Gynaecologists, London

Shirley, Blackwell, Cusick, Farman, Vicroy 1978 A user's guide to diagnostic ultrasound. Pitman Medical, London

Wald N et al 1988a Maternal serum unconjugated oestriol as an antenatal test for Down's syndrome. British Journal of Obstetrics and Gynaecology 95 (April): 334–341

Wald N et al 1988b Maternal serum screening for Down's syndrome in early pregnancy. British Medical Journal 297 (8 October): 883–887

42

The use of drugs by the midwife

SARAH ROCH

Legislation governing the use of drugs and medicines by the midwife in the UK

Administration of controlled drugs and prescription-only medicines by midwives working in hospital

Administration of medicines intravenously

'Topping-up' an epidural analgesic

The safety of medicines

SI Units

Many drugs are administered by midwives as an integral part of their professional practice and their use is governed by general drug legislation as well as the UKCC Midwives Rules (1991) and Code of Practice (1989).

All midwives bear a great responsibility when they administer drugs, as substances may act not only upon the mother but also on the fetus during pregnancy and labour, and on the baby in the early days of life.

Drugs used by midwives are concerned chiefly with the:

- relief of pain in labour
- resuscitation of the newborn baby
- prevention and treatment of haemorrhage
- prevention of infection
- management of minor problems in the prenatal and postnatal periods
- treatment of medical disorders.

LEGISLATION GOVERNING THE USE OF DRUGS AND MEDICINES BY THE MIDWIFE IN THE UNITED KINGDOM

Midwives must be familiar with the laws that govern the administration of those Controlled Drugs and prescription-only medicines that they are permitted to use on their own authority without a doctor's prescription. All midwives must also observe the regulations which govern the giving of drugs prescribed by a medical practitioner and the local policies for administration.

They must understand that should a drug error lead to litigation or disciplinary measures, ignorance of the law is no excuse.

Midwives must observe both the Statutory Acts and Regulations governing the giving of drugs and the government memoranda concerned with drugs issued by the UK Health Departments (e.g. Department of Health (DH) in England, and the Scottish Home and Health Department).

Legislation and regulations affecting midwives

- Misuse of Drugs Act (1971)
- Misuse of Drugs Regulations (1985)
- Misuse of Drugs Act (1971) Modification Order (1985)
- Medicines Act (1968)
- Medicines (Prescriptions Only) Order (1983)
- Midwives Rules and A Midwife's Code of Practice (UKCC 1991, 1989)
- Standards for the Administration of Medicines (UKCC 1992b).

Controlled drugs

Misuse of Drugs Act (1971)

This act is concerned with preventing the abuse of addictive drugs and applies to persons who legally import, export, produce, distribute, supply, have custody of and possess Controlled Drugs.

The supply, possession and use of drugs of dependence such as pethidine, morphine, diamorphine, pentazocine and other synthetic morphine-like compounds is prohibited except as provided by the statutory Misuse of Drugs Regulations and Orders:

Misuse of Drugs Regulations (1985) (Statutory Instrument No. 2066)
Misuse of Drugs Act (1971) Modification Order (1985) (Statutory Instrument No. 1995)
Misuse of Drugs (Northern Ireland) Regulations (S.R. 1986 No. 52)

These regulations stipulate the conditions under which Controlled Drugs can be used by medical practitioners and certain others such as midwives.

Since the introduction of the 1985 Regulations there are now five Controlled Drug schedules:

Schedule 1
Potent substances such as cannabis and hallucinogens, which are rarely used in conventional medicine.
Schedule 2
Extremely addictive drugs such as diamorphine, pethidine and morphine.
Schedule 3
Includes some barbiturates, and pentazocine (Fortral).
Schedule 4
Contains 33 benzodiazepine tranquillisers including diazepam (Valium), nitrazepam (Mogadon), lorazepam (Ativan) and temazepam (Euhypnos).

N.B. There is no legal requirement for drugs in Schedules 3 and 4 to be kept in the Controlled Drug cupboard or entered in the Controlled Drug register.
Schedule 5
Medicines containing only a very small amount of Controlled Drug and therefore subject to few restrictions, e.g. some cough linctus and antidiarrhoeal preparations.

A Registered Midwife who has, in accordance with the provisions of the Nurses, Midwives and Health Visitors Acts (1979 and 1992), notified her intention to practise to the Local Supervising Authority is authorised to possess and administer Controlled Drugs, as far as is necessary for her professional practice.

In practical terms, the only Controlled Drugs a midwife may use are pethidine (Schedule 2) and pentazocine (Schedule 3), as these are the only two permitted under the Medicines Act (1968).

Supply of Controlled Drugs to midwives

In order to obtain Controlled Drugs the midwife has to:

1. obtain a signed Midwives' Drug Supply Order from her Supervisor of Midwives, who will

require to see the midwife's drug register and record of 'booked' cases. She may also wish to see the midwife's remaining stock of Controlled Drugs.

2. take the Drug Supply Order to a pharmacy where she has made arrangements to obtain Controlled Drugs.
3. check the drugs before leaving the pharmacy.
4. enter the following details in her drug register:
   — name and quantity of drug
   — name and address of pharmacist
   — date drug supplied.
5. store the drugs safely in a fixed locked cupboard which can only be opened by her.

In some areas it is local policy that midwives obtain their supplies of Controlled Drugs and/or prescription-only medicines from the hospital pharmacy.

Surrender of Controlled Drugs

The 1985 Regulations not only outline the safe custody of Controlled Drugs but also the procedure by which midwives may surrender or destroy stocks of unwanted Controlled Drugs.

Midwives may *surrender* unwanted Controlled Drugs to an 'authorised' person, such as an approved medical officer, or to the person from whom the drug was obtained, e.g. the pharmacist.

Destruction of Controlled Drugs

The midwife may *destroy* unwanted drugs before an 'authorised' witness who, under the regulations, may be one of the following:

- Supervisor of Midwives in England, Wales or Northern Ireland
- Regional Pharmaceutical Officer (England)
- Pharmaceutical Adviser (Welsh Office)
- Chief Administrative Pharmaceutical Officer (Health Board, Scotland)
- Inspector appointed by DHSS (Northern Ireland)
- Medical Officers of Regional Medical Services (England/Scotland/Wales)
- Inspector of the Pharmaceutical Society of Great Britain
- Police Officer
- Home Office Drugs Branch Inspector.

Home confinement

Where Controlled Drugs are supplied directly to the woman on the prescription of a general medical practitioner, any unused drugs legally belong to the woman. The midwife can only advise her to destroy them and may suggest that this should be carried out in the midwife's presence.

Prescription-only medicines

Medicines Act 1968

This Act is concerned with regulating the legitimate use of medicinal products. Under Part III of this Act certain medicines, which are normally only issued on a medical prescription, may be supplied to midwives *for use in their community-based practice.*

The following preparations for use by midwives are listed in Schedule 3 (Parts I and III) of the Medicines (Products other than veterinary drugs) (Prescriptions Only) Order (1983) (Statutory Instrument No. 1212).

Part I
Ergometrine maleate (tablets)
Chloral hydrate derivatives, e.g.
   chloral hydrate
   syrup of chloral
   triclofos sodium.

Although Welldorm (originally dichloralphenazone) is still listed in Schedule 3 as a preparation suitable for use by midwives, it is now contra-indicated for use in midwifery because the chemical composition has been changed to a slightly different chloral derivative (chloral betaine) which is not recommended for use in pregnancy. This information was communicated to midwives in the UKCC Registrar's Letter 6/1991.

Part III (for parenteral use)
Promazine hydrochloride (Sparine)
Lignocaine hydrochloride
Phytomenadione (vitamin K_1)
Pentazocine lactate ⎫
Pethidine hydrochloride ⎬ Controlled Drugs
Naloxone hydrochloride
Oxytocin
Ergometrine maleate.

In Scotland, only ergometrine, Syntometrine, naloxone and lignocaine may be administered by a midwife without a medical prescription.

ADMINISTRATION OF CONTROLLED DRUGS AND PRESCRIPTION-ONLY MEDICINES BY MIDWIVES WORKING IN HOSPITAL

Drug Supply Orders are *only* issued to community midwives, and *not* to midwives practising in the hospital setting.

The Aitken Report (1958) in England, and the very similar Roxburgh Report in Scotland, stated that midwives working in hospitals were subject to the same regulations for the administration of medicines and Controlled Drugs as nurses, i.e. that these preparations must be prescribed by a doctor and obtained from the institution's pharmacy.

Following this, and in response to the concern of midwives to enable women to receive drugs such as analgesics and oxytocics *without delay*, the then DHSS issued a 'Dear Doctor' letter (DHSS Circular G.M. 152) in 1972 which permitted doctors to authorise standing orders for the range of drugs used by midwives in their usual practice, and this custom is now widespread in maternity units.

However, the DH report on the 'Safe and Secure Handling of Medicines' (Duthie Report 1988) indicated in Section 16.7.1.1 that in respect of the administration of medicines, it can be local policy to allow midwives working in the hospital setting to follow the same practice as midwives working in the community.

In hospitals, the pharmacist is responsible for obtaining and issuing supplies of Controlled Drugs and prescription-only and other medicines, and also for maintaining full drug records. The midwife in charge of the ward or department is responsible for the safe custody of drugs and for checking and recording the stock of controlled and other drugs according to the locally agreed drug policy.

Controlled Drugs must be kept in a locked compartment within a fixed locked cupboard and the keys should be the responsibility of the midwife in charge.

UKCC Midwives Rules (1991)

The Midwives Rules (1991) are contained within the following Statutory Instruments:

1. Part V of the Nurses, Midwives and Health Visitors Rules 1983, SI 1983 No 873 which was repealed. However the citation and interpretation in this Statutory Instrument, which is also known as the 'principal Rules' remain a relevant part of the Midwives Rules. The numbering of the Midwives Rules commences with Rule 27 which is sequential to Part IV of the principal Rules
2. SI 1986 No 786 — The Nurses, Midwives and Health Visitors (Midwives Amendment) Rules Approval Order 1986
3. SI 1989 No 1456 — The Nurses, Midwives and Health Visitors (Registered Fever Nurses Amendment Rules & Training Amendment Rules) Approval Order 1989
4. SI 1990 No 1624 — The Nurses, Midwives and Health Visitors (Midwives Training) Amendment Rules Approval Order 1990.

The following are also relevant:

A Midwife's Code of Practice (UKCC 1989)
Standards for the Administration of Medicines (UKCC 1992b).

The Midwives Rules (UKCC 1991) state that 'a practising midwife shall not on her own responsibility administer any medicine, including analgesics, unless in the course of her training, whether before or after registration as a midwife, she has been thoroughly instructed in its use and is familiar with its dosage and methods of administration or application'.

The UKCC Rules also lay down that a midwife may only administer inhalational analgesia if the apparatus she uses is approved by the UKCC and is properly maintained.

At the present time midwives on their own responsibility may administer a 50% nitrous oxide/50% oxygen mixture via a face mask or mouthpiece using one of four approved models:

- BOC Entonox apparatus
- PneuPac apparatus
- SOS Nitronox — midwifery model
- Peacemaker apparatus.

The legislative position related to Rule 41 of the UKCC Midwives Rules (1991) is clearly stated together with the mechanism for approving an apparatus in UKCC Registrar's Letter 14/1990.

The UKCC paper *Standards for the Administration of Medicines* lays down the expected standard of practice for all nurses, midwives and health visitors in relation to the prescribing, administration and recording of medicines, together with useful background information on the relevant legislation. It stresses the importance of properly negotiated local policies and states that professional judgement and responsibility should always be directed to the best interests of the client.

ADMINISTRATION OF MEDICINES INTRAVENOUSLY

The giving of intravenous injections is a procedure within the province of a midwife, provided that she has been properly instructed. Some employing authorities require a certificate of competence but the midwife herself is responsible for maintaining that competence (UKCC 1992a).

Midwives are permitted to administer ergometrine intravenously in the emergency treatment of postpartum haemorrhage. The administration of other intravenous (i.v.) medicines is outside the limits of normal midwifery practice and midwives should receive specific instruction before undertaking this procedure.

Medicines administered intravenously may be given directly through an indwelling cannula inserted by a doctor or added to i.v. infusion fluid but *not* to blood or plasma. The drug prescription, including full instructions, must be written up beforehand and the midwife should ensure that the drawing up of the dose and its administration are witnessed by a second trained member of staff.

The doctor delegating this responsibility to a registered nurse or midwife, should satisfy himself that she is competent to undertake this procedure. *Nurses in training must not add medicines to i.v. fluids.*

The midwife must remember that personal professional responsibility cannot be relinquished to any other practitioner.

Intravenous therapy — the midwife's responsibility

All midwives administering i.v. drugs should be responsible for:

- obtaining theoretical and practical instruction on the pharmacology, storage, inspection and administration of drugs and the infusion fluids to which they are added, including the potential hazards of drug/i.v. fluid incompatibility
- achieving competence in adding medicines to i.v. fluids
- limiting the drugs used to those within the scope of locally agreed policy
- reading instructions carefully
- carrying out the necessary aseptic technique and other instructions laid down by her employing authority
- confirming:
  — that the pharmacological name of the medicine to be administered is written clearly in capital letters
  — that the prescribed dose, amount of fluid and other instructions (e.g. infusion rate), have been written and signed by the doctor
- checking:
  — drug dosage, amount of i.v. fluid and infusion rate with a second registered nurse or midwife
  — that the drug and i.v. fluid are properly mixed by inverting the container several times
- reporting:
  — flaws or cracks in the i.v. fluid container
  — presence of cloudiness or particulate matter in the fluid
  — turbidity, change of colour or precipitation in the fluid upon addition of the drug

- ensuring that:
  - — air is expelled from the syringe
  - — the i.v. line is patent
  - — flow is at the prescribed rate
  - — the injection site shows no evidence of infection or displacement of the needle or cannula
- observing the condition of the mother, and the effect of the drug infusion (e.g. oxytocin) on fetal heart rate, uterine contractions, blood pressure and pulse rate
- maintaining accurate, legible records, and applying labels to i.v. fluid containers which state the drug content, dosage and time of administration.

Potential hazards

Medicines should not be injected into the following infusion fluids: blood, plasma, amino acids, lipids, mannitol and sodium bicarbonate. No more than one medicine should be added to an i.v. infusion fluid.

Overdosage

The following can all lead to error in administration of a drug which may result in fatality:

- Illegible writing
- Incorrect interpretation of dosage in SI Units
- Administration of a bolus dose of the drug through a needle or tubing, when it should have been added to the infusion fluid and given slowly
- Running the infusion too rapidly. (This not only causes overdosage but may also upset the fluid and electrolyte balance.)

Medicines may be incompatible with the infusion fluid and lists of drug/infusion fluid compatibilities should be available in all maternity departments.

Discontinuation of i.v. fluids

A midwife who removes i.v. apparatus on the completion of therapy must ensure that the cannula is complete. She must record the amount of fluid administered.

Intravenous medicinal therapy in neonatal units

The umbilical blood vessels are rarely available after the first week of life; one of the peripheral veins is more commonly used on the hand or foot (see Ch. 36). If a scalp vein is used, swelling of the scalp should be reported immediately as this indicates that the needle is displaced.

Disposable scalp vein sets with a wing which fixes the needle to the scalp are used. To prevent the flow being too rapid and the volume infused excessive, a subsidiary chamber containing 30 ml or more of infusion fluid is connected to the main infusion bottle by a 'shut off' valve. Servo-controlled electronic 'drip counters' and high-precision roller pumps are used to control the flow. This avoids over-burdening the baby's circulation and upsetting the fluid balance.

Midwives must find out whether the medicine is to be added to the infusion bottle or to the drip chamber from which the drug will be administered in a more concentrated form.

'TOPPING UP' AN EPIDURAL ANALGESIC (see also Ch. 28)

Midwives are allowed to give a 'topping up' dose provided the following safeguards are observed:

- The ultimate responsibility for such a technique should clearly rest with the doctor.
- *Written instruction as to the dose should be given by the doctor concerned.*
- *The dose given directly by the midwife should be checked by one other person.*
- *Instructions should be given by the doctor* as to the posture of the patient at the time of injection, observations on the blood pressure and measures to be taken in the event of any adverse side-effects.
- The midwife should have been thoroughly instructed in the technique and have satisfied the locally agreed criteria for competence in this procedure.

Each National Board issues regularly updated guidance on epidural 'top-up' by midwives and this must be used to inform local policy, which should be agreed between medical staff and midwives.

The epidural 'top-up' procedure may vary between institutions and, when this procedure involves the administration of a substance drawn into a syringe or container by another practitioner when the midwife taking responsibility for the mother was *not* present, then the following guidelines for safe practice should be established:

- confirmation of a valid prescription and instructions from medical staff
- evidence that a responsible practitioner has signed for the syringe or container containing the checked and validly prescribed drug
- clearly labelled syringe or container duly dated and signed
- a rigorous and detailed handover procedure.

Such good practice should also be applied to the administration of substances by the intravenous route, including central venous lines, and by arterial lines.

The importance of accurate, contemporaneous recording of all drug administration by midwives cannot be over-emphasised and it is a clear and specific requirement within the UKCC Midwives Rules.

THE SAFETY OF MEDICINES

New medicines are subjected to rigorous tests before being released for clinical use. Following the thalidomide tragedy in 1962, when hundreds of babies were born with absent or vestigial limbs, the Government set up The Committee on Safety of Medicines. Every new drug is now tested for activity, potency and toxicity; most are also tested on pregnant laboratory animals. The Committee reviews evidence on toxicity tests as well as on animal and human pharmacology before approving drugs.

Teratogenic effects

The fetus in utero is especially vulnerable to the effect of medicines. Some medicines that are harmless to the pregnant woman herself can have an adverse effect on the fetus. A number of medicines (teratogenic drugs) cause fetal abnormalities and this damage generally occurs during the first 12 weeks of pregnancy. The embryo is particularly at risk during the main period of organogenesis which is the initial 8 weeks of development.

Medicines found in the home and considered innocuous, such as aspirin, anti-emetics and mild sedatives, should be considered potentially dangerous during pregnancy. It is safest to assume that all medicines given to the pregnant woman are also given to the fetus, as the placenta is *not* a barrier to most drugs. It must also be remembered that many drugs pass into breast milk and can affect the neonate.

As far as possible all medicines should be avoided during the first trimester and this message should be stressed in pre-conception and postnatal education. If medicines are essential for pregnant or breast-feeding mothers, they should be prescribed by a doctor.

Pre-conception (pre-pregnancy) care

Pre-pregnancy care and education should be made more widely available to all young men and women, and information about the dangers of taking medicines in early pregnancy should be a major topic. It should be taught in senior schools and by health service personnel within both hospital and community.

Effects of drugs on the fetus during labour

It is well known that narcotic drugs such as morphine and diamorphine have a depressive effect on the fetal respiratory centre. Pethidine can also depress respiration at birth, and is best avoided during the last 2 or 3 hours of labour, especially if a second or subsequent dose is being considered.

Neonatal drug therapy

Neonatal drugs should be checked by two professionally qualified members of staff. Medicines given to the neonate should be dispensed in paediatric dosage by the manufacturer or pharmacist in order to avoid the errors that can occur when calculations are made from adult doses.

Naloxone (Narcan Neonatal) should be the only stimulant drug used to counteract narcotic drugs and initiate respiration. Although some of the older preparations are still legally available for use by midwives, they are not *pure* narcotic antagonists and may actually harm the newborn baby.

Some drugs can cause damage to the neonate when given in large or repeated doses. Streptomycin and gentamicin can affect the auditory nerve and cause deafness, and tetracyclines can stain the teeth yellow and lead to liver damage.

When giving medicines to babies intramuscularly, the needle must be inserted on the slant, and *not* at right angles, because the tissues are so shallow, and it is all too easy to penetrate periosteum or bone. To avoid injury to the sciatic nerve or hip joint, the upper, outer quadrant of the buttock should be used whenever possible (Fig. 42.1). The anterior area of the thigh may be used but the needle must point downwards towards the knee to avoid damaging blood vessels in the groin. Intramuscular injections should not be given into the arm of a baby.

Drug interaction

When two potent drugs are administered together, the action of one may lead to an increase, reduction or modification of the effect of the other drug, for example, monoamine-oxidase inhibitors such as phenelzine (Nardil) can potentiate the action of pethidine or morphine and may induce coma. Alcohol will increase the sedative effects of most central depressant drugs and in high doses may cause severe respiratory depression. It can also damage fetal brain cells during pregnancy (see fetal alcohol syndrome, Ch. 38).

Expiry date and storage of drugs

Midwives should be vigilant in noting the expiry date on all drugs and infusion fluids.

Some liquid medicines when stored for a long period can evaporate. This increases the concentration and can cause serious or fatal overdosage. Drugs such as ergometrine and Syntometrine should be kept in a cool place and not exposed to light over long periods.

The manufacturer's instructions regarding the correct storage conditions for drugs should always be followed.

Drug prescribing

Drugs should be prescribed by their pharmacological names. Pharmaceutical drugs, proprietary or trade names should be written with a capital letter and sometimes italics are used in printed material. The sign '®' after a proprietary name indicates a registered trade mark.

Pharmacological name	Proprietary name
promazine	Sparine
naloxone	Narcan
methyldopa	Aldomet
pentazocine	Fortral

SI UNITS (SYSTEME INTERNATIONAL D'UNITES)

SI units are an internationally agreed version of the metric system which has been used in scientific work and in industry since 1960. The British medical profession accepted the SI system in 1977 in order to unify and simplify practice in

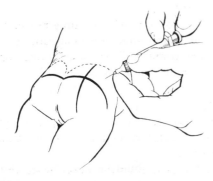

Fig. 42.1
Injecting upper outer quadrant of the buttock.

medical measurement and conform to the widely accepted international system.

Midwives must be able to use the SI system (Système International d'Unités or International System of Units). They should also be aware that in certain areas alternative measurements may still be used, with or without the SI equivalent, and conversion to SI units may have to be made.

Medicines are administered in milligrams, grams, and millilitres: intravenous solutions in litres.

Babies are measured in centimetres, weighed in grams. Adults are measured in metres and centimetres, weighed in kilograms.

Temperature is recorded in degrees on the Celsius scale, °C.

In laboratory reports, millimoles may replace milligrams, e.g. blood glucose is now recorded in millimoles per litre (mmol/l) instead of mg/100 ml. Bilirubin is recorded in micromoles per litre — micromole/l (μmol/l) instead of mg/100 ml.

SI BASIC UNITS
There are 7 units that form the basis of the SI system:

Physical quantity	SI unit	Symbol
length	metre	m
mass	kilogram	kg
time	second	s
electric current	ampere	A
thermodynamic temperature	kelvin	K
amount of substance	mole	mol
luminous intensity	candela	cd

SUBMULTIPLES AND MULTIPLES
These are denoted by the addition of prefixes

Prefix	Symbol	Submultiple or multiple	
deci	d	one tenth	10^{-1} or 0.1
centi	c	one hundredth	10^{-2} or 0.01
milli	m	one thousandth	10^{-3} or 0.001
micro	μ	one millionth	10^{-6} or 0.000 001
deca	da	ten times	10^{1}
hecta	h	one hundred times	10^{2}
kilo	k	one thousand times	10^{3}
mega	M	one million times	10^{6}

The kilogram
The kilogram is the basic unit of mass (2.2 lbs)
One kilogram (kg) = 1000 grams (g).
One gram (g) = 1000 milligrams (mg).
One milligram (mg) = 1000 micrograms (μg).
The word microgram should be written out in full.

The metre
The metre is the basic unit of length (39.3 inches)
One kilometre (km) = 1000 metres.
One decimetre (dm) = 0.1 metres (one-tenth metre).
One centimetre (cm) = 0.01 metres (one-hundredth metre).
One millimetre (mm) = 0.001 metres (one-thousandth metre).
One micrometre (μm) = 0.000 001 metres (one-millionth metre).
There are 10 millimetres in one centimetre (as on a ruler).
There are 2.5 centimetres in one inch.

The mole
The mole is an additional SI unit and is the unit of 'amount of substance' (weight)
One decimole (dmol) = 0.1 moles (one-tenth mole).
One millimole (mmol) = 0.001 moles (one-thousandth mole).
One micromole (μmol) = 0.000 001 moles (one-millionth mole).

The reporting of analyses in clinical chemistry laboratories is now made in millimoles per litre (mmol/l) instead of milligrams per 100 millilitres (mg/100 ml).

In laboratory work the mole replaced mass units such as the gram and milligram. The mole also replaced the milliequivalent for certain constituents of intravenous fluids.

The litre
The litre, which is a non-SI unit, is accepted as the reference unit of volume for all concentrations and cell counts.
One decilitre (dl) = 0.1 litres (one-tenth litre).
One decilitre (dl) = 100 millilitres.
One centilitre (cl) = 0.01 litres (one-hundredth litre).

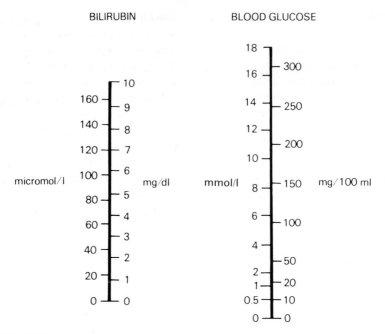

Fig. 42.2
Conversion from mg/dl to SI units for bilirubin and blood glucose.

One millilitre (ml) = 0.001 litres (one-thousandth litre).

Haemoglobin is recorded in grams per decilitre (g/dl).

SI derived units

There are 18 derived units, three of which are of interest to midwives.

Celsius temperature scale (°C). The centigrade temperature scale is known as Celsius (°C). Freezing point is 0°C and boiling point is 100°C.

On the Fahrenheit scale, freezing point is 32°F and boiling point is 212°F.

To convert Celsius to Fahrenheit, multiply by 9, divide by 5 and add 32.

To convert Fahrenheit to Celsius, subtract 32, multiply by 5 and divide by 9.

Pressure. The action of force on an area has been given the name pascal (Pa). The partial pressure of blood gases pO_2 and pCO_2 are expressed as kilopascals (kPa). 1000 pascals (Pa) = 1 kilopascal (kPa).

Blood pressure continues to be measured in mmHg; the changeover to kilopascals has not yet taken place.

The Joule (J). This term is used in nutritional science instead of the calorie and denotes the quantity of heat and energy released when food is utilised (burned) by the body or the heat and energy produced by fuel. The large or kilocalorie equals 4.184 kilojoules (approximately 4). 1000 joules (J) equals one kilojoule: 1000 kilojoules

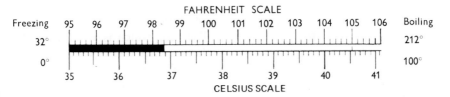

Fig. 42.3
Conversion from Fahrenheit to Celsius scale.

(kJ) equal one megajoule (MJ) which is one million joules.

When dealing with large numbers they are written as powers of ten and the raised number corresponds to the number of zeros.

100 (2 zeros) is written as 10^2 (10×10)

1000 (3 zeros) = 10^3 ($10 \times 10 \times 10$)

1 000 000 (6 zeros) = 10^6 ($10 \times 10 \times 10 \times 10 \times 10 \times 10$).

When the amount is less than one, a minus sign is placed before the raised number. The number of zeros still corresponds to the raised number, one before the decimal point and the rest after.

0.1 (1 zero) = 10^{-1} or one-tenth

0.01 (2 zeros) = 10^{-2} or one-hundredth

0.001 (3 zeros) = 10^{-3} or one-thousandth

0.000 001 (6 zeros) = 10^{-6} or one-millionth.

Midwives should be aware of the danger of confusing the symbols for microgram (μg) and milligram (mg). One mg (milligram) is the equivalent of 1000 micrograms: the symbol for micro being the Greek letter μ (mu).

The prefix micro should always be written out in full, e.g. microgram, micromole, when prescribing or labelling drugs.

Points to be noted

Plural units. The symbol for a unit does not have an 's' added when plural. Kilograms = kg (not kgs). Decilitres = dl (not dls).

The use of small and capital letters. There is a vast difference between small and capital letters used as symbols. Capital 'M' is the symbol for Mega which is one million times. The small letter 'm' signifies milli which is one-thousandth part: a millimole (mmol) is one thousandth part of a mole: a millilitre (ml) is one-thousandth part of a litre. The small letters, kg, are the symbol for kilogram. The use of Kg, KG, or kG is wrong. A small letter 'l' is used for litre.

The sign for 'per'. A sloping dash, /, is the sign for 'per', i.e. grams per decilitre = g/dl: millimoles per litre = mmol/l. The dash should be used once only in each unit.

Decimal points. When denoting figures less than one, the decimal point should always be preceded by a zero: 0.5 (not .5). The dot may otherwise be ignored and 10 times the dose given. A full stop is not used following symbols for units, e.g. 0.5 (not 0.5.); 10 g (not 10 g.) unless to end a sentence.

REFERENCES

Briggs G, Freeman R, Yaffe S 1990 Drugs in pregnancy and lactation, 3rd edn. Williams & Wilkins, Baltimore

Department of Health 1988 Guidelines for the safe and secure handling of medicines. (Duthie report), DH, London

Department of Health and Social Security 1958 Aitken report HM(58) 17. DHSS, London

McCracken G H 1986 Aminoglycoside toxicity in infants and children. American Journal of Medicine 80 (Suppl 6b): 170–8

Nurses, Midwives and Health Visitors Acts 1979 and 1992 HMSO, London

United Kingdom Central Council Registrar's letter 14/1990 Approval of apparatus for the administration of inhalational analgesia by midwives. UKCC, London

United Kingdom Central Council 1989 A midwife's code of practice. UKCC, London (Reprinted 1991)

United Kingdom Central Council 1991 Midwives rules. UKCC, London

United Kingdom Central Council 1992a The scope of professional practice. UKCC, London

United Kingdom Central Council 1992b Standards for the administration of medicines. UKCC, London

43

Vital statistics

V. RUTH BENNETT LINDA K. BROWN

In the mid-19th century it became evident that it would be useful to collect details of all births and deaths and on 1 July 1837 The Registration of Births and Deaths Act came into effect. This Act is still in force today. There are many subsequent Acts which govern the collection of statistical data. Causative factors, trends and their interaction can be studied. Analysis of the information gives national and local planners a sound basis for providing the right health care facilities.

The midwife holds a responsibility in supplying details of any births or deaths occurring within her practice.

NOTIFICATION OF BIRTH

Legislation
Provision for the early notification of birth was first made in 1907 but it did not become a statutory requirement until 1915. When these Acts were repealed the legislation was included in The Public Health Act 1936 and slightly amended by The National Health Service Act 1946.

Notification
It is the duty of the father or any other person in attendance or present within 6 hours after the birth to give notice in writing to the appointed medical officer in the district in which the child is born. This must be done within 36 hours of birth

for any child born after 24 completed weeks of pregnancy, whether alive or dead. The health authority supplies prepaid addressed envelopes and forms for the notification of birth. It is usual for the midwife to undertake completion of the form. In addition to biographical information about the mother and her baby, the midwife will record the period of gestation, any congenital malformation and factors which may put the baby at risk.

The purpose of notification is to enable the health visitor to call at the home as soon as the midwife ceases to visit. An 'at-risk' register (see Ch. 45) is compiled from the details on the cards and is used for providing appropriate care for the children concerned. The birth information is also made available to the Registrar of Births and Deaths of the district in which the birth took place.

REGISTRATION OF BIRTH

Every birth must be registered. A period of 6 weeks is allowed for registration to take place (3 weeks in Scotland). The responsibility to inform the Registrar falls primarily on the mother; if the parents are married, either of them may register the birth. If the parents are not married to each other, the father may still register the birth if he produces a statutory declaration by the mother, which states that he is the baby's father, or one of a number of legal documents which establish his paternity such as certain court orders.

If an *unmarried couple* wishes the father's name to be entered on the certificate they must make a joint registration; if the father is unable to accompany the mother she must produce a statutory declaration to the effect that he claims paternity. The form for this is provided by the Registrar of Births and Deaths.

At the time that the parents register the birth, the Registrar also collects further information which is used for statistical purposes but which is kept confidential and is not entered on the Birth Certificate. This relates to dates of birth and marriage of the parents and previous children borne, live or still. The Registrar General compiles statistics from details of birth registrations.

Place of registration

The birth must be registered in the district in which it took place. Many hospitals are able to arrange for the Registrar to visit the maternity wards regularly in order to provide the facility for mothers to register their babies.

If the mother is resident in a different registration district in England or Wales, she may go to her local Registrar and make a declaration. This will be forwarded to the Registrar of Births and Deaths in whose District the birth occurred and, after registration, he or she will issue a birth certificate in the usual way. This will be sent to the parent with a card bearing the National Health Service number which will enable the child to be registered with a family practitioner. This cannot, however, be done in the case of a stillbirth, which must be registered in the registration district in which it took place.

Birth certificates

A short Birth Certificate is issued free of charge at the time of registration. It gives details of the name of the baby, sex, date and place of birth, the place being the registration district.

A full Birth Certificate (Fig. 43.1) may be obtained at the same time on payment of the prescribed fee. This certificate contains details of the complete birth entry.

If the parents fail to register the birth for some reason, the midwife who was present at delivery is one of the people qualified to register the birth and may be requested to do so. Others who may be called upon are the 'occupier of the house' (who, in the context of a hospital, will probably be an administrator), any person present at the birth or anyone taking charge of the child. In general it is best if the parents themselves register the birth because they will be able to give the most accurate information. If the registration is not carried out within the stated period, there is a penalty of £50.

Legislation

The original Act was passed in 1837 but updated in the Births and Deaths Registration Act 1953.

VA 104830

The fee for this certificate is 8s. 0d.

CAUTION.—Any person who (1) falsifies any of the particulars on this certificate, or (2) uses a falsified certificate as true, knowing it to be false, is liable to prosecution.

CERTIFIED COPY OF AN ENTRY
Pursuant to the Births and Deaths Registration Act 1953

NHS Number	**BIRTH**	Entry No.

Registration district   Administrative area

Sub-district

Date and place of birth   **CHILD**

SPECIMEN

2. Name and surname   3. Sex

4. Name and surname   **FATHER**

5. Place of birth

6. Occupation

7. Name and surname   **MOTHER**

SPECIMEN

8. Place of birth

9. (a) Maiden surname   (b) Surname at marriage if different from maiden surname

10. Usual address (if different from place of child's birth)

INFORMANT

11. Name and surname (if not the mother or father)   12. Qualification

13. Usual address (if different from that in 10 above)

14. I certify that the particulars entered above are true to the best of my knowledge and belief

....of informant   Signature

15. Date of registration   16. Signature of registrar

SPECIMEN

* See note overleaf

17.* Name given after registration, and surname

B. Cert.   Certified to be a true copy of an entry in a register in my custody.

S.R.   ....Superintendent Registrar..................Date

Fig. 43.1
Specimen copy of a full birth certificate. (The design of the birth certificate is Crown copyright and is reproduced with the permission of the Controller of Her Majesty's Stationery Office.)

Stillbirths

Definition of stillbirth

A stillbirth is defined in the Births and Deaths Registration Act 1953.

A baby who has issued forth from its mother after the 28th week of pregnancy and has not at any time after being completely expelled from its mother breathed or shown any sign of life is a stillborn baby. (UKCC: A Midwife's Code of Practice 1989)

This definition was changed in the Still-birth (Definition) Act 1992 so that the words '28th week' became '24th week' in the above and other relevant Acts.

Registration of stillbirths

In order to register a stillborn baby, the informant must have a medical Certificate of Stillbirth. A medical practitioner or midwife who is present at a stillbirth or who examines the body of a still-born child may be asked for this certificate. In practice it is usual for the doctor to complete the certificate. A midwife would be unwise to offer to complete a stillbirth certificate unless she had personally witnessed and attended the birth.

The informant will take this certificate to the Registrar in order to register the stillbirth. The Registrar will give the informant a Certificate for Burial or Cremation of the fetus. The latter must be produced before the body of the baby can be buried or cremated. In cases where there has been an inquest, the coroner will issue the order.

Since 1983 parents have been able to register the forename and surname of their stillborn child.

Burial of a stillborn baby

Parents may make private arrangements for the baby to be buried or cremated but it is also possible for the hospital to undertake this on their behalf. Midwives who counsel the mother and father should encourage them to think about this carefully and to choose the arrangement which suits their need. See Chapter 49 for discussion of support to the grieving parents.

Duties of a midwife concerning stillbirth

Notification of stillbirth is the same as is required for live birth.

Certificate of stillbirth. The midwife will ensure that this has been completed, usually by the doctor (see above).

Registration of stillbirth. The midwife explains to the parents that the birth must be registered and the procedure for burial or cremation. In cases where the parents wish to make private arrangements for the funeral, the midwife may need to explain that no death grant is payable for a stillbirth.

The Supervisor of Midwives must be notified of the stillbirth by the midwife responsible for the care of the woman and her baby (UKCC: A Midwife's Code of Practice 1989).

THE CONCEPT OF VITAL STATISTICS

The word 'statistics' pertains to the systematic collection of numerical figures in order that they may be summarised and studied. In this context the term 'vital' means that the figures relate to life and death events. In measuring health there are difficulties in finding objective data to quan-

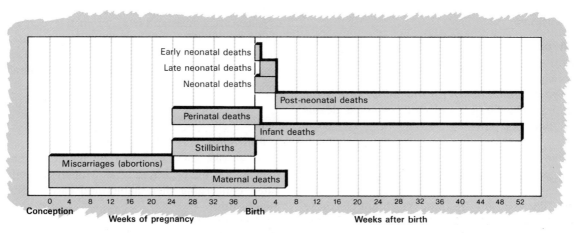

Fig. 43.2
Subdivision of deaths occurring during pregnancy and within 1 year of birth.

tify, therefore it is pertinent to study the numbers of deaths occurring at different ages and their causes. This may help to explain why there are so many types of death rate. The statistics of special interest to midwives are:

- birth rate
- stillbirth rate
- perinatal death rate
- neonatal death rate
- postneonatal death rate
- infant death rate
- maternal death rate.

Definition of 'rate'

Crude figures give little idea of the real frequency of events. If they are related to a specific number within the population, it becomes possible to compare one year's figures with another. If a particular group is studied, for example women in the fertile years, it is possible to identify the degree of risk in relation to certain events.

To calculate the rate of, for instance, stillbirth, the number of stillbirths is compared to the number of total births (both live and still). This comparison is then related to a group of 1000 of those total births. The mathematical formula is as follows:

$$\frac{\text{No. of stillbirths}}{\text{No. of total births}} \times 1000 = \frac{\text{Stillbirth rate per}}{\text{1000 total births}}$$

PERINATAL DEATH

Definitions

A perinatal death is either a stillbirth or a death occurring in the first week of life (early neonatal death).

The perinatal death (or mortality) rate is the number of stillbirths and early neonatal deaths per 1000 total births.

Causes and predisposing factors

The perinatal death rate is often taken as the primary indicator of success or failure in obstetric care. These deaths are those which are closest to the event of delivery and some of them are caused by such factors as hypoxia in labour and intracranial trauma during birth. Others may be the result of genetic factors or of events in pregnancy. The main identifiable causes are:

- low birthweight (preterm and small for gestational age)
- intra-uterine hypoxia
- asphyxia at birth
- intracranial injury
- congenital abnormality.

It may be impossible to attribute a perinatal death to any one of the listed causes but a combination of predisposing factors increases the risk of death. These include:

- socio-economic disadvantage
- poor maternal health (including effects of smoking, alcohol consumption, drug abuse and poor diet)
- multiple pregnancy
- antepartum haemorrhage
- pre-eclampsia
- breech presentation.

Trends

When new figures are published each year, small improvements are welcome but real encouragement is found in viewing the decline in rates over a number of years. These are often plotted in graph form (Fig. 43.3). In looking for reasons for these trends it is important to take account of a wide range of factors such as the establishment of the National Health Service in 1948 and the passing of the Abortion Act 1967.

Rates are consistently higher than average in social classes IV and V as defined by occupation of a parent, usually the father. Black women, especially those born outside the UK, are generally more likely to lose their babies (OPCS 1992).

Reasons for improvement

Improved care in pregnancy identifies the fetus at risk so that it can be monitored and delivered at the optimum time. Mothers are educated concerning diet, habits and care of their own health.

Improved care in labour aims at maintaining the mother and fetus in good condition. It also

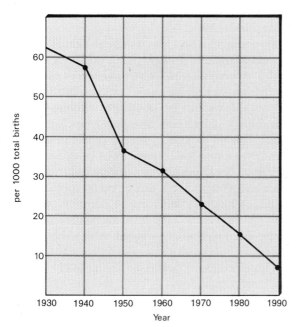

Fig. 43.3
Graph showing the perinatal death rates from 1930–90.

early neonatal deaths which occur in the first 7 days of life and late neonatal deaths which occur during the next 21 days. The reason for this is that the causes of early deaths are more similar to those of stillbirth while the causes of later deaths are different. The rates of neonatal deaths are calculated per 1000 live births.

Causes of late neonatal death

Some of the causes are similar to the earlier deaths because babies whose deaths are attributable to birth trauma or perinatal events may survive beyond the first week. After this time there is a greater likelihood of death occurring due to infection, intraventricular haemorrhage, necrotising enterocolitis and iatrogenic disorders.

Funeral arrangements

In the case of a neonatal death the funeral arrangements are the responsibility of the parents. There is a small death grant payable on the death of a child under 3 years but this will in no way offset the costs incurred. If there is hardship the midwife may refer the family to the social worker. Midwives should also be familiar with local policy as in a few cases the hospital administrator may agree to meet some of the cost.

Both a Birth Certificate and a Death Certificate are required. The midwife will need to make sure that the parents are aware of this in order to spare them unnecessary distress.

reduces the length of labour and offers safe intervention. This should not be taken to mean that more technological aids in themselves lead to better care. There is increasing realisation that skilled midwifery care contributes to safety in labour.

Improved neonatal care results in more survivors and in a better quality of life for those who do survive. Intensive neonatal care helps babies born after less than 28 weeks of pregnancy to survive, whereas in earlier years they were simply abortions and as such did not enter the perinatal figures.

Better socio-economic conditions result in improvement in both survival and health of babies. Health professionals must be wary of assuming, however, that improvement is continuous. The level of unemployment, for example, may rise and have unhappy effects for the family.

NEONATAL DEATH

Definitions

A neonatal death is one occurring in the first 28 days of life. Neonatal deaths are divided into

INFANT DEATH

An infant death is one occurring in the first year of life. By definition this includes all neonatal deaths and the remainder are termed postneonatal deaths. The infant mortality rate is calculated per 1000 live births. This rate is taken as one of the best measures of a nation's health.

Causes of postneonatal death

Some of the important causes that a midwife should be aware of are non-accidental injury, infection and, in the older babies, accidents in the home. Sudden infant death also accounts for a significant number; these are unexpected deaths in which no cause is identified.

Trends and reasons for improvement

There has been a dramatic reduction in the number of infants who die under the age of 1 year since the beginning of the century. In 1900 the infant mortality rate was between 140 and 160 per 1000 whereas in 1985 the rate was 9.4 per 1000 in England and Wales. By 1990 this had fallen further to 7.9 per 1000 live births.

Improvement has been due to a multiplicity of factors including:

- better housing and standards of living
- immunisation
- antibiotics and chemotherapeutic agents
- prevention of cross-infection
- health education
- intravenous therapy
- appointment of paediatricians and neonatal specialists.

Confidential enquiry

A confidential enquiry into stillbirths and deaths in infancy (CESDI) was commenced in early 1993 in England, Wales and Northern Ireland by the Department of Health. Three categories of death will be investigated, late fetal losses (20–23 weeks), perinatal deaths, and all other deaths under 1 year of age. A sample of sudden, unexpected infant deaths from two or three regions will be examined in greater detail. It is hoped that the information obtained will contribute to a further reduction in mortality.

MATERNAL DEATH

The International Federation of Gynaecologists and Obstetricians (FIGO) defines maternal death as one occurring during pregnancy or labour or as a consequence of pregnancy within 42 days after delivery or abortion. The maternal mortality rate is calculated as the number of deaths occurring per 1000 total births. It includes deaths due to abortion although abortions are not included in the number of total births.

The Report on Confidential Enquiries into Maternal Deaths

This triennial report on maternal deaths in the United Kingdom (formerly only in England and Wales) analyses details of virtually every maternal death. The information is entirely confidential so that factors can be examined without fear of recrimination. Practice in respect of each complication can be assessed and the report makes recommendations which have been most valuable. Any individual obstetrician, midwife or general practitioner is unlikely to see many mothers die in his or her care and cannot therefore rely on personal experience; the availability of a national report shares the knowledge which has been gained.

Three groups of deaths are defined: (1) 'True' maternal death may be regarded as the *direct maternal death*, which is one 'resulting from obstetric complications of pregnancy, labour and puerperium', from interventions, omissions, incorrect treatment, or from a chain of events resulting from any of the above. (2) *Indirect obstetric deaths* are 'those resulting from previous existing disease, or disease that developed during pregnancy which was aggravated by pregnancy'. (3) Deaths from other causes which happen to occur in pregnancy are defined as *fortuitous deaths* (DH et al 1991).

The report identifies the causes of maternal deaths and reveals the trends in incidence. It reveals substandard care and names the disciplines which are responsible. Where shortage of resources has contributed to the death, this is mentioned. The authors of the report are careful to stress that avoiding the elements of substandard care which are discussed would not necessarily have averted the death concerned.

Causes

In the Report relating to the years 1985–87 (DH et al 1991), the five main causes of direct maternal death in the UK were as follows:

- thrombosis and thrombo-embolism
- hypertensive disorders of pregnancy
- early pregnancy deaths including abortion
- antepartum and postpartum haemorrhage
- amniotic fluid embolism.

Table 43.1
Direct maternal deaths by cause, rates per million estimated pregnancies, England and Wales 1970–87 (rates for the United Kingdom were not available as there was no information on pregnancies for Scotland and Northern Ireland). (Adapted from Report on Confidential Enquiries into Maternal Deaths in the United Kingdom 1985–87, DH et al 1991.)

	Cause of direct maternal death										
Triennium	Hypertensive diseases of pregnancy	Pulmonary embolism	Ectopic pregnancy	Haemorrhage	Amniotic fluid embolism	Abortion	Sepsis excluding abortion	Anaesthesia	Ruptured uterus	Other direct causes	All deaths
1970–72	14.9	17.6	11.5	10.4	4.8	25.3	10.4	12.8	3.8	6.9	118.7
1973–75	13.2	12.8	7.4	8.1	5.4	10.5	7.4	10.5	4.3	8.5	88.0
1976–78	12.5	18.5	9.0	10.3	4.7	6.0	6.5	11.6	6.0	8.2	93.4
1979–81*	14.2	9.0	7.9	5.5	7.1	5.5	3.1	8.7	1.6	7.5	70.0*
1982–84	10.0	10.0	4.0	3.6	5.6	4.4	1.0	7.2	1.2	8.4	55.0
1985–87	9.4	9.1	4.1	3.8	3.4	2.3	2.3	1.9	1.9	7.5	45.6

* Includes two other direct deaths omitted in the 1976–78 Report.

Table 43.1 shows the causes of maternal deaths in England and Wales for the seven triennia from 1970 to 1987. The latest Report refers to all four countries of the UK for the first time. The Reports began in 1952 and they constitute the longest uninterrupted series of clinical audits in the world.

Trends
Broadly speaking the maternal mortality rate has fallen by about 20% in each triennium and, in the 1985–87 triennium, the rate was 7.6 per 100 000 total births. The rates in Africa are about 640, in Latin America 270 and in Europe less than 10 per 100 000. The huge disparity between the developed and the developing world has led to the setting up of the Safe Motherhood initiative by the World Health Organization (see Ch. 1).

Thrombo-embolic disorders, including pulmonary embolism after abortion, caused the highest number of deaths in the triennium 1985–87. Some women who died antenatally had silent deep vein thrombosis. Hypertensive disorders of pregnancy continue to account for a high proportion of maternal deaths in spite of improvement in the management of hypertension. Haemorrhage reappears as one of the top four causes of death for the first time since the 1976–78 Report.

While the actual number of deaths from sepsis is relatively low, midwives should realise that deaths do still occur from this cause which may be insidious in onset. High standards of hygiene and asepsis will help to prevent infection.

In many instances of maternal death where substandard care was given, the Report stresses that failure of communication of potential problems to more senior members of staff including midwives was a relevant factor. This highlights the need to summon assistance at an early stage in any developing emergency.

Reasons for improvement
The Confidential Enquiry has itself had a significant effect in reducing the number of maternal deaths over the 30 years of publication. During that time many medical advances have been seen and some would claim that increased hospital delivery has contributed to saving maternal life although this is debated (e.g. Tew 1990, Campbell & Macfarlane 1987). The Report has often suggested protocols for action in emergency situations such as haemorrhage or retained placenta. Some improvements of note are:

- Improved early recognition and treatment of pre-eclampsia
- Closer co-operation with specialists in the management of diabetes and renal and cardiac disease
- Monitoring and screening of women at risk
- Early hospitalisation for complications of pregnancy
- Advances in knowledge of blood coagulation disorders
- Better social conditions.

Conclusion

The study of national statistics may seem a dry subject to the midwife and perhaps not easy to relate to her own practice but she should make herself familiar with the figures collected at her own unit and try to identify reasons for changes. Midwives should discuss such changes with the obstetricians and point out any relationships which may be apparent. It may be appropriate to suggest subjects for research (see Ch. 50) and possible changes in practice which would lead to improvements for mothers and babies.

Acknowledgement

The chapter authors are grateful to Mrs M. McGowan, Registrar of Births, Deaths and Marriages, Elstree and Potters Bar Registration District and to Mr A. C. Major, former Superintendent Registrar for the Swindon Registration District for advice and assistance in the preparation of this chapter.

REFERENCES

Campbell R, Macfarlane A 1987 Where to be born? The debate and the evidence. National Perinatal Epidemiology Unit, Oxford

Department of Health, Welsh Office, Scottish Home and Health Department and Department of Health and Social Services, Northern Ireland 1991 Report on confidential enquiries into maternal deaths in the United Kingdom 1985–87. HMSO, London

Office of Population Censuses and Surveys 1992 Mortality statistics, perinatal and infant: social and biological factors 1989 (series DH3 no. 23). OPCS, London

Tew M 1990 Safer childbirth? A critical history of maternity care. Chapman & Hall, London

United Kingdom Central Council for Nursing, Midwifery and Health Visiting 1989 A midwife's code of practice. UKCC, London (Reprinted 1991)

44

Sociology related to midwifery

JEAN DAVIES

Macrosociology and microsociology

Sociology and midwifery

The ways in which a society copes with the major events of birth, illness and death are central to the beliefs and practices of that society and also bear a close relationship to its other major social, economic and cultural institutions. (Stacey, 1988)

This chapter looks at the part that sociology plays in the understanding of how people and societies function, with particular reference to midwifery.

Sociology provides the theoretical framework for studying social phenomena. It also provides the tools for assessing and planning, and for evaluating the implementation of plans. As with any tool, sociology needs to be used rigorously and with precision and care (Cox & Mead 1975).

Sociology is to society what anatomy and physiology are to the body. It looks at structures and examines the interrelationship of the different parts. It imposes some order on the diversity of human activity. It enables people to be studied in a systematic way, so that patterns of behaviour can be identified. It is multidisciplinary in that it encompasses many subjects: history, politics, economics, psychology, art and religion.

We are all members of society and have opinions about the world we live in. Some are informed, but a lot are based on prejudice. Prejudice is derived from a word meaning prejudged and only through the systematic study of social phenomena is it possible to establish what is fact. Because sociology deals with subject matter that is everyone's business, people tend to feel that it merely points out the obvious and that it can be done, almost as an afterthought.

Evaluation is an integral part of the nursing process, but the reader should be aware that it is not synonymous with evaluation through sociological research. Clinical work should be research based if the care is to be rational and midwives should be doing research but it is often assumed that anyone can 'do research'. However, it needs a theoretical framework, which has been developed by the thinkers who have studied society and developed theories about its construction.

MACROSOCIOLOGY AND MICROSOCIOLOGY

Sociology falls into two approaches:

- Grand theory — the macrosociological approach, where the question asked is 'why?'
- Empirical — the microsociological approach, where the question is 'what?'.

Macrosociology looks at grand theories regarding social structure.

Everyone develops as a result of their social circumstances and cultural background. Grand theories reflect the *structuralist* approach, which recognises the social framework and its structure, and that what occurs outside a structure may affect how it functions. It has a philosophical foundation which reflects the holistic ecological approach and the humanities are an integral part.

Microsociology reflects more the empirical, scientific approach. It quantifies and deals with facts and figures. It reduces things to their component parts, the *reductionist* approach. It involves measuring and producing statistics, often putting them into graphic form. It looks at parts of the social structure and at their interactions.

History of sociology

Marx, Weber and Comte were founding fathers and their backgrounds were in economics, history and political philosophy. Durkheim, another of the masters, is best known for his classic study on suicide, which tests data scientifically and which combines the humanities and science into sociology. The influence of these men can be traced into present day sociology. Marxism is the theory that the history of mankind is written in the conflict between the oppressed and the oppressor in the creation and division of wealth. It has changed the way that society is analysed and has had global political impact (Aron 1965).

Structural functionalism is another grand theory and Parsons and Lévi-Strauss were the thinkers who developed its theories. Good sociology should combine both the grand philosophical theory and the systematic study of groups and systems; micro studies done within the framework of macro theory (Badcock 1975).

Methodologies

There are many ways in which sociologists collect and analyse data and they are referred to as methodologies. (See Ch. 50 for information about research methods.)

To study any phenomenon it is necessary to have categories that are exclusive and share common attributes. It would not be possible to analyse perinatal mortality rates without clear definitions of stillbirth and neonatal death. That definitions may vary between countries makes comparative studies difficult.

Epidemiology looks at health geographically, as a social phenomenon. It played a vital role in the eradication of smallpox from the world. Data collection plays the most important role in epidemiology. It is important to midwifery. Semmelweis was an early epidemiologist who identified the fact that puerperal fever was transmitted by doctors going straight from dissection to the labour wards. By gathering and comparing data he showed that the use of disinfectant resulted in fewer deaths. He was persecuted for his findings by his medical colleagues and committed suicide, but he was vindicated by history.

Epidemiology has highlighted the fact that women in under-developed countries have high perinatal mortality rates and that in the developed countries women with low incomes have poor outcomes of pregnancy compared to those of the well-off.

Anthropology is also of importance to midwifery. It explores the cultures of the people studied. Given that birth is one of the important 'rites of passage' that define and affirm culture, those who are present have an important social role. It is perhaps time that there was an anthropological study about the part midwives play in this rite (Van Gennep 1906).

Anthropology originated from attempts to understand so-called primitive tribes in small-scale studies. The approach is used more broadly now, to study any identifiable group of people. It involves detailed observation and recording, known as *ethnomethodology*. Observation may be participant observation, in which the researcher is also an actor, but recognition must be given to this.

Statistics provides the tool for analysing the data that any study generates. A sociologist needs to gather data in a systematic way, so that it is representative without getting so prolific that it is impossible to handle. Statistics has a bad press but its methods are the mathematical means of organising and analysing data, enabling correlations and the significance of information to be assessed.

Social administration is where sociology has practical application. It is the foundation of British sociology. Work on poverty, the reports on health (Townsend & Davidson 1982; Townsend et al 1988) and the work done by the National Perinatal Epidemiology Unit and the Office of Population Censuses and Surveys (OPCS) are all built on it. It is used widely in the planning of services. Increasingly, information technology is engaged in social administration in the hope of providing rational organisation and resource management. Booth, Seebohm and Rowntree were founders of social administration and their work grew from the study of poverty, the major concern of social administration.

Ethics

All research demands that participants be protected from exploitation. They should be fully informed about any research which involves them. Informed consent should be given before any individual is included in any research. Recent changes in the legislation relating to midwifery in New Zealand resulted from the political backlash caused by public concern that gynaecologists had done research which had denied some women life-saving treatment for cancer. It caused the public to question medical motives and ideals and assisted the campaign to legalise independent midwifery.

Change is part of the dynamic of humankind. Research can be part of the change process as knowledge gives impetus to progress in practical politics. The impetus for sociology is the desire to understand how people in a society function; its aim is usually philanthropic and seeks to make improvements.

The skill of the sociologist lies not just in the gathering of information but in its analysis. It has an important part to play in analysing interactions within the political arena in order to explore what is appropriate and what is irrational. There is a need to get a balance between quantitative data which does not provide qualitative information, and qualitative work that fairly illustrates the meaning of the figures.

SOCIOLOGY AND MIDWIFERY

Sociology is relevant to midwifery in two ways:

- by establishing exactly what the profession of midwifery means; this is the *sociology of midwifery*
- by incorporating research into clinical practice and resource management; this is *sociology in midwifery*.

(Turner 1987.)

Sociology of midwifery

This is the analysis of the roles of the midwife, the mother and medicine, putting them into their political and economic structures in order to study behavioural patterns and social interaction.

Analysis could look at who is central in a situation, how this occurred, if it is likely to change and how this affects interaction. It asks if the mother, the midwife, the consultant obstetrician, the baby, the Unit General Manager, or even God is the most important person. How do they all interact? From what angle is this interaction viewed, financial, medical, or cultural? How does this affect not only data collection, but analysis?

A lot has been written about the socialising effect of medicine and the medicalisation of society (Ehrenreich 1978). Disease has a biological reality but biology may have been affected by social phenomena, for example smoking, a lack of sanitation or economic hardship. How illness is treated, by whom and where, are the result of politics and economics. The relationships between doctor, nurse and patient have developed as part of the health care structure of any society and the behaviour of each to the other is prescribed by the position and power of the participants.

Maternity care is primarily about healthy women giving birth. However, it is undeniable that it has become medicalised in the developed countries. Sociology has a part to play in the understanding of how this has occurred and what effects it has had and might be having not just on mothers and midwives but on society (Haire 1978).

Sociology in midwifery

This relates to the practical application and implications of sociological findings, be they reports of clinical research or the use of data analysed for purposes of resource management. It should play an important role in the process of planning the delivery of care, both clinically and managerially.

Each time a midwife delivers a baby the birth is notified and this becomes one datum both locally and nationally. It is part of the data base of official statistics, in the United Kingdom held by OPCS. OPCS publishes the perinatal and maternal mortality rates which are used as the measurement of the effectiveness of maternity services. Census data collected also provide a lot of sociological material.

The empirical study of practice in clinical trials is also an important way that sociology in midwifery is used. Practices may be developed or abandoned as research findings are implemented. Descriptive, qualitative data are also important if maternal perceptions are to be understood.

The cultural aspects of birth

Birth is a fundamental act, a crucial 'rite of passage'. All rites have people in attendance on the participants who guide, or coerce, the individuals through the transitional period into their new position in society. Midwives have always been present at births, either as traditional birth attendants or as trained midwives. At this time not only does the woman give birth but she assumes the role of mother and will experience a change in social status that will affect the way others relate to her and how she herself behaves.

The way birth is managed is symbolic and reflects the society in which it occurs (Kitzinger 1978). In Britain, it affirms society as highly medicalised and because of this it is specialised and hospitalised. This is not chance but part of an historical process (Tew 1990).

Childbirth changes a woman. How it is experienced can affect her self-perception thereafter. A midwife who has the responsibility for being a guide at this time should be aware, not just of the physical needs of the woman, but of her psychosocial needs as well. This needs more than empathy, it requires some understanding of cultural diversity and an awareness of interrelationships during the period in which support is given. A sociological perspective increases this understanding. Transactions at birth operate within the *double hierarchies* of occupation and gender status. Where there are social organisations there will be hierarchies which show the stratifications of importance and power; these may be demonstrated publicly by who has the biggest room, who speaks to whom first, who touches whom. Power is not intrinsic, but maintained by ritualistic performance and through people conforming to patterns of behaviour. An antenatal clinic is an organisation where *social interaction of hierarchy* could be examined.

In the study of any society, culture is an essential definer. Eating is universal, manners are cultural; clothes are universal, costume cultural; birth is universal, its organisation and conduct are cultural and reflect the society in which it occurs. Culture is belief expressed by people through their public behaviour.

Rites and rituals

The term sociology was coined by the French philosopher Auguste Comte who described societies as being held together by common beliefs. Patterns of behaviour grow from the cultural inheritance of the past and culture is transmitted through ritual that often relates to rites of passage.

Rites of passage are the events signifying moving from one social status to another, such as birth, coming of age, graduating, marriage, childbirth and dying. Van Gennep's (1906) theory was that all rites involve:

- *separation* from the original status
- *transition* through ritual into vulnerable destabilisation
- *incorporation* into the new status.

Rituals usually mark these rites, affirming the person in the new position and, through repetition, they reinforce cultural integrity. They facilitate social change without disruption.

At a coronation a monarch is crowned with pomp and ceremony, that is with ritual. Positions of power are publicly demonstrated at their most colourful and graphic through protocol. This is common to all public rituals.

Roles

Roles are the behavioural patterns that people assume in the performance of certain social acts which define their position in a cultural system. The behaviour is expected and the person socialised into performing accordingly. This is not necessarily benign; class systems create distinct social division, and economics and patriarchy have combined to create socially inferior roles for women wherever they are in the class structure.

Socialisation is an integral part of child care. It is not only the way in which roles are learned, it is also the means by which culture is assimilated. Individuals exist throughout the world but the *individualism* of the capitalist West is a political philosophy, which affects behaviour and child care as much as the *collectivism* of communist China. Both philosophies have an effect on family size and on the way children are raised. The roles learned reflect the very different cultures of each society.

Woman's role

Biology has always defined a woman's role. Childbirth has always been a central issue in the position of women in society (Davies 1915, Shorter 1982). The horrors of frequent childbirth in the past are well documented and descriptions of some of the early obstetric interventions show how, in many cases, they exacerbated problems. The relationship between midwives and medical men illuminates the position of women (Donnison 1988). Not only were physical appliances developed but they were used under circumstances which highlight the control and treatment of pregnant women (Ehrenreich & English 1979).

The way in which pregnancy and childbirth are managed is a very clear indicator of the status of women in any society (MacCormack 1990). A woman in a non-industrialised country would benefit from access to the water and electricity that are taken for granted in the developed world. Shorter (1982) argues that it is modern obstetrics that has liberated women. However, few would claim that antenatal clinics are monuments to women's liberation. Women's lives have probably been more affected, physically and socially, by the introduction of tapped water.

The increased safety of childbirth is of course liberating. However, it is possible that this could have been achieved without the transitional period of birth being controlled in such a way as to maximise the vulnerability of women by reinforcing their status vis-à-vis the medical profession which is overwhelmingly male.

Oakley (1980) has developed a sociology of childbirth in which the power relationships are explored. She believes power is held by medical men and what they think women want does not correspond with what women really want. The maternity services introduce women to the role of quiescent citizens. Women go through an enormous transition during birth: that its organisation encourages passivity is worthy of study; its consequences might affect child care.

The role of the family

The management of birth is where anyone studying the changes in the family should begin looking. Advances in science and technology in the fertility field have had a radical cultural effect on the family. Contraception, infertility treatment and neonatal paediatrics are pushing the boundaries of procreation into new areas. Social mores are changing as rapidly as the advances in science. This is not to say that one causes the other but a correlation is not ruled out.

Family is a concept that everyone presumes to understand. Social change is so rapid that a large proportion of people live outside what was, until recently, considered the norm of the nuclear family, father, mother and children. The numbers of lone parents and step-families are escalating and are indications of a cultural shift. Two decades ago an unmarried mother in the maternity hospital would have tried to conceal her single status. Now hospital notes refer not to husband but to partner, which, in some cases, might mean another woman. In the past this would have been quite unthinkable, or at least unmentionable.

It is only about 30 years ago that teachers and nurses had to leave work when they got married. Continuing to work as children arrived was the exception, rather than the expectation that it is today. The way families function has undergone a radical change which reflects economic and political changes. Each year OPCS publishes its report *Social Trends* and it is an excellent source of information about these changes.

Race, nationality and ethnicity are not just based on place of birth but are affirmed by rite and ritual, and diverse roles are indicators of cultural differences. Women in the United States, the CIS and Africa all have different cultures which will be reflected in their expectations and experiences of birth. Those attending them would also have different expectations, different equipment and different status. In a multicultural society midwives might meet the physical needs of a woman but be unable to meet her need for a coherent cultural transition because of language, accent and rhythm. Hospitalisation has made birth culturally medical.

Ignorance of the cultural norms of the woman giving birth on the part of those attending her could undermine her essential sense of self at a very crucial time and might even affect the biological process if the woman feels alienated and alone. This highlights the needs for the woman to 'know her midwife' (Flint & Poulengeris 1987) so that the midwife has some chance of being aware of the woman's fundamental beliefs and of being sensitive to them, in recognition that birth is more than a medical process.

Religion. Ritual often has a religious origin; belief galvanised into action. Shared belief creates ethics and morality. In some societies magic and the supernatural are the cornerstone of culture, in others it is religion in its many manifestations. It has been argued that in industrial societies technology has superseded religion as having the greatest cultural impact. However, Weber theorised that industrialisation was born of the Protestant ethic (Tawney 1922). He illustrates the effect of religion, hard work and philanthropic work conditions on the growth of capital. This has been instrumental in the development of the economic structures that exist throughout the world, controlled by the canons of capital.

The efforts of missionaries to spread religion world-wide have been responsible for as much change in the world as the influence of trade, not least medical change, as many missionaries were and are medical men and women.

Economics and politics

Poverty

Analyses of poverty have been attempted with the primary aim of its eradication. Sociology looks at poverty within the structure of politics, which affects the economy of any country. Economics needs to be examined in the light of the social realities affected by it.

Poverty and childbirth. There is overwhelming evidence of the effect of poverty on childbirth (Townsend & Davidson 1982). Maternal mortality is almost eradicated in developed countries, and the perinatal mortality rates continue to fall. The wealthier the country the better the figures. However, within these countries there is a disparity between those with high and those with low incomes. This disparity is acknowledged as it has been exposed many times. However, it is rare that specific steps are taken to address the problem. In Newcastle-upon-Tyne the Community Midwifery Care Project was set up in order to study the effect, if any, of giving additional midwifery care to women considered to be at risk because of their low incomes. A sociological analysis of the work (Evans 1987) showed that the women did benefit, not least because they used the service more effectively and found the experience of birth better. There was also evidence of improved clinical outcome for low birthweight and preterm babies. It is of political interest that there was consistent medical resistance to this essentially midwifery project.

Political and economic systems have evolved throughout the world. Religion often provides the cultural framework which leads to the socialisation and the ideologies that form organisations. It has been suggested that medicine is now the arbiter of ethics and morality in the West rather than the church (Davies 1992). Whether the positions of women and midwives have changed concurrently is a fundamental question in political and economic analyses.

The varying rates of obstetric intervention world-wide are not due to biological differences in women but to the economics that make such intervention possible. Both politics and economics are involved. A 20% caesarean section rate reflects an economic structure in which this amount of intervention can be afforded. It also reflects obstetrically structured maternity care. It shows how medicalised society has become, what is considered important, who is in control and where their priorities lie. Developments in neonatal paediatrics depend on economic decisions made in the political arena.

It is within the economic and political realities of the world that there are 500 000 maternal deaths annually, and that 99% of these occur in developing countries. 50% of women who give birth do so without trained assistance. It is a reflection of women's cultural and economic status as well as their biological reality. The apportionment of spending on services within a society is a political decision. Preventive health is low on the agenda, exciting technological development high. This is a reflection of the power spectrum. Sociology has a part to play in exploring interactions to see where change is possible and whether it is desirable.

Finally, however competent the sociological study, however interesting the analysis, unless the findings are implemented, it is of no benefit.

Reader Activities

1. A *sociogram* is a graphic representation of interrelationships. Draw a diagram of the maternity services in your area in which you display the main participants and show how they interact with each other, putting yourself at the centre. Who else is included? What does this tell you about the sharing of responsibility or about hierarchy?

Now redraw your sociogram putting the mother at the centre. Does this make you include different people? Does it appear to change the balance of power in any way?

What is the effect if the obstetrician is at the centre? the GP? the woman's partner?

2. Find a detailed map of the locality which is served by your local maternity services. Make enquiries about the social background of the clientele, such as the industries they work for, the type of housing that they live in and the facilities available for their use in each district. Mark these on the map. Take note of the clinics run by midwives and GPs in each area. What parent education is offered? Discuss with colleagues what the map reveals about provision for women and their families.

3. *Data collection and analysis*. Analysing through counting and averaging is where statistics starts. This simple diagram is an example of classifying groups in order to be able to begin to analyse them.

Babies born in 1993 in Newtown	Male	Female	All
Under 2500 g	6	15	21
Over 2500 g	14	65	79
Total	20	80	100

What percentage of the males are under 2500 g? _____

What percentage of the females are under 2500 g? _____

What percentage of all are under 2500 g? _____

In statistics you set out to find grounds for refuting a null hypothesis, which states that there is no difference between groups; in this case that there is no difference between boys and girls in Newtown. The next step would be to establish the expected distribution of birthweights, and compare it with Newtown's. Was the null hypothesis upheld; that there is no difference? Or have statistics been able to show that there is something significant?

There is a long way to go, into chi-squares and *t* testing, but a first step is knowing that you are not proving but refuting.

4. *Observation.* Become a 'fly on the wall' with note pad in hand, and write down everything that happens within the area you are wanting to investigate, for example an antenatal clinic. Write down everything a woman does and says, and what is said to her, and by whom, and time it. A vast amount of data will be collected. Post-coding is a process of categorising data into sections which can then be handled, and counted.

Do the same for a student midwife, which will illustrate the difference in perspective.

5. *Survey or questionnaire.* Compile a questionnaire about something that interests or puzzles you. How questions are asked can affect the answers. Try it out on your colleagues; doing a pilot study is always a good idea as it helps you to minimise ambiguities in the questions. A recent study by midwives of the pain produced by scalp electrodes is an example of trying things out with the peer group. Questions can be closed, with a limited number of responses; or open, which again involves post-coding for any analysis.

Anybody can ask anyone a question, but if the questioner is a professional the ethics of asking questions of someone receiving attention must be considered. Positions of power should not be exploited in order to gain data, and people must be informed and have the opportunity to refuse to give information.

REFERENCES

Aron R 1965 Main currents in sociological thought 1. Pelican, Harmondsworth

Aron R 1967 Main currents in sociological thought 2. Pelican, Harmondsworth

Badcock C R 1975 Lévi-Strauss structuralism and sociological theory. Hutchinson, London

Cox C, Mead A 1975 A sociology of medical practice. Collier Macmillan, London

Davies Llewellyn M 1915 Maternity — letters from working women. Republished 1978, Virago, London

Davies J 1992 Obstetrics in the 1990s — current controversies. Mackeith Press. Blackwell Scientific, Oxford

Donnison J 1988 Midwives and medical men, 2nd edn. Historical Publications, London

Ehrenreich E, English D 1979 For her own good. Pluto Press, London

Ehrenreich J 1978 (ed) The cultural crisis of modern medicine. Monthly Review Press, New York

Evans F 1987 An evaluation report — the Newcastle-upon-Tyne community midwifery care project. Newcastle Health Authority, Newcastle-upon-Tyne

Flint C, Poulengeris P 1987 The 'Know Your Midwife' report. Privately printed; available from 47 Peckarman's Wood, Sydenham Hill, London SE26 6RZ

Haire D 1978 The cultural warping of childbirth. In: Ehrenreich J (ed) The cultural crisis of modern medicine. Monthly Review Press, New York

Kitzinger S 1978 Women as mothers. Fontana\Collins, Glasgow

MacCormack C (ed) 1990 Ethnography of fertility and birth. Academic Press, London

Oakley A 1980 Women confined — towards a sociology of childbirth. Martin Robertson, Oxford

Shorter E 1982 A history of women's bodies. Allen Lane, London

Stacey M 1988 The sociology of health and healing. Unwin Hyman, London

Tawney R H 1922 Religion and the rise of capitalism. Penguin Books, London

Tew M 1990 Safer childbirth? A critical history of maternity care. Chapman & Hall, London

Townsend P, Davidson N 1982 Inequalities in health: the Black report. Penguin, Harmondsworth

Townsend P, Phillimore P, Beattie A 1988 Health and deprivation — inequality and the North. Croom Helm, London

Turner B S 1987 Medical power and social knowledge. Sage Publications, London

Van Gennep A 1906 Rites of passage. Republished 1965, Routledge & Kegan Paul, London

45

Community health and social services

JANET ASHERSON

The community health and social services embody an area of social policy in which the state endeavours to reduce the differences in life-chances and enhance the well-being of its people.

BENEFITS

The benefits available to a pregnant woman may be considered under the headings of monetary and non-monetary.

Monetary benefits

These constantly change as a result of new legislation and with inflation, so an outline of the present scheme is given here, and the reader is advised to consult the leaflets produced by the DSS with every change. Parts of the monetary benefits system are extremely complex, notably the details of paid maternity leave, and these are merely outlined here.

Timing is very important in the claiming of these benefits and the midwife must be clear and accurate in her advice to her clients in the antenatal clinic. She must be careful to offer the relevant forms at the appropriate times and must be able to direct the woman to other health professionals or local advice centres for further guidance when necessary so that optimum benefit may be obtained.

Social fund

Only those women receiving income support or family credit receive this grant. It is means-tested and is payable up to a maximum of £100 for each baby expected, born or adopted. The total will be reduced if the family has savings over £500. It is paid from the social fund. Women receiving income support may apply for help towards buying maternity clothing.

The social fund payment is payable from 29 weeks' gestation and must be claimed before the baby is 3 months old. It is payable when delivery occurs after 29 weeks' gestation whether or not the baby is born alive. In the case of multiple pregnancy it is payable for each additional infant and the mother makes a claim in the usual way.

Application is made on the social fund claim form. This must be accompanied by form Mat B1 (certificate of expected confinement) which is supplied and signed by the midwife or doctor. Following delivery, form Mat B2 is required; this is a certificate of confinement of very similar format to the Mat B1 and it is also supplied and signed by the midwife or doctor.

Maternity allowance

Maternity allowance is available for women who are not entitled to Statutory Maternity Pay: the self-employed and those who have recently given up their jobs or changed jobs. These women may claim a basic rate of maternity allowance from the Department of Social Security (DSS) if they have paid their national insurance contributions for 26 of the 52 weeks ending in the 15th week before the *expected week of confinement*. The expected week of confinement begins on the Sunday of the week in which the baby is due.

The maternity allowance is paid for 18 weeks which is flexible but must include a *core period* of 13 weeks beginning 6 weeks before the baby is due. The remaining 5 weeks may be taken according to the mother's choice. She can take some before and some after the core period or all before or all after. It is not payable for any week or part of a week in which a woman works.

Application is made on form MA.1 after the 26th week of pregnancy and must be accompanied by form Mat B1. Late application may result in loss of allowance.

Statutory Maternity Pay (SMP)

This scheme is operated by the employer. Any woman who has worked for the same employer for the first 6 months of her pregnancy is entitled to SMP provided that her earnings average more than the *lower earnings limit* between the 18th and 26th week of pregnancy. The lower earnings limit is the level of pay at which people begin to pay national insurance contributions. There are two rates of SMP, both payable for 18 weeks. The lower rate is equivalent in amount to Statutory Sick Pay. Women who have worked for the same employer for at least 16 hours a week for 2 years, or for at least 8 hours a week for 5 years, are entitled to a higher rate of SMP for the first 6 weeks. This is equal in amount to 90% of their average earnings. The lower rate of SMP is paid throughout the SMP period if a woman has worked for less than 2 years.

The period of 18 weeks is flexible in the same way as for maternity allowance. The woman must tell her employer at least 3 weeks before she intends to leave work. Payment of SMP does not depend on returning to work. SMP is subject to all deductions usually taken from wages.

Women in paid employment should always be advised to discuss arrangements with their employers early in the pregnancy as some firms operate schemes which provide better terms than the minimum requirements.

Family benefits

The family whose income falls below a certain level is eligible for certain financial and non-monetary benefits. The birth of a baby may render a family eligible for these benefits, either by virtue of a fall in income, or because there is another mouth to feed.

Income support is a non-contributory benefit. It is paid to top up other benefits or a low income earned from working less than 24 hours a week. It is made up of personal allowances and includes housing mortgage interest payments. Recipients automatically qualify for NHS benefits and may qualify for housing benefits, Social Fund payments and assistance with fares to hospital for antenatal appointments. It is usually only available to those over 18 years of age but younger, single parents may qualify.

Family credit is paid to a family where one parent is working at least 24 hours a week. Members of the family are allocated 'credits' and these are paid in full if income does not reach Income Support level. Recipients of Family Credit will also be entitled to NHS benefits and will be able to apply to the Social Fund.

Child benefit is a non-contributory, tax-free benefit paid to anyone responsible for a child.

It is paid for any child under 16 years of age, or older if he or she is in education. It is paid on a weekly or monthly basis. The mother of a new baby must obtain the claim form and state whether the baby is her first-born or a later child. The form has to be accompanied by the baby's birth certificate. Benefit can be back-dated up to 6 months.

Single parent benefit. A single parent can claim this additional supplement to child benefit for a first-born child.

Non-monetary benefits

Free prescriptions. All pregnant women eligible for treatment under the National Health Service may claim exemption from prescription charges. This exemption then applies until the baby is (or would have been) 1 year old. Form FW8 is supplied by the doctor or midwife and is completed as soon as possible in pregnancy.

Free dental treatment. This applies in the same way as prescription charge exemption. However, it is not an all-embracing service and the dental practitioner is entitled to charge for non-essential treatment.

Vitamins and milk. Vitamin tablets for pregnant and nursing mothers and formula milks for infants may be purchased at subsidised or cost price in clinics and health centres. For those with a Family Credit order book and a child under a year old, formula milk can be purchased at a reduced price. In families on Income Support, free vitamins and milk are available to pregnant women and children.

Antenatal care may be regarded as one of the non-monetary benefits provided in the UK. It is freely available to every pregnant woman and the aim is to give comprehensive care and surveillance in the interests of a healthy mother and baby.

Delivery in hospital is available to almost every woman in the UK and the provision of midwifery services to every woman in labour is mandatory. Indeed, it is illegal for a person other than a midwife or medical practitioner to conduct a delivery except, of course, in an emergency.

The rights of the pregnant woman at work

Pregnant women in paid employment outside the home have certain rights in addition to monetary benefits. These are:

- the right to paid time off for antenatal care
- the right to retain a job while pregnant
- the right to return to work after the pregnancy.

Antenatal care. This may include any aspect of care given during the pregnancy such as visits to the antenatal clinic, the midwife's visits to the home and attendance at parent education sessions. The employer is entitled to request evidence that the woman has a genuine appointment.

Retention of a job. A woman cannot be dismissed for being pregnant. If she is unable to do her job or if it is dangerous for her to continue while pregnant the employer must offer her alternative employment. In the absence of a suitable alternative post she may be dismissed fairly but still retains the right to return to work after her baby is born.

Return to work. After delivery of her baby a woman has the right to return to her previous job provided she complies with certain regulations. These entail informing her employer of her intentions to leave and return well in advance of the time.

Any large firm will have a personnel department which should be acquainted with the details of these rights and be able to advise the woman accordingly.

THE HEALTH VISITOR

Background and training

Health visiting has its roots in the 19th century when the Industrial Revolution resulted in the growth of slum areas in the inner cities, with parents and older children working long hours for a mean wage. Ignorance and poverty took their toll, and infant mortality was high. Understanding of the nature and spread of infection was growing and the first health visitors, who were not nurses, were sent out to instruct mothers on very basic matters of health and hygiene.

In 1919 the first training scheme for health visitors was set up. The course lasted 2 years but trained nurses could qualify after 1 year.

In 1956 the Jameson report recommended that health visitors should broaden their scope to include mental health, hospital after-care and the care of the elderly. Child health was to continue as an important part of their role and health education was to have a high priority in all their dealings with clients. Every health visitor was to be a registered nurse and either be a qualified midwife or have undertaken a special course in obstetrics prior to her health visitor training.

The Jameson report led to the passing of the Health Visiting and Social Work (Training) Act of 1962 and the development of the Council for the Education and Training of Health Visitors. In 1979 the Nurses, Midwives and Health Visitors Act set up the United Kingdom Central Council for Nursing, Midwifery and Health Visiting. This, in association with the four National Boards, is now responsible for education and training. To train as a health visitor today, a person must have five 'O' levels and be a registered nurse: obstetrics is included in the course.

The working situation

Health visitors work either as members of primary health care teams within GP practices or they can be community based and work in defined geographical areas.

The role of the health visitor

The health visitor is a nurse who focuses her practice on the promotion of health through home visiting and community action. Her work is considered to be 'pro-active' in that it searches for health needs (rather than responding to symptoms of 'dis-ease') and raises awareness of those needs. Health visiting facilitates participation of individuals, families or groups in planned activities which enables people to improve their own health or personal situations. In its broadest sense, health is a complex mixture of physical, psychological, social and environmental factors. A health visitor could therefore justifiably see her role as being involved in almost any activity, in any age group of the local population. Although the principles of health visiting are not under question, the way in which the service is delivered to the public often is. The professional debate is continuous and the health visitor's role changes in response to the latest research, political climate and requirements from employing authorities.

Prevention. Preventive measures are seen as a vital part of health visiting.

- Primary prevention involves action taken to prevent problems ever occurring. It includes health promotion activities, such as lobbying for 'no smoking' policies, and health education about balanced diets and how to reduce home accidents.
- Secondary prevention concerns itself with the early discovery of disease through screening and identifying 'at risk' groups.
- Tertiary prevention is the supportive care necessary to maintain an optimum situation, for example self-help groups.

Defining priorities. Where there is infinite need with finite resources, priorities must be defined. Caseload or community profiles are designed to do this. They provide analysis of the available services and relevant health data for the area in which the health visitor works and the clientele she visits. In this way a specific health need may be highlighted and the health visitor can target her practice to meet that need. Occasionally priorities depend on the health visitor's perception of her own skills as well as her job description: some health visitors combine their role with that of midwife or school nurse; some liaise between hospital and community or carry responsibility for a specialist area.

Teamwork. Health visitors are part of the primary health care team. This may be defined as the group of health professionals responsible for delivering first-line health care to the public, which may be either preventive or curative. The primary health care team has a central core, consisting of the general practitioner, the district nurse, the community midwife and the health visitor. The team may be extended to include members of any professional discipline giving care in the community such as the speech therapist. The health visitor often considers local voluntary, charity or community workers to be part of the team if she organises programmes of care jointly with them. Administrative staff are indispensable for the day-to-day running of the primary health care team.

Referral to various agencies. The health visitor needs to have a comprehensive and clear knowledge of the wide spectrum of voluntary and statutory agencies available to herself and clients for practical help, advice and support. Functioning alongside these agencies is also an aspect of teamwork.

Organisation of work. The health visitor has to organise her work in the context of the broad aims of professional training, the latest research of health visiting practice, the specific targets of her employing authority and her own talents. Organisation of work carried out with clients involves the health visiting process of assessment, planning, implementation and evaluation.

Her public image. It is the responsibility of the health visitor to explain her role to the public and to colleagues. The wearing of uniform was largely abandoned some years ago, in an attempt to shed the 'authoritarian' image. It enables health visitors to work more closely with people in a variety of settings. It is often thought that health visitors have a statutory duty to visit but this is incorrect. The statutory duty is on the health authority to provide the service, not any specific visit nor the acceptance of that visit by the client (Robertson 1988).

The health visitor and the 0 to 5s

The health visitor is trained to work with all ages, but historically her work has been associated with women and children. It is in this capacity that a health visitor works most closely with her midwife colleague.

The antenatal period. Alongside the midwife, a health visitor can offer health education through formal preparation for parenthood classes, working with outreach groups or meeting women in their own homes. Early contact provides an opportunity to establish a good working relationship and put the mother in touch with the supportive services available to her. This anticipatory guidance can be particularly important once the baby is born.

The 'primary' visit. The health visitor performs this visit when the community midwife discharges the new mother and baby from her care. This is frequently as early as the 10th day but some midwives continue visiting until 28 days. The primary visit is also the only visit which is a result of a systematic referral to the health visitor. The Birth Notification, which is completed by the midwife (most commonly) or some other person present at delivery, provides information for a set of *child health records* and also informs the Registrar of Births and Deaths that a baby has been born. The child health records are designed for use by the health visitor and doctor. Frequently the school nurse uses them until school-leaving age. These records are sent out from the Health Authority's child health records department to the health visitor concerned. It is therefore very important that all information should be written clearly and correctly on the Birth Notification form.

The mother is offered information about the services available and care will continue as a combination of home and clinic visits. If a good rapport can be established between health visitor and mother, self-referral for advice and support will usually follow.

Special programmes of visiting. Certain methods of health visitor intervention have been shown to be effective in reducing the incidence of sudden infant death (Carpenter et al 1983). The Child Development Programme looks at working with parents as partners to build on existing parenting skills (Tissier 1990). It involves a highly structured home visiting service, but it has been shown to reduce the incidence of behavioural and emotional problems and non-accidental injury. Improvements in child health and development have been noted.

Child Health Clinics. These are run in every imaginable setting, from purpose-built health centre to draughty church hall. Services available include baby weighing, consultation with the health visitor, immunisations and routine medical and developmental checks by the doctor. Mothers can buy, at a subsidised rate, baby milks, vitamin drops for babies and children, and vitamin tablets for themselves when pregnant and nursing. The medical checks may be performed by the general practitioner or by a Clinical Medical Officer employed by the health authority.

Developmental assessments. Development is considered in the areas of gross motor movements, vision and fine motor movements, hearing and language, social behaviour and play. It is looked at within the context of family health and family dynamics. Assessment of development, either formally or informally, provides an opportunity for the mother and health visitor to consider the progress of the child and think about possible remedial help if it is needed. The early identification of developmental delay and appropriate intervention can reduce the effects of an otherwise handicapping condition. Assessment of a child's development is usually carried out at specific ages, in conjunction with medical examinations by a doctor. The exact timing and use of personnel vary from one health authority to another.

Screening. Certain screening tests are included in the care of the 0–5 year age group. The hearing test is usually performed by the health visitor on every baby at 7 months of age. The test for congenital dislocation of the hip is usually repeated at least once, even though the midwife and doctor may both have performed it in the first days of life. The health visitor may be asked to repeat the blood test for phenylketonuria and hypothyroidism if the result of the original one was abnormal or undetermined.

Advice and support. The health visitor's role is to help the client to find ways of overcoming problems by offering counselling or advice. Where there is no solution she may be able to offer emotional support by strengthening support systems for clients. This may mean initiating a group or introducing a client to an established network that exists because of a common bond. An example could be the National Childbirth Trust local postnatal support groups.

Referral to and liaison with agencies. There are many agencies, statutory and voluntary, with whom the health visitor may have contact in her work of caring for mothers and babies.

IMMUNISATIONS

These are an important part of the preventive measures designed to improve the nation's health and to reduce morbidity and mortality. Health professionals can positively influence the immunisation rate by giving consistent accurate information, knowing the true contra-indications, being enthusiastic in their approach and adopting a policy of immunising whenever a suitable opportunity arises.

As a general rule, immunisations should not be given to children who are in the acute phase of an illness, who have had a severe reaction to a previous dose, or whose immune system has been affected by disease (e.g. malignancy) or by treatment (e.g. chemotherapy). Live vaccines should not be given to a pregnant woman because of possible harm to the unborn child. Sometimes, extensive media coverage of the rare adverse effects of vaccination has led to a high level of parental and professional anxiety with subsequent low acceptance rates. This has been the case with pertussis immunisation. Current policy states that absolute contra-indications to pertussis vaccine are as mentioned above. The signs and symptoms which are regarded as severe are: an extensive, red, hard, swollen area at the site of injection, fever of 39.5°C or more within 2 days of receiving vaccine, collapse, prolonged incessant screaming, convulsions occurring within 72 hours or anaphylactic shock. Special attention should be paid to those parents whose children have a personal or family history of cerebral damage or convulsions. They will need help to understand that while their children are at greater risk of experiencing a febrile convulsion after receiving the pertussis or measles vaccine, they are not at greater risk from suffering long-term adverse effects of vaccine. For this reason it is recommended that when these children are immunised, parents are instructed in the management of temperature control by sensible dressing, tepid sponging and appropriate administration of paracetamol elixir.

The decision by a parent not to immunise a child because of possible reactions to a vaccine, should be balanced with consideration of the

Table 45.1
Immunisation schedule

Vaccine	Dose	Age	Comments	Route
Tuberculosis (BCG)		Birth	For those likely to be in close contact with a case of tuberculosis	i.d.
Hepatitis B	1st	Birth	For infants whose mothers are carriers of hepatitis B surface antigen	deep s.c. or i.m.
Hepatitis B	2nd	4 weeks		
Diphtheria, tetanus, pertussis (DTP)	1st	8 weeks		deep s.c. or i.m.
Oral polio (OPV)	1st	8 weeks		oral
DTP	2nd	12 weeks		
OPV	2nd	12 weeks		
DTP	3rd	16 weeks		
OPV	3rd	16 weeks		
Hepatitis B	3rd	26 weeks		
Measles, mumps, rubella (MMR)		12–18 months		deep s.c. or i.m.
Diphtheria, tetanus	Booster	4–5 years		deep s.c. or i.m.
OPV	4th	4–5 years		
MMR		4–5 years	If not given between 12–24 months	
BCG		10–14 years	If tuberculin negative	
Rubella		10–14 years Adult	Girls who have not already had MMR Offered to non-immune women following childbirth or as part of preconception care	
Tetanus		15–18 years		deep s.c. or i.m.
OPV		15–18 years		

Key: s.c. = subcutaneous; i.m. = intramuscular; i.d. = intradermal

possible severe complications following the disease itself, information often unacknowledged by many parents today.

Immunisation programmes are designed to stimulate the baby's immune system to produce specific antibodies. His inherited protection (provided by maternal antibodies) diminishes at about the time that his own defence mechanisms mature and immunisation is timed to coincide with this point in order to minimise the period when he is particularly vulnerable to infection. The spacing of immunisations is important and parents are encouraged to bring their children for immunisation at the appropriate times.

THE SOCIAL WORKER

The history of social work may be traced back to the Poor Law of 1834 and the workhouse. Prompted by the poor living conditions of both the inner city and the rural populace various attempts to alleviate distress and reform conditions were made by the church and the great humanitarians of the 19th century. They tackled a wide variety of social ills, for example the plight of orphans and conditions in the factories, mines and prisons. Although the Poor Law and its provisions created a stigma by defining and putting emphasis on the poor, it was at least some kind of attempt to recognise and meet their needs. Provisions set up in the last century have changed and evolved as needs have changed. Thus Dr Barnardo's homes and the Church of England children's homes have developed from large scale orphanages to small group homes, often catering for children with special needs.

Many functions performed by the voluntary sector, such as adoption, have been taken over by the state to a great extent. However, there are still some voluntary agencies which function independently and a mother considering adoption will often approach such an agency, especially if she wishes her child to be placed with adoptive parents of a particular religious persuasion. The British Agencies for Adoption and Fostering (the BAAF) will provide details of these on request.

Important milestones for social work include the Beveridge report of 1946 which led to the setting up of the National Health Service in 1948. At this time social workers were involved in a variety of areas; each was highly specialised. Their areas of responsibility included child care, mental health and the elderly. The 'almoner' was the hospital social worker. In an attempt to unify this diversity and to give the social workers a professional identity, the Seebohm report of 1968 recommended that all social workers become generic. This report led to the Social Services Act of 1970 and resulted in a reorganisation of the entire service.

The social worker's role is to assess people who have to cope with special problems and to arrange for their appropriate social care from community resources. They also support clients at specific times of stress and help them to gain insight into the nature of their difficulties. Such people may include the elderly, the mentally or physically handicapped, the poor and those whose family relationships have broken down. Social workers are assisted in decision-making by their team leaders. They organise their work in terms of casework or fieldwork (with individuals) or community work (in local neighbourhood groups).

The social worker's practice is influenced by various Acts of Parliament, for example:

- in child care:
  the Children and Young Persons' Act of 1969
  the Children Act of 1975
  the Children Act of 1989
- in mental health:
  the Mental Health Act of 1983
- in the care of the elderly:
  the National Assistance Act of 1948
- in the care of the handicapped:
  the Chronically Sick and Disabled Persons' Act of 1970.

Many older practising social workers have no formal qualifications but do have a wealth of experience. Younger social workers may elect to undertake a 2-year course leading to the Certificate of Qualification in Social Work (the CQSW). A student with a university degree in a related subject such as sociology or social administration may take a shorter, 1-year course leading to the CQSW. Some university degrees incorporate the CQSW.

The midwife works closely with social workers in both hospital and community. Many primary health care teams now include a social worker.

VIOLENCE IN THE FAMILY

Child abuse

From earliest times children have been ill-treated, neglected or left to die. The value adults place on a child changes with time and between cultures. Much of what is perceived as right or wrong in terms of child care is opinion. In spite of this, each society usually holds some strictly kept rules of acceptable and unacceptable behaviour with regard to its treatment of children. Breaking of these rules is one of the greatest social taboos. There is nothing new about child abuse: what is a new phenomenon of the late 20th century is society's concern about it. Much energy has been devoted to defining it, studying the causes and considering methods of dealing with it.

Today child abuse is classified in the following ways:

- physical abuse — non-accidental tissue damage
- sexual abuse — involvement of children in sexual activities where they are unable to give informed consent
- emotional abuse — intentional methods of reducing a child's self-esteem leading to inappropriate behaviour

- failure to thrive — a child failing to grow at the recognised 'normal' rates consequent on emotional neglect
- neglect — failure to provide conditions for suitable development or protection of the child.

In spite of increased information, child abuse often remains difficult to prove. Solutions to the problem are often felt to be unsatisfactory. For these reasons, professional attention largely focuses on the area of prevention which includes increasing everyone's understanding of the basic needs of children; providing either personal or community based support systems (such as help with child care) when family tensions become too strained; preventing deterioration of an existing abusive situation. Ultimately, protection for a child may necessitate providing alternative accommodation and enforcing this with legal care proceedings.

Abused children and their families present with a range of signs and symptoms. Commonly it is noticed that physical injuries could not have occurred in the way in which the parents describe; there may be a delay in seeking treatment for the child; children may appear either unusually passive, expressing no emotion whatsoever, or be excessively cowed, withdrawn or overly friendly to strangers. There can also be inappropriate age-related behaviour. A child who has been sexually abused for instance, can act in a sexually provocative manner. The child may also be abnormally small with an unusual distribution of body fat. This non-organic cause of failure to thrive is sometimes accompanied by features of general uncleanliness and unkempt appearance. Hands and feet may look puffy and mottled and feel cold; hair may be dry, sparse and coarse. All forms of abuse in a family are usually accompanied by feelings of inadequacy, guilt, fear and shame. There is often a history of family collusion, especially in sexual abuse.

The National Society for the Prevention of Cruelty to Children (NSPCC) is a voluntary body with an important role to play in supporting and treating 'at-risk' families. They, and the social services, will take referrals from any individual regarding suspected child abuse.

There are now carefully laid down procedures in every area for dealing with actual or suspected child abuse. As soon as possible, a 'case conference' is held which includes every professional, and there may be several, involved with the family. All knowledge is then pooled and a *key worker* appointed. This is usually the social worker. Recommendations are made as to what action will be taken.

A family which is felt to be 'at risk' may be discussed at a case conference and the procedure described above may be followed in order to try to prevent child abuse occurring. Child abuse is a multi-factorial problem and the need for preventive measures far exceeds the resources available. Definable risk factors include the following:

Table 45.2
Factors increasing the risk of child abuse

In the baby
- prematurity, especially if the baby was in the Special Care Baby Unit
- chronic illness
- abnormality
- multiple or problem pregnancy
- excessive crying (as defined by the parents)
- poor sleep habit

In the mother
- single parent
- under 18 years old
- lower social classes
- prolonged or difficult labour
- lack of parent–child attachment
- poor experience of mothering — the 'cycle of deprivation'
- social isolation, poor family support
- acute or chronic illness
- postnatal depression
- psychiatric illness, mental handicap
- sees baby as a solution to her problems

Family and social
- unemployment
- housing or financial problems
- unwanted pregnancy or baby of the 'wrong sex'
- marital problems
- unrealistic expectations of baby
- recent bereavement
- alcohol or drug abuse
- history of child abuse in either parent (either as victim or inflictor)
- step-parents or -children
- criminal record — either parent
- chaotic lifestyle — numerous moves

Most families will encounter one or more of these problems when a new baby is born and will cope well, emerging unscathed. An already stressed family may not be able to cope with a single added stressor; a cluster of these 'risk factors', many of which are interrelated, may provide a warning signal in any family. (See also Ch. 44.)

Marital violence

This is another problem of unknown proportions. Either partner may be the victim of the violence, but it is the 'battered wife' who receives more recognition and sympathy. There are voluntary agencies which run hostels in the bigger cities, where the 'battered wife' and her children may seek refuge. Children may need to be taken into local authority care.

CHILD CARE PROVISIONS

These will be considered under the categories of day care, residential care and adoption.

Day care

Day nurseries are run during the week from Monday to Friday. Pre-school children and babies are admitted and full care, including the provision of meals, is given.

They are run either by local authorities or privately. In either case, the nursery is controlled and regulated by legislation and the local authority oversees this. Places are relatively limited. Most nurseries have policies governing the type of placement they offer, for example children in 'special need' and children of working or single mothers may be given priority. Provision of a place in a day nursery invariably relieves some of the stresses of family life and may even reduce the risk of family breakdown. Most nurseries charge a fee, although financial help may be offered where necessary. Staff usually have teaching or nursery nurse training and are assisted by untrained helpers.

Family centres are set up to try to help the whole family. Support and help is given to parents in order to try to establish positive interaction within the stressed family. Parents are positively encouraged to participate in the activities of the centre. In this way they often acquire additional skills, particularly in the area of constructive play and management of behaviour problems. The Children Act 1989 advocates that every local authority provides a family centre as it sees appropriate. They are usually run in association with a voluntary organisation.

Nursery schools and classes are run during school hours and may be on the same site as the infants' school. They are provided by the Education Authority but are not a statutory provision and the number of nursery school places available will depend on local policy and priorities. Staff will be qualified nursery teachers and nursery nurses who work together with untrained helpers. Ideally there is a high ratio of staff to children. Nursery schools have both an educational and a social function. Priority may be given to children with special needs but nursery school places are available to any pre-school child on a basis of first come, first served.

Workplace nurseries and crèches. It is anticipated that there will be a rapid growth of this particular day-care provision as the demand for women to rejoin the labour market increases. They are a new phenomenon in Britain and it remains to be seen how effectively they will operate. The local authority will be responsible for their registration and annual inspection.

Playgroups are an informal or voluntary provision. A voluntary body, the Pre-school Playgroups Association, gives advice and help to playgroup leaders, who often have no formal training but who have small children of their own, and plenty of energy and enthusiasm! Playgroups offer socialisation training for children and an opportunity for supervised and constructive play. They also provide social contact and support for mothers, who may be drawn in to help if they wish. Children are usually admitted from 3 years of age.

Opportunity playgroups. These take mentally and physically handicapped children, often alongside their normal siblings and other normal children, and have a higher ratio of helpers to children.

Child minders. A child minder cares for other people's children regularly in her own home, usually for payment on a sessional basis. Child minders should apply for registration with the local authority, even if they do not charge for their services. Before registration is granted, premises and facilities are inspected and a limit placed on the number of children who may be cared for at the same time. Obviously child minding may be an informal, neighbourly arrangement and so it is difficult to control.

Sponsored child minding. This is an interesting provision, an example of which is found in Bristol. Child minders are appointed and paid by the local authority to care for children from families at risk. The hope is that as well as giving mother and children a break from each other, a trusting and supportive relationship may grow up between parents and child minders and possibly some help may be given with family dynamics. Another great advantage is that it provides continuity of supervision and the child minder can make helpful suggestions when the family's situation and progress are reviewed at the case conference.

Home visiting services. An example of this is Homestart. A charitable organisation, it may be considered to contribute towards child care provision in that a volunteer, herself an experienced mother, shares her time and skills within a family's home. In this way she can alleviate some of the overwhelming responsibility felt by some mothers who may have limited access to other types of facility.

Residential care

Reception or assessment centres. A child may be admitted to one of these for assessment so that the best means of care may be decided for him or her.

Community homes are run collaboratively by local authorities and voluntary organisations such as Dr Barnardo's or National Children's Homes. These endeavour to run on a small group basis with house parents and integrate, as far as possible, into the community. They are said to receive those children 'in care' (i.e. those subject to a care or supervision order) or provide 'accommodation' for those children who come into care voluntarily.

Special units. These are reception, assessment and treatment centres for children and young people referred by the Juvenile Courts. They were formerly known as remand homes and approved schools. They are sometimes referred to as CHEs, Community Home with Education.

Special schools. These are provided by the Education Authority and cater for the following categories of children:

- maladjusted, difficult or delinquent children
- children with learning difficulties
- 'delicate' children (this is much less common nowadays)
- children with specific handicaps, e.g. blind or deaf children
- the physically or mentally handicapped; the policy is increasingly to educate these children in normal schools as far as possible, even if this is only feasible for a short period of time.

Some of these schools are run by voluntary agencies or commercial ventures and the local authority may sponsor individual children.

Foster care. The foster care of children is another form of residential care and is likely to provide better support and security for the child who is socially and emotionally deprived. It may be a long-term or short-term measure. Foster parents are registered with the Social Services department and are selected carefully. They are usually very ordinary people and must be able to provide a warm, secure family life for the children concerned. Foster parents receive social work support as necessary and the children are carefully selected, since the strain on the foster family's life can be considerable. Foster parents receive financial help, which may be at enhanced rates for handicapped or difficult children, but they do not have the parental rights of adoptive parents. The situation is less secure for all concerned since it may, in theory, change at any time.

Private fostering. A child is considered privately fostered if cared for by a person who is not a relative, or who does not have parental responsibility, and provides the child with accommodation for more than 28 days. In these cases the local authority has to satisfy itself that the child's welfare is safeguarded.

Adoption

Adoption is a much more limited option for childless couples than it was a generation ago.

Relatively few babies are available for adoption at birth. Many unwanted pregnancies are now terminated. A single mother is much more socially acceptable and receives some support at least initially. Plenty of older children need adoptive parents, including those who are from ethnic minorities or who are handicapped or have some kind of emotional problem. These children may impose great strains and stresses and are not easily placed. Private adoption through a third party is no longer legal and few voluntary adoption agencies exist nowadays. The majority of children are placed for adoption by the local authority.

Control of adoption has become centralised under the Social Services. Admission of childless couples to the list of would-be adoptive parents is stringently controlled and the wait can be long and disheartening. Even when a child is placed with a couple with a view to adoption, there is a stressful period ahead, awaiting finalisation through the courts, with the ever-present possibility that the natural mother may exercise her rights and reclaim her child.

An outline of the adoption procedure is as follows:

1. The baby may be taken by a social worker from hospital to *short-term foster parents*, usually for about 6 weeks. Alternatively the baby may be taken directly to the prospective new family. The natural mother may request that this be done in her baby's best interests.

2. Application for an *Adoption Order* is made to the Courts by the would-be parents. Once the papers are lodged the child cannot be removed from the adoptive parents without the permission of the Court, even if the natural mother requests the baby's return.

3. The child must remain with the adoptive parents for 3 months before an Adoption Order may be made, and this may not be done before the child is 19 weeks old.

4. Both the natural mother or parents and the adoptive parents will receive social work support and counselling. The Court will appoint a *Reporting Officer* whose function is to counsel the natural mother, ascertain that adoption is, in her view, the best course of action, and to obtain her formal consent. The reporting officer is usually a local authority social worker or a probation officer.

5. If the adoption is disputed by the natural parents or is complicated for some other reason the Court will appoint a *guardian ad litem* who will oversee the child's best interests, make a full report on all aspects of the case and give this report at the Court hearing.

The natural mother must understand clearly that she hands over all parental rights when the adoption is finalised. This means that she has no access to, or control over, her child and at the present time there is no formal provision made whereby she may trace her child, though many adoption agencies maintain a register of mothers and babies. The Children Act of 1975 made provision for adopted children to obtain access to a copy of their original birth certificate, once they reach the age of 18. This may enable a young person to trace his or her natural mother.

Legislation. The laws governing adoption are complex and detailed but are designed to protect both the child and his natural mother. The mother must be given time to make a reasoned and thoroughly considered decision which she will not regret, since it eventually becomes final and irrevocable. The legislation concerned includes parts of the following:

The Guardianship Act 1973
The Children Act 1975
The Adoption Act 1976
The Adoption Agencies Regulations 1983
The Children Act 1989

OTHER PROVISIONS

Home helps and home aides. Although services are stretched and budgets tight, a *home help* may sometimes be available to the new mother if, for example, she has had a caesarean section or has no family support. However, such provisions will vary with different local authorities. For the woman needing more constant support or supervision, a *home aide* may be available in some areas. The home aide has received a brief training and will give more intensive help to the family; this intensive help may be for a limited period.

Child and family guidance service. This is usually jointly funded by the health, social and education services. It can provide help for a family who perceive their child to have 'problems', or for adults who have personal difficulty in coping with a specific aspect of their child's behaviour. A team of specialists, such as psychiatrists, psychologists, play therapists and social workers, helps the family make improvements in their situation through appropriate counselling or behaviour modification.

Family support services. Social Service departments have a budget for offering intermittent residential care for the handicapped. This may be on a regular periodic basis so that the family is better able to cope with its handicapped member while he or she is at home. Alternatively it may only be offered at times of crisis, such as parental illness or bereavement. Many families are placed under great stress by a physically or mentally handicapped child and as policy directs towards more community-based care, such provisions are very important.

In some areas an informal provision may exist by which a family with a handicapped child will be linked with another family who will offer short-term care or perhaps baby-sitting services when required.

Education for schoolgirl mothers. Every child in the UK is legally required to attend school until the age of 16 years. The Education Authority therefore has a responsibility to educate the pregnant schoolgirl. Generally speaking there has been a reluctance to keep a girl at school in advanced pregnancy and some head teachers prefer girls to leave before their pregnancy becomes obvious. Home tutoring is the usual solution to the problem but there are a few 'schoolgirl units' with crèche facilities, where the girl may continue her education before and after her baby is born, rather than having to face the problems of 'being different' at her former school. These units also attempt to meet the girls' own specific needs as mothers, with an emphasis on applied learning in home economics, maths related to house-keeping, health education and baby care, alongside preparation for formal examinations.

Residential mother and baby homes also exist for the girl who is no longer welcome at home. These may be voluntary homes but are usually assisted financially by the Social Services department. They offer support, shelter in pregnancy and accommodation for mother and baby for a limited period following delivery. Social work help is given in finding housing and with financial benefits. Some homes will give longer-term help for example to the educationally subnormal girl, who needs an intensive period of child-care teaching and supervision.

Yet another type of provision has arisen in some areas from within the health service. In an attempt to maximise uptake of antenatal care by an at-risk group, staff at some antenatal clinics have developed a teenagers' clinic, or at least special antenatal preparation classes, in order to try to meet their particular needs and to offer them professional support as well as peer group support. Girls may be offered this facility, though the older teenager may prefer not to be singled out in this way.

Translation facilities. As ethnic minorities become a feature of every city and many smaller towns, cultural barriers and communication difficulties become more common. Most cities have some kind of facility for linking up translators and clients but these vary in quality and diversity. Some areas have schemes such as the 'English for pregnancy' scheme. The immigrant woman meets an individual who befriends her, helps her to acquire a grasp of the relevant English and to become familiar with the British health system and who often accompanies her on clinic visits to offer support and assistance. Some health authorities have *link workers*, with similar functions.

At most antenatal clinics information and health education leaflets are available in a variety of languages and dialects.

Informal support groups. With the disintegration of the extended family there has been an enormous growth in support groups for almost any social situation or medical condition. The sense of well-being they often bring to a family cannot be underestimated. At a local level they offer practical help and exchange of information and reduce social isolation. At a national level, they are excellent forums to raise the profile of their cause and champion changes in social law. Many have charitable status but members are active in generating the funds necessary for their survival.

Mother and toddler groups provide play opportunities for the under-3s and a social outlet for mothers. Many churches run *Young Wives* groups or *Pram clubs*.

Baby-sitting circles are often set up by a group of mothers; this tends to be a fairly middle class institution but it fulfils a very useful function and there is no reason why it has to be middle class!

At local level, the National Childbirth Trust (NCT) runs a wide range of support groups, offering postnatal support, postnatal depression support and caesarean section support. Their breast feeding counselling service and that of La Leche League are also important support services which provide one-to-one support, rather than a group meeting.

Nationally, there are groups such as the Cleft Lip and Palate Association (CLAPA) and the Compassionate Friends (for parents who have suffered a stillbirth or neonatal or infant death).

Information on these groups can be found in libraries, advice points and publications for parents and/or professionals.

USEFUL ADDRESSES

Gingerbread (Association for One Parent Families)
35 Wellington Street
London WC2

Home Start Consultancy
140 New Walk
Leicester LE1 7JL

National Childbirth Trust
9 Queensborough Terrace
London W2 3TB

National Society for the Prevention of Cruelty to Children
67 Saffron Hill
London EC1N 8RS

Pre-School Playgroup Association
61/63 Kings Cross Road
London WC1X 9LL

The Foundation for Sudden Infant Deaths
4/5 Grosvenor Place
London SW1X 7HD

Reader Activities

Midwives and health visitors both have a professionally active and valuable role with pregnant women. Use the following exercises to explore how the two services are organised in your area.

- Ask first a midwife and then a health visitor what objectives for care have been agreed locally. Are they similar?
- Ask a midwife to describe the role of a health visitor in the antenatal period. Make notes as she or he talks. Ask a health visitor to look at your notes and talk about how it varies from what the health visitor thinks her role is.
- Do the same exercise the opposite way round.
- Ask a pregnant woman who has at least one child already to say what she thinks the role of the midwife and the role of the health visitor are during her pregnancy. Do they overlap? Are some of her needs not adequately dealt with?
- Suggest one change you would like to make locally and say why. Could you propose this change to your manager?

REFERENCES

Carpenter R G et al 1983 Prevention of unexpected infant death. Lancet (2 April): 723–727
Robertson C 1988 Health visiting in practice. Churchill Livingstone, Edinburgh, ch 4, p 52
Tissier G 1990 Hand back the child. Community Care (14 June): 14–16

FURTHER READING

Baker G, Bevan J M, McDonnell L, Wall B 1987 Community nursing research and recent developments. Croom Helm, London
Barnes A 1987 Personal and community health, 3rd edn. Baillière Tindall, London
Byrne T, Padfield C 1990 Social services, 4th edn. Made Simple Books, Oxford
Department of Health 1990 Immunisation against infectious disease. HMSO, London

Department of Social Security Leaflet 1990 Babies and benefits FB8

Department of Social Security Leaflet 1990 Which benefit FB2

Drennan V (ed) 1988 Health visitors and groups. Politics and practice. Heinemann, London

Hall D B M, Hill P, Elliman D 1990 The child surveillance handbook. Radcliffe Medical Press, Oxford

Lakhani B, Read J, Wood P 1989/90 National welfare benefits handbook, 19th edn. Child Poverty Action Group

Rowland G, Kennedy C, McMullen J 1989/90 Rights guide to non-means-tested benefits, 12th edn. Child Poverty Action Group

Whitfield C (ed) 1990 People who help. Profile, London

46

Organisation of health care in the UK

ROSEMARY JENKINS

The main source of health care in the United Kingdom is the National Health Service (NHS), although there is a small private sector. The Health Service was set up by an Act of Parliament and subsequent changes have also been introduced as a result of new statutes. NHS care is funded out of general taxation so that levels of funding are decided by the parliamentary process.

Not all health-related services, however, are provided by the NHS. Social and environmental services are the responsibility of local government. These include education, environmental health, social services and housing.

CENTRAL GOVERNMENT

The United Kingdom has a dicameral parliament. Its two chambers are the House of Commons and the House of Lords.

The House of Commons consists of democratically elected Members of Parliament (MPs) who each represent one constituency. The Prime Minister, chief executive of the government, is the leader of the largest party in the House of Commons and the legitimate spokesperson for the party's MPs. The Prime Minister of the day determines which of several hundred MPs should serve as Cabinet Ministers. Some 60 MPs are appointed to junior posts outside the Cabinet, either as ministers of state in charge of minor departments or in subordinate posts within departments as parliamentary secretaries or as under-secretaries of state. Collectively, these ministers constitute the *front bench* of the governing party.

A Cabinet Minister heads a particular ministry or department. The heads of the Departments of Health and of Social Security (DH and DSS) are assisted by ministers. These ministers are advised by paid officers such as the Chief Medical Officer and the Chief Nursing Officer. As part of this team there is a Midwifery Officer. It is the DSS which deals with social security benefits in England including the maternity benefits.

Health matters in Wales are dealt with by the Welsh Office, in Scotland by the Scottish Home and Health Department and in Northern Ireland by four Health and Social Services Boards under the Secretary of State for Northern Ireland. Each of these has a Chief Nursing Officer and a team of nursing and midwifery officers.

The House of Lords is made up of bishops, senior judges and peers of the realm who may be life peers or hereditary peers.

Legislation

One of the functions of parliament is to pass legislation. This may be in the form of an Act of Parliament (primary legislation) or a Statutory Instrument (secondary legislation). The Midwives Rules are a Statutory Instrument under the Nurses, Midwives and Health Visitors Act 1979.

How a law is passed

The actual process of enacting legislation is complex. A bill is introduced to the House of Commons by a Minister, given a first reading and published without debate. At the second reading, the general principles of the bill are debated. Major bills are then usually referred to the committee of the whole House; lesser bills are considered by standing committees containing a fraction of the House. The committee reports to the full House (the report stage) and all MPs are given a chance to discuss the bill once again. A third reading debate is the final stage.

The bill can then proceed to the House of Lords, where it goes through the same process. If it is passed it receives the Royal Assent and becomes an Act of Parliament. If the House of Lords makes amendments or votes against a bill, it returns to the Commons for further consideration.

This process does not apply to the enactment of secondary legislation, revisions of which will be placed before the House by a Secretary of State, for ratification. Thus many Acts of Parliament contain enabling legislation to allow for subsequent Statutory Instruments to be revised quickly as circumstances require.

LOCAL GOVERNMENT

Local government in Britain is the responsibility of elected local authorities which provide local services under specific powers conferred by parliament. The concept of a comprehensive system of councils was first incorporated in statute law in the late 19th century. At that time the local authorities' functions involved public health, highways, the police and regulatory duties. They have since become responsible for education, housing, most of the environmental health services, personal social services, traffic administration, planning, fire services, libraries and many minor functions. Local government in Greater London was re-organised in 1965 and in the rest of England and Wales in 1974. A similar reorganisation was completed in Scotland in 1975. Changes in the structure and function of local government in Northern Ireland were made in 1973.

The Local Government Act 1985 abolished the Greater London Council and the six Metropolitan Councils.

Local authorities consist of various types of council (see Fig. 46.1). These are in three tiers, at county, district and parish level. Parish councils only exist in small towns and rural areas; in Wales these are known as community councils. Scotland has a two-tier structure while Northern Ireland has a single tier, with fewer functions than those in Great Britain.

Financing of local authorities

Services are paid for by three types of revenue:

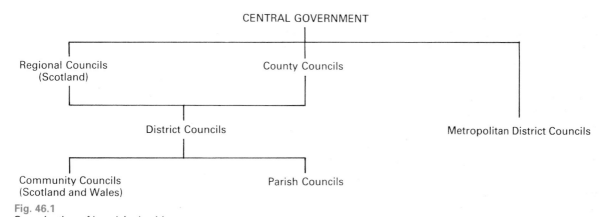

Fig. 46.1
Organisation of Local Authorities.

- council tax or domestic rates (Northern Ireland)
- grants from central government
- exchequer grants for specific projects, e.g. education, housing.

THE NATIONAL HEALTH SERVICE

The National Health Service (NHS) came into operation on 5th July 1948 in accordance with the National Health Service Act 1946. It established a system of health care, free at the point of delivery, to combat the 'Giant of Sickness'. The Welfare State was set up to overcome the five giant evils of *want*, *squalor*, *poverty*, *ignorance* and *idleness*. The aims of the 1946 Act were:

- that the state should provide health care at the point of delivery for those in need
- that the health service should promote the improvement of the physical and mental health of the people of England and Wales
- that health services should be available without charge upon determination of need by professionals providing the service
- that the service provided should be, as far as possible, of a uniform standard for all.

The Act set up a tripartite system of health care, with acute services provided by Hospital Management Committees, some services — notably district nursing and midwifery and ambulances — run by local authorities and with general practitioners contracted to a Medical Executive Com-

mittee who paid them fees for services given to the NHS. This system continued until 1973.

The National Health Service Reorganisation Act 1973

This Act abolished the tripartite system and integrated all health services under a single management structure (shown in Fig. 46.2). General practitioners continued to be contracted to the health service rather than be employed by it. A committee of the Health Authority, the Family Practitioner

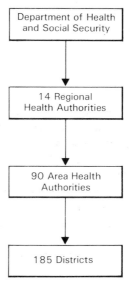

Fig. 46.2
Simplified structure of the National Health Service in England 1974–82.

Committee, administered the NHS contracts of GPs, dentists, opticians and pharmacists.

The Health Services Act 1980

The Department of Health and Social Security published, in December 1979, *Patients First*. This document aimed to encourage decision-making in the locality rather than at the centre and recommended that a tier of administration should be removed.

After consultation, the Health Services Act 1980 was passed and on 1st April 1982 Area Health Authorities and health districts were replaced by District Health Authorities (DHAs), which would be served by a team of officers. The Regional Health Authorities (RHAs) remained.

Regional Health Authorities each consisted of about 16–20 members and a chairman appointed by the Secretary of State. The RHA was served by a team of officers consisting of:

Regional Medical Officer
Regional Nursing Officer
Regional Works Officer
Regional Treasurer
Regional Administrator.

The RHA in England is the Local Supervising Authority for midwives.

The District Health Authority was served by a team of officers consisting of:

District Medical Officer
District/Chief Nursing Officer
District Finance Officer
District Administrator
A hospital consultant   representing the district
A general practitioner   Medical Committee.

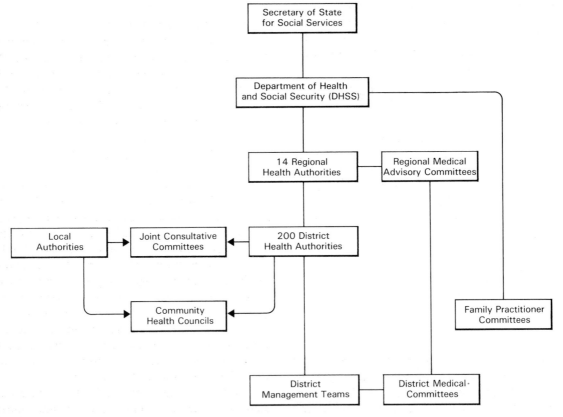

Fig. 46.3
Structure of the National Health Service in England after 1982.

The Regions were the policy and strategy making bodies whereas Districts were responsible for operational management. Some large districts were sub-divided into smaller operational units — health districts. Management decisions were reached through consensus agreement of the officer teams working with the Health Authority.

Health Services in Scotland

The central governing body is the Scottish Home and Health Department (SHHD) under the Secretary of State for Scotland. There is a management executive at this level.

There are 15 Health Boards which are directly responsible to the Secretary of State. These, not DHAs, are the units of management in Scotland and they are also the Local Supervising Authorities for midwives.

Health Services in Wales

Overall responsibility for health services in Wales rests with the Secretary of State for Wales. The structure is similar to that of England, except that there is no RHA. There is a management executive at this level. The country is divided into 9 districts. These DHAs form the Local Supervising Authorities for midwives working in Wales.

Health Services in Northern Ireland

Health care services are provided by four Health and Social Services Boards and a management executive responsible to the Secretary of State for Northern Ireland. These Boards are the Local Supervising Authorities for midwives working in Northern Ireland.

THE 'GRIFFITHS REPORT' 1983

Implementation of general management in the NHS

Sir Roy Griffiths, Chairman of a large supermarket chain, was invited to examine the efficiency of the NHS. Following his investigations he recommended the widespread introduction of general management.

To head the management function of the NHS, a Health Services Supervisory Board, chaired by the Secretary of State, and a National Health Service Management Board, chaired by a Chief Executive, were set up. The latter was to be multi-disciplinary, under the direction of the Supervisory Board and accountable to it. The role of the NHS Management Board includes:

- implementation of policies approved by the Supervisory Board
- giving leadership to the managers of the NHS
- control of performance
- achievement of consistency and drive over the long term.

Griffiths also recommended that Regional and District Health Authorities should reorganise their management structures and appoint a general manager at each level. Although they were allowed flexibility in this, the new arrangements were subject to approval by the Secretary of State.

Regional and District levels

The Health Authority Chairman at each level was responsible for the appointment of the general manager. The objective was to extend the accountability process down to unit level. The general manager was charged with the responsibility for achieving the objectives set by the Authority and with initiating and implementing major cost improvement programmes.

Units of Management. Each Health District is divided into Units of Management, which may consist of several care groups or sites within the District. A unit has its own Unit General Manager (UGM) whose responsibility is to propose the management structure of the Unit and to plan for day-to-day decisions. He or she should involve clinicians in the management process more closely than was formerly the case. Management budgeting was introduced as a new development.

The implementation of general management in the NHS has therefore replaced consensus management by the placing of responsibility upon one identified person at each level. This person must plan and implement strategies for the efficient running of the service and must monitor and control performance.

THE NATIONAL HEALTH SERVICE AND COMMUNITY CARE ACT 1990

1987 saw widespread criticism of the level of government spending on health care with stories of bed closures and failure to provide services. To counteract this, a Cabinet level review of the NHS was announced and the recommendations of this review were published in 1989 as the White Paper, *Working for Patients*. Also that year, Sir Roy Griffiths was asked to undertake a review of community services for those requiring long-term care. These recommendations were then published as a second White Paper, *Caring for People*. Both of these White Papers were incorporated into the National Health Service and Community Care Act 1990. Changes in community care were introduced on 1st April 1993; the NHS changes were introduced in September 1990 and April 1991.

Working for Patients introduced changes into health care that are almost as profound as the original change brought about in 1948. Although the service is to continue to be provided by the state and funded out of general taxation it aims to bring something of the 'free market economy' to the system. The users of the service will still obtain care along the same lines as envisaged by the 1946 Act, but an 'internal' market will operate inside the NHS with some NHS bodies charged with 'purchasing' health care and others with 'providing' it. Decision-making is to become even more decentralised and systems are to be introduced which will make clinicians — doctors, nurses, midwives and others — more accountable for the resources they use. Paramount to the way health services are to be provided in the future will be patient choice. This was particularly confirmed in the foreword to the White Paper, written by the Prime Minister. The roles of RHAs, DHAs and service providers are also radically changed.

The purchasers of care

District Health Authorities
The 1990 Act changed the composition of DHAs. The old authorities were disbanded on 31st August 1990 and the new took over on 1st September. Each authority consists of:

- a chairman appointed by the Secretary of State
- five non-executive members (i.e. lay members) appointed by RHAs in England and the Secretary of State in the other countries
- five executive members who are also employees of the health authority. The District General Manager and District Treasurer are statutory appointments to the DHA; the other three positions are appointed by the eight members already on the authority.

The authority is advised by a team of officers which includes the Chief Nurse Adviser and Director of Public Health. Both of these officers may or may not be on the authority.

The new role of the DHA commenced on 1st April 1991. From that date the DHA's prime objectives are to:

- ascertain the health care needs of the population living within its boundaries
- draw up service specifications for the care it wishes to purchase, taking into account the priorities it has set
- purchase health care to meet those needs from the providers of care.

Fund-holding general practitioners
Practices with over 7000 patients may apply to receive a fund from government with which to buy health care needed by their patients.

The providers of health care

All services offering care are now providers of care in the NHS 'internal market'. This includes hospitals, community services, maternity services and ambulance services. Until 1st April 1991 all these services, with the exception of the ambulance services in England, were managed by DHAs. The 1990 Act allowed these services to apply to become *NHS Trusts*. An NHS Trust, which may be based on a single hospital, a community service or a group of services is a management unit separate from the DHA. It is able to make its own decisions on how to provide a service and what to provide, except for a few facilities, such as accident and emergency, which it will be required to provide if appropriate. Its autonomy and the break from central control is such that it is even able to make decisions on the type of staff it will employ and the terms and conditions for those staff.

To become a Trust, the organisation must apply to the Secretary of State and this must be approved. In 1991 over 50 NHS Trusts came into being and a greater number are expected to be set up as time goes on. For some time provider units will continue to be either directly managed by the DHA (a directly managed unit — DMU) or an NHS Trust.

A third potential provider of health care is the private sector.

An NHS contract

The Act set up a system whereby a formal agreement must be reached between a DHA and a provider of care for the amount and level of care needed. The DHA may enter into an agreement with any provider that can offer the service it wants to buy. Thus there is some element of competition between the providers. Providers and purchasers alike are expected to ascertain consumers' views when entering these contracts. Once the contract is agreed the DHA will pay the provider unit for the service. These contracts are not enforceable in law but the Secretary of State is ultimately responsible for arbitrating in any dispute arising from a contract. He does this through the RHA.

Regional Health Authorities after 1991

The composition of the RHAs also changed in September 1990 and is the same as for the DHA.

It is envisaged that planning and development of the service will be led by the operation of the NHS contract. The Region's role in planning is therefore diminished. RHAs have a duty to oversee the operation of the contracts to ensure that they work in the interests of the consumer and are efficient. On behalf of the Secretary of State they also arbitrate in any dispute arising from the contract agreement. In England they continue to be the Local Supervising Authorities for midwives. A major new function of RHAs is to determine the manpower needs of the Region and finance the appropriate levels of basic education (for midwives, pre- and post-registration programmes) in order to meet the manpower requirements.

Audit and Resource Management

For a contract to work smoothly and efficiently, measures must be introduced to determine the standard of service and the cost. *Working for Patients* stated that a system of medical audit, based on peer review, must be introduced into health care. The Department of Health is also encouraging the introduction of schemes of nursing and midwifery audit. Pilot projects to introduce computerised costing of care, which is then made available to clinical staff, have also been started under the title Resource Management. It is anticipated that this computerised information will become widely available throughout the NHS.

Clinical Directorates

Although this change was not explicit in the 1990 Act, many services are now introducing this system of operational management. A Clinical Director, often but not necessarily a senior consultant, heads a clinical specialty. He or she will have the support of a business manager and if appropriate a senior nurse or midwife. He or she, with the others, will be responsible for running the unit, particularly ensuring that care is given within the resources allowed.

Health Services Committees

Standing Advisory Committees
These committees advise the Secretary of State on the views of the various professionals. The one which affects midwives is the Standing Nursing and Midwifery Advisory Committee (SNMAC). Others represent the interests of doctors, dentists and pharmacists.

Professional Advisory Committees
These Regional and District committees are set

up by the professions themselves. Nursing and Midwifery Professional Advisory Committees are composed entirely of nurses and midwives who represent those working in administration, clinical practice and teaching. They advise the Health Authorities and Health Boards at all levels in the four countries of the UK.

Family Health Service Authorities

The 1990 Act disbanded the Family Practitioner Committees of the DHAs and set up a network of new authorities, Family Health Service Authorities (FHSAs). Each FHSA has a general manager. The main task of these is still to administer the family practitioner services. Like the other authorities the membership consists of a chairman, five executive and five non-executive members.

The FHSA arranges for family practitioner services to be provided. It issues contracts and investigates any complaints which a person may make against an individual practitioner.

The FHSA issues medical cards. It publishes lists of practitioners who undertake NHS work including those general practitioners who offer maternity care. These lists are available at local post offices.

District Medical Committees

District Medical Committees represent the views of medical staff and co-ordinate the medical aspects of health care at District level. Ten members represent the interests of hospital medical staff, GPs, pharmacists, ophthalmologists and the local authority (for public health). A hospital consultant is usually chairman.

The equivalent committee at Regional level is the Regional Medical Advisory Committee.

Maternity Services Liaison Committees

The government report, *Maternity Care in Action: Part 1 — antenatal care* suggested that each health authority should consider setting up a Maternity Services Liaison Committee. The membership should include representatives of the professional groups concerned with giving maternity care and preferably a consumer representative. The aim of such committees is to facilitate co-ordination of the services between obstetrician, GP and midwife and between hospital and community services. The way these committees function varies from authority to authority.

Community Health Councils

Community Health Councils (CHCs) are the voice of the people on matters concerning the Health Service. There is one in each DHA. Members are appointed by the Regional Health Authority, the local authority and local voluntary organisations.

CHC meetings are held at least once a month and are open to the public. They discuss local policies and can set up enquiries into complaints such as poor hospital food, long waiting lists and lengthy delays at outpatient clinics. They may not investigate clinical aspects of health care but they do inspect NHS premises and have access to NHS policy documents in their own Health District.

Each CHC elects its own chairperson and appoints a full-time paid secretary. It communicates with the District Health Authority and must publish an annual report.

OTHER PROFESSIONAL PEOPLE AND TEAMS WITHIN THE NHS

Director of Public Health or District Medical Officer

The post of Director of Public Health is held by a specialist in community medicine of consultant status. This post is fundamental to the new role of District Health Authorities. The Director is responsible for assessing the health care needs of the population and his department will collate the epidemiological and demographic statistics that will be necessary for the health authority to make decisions on the health care it will need to obtain.

Primary health care teams

The primary health care team is usually based on a health centre or a general practice surgery. It forms the first line of defence against disease in the community. Much of its work involves prevention, for example child immunisation programmes (see Ch. 45). The team comprises general practitioners, district nurses, practice nurses, a health visitor, a midwife and sometimes a social worker. The practice is supported by administrative and secretarial staff.

Members of the team are responsible for giving care in the community setting by receiving patients at the surgery or health centre or visiting them in their own homes. The midwife who is part of an integrated midwifery service enjoys close liaison with her hospital colleagues as well as with other members of the primary health care team.

General practitioner obstetrician (GPO)

The registered medical practitioner may offer maternity care to any woman on his own list without further training in obstetrics. However the GP may choose not to offer care although he is bound not to refuse in cases of emergency. Some GPs offer obstetric care and may give this care to women other than those on their own list. To do so they must be entered onto the local obstetric list. Admission to this is decided by a local committee of the Family Health Service Authority. Although the Diploma of the Royal College of Obstetricians and Gynaecologists is desirable the minimum requirement is that the GP has completed 6 months' working in a recognised training post in obstetrics. This list is kept by the Family Health Services Authority and is available at post offices. The GPO can give care to women during pregnancy, labour and the puerperium and works in partnership with the community midwife and the hospital obstetric team.

The ombudsman

As Health Service Commissioner, the ombudsman is appointed to investigate complaints regarding the Health Service made by members of the public whose complaints have not been satisfactorily resolved at local level. Complaints involving a question of clinical judgement are not dealt with by the ombudsman.

OTHER SERVICES PROVIDING CARE

Family planning service

District Health Authorities assumed responsibility for family planning services in April 1982. These services are provided free within the National Health Service. Couples may obtain free advice and supplies from various sources:

- hospitals — gynaecological wards and clinics, maternity wards and postnatal clinics
- family planning clinics in the community
- a general practitioner
- domiciliary family planning service.

The Family Planning Association also provides clinics but these are outwith the National Health Service and therefore fees are charged. Certain supplies are also available for purchase at chemists.

Well woman clinics

Well woman clinics which are run within the NHS mainly provide a service for the early detection of cervical and breast cancer. Some do provide a more extensive service of health advice and screening and also counselling. They are attractive to women who 'just want a check-up' but are not complaining of a specific problem. A few areas have opened well man clinics.

All mothers attending for maternity care have the benefit of preventive health care.

In many areas, well woman facilities are limited and the only opportunity for screening for health — as opposed to sickness — is to attend a private clinic.

Preconception care

Preconception clinics are beginning to be set up in the community and in hospitals. These clinics aim to achieve optimum health prior to the onset of a pregnancy in order to reduce the risk of complication for mother and fetus. The advice and counselling which are offered also aim to teach healthy living patterns which will continue into the pregnancy. In this way health can be improved in the vital first trimester which is often almost over before the mother attends an antenatal clinic.

At present there are few such clinics within the Health Service but preconception advice is frequently given in the GP's surgery and at family planning clinics. Midwives have an opportunity to give this advice during the period of postnatal care in preparation for a subsequent pregnancy.

There are also preconception clinics in the private sector.

Reader Activities

- Find out how many NHS Trusts there are in the Region or country where you work.
- Health Authority meetings have open sessions. Arrange to attend one of these.
- Attend a meeting of your local Community Health Council and find out the name of the secretary to the Council.
- Find out who your local MP is and when he holds his constituency 'surgery'. These are usually advertised in the local paper.

REFERENCES

Consultative paper on the structure and management of the National Health Service in England and Wales 1979 HMSO, London
Department of Health 1989 Working for patients. HMSO, London
Department of Health 1989 Caring for people: community care in the next decade and beyond. HMSO, London
Department of Health and Social Security and Welsh Office 1979 Patients first. DHSS, London
Maternity Services Advisory Committee 1982 Maternity care in action: Part 1 — antenatal care. HMSO, London

FURTHER READING

Allsop J 1984 Health policy and the National Health Service. Longman, London
Rose R 1980 Politics in England, 3rd edn. Faber, London
Thunhurst C 1982 It makes you sick — The politics of the N.H.S. Pluto Press, London

47

The education and practice of midwives in the 20th century

E. ANNE BENT

This chapter outlines the struggle for legislation to control the practice of midwives in the 19th century which resulted in the first Midwives Act in 1902. The provisions of this Act and subsequent legislation are considered, culminating with the Nurses, Midwives and Health Visitors Acts 1979 and 1992. Their effect on the development of the midwifery profession and the maternity service during the 20th century through improved training and practice are described. The chapter ends with a brief look at international matters and future trends.

The majority of midwives in Britain at the beginning of the 20th century were uneducated and responsible for the midwifery care of the lower social classes who frequently could not afford the small fees which they were charged. The picture of Sairey Gamp in Charles Dickens' *Martin Chuzzlewit* was sadly true. Now, towards the end of this century, a very different picture is seen. It is that of a well-educated midwife practising as a member of a profession which is respected both nationally and internationally and responsible for the delivery of midwifery care to women in all levels of society.

To try to describe in one chapter the way in which this transformation has occurred is to attempt to put a quart into a thimble! It is therefore only possible to give a brief outline of the way in which the midwifery profession and the midwifery service have developed in the 20th century and to indicate further reading.

Before considering this outline of midwifery practice and education in the 20th century it is necessary to take a brief glimpse at midwives from earliest times and the struggle for legislation in the 19th century. This has been well documented in recent years particularly by Towler & Brammall (1986) and Donnison (1977, 1988).

BACKGROUND

Prehistoric age to 1500 AD

In prehistoric times evidence would suggest that although the healing of the sick was practised by witch doctors and medicine men and later priests and men of learning, midwifery remained in the hands of uneducated midwives. Tribal customs during labour were based on belief in magic, charms and incantations being used to warn off demons.

Hippocrates, 'The Father of Medicine' (470–370 BC) inaugurated the scientific approach to the healing of the sick. He believed that disease was due to natural causes and discarded methods based on superstition, magic or religious rites. Although Hippocrates took some part in the management of childbirth, midwifery remained the province of midwives who, in difficult cases, sought the advice but not the assistance of physicians and surgeons.

In biblical times midwives appear to have been responsible members of society. They are mentioned several times in the Old Testament. The best known reference is Exodus 1, v 15–21. Here Pharoah, the King of Egypt, commanded the midwives to slay all Jewish newborn male babies. The midwives disobeyed because they feared God and said to Pharoah, 'the Hebrew women are not as the Egyptian women; for they are lively and are delivered ere the midwives come unto them'. And so the story of Moses came to be told.

From the 1st to the 15th century it would appear from available literature that midwives in Europe remained responsible for caring for women in childbirth but their status in society varied from time to time.

British midwifery 1600–1902

In the 17th and 18th centuries in Great Britain and Ireland the majority of midwifery practice was still undertaken by uneducated midwives. Following the Reformation the Bishops of the Church of England accepted responsibility for issuing licences to midwives to practise their profession. The only qualification required was to be of good moral character. Royalty and the upper social classes employed midwives and such midwives received reasonable recompense and lived comparatively comfortably. This was not true for the majority of midwives who cared for those in the lower classes and who were paid very little, and frequently nothing at all, by their clients.

The 19th century saw an increase in medical men involved in midwifery, although it was not a compulsory part of medical training until 1886, and gradually doctors took over the care of childbearing women in the upper classes. The midwives' practice therefore became limited to the lower classes with resultant loss of remuneration and status. With the opening of maternity hospitals and maternity beds in general hospitals midwives began to work in hospitals where they were subservient to the doctors.

The need to raise the standard of the midwives' practice became apparent and this was tackled in two ways, by education and by legislation.

Early education of midwives

The first chair of midwifery was created in Edinburgh in 1726 for the purpose of giving instruction to midwives although nowadays lectures are exclusively for medical students. The magistrates in Edinburgh, who controlled the University, insisted on midwives holding a certificate of attendance at a course of instruction signed by a physician or surgeon before allowing them to practise in the city. Hospitals in the other major towns and cities in Scotland later offered 6-month courses and awarded certificates.

In England, Wales and Ireland courses of instruction were also given in some hospitals. Educated women, many of whom had taken some nurse training, undertook these courses and formed the core of midwives who were later in the forefront of the battle to obtain the statutory control of the practice and education of midwives.

The Ladies Medical College was founded in 1865 by the Female Medical Society and the educated daughters of professional men attended and subsequently practised midwifery. The aim of the College and Society was to put midwives under the control of medical men. This was unsuccessful as the medical profession was opposed to the idea and the Society and College had foundered by 1874.

The Obstetrical Society of London constituted an Examining Board in 1872 and awarded certificates to successful candidates which testified to their competence to attend normal confinements. The only specification in relation to training was the conducting of five deliveries under supervision and attendance at 15 others. The examination apparently varied in relation to the level of knowledge required and was normally taken by midwives who already held hospital certificates.

The emergence of medical men involved in midwifery occurred during the 16th to 19th centuries. A number of them contributed enormously to the practice of midwifery and obstetrics. Such men included the following:

William Harvey (1587–1657), the discoverer of blood circulation, wrote a book on midwifery which was translated into English in 1653. It contained details of the development of the embryo and fetus and the management of labour.

Dr Percival Willughby, a Middlesex physician, assisted his midwife daughter at a breech delivery under cover of towels and unbeknown to the woman giving birth. He later wrote a text about midwifery for midwives and physicians which included 150 case histories. Unfortunately this was not published until 200 years later in 1863.

The Chamberlen family (1569–1683). Four generations of this family practised medicine in England and invented midwifery forceps which they used successfully. These were kept secret until 1813 when they were discovered in an attic where they had been hidden in 1683 on the death of Dr Peter Chamberlen, the last of the line.

William Smellie (1697–1763), was a Lanarkshire doctor who later practised in London. As a result of his concern at the high death rate of babies at midwives' deliveries, he studied obstetrics and taught the subject widely to doctors.

Sir James Young Simpson introduced analgesia for pain relief in labour in 1847, using chloroform for this purpose.

Ignatius Philipp Semmelweiss (1818–1863) was a pioneer in the treatment of puerperal sepsis. He observed the high incidence of infection in women attended by medical students and in 1847 advocated the use of hand washing with chloride of lime prior to attendance on women in childbirth. Maternal mortality from this cause was dramatically reduced in his unit. There was considerable opposition from the medical profession to his work and his paper on the aetiology and prophylaxis of puerperal fever was not published until 1860.

Introduction of midwifery legislation

In European countries legislation governing the control of midwives had been adopted: in Austria, Norway and Sweden in 1801; in France 1803; in Belgium 1818 and in Russia, Holland and Prussia in 1865 (WHO 1954). It is significant that in these countries the legislation had been initiated by the respective governments. In Britain the first midwifery legislation was introduced through private members' bills on pressure from individuals and organisations and at no time did the Government take the initiative.

The earliest attempt to introduce statutory control of midwives in Britain was made by the Apothecaries Society in 1815 by including it in the Apothecaries Bill. This insertion was rejected by Parliament.

Between 1879 and 1884 Parliamentary Bills for control of midwives were drafted but not introduced.

The main thrust for legislation came from the Midwives Institute later named the College of Midwives and in 1947, on obtaining a Royal Charter, the Royal College of Midwives (RCM). The Institute was founded in 1881 as the Matron's Aid Society by a small group of educated midwives. Its objectives were to raise the standard of efficiency and status of midwives and it recognised that education was essential for both of these to be achieved. These pioneer midwives pressed for legislation to register midwives and control their practice and raised £1000 for a guarantee bond in order to have the Bills introduced into Parliament.

Three of these midwives were:

Mrs Zepherina Smith née Veitch who in 1876 had married Professor Henry Smith. In order not to embarrass him she gave up active midwifery practice but continued to work hard on behalf of midwives and was the first President of the Institute until her death in 1894.

Miss Jane Wilson who succeeded Mrs Smith as President.

Miss (later Dame) Rosalind Paget (1855–1948) who joined the Institute in 1886. She was the initiator of its educational focus.

From 1889 eight Bills were introduced but did not succeed. The reasons for this included:

- opposition from the medical profession as doctors thought that midwives would encroach upon their practice
- opposition from the nursing profession which, led by Mrs Bedford Fenwick, had wanted nurses to be included in the legislation
- lack of interest by members of Parliament
- lack of Parliamentary time.

Eventually in July 1902 the Midwives Act was passed. This legislation was designed to protect the mothers and babies of the poor and, unlike other laws regulating professions, was not designed to protect legitimate practitioners from unqualified rivals. Nevertheless it signalled a new era for the midwifery profession and for the care of mothers and babies in Britain. Legislation for nurses was achieved in 1915.

THE MIDWIVES ACT 1902

The Midwifery Statutory Bodies

The Midwives Act 1902 established the Central Midwives Board (CMB) with jurisdiction over midwives in England and Wales. This was followed by the Midwives (Scotland) Act 1915

and the Midwives Act (Ireland) 1918 which established similar Boards in Scotland and Ireland. After the partition of Ireland in 1922 the Republic of Ireland continued with the Central Midwives Board for Ireland until legislation established An Bord Altranais in 1951 which became responsible for the statutory control of both nurses and midwives. In Northern Ireland the Joint Nurses and Midwives Council (Northern Ireland) Act 1922 made provision for a Joint Council to take over responsibility for nurses and midwives and the Nurses and Midwives (Northern Ireland) Act 1970 established the Northern Ireland Council for Nurses and Midwives (NICNM).

Initially the statutory bodies were responsible to the Privy Council but this responsibility was transferred to the Ministry of Health when it was established under the Ministry of Health Act 1919.

Although prior to 1983 four separate statutory bodies responsible for midwives existed in the United Kingdom and Republic of Ireland, there was reciprocity between them. It was necessary for midwives moving from the area of one statutory body to another to enrol with the host body. In order to maintain a common approach to midwifery education and practice which was essential to reciprocity the bodies normally met annually to discuss matters of concern and interest.

As there is a generally similar pattern in the development of midwifery education and practice across the four countries of the UK this chapter will mainly describe that which took place in England and Wales. Significant differences in Scotland and Northern Ireland will be mentioned.

Membership of the Central Midwives Board (CMB)

The first CMB had nine members which did not mandatorily include any midwives probably because it was considered that the profession being regulated could not be represented officially. The Midwives Institute which had worked so hard to gain legislation was allowed to nominate a doctor. However, three members of the Institute were nominated by other bodies. They were Rosalind Paget (Queen Victoria's Jubilee Institute for Nursing); Jane Wilson (Privy Council) and

Dorothea Oldham (the Royal British Nurses Association). The first chairman was Dr (later Sir) Francis Champneys who retained the appointment until his death in July 1930. He was a friend to the midwife and played a large part in laying the foundation of the present educated midwifery profession. He was also a founder member of the (Royal) College of Obstetricians and Gynaecologists in 1929.

In 1921 the RCM was allowed to nominate two midwife members and from 1952 this was increased to four but it was not until 1973 that a midwife chairman, Miss M. Farrer OBE, was elected and subsequently Miss N. Hickey OBE.

When the midwife nominations to the Central Midwives Board for Scotland were increased to four the midwifery profession in Scotland elected their nominees. The Board had two elected midwife chairmen: Miss S. Bramley, 1977–78 and Miss M. Turner, 1978–83.

At no time did the midwifery statutory bodies have a majority of midwives but they were dominated by doctors who also held the chairmanships until the last decade prior to dissolution in 1983.

The provisions of the Midwives Act 1902

The provisions of the 1902 Act were substantially the same in the later Scotland and Ireland legislation. The main provision was to establish the functions of the Central Midwives Board which included:

- certification of all midwives and maintenance of a roll of all certified midwives
- establishment of Local Supervising Authorities (LSAs) to supervise the practice of midwives within the geographical area of each Authority
- framing of rules regulating, supervising and restricting within due limits the practice of midwives
- arranging for the training of midwives and the conduct of examinations
- professional conduct proceedings and the removal from the Roll of any midwife found guilty of misconduct and restoration of the name of any one so removed.

The certification of midwives

Certification for midwives under the 1902 Act was possible in two ways:

1. compliance with the rules of the CMB relating to training and examinations
2. before 1st April 1905 midwives who held certificates of the London Obstetrical Society or other midwifery certificates approved by the Board could apply for certification; midwives who had been in bona fide practice for one year and were of good character could also apply. The latter were known as bona fide midwives and some remained in practice until 1947 when they were compulsorily retired.

By 1905, 22 308 women had been certificated and admitted to the CMB Roll. 7000 held certificates of the London Obstetrical Society; 400 certificates from the Rotunda Hospital, Dublin; 300 from Queen Charlotte's Hospital and others held certificates from 13 other approved hospitals.

The Act made it illegal from 1st April 1905 for anyone to use the title of midwife or imply certification as a midwife unless on the CMB Roll. However, for another 5 years it was possible for a person to act as a midwife as long as she did not purport to be certificated or use the title of midwife.

By 1st April 1910 the only persons allowed to attend a woman in childbirth *habitually or for gain* were a woman holding a certificate of the CMB and a qualified medical practitioner. It was, however, acceptable for any person to render assistance in an emergency. This restriction was one of the major items of concern in the evidence given to the Departmental Committee of the Privy Council which was set up in 1908 to consider the working of the Midwives Act 1902. The concern centred around the shortage of midwives, particularly in rural areas, because some pupil midwives were unable to meet the requirement of the CMB to conduct 20 deliveries under supervision. Rosalind Paget and others, in their evidence to the Committee, spoke strongly against making concessions and reducing the number of deliveries where difficulties existed, as in their opinion this would result in two grades of midwife.

Women who were not certified midwives continued to attend women in childbirth after April

1910 nominally under the direction of a doctor. This was particularly the case in rural areas where it was common for the doctor not to be personally present unless summoned by the woman in attendance. This was rectified in the Midwives Act 1926 when unqualified persons could only attend women in childbirth under the direction and *personal supervision* of a doctor which made the presence of the doctor mandatory unless a certified midwife was present. This Act also allowed pupil midwives and medical students to attend women in childbirth.

Rules regulating the practice of midwives

The first practice rules were issued in 1903 at a cost of 6d ($2\frac{1}{2}$p) or 7d by post and lasted 3 years. They were written in simple English with considerable details about midwifery practice and the midwife's personal hygiene, information which was essential as the majority of midwives were untrained and uneducated. Many midwives needed help to read the rules and sign their names. In subsequent revisions the details of midwifery practice, Section E of the CMB rules, were reduced. In 1947 the majority were extracted and put into a series of *notices concerning a midwife's code of practice.* However the Code still remained fairly prescriptive even in its last CMB edition in February 1983 and some paragraphs dealt with matters which were more appropriately the responsibility of health and/or local supervising authorities. The term 'pupil midwife' was used in the rules and was therefore the correct legal term until the 1981 revision of the rules when the term 'student midwife' was substituted.

The CMB for Scotland and the NICNM, although reducing the detail in the midwives' practice rules, did not produce a Code of Practice. At the handover of functions of the three midwifery statutory bodies in July 1983 the United Kingdom Central Council for Nursing, Midwifery and Health Visiting (UKCC) took over the three sets of rules and for England and Wales also the Code of Practice.

The rules have at all times identified the sphere of practice of the midwife as being related to midwifery care of a woman in whom there are no complications.

Local Supervising Authorities

In accordance with the 1902 Midwives Act LSAs were appointed to supervise the practice of midwives and ensure that the midwives obeyed the midwives' rules. Initially they were County and Borough Councils but County Councils were allowed to nominate viable District Councils for approval by the CMB. Local government bodies, although geographical boundaries were adjusted, remained LSAs until the re-organisation of the National Health Service (NHS) in 1974. At that time the Regional Health Authorities in England, Area Health Authorities in Wales, Area Health Boards in Scotland and Health and Social Services Boards in Northern Ireland became the LSAs.

The LSAs were given powers to appoint Inspectors of Midwives. In the early days they were employees of the local government authorities, usually medical officers. Non-medical persons were also appointed and included sanitary inspectors, clerks and later health visitors. Some authorities and their executive officers appreciated the importance of supporting, assisting and educating the midwives whilst others were oppressive.

With the introduction of a salaried domiciliary midwifery service in 1936 the title *Inspector* was changed to *Supervisor of Midwives.* It was also made mandatory for all non-medical supervisors to be experienced, practising domiciliary midwives and they also became the organisers of the domiciliary service. Supervisors of midwives initially had no jurisdiction over the hospital service. In 1942 it became mandatory for institutional midwives to notify their intention to practise to the LSA and as there were no supervisors in institutions the notifications were made to the domiciliary non-medical supervisor. A circular to the LSAs from the Ministry of Health in 1937 stated that the supervisor of midwives should be the counsellor and friend of midwives.

Following the re-organisation of the NHS in 1974 and the integration of the hospital and community services the category of medical supervisor of midwives was discontinued and The Midwives (Qualifications of Supervisors) Regulations 1977 specified that supervisors of midwives should be practising midwives with appropriate experience and preparation for their role. It was recommended by the CMB that the heads of midwifery services, who were normally hospital-based, should be designated by the LSAs as supervisors.

Practising midwives have been required to give notice of intention to practise to the LSA since the inception of the CMB. It was not uncommon at the beginning of the century for a midwife unable to write to use her thumb print or ask a proxy to sign the notification. Approximately every 10 years the midwifery statutory bodies wrote to those midwives who had not notified intention to practise for 10 years or since the preceding survey and asked if they wished to remain on the Roll of midwives. A midwife who replied negatively or did not respond had her name *purged* from the Roll but could have it replaced on payment of a fee. Midwives did not pay fees for enrolment on qualification or subsequently as the CMB was considered to be a public service. The Board was financed by a levy on the local supervising authorities on a population per capita basis and from examination and student registration fees.

Education and training

The way in which midwifery education and training developed from 1902 is described later in this chapter.

Professional conduct

In the early years of the CMB many midwives were reported to the Board and their names were removed from the Roll. In the first 5 years 235 midwives were reported and 138 removed; in 1911 there were 128 reported and 74 removed from the Roll. In the last report of the Board in 1983, which covered a 2-year period, 60 cases were dealt with and 21 names were removed from the Roll.

Midwives charged with professional misconduct whose names appeared on the Registers and/or Rolls of other statutory bodies in the UK were obliged to appear before the disciplinary committee of each body. There are several instances of a midwife having to appear before the two CMBs and the two General Nursing Councils.

THE DEVELOPMENT OF THE MIDWIFERY SERVICE

Between 1902 and 1936 the majority of women gave birth at home and booked either a doctor or a midwife. A few women entered voluntary or private hospitals and those who could not afford even the midwife's fee entered a Poor Law hospital which was under the control of the local Board of Guardians. This latter was held to be a social stigma and was avoided if at all possible. The majority of midwives practised as self-employed domiciliary midwives and were paid by their clients. *Monthly nurses* were employed by women following childbirth to stay in the home for a month and undertake nursing and domestic duties. Only the very rich could afford to pay a midwife in this capacity.

Financial problems of midwives

Problems arose for midwives when it was necessary for them to call in medical aid since the woman frequently could not afford the doctor's fee and the doctor in many cases would not attend without one. All too often the midwife paid the doctor's fee which could well be more than she received for her own services. There was also a continuance of the rivalry between doctors and midwives which had existed in the 18th and 19th centuries.

The difficulties over doctors' fees were a cause of great concern as it made midwives reluctant to call in medical aid and therefore the expected improvement in maternal mortality following the implementation of the Midwives Act 1902 was to some extent inhibited. The CMB recommended to the Privy Council in 1907 that provision should be made out of public funds for payments to doctors and suggested that this could be a duty of the Boards of Guardians. The Committee of the Privy Council set up in 1908 and referred to earlier considered the situation and recommended that the Poor Law authorities should be responsible. However, no action was taken until the

Midwives Act 1918 provided for LSAs to pay the fees of doctors called by midwives to a woman in an emergency. The LSAs could reclaim all or part of the fee from the woman, her husband or her family.

Maternal mortality and the midwife

It had been expected that maternal mortality would decrease as a result of the statutory control of midwives. Unfortunately this did not happen although other mortality rates were declining. Because of this reports were commissioned by the government in 1924 and 1929. The first, by a civil servant Janet Campbell (later Dame), reported that 50% of births were being attended solely by midwives and that there was a need for an increase in their numbers and their competence (1924). It is significant that Janet Campbell identified several problems which to a greater or lesser extent were noted by subsequent committees and working parties. These difficulties included the maintenance of a regular income, recruitment into midwifery training, the availability of training facilities and relationships with health visitors, doctors and nurses. It must be realised that midwives paid for their training and that when qualified their annual earnings ranged between £30 and £350.

The Departmental Committee on the Training and Employment of Midwives (1929), established to consider the working of the Midwives Act 1902, reported that there were still 3000 maternal deaths annually and considerable maternal morbidity. The Committee observed that:

the midwife occupies an exceptionally responsible position in the life of the community compared with women in allied branches of the nursing profession.

It pointed out that any failure on the part of a midwife could result in disaster, disciplinary action by the CMB and possibly removal from the roll of midwives and loss of livelihood. The Committee came to the conclusion that the shortage of midwives was due to an excessive number practising in the urban areas and none at all in some rural areas where doctors still allowed handy women to attend women in childbirth when they were not present. Before starting its

enquiry the Committee considered the form that a maternity service for the country should take and the midwife's role in it. It came to the conclusion that only a state maternity scheme in which the woman had the right to engage a doctor and a midwife without charge would curtail the practice of midwifery by unqualified persons and so improve the maternal mortality rate.

Effect of the Local Government Act 1929

The Registrar General's statistical review of England and Wales in 1937 reported:

For England and Wales as a whole the number of live births recorded as occurring in institutions in 1937 was 212 286 or 34.8% of the total. This compares with 147 170 or 24% of the total in 1932 and 97 933 or 15% in 1927.

This increase in institutional births had probably been due to the Local Government Act 1929 which did away with Boards of Guardians and their Poor Law Hospitals became local authority hospitals. Large and efficient maternity departments were created and maternity hospitals and homes were erected or improvised. The domiciliary midwives could not compete with the hospitals as the birth rate was also falling. Eventually there were too many midwives chasing too few confinements and it became increasingly clear that action would need to be taken to preserve a domiciliary midwives' service.

A salaried domiciliary midwifery service

The Midwives Act 1936 made it mandatory for LSAs to provide a salaried domiciliary midwifery service either directly or indirectly through voluntary agencies which acted on their behalf. The Act was unique in that it also provided compensation for midwives, who, as a result of this legislation, were compulsorily retired or took voluntary retirement. Midwives who were considered to be incapable of continuing their profession efficiently because of age (some were over 80 years old) or infirmity had to retire and were given the equivalent of 5 years' earnings which for some was very little. Midwives who were not offered employment by the LSAs and did not wish to be self-employed or to take posts in institutions were allowed to retire voluntarily. They were paid 3 years' earnings. In many cases they received more than those who were compulsorily retired, as they were more active and conducted more deliveries annually. Some of those who retired voluntarily were called back into practice during the Second World War because of the shortage of midwives. The salaried domiciliary midwifery service was not completely implemented until 1947. It was a success in spite of opposition from many midwives who thought that a midwife who was paid a salary could not be as conscientious as a midwife who earned a fee.

The inception of the salaried midwifery service enabled domiciliary midwives to deliver a full range of antenatal care as remuneration was received for a total service. The CMB in 1935 had advised midwives that they should conduct antenatal clinics and encourage women to be examined by a doctor early in pregnancy and again towards the end of it. This advice could not be made a mandatory directive because at that time a self-employed midwife would not have been paid a fee by the pregnant woman for delivering antenatal care. The doctor would also charge a fee for examining the woman.

The Second World War had two major effects on the domiciliary midwifery service. It further increased the demand for hospital confinement as the majority of people became involved in the war effort and women did not have the support of relatives and friends. The pressure on institutional beds was so great that some women tried to book a bed in advance of pregnancy when they knew the date of their husband's leave. The war also increased the take-up of antenatal care by pregnant women as they became eligible for an extra half food ration on production of a certificate of expected confinement provided by a midwife or doctor.

The Stocks Report

In 1947, following a report of a shortage of midwives, the government set up a working party under the chairmanship of Baroness Stocks to once again review midwife training and employment. The working party report (1949) made 62 recommendations. It highlighted problems, some of which remain today, including the difficulty of retaining midwives in practice after qualification. Although at that time one-third of midwives in practice were direct entrants to midwifery only 4% of midwives in training did not hold a nursing certificate. The Stocks working party stated that there was a fundamental difference between nursing and midwifery and considered that even though midwives needed some nursing skills it was neither necessary nor desirable for a midwife to have to undertake a full nurse training. The report proposed that all posts in midwifery should be open to singly qualified midwives.

The working party discussed the relationship of the doctor and midwife and concluded that the midwife was the practitioner of normal midwifery and should continue to give care for at least 1 month after delivery. This latter has been implemented in some parts of the country but in most areas the midwife hands over care of the mother and baby to the health visitor as soon as is practicable after 10 days postpartum. The 1929 Departmental Committee had acknowledged the overlapping roles of midwife and health visitor and stated that the two professions should respect each other's roles and work together for the good of mothers and babies.

The Midwifery Service since the National Health Service Act 1946

The implementation in 1948 of the NHS Act 1946 had a profound effect on both the institutional and domiciliary midwifery services. Suddenly any pregnant woman could have the free services of a general practitioner, a privilege for which she would formerly have had to pay. Consequently women began to book with a general practitioner who may not have been undertaking midwifery previously and who all too often did not inform the community midwife until the woman went into labour. This caused increased friction between midwives and general medical practitioners. The system encouraged doctors to undertake maternity cases as they were paid an extra fee. If they were experienced in obstetrics they could apply for inclusion on the general practitioner obstetric list and they were then paid a higher fee. Over the years it became common for a pregnant woman to go to her general practitioner for diagnosis of pregnancy and discussion about the place of confinement. No longer did the domiciliary midwife book a woman for midwifery care and if the woman wanted a home confinement this was frequently a matter for negotiation.

In the hospitals the implementation of the NHS Act led to an increase in the number of junior hospital doctors and consultants which in turn resulted in considerable loss of autonomy for the hospital midwife. The introduction of blood transfusions and antibiotics and the consequent reduction in the maternal mortality rates were possibly among the factors leading to a further increase in the demand for hospital confinement. This caused a corresponding decrease in the number of home confinements. As a result the then Ministry of Health Standing Medical Advisory Committee established a sub-committee under the chairmanship of Sir John Peel, the eminent obstetrician, to examine the need for domiciliary midwifery and maternity beds. The Committee reported in 1970 and recommended that facilities should be available for 100% hospital confinement. The subcommittee also addressed itself to the problem of the tripartite administration of the maternity service.

The NHS Act had retained the tripartite system for the delivery of health care. The domiciliary nursing, midwifery, health visiting and related services were under the control of local health authorities administered by local government and were separate from both the hospital and general practitioner services. This had particular problems for the maternity service and was detrimental to good maternity care. This was acknowledged in several official reports, notably Cranbrook (1959) and Peel (1970), and attempts were made to improve communications, as a woman could be under the care of at least two and frequently all three parts of the service.

National Health Service Re-organisation Act 1974

This Act brought the hospital and local health authority services under one administration which went some way towards solving the problems of communications in the midwifery service. Most health authorities integrated the hospital and community midwifery services and appointed a head of midwifery services who was also the supervisor of midwives and was responsible to the Chief Nursing Officer of the authority. The subsequent re-organisation of the NHS in 1982 and the implementation of general management in 1985 has in some cases put the management of the midwifery service at a lower level.

NHS and Community Care Act 1990

The level of management by practising midwives of the midwifery service appears also to have been adversely affected by the implementation of the above Act. It separated out the purchasing of health care by health authorities from the provision of health care by hospital and community services, many of which became Trusts responsible directly to the relevant government health department.

EDUCATION AND TRAINING OF MIDWIVES

Basic midwifery training

Midwifery training has always been linked with practice and the length of training and its content has increased over the years. It has also been influenced by the need to reduce maternal mortality and, in recent years, perinatal mortality. There was a firm belief that if the practice of midwives was improved, mortality would decrease in spite of evidence that maternal mortality rates were higher in hospitals where doctors were in attendance.

In 90 years the length of midwifery training has increased from 3 months to 3 years and a remission of training for entrants with a nursing quali-fication was instituted in 1916. Increases in the length of training are illustrated in Figure 47.1.

The Departmental Committee in 1929 advo-cated the division of training into two parts as it was concerned that training facilities should be used primarily for medical students and those pupil midwives who intended practising mid-

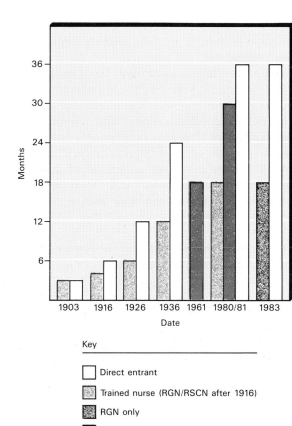

Fig. 47.1
Length of training for certification or registration as a midwife.

Key
- ☐ Direct entrant
- ▨ Trained nurse (RGN/RSCN after 1916)
- ▨ RGN only
- ▨ Trained nurse other than RGN/RSCN

wifery on qualification. Many trained nurses undertook midwifery training in order to obtain senior posts in nursing or in order to take health visitor training for which it was a pre-requisite. The training was divided into two parts in 1938. Part 1 was 18 months except for registered general and sick children's nurses for whom it was 6 months. All entrants were required to have at least 3 months' experience on the district in Part 2 but the 6 months' training could be completely district-based. It was not uncommon for a pupil midwife to conduct approximately 60 home confinements in this period of her training. Successful completion of Part 1 was approved as sufficient preparation for health visitor training.

The division of training was not satisfactory as the pupil midwives experienced mainly abnormal midwifery during the hospital-based first part and training was too theoretical. As a result of this in 1968 Scotland and two Regions in England introduced a single-period training and gradually all training schools throughout the UK offered a 1-year training for registered general and sick children's nurses.

Pre-registration midwifery training for direct entrants has in recent years only been available in England and Wales. The number of training schools offering this type of training decreased until in 1983 only two such training schools remained, both in England. This decrease was due to several factors including the difficulty in containing the required theoretical and practical experience in 2 years, the difficulty of obtaining the nursing content after the 6 months' preliminary nurse training schools had been discontinued and lack of career structure for singly qualified midwives.

In 1961 enrolled nurses were allowed, as were psychiatric, mental handicap, tuberculosis, orthopaedic and fever-trained nurses already, to take Part 1 midwifery training in 12 months. When single-period training was reintroduced the length of training for these categories was 18 months.

With the increase in scientific knowledge and the introduction of technology into maternity care in the 1970s, it became apparent that a longer training was needed if the midwife, on qualification, was to be competent and confident to practise. Implementation of a longer training was delayed until the EEC Midwives Directives were signed in January 1980. An 18-month training for registered first level nurses, SRN or RGN, was introduced in Northern Ireland in January 1980, in Scotland in August 1981 and in England and Wales in September 1981. Pre-registration training was extended to 3 years. There has been a considerable increase in the number of 3-year pre-registration courses since 1989. In England alone 25 such programmes had been approved by July 1992.

Obstetric nursing and maternity care experience

A 12-week obstetric nursing module was introduced into general nurse training for female students in 1961 and opened to male students in

1974 when it was reduced to a minimum of 8 weeks. With the implementation of the EEC Nursing Directives (1977) in 1979, the minimum length and content of the module was further reduced to a minimum of 4 weeks' maternity care experience.

Postbasic midwifery education

Postbasic midwifery education owes a great deal to the foresight of Janet Campbell and the pioneer initiatives of the RCM. Janet Campbell recommended that midwives responsible for teaching pupil midwives should have a thorough knowledge of midwifery theory and that practising midwives should be regularly updated. As a result the RCM introduced a *Midwife Teachers Diploma (MTD)* course and awarded a certificate in 1926. The 1936 Midwives Acts gave power to the CMBs to approve such courses and hold examinations. The courses predominantly consisted of midwifery theory and all midwives who wished to progress in the clinical and management fields as well as in teaching studied for the diploma.

The CMB for Scotland and the NICNM also approved a course for midwife clinical teachers and midwives holding the qualification became members of the training school team. The CMB did not approve a similar qualification and all teaching staff in the training schools in England and Wales held the MTD.

When all the MTD courses became 1 year full-time in the early 1970s the Boards and NICNM introduced *advanced diplomas in midwifery* for midwives wanting to enlarge their midwifery knowledge but not enter full-time teaching. This diploma also became the pre-requisite for entry into a teaching course for intending midwife teachers.

The Midwives Acts 1936 also gave power to the Boards to introduce *statutory refresher courses* but this was delayed, because of the war, until 1947.

With developments in the midwife's role, other postbasic training courses became necessary. One of the earliest of these was for the administration of inhalational analgesia. More recent ones include parent education, family planning, special and intensive care of the newborn, elementary principles of teaching for midwives in the clinical situation in training schools, research appreciation and counselling.

Three developments of significance have taken place in recent years in the education of the midwife. These are the steady movement of basic and postbasic education into higher education, the availability of degree programmes leading to registration as a midwife and degrees in midwifery studies for qualified midwives and the development of distance and open learning materials, notably for an advanced diploma in midwifery and for midwifery updating.

SEX DISCRIMINATION ACT 1975

All the midwifery legislation from 1902 applied only to the certification of women as midwives and it was illegal for a man to train or practise as a midwife in the UK. During the passage of the Sex Discrimination Bill through Parliament there was considerable opposition from both the midwifery and medical professions to the opening of midwifery training and practice to men. Mrs Barbara Castle, the then Minister of Health, did not support the request to include midwives in the categories of workers and professions exempted from the provisions of the Act. Before the Bill was passed, it was agreed that the training of male midwives and their subsequent practice should be restricted to two midwifery training schools until the results of these two experimental schemes had been evaluated. One school was opened in London and one in Scotland. Subsequent evaluation showed that the problems envisaged had not been demonstrated to the extent expected and all restrictions were lifted by Parliamentary Order in September 1983. To have maintained restrictions would also have been in contravention of the EEC Midwives Directives which, like other EEC legislation based on the Treaty of Rome, are non-discriminatory.

It is interesting to note that very few men have in fact entered midwifery training and of those who have qualified only a small percentage have taken up practice in this country. This is in line with the experience of other European countries who have had entry open to men and women for many years.

THE NURSES, MIDWIVES AND HEALTH VISITORS ACTS 1979 AND 1992

The Midwives Act 1951 and the Midwives (Scotland) Act 1951 were primarily consolidating Acts drawing together the 1902, 1918, 1926 and 1936 Midwives Acts. The midwifery profession in the 1960s was aware that the legislation under which the midwifery statutory bodies were working was in need of radical revision if the much-needed progress was to be made in the practice and education of the midwife. The main constraints to progress lay in the method of funding the CMBs and in the philosophy of the legislation which originated from the unsatisfactory situation at the beginning of the century. The midwifery profession also considered that it was time for it to be in control of its own practice and education in the same way as were the nursing and medical professions.

The Committee on Nursing, established by the government under the chairmanship of Asa Briggs (later Lord), reported in 1972. After lengthy discussions and pressure from the nursing professions the government adopted, with some modifications, the recommendations of the Committee in relation to the statutory structure. This was incorporated in the Nurses, Midwives and Health Visitors Bill and brought together nurses, midwives and health visitors in one structure for the whole of the UK. It also gave the new bodies control over postbasic education for the three professions.

The Bill was strongly opposed by the CMB but not by the CMB for Scotland nor the NICNM. The RCM realised that the existing legislation was inhibiting progress and new separate legislation for midwives was not government policy. It was concerned to ensure that relevant specific legislation relating to midwives was carried over from existing legislation in order to ensure that midwives remained legally practitioners in their own right. The RCM, midwives and consumer pressure groups lobbied members of Parliament.

At the height of the controversy during the House of Commons Committee stage Mr Roland Moyle, the then Minister of Health, introduced a new clause giving midwives control over their practice. This is now Section 4(4) of the Act and its effect is described in Chapter 48.

In 1989 the Health Departments commissioned Peat Marwick McLintock, management consultants, to review the working of the 1979 Act. The majority of their recommendations are embodied in the Nurses, Midwives and Health Visitors Act 1992. Under the 1992 Act midwives retained the control over their practice which they had gained under the 1979 Act.

INTERNATIONAL MATTERS

Midwives trained in Britain have travelled and practised in all parts of the world, particularly in the old and new Commonwealth countries. Initially many of these countries adopted similar midwifery statutory structure and training programmes to those of the CMBs. In recent years however they have been combining nurses and midwives under one statutory structure and organising training programmes which suit the delivery of health care in situations which are very different from those in the UK.

The International Confederation of Midwives has in membership midwives' associations from more than 50 countries. Its headquarters are in London. A Congress is organised triennially, each time in a different country. In recent years the majority of papers have been presented by midwives, which demonstrates the active interest that midwives worldwide have in the care of mothers and babies.

Membership of the EEC by the UK since 1973 has enabled members of the professions who are nationals of and have trained in a member state to have freedom of movement within the Community. With the exception of the Republic of Ireland there has been very little migration of midwives between the UK and member states either before or since the implementation of the EEC Midwives Directives in January 1983.

FUTURE TRENDS

The midwife is still the most senior professional present in over 70% of births in the UK. Approximately 99% of births take place in institutions. In recent years there has been a growing demand for home confinement and for the services of a midwife for total midwifery care. Consequently in some areas a few midwives have become self-employed in private practice. Various patterns for the delivery of midwifery care are developing in the NHS in order to improve the continuity of care to mothers and babies, for example women being cared for by small teams of midwives.

It remains to be seen what the long-term effects of the 1974 and 1990 NHS Acts will be on the midwifery service. However, any adverse effects could be outweighed by the report in 1992 of the Parliamentary Health Committee on the maternity services which recommended that the midwife should have a key role in the organisation and delivery of maternity care.

With these developments and the increasing availability of pre-registration midwifery education it will be interesting to watch how far the pendulum swings back towards the pattern of practice of the mid-20th century.

Reader Activities

- How much has the role of the midwife and the maternity service changed in the last 30–40 years in the area in which you are working?
- How does it compare with other countries?

To help in your understanding of these changes talk with senior midwives and older men and women in the community and look at hospital and community health reports in the nursing, medical or general libraries. If you work outside the United Kingdom compare your maternity service and the role of midwives with what has been described in this chapter.

REFERENCES

Campbell J M 1924 Maternal mortality (Reports on Public Health and Medical Subjects No 25). HMSO, London
DHSS and Welsh Office Central Health Services Council, Standing Maternity and Midwifery Advisory Committee 1970 Domiciliary midwifery and maternity bed needs, (Peel) Report of a sub-committee. HMSO, London
Donnison J 1977 Midwives and medical men, Heinemann, London
Donnison J 1988 Midwives and medical men: the history of the struggle for the control of childbirth. Historical Publications, London
EEC Midwives Directives 1980 Official Journal of the European Communities No L33 of 11.2.80
EEC Nursing Directives 1977 Official Journal of the European Communities No 20: 176
House of Commons 1992 Health committee, 2nd report, Maternity services Vol 1. HMSO, London
Report of the Departmental Committee on the Training and Employment of Midwives 1929 HMSO, London
Report of the Committee on Nursing (Briggs) 1972 HMSO, London
Report of the Maternity Services Committee (Cranbrook) 1959 HMSO, London

Report of the Working Party on Midwives (Stocks) 1949 HMSO, London
Review of the United Kingdom Central Council and the four National Boards for Nursing, Midwifery and Health Visiting by Peat Marwick McLintock, management consultants. 1990
Towler J, Brammall J 1986 Midwives in history and society. Croom Helm, London
World Health Organization 1954 Midwives, a survey of recent legislation. WHO Geneva, Introduction, p 434

FURTHER READING

Central Midwives Board 1983 Evolution to devolution 1902 to 1983, Milestones in the history of a statutory body. CMB, London
Cowell B, Wainwright D 1981 Behind the blue door: The history of the Royal College of Midwives. Baillière Tindall, London
Rivers J 1981 Dame Rosalind Paget DBE ARRC 1885–1948. Midwives Chronicle
Rhodes P 1977 Doctor John Leake's Hospital: a history of the General Lying-in Hospital, 1765–1971. Davis-Poynter

48

Statutory control of the practice of midwives

E. ANNE BENT

This chapter outlines the current statutory control of the practice of midwives by the United Kingdom Central Council for Nursing, Midwifery and Health Visiting (UKCC or Council) and the four National Boards in accordance with the Nurses, Midwives and Health Visitors Acts 1979 and 1992. It lays particular emphasis on the ways in which midwives are enabled by the legislation to have control of their own practice. The Midwives' Rules, Code of Practice, supervision of midwives and their education and training, the EEC Midwives Directives together with the UKCC's responsibility for maintaining standards of professional conduct are all covered.

INTRODUCTION

Most midwives are car drivers. Even those who are not drivers are no doubt very familiar with road traffic laws and the Highway Code. No-one would dare to drive without familiarisation with what is virtually statutory control of vehicle drivers and good drivers make it their business to keep up to date with changes and developments in road traffic legislation.

Midwives must be conversant and up to date with the statutory structure, legislation and codes of professional conduct and practice which form the basis of the statutory control of the practice of midwives. This chapter endeavours to explain these and to help the reader to find that what she may have considered to be a bureaucratic, complex and dull subject is less intricate than she envisaged, is relevant to professional practice and is quite interesting.

It may be helpful before going further to clarify the difference between *primary* and *secondary legislation* into which all legislation is divided. Primary legislation is enshrined in Acts of Parliament which have been debated in the House of Commons and the House of Lords before receiving the Royal Assent. Such legislation is expected to last at least one or two decades before being revised. With the pressure which exists on parliamentary time Acts of Parliament are frequently designed as *enabling legislation*, i.e. a framework on which secondary legislation is based. Secondary legislation is contained in rules which must directly relate to the provisions of the relevant Act. Such rules are normally approved by Parliament without debate or by the appropriate Secretary of State. All secondary legislation is published in Statutory Instruments (SIs). Although requiring considerable time in preparation, secondary legislation does not normally require parliamentary time and can therefore be amended, revoked and formulated more frequently than primary legislation.

The primary legislation in the context of the statutory control of the midwife is the two Nurses, Midwives and Health Visitors Acts 1979 and 1992 (1979 Act and 1992 Act). An example of secondary legislation is the Midwives Rules.

BACKGROUND

On 1 July 1983 the statutory control of the practice of midwives became the responsibility of the UKCC and four National Boards for Nursing, Midwifery and Health Visiting (Boards), one in each of the four countries of the UK. These five bodies are referred to as *statutory bodies* as they are established in accordance with the 1979 Act.

Two underlying principles of the Acts are the protection of the public and the government of the three professions *by* the three professions *for* the three professions. In order to achieve

the latter principle a majority of the Council and National Board members are nurses, midwives and health visitors. The majority of such members on Council are elected by the three professions from the four countries of the United Kingdom.

The 1992 Act amended the 1979 Act. The UKCC became the elected body whereas formerly elections had been to the National Boards which then nominated members to the Council. Responsibility for investigation of alleged professional misconduct was transferred from the Boards to the Council. Funding for training was moved from the Boards to health authorities. The National Boards became smaller, executive bodies concerned with the approval and monitoring of training institutions and retained responsibility for the supervision of midwives in accordance with UKCC rules.

During the passage of the 1979 Act through Parliament midwives were concerned lest nurses would be in control of the practice of midwives, since nurses are a larger profession numerically and would therefore have a majority professional representation on the five statutory bodies. The Act, however, has safeguards built into it to allow the midwifery profession to take responsibility for matters directly related to the control of the practice of midwives. All practising midwives have some responsibility in this matter and so must be aware of these provisions.

THE UNITED KINGDOM CENTRAL COUNCIL (UKCC)

Membership

The 1992 Act allowed the UKCC a maximum membership of 60, in multiples of three, of whom two-thirds are to be elected by the three professions and subsequently appointed to the Council by the Secretary of State. The remaining members are appointed by the Secretary of State from nominations invited from relevant organisations. Those appointed include members of the three professions to ensure that adequate representation on Council includes a broad spectrum of expertise and representation from the main geographical areas in the United Kingdom. This is particularly important if the election scheme allows for equal representation from the four countries of the United Kingdom, in view of the geographical and population size of England. The appointments also include persons with qualifications and experience of value to the Council, for example from higher education, medicine, business and finance.

Both Acts require the Secretary of State to ensure that the members of the UKCC include adequate representation of nurse, midwife and health visitor teachers. This makes sure that there is a practising midwife teacher on the Council.

Elections

The UKCC must hold an election for its Council members at least every 5 years. The election scheme, which may be varied from time to time, is enshrined in secondary legislation and therefore approved by the Secretary of State. The first direct elections to Council in accordance with the 1992 Act were held in early 1993. At that election seven nurses, two midwives and one health visitor were elected from each country of the United Kingdom making a total of 40 members. A maximum of 20 more members were appointed by the Secretary of State.

In the 1993 election, as in previous elections, there were separate electoral categories for nurses, midwives and health visitors. Candidates were required to be practising nurses, midwives or health visitors and to declare in which of the three professional categories they wished to be included. Members of the three professions were allowed to choose one category in which to vote. This meant that the majority of practising midwives voted for midwives and similarly practising nurses for nurses and health visitors for health visitors.

President and vice-president

The president and vice-president of the UKCC are elected from among its members. Although not specifically stated in the Acts it is customary for both these persons to be members of the nursing, midwifery or health visiting professions.

Functions of the UKCC

The principal function of the Council is defined in the 1979 Act, Section 2(1). It is to establish and improve standards of training and professional conduct for nurses, midwives and health visitors. Its other functions, defined in the 1979 and 1992 Acts, are listed below:

- Establish and improve standards of training
- Make rules for entry to training and for the kind and standard of training to qualify for registration; make rules for recording additional qualifications
- Maintain a professional register
- International matters including compliance with relevant European Community Directives
- Establish and improve standards of professional conduct:
  — advise the three professions
  — investigate reports of alleged professional misconduct
  — hold hearings for alleged professional misconduct and unfitness to practise for reasons of ill health with a view to removal of a person from the register
- In relation to midwifery:
  — make rules for the practice of midwives
  — make rules to lay down the standards to be observed by the National Boards when giving advice on the supervision of midwives to the Local Supervising Authorities.

The UKCC has the power to make statutory rules relating to its functions which are approved by the Secretary of State and have the force of law. In addition to the rules relating to midwifery and midwives they include education and training rules, registration and elections to Council. Rules relating to professional conduct proceedings are also statutory but are approved by the Lord Chancellor for England and Wales, the Chief Justice in Northern Ireland and the Lord Advocate for Scotland. The Council is required to consult any interested parties before making rules.

Establishment of committees

In order to carry out its functions the UKCC, in accordance with the 1979 Act, may establish committees as required. However, the 1979 Act specifically requires it to establish:

- a Finance Committee
- a Midwifery Committee.

Since the 1992 Act these are the only two mandatory committees as it repealed the requirement in the 1979 Act for the Council to establish a joint committee for health visiting with the National Boards. The power to establish other joint committees was similarly repealed.

UKCC MIDWIFERY COMMITTEE

Functions

The proportion of elected midwives to the total Council membership is comparatively small, eight out of 60. Therefore the Midwifery Committee is very important in the control of the practice of midwives. The function of the Committee is defined in the 1979 Act, Section 4(2) as follows:

The Council shall consult the (Midwifery) Committee on all matters relating to midwifery and the committee shall, on behalf of the Council, discharge such of Council's functions as are assigned to them either by the Council or the Secretary of State

The Midwifery Committee also has particular powers relating to the formulation of the midwives' rules which will be considered later.

Membership

The Midwifery Committee must have a majority of members who are practising midwives in accordance with Section 4(2) of the 1979 Act. It is expected that all the practising midwife members of Council will be members, together with other Council and non-Council members. They will normally include an obstetrician and at least one other medical practitioner who may be a paediatrician or a general practitioner. Persons, including practising midwives, who are not members of Council are appointed to the Committee by Council from nominations received from the appropriate professional organisations, trade unions and other interested bodies.

Practising midwife members on Council are also required to participate in other Committees of Council.

MIDWIFERY LEGISLATION

Primary midwifery legislation

Specific provisions relating to midwifery in primary midwifery legislation are enshrined in Sections 15, 16 and 17 of the 1979 Act and Section 12 of the 1992 Act. These provisions, which were taken over from the former Midwives Act 1951; Midwives (Scotland) Act 1951 and the Nurses and Midwives Act (Northern Ireland) 1970, are as follows:

Miscellaneous provisions about midwifery. **Section 15.** The Council is required in this section to make rules regulating the practice of midwives, i.e. secondary legislation, and particular matters are specified which might need to be included. These are:

- to determine the circumstances in which midwives may be suspended from practice
- to require midwives to give notice of intention to practise to the local supervising authority (LSA) in the area in which they intend to do so
- to require midwives to attend refresher courses.

Local supervision of midwifery practice. **Section 16.** The duties of the LSA, referred to above, are specified as follows:

- to exercise general supervision over all midwives practising in its area including those working in the private sector and self-employed midwives. This supervision is related to the midwives' practice rules and should not be confused with the management of the maternity service.
- to report any prima facie case of misconduct on the part of a midwife which arises in its area to the UKCC.
- to have powers to suspend a midwife from practice in accordance with the Council's rules.

The LSAs are designated in this section of the Act as:

- England   Regional Health Authorities
- Wales   Area (now District) Health Authorities
- Scotland   Health Boards
- Northern   Health and Social Services Ireland   Boards

The responsible officer in each LSA is normally the chief nurse who does not necessarily hold a midwifery qualification. Each LSA is therefore empowered to appoint supervisors of midwives in its area who are qualified in accordance with the Council's rules.

The National Boards are also authorised in Section 16(4) to give advice and guidance to LSAs with regard to supervision of midwives. The 1992 Act Section 12 allows the UKCC to make rules prescribing the standards which National Boards must observe when they give this advice and guidance to LSAs.

Attendance by unqualified persons at childbirth. Section 17. This section is extremely important as it permits a midwife to give care to a woman in childbirth on her own responsibility. It does so by prohibiting any other person than a registered midwife or a registered medical practitioner from attending a woman in childbirth. Childbirth in this context is defined as the three stages of labour. The two exceptions to this provision are when:

— the attention is given by another person in a case of sudden or urgent necessity
— a person is undergoing training to be a midwife or medical practitioner and is undertaking a course of instruction approved by a National Board or the General Medical Council.

There is provision in the Act for a fine of not more than £500 for a person who is convicted of contravening this legislation.

The Secretary of State by Order in January 1984, in accordance with the Sex Discrimination Act 1975, (para. 3(1) of schedule 4), removed all restrictions on male registered and student midwives from attending women in childbirth.

Secondary midwifery legislation

Formulation of the midwives' practice rules

The midwives' practice rules are the major element in the control of the practice of midwives. It is therefore important if the principle of the Acts, government of the profession by the profession, is to be achieved that the practising midwife members of the Central Council must have control over the formulation of the midwives' practice rules. The Acts enable all the practising members of the midwifery profession to have this control by:

- election of practising midwives to the UKCC
- mandatory establishment of a midwifery committee with a majority of practising midwives
- making it mandatory for the Council to consult its midwifery committee on all matters relating to midwifery
- specifying that the Council assign to its midwifery committee any proposal to make, amend or revoke midwives' practice rules (Section 4(3))
- requiring Council to consult interested parties which in the case of midwives' rules would include the midwifery profession (Section 22(3)(a))
- making it mandatory that the Secretary of State does not approve and sign midwives' practice rules unless satisfied that they have been framed in accordance with the recommendations of the Council's midwifery committee (Section 4(4)).

This last provision is perhaps seen to be the most important safeguard to the control of the practice of midwives by midwives but it should be noted that all practising midwives have responsibility for the election of practising midwives to the UKCC.

Current midwives' practice rules

The Nurses, Midwives and Health Visitors (Midwives Amendment) Rules 1986 were approved by the Secretary of State in May 1986 and are currently in force (UKCC 1991). They were formulated through the process described above.

This included an extensive consultation of the midwifery profession and LSAs and in the final stages the General Medical Council. These 1986 rules superseded the midwives' practice rules approved in 1983 when the Council took over the existing midwives' practice rules of the former statutory midwifery bodies.

Compliance with the rules is the responsibility of any midwife practising in the United Kingdom whether employed within or outwith the National Health Service or self-employed. Failure to do so is likely to result in an allegation of professional misconduct. A midwife registered with the UKCC but practising midwifery outside the UK is required to comply with the midwifery legislation in the country in which she is practising.

Summary of the Midwives' Rules

As every midwife practising in the United Kingdom must be familiar with and have a copy of these rules they are only summarised below. The UKCC publishes the practice and education rules in a handbook (UKCC 1991) which is available free of charge. The practice rules only are dealt with in this section.

Interpretation — Rule 27

This is frequently overlooked but it defines some of the terms used in the rules and must be referred to when reading them. The interpretations avoid the use of lengthy explanations. Two of particular importance are:

- *mother and baby*. It is necessary to define this because several rules refer to mother and baby when the intent is the pregnant woman and fetus.
- *postnatal period*. This defines the period for which a midwife is required to attend the mother and baby after the birth of the baby which is at least 10 days and not more than 28 days. A midwife who made her final visit earlier than the 10th day after the birth of the baby would be in contravention of the law.

Responsibility and sphere of practice — Rule 40

This rule defines the parameters within which a midwife may practise. It firstly defines quite clearly that a practising midwife is responsible for providing midwifery care for a mother and baby during the antenatal, intranatal and postnatal periods and for calling in a registered medical practitioner in the presence of any deviation from the norm. Secondly it prohibits a midwife, except in an emergency, from undertaking any treatment which she has not at any time been trained to do or which is outside her sphere of practice.

Administration of medicines and other forms of pain relief — Rule 41

Practising midwives in the UK are permitted, in accordance with the Misuse of Drugs Act 1971 and the Medicines Act 1968, to obtain and administer certain medicines, including Controlled Drugs, on their own responsibility. This rule requires that a midwife does not administer any medicine on her own responsibility unless she has been instructed in its use and is familiar with its dosage and method of administration or application.

The rule also restricts the midwife to using only that equipment for inhalational analgesia or other forms of pain relief which has been approved by the UKCC. The midwife is required to ensure, if using such apparatus, that it has been properly maintained.

Records — Rule 42

The midwife is required by this rule to keep detailed records of observations, care given and medicines or other forms of pain relief administered by her to all mothers and babies. It further specifies the form in which such records must be kept, forbids a midwife to destroy her official records and places a responsibility on her for their safe storage.

Inspection of premises and equipment — Rule 43

In order to ensure that a midwife's methods of practice are satisfactory and her records and equipment are kept in good order this rule requires her to give every facility for inspection by the supervisor of midwives, the LSA and the relevant National Board. If necessary, this inspection may be extended to any part of the midwife's residence which she uses for professional purposes.

Notification of intention to practise — Rule 36

All midwives who wish to practise must give notice of intention to do so on the approved form to the supervisor of midwives who acts on behalf of the LSA. If she practises in an emergency the midwife must make a retrospective notification within 48 hours of so doing. After the first notification of intention to practise the midwife must notify annually in March if she continues to practise. The notifications are forwarded by the LSA to the UKCC and are recorded on the register.

Refresher courses — Rule 37

The previous chapter outlined the development of refresher courses for midwives. All midwives are required to attend refresher courses at regular intervals so long as they continue in practice. The National Boards approve suitable courses or may consider alternative evidence of appropriate professional education submitted by the midwife. A midwife who returns to practice after an absence of 5 years or more or who has not practised for more than 12 weeks in the previous 5 years is required to undertake a theoretical and practical midwifery course of at least 4 weeks.

Suspension from practice by an LSA — Rule 38

This rule should not be confused with suspension from employment although a midwife suspended from practice in accordance with this rule may also be suspended from employment or vice versa.

The power to suspend from practice is given to the LSA and is allowed in two circumstances:

— for prevention of spread of infection
— when the midwife has been reported to the UKCC for investigation of alleged professional misconduct or has been reported to its Health Committee.

Duty to be medically examined — Rule 39

The provision to suspend a midwife from practice to prevent the spread of infection may necessitate the midwife undergoing a medical examination. This rule requires the midwife to allow this if the LSA considers it to be necessary.

Supervisors of midwives — Rule 44

The qualifications of supervisors of midwives appointed by the LSA are laid down in this rule. The supervisor must be experienced and eligible to practise as a midwife and undertake initial and periodic courses of instruction in the duties of a supervisor of midwives.

As a result of the 1992 Act some minor amendments to these practice rules were made but the substance remains basically the same. Later the required frequency of professional updating, such as refresher courses, may be increased to 3-yearly intervals as proposed by the UKCC in its Post-registration Education and Practice Project (PREPP).

A MIDWIFE'S CODE OF PRACTICE

This code is issued by the UKCC as guidance to the midwife and is applicable to all midwives practising in the UK. It is compiled by the Council's Midwifery Committee in a similar way to the practice rules to which it is complementary. As the code of practice is not secondary legislation it can be reviewed and revised as frequently as necessary.

It is significant that *A Midwife's Code of Practice*, which was issued in May 1986 concurrently with the rules and revised in 1989 (UKCC 1989), is not prescriptive in relation to details of midwifery care. It takes into account that the midwife has undergone a comprehensive course of training and is accountable for her own practice.

The code is formulated in four parts:

1. an introduction including the EEC and WHO definitions of the activities of the midwife
2. matters directly related to and amplifying the midwives' rules
3. guidance on other matters of midwifery practice not included in the rules, e.g.

— home confinements
— arranging for a substitute
— equipment to be carried by a midwife in the community

4. other legislation relevant to the practice of a midwife:
    — Congenital Disabilities (Civil Liabilities) Act 1976
    — relevant parts of Births and Deaths Registration Acts and Public Health Acts
    — exemption from jury service.

STATUTORY SUPERVISION OF THE PRACTICE OF MIDWIVES

The statutory supervision of the practice of midwives is distinct from management of the maternity service although the majority of supervisors of midwives are heads of the midwifery services in district health authorities and some of the duties of a supervisor are consistent with the responsibilities of a good manager. The supervisor acts on behalf of the LSA to which she is accountable in respect of her statutory duties and to which she has direct access.

Duties of supervisors of midwives. In her area of jurisdiction a supervisor of midwives has a duty to:

- receive notifications of intention to practise
- forward to the LSA in April the annual notifications received in March, and monthly those notifications received during the year
- ensure that midwives are familiar with and have copies of the midwives' rules and code of practice
- ensure that all midwives have attended appropriate refresher courses or obtained appropriate alternative professional education
- specify equipment to be carried by a community midwife on behalf of the LSA
- inspect methods of practice, records and equipment of practising midwives
- advise midwives as appropriate in respect of their practice particularly concerning difficult situations such as home confinements
- issue a supply order for controlled drugs to a midwife if authorised to do so

- witness the destruction by a midwife of unwanted controlled drugs supplied to her
- advise midwives working outwith the NHS on appropriate forms for record-keeping
- report to the LSA and advise in respect of suspension from practice in accordance with Rule 38 (see above)
    — alleged professional misconduct by a midwife
    — midwives considered to be unfit to practise by virtue of ill health.

    It is the responsibility of the LSA to refer the report to the Council.

This list is not exclusive and a midwife is advised to consult her supervisor of midwives on any matters relating to her practice about which she is concerned or experiencing difficulty.

THE EDUCATION AND TRAINING OF THE MIDWIFE

The statutory control of the practice of midwives could be said to start with education and training. The midwives' training rules were amended and co-ordinated at the same time as the revision of the midwives' practice rules in 1986 and are to be found in the same statutory instrument. Some of these rules have been subsequently amended and all are published in the current UKCC handbook of midwives' rules (UKCC 1991).

The programmes of midwifery education which are offered by the training institutions approved by the Boards must meet the kind, standard and content specified by the UKCC training rules. The UKCC has also to ensure that the training rules meet the requirements of the EEC Midwives Directives. The training rules allow midwives to qualify through a 3-year programme (pre-registration) or through an 18-month post-registration programme for first level nurses in general care who have obtained their qualification in accordance with the EEC Nursing Directives. Since 1990 there has been an increase in pre-registration programmes and, in 1992, 25 had been established in England.

THE PROFESSIONAL REGISTER

The maintenance of the register of nurses, midwives and health visitors is the responsibility of the UKCC.

Registration of qualifications

Midwives who qualify in the UK on successful completion of a programme of midwifery education approved by a National Board may register with the UKCC on payment of a fee. This is not obligatory but a qualified midwife may not practise unless she is registered as a midwife.

Applications for registration from midwives qualified in countries outside the UK are considered by the UKCC on an individual basis except for those midwives who are eligible for registration in accordance with the EEC Midwives Directives. Midwives making application for registration are frequently required to obtain further training or experience.

Midwives who are nationals of, and undergo midwifery training in, one of the member states of the European Community are registered without further training or experience if they have completed:

— training in accordance with the EEC Midwives Directive or
— 3 years' practice as a midwife in the 5 years preceding application for registration.

Recording of qualifications

The UKCC approves certain qualifications obtained by nurses, midwives and health visitors for recording against the person's data on the professional register. For midwives these qualifications include:

— advanced midwifery diplomas
— teaching qualifications
— clinical course certificates awarded by a National Board such as special and intensive nursing care of the newborn.

It is advisable for a supervisor of midwives to check the registration details of a midwife with the UKCC when she receives her initial notification of intention to practise.

PROFESSIONAL CONDUCT

The Council fulfils its functions to establish and improve standards of professional conduct by:

- providing professional advice on standards of conduct
- investigating cases of alleged professional misconduct
- hearing cases of alleged professional misconduct
- dealing with cases of unfitness to practise by virtue of ill health.

The advice on standards published by the UKCC for the guidance of registered nurses, midwives and health visitors can be classified under two headings:

- General
  — Scope of Professional Practice
  — Code of Professional Conduct
- Specific
  — advertising
  — administration of medicines
  — confidentiality
  — accountability.

These have been issued as a series of booklets and the UKCC is likely to add to them in the future. This guidance is applicable to midwives and complementary to midwives' practice rules and code of practice.

Allegations of professional misconduct

In accordance with the Acts, this is a two-tier procedure and remains so even though, since the 1992 Act, the Council **both** receives and investigates reports of alleged professional misconduct **and** conducts hearings. Members of Council who consider the case at the investigation or preliminary proceedings stage may not sit on the Professional Conduct Committee when the case is heard.

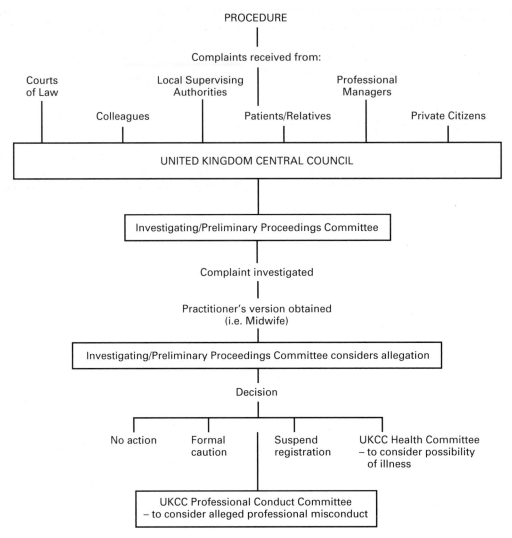

Fig. 48.1
Possible decisions of the Investigating/Preliminary Proceedings Committee.

The rules of procedure are laid down in secondary legislation. The 1979 Act requires that membership of committees dealing with alleged professional misconduct should be constituted with due regard to the professional field in which the defendant works. This ensures that when a practising midwife is the subject of an investigation or hearing there will be practising midwives on the relevant committee. Meetings of the Investigating/Preliminary Proceedings Committee are not open to the public but the public is ad-mitted to Council's Professional Conduct Committee meetings.

The 1992 Act, in addition to making the UKCC entirely responsible for dealing with all matters relating to professional conduct, gave it three further powers, which are:

- to administer a formal caution; this may be implemented by the Council at both levels
- to suspend a practitioner's registration; this is likely to be used rarely and is expected to be

used by the Investigating/Preliminary Proceedings Committee where it considers it to be in the interests of the safety of the public

- to allow committees dealing with professional conduct proceedings at both levels to include non-Council members as part of the Committee. When this power is used, the majority of members of the Committee must be Council members.

Health Committee membership will be composed entirely of Council members.

The procedure of the Council and possible decisions of the Investigating/Preliminary Proceedings Committee are outlined in Figure 48.1 and that of the Professional Conduct Committee in Figure 48.2.

Allegations of unfitness to practise by virtue of ill health

Experience over many years demonstrated that many nurses and midwives who came before the disciplinary committees of the former statutory

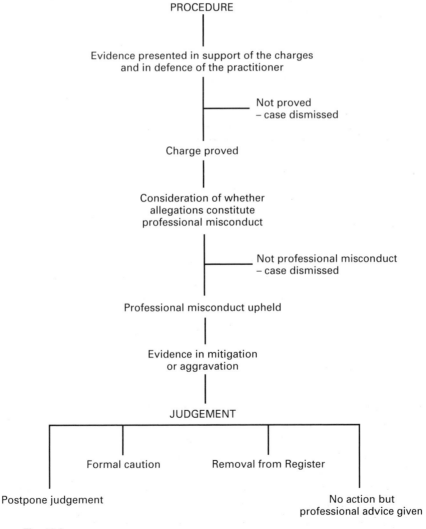

Fig. 48.2
Possible decisions of the Professional Conduct Committee.

bodies were suffering from an underlying health problem which put the public at risk. In order to deal with such people in a way that would not exacerbate an existing health problem and also be able to minimise risk to the public by consideration of the problem before professional misconduct had occurred the UKCC established a Health Committee. All matters relating to a person who is subject to this procedure are dealt with confidentially and meetings of the Committee are held in camera. The procedures and possible outcomes of cases referred to the Health Committee are outlined in Figure 48.3.

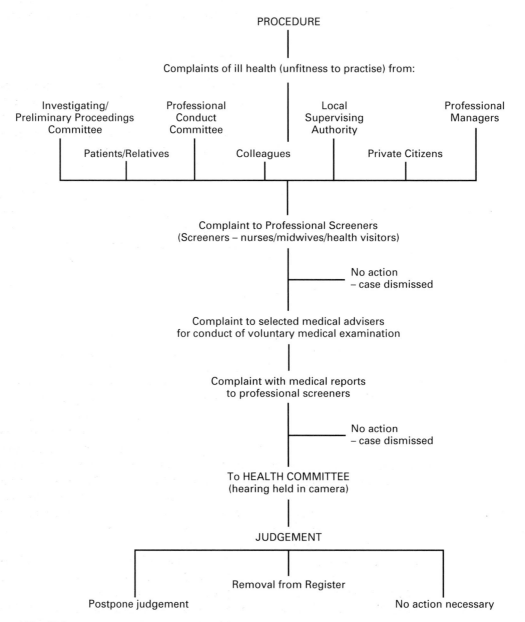

Fig. 48.3
Procedures and possible outcomes of cases referred to the Health Committee.

THE NATIONAL BOARDS

The National Boards for Nursing, Midwifery and Health Visiting were established in 1983 under the 1979 Act. They had cross-representation with the UKCC and were interdependent. With the passing of the 1992 Act, as has been seen earlier in this chapter, some of their responsibilities were transferred to the UKCC and some to the health authorities.

Functions

- Collaborate with UKCC in promotion of improved training methods
- Approve and monitor institutions for the provision of courses which meet the UKCC requirements for registration or for recorded additional qualifications. Arrange for examinations for registerable and recordable qualifications
- Give guidance to Local Supervising Authorities on supervision of midwives in accordance with UKCC rules
- Any other functions relating to nurses, midwives or health visitors which the Secretary of State may prescribe.

The National Boards are also required to ensure that they function within any UKCC rules which may be applicable and take account of any differences applying to the different professions.

Membership

The majority of the members of the National Boards must be members of the nursing, midwifery and health visiting professions. All members are appointed by the Secretary of State in the country of the Board, including the Chairman who is required to be a nurse, midwife or health visitor. It is expected that the Boards will be constituted with a Chairman and an equal number of executive and non-executive directors similar to the health authorities since 1991, approximately five of each, the executive members being Board Officers. The Chief Executive Officer of the Board is the only officer who must be a member of the Board.

During the passage of the 1992 Act through Parliament the midwifery profession lobbied members of both Houses to have a specific requirement that there should be a practising midwife on each National Board. This was not agreed but assurances were given that it would be taken into consideration when appointments were made.

Committees

Although the 1992 Act repealed all the statutory committees of the Boards established by the 1979 Act, it does not prevent a Board setting up Committees in order to carry out its functions. The Secretary of State may also make an order setting up a committee(s) where necessary. It will also be possible to have non-Board members in membership of these committees. This is important for midwives if there are midwifery matters for which a Board may need to establish a permanent or temporary committee.

EEC MIDWIVES DIRECTIVES

The control of the practice of midwives is influenced to some extent by the EEC Midwives Directives. The Directives allow freedom of movement within the Community to midwives who are nationals of, and have trained in, member states. They were implemented in January 1983. These Directives were the first of the Directives relating to professions which specified the minimum activities of a member of the profession (Article 4 80/155/EEC). The reason for this is to ensure that the midwife is trained to undertake these activities. Member states may, however, define the parameters of the practice of the midwife once trained.

The UKCC is the Competent Authority for both the Nurses and Midwives Directives and any subsequent Directives relating to the three professions. Its responsibility is to ensure that the requirements of the Directives are fulfilled. This includes:

— ensuring that training programmes include the minimum requirements of the Directives

— registration of midwives from other member states who qualify in accordance with the Directives

— provision of necessary certification of midwives who are nationals of a member state and who have trained and qualified in the United Kingdom. This includes certification of one year's practice in the activities of a midwife for those midwives who qualified on completion of the 18-month training for registered nurses in general care.

The EC Advisory Committee on the Training of Midwives

This Committee is established in accordance with Directive 80/156/EEC and consists of three persons from each member state representing the Competent Authority, training institutions and the midwifery profession and an alternate to each representative who may attend meetings. The UK delegates are normally all practising midwives. This Committee is extremely important as it advises the European Commission on matters relating to the training of midwives. The Directives specifically require it to advise on the co-ordination of the length of training for first level nurses which is currently either 18 months with 1 year's post-qualification practice or 2 years. It is also required to advise on the educational entry qualification to training.

CONCLUSION

This chapter gives an outline only of the control of the practice of the midwife and many midwives will wish to explore the subject further. Whilst being the responsibility of the UKCC, National Boards and LSAs by virtue of primary and secondary legislation, the control of the practice of midwives is also influenced by practising midwives themselves. It is imperative that all midwives keep up to date with any proposals for change and participate in elections for, and consultations of, the statutory bodies.

Reader Activities

For students and midwives in the United Kingdom
Ascertain which persons are:

- the elected practising midwives on the UKCC from the country in which you are working
- the members of the UKCC midwifery committee
- the members of the National Board in your country; identify any practising midwife member
- the supervisor(s) of midwives in your locality.

For students and midwives working outside the United Kingdom
Find out as much as possible about the statutory (legal) control of the training and practice of midwives in your country and compare it with that of the United Kingdom.

REFERENCES

The EEC Directives on the activities of the nurse responsible for general care 1977. Official Journal of the European Communities 20: 176 (obtainable from HMSO, London)

The EEC Midwives Directives 1980 Official Journal of the European Communities 23:33 (obtainable from HMSO, London)

Nurses, Midwives and Health Visitors Act 1979 HMSO, London

Nurses, Midwives and Health Visitors Act 1992 HMSO, London

Nurses, Midwives and Health Visitors Rules Approval Order 1983, Statutory Instrument 1983 No. 873. HMSO, London

Nurses, Midwives and Health Visitors (Midwives Amendment) Rules Approval Order 1986, Statutory Instrument 1986 No. 786. HMSO, London

Nurses, Midwives and Health Visitors (Registered Fever Nurses Amendment Rules and Training Amendment Rules) Approval Order 1990, Statutory Instrument 1989 No. 1456. HMSO, London

Nurses, Midwives and Health Visitors (Midwives Training) Amendment Rules Approval Order 1990, Statutory Instrument 1990 No. 1624. HMSO, London

United Kingdom Central Council 1989 A midwife's code of practice, 2nd edn. (Reprinted March 1991), UKCC, London

United Kingdom Central Council 1991 Midwives rules. UKCC with permission of HMSO, London

49

Counselling skills in midwifery practice

VALERIE J. TICKNER

The role of the midwife involves relating to people who are usually healthy and who are facing a natural, exciting change in their lives. Yet for some, childbirth may be less exciting; it may be a time of anxiety, depression or fear. However a couple feel when their baby is about to be born or, in the case of adoptive parents, received into their home, it means that they are facing a change in life. This change is inevitable no matter what circumstances surround the event.

The midwife needs to be alert and sensitive to the consequences of such change and be ready to offer the most appropriate helping skills out of the range of skills available.

This chapter is about the midwife developing and using the skill of counselling. It is *not* about the midwife becoming a counsellor as opposed to or as well as being a midwife.

DEFINITIONS

Most books on counselling begin by defining the meaning of the word. As a result there are hundreds of definitions from which to choose.

Two useful definitions are:

1. a *process* through which one person helps another by purposeful conversation in an understanding atmosphere. It seeks to establish a helping relationship in which the one counselled can express his thoughts and feelings in such a way as to clarify his own

situation, come to terms with some new experience, see his difficulty more objectively and so face his problems with less anxiety and tension. Its basic purpose is to assist the individual to make his own decisions from among the choices available to him. (SCAC Steering Committee 1969)

2. a way of helping another person to learn to cope more effectively with their life or work. (Egan 1986)

The basic meaning of counselling then is to do with helping someone to help themselves.

This form of helping is very appropriate in midwifery practice as a midwife seeks to enable a new mother to become confident in her own unique style of mothering.

Counselling as stated in the first definition is a process, an encounter between two or more people which has a purpose and requires knowledge and skill on the part of the helper. Counselling is not a casual encounter between two people, nor is it a conversation or gossip session.

The essence of the counselling relationship described by Nurse (1977) is that it is a partnership where both helper and client are attempting to understand and explore together and both are open to learn.

HELPING SKILLS

The midwife uses many helping skills as she seeks to support a woman and her partner through childbirth and parenting. It is therefore appropriate to explore the difference between these various forms of helping and to identify the difference between counselling skills and other helping skills.

Hopson (1978) described a number of helping skills used by people in the caring professions. The following list has been adapted and extended from his original work.

- Teaching
- Advising and guiding
- Taking direct action
- Managing
- Counselling.

Table 49.1 gives examples of helping skills applied to a situation in midwifery practice.

Human qualities

A counselling relationship is one in which two people work together in mutual respect. The quality of the relationship is dependent upon the sharing of human qualities by the helper. Rogers (1983) identifies three human qualities as being essential in the counselling helping relationship:

1. empathy
2. genuineness
3. non-possessive warmth.

These qualities will be explored in relationship to the role of the midwife.

Empathy

Empathy is the basic quality required for helping in the counselling relationship. To be empathic means seeing the world through another person's eyes or feeling what another person's world is like by walking in their shoes. The empathic midwife then communicates to the woman the 'living picture' of the world as it is understood by the midwife in order that the woman may be helped by this understanding.

Mayeroff (1972) describes empathy as follows:

To care for another person I must be able to understand him and his world as if I were inside it. I must be able to see, as it were, with his eyes what his world is like to him and how he sees it himself. Instead of merely looking at him in a detached way from outside, as if he were a specimen, I must be able to be with him in his world, 'going' into his world in order to sense from 'inside' what life is like for him, what he is striving to be and what he requires to grow.

Empathy is more than a definition; it is an experience. The midwife needs to be able to put aside her own thoughts, feelings and experiences and to 'be with' someone in their experiences. The midwife responds to a new mother and father from where they are in their difficulty or distress rather than from the place where the midwife thinks they ought to be.

Empathy is not automatic; it has to be developed. When the midwife relates to and communicates with a pregnant woman or her partner the midwife's attitude may be influenced by her own feeling of tiredness or emotional reactions or

Table 49.1
The examples of various helping strategies applied to one situation in midwifery practice

The skill	The application of the skill	The example in clinical practice
Teaching	Helping someone acquire knowledge and skills appropriate to need	The midwife explains the theory of successful breast feeding and teaches the mother how to hold her baby in the most appropriate position. Mother learns from the teaching how to feed baby herself.
Advising	Making suggestions about courses of action another person can take, looking at it from the midwife's point of view	Baby is having difficulty in suckling at the breast. The midwife advises mother to try holding baby closer in order to assist baby to 'fix' firmly onto mother's breast.
Direct action	Taking action yourself to provide for someone else's need	The mother and the baby look uncomfortable. The midwife adjusts mother's position in order to support her back and puts a pillow on the mother's lap to raise baby closer. Comfort is achieved.
Managing	Organising the environment and work force in such a way as to enable people to be comfortable, satisfied and function effectively	The midwife has planned her duties in order to be available to the new mother at feeding time. The midwife has organised a special low chair to be brought into the room for mother to sit on when feeding baby.
Counselling	Helping someone to explore the problem so that she can decide what to do about it	During feeding time mother begins to express her feeling about breast feeding. Eventually mother expresses her deep fear that her breasts may become misshapen. The midwife gives full attention as the new mother has begun to look agitated and tearful. The midwife may gently enquire what the origin of the fears \ may be. As the mother talks, she realises that she knows lots of women who look perfectly normal in spite of having breast fed. As the midwife listens and responds supportively, the mother's anxiety is released and she relaxes. The midwife arranges to continue support for feeding until the mother feels confident.

by memories of experiences which have occurred in her own life. In counselling the focus is on the needs of the one being helped, not on the helper, for example:

A young unmarried woman (Miss S.) is expecting a baby for the second time: her first pregnancy ended in an abortion. It is the first booking interview with the midwife.

Miss S.:   'I am scared that this baby won't be all right.'

Midwife: 'You sound nervous about this baby.'
             or
             'You are scared that this baby won't be all right?'

The midwife has picked up the word which expresses the feeling so that Miss S. could hear it again and respond.

Miss S. might go on to say: 'Yes, I am afraid that what happened last time with the miscarriage might affect this one . . .'

The midwife listened carefully and accurately to what Miss S. said and she tentatively repeated it , using Miss S.'s own words, or she used another word which did not change the meaning.

As the relationship continues, the midwife will continue to respond empathically in order to see the world (or situation) as Miss S. sees it and help Miss S. to respond in a way that is appropriate for her.

The midwife seeks to understand and accept the situation as Miss S. sees it without making judgements or wielding professional power.

Genuineness

Genuineness, as Rogers (1983) describes the

quality, means being truthful, real and open with a person (Rogers uses the term *congruent*). This quality enables trust to develop in a relationship and provides a safe place for the client to explore and express her feelings.

Genuineness is about respecting and valuing another person enough to be honest with her. It is not about hiding behind the professional role but rather about being spontaneous, non-defensive and yet thoughtful.

Very often genuineness is *shown* in the way the words are expressed rather than in what words are spoken. There is no room for pretence in a genuine relationship.

Midwives are partners in care with mothers and fathers. All are working towards getting the best out of the experience of childbearing and parenthood.

It is helpful if the midwife is seen by the parents and other relatives as trustworthy, dependable, thoughtful, warm and caring if they are to be enabled to become the parents they want to be. It must be recognised that this is not always easy to achieve and someone else may need to provide support.

Non-possessive warmth or acceptance

This quality is also essential in the counselling relationship. When a person feels that she is accepted for her own self she becomes more confident and less afraid to express how she really feels about the difficulty or confusion which is causing her distress.

It is the capacity to be genuine and to feel warm towards people without needing to be possessive of them which is vital for the midwife in her relationships with parents. To develop the quality of caring for individuals or working with people without needing to possess them is not always easy but it is possible if the focus of attention is on the person in need and not on the needs of the person helping.

Self-awareness (or self-knowledge)

Besides empathy, genuineness and non-possessive warmth there are many human qualities which are helpful in the counselling relationship, for example:

- trust
- sensitivity
- gentleness
- patience.

A midwife can acknowledge that she already possesses many of these qualities. Cultivating self-awareness is particularly helpful in this discovery.

In order to be aware of the needs, strengths and gifts of others the midwife needs to be aware of her own needs, strengths and gifts. Being caring and supportive of others means that the midwife must be caring and supportive of herself. This is a difficult concept to apply, particularly when there are so many professional and social demands, but it is fundamental to the counselling aspect of the midwife's role.

Self-awareness as defined by Burnard (1985) refers to the gradual, continuous process of noticing and exploring aspects of the self, whether behavioural, psychological or physical, with the intention of developing personal and interpersonal understanding.

The midwife who is self-aware is able to listen to herself, her own thoughts and feelings, and to accept that they are a reality and an important part of being human.

Sometimes the imaginary and not the real self interferes with the process of helping others. The midwife may forget during the course of her work that she is also a person with thoughts and feelings which are sometimes rational and sometimes irrational, particularly in times of change or stress.

The more the midwife understands and accepts herself, the less likely she is to make judgements or impose her own views on others.

COUNSELLING SKILLS

Having established the meaning of counselling in the context of midwifery, explored the qualities of the counsellor and considered the importance of self-awareness, this chapter now sets out the development and practical use of counselling skills by the midwife.

Firstly it is useful to consider some situations that a midwife may encounter in which a person might be most appropriately helped by counselling skills. These include:

- apprehension about having a first baby
- anxiety about partner's reactions to a demanding baby
- unwanted pregnancy
- infertility
- fetal death in utero
- miscarriage, stillbirth or neonatal death
- abnormal or handicapped baby
- marital incompatibility or breakdown
- child or adult sexual abuse or rape
- unemployment, poverty
- drug or alcohol abuse
- HIV positive results
- racial harrassment or cruelty
- depression.

This list could be added to from a midwife's own experience.

In any one of the situations listed, the person with the difficulty will need to be helped to work through a process defined by Egan (1990) comprising three basic phases: exploring, understanding and then acting. Counselling skills used appropriately will enable a person to work through this process in order to cope more effectively. The integration of the process and the skills creates a helping relationship which at best takes place in a supportive, caring environment.

The process

A person in difficulty or distress will need opportunity to *explore* the difficulty, and express how she feels about it. This may take a little while as it is difficult to find words to express feelings adequately. Also it is painful to, as it were, 'look at feelings' and 'speak them out'. This exploration of feelings may include being enabled to cry or sob in sorrow or to shout in anger.

As feelings are expressed some *understanding* of the difficulty emerges. It is as if the release of feelings makes the picture clearer and the energy that was dealing with the pain and distress has been re-directed in order to allow understanding or awareness to emerge. Once a person has come to understand why she feels the way she does about

a difficulty she is then able to take appropriate *action*. She may, for example, decide to change jobs or move house or make some other major change in her life. She may be able to accept the situation as it is because she has seen it differently or because the situation is out of her control. Whatever the outcome, it is to do with an individual learning to cope more effectively with her (or his) difficulty or distress.

Often this process of exploratory understanding and action takes a long time; hours, months or years. Sometimes it is possible to work through a difficult situation fairly quickly.

The skills

The basic skills required to help this process are, attending, listening and responding (see Fig. 49.1).

Attending

Attending is an active, rather than a passive, skill. It involves blocking out all distractions and giving total attention to the person speaking.

The midwife using this skill in the course of her work will enable a new mother to feel as if she is the only person who matters at that moment in time. The midwife using the skill of attending would be focused physically and psychologically on the client or person in need.

Listening

This skill cannot be separated from the skill of attending. Listening is the beginning and end of helping. However, it is possible to listen but not

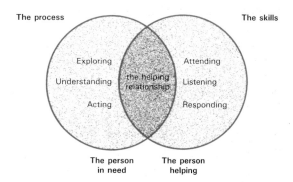

Fig. 49.1
The model of helping (adapted from Egan (1986)).

hear what a person is saying. Listening involves using the mind and senses as well as the ears, and the midwife needs to be alert and free to concentrate on two levels of communication, that which is being spoken and that which is not.

Listening is hard work and takes a lifetime to learn. It requires the use of all the senses.

Responding

The ways in which a midwife will respond to a person are varied and at many levels. Responses may be spoken or not spoken, for example a smile or a grimace is a response. These messages are important in helping someone to explore a difficulty and express how she feels. A person in distress or difficulty is more likely to express how things are for her if she receives a non-verbal message of warmth and interest 'spoken' as it were through ways of sitting, or looking. Body language gives a number of messages to the recipient by movement, eye contact, posture and so on.

Touching. A midwife may also respond to a person by touching her. This may be the most appropriate response in situations where there is deep distress and words seem to be inadequate. Care for a person may be communicated by a hug or holding a hand or by stroking. Sensitive use of touch can help a person to relax and focus her thoughts more steadily on a situation in which she feels confused or afraid. It is important, however, for the midwife to be aware of how her touch is received. Some people find touch difficult; others may feel personally invaded by touch. In both these situations signals are given out by the person on the receiving end. She may become tense and withdraw either physically or verbally or she may speak out her feelings by saying, 'Get away' or, 'No, don't touch me'. It is important for the midwife not to feel rejected by this behaviour but rather to understand it as a message from a person in distress who may not be able to cope with the touch of another human being at that point in time. The same person later in time may be helped and comforted by touch, so again it is important for the midwife not to make a judgement that she is a person who does not ever wish to be comforted by the skilful use of touch.

Whatever ways of responding are used by the midwife they need to be genuine or congruent. If the midwife does not find it natural or easy to comfort by using touch, then such a response would probably be inappropriate. It is wise for the midwife to show care in ways that are natural and comfortable for her, whilst at the same time being aware of the client's reception of thoughtful responses.

Questioning is the most obvious way of seeking information and a useful way of enabling a person to hear herself tell about a situation. Asking questions is as much about *how* they are said as *what* is said, therefore voice tone, speed of speech and attitude in asking a question influences how a question is heard.

A question may be spoken in an authoritative or demanding way or it may be gently or tentatively put.

Two basic questioning responses are open and closed questions, for example:

Open   — How do you feel about being pregnant?
Closed — Did you feel shocked when you knew you were pregnant?

Allowing responses give the person permission to express herself in ways congruent or true for herself. It is important that the midwife follows the 'cues' of the person in difficulty and responds at her pace in an encouraging, open and supportive way. To invade or manipulate the feelings or expressions of the person is not helpful. An example of allowing a response might be:

Mrs W.:   'It's just so difficult, what with the new baby, little Tommy and then Bill expects everything to be the same as before . . .' (breaks off)

Midwife: 'Are you able to say more about . . .'
or
'Do go on . . .'

Reflecting responses are to do with being like a mirror for the person in difficulty in order that they might see and hear what they are saying. The skill is to offer back to the person what they are expressing. The person will then pick up the message that she is hearing and take it on further in the way in which she wants to go in her own exploration of the difficulty. The attentive, caring midwife will listen and follow the exploration without interruption, only picking up the expressions made and reflecting them back as appropriate, for example:

Mrs W.: 'I feel like I am being torn in bits with Tommy, the new baby and Bill wanting me to do things.'
Midwife: (reflectively) 'It seems as if there are a lot of demands in your life.'
Mrs W.: 'It isn't as if I don't love them all, it's just that I'm not sure I have enough for everyone all the time.'
Midwife: 'It sounds as if you are looking for time for yourself.'

The midwife may reflect back words or feelings expressed so long as they are Mrs W.'s words and feelings, not what the midwife thinks she should say.

Clarifying. When a person is in distress or difficulty, the emotional turmoil very often makes the situation unclear. As a result the expression may be jumbled or disjointed. It is important for the midwife to make a clarifying response in this situation rather than pretend that she has understood, for example:

Mrs W.: 'I just feel so muddled and worn out about it all.'
Midwife: 'Can you explain the muddled, worn-out feeling?'
or
'I am not sure I understand . . .'

Supporting. The value of supportive responses is that they may give a person courage to go on working at her difficulty even when she is 'hurting' inside. It is important, however, for the midwife not to use supportive responses in a manipulative way. The skill is to offer these responses in order to show warmth and respect, particularly at the beginning of a counselling session when the helping relationship is being formed on a basis of trust.

Support in counselling is always offered in order for a person to have the emotional energy and strength to help herself; it is not taking the issue out of the hands of the person in distress to satisfy the needs of the helper, counsellor or midwife.

Non-verbal responses. Responding with body language, posture, facial expression and eye contact all give messages to the person that will either enable her to go on exploring her difficulty or may block that process.

Sometimes, particularly when a person is trying to sort out a difficulty or face a painful emotional experience, there are silences. Often these are 'working' silences where the person is struggling with feelings or the words to express those feelings. The midwife needs to be sensitive to what is happening in these times of silence. Sometimes it is difficult just to be with someone in her silence. The midwife must take care not to disturb the process simply in order to meet her own need to talk or explain. The focus of attention and support should always be on the person in need.

To enable someone to return from silence requires a gentle and sensitive response like, for example:

Midwife: 'It must be difficult to come to terms with . . .'
'You were saying about . . .'
or
'Would you like to explain further . . .'

SPECIFIC ISSUES RELATED TO COUNSELLING

Finally this chapter will focus on four issues which may emerge as the midwife develops skills of counselling:

- referral
- confidentiality
- evaluation
- personal support.

Referral

The midwife may encounter a situation where the person in difficulty is obviously in need of specialist counselling or medical help.

Sometimes the person in need recognises this for herself. In this situation the midwife will help the person make her own application or referral. Occasionally the midwife will need to assist a person in need to accept appropriate help or expertise. Maybe the midwife recognises that the difficulty would take more time than she has available, or that she has not the necessary skill to offer help in this particular area.

In order to assist an individual to make a choice regarding appropriate help and to act upon that choice the midwife will need to be familiar with the services available, particularly locally but also nationally. The type of information required might be about:

- marriage guidance counselling service
- genetic counselling service
- self-help or client support groups such as
  - Alcoholics Anonymous
  - family planning service
  - drug abuse centre
  - Stillbirth and Neonatal Death Society.

Such information should be available in the maternity ward, clinic or GP surgery or from the community midwife in the woman's own home.

It is important for the midwife to let the person know that referral is part of her overall care and concern and the midwife should continue to support her until the referral is completed.

Confidentiality

In a counselling or helping relationship an individual may share aspects of herself or her difficulty for which trust between the person in need and the midwife is fundamental. Usually there is no difficulty in keeping confidentiality. If, however, information is disclosed during the encounter which is against the law or puts life in danger, the midwife is faced with a moral dilemma. On the one hand the midwife agrees to respect and treat as confidential any information which the person discloses: on the other hand the midwife has a duty as a citizen and a professional to report or take action when she becomes aware of information which contravenes the law of the land or the Midwives' Rules.

The Code of Professional Conduct (UKCC 1992) states that the nurse, midwife or health visitor must:

protect all confidential information concerning patients and clients obtained in the course of professional practice and make disclosures only with consent, where required by the order of a court or where [she] can justify disclosure in the wider public interest.

It is always important to make clear to the person that matters disclosed by her will be kept as confidential and will not be disclosed to others without her prior knowledge or permission. If the midwife is presented with the dilemma of needing to break confidentiality, she may need to spend some time talking and explaining to the person why it is important to disclose the information to someone else. It is best if the individual concerned can be encouraged to disclose the information herself.

Evaluation

Knowledge and theories about counselling are valuable and enable a midwife to understand and accept that counselling is truly a human-to-human partnership. Nurse (1980) states 'The counsellor does not know all the answers; she is a fallible human being like everyone else'.

The following checklist is offered to help the midwife to assess her own use of personal qualities and counselling skills to the benefit of the person in need.

Checklist: questions the midwife might use to assess her development in using counselling skills:

- Was counselling the most appropriate form of helping in the situation; did I use any other helping strategy like advising, guiding, or teaching?
- Did I really hear what the person was saying?
- Did I talk more than the person in need?
- Did I see the world through the person's eyes?
- Did my behaviour and responses demonstrate that I was interested in what she was saying?
- Did I feel warmth and compassion towards that person?
- Was I able to be truthful and genuine?
- Was I able to put the other person's needs first or did my own needs keep getting in the way?
- What emotions am I now feeling towards that person; how will these influence my future actions towards her?

• Did I manage to establish a relationship that enabled the person to feel safe enough to begin to work through her own situation herself?

This is not a definitive list: there may be many more questions that the midwife may wish to ask or to discuss with a colleague.

Occasionally the very knowledge that the midwife has also experienced a similar kind of sorrow or distress may help a mother to share her own feelings more freely. However, self-disclosure must be used carefully by the midwife as the focus of attention and support must always be on the mother's need and not the need of the midwife.

There are times in the midwife's own life when she will not have the space for others' difficulty or distress no matter how caring she is. It is important for the midwife to take care of herself in order to take care of others effectively.

A midwife will need to *learn* counselling skills. They do not automatically come with the role, but it *is* possible to learn the skills. Midwives wishing to explore the subject further might wish to contact The British Association for Counselling UK for information about resources and courses (see end of chapter for BAC address).

The qualities and skills required in relating to other human beings may take a lifetime to learn.

BEREAVEMENT AND MIDWIFERY PRACTICE

This section is not specifically about counselling skills. It is about the knowledge and skills which the midwife requires in order to provide effective care for parents and relatives who are bereaved. Counselling skills are needed in all normal life situations but particularly at times of grief and loss. Although the focus of this part of the chapter is on bereavement, the reader is invited to draw upon relevant information from the section on counselling skills.

Midwifery is a profession concerned with new life and hope, joy and expectation. When death occurs, the impact is particularly devastating and the loss may be felt by parents, relatives and maternity care staff.

The devastation of loss caused by death is its perceived permanency and the stark reality of one's own human frailty. For the midwife this experience is compounded by the feeling of professional responsibility as it is the midwife's normal role to help to create a suitable environment for the preservation of life.

The parents of a baby who has died experience feelings of distress, disappointment or frustration at unfulfilled expectations. The parents of a sick, preterm or abnormal baby may experience another form of loss, the loss of the perfect, longed-for baby, and their feelings will be similar.

The midwife needs to have sufficient insight into her own reactions and needs in situations of loss and grief if she is to be effective in taking appropriate care of others.

A midwife may be involved in the care of a woman and her partner at any stage in their experience of grief. It may be that they have just received news that they will never be able to have a child, or that their baby has died in utero. The midwife may have delivered their stillborn baby or cared for their baby who at birth was ill, premature or showed signs of abnormality. On rare occasions the midwife may have to support a husband whose wife has died during or following childbirth. Whatever the situation at home or in hospital the midwife is most often the main contact and support to parents in their bereaved state.

Bereavement situations which a midwife may encounter in practice are:

• infertility
• abortion (miscarriage)
• maternal or paternal death
• stillbirth, perinatal or neonatal death
• abnormal or handicapped baby
• giving a baby for adoption or fostering
• forced removal of a baby or child into care
• cot death
• child abuse (non-accidental injury) resulting in death.

In each of these potentially tragic situations the mother, father or both will experience emotional pain.

Although the experience or process of grief is common, the ways in which people cope with their own individual grief experience will vary. Reactions to loss caused by death, or absence of life in the case of infertility, are largely dependent on the value of the relationship or the quality and meaning of the life which was to be created or the life which was lost. A person can feel very deeply the loss of a friend or relative who was known only for a short time if the quality of the relationship was deep and loving or if it met a fundamental need. Support from family, friends and maternity care staff in both hospital and community can make a considerable contribution to helping a person to come to terms with death.

A grief which has been worked through allows for the development of new relationships, a greater acceptance of self and a deeper understanding of life.

The basic experience of grief involves accepting the fact or reality of loss and experiencing the emotional pain of bereavement. It involves adjusting to the loss and working through it to an understanding of the situation and a more focused view of life. There are no short cuts.

It is essential for the midwife to have a basic knowledge and understanding of normal grieving in order that she may assist the person in her care to work through it to healthy acceptance.

The normal grieving process

The normal grieving process identified by Kübler-Ross (1978) has been adapted in this chapter to apply to situations which a midwife may have to face.

Although the process is presented in phases, it must not be interpreted too rigidly. Individuals vary in their reactions and the time at which their reactions to grief occur. Research, particularly that of Kübler-Ross (1978) and Murray-Parkes (1986), has revealed common threads experienced by most people. This will help the midwife to understand the needs of her clients who are grieving.

First phase

Shock, denial and numbness are common early signs of grief. The woman who has just given birth who is told that her baby is dead may react by shouting, 'No, oh no, my baby cannot be dead' or she may remain silent and appear dazed or stunned at the news. Sometimes a woman will 'act out' distress but the reality of the loss has not reached her innermost feeling.

Second phase

Pining, anger, guilt, bargaining, depression, emptiness; any or all of these may be experienced as part of the emotional working towards acceptance of the situation.

Pining. As the shock and numbness wear off, the pain of loss emerges. The longing and loneliness of these emotions may feel very intense. A woman whose baby has died may experience physical pain in her breasts or arms as she longs or pines to hold and feed her baby.

Anger is a very common emotion in grief and is usually misplaced and directed against the service or the providers of care. The midwife needs to understand that although the anger may be directed at her it is not usually meant to be a personal attack. This is not an easy task when the force of such anger is so real. It is helpful if a midwife can accept and indeed enable anger to be expressed in a safe place.

Guilt is also a common emotion felt by a person in grief. A husband whose wife has died in childbirth or soon after may experience a profound sense of guilt: 'If only she had not got pregnant I would not have to be without her now . . . it's all my fault.' On the other hand he may just think these thoughts or feel these feelings and find them too painful to express. Sensitive, skilled listening by the midwife may enable him to release these irrational, but none the less real, feelings. Sometimes women do not express such thoughts or feelings either. If they are expressed, it may be in some of the following ways:

'If only I hadn't smoked in pregnancy.'
'If only I had got to the hospital earlier.'
'If only I had decided not to have my pregnancy terminated . . .'

Guilt may also be experienced by the mother or father of a handicapped or abnormal baby.

They may blame themselves or each other for the tragedy. Guilt takes many forms and there may be deep, hidden, personal guilt feelings which only emerge at a time of bereavement. The skill of the midwife is to help the person to acknowledge that feelings of guilt are a normal (though painful) part of grieving.

Bargaining is usually with God or with oneself, for example, a mother who is a heavy smoker and whose baby was born prematurely and then died, may bargain in this way, 'I promise I won't smoke again if my baby's life could be saved.' It is very important for the midwife not to judge the situation in terms of whose fault it is that a baby, mother or relative has died but to help the bereaved person to come to terms with this loss.

Depression and emptiness may show in physical as well as in psychological behaviour. Lewis (1961) describes the feeling, 'No one ever told me that grief felt so like fear. I am not afraid but the sensation is like being afraid. The same fluttering in the stomach, the same restlessness, the yawning. I keep on swallowing.'

The parents of a dead or dying baby may feel similarly too depressed or exhausted to care for themselves. For example, the particular difficulty for the woman who has been delivered of a stillborn baby is that the physiological sequelae of birth continue: her breasts fill with milk but she has no baby to feed; her perineum may be sore or uncomfortable but she has no live baby to show for the discomfort. The midwife in continuing to care for such a mother will need to be particularly sensitive to her physical as well as to her emotional needs, and work with the mother towards her acceptance and freedom from grief in her own way.

Third phase

This is a phase of acceptance and readjustment; when this stage is reached it can be said that the task of mourning is completed. The time that it takes to work through grief completely is difficult to state with any degree of accuracy. It may take anything from 2–3 years. It would be a sign of abnormal reaction to grief if the years passed without any evidence of progress or change.

The sadness and the profound impact of the death of a baby or spouse is understandably never forgotten. Special occasions, particular happenings in the family and anniversaries will renew memories of a dead baby or spouse. Although such memories will continue, the pain of grief grows less.

Provision of care for the bereaved

Breaking the news

Parents are usually informed immediately a diagnosis of death or abnormality is confirmed. It may be the first time in their lives that they have faced such a devastating experience either alone or together.

The shock of bad news often causes people to forget what has been explained to them and it is helpful to have more than one person present at the time. The midwife may need to repeat the information on several occasions before the parents are able to accept or understand.

Breaking bad news requires all the skill and support that a midwife can give even though she herself may feel afraid and distressed at the situation. Counselling skills, particularly the skills of attending and listening, are extremely useful. Touch may also be an appropriate empathic response. Sensitive stroking of the bereaved person's arm, holding her hand or giving a gentle hug may provide comfort and release from emotional pain. A person experiencing deep grief or distress is not always aware of feeling the comfort of human contact so moving the place of touching from time to time may assure her of a comforting human presence.

Supporting people in distress when they receive sad news is not easy. Midwives need not be afraid to show that they care and are distressed too, provided that they are not self-indulgent, as their primary responsibility is to take care of the person in distress.

Special needs

Sometimes the needs of the husband may be missed as the focus of attention is on his wife. It is important for the midwife to observe his behaviour and be sensitive to his needs. He may wish to stay with his wife, and many units provide suitable facilities such as a double room (see Ch. 16). If he is at home he may wish to walk outside for a little while to escape from the intensity of the situation. If he has to travel, the midwife may suggest that someone accompanies him on his journey. She should try not to let him go home alone unless it is his expressed wish to do so.

Women who suffer the loss of one twin require especially sensitive care (Wilson *et al* 1982). People tend to assume that thankfulness for the survival of one baby offsets the grief at the death of the twin but this is not the case and parents should be encouraged to grieve.

Privacy

For the couple who are bereaved, privacy is desirable but it is helpful for the parents to know that the midwife is near or within calling distance. The midwife needs to be very sensitive and aware in order to assess whether to stay or to leave them alone for a while.

Sedation and analgesia

In the report *Midwives and Stillbirth* (HEC/RCM 1985) the use of analgesia for known intra-uterine fetal deaths or expected stillbirths was seen as a matter of individual choice. It was identified in the report that staff sometimes encouraged the use of analgesia, not for the mothers' benefit but for their own. It was noted that emotional and physical pain might need to be distinguished when helping parents to make a decision about analgesia. It is important for a mother and father to know that the birth of their baby was a reality.

Presentation of the baby

In the event of stillbirth or neonatal death, parents may wish to see and hold their dead baby. Some parents will wish to see their baby immediately, whilst others will wish to delay the event and a few may not wish to see or hold the baby at all. Parents need to be given time in this situation to come to the point of being able to look at and touch their baby. In either case, but

particularly when the baby is abnormal, it is suggested that the midwife shows the parents the normal parts of the baby first and then helps them to explore further if they wish. The way in which a mother perceives her baby as she looks at him is different from the perception of the midwife. Parents are likely to watch the midwife's behaviour towards their baby. The midwife should handle the body of the baby respectfully as though he were alive.

Mementoes

Some parents may wish to have a photograph of their dead baby to keep as a memento reminding them of the real little person who belonged to them. The practice in some areas is to take a photograph of each dead baby and keep a copy in the woman's notes in case the mother changes her mind and wishes she had decided to request a photograph to keep.

Work done by the medical photographer Shamus K. Reddin at Peterborough District Hospital demonstrates how a photograph which offers a good memory may be achieved (Figs 49.2–49.4).

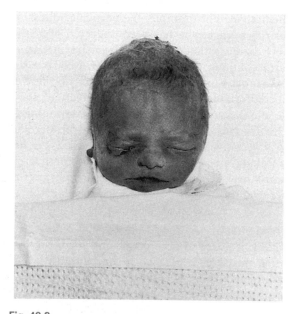

Fig. 49.2
A frontal photograph of baby. Note that the sheet and blanket have been left straight and flat, and no attempt has been made to hide facial bruising.

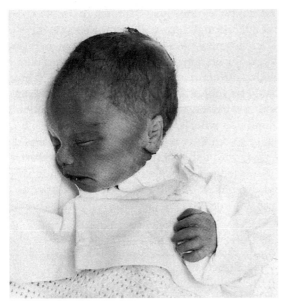

Fig. 49.3
A photograph of the same baby as in Figure 49.2. Note that baby's head has been turned slightly to one side to hide facial bruising.
By making folds in the blanket and exposing a little arm and hand the picture looks as if there has been movement and so appears less 'cold' and flat.

Other mementoes which may be offered to enhance the memory might be:

- a lock of hair
- a blessing certificate
- the baby's name label or cot card
- a memorial anniversary card
- entry in a book of remembrance
- a memorial plaque at the grave
- planting a shrub or tree in their own garden.

Parents need to be helped in a sensitive way to talk about the event and to decide for themselves whether or not they would like a memento.

Religious ceremonies and burial arrangements

All parents need to know where their baby is buried irrespective of the gestational period. It is important that the religious needs of the parents are met. Both Speck (1978) and Jolly (1988) offer information and practical suggestions about meeting cultural and other needs at this time. Most authorities and communities have policies and guidelines which are designed to assist maternity care staff in helping parents to cope. A most useful document for midwives and parents alike is the Stillbirth and Neonatal Death Society's publication, *When a Baby Dies* (Kohner & Henley 1991). There is also a book for professionals

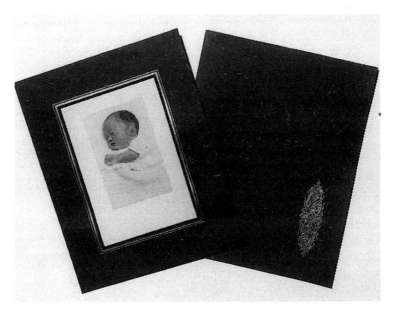

Fig. 49.4
The photograph looks even better framed. (© Journal of Audiovisual Media in Medicine.)

(Henley & Kohner 1991). It provides all the basic information required after stillbirth and neonatal death.

The midwife's role is to make sure the parents are adequately informed and have their needs met which means that the midwife should be familiar with the administrative procedures at such a time.

Aftercare

If the mother has had her baby in hospital no assumptions should be made about the length of time that she should stay. Some mothers wish to go home immediately; others wish to stay longer to rest and adjust to the loss. Some mothers wish to be near other live babies; others wish to be alone and quiet. The mother should be able to choose where she would like to be initially, and have the option of changing her mind as her feelings change.

Whether the mother is at home or in hospital it is important for the midwife to make contact and communicate with the parents. To 'be with' a mother, a father or both parents in their grief requires personal sensitivity on the part of the midwife and a willingness to exercise the skill of listening. Practicalities such as registration and burial are also important and the midwife needs to be able to provide information about local arrangements or to know to whom the parents may be referred.

It is not possible within the confines of this chapter to address all the different issues which may relate to the subject. Questions like 'When should I try again for a baby?' are difficult to cope with. A guideline response might be, 'When you feel physically recovered and emotionally healed then you will know the time is right.' Some couples will require advice about where to obtain genetic counselling following the birth of an abnormal or handicapped baby. It may be appropriate for the couple to discuss this with their medical consultant with possible referral to the Regional Genetic Counselling Service.

Bereavement is a family affair. The midwife needs to be aware that siblings, grandparents and others will need support. Questions from parents like 'How shall we tell the children?' may be asked.

The midwife may help parents to think about and talk through how to break the sad news.

Bereavement is also a lonely experience and physical isolation may intensify if a woman is separated from human contact in her grief. Visitors should be supported and made especially welcome; visiting a person who is grieving can feel difficult. A midwife who is able to 'be with' a person in her grief without needing to talk or invade the silences with her own needs offers real comfort.

Knowledge and experience of counselling skills and awareness of the grieving process provide a basis for the midwife to offer effective comfort and care.

Reader Activities

Questions for consideration or discussion:

- Should the parents know if their baby has died in utero or is likely to be abnormal?
- Who should tell parents that their baby will be born dead or has died at, or after, birth?
- What would be the 'ideal' way, and the 'ideal' place to break such news?
- Should parents see or hold their dead or abnormal baby and how will a midwife arrange for this to happen?
- In the case of a dead baby or mother, what are the needs of the father and how may these needs be met?
- What acts of remembrance might be suggested or arranged?
- What do I say first when meeting a mother or father whose baby has died?
- Does it matter if the midwife cries?
- How does the midwife take care of her own fears and associations about death?

USEFUL ADDRESSES

British Association for Counselling
1 Regent Place
Rugby, Warwickshire
CV21 3PJ

SANDS (Stillbirth and Neonatal Death Society)
28 Portland Place
London W1N 4DE

REFERENCES

Burnard P 1985 Learning human skills. Heinemann, London

Egan G 1986 The skilled helper, 3rd edn. Brooks/Cole Publishing, Monterey, California

Egan G 1990 The skilled helper, 4th edn. Brooks/Cole Publishing, Monterey, California

Henley A, Kohner N 1991 Miscarriage, stillbirth and neonatal death: guidelines for professionals. SANDS, London

Hopson B 1978 Counselling — a case for demystifying and deprofessionalising. Nursing Times 12 January: 50–51

Jolly J 1988 Missed beginnings. The Lisa Sainsbury Foundation Services Austen Cornish

Kohner N, Henley A 1991 When a baby dies. SANDS, London

Kübler-Ross E 1978 On death and dying. Tavistock Publications, London

Lewis C S 1961 A grief observed. Faber, London

Mayeroff M 1972 On caring. Harper & Row, New York

Murray-Parkes C 1986 Bereavement: Studies of grief in adult life, 2nd edn. Tavistock Publications, London

Nurse G 1977 Counselling and the nurse. HM&M, Chichester

Nurse G 1980 Counselling and the nurse, 2nd edn. HM&M, Chichester

Rogers C 1983 Freedom to learn for the 80s, 2nd edn. Charles E. Merrill

Royal College of Midwives/Health Education Council Report 1985 Midwives and stillbirth. RCM, London

Speck P 1978 Loss and grief in medicine. Baillière Tindall, London

Sutherland J D 1971 Address to the Inaugural Meetings of the Standing Conference for the Advancement of Counselling. October

Tschudin V 1987 Counselling skills for nurses, 2nd edn. Baillière Tindall, London

Wilson A L, Fenton L J, Stevens D C, Soule D J 1982 The death of a newborn twin: an analysis of parental bereavement. Paediatrics 70: 587–591

United Kingdom Central Council 1992 Code of professional conduct. UKCC, London

FURTHER READING

Forrest G 1989 Care of the bereaved after perinatal death. In: Chalmers I, Enkin M, Keirse M J N C (eds) Effective care in pregnancy and childbirth. Oxford University Press, Oxford

Rogers C 1961 On becoming a person. Constable, London

Stillbirth and Neonatal Death Society 1990 Mainly for fathers. SANDS, London

Warden J W 1992 Grief counselling and grief therapy, 2nd edn. Routledge, London

50

Research and the midwife

TRICIA MURPHY-BLACK

Research design

The research process

Application of research findings

Initiating research projects

Midwifery research is still in the early stages of development, but it is growing in size and strength. The eagerness with which midwives have seized the opportunities for research presented to them is very encouraging. Although there is still much of midwifery practice that needs a research base, the increase in research, both in the UK and elsewhere, is encouraging. With the introduction of diploma and degree level midwifery programmes in the UK, as well as the development of midwifery education at a tertiary level in other parts of the world, midwives will have the opportunity to learn about research from the start of their studies. The questioning approach that will result will help the 'baby' of midwifery research grow into a strong and vigorous 'child' to give midwives a research base for their practice for the benefit of mothers and babies.

Research is a means of objective information gathering about any environment to describe or document a change in practices which are or could be beneficial. Practices, which may be national or local, often develop in response to a variety of circumstances, such as current fashion, the likes and dislikes of a particular midwife or consultant, the introduction of new equipment or the demands of a group of mothers. After a while, these practices can become enshrined in tradition, with generations of midwives carrying out practices in the belief that they are doing the right thing, which is not supported by any evidence or indeed for which there may be opposing evidence. Two examples of such practices were the pre-delivery shaving of pubic hair (Romney 1980) and the administration of enemas (Romney & Gordon 1981). Both of these studies contributed to a change in practice, reducing in incidence of procedures which had little or no benefit, produced considerable discomfort for mothers and which were time-consuming for midwives.

Research has been defined as 'an attempt to increase available knowledge by the discovery of new facts or relationships through systematic enquiry' (Macleod Clark & Hockey 1989). This chapter will outline some different types of research and briefly describe each of the stages of the research process. Then suggestions for applying research findings and how to evaluate research reports are discussed. This is followed by a section on how to get involved in research.

RESEARCH DESIGN

There are many different ways of doing research, which can involve a variety of approaches and methods. The overall plan or framework is known as the research design (Polit & Hungler 1985), some examples of which are given below.

Historical research examines past events using primary sources, i.e. original documents such as Florence Nightingale's letters, to increase understanding and knowledge of the present situation.

Empirical research, which is based on experience in the real world, may use different designs to collect information.

A descriptive study looks at what is happening and records this systematically; for example, it may be a survey of a large number of mothers or a case study, which has relatively few subjects but describes a situation in depth. If the study is looking back at recent events, e.g. the mothers who delivered last year, it is known as a retrospective study, while a prospective study starts from a set date until the end of the data collection period.

Experimental research involves the deliberate manipulation of circumstances, with measurements made before and after on both the experimental and matched control group. Although this design

has been derived from biological research, there are occasions where similar designs are used in social research.

A controlled trial uses many of the methods used in experimental research but may have limitations which are imposed on it because the subjects are people in the real world rather than in laboratory conditions where external influences can be controlled. This design is considerably strengthened, (i.e. a better experiment) if the two groups are chosen randomly from the available subjects.

Evaluation research determines the value and/or effect of a policy, practice, education or a change in a particular setting. The researcher may have little or no control of the process but provides information for others to make decisions.

Action research is used to solve local problems and cannot be generalised to other situations. The researcher may initiate change during the study period as well as measure it.

THE RESEARCH PROCESS

The stages of the research process apply to all disciplines, not just midwifery. Those who want to do research need to consult textbooks on design and methods (such as Cormack 1984, Polit & Hungler 1985, Treece & Treece 1986, although there are many others) as well as seeking help from experts, possibly undertaking a course on research methods and having a supervisor while carrying out a research project. The stages of the research process are shown in Table 50.1. Although there is an order to these steps, much of the work of each step overlaps the others. For instance, the decisions about which method to use may depend on the research question, but may be limited by the skill of the researcher or the time and money available. Designing the research and planning the practical details as well as how to analyse the data collected, needs advice right from the start. The steps in Table 50.1 are used to ensure that the findings have come from systematic enquiry. Each of these steps is discussed in turn.

Table 50.1
The stages of the research process

1. Defining the problem
2. Reviewing the literature
3. Formulating a research question or hypothesis
4. Choosing the method
5. Collecting the data
6. Analysing the data
7. Writing the report
8. Disseminating the findings
9. Implementing the findings

1. Defining the problem

The first step in the process is to be clear about what is to be investigated. The problem area needs to be defined, turned into a research question or hypothesis and examined to see how it can best be investigated. Some research is designed to produce a hypothesis to test, rather than starting from a hypothesis which is then tested (Field & Morse 1985). The choice of subject for research depends on a variety of circumstances: it may be a topic of burning interest to the individual; something which has arisen as part of everyday practice in the hospital or community; the requirements for a course or training; or part of a large scale project which an investigator has been employed to research. Initially the problem area may be very wide and too big for a single research project and will have to be narrowed down to something which is manageable. If the problem is too large and ambitious it may never be completed or end up as a poorly conducted project which would have been better not attempted.

2. Reviewing the literature

Reading, analysing and criticising the previous research on the topic is an essential, if time-consuming, part of the process. This gives more information about the problem; may, in fact, define it, or may guide the choice of method, suggest ways of clarifying the questions, or reveal gaps which have not been researched. It may also indicate studies which need to be replicated, i.e. studies which repeat the work done by others to see if the same results are obtained, or alternatively

indicate areas already well covered which may act as a basis for further research. Searching for relevant articles and books is the first task. Midwives are fortunate to have a number of services which can help them with a literature search. In the UK there is the Current Awareness Service (CAS) distributed by the Royal College of Midwives (RCM); the RCM also have a Midwifery Index (Ayres 1987, 1992); the Midwives Information and Resource Service (MIDIRS) is an abstracting service and the Midwifery Research Database (MIRIAD) lists research projects relevant to midwifery. The International Clearinghouse of Maternity Nursing Research at the University of Calgary, Canada, is a computer-based compilation of completed and in-progress studies, and the WHO Safe Motherhood Initiative (based in Geneva, Switzerland) publishes regular reviews of work in maternity care from a global viewpoint. (See addresses at the end of this chapter.)

Other methods of literature searching, such as using an on-line computer or CD ROM (a collection of references and abstracts on a compact disc which can be searched by a computer, using keywords) are available to all researchers and can be found in libraries. There are guides to literature searching (e.g. Polit & Hungler 1985, Ch. 4; Moorbath 1988a) as well as writing references (Moorbath 1988b, Bennett 1991). Librarians are very helpful; do not be afraid to ask for guidance round your library, the classification system and how to choose keywords.

Details of the references, with the author and source, should be noted and stored carefully. Librarians will also give guidance on this.

3. Formulating a research question or hypothesis

Both defining the problem and the information from the literature review help towards clarifying the research question or hypothesis. A hypothesis is usually worded in such a way as to suggest a relationship between two variables but can be expressed negatively, i.e. that there will not be a relationship between the variables measured. As research is looking for associations and relationships between facts, it is usual to refer to accepting or rejecting a hypothesis rather than proving or disproving a relationship.

Research which is dealing with people, as in midwifery, rarely demonstrates cause and effect such as are found in a laboratory experiment. For instance, if a lighted candle is placed in an up-turned jam jar, the flame will go out when the available oxygen is used up. The effect is the flame going out; the cause is the lack of oxygen. The conditions may vary; it will burn longer in a bigger jam jar, but the result will be the same in the end. Such certainty is rarely, if ever, found in research on people.

4. Choosing the method

Social and biological research, although using the same stages of the research process, may use different methods of data collection. This difference can start with the problem. If the hypothesis is to be tested, quantitative methods (quantity usually associated with large numbers) will be used. Qualitative methods (quality, small numbers studied in depth) are used when the hypothesis is to be developed. The choice of which method to use is dependent on the nature of the problem and the facilities available. All methods have advantages as well as disadvantages and this may guide the choice. Some projects combine one or more methods to try to overcome some of the disadvantages.

5. Collecting the data

Some methods of data collection

Questionnaires can be sent through the post, handed out personally, or filled in on site by the researcher to collect information from a large number of people. A questionnaire may use different types of questions, e.g.

Closed questions: 'Is this your first pregnancy? — Yes/No.'

Open questions: 'How do you feel about your pregnancy?' and leave a space for the answer, or use a variety of scales, e.g.

'I am pleased I am pregnant. Please tick one of the following:

Strongly agree, agree, not sure, disagree, strongly disagree.'

Closed questions can be analysed in large numbers with relative ease by giving respondents limited choices but the answers may not fully reflect their views, feelings or circumstances. Open questions allow for greater individuality in the replies but may present difficulties in the analysis and presentation of results. There are many scales for measuring attitudes and systems of ranking responses which have been designed and tested in different situations.

Interviews are usually conducted face to face, although some are done by telephone, with the interviewer asking the questions and recording the answers. The recording may be directly onto a data collection sheet, or by taping the replies. The interviewer can check if the question has been understood, probe the answer to get more details and build up a fuller picture of the situation, attitudes or feeling on a particular topic. Interviews may be structured, in that questions are asked in a particular form and order, or semi-structured in which the interviewer may prompt the respondent to expand on parts of the interview or particular questions. Unstructured interviews use open questions without prompting. Interviewing, however, is time-consuming and expensive, especially if tape-recorded replies have to be transcribed, and analysis is not as easy as with a questionnaire.

Observation is concerned with watching behaviour which may occur in its natural setting or a special place such as a laboratory. Observation may involve looking at an individual, e.g. reactions, facial expressions or speech; a group, e.g. mothers, babies, ward staff; or events, e.g. deliveries, community visits, ward organisation. Observation is often a more accurate way of documenting what is done rather than asking what people think is done (Crow 1984). As it is impossible for one person to observe and record everything going on in a room or ward at the same time, the behaviour to be observed has to be selected. Once selected, the details of the behaviour need to be defined and classified, so that the system used to record what is going on always records the same behaviours.

There are many existing systems for observation (see Crow (1984) for some references). The selected behaviour may be recorded by taping speech, video recording actions or noting observations on a data collection sheet.

Types of observation

The participant observer is a member of the group being observed and acts as a member of the group so that the data collected have to be recorded after the observation period. If the researcher is not normally part of the group, joining may alter the group's reactions. There are also ethical aspects to be considered, if the group do not know of the research and would not willingly behave in such a way if they knew they were being observed.

A non-participant observer joins the group but does not take part in the activities. This makes it easier to record the behaviour as it happens than for the participant observer but also demonstrates to the group that they are being observed, which may change their behaviour.

Observation through a one-way mirror is normally only possible in a laboratory. This is useful to observe the behaviour of those who would be distracted by an observer, e.g. young children. A similar method of observation might be to video-record actions in a ward or to pin a microphone to a midwife or patient to record conversations. It is unethical to use such techniques to observe behaviour if the subjects, or their parents, are not asked, cannot or will not give their consent.

Observation can be continuous, for instance during one shift, or the whole of a mother's labour. Activity sampling records behaviour or patterns of work, which occurs during specified time periods, perhaps 5 minutes every hour; these periods are usually chosen randomly.

Clinical trials

Much research in midwifery involves clinical trials. These studies involve objective measurements, rather than attitudes and the data are collected in a systematic fashion. Some of the issues involved in clinical research are discussed by Maxwell (1973). Mothers may not be expected to answer questions directly, but the consent of the individual must be obtained before inclusion in the study.

Validity and reliability

The questionnaire or interview schedule or form to record the observations or measurement scale is known as the research instrument. It has to be tested for validity and reliability. Validity is testing the instrument to see if it does measure what it is supposed to measure. A test for reliability checks that the instrument will always measure the same response or behaviour at different times, under different conditions and from a variety of respondents, so that the results are consistent.

Sampling

Once the method of collecting data has been decided, the people (the research subjects) from whom information will be obtained must be chosen. The majority of research projects have to use a smaller number, known as a sample, than those to whom the results will apply. For example, research into any one aspect of pregnancy cannot include every pregnant woman. A large sample, whether 2000 or 20 000, is still a sample as it does not include all pregnant women. Unless the research design in such that the results are not meant to be generalised, i.e. applied to those in a similar situation but not included in the research, the subjects included need to be chosen by sampling. One method of overcoming the problem of having an unrepresentative sample is to choose the subjects by random numbers. This might be from a list of mothers to send a questionnaire to or to interview; or in experimental research, where a double blind trial method is used — those to be included in the treatment and control groups will be allocated randomly to each group. Consult a statistician before deciding on how to select the sample size.

Phases of data collection

Collecting the data generally has two phases: the pilot and the main study.

A pilot study provides an opportunity to test the instrument, the questionnaires, the interview schedule, the observation system, and the practical details of carrying out the study. This testing may reveal difficulties: the wording of the questionnaire may be misunderstood or be too complex to answer, the interview may take too long to complete or the practical details of getting the names and addresses may not work as smoothly as planned. A pilot study is vital before starting the main study.

Storing the data in preparation for analysis, and the means of collation, should be planned before the main study. These will depend on the type of data to be collected, the number of subjects and type of analysis. Two methods of storage are Cope Chat cards or a computer. The Cope Chat cards hold the data of each individual and can be used for analysis (see Cormack 1984). Some filling systems are very sophisticated but others are simple, e.g. a shoe box. It is also important to check if the data stored on a computer will be subject to the Data Protection Act.

The main study is the period of time during which the questionnaires are sent out or distributed personally, the interviews are conducted, the observation is undertaken or the clinical trial is carried out. If the planning stages of the project have been followed carefully and the problems from the pilot study ironed out, the main study should proceed fairly smoothly. With all projects, however, there can be unforeseen difficulties. If these do occur, careful notes should be made at the time for two reasons:

1. these can affect/influence the results and therefore explain them
2. someone replicating the study needs to know of these problems to avoid them and/or to explain the differences in the results between the two studies.

6. Analysing the data

Data are analysed to demonstrate relationships between variables. The variables are the characteristics of the subjects which are being measured, e.g. a baby's birthweight; a mother's attitude to her care. In a study with small numbers, it is possible to sort the data by hand so that, for example, the number of primigravidae or multigravidae who give a certain answer can be tabulated. Larger numbers require a system such as

the Cope Chat cards or a computer. Some analysis, especially of qualitative data, is done as soon as possible after data collection from an individual, while other methods start analysis when the data collection is finished.

The first stage of quantitative analysis is to count the number within each group or category, known as the frequencies, then check and remove any coding errors. As these give only fairly simple information, the second stage is to look at relationships between the categories or variables. Tables which compare group counts are known as cross tabulations. The next step is to use statistical tests to see if there is a difference between the groups.

Statistical tests are used as the sample (e.g. 100 pregnant women) is always part of the whole population (all pregnant women) and if properly chosen will represent the population. Differences between groups, e.g. comparing the birthweights of babies born to primigravidae and multigravidae, are tested statistically to see if the difference between them could have occurred by chance if they came from the same underlying population. The result of such a test is expressed as 'the probability'. Probabilities are compared to significance level.

Probability at the end of a table of results is written as '$p = $'. The number is less than 1; the larger it is, the more likely the difference reported occurred by chance. If the result of a test is '$p = 0.9$' it would be reported as 'not statistically significant'. Figures which are frequently seen in such tables are $p = 0.05$ or $p = 0.01$. The $p = 0.05$ means that there is a 1 in 20 chance, also called the 5% level, while $p = 0.01$ means there is a 1 in 100 chance (or 1% level) of the measured change occurring by chance. For example, it is often said that babies of smokers have lower birthweights than babies of non-smokers. When the birthweight of babies of a group of heavy smokers were compared with a group of non-smokers, the average weight difference was reported as 255 g (Black 1982). This difference between the weights is reported as 'significant at the $p = 0.001$ level', i.e. the probability of the weight difference occurring by chance (and not related to smoking) is 0.1% or 1 in 1000. The statistical test used in this example was the Student's t test.

Two statistical tests which are seen frequently in reports of midwifery research are the Student's t test and Chi square test. They have different uses. The Student's t test is used with continuous data which has a normal (bell-shaped) distribution when recorded for a large number of people. Weight and length are examples of data which are usually normally distributed. An example of the use of the t test is with birthweights. Birthweights within two groups are compared, e.g. the babies of primigravidae against multigravidae, or girls compared with boys. The mean birthweight (i.e. the weights in each group added together and divided by the number of babies) of the two groups may not show a big difference; it might be 50 or 100 g but did this difference occur by chance or not? By using a Student's t test on the birthweights, the probability of the difference occurring by chance can be calculated. So the probability may be $p = 0.09$ (this difference has occurred by chance) or $p = 0.001$ (the probability of this occurring by chance is 0.1%). Chi square tests (also written as χ^2) are used on data which are in categories, e.g. to compare the answers given by married midwives with single midwives on a question about working shifts. The answer is again given as the probability. To find how to do these tests, refer to a statistical textbook (e.g. Swinscow 1976, Robson 1983, Siegal & Castellan 1988). There are computer programs which will do the work, some of which can be used with personal computers.

The type of statistics used depends on many of the factors of the study. The statistics may be descriptive, i.e. used to describe or summarise observations, or inferential, used to make an estimate or prediction (Rowntree 1981). Parametric statistics are used to test normally distributed data while non-parametric statistics are used for data which are not normally distributed (Siegal & Castellan 1988).

7. Writing the report

When all the data have been analysed, the report has to be written to make the findings known to others. This may be in the form of an article for one of the midwifery or nursing journals. A report will almost certainly be required by the funding body or if the research has been done as one of the requirements of a course a report will be a prerequisite. Most reports follow the outline provided in Table 50.1, replacing stage 9 with conclusions and recommendations for action, change in policy or practice or further research.

8. Dissemination

As well as writing a report and having the results published, there are other means of letting people know what has been found and recommended. A project which is locally based, say in a hospital or one Health Authority, especially one which is concerned with a local problem, needs to be discussed locally. A meeting of the relevant staff, the ward and/or community midwives, teachers and managers, is a suitable way of letting them know the results. It is good public relations to make the results of research available to those people such as ward sisters who have helped to collect the data. This could be by giving a talk at a meeting. A summary of the whole report, giving an outline of the study with the conclusions and recommendations should be distributed to all in the wards or community. The results could also be presented as a session during a study day, perhaps organised by inservice training. Conferences — local, national or international — are another means. Sometimes speakers are invited but might have to submit an abstract of the proposed paper for consideration by those planning the conference.

9. Implementation

The final step of the research process is putting the results into action, where this is possible. Some research projects have change built into them, for instance, an experimental design may be testing a different treatment, practice or policy on a small group. If the results show the change is favourable, then it can be applied to a larger group. Other projects have results which show a need for change, e.g. of attitudes or improvement of teaching or communication skills. In these cases, implementation takes longer. It may be necessary to arrange for training in such skills and it will take time before all members of staff can be trained.

APPLICATION OF RESEARCH FINDINGS

The person to initiate change in the ward or community may be the midwife who works there or a manager who wants to involve the midwives. Change in educational ideas (a new course or training) will obviously involve the midwife teachers but may also have implications at a higher level, for instance a National Board. Organisational change, or change in policy for a ward or hospital will require considerable consultation before implementation.

Critical evaluation of a research report is essential before deciding to implement the findings. The questions which start research — who, what, when, why, where, how — can also guide the examination of a report to decide whether or not it should be used. Some of the questions to consider are listed below:

1. *Who*
    — who did the study? midwives, sociologists, midwife teachers, doctors? are they appropriate?
    — who were the subjects? mothers, babies, midwives, students, wards, managers?
2. *What*
    — what was the problem?
    — what was the research question or hypothesis? was there a hypothesis? was it clearly stated? is it understandable? does it make sense? does it relate to a problem or situation locally?
3. *Why*
    — why was the study done? was it a problem which grew out of practice? did it come from a complaint from the mothers? was it done as a requirement for a course?
4. *When*
    — when was it done? recently or 10 years ago? does it still apply (e.g. the physiology of breast feeding is unlikely to change over

10 years but the attitudes of mothers or midwives to it might change considerably)?
5. *Where*
    — where was it done? in a similar hospital or area to one's own or one completely different? will this make any difference?
6. *How*
    — how was it done? what methods were used? was it an appropriate method for the question and was it used correctly? how big was the sample? were the statistical tests appropriate? how was the sample chosen? was it representative of the population? can it be generalised to this hospital?

If after this critical evaluation, it is decided that this research is of some value to a group of mothers, babies, or midwives or to a hospital, the next decision is what to do with the findings. Should the study be replicated to see if there will be the same results? Or should the practice be changed in view of the findings? If so, who has to change what and how will it be done? These questions cannot be answered in a textbook but have to be discussed with those who will be most closely involved with the process of change.

INITIATING RESEARCH PROJECTS

The ultimate aim of research in midwifery should be to improve conditions for the clients of the maternity services, the mothers and babies. From this it follows that all aspects of midwifery can and probably should be researched, such as what the midwife does, how she does it, how she is trained to do it and the organisation in which she carries out her work. In order to consider what research should be done, it is essential to have a questioning approach. Research is initiated by asking such questions as why, what, when, where and how. All can question their practice but not all midwives will, or can do research. Research is a skilled activity, which can be learnt as midwifery can be learnt, but should not be attempted by those who do not know how to do research unless they are closely supervised by someone experienced in research.

Learning in training is perhaps the most

common contact with research methods. This may be as a student midwife or during a post-basic course. Sometimes it is called 'doing a project' rather than research, as it may only involve part of the process, perhaps steps 1–3 in Table 50.1. In other cases, all the steps of the process are followed but with very few subjects. In these cases the purpose of research is to understand how it is done rather than to produce findings which will alter practice, although such a by-product is possible. With small numbers, it may not be possible to do many statistical tests and the results should not be generalised to a larger group.

Research as part of a job, which may be descriptive, experimental, evaluative or action research, usually grows out of a particular practice within one hospital, or community. Such research may also be a replication of a prior study, for instance to find out if a change of practice which is beneficial in an urban area may be of value in a rural area. There are courses in research methods, which may be local or national, and before embarking on research, it is worth getting training as well as help from others. Anyone doing research while continuing their normal duties will find it both expensive and time-consuming. It may be possible to arrange locally for funding to help with typing, photocopying and postage while a sympathetic manager may be able to arrange to release one day a week to concentrate on the research. Research scholarships for small amounts are useful to fund this type of research. There may be NHS funds available for nurses and midwives, so it is always worth asking.

To do full-time research there are three approaches. For those with little or no research experience, a research training fellowship is one method. These fellowships, funded by the Department of Health (DH) and Scottish Home and Health Department (SHHD), are awarded annually and the successful candidate has a salary as well as a placement within a formal setting, such as a university, for research training. Supervision is provided and there is the possibility that the research might be submitted for a degree.

The second approach is to apply for a post as a research associate or research assistant, sometimes called research midwives or nurses, and become part of a research team. These teams may be multidisciplinary and include obstetricians, paediatricians and others. Some of these posts will have research training built into them and the successful candidate will be involved in the planning and design as well as other phases of the project. Other posts will demand only data collection and employment will start after the planning phases. Posts like these will pay a salary but will almost certainly be on short-term contracts.

The third approach is to seek funding for a research project. This may be from the DH, SHHD, Regional Health Authority or Health Board, a charity which exists to give research grants (such as Birthright) or other foundations such as the Iolanthe Trust. Each funding body will have specific requirements and it is essential to find these out in advance of formal application. A request for research funding is known as a research protocol; guidance for preparing this can be found in Bond (1984). The majority of funding bodies will require evidence that the project leader has some experience in research and is capable of carrying it out competently, or that the research will be suitably supervised.

Access to the site or the group of people involved in the research will vary according to the type of research. Permission to do research in a hospital or community, or using a particular group of mothers, will have to be obtained from those who have overall responsibility for that area, or group of subjects. It is not sufficient to assume that a midwife will have permission to do research in a place just because she is working there. Permission to carry out a research project is not the same as getting the consent of the research subject.

Ethical aspects of research need serious consideration. Research, while it may advance knowledge, should not do this at the expense of causing patients or mothers or babies or midwives any harm or inconvenience. The researcher needs to consider the effects of doing the research on the subjects, and may have to modify the research design from the ideal which may be unethical. One safeguard is that most health authorities will require the project to be approved by a research ethics committee before permission will be given to undertake the research. Prospective researchers should find out the requirements of the committee in advance. They will ask for a research protocol which they may require on a special form or to follow certain guidelines.

Informed consent of the subjects is one aspect of the protocol the ethical committee will ask about. The subjects of the research need to know enough about the project to be able to understand why it is being done and what benefits or harm, if any, will accrue to themselves as a result of involvement in the research. When the subjects know about the project, they must be given the option to say they will not take part or to withdraw from the project at any stage. Research which involves intrusive procedures (taking blood, giving drugs) requires a signed record that the research subject understood and consented.

Conclusion

Research can be very rewarding, both while doing it and seeing the results produce a change which is beneficial. Some research findings are put into practice quickly, while other studies take years between recognising a problem, researching it and producing change in the work of practitioners. However, this process will be assisted if all midwives are willing to question the work they do and seek to base their practice only on research-based evidence.

Reader Activities

Think of an everyday part of your work:

- how did you come to do this aspect of your work in the way you do it?
- who influenced/taught you?
- what constraints are there on you that you must do this work in a particular way?
- do you think you are acting in a way that is the best for the people you are caring for?
- what research can you find to support this?
- how do the relevant research articles stand up to critical evaluation?
  (use the questions given in this chapter)
- do you see where research is needed in this aspect of your work?

USEFUL ADDRESSES

Birthright
Royal College of Obstetricians and Gynaecologists
27 Sussex Place
Regent's Park
London NW1 4SP

Current Awareness Service
The Librarian
Royal College of Midwives
15 Mansfield St
London W1M 0BE

Iolanthe Trust
c/o Royal College of Midwives
15 Mansfield St
London W1M 0BE

International Clearinghouse of Maternity Nursing Research
The Faculty of Nursing
University of Calgary
Calgary
Alberta
Canada T2N 1N4

MIDIRS — Midwives Information and Resource Service
Institute of Child Health
Royal Hospital for Sick Children
St Michael's Hill
Bristol BS2 8BJ

MIRIAD — Midwifery Research Database
National Perinatal Epidemiology Unit
Radcliffe Infirmary
Oxford OX2 6HE

Safe Motherhood Initiative
World Health Organization
1211 Geneva 27
Switzerland

REFERENCES

Ayres J (ed) 1987 Midwifery index: a source of journal references on midwifery and related topics, 1980–86 (with selective coverage of 1976–1979). Royal College of Midwives, London.

Ayres J (ed) 1992 Midwifery index. Vol. 2, 1987–1991. Royal College of Midwives, London

Bennett V R 1991 Referencing: a step-by-step guide for beginners. Royal College of Midwives, London

Black P M 1982 The effects of low tar cigarettes on birthweight. In: Robinson S, Thomson A (eds) Research and the midwife conference proceedings. Kings College, University of London.

Bond S 1984 Preparing a research proposal. In: Cormack D F S (ed) The research process in nursing. Blackwell Scientific, Oxford

Cormack D F S (ed) 1984 The research process in nursing. Blackwell Scientific, Oxford

Crow R 1984 Observation. In: Cormack D F S (ed) The research process in nursing. Blackwell Scientific, Oxford.

Data Protection Registrar 1985 Guideline No 1, an introduction and guide to the Act. Office of the Data Protection Registrar

Field P A, Morse J M 1985 Nursing research: the application of qualitative approaches. Croom Helm, London

Macleod Clark J, Hockey L 1989 Further research for nursing: a new guide for the enquiring nurse. Scutari Press, London, p 4

Maxwell C 1973 Clinical research for all. Cambridge Medical Publications, Cambridge

Moorbath P 1988a A guide to nursing research literature. Senior Nurse 8(1): 35–36

Moorbath P 1988b Writing references: a guide. Senior Nurse 8(7/8): 22–23

Polit D F, Hungler B P 1985 Essentials of nursing research: methods and applications. J B Lippincott, Philadelphia

Robson C 1983 Experiment, design and statistics in psychology, 2nd edn, Penguin Books, Middlesex

Romney M L 1980 Predelivery shaving: an unjustified assault? Journal of Obstetrics and Gynaecology 1: 33–35

Romney M L Gordon H 1981 Is your enema really necessary? British Medical Journal 282: 1269–1271

Rowntree D 1981 Statistics without tears: a primer for non-mathematicians. Penguin, Harmondsworth

Siegal S, Castellan N J 1988 Non-parametric statistics for the behavioural sciences, 2nd edn. McGraw-Hill, New York

Swinscow T D V 1976 Statistics at square one. British Medical Association, London

Treece E W, Treece J W 1986 Elements of research in nursing, 4th edn. Mosby, New York

51

Ethics in midwifery

ANNE THOMPSON

Facing up to ethics

Identifying the problems

Structures and strategies

Professional ethics are among the sinews of a free society; they sustain and extend (when they do not abuse) reliance on trust; they limit coercive regulation and state control where human interests are best served by free, privileged communication. (Dunstan 1987)

FACING UP TO ETHICS

Ethics is rarely thought of as a practical subject or an easy one to tackle. Many people question its legitimacy as a subject within the curriculum, largely because their view is that ethics or morality is a personal matter to be determined by the individual alone according to his or her personal lights. For simplicity's sake I follow Baroness Warnock in making no distinction between the two terms, while realising that for many theologians and philosophers they have different meanings. In the professional field, discussion of ethics in the early decades of this century was often limited to prescriptions relating to interdisciplinary etiquette and the duty of obedience owed by nurses and midwives to doctors. Three decades of great technological and sociological change have altered that dramatically (see Fig. 51.1). Improved access to education and increased levels of information and debate through the media have meant that women in many parts of the world are challenging decisions which once they would have accepted simply on the authority of their caregivers. A large

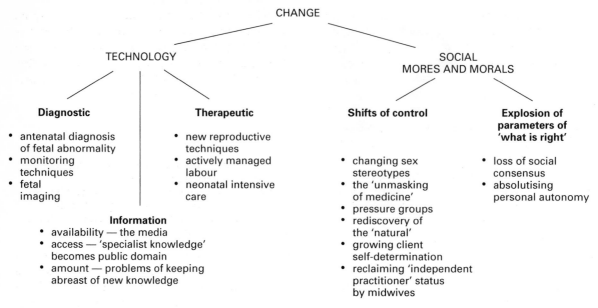

Fig. 51.1
Some elements of change in relation to midwifery practice.

part of today's debate in midwifery centres on the issues of power and control, as women claim a voice in the decisions which are made about their care.

These two concepts will provide the framework for this chapter as it examines what is meant today by ethics in midwifery practice and why it has become an important area for reflection. In moving on to look at some of the problems which cause concern a number of case studies will be used to identify the main issues in practice. The values which underpin many of the decisions and choices in midwifery are frequently a source of conflict, as mothers, midwives and doctors necessarily view childbirth from different perspectives. Strategies for resolving such conflict constructively will be discussed and there will be a brief examination of some of the classical moral frameworks which are used to achieve consistency and coherence in decision making. Throughout the chapter readers will be invited to explore their own experience, beliefs and values for, while being an intensely practical discipline in the way that it guides and determines our actions, the root of ethics lies at the core of the individual person. In sharing an honest account of their own values and beliefs while attempting to listen without pre-

judice to people whose stance is very different midwives can carry forward the work of the 'reflective community', the development of a social sense of what is right and acceptable for our times and our world, which people have engaged in throughout history (Engelhardt 1986).

What is ethics?

The current concern for ethics in health care has been described as 'a product of the collision of an exquisite technology with an age which has achieved total communication saturation' (Stenberg 1979). Many will sympathise with her additional comment that the technology 'moves inexorably forward without answering any of the questions inherent in its use'. None the less, the accelerating rate of technological development in the fields of prenatal diagnosis, assisted reproduction or life support for the very sick neonate is only one aspect of the ethical problem. Schröck (1980) illustrated this very clearly in relation to nursing care. Despite the new technologies' high profile in the media and even in some professionals' minds, it is the ordinary events of daily practice which offer the practitioner the greatest scope for the exercise of ethical judgements. The midwife who is sensitive to the way in which the power inherent in professional status and the health care framework can undermine her clients' ability to express their views will seek out ways to shift the balance so that the people in her care can have their voices heard (Wagner 1986).

Ethics claims to be a discipline of systematic reflection and analysis designed to enable people to identify the answers to questions about what ought to be done in some sort of consistent and coherent manner. 'Ought' is a value-laden word, heavy with a weight of moral constraint. Kant, an 18th century philosopher who had a great impact on modern thinking, talked about 'imperatives', in the sense that once it has been determined what ought to be done one is then compelled to do it (Paton 1947). The criteria by which the 'ought' is determined are rooted in the systems of moral theory. Whichever of the many theories are chosen as a guide for action, they are all concerned, in one way or another, to identify the 'right' course, the 'good' decision, the 'best' pathway. What exactly constitutes that good, or best or right depends largely on which of the frameworks one usually chooses to work by.

Examples of such frameworks include those specific to a particular religious tradition, such as the Ten Commandments; precepts designed for a group of practitioners, such as the UKCC Code of Professional Conduct; or a more universally applicable utilitarian consideration of how to achieve the maximum benefit for the greatest number of people. Some of the more important ethical frameworks will be discussed in more detail towards the end of this chapter.

The choice of framework is certain to be coloured by the individual's early experience, upbringing and culture. The fact that ethics claims to be a system of rational enquiry should not disguise the fact that the decisions that the system leads to are made by human beings with hearts that are at least as powerful as their heads (Midgely 1981). Although some philosophers would much prefer ethical reflection to remain uncluttered by messy human emotion, the reality of life in the health care system is that very many of the situations which arise are highly charged with positive or negative feelings which should not be ignored. Childbirth is one of the most significant of human events for everyone involved, and as such quite properly engages people's emotions. The process of ethical reflection must take account of this and allow due weight to the fact that we are only able to make decisions as whole people if our hearts are permitted to inform our heads.

The uses of power

'Membranes will be ruptured at three centimetres dilatation' (delivery suite protocol).
'It would be much better if you let me give him a top-up' (midwife to mother with hungry baby).
'I'm going home anyway' (mother discharging herself against medical advice).

Midwives will not find it difficult to think of examples which illustrate just how much control is exercised over people who make use of the maternity services. On one level this is inevitable. Large institutions need rules and regulations to maintain an acceptable standard of smooth functioning. Protocols, policies and guidelines are developed to ensure some degree of consistency and order in the managing of situations. The difficulty arises when there is conflict between the needs and values of the individual client or practitioner and those of the organisation. The midwife is likely to be as unhappy as the mother with a rigid protocol. The heart of the problem seems to be that an externally determined, formally imposed set of rules is substituted for individual decision-making processes which can take into account the particular features of a given situation.

As with so many other human situations, a certain amount of common sense is called for in trying to arrive at a way of working which creates the conditions necessary for dialogue. In recent years midwifery care has often been described as a partnership. This is a concept which embraces equality and dialogue. Where these characteristics exist there is no inappropriate use of power by one partner over the other. Rather, trust is established between them. Trust is a quality often mentioned when midwives speak about the women they care for. For most midwives it remains a recurring source of wonder that they are so readily trusted by the great majority of their clients. To trust renders a person very vulnerable and puts the trusted individual in a position of great personal power. Add this to the power midwives already hold by virtue of their professional qualification and status and it is obvious that, unless they take care, the partnership they want to establish with women will be ineffective, because unequal.

Nevertheless, it would be unrealistic to deny the usefulness of formal policies and guidelines, properly established and appropriately used. 'Properly established' should mean that midwives are actively involved in designing Unit protocols and that the people to whom policies apply should in some way be consulted about them. Few people like committee meetings but failure to get involved means that someone else will do the deciding. 'Appropriately used' must mean that, in the ordinary run of day-to-day events, policies do not become a substitute for thought. When, some years ago, the authors of the confidential enquiries on maternal mortality (DH 1989) recommended that each delivery suite in the country develop its own protocols for the management of catastrophic haemorrhage, it was a totally appropriate suggestion. Such situations demand urgent, co-ordinated and effective action. A team needs to be able to move into action smoothly and swiftly. Such a moment is not the time to enter into debates about values and beliefs. Used in such circumstances, policies like this can save lives. However, this does not eliminate the need to identify clients' wishes. In a case when a team of obstetricians were faced with a Jehovah's Witness giving birth to twins, they respected her request not to have a blood transfusion. They refrained from using their professional power to override her clearly stated, deeply held beliefs. As a consequence the mother died. Many would argue that the doctors' duty was to save her life. The team evidently felt that this duty did not warrant violating the conscience of a self-determining rational adult.

IDENTIFYING THE PROBLEMS

Central issues in caring

When midwives were asked to identify the main sources of moral conflict in their practice, the level of obstetric intervention in the delivery suite accounted for nearly 50% of the items listed (Thompson 1987). 'Bioethical issues', (e.g. termination for fetal abnormality, life support for the very low birthweight or grossly handicapped baby) was the only other category to achieve a two figure score (14.2%). This perception is echoed in much of the contemporary literature on childbirth where the extent of the medical profession's control is constantly challenged (Overall 1987, Katz Rothman 1986, Tew 1990).

One of the anxieties which flows from this situation is that the legitimate concern about levels or intervention too readily becomes an extreme attitude. Without timely intervention many mothers and babies would have died over recent decades and would continue to do so. Women and their babies could suffer if too simplistic an approach to the problems of childbearing caused them to lose faith in their practitioners and reject sound advice. There have been healthy and successful challenges to intervention levels such as the induction rates of the late 1970s, but it is vital that challenge is well founded, that evidence is clear and that alternative approaches can be demonstrated to be at least as safe as those which are being challenged. Part of the problem here lies in the inequality which has already been discussed. Partnership in care, true interdisciplinary co-operation, can only be achieved in a climate of mutual respect and confidence, conditions which do not always prevail. Midwives are key partners in the obstetric team and women need the services of the whole team, functioning in a spirit of competent interdependence.

Choice and control

Choice is another issue which has received much attention in recent years. Gilligan (1977) comments that 'the essence of the moral decision is the exercise of choice and the willingness to accept responsibility for that choice.' In a study on why women make the choices they do regarding abortion she tries to show that, where women have control over the domain in which the choices are made, their moral decision-making processes are just as principled as those of men. Women just formulate their experience 'in a different voice', as she puts it. Arguing that her data demonstrated that responsibility and caring were the main motivators of their decisions, Gilligan continues: 'Women's judgements are tied to feelings of empathy and compassion and are concerned more with the resolution of "real-life" rather than hypothetical dilemmas.'

The freedom of women to make choices about their childbirth experiences, particularly if the birth itself is to take place in hospital, is largely dependent on the willingness and co-operation of midwives and obstetricians. Many centres, both in the UK and overseas, have taken seriously the challenge of providing women with authentic choice. There can be problems at times when the difference of perception which Gilligan notes comes into play and women's choices do not coincide with the established policies. Wilson (1986) points out that the attempt to provide professional services which respect the autonomy of the client requires the development of strategies which will encourage the free flow of communication. Recent reorganisation of midwifery care in order to achieve more continuity is one way in which this can be done. The development of birth plans and increasing the number of women who are visited antenatally in their own homes could also help.

Conflicting loyalties

One of the consequences of working in a multidisciplinary team is that the potential for conflict is increased. This is illustrated in the following case study.

> A manager refused to allow a midwife to come in on her day off to deliver a particularly nervous young mother with whom she had built up a good relationship. The woman was tense and anxious throughout a difficult labour, cared for by a midwife she did not know. The outcome was a traumatic instrumental delivery. The couple later tried to book the first midwife privately for the next confinement. She declined the request 'reluctantly'.

This is only one of many possible examples of instances where the individual's professional judgement is in conflict with either her client's or other professionals' views. It is a very painful situation and there are no 'blanket' remedies. The very fact that such a situation can arise between a midwife and her manager or an obstetrician is sufficient for some people to contest the midwife's claim to be an autonomous practitioner. Such an argument fails to recognise that all moral decisions are set in a given context, a particular cultural, social or professional framework, and that decisions are not made in some form of neutral, impersonal moral vacuum. Ethics, of its nature, is interpersonal and hence complex. Precisely because 'no man is an island' people are accountable for their actions and professionals are accountable in a public, formal manner, first of all to their clients and then to their profession.

Among the strategies that midwives can develop in order to handle situations of conflict without compromising their own personal integrity Joyce Thompson (1984), an American midwife, identifies what she calls 'professional maturity'. Arguing that to be professional is to be ethical, she describes the characteristics of such maturity as:

- knowledge and acceptance of all the responsibilities inherent in midwifery practice and education
- mutual trust and respect in relationships between clients and different practitioners
- maintenance of competence and ongoing learning
- a knowledge of history, to avoid repeating past mistakes
- risk-taking with responsibility for outcomes
- reasoned decision-making in all domains
- the ability to live with uncertainty.

The recognition of one's personal and professional limitations should be added to complete the list. Although this sounds self-evident, it is frequently as difficult for a practitioner to admit to this as it is to acknowledge uncertainty. Professional training and social expectations combine to put considerable pressure on her to provide an answer. In the moral domain, above all, it will usually be quite inappropriate for the midwife to attempt to supply such answers. Her role will be to act as a catalyst to enable her clients to reach their own solutions. The response 'if I were you ...' short-circuits the hard work of reflection and analysis which they will need to engage in order to reach decisions which are truly their own. Her respect for their autonomy lies in refraining from bringing the power of her professional status to bear on their choice. This in no way means that she may abdicate her responsibility for ensuring that her clients are in possession of the best possible information before they make their decisions. It simply implies that she will not assume that her professional position automatically gives her the right to decide what is best for her clients.

Values

Few words have been subjected to such a variety of usage, by economists, philosophers, social scientists of various persuasions and recently by educators at large ... there can be no confidence that two authorities who discuss values are referring to the same range of phenomena. (Kitwood 1977)

Despite Kitwood's gloomy account of the uselessness of the word 'values', it is nearly impossible to discuss ethics without it. Here the word will be used in the sense of those action-guiding criteria which people adopt for their standards of per-

formance in relation to other people or situations. Hall (1973) describes a value as a stance that is taken and expressed through behaviours, feelings, imagination, knowledge and actions. Values are inherent in what matters most to individuals, in what has meaning for them and in what they hold most dear. Once this is accepted, it is easy to see that to ignore, dismiss or affront another's values, even unintentionally, can be an assault on her personal integrity.

Organisations, as well as individuals, function from a chosen set of values which become part of their corporate image. In the study mentioned earlier (Thompson 1987), midwives identified five major areas of potential value-conflicts which they experienced (Fig. 51.2). It would be possible to get women and their partners to draw a similar picture from their perspective. Midwives and mothers alike have to develop communication and negotiation skills in order to safeguard their own values to a reasonably satisfactory level.

When midwives were asked what mattered most to them in their practice their replies focused on maintaining a high standard of care with confidence and flexibility, on being able to ensure a satisfactory experience for the women they care for and on achieving a level of personal satisfaction from recognising that their work had been worthwhile. These responses seem concerned with

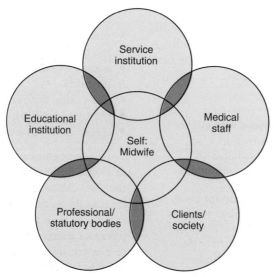

Fig. 51.2
Potential sources of values conflict in midwifery practice.

realising a 'best' outcome for midwives and mothers alike. As such they meet the criteria for a morally responsible service. Nonetheless, the questions concerned the ideal rather than the real and the constraints imposed by some of the systems noted in Figure 51.2 can alter the picture quite dramatically.

On a more personal level, problems can arise from different interpretations of concepts such as respect for life, fetal rights, quality of life and many other controversial issues. The following case study highlights the difficulties raised by the differing personal stances held by the people involved.

A midwife took over the care of a woman with a 36 week pregnancy. Labour was being induced at the woman's request. The fetus had recently been diagnosed in her country of origin as suffering from Down's syndrome and a cardiac abnormality. The midwife was disturbed to find that none of the customary measures for monitoring fetal well-being were being taken. Discussion with the mother made it clear that she would be happier if the baby did not survive its birth, because her family life would be disrupted and such handicaps were poorly accepted in her country. The midwife was unable to accept what she felt was a level of tacit collusion designed to give the baby minimum chances of survival and, after further discussion, started fetal monitoring and requested the presence of a paediatrician at delivery. The baby responded well to resuscitation and went to the Neonatal Intensive Care Unit. Surgery was later performed successfully. The mother was extremely distressed by the course of events, and the midwife was criticised by the obstetrician, many of her peers and the consultant paediatrician.

It could be valuable to analyse this case, either alone or with others, suspending personal judgement while trying to enter into the minds of the people involved. It helps one to keep the issues distinct if the responses of only one person at a time are examined. In the process of analysis, and in the absence of any of the people concerned, it is legitimate to speculate on the values which motivated their responses. Which principles underpinned their choices? Who stood to gain from the decisions made? At cost to whom? Which principles clash and on what basis is it decided which should take priority in this situation? Whose decision is it anyway? Is it possible to respect the views of more than one person in the outcome? Indeed, is ethics properly concerned with outcomes only? Does the quality of the process which precedes decision-making have a value in itself?

Questions multiply around a situation like this. If responses are to carry more weight than 'gut feeling', which should, however, not be ignored, or simple opinion; if the decision is to be based on one principle rather than another; if the choice is to lay claim to being rational and coherent; then the moral frameworks which guide principled thinking will have to be used, even if they are only visible when, as in this case, the argument is examined with hindsight.

STRUCTURES AND STRATEGIES

Moral frameworks

One of the features of the study of ethical theory is that nearly every text will provide a different version of the structure and content of a range of moral frameworks. There is a sense in which this diversity is a healthy and honest reflection of the way human beings are when they come to thinking about the things which matter most to them. If the world's greatest minds, over a period of some 3000 years of documented thought, have failed to agree about what constitutes the 'right' course of action or the 'best' decision in any given set of circumstances, it should be no surprise to us that we find it a challenge to our thinking.

Nevertheless, some general frameworks do exist and they act rather like maps to guide people through the little-known and hazardous terrain of human experience. Like maps, they can be used to identify the features of an unexpected and difficult journey just completed as well as to plan a route through anticipated rough territory. This is important in the professional situation since, so often, events evolve at a speed which leaves little opportunity for planning or reflection. In this case, two things tend to happen. People respond using a habitual frame of reference, appealing to their usual action-guiding criteria. Later, though not always, they may review that decision in the light, not only of its outcome, but of the process and the foundations upon which the choice was made. This exercise of reflection, free of the pressures of an emergency, permits the consideration of alternative moral frameworks and may help people to appreciate and respect other responses than their own.

Ethical frameworks can broadly be grouped according to whether they are goal-based or rule-based.

Goal-based theories originate from the secular utilitarian tradition (generally, maximising the benefit to be achieved). These are sometimes known as *teleological* or *consequentialist* theories and, with their emphasis on the goal to be achieved, on the outcome to be expected from a chosen course of action, they have considerable appeal in a world of practical decision making such as the NHS.

Rule-based theories. This group of theories stems largely from a range of classical and theological traditions and includes concepts such as Natural Law, agapeistic theory and deontological ethics.

Natural law has a very long history in European thought and provides the foundation for the legal codes of a number of nations as well as much of the theology of the Roman Catholic Church. It has its roots in belief in a universal rational order written into creation and governing right action between people. This order, supposedly perceivable by all right-minded rational people, is held to be inviolable, for to violate it would be to introduce chaos into society by ignoring divinely instituted moral precepts.

Agapeistic theory comes more directly from the christian gospels and subsequent tradition. Downie and Calman (1987) note that the story of the Good Samaritan is one of the most powerful illustrations of the type of love meant by the Greek word *agape*. They describe it as 'an attitude which combines a regard for others as self-

governing with a compassion for them in the pursuit of their end'. Agapeistic theory in recent years has been linked with the development of what some have called 'situation ethics', where the central question to be asked in any dilemma is 'what is the most loving thing to do?' Problems arise when there is failure to reach agreement on what are the criteria by which one can identify the most loving action. Immanuel Kant, the 18th century philosopher mentioned earlier in this chapter, tried to establish criteria by which moral rules could be judged to be binding.

Deontological or duty-based theory is closely linked with his name. Thompson et al (1983) note that Kant maintained that a moral principle must be universal, unconditional and imperative before it can be considered moral and therefore binding. Before an action can be considered good or moral it has to pass the test by which one could will that same action to become universally applicable. A further development of his thinking led him to state that right action never permits the use of people as means to achieve an end, a consideration which has been very influential in deciding what constitutes respect for persons. One clear instance of the application of the rule is seen in the core statement of the Children Act 1976 that all legal decisions must be determined by the child's best interests. Unfortunately there is no space to do justice to his complex theories here.

Intuitionism lies somewhere between goal-based and rule-based theories of ethics. Intuitionists not only hold that moral judgements are arrived at by the subjective and personal insights of individuals, by intuition, but they also maintain that there are 'several distinct moral duties that cannot be reduced to one basic duty, in contrast, for example, to utilitarianism' (*Pan Dictionary of Philosophy* 1979). While intuitionism probably gives more weight to the emotions in the process of forming an ethical judgement than either of the other main systems, it is by no means merely a question of the individual's response to 'gut feeling'. The rational processes of information gathering, reflection, and analysis all have their part in establishing the intuitionist's moral framework.

Principled thinking

All the ethical frameworks which have been considered provide a structure within which ethical principles can be brought to bear on the human situation. They are very frequently listed as respect for persons (sometimes discussed as autonomy), benevolence, non-malevolence (the duty to do no harm), justice and utility. Downie and Calman (1987) see respect for persons as the great over-arching principle which is served by the four subsidiary principles just mentioned. These are identified as the most 'morally appropriate ways of treating autonomous people'. Engelhardt (1986) sees the principles of respect for autonomy and benevolence (doing what is best for the client) as creating a fundamental tension which health care workers must grapple with in attempting to make moral decisions. He uses the expression 'the morality of mutual respect' to describe the practical application of the principle of autonomy within the professional situation. There remain a host of other moral principles which play a subsidiary role to the ones we have just mentioned. These include truth-telling, promise-keeping and confidentiality, all of which have obvious application to midwifery practice. The problem with lists of moral principles is that the longer the list gets the greater the potential for conflicting priorities among those principles. Since most people use an amalgam of ethical frameworks in their day-to-day decision-making, what is of more importance, perhaps, than such lists is some way of evaluating the efficacy of the frameworks.

Using the frameworks

Benjamin and Curtis (1986) follow John Rawls in using a method of 'wide reflective equilibrium' to do just this. This method uses three elements to construct the 'equilibrium' (Fig. 51.3). They are, firstly, our secure, pretheoretical moral judgements (e.g. causing unnecessary pain to newborn babies is wrong), secondly, our background beliefs and theories (our basic knowledge and beliefs about how the world and people function) and, thirdly, the ordered sets of moral principles which constitute the framework in question. The appropriateness and validity of the chosen framework are judged by estimating the extent to which the sets of principles do effectively 'give consistent and comprehensive guidance while cohering with two other sets of beliefs'. The three components need to maintain an equilibrium, to be mutually

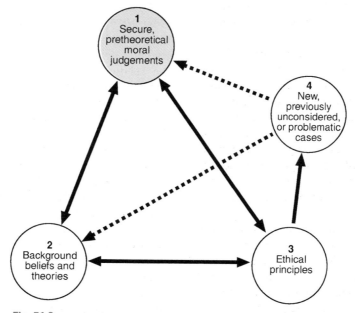

Fig. 51.3
A method of wide reflective equilibrium. (After Rawls J 1986 In: Benjamin M, Curtis J (eds) Ethics in nursing, 2nd edn. Oxford University Press, Oxford.)

supportive. No one of the elements is permitted to dominate over the others. It may transpire that one form of ethical framework actually maintains this balance better than others. When new situations for which we seek a resolution arise they have to be incorporated into the dynamic which seeks to maintain the three main elements in equilibrium. If there is dissonance then some form of modification of one or other of the elements may need to take place, to accommodate the demands of the new situation. The developments surrounding in vitro fertilisation are a good example of new situations which (a) seem not to be explicitly provided for in any previous code of ethics (unless, in deontological terms, one subscribes to the theories of Natural Law), (b) require a revision of our previously held background beliefs and theories about the way humans are conceived and (c) put a question mark over our previously secure, pretheoretical moral judgement about what is 'right' or permissible in the field of human reproduction.

This may seem a complex exercise which is for the academics. In reality, much of it is what we do, albeit unconsciously, when we look at a new situation and feel uneasy about it, when we swap ideas about it in the coffee room and try to find out how others react. By those acts we are trying to validate our own response. Where others react differently we may be pushed into looking more closely at why we respond as we do and so become more aware of the origins of our own ethical stance. Sometimes this can be quite disturbing — most of us prefer to have our foundations left unshaken. More frequently, such a process is experienced in the long run as growth and affirmation. The analysis and questioning involved provide an occasion for self-discovery as well as a greater awareness of the perspectives held by others. It is important that ethical reflection should not be constrained by too limited a use of a certain range of abstract concepts. It is by the careful analysis of situations and the different approaches which people bring to them that midwives will effectively develop their sense of what constitutes good practice.

This is why this chapter has placed far less emphasis on those concepts which traditionally constitute the domain of 'medical ethics' and has focused instead on the use and abuse of power in professional practice, on how midwives can safeguard the autonomy of the women in their care and how they can meet the challenge of maintaining their personal integrity at the heart of a complex network of sometimes conflicting values.

Wilson (1978) claimed that 'reciprocity is the fundamental attribute of a mature moral transaction'. Midwifery is largely based on a continuous dialogue with women and their families. Without such an exchange the service cannot hope to meet their needs, since it will only have its own view of what those needs are. At a much deeper level, that dialogue is the only clear way of honouring the autonomy of the women, giving them a voice which can effect the changes which they see as important. Midwives have spoken a lot in recent years about the duty of 'empowering' women. This cannot be done without the establishment of the trust relationship discussed at the beginning of this chapter.

Covenant

These qualities of reciprocity, mutual respect and dialogue are enshrined in the covenant concept (May 1975, Stenberg 1979, Campbell 1984, 1987). Covenant has its roots in the Judaeo-Christian tradition, where it was frequently used to describe the relationship between God and his people, Israel. Writers in the health care field have been attracted to the concept because it has a flexibility and dynamism that is missing from similar structures such as codes and contracts. Covenant partners value each other. There is a mutual commitment, a reciprocal obligation. Both partners give and receive. May argues that the covenant model frees the professional relationship from the one-sided, paternalistic element of philanthropy inherent in models such as codes of conduct or advocacy. It seems a useful framework for the sort of morally responsible professional relationship which midwives and mothers engage in. Its reciprocal nature levels out the inequalities usually present in the client–health care worker relationship. In stressing the self-determination of the client, it reduces the emphasis on the practitioner's role as advocate (cf. UKCC 1989). With its dynamic, reciprocal qualities, which require the establishment of a true partnership, covenant offers potential which midwives may well find corresponds with the demands of their practice. To those who are fearful of the level of commitment required by a professional covenant relationship, May offers the reminder that covenant ethics retains realism about human ability by shying away from the idealistic (and arrogant) assumption that professional action should be wholly gratuitous as well as from the contractualist tenet that every exchange should be governed by self-interest. Stenberg (1979) offers a seven-point outline of the characteristics of covenant, which have been adapted for midwifery in Box 51.1.

Despite its comprehensive nature, Stenberg's account of covenant seems insufficiently to stress the quality of mutuality, the active role of the woman in determining how she wishes to structure this event as a partnership. In midwifery practice where mothers have months to prepare for childbirth, the gradual and carefully thought through establishment of birth plans can provide a valuable means of clarifying the 'term of the covenant' with her midwife.

Box 51.1
Elements of a convenant framework (after Stenberg 1979)

Covenant requires:
* fidelity in both promises and truth-telling
* proficiency — a woman's faith is based on belief in the midwife's competence
* safeguarding the woman's self-concept, her personhood
* care that goes beyond the level of utility to that of ultra-obligation
* control of her person and her environment offered to the woman where possible
* freedom for the woman from fear, pain and the possibility of abandonment
* the encouragement of realistic hope.

The idea of promise-keeping, of fidelity, is central to convenant. The ethical implications of such a stance are evident and widen out from the central commitment to include issues of truthfulness and competence. Midwives, committed to being 'with women', could find this a powerful and relevant model for their practice. Attempts to structure their practice within a covenant relationship could well result in them discovering with

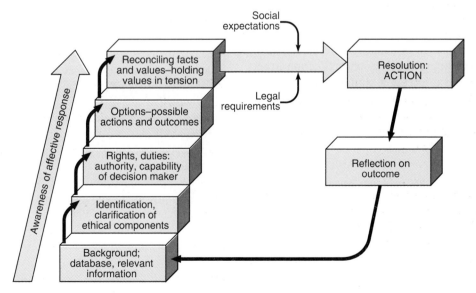

Fig. 51.4
Steps in ethical decision-making. (After Curtin L 1982 In: Curtin L, Flaherty M J (eds) Nursing ethics, theories and pragmatics. Brady Communications, Maryland.)

William May (1975) that 'covenants have a gratuitous, growing edge to them that nourishes rather than limits relationships'.

Making decisions

Whichever ethical framework the midwife chooses to adopt, she will find it helpful at times to use some form of systematic approach to the analysis of her decisions. Many are available, but the grid developed by Curtin & Flaherty (1982) and expanded here to incorporate elements such as affective response and the possibility of it being a reflective process is shown in Figure 51.4. It can be useful in group discussions and case reviews as well as in the process of personal reflection.

Rebecca Bergman, one of the early writers on nursing ethics, states:

There is, in total, a new, evolving ethic; it is one of personal responsibility for nursing practice; it is one of social commitment ... to speak up and be counted when an issue is at stake; it is one of accountability ... to take considered action and to present it for scrutiny to those concerned; it is an ethic from dependence to independence to interdependence; from separateness towards togetherness with colleagues and community. A code of ethics should not be a shield, or even a crutch; it should be a firm launching pad from which to project into the future (Bergman 1976).

Her words ring just as true of midwifery and its responsibilities. It may be that we constantly raise more questions than we answer in our practice but if, in the process of careful, honest and painstaking fact-gathering, analysis and reflection it becomes possible to create a climate of confidence within which people can act with greater freedom, then much will have been achieved.

REFERENCES

Benjamin M, Curtis J 1986 (eds) Ethics in nursing, 2nd edn. Oxford University Press, Oxford

Bergman R 1976 Evolving ethical concepts for nursing. International Nursing Review 23(4): 116–117

Campbell A 1984 Moderated love — a theory of professional care. SPCK, London

Campbell A 1987 (ed) A dictionary of professional care. SPCK, London

Department of Health 1989 Report on confidential enquiries into maternal deaths in England and Wales 1982–84. HMSO, London, p 28

Downie R S, Calman K C 1987 Healthy respect — ethics in health care. Faber and Faber, London, p 56

Dunstan G R 1987 In: Campbell A (ed) A dictionary of professional care. SPCK, London, p 83

Engelhardt H T 1986 The foundations of bioethics. Oxford University Press, New York

Gilligan C 1977 In another voice — women's conceptions of self and of morality. Harvard Education Review 47(4): 487–517

Hall B P 1973 Values clarification as a learning process. Paulist Press, New York

Katz Rothman B 1986 The tentative pregnancy — prenatal diagnosis and the future of motherhood. Pandora, London

Kitwood T 1977 What does 'having values' mean? Journal of Moral Education 6: 81–89

May W F 1975 Code, covenant, contract or philanthropy. Hastings Centre Report 5: 29–38

Midgely M 1981 Heart and mind — the varieties of moral experience. Methuen, London

Overall C 1987 Ethics and human reproduction — a feminist analysis. Allen and Unwin, Boston

Paton H J 1947 The moral law. Hutchinson, London, In: Flew A 1989 An Introduction to western philosophy. Thames and Hudson, London

Schröck R A 1980 A question of honesty in nursing practice. Journal of Advanced Nursing 5: 135–148

Stenberg M S 1979 The search for a conceptual framework as a philosophic basis for nursing ethics: an examination of code, contract, context and covenant. Military Medicine 144: 9–22

Tew M 1990 Safer childbirth? — a critical history of maternity care. Chapman and Hall, London

Thompson A 1987 Teaching ethics in midwifery education. Unpublished dissertation for BEd (Hons) degree, Southbank Polytechnic

Thompson I E, Melia K M, Boyd K M 1983 Nursing ethics. Churchill Livingstone, Edinburgh, p 137

Thompson J 1985 Professional maturity or independence. Journal of Nurse Midwifery 31(2): 92–102

UKCC 1989 Exercising accountability. United Kingdom Central Council for Nursing, Midwifery and Health Visiting, London

Wagner M 1986 Birth and power. In: Phaff J M L (ed) Perinatal health services in Europe. Croom Helm, London

Wilson J 1986 Patients' wants versus patients' needs. Journal of Medical Ethics 12: 127–130

Wilson R W 1978 A new direction for the study of moral behaviour. Journal of Moral Education 7(2): 122–129

52

Quality assurance in maternity care

JEAN A. BALL   DEBORAH HUGHES

Concern about the quality of care is as old as medicine itself but an honest concern about quality, however genuine, is not the same as methodological assessment based upon reliable evidence (Maxwell 1984).

WHAT IS QUALITY ASSURANCE?

In 1982 The World Health Organization urged all its member states to introduce regular assessment of the quality of their health services and to establish principles for the development of quality assurance programmes (Vuori 1985). If the term *quality* means 'essential or distinguishing characteristic, degree of goodness or value' and *assurance* means 'formal promise, pledge, certainty, confidence', then the term *quality assurance* suggests:

1. a need for defining and describing the special characteristics and values of good quality care or service
2. setting up a means of regularly achieving those defined standards within a health care organisation.

Shaw (1986) puts this process into a nutshell when he says: 'Quality Assessment is the measurement of provision against expectation. Quality Assurance is the same but with the declared intention and ability to correct any demonstrated weaknesses.'

A number of factors and developments are involved in setting up a quality assurance system. They are shown in Figure 52.1 and may be summarised as:

- defining and describing quality of care and how it is to be achieved
- promoting quality in various ways within the organisation
- measuring the degree of quality being achieved
- publishing the results and using them as a spur for further improvements.

The term *total quality management* is sometimes used to describe the processes involved in making quality assurance an integral part of the decision-making processes of an organisation. This chapter outlines the main principles and processes of developing quality assurance.

Why quality assurance has become so important

The need for quality assurance has arisen because of:

- the rising expectations of consumers of the service
- increasing pressure from international, national government and other bodies to demonstrate that the allocation of funds produces satisfactory results in terms of patient care, disease reduction etc.
- the increasing complexity of health care organisations.

Quality and organisations

Quality assurance first began in manufacturing industry. As this became increasingly mechanised, many different processes and people were involved in the production of a single item. In order to make certain that the finished product was satisfactory it became increasingly necessary to ensure that each part of the process met a required standard of quality. The same need can be recognised within the complex organisation of health care, where many different people and processes are involved.

However, while the quality of manufacturing processes and products is comparatively easy to assess and control, this is not true of the complex organisation needed to provide health services. Not only are many different people and processes involved in providing care but each client has a variety of needs to be met and his or her own opinion about the acceptability of the care offered. This means that although the purpose behind quality assurance is the same in industry and in health care, the concepts to be used within the

1. WHAT IS THE ORGANISATION THERE TO PROVIDE?
   What kind of health benefits? How can they be achieved for local needs?
   Define
   Access to care, acceptability, appropriateness Effectiveness, efficiency, equity
   Draw on
   Relevant research, consumer reports, government reports, public opinion
2. HOW CAN THESE STANDARDS BE ACHIEVED THROUGHOUT THE ORGANISATION?
   Managers, professionals, quality groups produce objectives and standards which will describe and promote the quality to be achieved
   Describe quality
   Mission statement, philosophies, objectives
   Standards of practice
   Standards of performance
   Promote quality
   Structure, processes needed to provide defined level of quality: resources, education, guidelines, research etc.
3. START THE QUALITY CYCLE
   Monitor quality, collect information
   Develop monitoring processes, measuring instruments
   Produce information about current level of quality
   Take action on results
   What is good? — applaud achievement
   What needs improving? — set action plans
   What needs further resources to achieve? — set longer term plans for improvement
   Publish results
   Produce reports for management, consumers, public
   Debate issues with professional colleagues, quality circles, groups
   Implement results in staff education, initiate further research
   Make new plans
4. OUTCOME OF PROCESS
   Quality performance known and published
   Quality activities part of the continuing policies of organisation
   Quality assurance information becomes integral part of making clinical and service management decisions

Fig. 52.1
Model of the processes of developing quality assurance within an organisation (copyright © J A Ball).

health services must be developed to suit its particular pattern of work.

Factors affecting quality

The quality of a service is affected by a number of factors including:

1. The extent and variety of the *needs* of the population that is served. These will include the numbers of clients, social factors, age range, disease patterns etc.

2. The *values* which determine the style and range of services will arise from:

   a. the knowledge and aspirations of the professional groups concerned
   b. the political will and aspirations of the population
   c. the attitudes and expectations of those who manage and control the service
   d. the expectations of the individual clients and consumer groups.

3. The *capacity* of the service, i.e. the resources of knowledge and skills, facilities and equipment, staff and finances which are available.

4. The *way* in which care is *planned, organised and led.*

Strategic and operational quality

In order to provide the appropriate pattern of care for any population, there will be need to consider both *strategic* and *operational* issues.

Strategic quality is concerned with the overall planning and conduct of large-scale methods for achieving objectives of care.

Operational quality is concerned with the day-to-day organisation of care for individuals and groups.

STRATEGIC QUALITY ISSUES

For many years the maternity services have been setting strategic quality targets for reducing the incidence of deaths and handicap of mothers and babies. The achievement of these objectives has been assessed by the consistent measurement of outcomes in terms of maternal and perinatal mortality statistics. Results have been followed by action in providing improved or extended services. Some of the ways in which the strategic quality of maternity care has been controlled are:

Control of midwifery education and practice. 1902 saw the first registration of midwives with statutory restriction of practice.

Provision of free midwifery care. In 1936 a free domiciliary midwifery service was introduced, and resulted in dramatic falls in both maternal and perinatal mortality.

Confidential enquiries into maternal deaths. In 1949 a further and more detailed evaluation of the causes of maternal deaths came into being when the confidential enquiries into maternal deaths were set up. In this triennial survey the details of each maternal death are investigated by eminent obstetricians, histopathologists and anaesthetists, in order to identify avoidable and unavoidable factors associated with each death. The results of these enquiries have had a major influence on policies for maternity care. The most recent report (DH 1991) shows that maternal deaths halved every 10 years between 1955 and 1984, showing a clear improvement in the effectiveness of the service and in the general health of women. It is important to realise that such stringent review of the outcomes of care is unique. However the confidential enquiry approach was used as the basis for a study of peri-operative deaths, that is, deaths occurring within 1 month of planned or emergency surgery (Buck et al 1987) and all health authorities are now required to investigate such deaths.

International strategies for maternity care

The World Health Organization is currently mounting the Safe Motherhood campaign designed to reduce the high level of maternal deaths in developing countries. This has been described (Maine 1986) as the equivalent of a jumbo jet crashing every 4 hours, every day, whose passengers are all women in the prime of their lives!

A number of factors were identified as being linked to maternal deaths. In many cases lack of facilities was compounded by the large distances which women in distress had to travel before reaching care. Research in nine countries showed that many of these deaths could have been avoided given the standards of care which it was realistic to expect in the country concerned. For example, it was judged that in Turkey 51% of deaths should have been avoided within the existing health system, (better *operational* quality) while a further 24% could have been avoided within an improved maternity service (better *strategic* quality) (Maine 1986).

OPERATIONAL QUALITY

Operational quality is concerned with the way a service performs and the quality of care it provides. Maternity care is provided by many people, working with different skills and undertaking different activities. All of these activities contribute in some way to the delivery of care. The larger the number of people involved with the care process, the greater is the need for providing a framework for defining the quality to be achieved. Unless all the people involved are working towards the same end, with clear objectives and standards, it will be difficult to 'assure' the quality of service. There have been a number of government and consumer reports which have made recommendations about the operational quality needed for maternity care.

Reports on maternity care

Since the 1950s numerous reports have made recommendations for changes in the organisation of maternity care in the United Kingdom. The Peel Report (DHSS 1970) accelerated the change to hospital-based births. 10 years later the Short Report (DHSS 1980) discussed the need for further improvement in the availability and uptake of appropriate maternal and neonatal care and emphasised the need to provide for the emotional as well as the physiological needs of the mother. This report was primarily concerned about the operational quality of the service; the resources which should be available, the processes of care and the need for flexibility in providing for the different needs and aspirations of mothers. It also drew attention to the importance of ensuring *consumer satisfaction* as a means of increasing the uptake of the service. The report produced 153 recommendations for changes in the provision and organisation of maternity care. The Short Report led to the setting up of the Maternity Services Advisory Committee who produced three Maternity Care in Action reports (MSAC 1982, 1984, 1985). These set standards for antenatal, intrapartum, postnatal and neonatal care. Each report includes a series of check-lists for different aspects of care, which are designed to enable maternity services to monitor their performance against the standards listed. Sadly many of these standards have not yet been established in all maternity services. The process of changing aspirations into reality is what quality assurance is all about!

Consumer reports and action

The last decade has seen vigorous consumer activity within the maternity services. The publication of the Good Birth Guides (Kitzinger 1979, 1983) gave a consumer view of almost every maternity hospital in the country. The work of the Association for Improvements in the Maternity Services, the National Childbirth Trust and numerous reports, including many from community health councils, have all fuelled the consumer debate.

The publication of the Short Report, the Maternity Care in Action reports and pressure from consumer groups have marked the move towards focusing upon the operational aspects of the quality of maternity care.

MODELS FOR DEVELOPING QUALITY ASSURANCE IN HEALTH CARE

Quality assurance has four main components:

- Defining quality; statements and descriptions of what is to be accomplished
- Promoting quality; education, guidelines, facilities etc. needed
- Monitoring quality; measuring performance against desired standards

- Taking action; acting on the results to acknowledge and praise good work and setting targets for improvement of shortfall.

These components form the basis for the *quality cycle* which is shown in Figure 52.2.

Defining the quality of care

Defining and describing the quality of care needed for a particular population or care group are best begun by asking:

- What type of care or service is needed to achieve the desired health benefit?
- How can this definition of quality be described in terms of the necessary organisation and practice of a health care organisation?

For example, it is considered that providing antenatal care as early in the pregnancy as possible can improve the outcome in terms of maternal and neonatal well-being. Antenatal care also provides an opportunity for building relationships, planning care and providing information. These

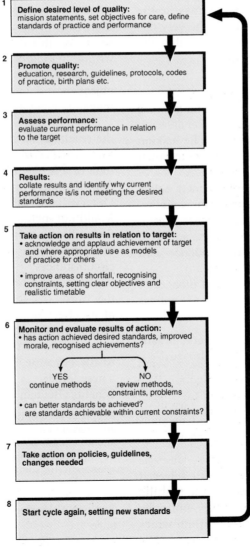

Fig. 52.2
Stages of the quality cycle (copyright © J. A. Ball).

activities might not have a direct effect upon *outcome* but can be described as *health benefits*. Therefore a standard might be set of ensuring that all expectant mothers should have been seen by a midwife and/or doctor by the 12th week of pregnancy and have received a full health check.

In the United Kingdom the uptake of early antenatal care will depend upon providing readily accessible clinics, home visits by midwives, attractive facilities, good advertising of facilities and the importance of care, courteous staff, convenient appointments and running special clinics for teenagers. However, in the developing countries, although the need for antenatal care may be the same, the means of providing it may be very different and not immediately available within the current resources for maternity care.

Concepts of quality in health care

During the past decade there has been a growing understanding of ways in which the quality of health care can be defined and assessed. The section which follows outlines the most widely accepted texts.

The definitions and concepts outlined below are capable of forming a framework for defining, evaluating and improving the quality of health care. They can be applied to different services and used to develop specific standards of practice and performance.

Donabedian is a doctor who was a pioneer of quality assurance in the United States. He defines the components of health care as:

- *Structure.* The physical, financial and organisational resources provided for health care.
- *Process.* The activities of a health system or practitioner in the provision of care.
- *Outcome.* A change in the patient's current or future health that can be attributed to antecedent care. (Donabedian 1980, 1986.)

Donabedian's model is primarily a *strategic* model. It maintains that the quality of care achieved depends upon the quality of the structure and the processes such as the resources, values and skills of the health system and practitioner. Both structure and process may affect the outcome. His definition of outcome is related to the effect on

the health of the client, which 'can be attributed to antecedent care'. Such outcomes are readily measured in terms of mortality rates, and rates of the incidence and prevalence of disease. It is easy to see how his model fits with the research findings on maternal deaths in Turkey discussed above. Some deaths were due to problems in the *structure* of the service, others to deficiencies in the *processes* within the existing structure.

Donabedian's model is widely used in nursing practice and is a helpful model in identifying factors which affect the delivery of care. However, caution must be exercised in its application to operational settings. Donabedian's model has been used to provide a framework for defining standards but this can be cumbersome. Insisting on writing standards which describe the structure, process and desired outcome of a particular objective and intervention is not necessary and may not be helpful.

The term *outcome* is sometimes used to describe the results of an interaction between a client and care provider which can be seen to meet the criteria of a health benefit, such as comfort, reduction of anxiety or maintenance of breast feeding. Donabedian's definition of outcome, however, would not include such results. In the opinion of the authors it is better and quite legitimate to use the term *results* rather than outcome in these circumstances.

There may also be a danger of assuming that the 'worth' of a service can only be judged in terms of its effect or otherwise upon health outcome. Health care, however, consists of numerous processes, many of which do not contribute directly to the outcome but are essential in themselves. These processes are usefully defined as health benefits (Buchan et al 1990):

People in need of health care . . . are those for whom an intervention produces a benefit at reasonable risk and acceptable cost. The benefit may not necessarily be improved outcome. It may relate to information or reassurance or some other aspect of the care process.

Setting objectives for the delivery of health care

One of the dangers to be guarded against is that of simply measuring the quality of the current levels and patterns of service and not questioning whether those patterns are the most effective or efficient method of providing health care. Defining different and interactive dimensions or targets which contribute to the quality of the service can be helpful in defining and measuring the quality of care to be achieved for a particular group of clients or by a particular section of the service. The items listed below are to be found in the work of Maxwell (1984), the World Health Organization (Vuori 1984) and Shaw (1986). They can easily be remembered as three As and three Es.

Three As

Access to health care. This comprises the availability of a service, its accessibility and promptness of response. 'Services are not compromised by undue limits of time or distance.'

Acceptability. This dimension is described as 'a service which meets the reasonable expectations of patients, providers and the community'. It is concerned with the *way* care is provided and includes all the aspects of courtesy, communication, comfort, confidentiality and preserving the dignity and self-esteem of the client.

Appropriateness and relevance to need. Shaw (1986) uses the term 'appropriateness', meaning that 'the service or procedure is what the population or individual actually needs'. Meeting this dimension will require providing specialist services, applying relevant research and questioning practices and beliefs about treatment or care processes. Maxwell (1984) uses the term 'relevance to need' which he describes as 'ensuring that service given matches the need of the individual or community'. Although this is similar to the term appropriateness, which is primarily about the care given to individual clients, Maxwell emphasises the need to plan different patterns and provision of care for specific client groups, rather than a general provision irrespective of different needs.

Three Es

Effectiveness. 'The service achieves the intended benefit for the individual and for the community.' This dimension describes the degree to which the interaction between the client and the service produces the desired result and finding ways of overcoming problems in doing so. Being effective will mean making sure that practice is research-based wherever possible. One example of research which has changed beliefs and improved the effectiveness of perineal care is that undertaken by Sleep (1990). It is also important to ensure that the organisation of care is effective, for example making certain that there are sufficient midwives on duty within a delivery suite to care properly for women during labour.

Efficiency. 'Achieving the desired result without unnecessary expenditure of resources.' Efficiency may not always be regarded as a measure of the quality of a service but Maxwell (1984) argues that being efficient will enable resources to be used as widely as possible. Being efficient means being competent, skilled and productive. Efficiency and effectiveness are closely linked and it could be argued that although it is possible to be effective without being efficient, it is *not* possible to be efficient without being effective. After all a service which wastes time, skills and resources upon unnecessary and ineffective activities cannot be described as being of the best quality.

Equity. 'Available resources are fairly distributed among all who have need of them.' 'Resources are not wasted on one service or patient, to the detriment of another.' Equity can be described as fairness in providing care, for example making sure that less vocal or less assertive clients do not receive less support than others and that there is consistency in the quality of care achieved for different client groups.

Producing a theoretical framework for the quality assurance process

These definitions are helpful because they provide a comprehensive and interactive set of issues to be addressed when setting quality objectives and standards in many different situations. This is vital if important issues are not to be overlooked during the process of developing quality targets within an organisation. An example of applying them to a particular service is shown in Table 52.1.

Table 52.1
Quality grid for linen service for postnatal wards (copyright © J A Ball)

Basis: Maxwell	Standards of practice	Standards of performance	Donabedian
Access to service	Daily deliveries of agreed supply Access to extra supplies out of hours/weekends Telephone contact available as needed	% times when agreed supply matched needs Agreed numbers and types of linen needed Telephone contact available	Structure Process Issues
Acceptability	Linen clean, in good repair Staff courteous and helpful Personal items get special attention	Staff and patient surveys Complaints	Process
Efficiency	Linen turnover adequate and swift Deliveries on time	Cost per item No need for storage on wards Need for special deliveries kept to minimum	Process Structure
Effectiveness	No risk of infection or allergies for patients Staff time well used Job satisfaction for porters	Infection rates low, complaints minimal Good staff retention	Outcomes
Relevance to needs	Different arrangements for different groups of patients, service matches population needs	As above but classified by different groups	Structure/process
Equity	Postnatal wards' demands do not reduce service to other areas	Success rate similar for all wards/services	Outcome Structure

Defining specific objectives and standards for quality within an organisation

The first task in setting up the quality cycle lies in deciding the objectives of care which a service wishes to achieve. They take several different forms depending upon the level of the organisation at which they are set.

Corporate vision. This is set by top management, a professional body etc. It is a description of the main purpose, values and aspirations of an organisation. Examples of corporate visions are the documents, *Towards a Healthy Nation* (RCM 1987) and *The Vision* (ARM 1986).

Mission statements are produced by health authorities, hospitals or specific care groups, such as a maternity service. A mission statement is a short statement which encapsulates the objectives and philosophy in an attractive way. An example is shown below. This statement and the service objectives which follow were produced by a group of midwives working on quality assurance

in Central Nottinghamshire Health Authority; some of the group can be seen in Figure 52.3.

Mission statement for antenatal care
Our aim is to ensure the optimum physical, psychological and emotional well-being of the woman, her unborn child and her family by offering support and guidance, so enabling participation in the planning and delivery of her care and the nurturing of parent–child relationships. (Midwifery Quality Project. Central Notts H.A.)

Service objectives and goals. Once the mission has been defined, the next stage is to define the objectives and to enable all staff members to work together to achieve the mission. These can be defined by managers and/or the staff working in a particular hospital, a unit of care, professional group, or working on a special focus of care, such as antenatal or neonatal care.

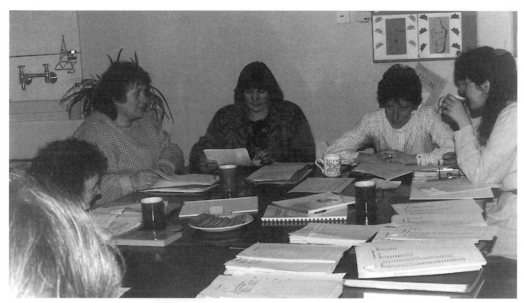

Fig. 52.3
Some of the members of the Midwifery Quality Assurance Group setting objectives for care at the Dukeries Maternity Unit, Kings Mill Hospital, Sutton-in-Ashfield, Nottinghamshire.

The term *objective* is used here to describe something which is to be achieved. Objectives generally describe long-term or continuing targets, goals describe particular or short-term targets. Objectives arise from the concepts outlined in the mission statement. One way of understanding this is to consider that the objective of a football club is to win the cup, and this is achieved by scoring goals at key matches. Examples of antenatal objectives for care arising from the mission statement shown above are given below.

Objectives for antenatal care
* To achieve and maintain the health of the mother and her baby.
* To reach and retain every member of the community who is entitled to and in need of antenatal care.
* To ensure that all expectant mothers receive relevant care.
* To enable the woman and her family to make an informed choice on all relevant aspects of her pregnancy, with an opportunity to discuss specific requirements relating to her care. (Midwifery Quality Project. Central Notts H.A.)

Standards of practice and performance
Most people associate the term 'quality assurance' with setting standards. One of the pitfalls of quality assurance is when standards are set without being related to the objectives of the organisation. Once the objectives of care or service have been defined, standards of practice and performance can be set which will enable the desired objectives to be met.

What is a standard? The Penguin dictionary (Garmonsway 1980) defines a standard as 'that which authority, custom or public opinion lays down as a good model, approved pattern of behaviour, desirable level of efficiency or value, criterion, test, grade of merit ... and rallying point, flag or banner.'

Standards are ways of defining very specific methods, values and actions which are designed to produce the necessary quality of care or service, and which can be measured in some way. They should be based upon research (where available), consumer reports, professional standards and government reports, such as the Maternity Care in Action reports (MSAC, 1982, 1984, 1985).

There are two kinds of standards; standards of

practice and standards of *performance*. The antenatal care objectives above show standards of *practice*, e.g. that the woman will have an opportunity to make an informed choice on all relevant aspects of her pregnancy and to discuss her specific requirements. In the Central Notts Health Authority Midwifery Service, this objective has led to developing pregnancy option plans, which include antenatal, intrapartum and postnatal care options.

A standard of *performance* is a predetermined measure of success in achieving the standard of practice, which is considered to represent good practice or satisfactory service. In the example being used, the standard of performance might be the number of women who completed a pregnancy option plan and might be set at a success rate of at least 85% of all women who are cared for by the maternity service. This provides the midwives with a target to aim for and encourages them to plan their work to ensure that every mother has this opportunity given to her.

Wilson (1987) provides good advice on setting standards and uses the mnemonic R.U.M.B.A. to describe effective standards: *R*elevant, *U*nderstandable, *M*easurable, *B*ehavioural (can be seen in action) and *A*chievable. This should be kept in mind when setting standards. For example a standard might be; 'Women in labour will receive the best possible care at all times.'

This standard is relevant and understandable, but is rather vague, and not easily measured. What is meant by 'best possible care'? The secret is to define the standard further in ways which reflect good care, for example 'The labour and delivery of a client will be conducted by a midwife whose experience and competence is appropriate for the individual client.'

This could be measured by assessing the skill mix shown on duty rosters, ensuring that a senior midwife was readily available to give help or advice, and midwives could be asked to assess whether they felt that clients had been allocated to them in ways which were appropriate to their skills and experience.

A further standard related to 'best possible care' might be 'Clients will be offered appropriate pain relief, based upon the choices made during preg-

nancy and listed in the pregnancy option plan.'

This could be measured by assessing (by client survey) how frequently the mother's choices were respected, whether an emergency situation had caused the options to be overridden, whether the mother (or her partner) had been consulted and whether the mother had been satisfied at the degree of pain relief she had obtained.

Summary. This section has described the important first events in setting up quality assurance. The process of setting objectives and standards leads to the challenging of existing patterns of care and to ensuring that a climate exists by which the desired quality of care is created.

Promoting quality within health care organisations

Health care organisations have a long history of action to promote and control the quality of services; some of them are outlined below.

Professional standards for the quality of the service

Professions have developed specific mechanisms for the education, examination and control of practice of their members. In many cases (but not all) these standards are enforced by law. Standards are set which relate to the skills, knowledge and competence which must be acquired during the period of education before the candidate is allowed to practise his or her profession and to the way in which education is to be provided and the skill and competence of those who teach. Only those institutions which meet the required standard receive accreditation to undertake professional education and training.

Control is also exerted over the practice of members of the profession. In many cases this is done via an agreed code of practice and disciplinary procedures to deal with those who transgress these standards.

The role of research in quality assurance

A profession must also make certain that its standards of knowledge and skill are based upon research. One factor in evaluating the quality of technical care is to have evidence that it is based upon relevant research. Secondly its practitioners should contribute to an expanding body of knowledge, thus continuing to increase and enhance the current level of knowledge and competence (Donabedian 1980).

Setting standards may highlight the need for new opportunities to explore research and disseminate its findings via study days etc. For example, when the midwives in Central Nottinghamshire were setting standards for intrapartum care, they found that the guidelines for dealing with stillbirth were out of date and that many staff were unaware of them. This led to the setting up of a series of study days for midwives and doctors about the emotional needs of bereaved parents and the best ways of providing support.

Other control mechanisms for quality

Accreditation systems. In the United States of America and Canada, hospitals operate within an accreditation system. Specific standards for different services (e.g. anaesthetics, surgery) are set by panels of professional experts and managers. A regular independent audit of those standards is carried out and only those hospitals who reach a satisfactory standard of performance receive government funding for providing health services. Similar methods are likely to be adopted in the United Kingdom as contracts develop between Health Authorities as *purchasers of health care* and hospitals as *providers of health care*.

Within the NHS a number of less formal methods exist for describing the standards to be met and these include guidelines and procedures, clinical protocols and care contracts.

Guidelines and procedures. Most hospitals have produced sets of guidelines, procedures or clinical protocols whose purpose is to make plain to all concerned a set of standards which describe the way care should be provided in relation to a desired objective. They should be grounded in appropriate research and updated as necessary.

Care contracts, birth plans etc. A further example of control mechanisms can be found in the birth plans, pregnancy option plans or care contracts drawn up between expectant mothers and their caregivers. The use of birth plans has arisen from the desire to provide an individualised service to women and from consumer pressure (Kitzinger 1983). One of the objectives of antenatal care listed earlier was to enable women to make informed choices about their care. If these plans are to be successful, they will need to be accessible, updated as necessary and used by the midwives and doctors who actually carry out the care but may not be the same staff who produced the care contract with the mother.

Promoting quality by the way care is organised

It is sometimes necessary to change the way care is provided in order to achieve the desired standard. The check-lists in the three Maternity Care in Action reports indicate what care is needed and how it should be provided, for example making it easier for women to receive antenatal care by providing community-based consultant clinics (Currell 1990). The desire to provide continuity of care has led to the formation of midwifery teams within hospital and community services (Flint & Poulengeris 1987).

However, it is not sufficient to change the organisation of care simply because it is thought to be a good idea; clear objectives should be set and the success of the change should be measured in a variety of ways. In one study, improved access to antenatal care (Evans 1989) was measured by improved perinatal outcome and reduced smoking among clients (health benefit) as well as by client satisfaction.

The essence of quality assurance is to ensure that policies and practices designed to promote quality are actually carried out and produce the desired results. This is achieved during the next two stages of the quality cycle: measuring or monitoring the quality achieved and acting on the results.

Monitoring quality

Midwives have many ways of assessing and monitoring their work and these continue to exist alongside the more comprehensive and methodological tools which are now being developed.

Measuring quality — a range of activities

A survey carried out in 1987/1988 ascertained how midwives assessed their care in the absence of researched audit methods (Hughes & Goldstone 1989). The results of that survey showed that gauging clients' opinions about the care they had received was the most widely used means of assessment. This took the form of intermittent questionnaires or surveys, comments on evaluation forms or care plans at discharge, inviting feedback from individual clients at postnatal classes and from user groups such as the National Childbirth Trust and Community Health Councils, investigating letters of complaint, talking to clients and receiving letters of appreciation. With the possible exception of questionnaires and surveys, which may have been developed via a research process, these methods are open to considerable bias. At best, they provide an insight into how *some* clients felt about *some* aspects of their care. The emphasis on client opinions also demonstrates the way in which consumer opinion has become central to any assessment of the quality of maternity care.

Other means used, though mentioned less often by respondents to the survey, were more service-orientated activities such as clinical audit (mainly in the form of workload assessments and bed occupancy statistics), checking the standard of record keeping, perinatal mortality meetings, unit meetings, quality circles, senior midwives supervising the work of others, the use of policies and protocols, infection control reports, procedure committees, some standard setting groups and maternity liaison committees. As has already been discussed in the section on promoting quality, all these activities generate information which can be used to maintain or improve the quality of care. Whereas clients can provide a lot of information about the *process* of care that they experienced, many of the other activities listed in this paragraph provide data about the *structure* and *outcome* or *results* of the service given. Whilst this is a somewhat crude division (clients can also tell us about the structure and outcome of the service and staff can assess much of the process) it demonstrates the number of different forms of enquiry and quality-related activities which can help to construct an overall picture of the care given.

The respondents also mentioned a number of other issues related to assessing quality, albeit less frequently than those listed above. These related primarily to midwives and consisted of such items as staff questionnaires, staff appraisal, talking among colleagues, evaluations by student midwives, midwifery working parties, the recruitment, retention and morale of midwives (open to extreme bias) and staff sickness levels. Midwives' perceptions and concerns about their work and its quality can be a useful indicator of the quality of the service they work in, and may be underused in terms of quality assurance at the present time. Such concerns, however, indicate the degree of knowledge and commitment which is needed for defining and promoting quality via quality groups or circles.

Experience in the maternity services indicates that a great deal of activity is going on, which directly or indirectly assesses some aspect of the quality of care given. The methods mentioned above do not constitute a complete list; no doubt you could add to it. What is important to remember is that quality assurance requires a multi-faceted and complex array of activities rather than a specific exercise.

Quantitative and qualitative techniques

Quality assurance may use both quantitative and qualitative techniques. Quantitative data are concerned with facts which have a finite range, and can readily be measured numerically. They tell us *what* has been done, for example the number and percentage of women who completed a pregnancy option plan. These data may be analysed by volume, percentage, mean averages, standard deviations, analysis of variance tests etc.

Qualitative methods deal with peoples' feelings, opinions, attitudes and perceptions. An example might be the woman's perception of the degree of relief from pain she had experienced. Such data are not finite, but can be classified into discrete categories and ranges. Qualitative data can be analysed by percentages, chi-squares and non-parametric methods, such as correlation co-efficients, Mann-Whitney tests etc.

Most quality assurance studies will use a combination of qualitative and quantitative techniques.

Tools for assessing quality

During the last few years, a number of quality assessment tools have been developed in nursing and more lately in midwifery. These can provide a great deal of information in a relatively comprehensive and systematic way but they are not meant to replace all other activity or obviate the need to pursue the various lines of enquiry listed above.

How tools measure care

All tools basically consist of a list of questions and the answering of these questions constitutes the audit of care. This process of auditing is, as has been emphasised, only one part of the quality assurance cycle. Each question or statement specifies or implies a certain standard of care to be achieved. Questions may be answered with a simple 'yes' or 'no' as in the Monitor series of quality assurance tools (Goldstone et al 1983). A 'yes' response indicates that the criterion for satisfactory care outlined in the question has been achieved. Alternatively a rating method can be used in which the respondent chooses from a number of possible responses which indicate different degrees of opinion.

For example, if we wanted to determine how frequently antenatal clients were kept waiting then we could ask:

When you attended the antenatal clinic, were you seen within 15 minutes of your appointment time? Yes / No

If you answered No to the last question, how long were you kept waiting after your appointment time?
(Please tick the time which is nearest to the time you were kept waiting.)
More than 15 minutes, less than half an hour
More than half an hour, less than an hour
More than an hour, less than an hour and a half
More than an hour and a half.

- If you were kept waiting for more than 15 minutes after your appointment time, did anyone give you an explanation?   Yes / No
or an apology?   Yes / No

If we wanted to know how our client felt about the time she spent in the antenatal clinic then a qualitative question could be added such as:

When you attended the antenatal clinic, how did you feel about the time you had to wait before you were seen?
(Please tick the appropriate response.)
Very satisfied   Satisfied
Dissatisfied   Very dissatisfied

Audit techniques are quite easy to use and, if standards are written in a form which facilitates this approach, results can be readily achieved. When using such methods care must be taken to ensure that:

- the sample size is sufficient to draw valid conclusions
  there is agreement that the questions used represent an accepted standard of quality
- the questions are not ambiguous and can be answered easily by 'Yes' or 'No', or by the rating method chosen.

One must point out, however, that no scoring system is sufficiently sophisticated to 'measure' every nuance of quality but all can provide an *indication* of the quality of care and enable midwives to identify areas of strength and weakness in the service they provide.

Tools for assessing the quality of nursing care

In recent years a number of quality assessment tools have been published. Among the better known are the Monitor series and Qualpacs.

Monitor (Goldstone et al 1983) was the first audit tool produced by British nurses and addressed the quality of care in medical and surgical wards. It has been extensively used (RCN 1988). Special versions appropriate to different groups of clients have now been published including Midwifery Monitor (Hughes & Goldstone 1990a, b and c).

The Qualpacs system (Wandelt & Ager 1974)

uses a rating scale for the assessment of nursing quality and is used during observation of direct nurse–patient interactions. It has 68 items, which span six areas for assessment and uses a five-point rating scale. The assessor is asked to rate the care being given from 'best care' to 'poorest care'. The judgement of the quality of the care is that of the nurse observer, the patient's views are not sought. However, as opinions about what constitutes 'best' or 'poorest' care may vary, it may be difficult to claim that the standards set are measurable or understandable. Qualpacs do, however, give a useful example of using rating scales.

Tools designed for maternity care

Midwifery Monitor Parts I, II and III (Hughes & Goldstone 1990a, b & c). This consists of three linked questionnaires concerned with (respectively) antenatal care, intrapartum care and postnatal and neonatal care. Each is based upon the checklists in the Maternity Care in Action reports, relevant research and consumer surveys. Each questionnaire has sections which are answered directly by the client, from client records, by the midwife and, occasionally, by direct observation by the assessor. The scores build up to a percentage rating of the number of desired standards of care which have been met (standards of performance). Midwifery Monitor can therefore be used in a very specific way for identifying where good quality is being achieved and the issues which require review and action in order to make improvements.

OPCS survey manual (Mason 1989). This is another valuable tool designed to help in the assessment of maternity care. It has been extensively validated and consists of two questionnaires, one for antenatal care, the other for postnatal care. It is primarily concerned with the consumer's assessment of the care received.

Advantages of published methods. When choosing a published method it is important to choose one which is appropriate to the service being evaluated, its clients and its resources and which will provide relevant and usable information. One of the advantages of published assessment tools is that they have been extensively tested for reliability and validity, and reduce the likelihood of producing data which are difficult to interpret, ambiguous or misleading. These tools also shorten the time required to produce validated methods. They can be used to supplement the questions generated by individual units, hospitals or groups of staff and can provide a model for the design of 'home grown' audit methods.

Other information needed during assessment of quality

Whatever method is used, it is important to collect additional data in the form of a client or hospital profile. These data help to explain how or why certain results are achieved. It may for example show that certain client groups fare less well in terms of the care they receive. Both Midwifery Monitor and the OPCS manual compare age, parity and ethnic group of respondents thus enabling service providers to discover whether the quality of women's care is affected because they belong to different groups.

This can enable the identification of 'unpopular' clients or problems such as teenage mothers receiving less information than older women. By using a dependency rating system (Ball 1992) it would also be possible to review whether women with complications in labour received a higher or lower standard of care than women who had no complications. It would also help to identify the specific areas of care which were, or were not, given. These issues will be very important when dealing with the final and key phase of the quality cycle.

Taking action

It cannot be overemphasised that the purpose of quality assurance is to take action to ensure the quality of care by defining, promoting and measuring quality, followed by any action needed to maintain and improve the quality demonstrated. Unless the fourth stage of the quality cycle is fulfilled it cannot be said that quality assurance is a reality.

Once the results of a survey are known, then judgements are made about the degree, nature and relevance of the quality shown by the results.

The judgement is made by the researcher or quality assurance assessor, the staff, managers and clinical leaders concerned.

Acting on the results

Two types of action are needed: first to applaud and praise staff for every good result achieved, secondly to consider why other results are disappointing and to plan what is needed to improve the situation.

Planning for improvement

Plans for improvement may be either short, medium or long term. In many cases, ways of improving quality may be obvious and easy to achieve, in others, changes in either the structure or the processes of the service may be needed. For example, there may be need for extending care facilities (structure) or changing the way care is given (processes). In some cases there may be need to liaise with other staff in order to achieve the desired quality of care.

Setting targets for improvement

Plans for improving the service should include a time scale during which it would be reasonable to achieve change. This helps the staff concerned to concentrate on one or two main issues over a certain length of time. The standards achieved are then re-assessed at the end of the agreed time span. If there is improvement, this is further cause for praise and satisfaction; if there has been no improvement, then further action is needed or the standard is re-appraised.

Setting new standards

At the end of the quality cycle, the standards being used should be re-appraised to ensure that they are still relevant. During the process of measurement it is likely that faults will have been found in the way standards were written and these should be amended in the light of experience. It may be that some standards prove too difficult to define and often it is found that producing suitable guidelines will overcome the problems.

Once the standard setting and assessing process is well understood and satisfactory standards of performance are being achieved, then further

standards may be set and the objectives of care extended to new horizons.

QUALITY ASSURANCE — FACT OR FICTION?

Developing quality assurance systems in health care is a comparatively new concept although, as has been seen, many of its principles have been in use for many years. It is reasonable to expect that, as lessons are learned, the theories which underpin quality assurance at present will develop further. Present experience suggests that the principles outlined in this chapter can be applied in many different health and social care settings. The secret of bringing quality assurance about will lie in the commitment of professionals and managers to the principles of quality which underlie all good health care, and to the resources of time and energy which are given to making quality assurance an integral part of the clinical, financial and general management of any service. This presents a considerable challenge and provides a spur to development and achievement. History shows us that those who care most passionately about the needs of mothers, babies and their families, are also those whose efforts, research and leadership are used to produce the best possible service.

Reader Activities

- Has your local Community Health Council produced a report on the local maternity services?
- If so, have you read it?
- What action has been taken to meet the recommendations made in it?
- Are some recommendations still not met? If so, what is being done about this?
- Does the Community Health Council plan to review the maternity services within the coming 12 months?

- What methods are used in your own area of work to assess the quality of care? (Quality assessment)
- How are the results of any such assessment used to improve the quality of care? (Quality assurance)

Acknowledgements

Many thanks are expressed to Pat Preston, Director of Midwifery; Marie Washbrook, Research Officer; the Quality Assurance Group Midwives, The Dukeries Maternity Unit, Kings Mill Hospital, Sutton in Ashfield; and to Dr Gillian Todd, District General Manager and Pat McAlman, Chief Nursing Adviser, Central Nottinghamshire Health Authority, for their colleagueship and permission to publish extracts of their work. A special acknowledgement to Mrs Chris Siggee, Community Manager, who died suddenly during the quality assurance project.

REFERENCES

Association of Radical Midwives 1986 The vision: proposals for the future of the maternity services. ARM, London

Ball J A 1992 Birthrate: using clinical indicators to assess case mix, workload, outcomes and staffing needs in intrapartum care and for predicting postnatal bed needs. Nuffield Institute for Health Service Studies, University of Leeds, 71–75 Clarendon Road, Leeds LS2 9PL

Buchan H, Muir G, Hill A 1990 Needs assessment made simple. Health Service Journal 100(5184): 240–241

Buck N, Devlin H B, Lunn J N 1987 The report of the confidential enquiry into perioperative deaths. Nuffield Provincial Hospitals Trust & Kings Fund, London

Currell R 1990 The organisation of midwifery care. In: Alexander J, Levy V, Roch S (eds) Antenatal care: a research-based approach. Macmillan, London

Department of Health and Social Security 1970 Domiciliary midwifery and maternity bed needs: report of the Subcommittee, Central Health Service Council Standing Maternity and Midwifery Advisory Committee. HMSO, London

Department of Health and Social Security 1980 The second report from the Social Services Committee on perinatal and neonatal mortality. HMSO, London

Department of Health et al 1991 Report of the confidential enquiries into maternal deaths in the United Kingdom 1985–87. HMSO, London

Donabedian A 1980 The definition of quality assurance and approaches to its measurement. Health Administration Press, Ann Arbor

Donabedian A 1986 Evaluating the quality of medical care. Millband Memorial Quarterly 64(3): 66–206

Evans F 1989 Partnership to tackle poverty. Community Care 792: iv–vi

Flint C, Poulengeris P 1987 The know your midwife report. 49 Peckarmans Wood, Sydenham Hill, London

Garmonsway G N 1980 The Penguin English dictionary. Penguin, Harmondsworth

Goldstone L A, Ball J A, Collier M M 1983 Monitor: an index of the quality of nursing care for acute medical and surgical wards. Newcastle-upon-Tyne Polytechnic Products, Newcastle-upon-Tyne

Hughes D J F, Goldstone L A 1989 Frameworks for midwifery care in Great Britain: an exploration of quality assurance. Midwifery 5(4): 163–171

Hughes D J F, Goldstone L A 1990a Midwifery Monitor I: Pregnancy care: an audit of midwifery care in pregnancy. Poly Enterprises, Leeds

Hughes D J F, Goldstone L A 1990b Midwifery Monitor II: Labour care: an audit of the quality of midwifery care in labour. Poly Enterprises, Leeds

Hughes D J F, Goldstone L A 1990c Midwifery Monitor III: Care after birth: an audit of the quality of postnatal midwifery care. Poly Enterprises, Leeds

Kitzinger S 1979 The good birth guide. Fontana Paperbacks, Glasgow

Kitzinger S 1983 The new good birth guide. Penguin, Harmondsworth

Maine D 1986 Maternal mortality: helping women off the road to death. WHO Chronicle 40(5): 175–183

Mason V 1989 Women's experience of maternity care: a survey manual. HMSO, London

Maternity Services Advisory Committee 1982 Maternity care in action Part I: antenatal care. HMSO, London

Maternity Services Advisory Committee 1984 Maternity care in action Part II: care during childbirth. HMSO, London

Maternity Services Advisory Committee 1985 Maternity care in action Part III: care of the mother and baby. HMSO, London

Maxwell R J 1984 Quality assessment in health. British Medical Journal 288(1): 470–471

Royal College of Nursing 1988 Nursing quality assurance directory. RCN, London

Royal College of Midwives 1987 Towards a healthy nation: a policy for the maternity services. RCM, London

Shaw C D 1986 Introducing quality assurance. Kings Fund project paper no. 64. Kings Fund Publishing House, London

Sleep J 1990 Postnatal perineal care. In: Alexander J, Levy V, Roch S (eds) Postnatal care: a research-based approach. Macmillan, London

Wandelt M, Ager J 1974 Quality patient care scale. Appleton-Century-Crofts, New York

Wilson C R M 1987 Hospital-wide quality assurance: models for implementation and development. W B Saunders, Canada

Vuori M 1985 The principle of quality assurance: report on a WHO meeting. Euro reports and studies 94. WHO, Copenhagen

Index